S0-ASL-554

VASCULAR SURGERY

THERAPEUTIC STRATEGIES

Mark K. Eskandari, M.D.
Associate Professor of Surgery, Radiology, and Cardiology
Division of Vascular Surgery
Department of Surgery
Northwestern University
Feinberg School of Medicine
Chicago, IL

Mark D. Morasch, M.D.
Associate Professor of Surgery
Division of Vascular Surgery
Department of Surgery
Northwestern University
Feinberg School of Medicine
Chicago, IL

William H. Pearce, M.D.
Violet R. and Charles A. Baldwin
Professor of Vascular Surgery
Chief, Division of Vascular Surgery
Department of Surgery
Northwestern University
Feinberg School of Medicine
Chicago, IL

James S. T. Yao, M.D., Ph.D.
Professor Emeritus
Division of Vascular Surgery
Department of Surgery
Northwestern University
Feinberg School of Medicine
Chicago, IL

2010
PEOPLE'S MEDICAL PUBLISHING HOUSE—USA
SHELTON, CONNECTICUT

People's Medical Publishing House–USA
2 Enterprise Drive, Suite 509
Shelton, CT 06484
Tel: 203-402-0646
Fax: 203-402-0854
E-mail: info@pmph-usa.com

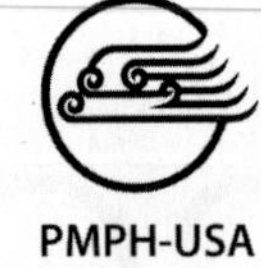

09 10 11 12 13/PMPH/9 8 7 6 5 4 3 2 1

13-digit ISBN 13: 978-1-60795-055-4
10-digit ISBN 10: 1-60795-055-3

Printed in China by People's Medical Publishing House of China
Copyeditor/Typesetter: Spearhead Global, Inc.; Cover Designer: Mary McKeon

LOC to come

Notice: The authors and publisher have made every effort to ensure that the patient care recommended herein, including choice of drugs and drug dosages, is in accord with the accepted standard and practice at the time of publication. However, since research and regulation constantly change clinical standards, the reader is urged to check the product information sheet included in the package of each drug, which includes recommended doses, warnings, and contraindications. This is particularly important with new or infrequently used drugs. Any treatment regimen, particularly one involving medication, involves inherent risks that must be weighed on a case-by-case basis against the benefits anticipated. The reader is cautioned that the purpose of this book is to inform and enlighten; the information contained herein is not intended as, and should not be employed as, a substitute for individual diagnosis and treatment.

Sales and Distribution

Canada
McGraw-Hill Ryerson Education
Customer Care
300 Water Street
Whitby, Ontario L1N 9B6
Canada
Tel: 1-800-565-5758
Fax: 1-800-463-5885
www.mcgrawhill.ca

Foreign Rights
John Scott & Company
International Publisher's Agency
P.O. Box 878
Kimberton, PA 19442
USA
Tel: 610-827-1640
Fax: 610-827-1671

Japan
United Publishers Services Limited
1-32-5 Higashi-Shinagawa
Shinagawa-ku, Tokyo 140-0002
Japan
Tel: 03-5479-7251
Fax: 03-5479-7307
Email: kakimoto@ups.co.jp

United Kingdom, Europe, Middle East, Africa
McGraw Hill Education
Shoppenhangers Road
Maidenhead
Berkshire, SL6 2QL
England
Tel: 44-0-1628-502500
Fax: 44-0-1628-635895
www.mcgraw-hill.co.uk

Singapore, Thailand, Philippines, Indonesia, Vietnam, Pacific Rim, Korea
McGraw-Hill Education
60 Tuas Basin Link
Singapore 638775
Tel: 65-6863-1580
Fax: 65-6862-3354
www.mcgraw-hill.com.sg

Australia, New Zealand
Elsevier Australia
Locked Bag 7500
Chatswood DC NSW 2067
Australia
Tel: +61 (2) 9422-8500
Fax: +61 (2) 9422-8562
www.elsevier.com.au

Brazil
Tecmedd Importadora e Distribuidora de Livros Ltda.
Avenida Maurilio Biagi 2850
City Ribeirao, Rebeirao, Preto SP
Brazil
CEP: 14021-000
Tel: 0800-992236
Fax: 16-3993-9000
Email: tecmedd@tecmedd.com.br

India, Bangladesh, Pakistan, Sri Lanka, Malaysia
CBS Publishers
4819/X1 Prahlad Street 24
Ansari Road, Darya Ganj, New Delhi-110002
India
Tel: 91-11-23266861/67
Fax: 91-11-23266818
Email:cbspubs@vsnl.com

People's Republic of China
PMPH
Bldg 3, 3rd District
Fangqunyuan, Fangzhuang
Beijing 100078
P.R. China
Tel: 8610-67653342
Fax: 8610-67691034
www.pmph.com

Contents

Preface

This book examines vascular surgery from multiple viewpoints. It is certain that the current health care system has many deficits and will certainly undergo revision by Congress and the current administration. Twenty years ago, vascular surgery was recognized as a separate and distinct specialty with complex operations that were reimbursed appropriately. However, in the past two decades, as new procedures have developed, standard open vascular surgery is almost a relic. As a result, many of the older open procedures, which are extremely time-consuming, are reimbursed at very low levels. For example, lower extremity bypasses, which require many hours in the operating room and postoperative care, are reimbursed at a rate less than laser vein ablation for varicose veins performed in the outpatient setting. Furthermore, vascular surgeons pay an extraordinary sum of money for malpractice insurance in many areas of the country. Because these expenses cannot be passed on to the patient and because of shrinking reimbursement, many vascular surgeons have limited their practices or moved to states in which tort reform has occurred.

By and large, most vascular surgeons would agree that they are working longer and doing more cases with less reimbursement. As a result of this climate, vascular surgeons have turned to the hospital for support. Unfortunately, the devices we use reduce hospital profits and, while we once represented a greater profit center, we now represent less than 5% of their revenue.

Vascular surgeons must maintain critical business management of their offices and practices. Vascular surgeons must educate CMS on the value of vascular surgery in the Medicare population and how we can reduce overall expenses compared to other specialties. CMS must understand that the majority of patients we see do not undergo surgical procedures but are treated conservatively. We only select those patients needing intervention and do so in a cost-effective manner. Finally, as part of the value proposition, vascular surgeons must determine which of the many endovascular procedures have true benefit. The endovascular treatment of aneurysms and particularly thoracic aneurysms has demonstrated significant benefit. However, other interventions may not be as efficacious. Vascular surgeons must take the lead in determining which procedures should be kept and which should be discarded.

The theme of this book is to develop therapeutic strategies in various clinical vascular areas. There are 12 sections on clinical categories including carotids, upper extremity, thoracic outlet syndrome, trauma, AV access, lower extremity, visceral vessels, venous problems, thoracic aortic problems, aneurysms of the abdominal aorta, and vascular laboratory. Fifty-six chapters, evenly distributed among these sections, highlight the clinical problems vascular surgeons encounter in their practices.

Management strategy is developed based not only on graft patency but also on quality of life, cost-effectiveness, and long-term results. Special emphasis is placed on the pros and cons of open versus endovascular approach and the need for a surveillance program for follow-up study. In the last decade, treatment of abdominal and thoracic aortic aneurysms has changed significantly and three sections address critical issues related to aortic aneurysms.

The advent of endovascular technology has changed the face of the practice in vascular surgery. Vascular surgeons must adapt to new endovascular technologies and develop a therapeutic strategy to provide optimal care to patients. It is our sincere hope that this volume, contributed to by many leaders in their chosen field, will help to achieve this aim.

Mark K. Eskandari, MD
Mark D. Morasch, MD
William H Pearce, MD
James S.T. Yao, MD, PhD

Acknowledgment

We thank the administrative staff of the Division of Vascular Surgery—Sara Minton and Jan Goldstein—for their support. Special thanks to Susan Parmentier of Greenwood Academic for reprocessing chapters of the last five Northwestern Symposia. We would also like to thank W.L. Gore & Associates for a generous education grant to support the Northwestern Vascular Symposium over the years. Finally, we thank Mr. Jason Malley of People's Medical Publishing House-USA and Mr. Harjeet Singh from Spearhead Global, Inc. for their expert assistance.

Mark K. Eskandari
Mark D. Morasch
William H. Pearce
James S.T. Yao

SECTION I

Carotids

1

Concurrent Carotid Revascularization and Coronary Bypass Strategies in the United States: The Roles of Carotid Stenting vs. Endarterectomy

Carlos H. Timaran, M.D. and Eric B. Rosero, M.D.

The presence of combined coronary and carotid artery disease is not infrequent. Approximately 22% of patients undergoing coronary artery bypass grafting (CABG) have moderate to severe carotid stenosis, whereas 30% of patients undergoing carotid endarterectomy (CEA) have "reconstructible" coronary artery disease, (CAD).[1] Stroke continues to be the major noncardiac complication of open cardiac surgery, with an absolute incidence of 2%. In patients with concurrent carotid artery disease, a fourfold increased risk of perioperative stroke following CABG has been reported.[1–2] Carotid revascularization could theoretically reduce the stroke rates in patients with concurrent lesions as suggested by reduced rates of post-CABG stroke after CEA.[2-4] To be beneficial in reducing stroke rates, however, carotid revascularization and CABG need to be performed with low cardiac and neurologic morbidity and mortality. Because of conflicting results, the management of concurrent severe carotid and coronary artery disease has not been established.

Systematic reviews and meta-analyses of combined open coronary and carotid revascularization procedures reveal rates of perioperative major adverse events (MAEs), that is, combined stroke, myocardial infarction (MI), and death in the 10 to 12% range.[2] No significant differences in outcome between staged and simultaneous procedures have been noted. Although single-center observational studies and systematic reviews of the literature have revealed acceptable outcomes of combined CEA and CABG,[2,5–6] community-based outcomes have been alarmingly dismal.[7] The timing and sequence of treatment of patients with combined coronary and carotid stenosis, therefore, remain unresolved, particularly for patients who require combined urgent reconstruction during the same period of hospitalization.

Patients with severe coronary and carotid artery disease may now be treated with carotid stenting under cerebral embolic protection, which is currently reserved primarily for patients at high risk for CEA.[8–9] Recent observational studies have shown that carotid artery stenting (CAS) may be performed prior to CABG with acceptable stroke and death rates.[10-13] To what extent CAS is currently being used for the management of combined carotid and coronary artery disease and the outcomes of concurrent procedures are not well known. Although CAS is a less invasive procedure than CEA, which may result in a reduction in the rate of myocardial events in patients requiring CABG, the need for dual antiplatelet therapy and the potential adverse hemodynamic depression associated with CAS may result in MAEs in patients with unstable CAD.

This review describes the nationwide trends and outcomes of carotid interventions performed in patients who undergo CABG in the United States. The results of CAS versus CEA performed in conjunction with CABG during the same hospitalization are assessed in terms of the risk of perioperative stroke and death.

IDENTIFYING CONCURRENT CAROTID INTERVENTIONS AND CORONARY BYPASS IN THE UNITED STATES

For this review, CAS and CEA procedures performed in conjunction with CABG in the United States were identified using the Nationwide Inpatient Sample (NIS) from the Healthcare Cost and Utilization Project (HCUP). The NIS is the largest all-payer inpatient database in the United States, representing a 20% stratified sample of inpatient admissions to U.S. academic, community, and acute care hospitals nationwide (about 1000 hospitals in 35 states; excluding federal and prison hospitals).[14] Typical discharge data collected include demographics, primary and 14 different secondary diagnoses, primary and 14 different secondary procedures per patient as identified by the *International Classification of Diseases, 9th Revision, Clinical Modification* (ICD-9-CM) codes, length of stay, charges, and outcomes. Sampling weights are provided for accurate calculations based on the complex survey design.

The NIS core inpatient files were used for data extraction and analysis for all concurrent carotid interventions performed in conjunction with CABG from 2000 to 2004. The ICD-9-CM procedural codes for CEA and CAS and procedural codes for CABG were linked.[15–16]

The symptomatic status of patients with carotid stenosis was determined according to ICD-9-CM discharge diagnosis. Patients were classified as symptomatic if discharge diagnosis was "carotid artery stenosis with stroke" or if diagnosis codes included transient ischemic attacks (TIAs) or amaurosis fugax. Patients with a discharge diagnosis of "carotid artery stenosis without mention of stroke" with no accompanying diagnoses for TIA or amaurosis fugax were classified as asymptomatic. Based on 15 diagnosis codes (ICD-9-CM) and the clinical classification software (CCS; Agency for Healthcare Research and Quality, Rockville, MD) coding system included in the data set, which limits and prevents overcoding,[17] comorbid medical conditions were defined and used further to calculate a comorbidity risk score based on the modified Charlson Comorbidity Index (CCI).[18] The CCI is a validated risk stratification measure for use with administrative data that correlates with in-hospital morbidity and mortality after surgical procedures, including elective carotid interventions.[19] Each of the indicated diagnoses is assigned a weight and summed to provide a patient's total score. The ability of CCI to predict in-hospital mortality was initially assessed. Once validated, the CCI was further used to define two surgical-risk based groups according to comorbidities (CCI ≤1 indicating low-risk versus CCI ≥2 indicating greatest comorbidity) for analyses.

In-hospital stroke and death after combined carotid and coronary revascularization procedures (i.e., stroke and/or deaths) that occur after CEA or CAS performed during the same hospitalization as CABG were assessed as the primary outcome endpoint of this cross-sectional population-based review. Postoperative stroke was defined as an ICD-9-CM secondary diagnostic code of "post-operative stroke (997.02)." Postoperative death was defined as any death occurring during the same hospitalization. Mortality data were available directly from the data set, which is noted as "died during hospitalization" and is coded from the disposition of the patient. HCUP quality control procedures are routinely performed to confirm that data values are valid, consistent, and reliable.[20] Weighted analyses for predictors of in-hospital stroke and death included demographic data, symptomatic status, preoperative comorbidities, and risk stratification, which was based on the comorbidity index, and hospital characteristics.

Weighted exact Cochrane-Armitage trend tests were used to determine if there were any trends in outcomes from 2000 to 2004. Because no significant changes in in-hospital stroke and death rates were evident, further statistical analyses included the whole data set using the revised trend sampling weights necessary for analyses that span multiple years to reflect increases in state participation. Descriptive statistics for categorical variables are presented as relative frequencies (percentages), which were compared with χ^2 test (χ^2 for independent groups, two-tailed P value). Continuous variables were expressed as medians and interquartile ranges (IQRs) and compared with nonparametric tests. In-hospital stroke and death rates were adjusted for patient age, sex, symptomatic status, and CCI for risk stratification using multivariate stepwise logistic regression analyses. Findings were considered statistically significant for the primary endpoint, i.e., in-hospital stroke and death, if the resulting P value was less than .05. Multivariate odds ratios (OR) are reported with 95% confidence intervals (95% CI). Relative frequencies of the primary outcomes were calculated for each year. SAS version 9.1 (SAS Institute, Cary, NC) was used for data analyses.

OUTCOMES OF COMBINED CAROTID REVASCULARIZATION AND CORONARY BYPASS

In the United States, the estimated number of concurrent carotid revascularizations and CABGs performed during the same hospitalization was 27,084 from 2001 to 2004. During this 5-year period, the proportion of patients undergoing CAS-CABG versus CEA-CABG has not significantly changed (P=.16). CAS-CABG was performed in 2.5% of all combined procedures in 2001 and in 2.9% in 2004. Most patients underwent CEA-CABG (96.7%), whereas CAS-CABG was performed in only 887 (3.3%) patients. Of these, 85.5% were elective combined procedures.

Most patients (96.4%) undergoing combined carotid and coronary revascularization underwent treatment for asymptomatic carotid stenosis. Of those with symptomatic carotid stenosis, 12% had TIAs and 88% had stroke listed as the principal or secondary diagnosis. Patients undergoing CAS-CABG had a significantly greater prevalence of acute MI, hypertension, and renal failure, whereas patients in the CEA-

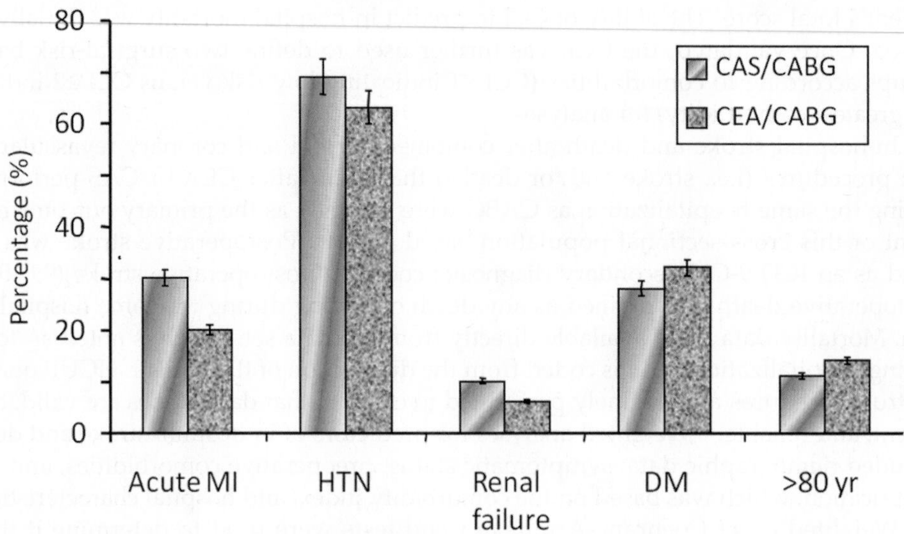

Figure 1-1. A higher frequency of acute myocardial infarction (MI), hypertension (HTN), and renal failure among patients undergoing CAS-CABG, whereas patients in the CEA-CABG group were older and had a greater prevalence of diabetes (P<.05).

CABG group were older and had a greater prevalence of diabetes (Figure 1–1). Overall, CAS-CABG patients had a higher surgical risk profile according to the CCI (48.8% with CCI ≥2 vs. 37.9% in the CEA-CABG group; P<.001). More octogenarians underwent CEA-CABG compared with CAS-CABG (14.4% vs. 11.4%; P=.01). The length of stay of patients undergoing CAS-CABG (median, 11 days; IQR, 8-15 days) was significantly longer than that of patients undergoing CEA-CABG (median, 10 days; IQR, 7-15 days; P=.002). A higher proportion of CAS-CABG procedures were performed in teaching hospitals (70.1% vs. 60.6%) compared with CEA-CABG procedures.

Patients undergoing CAS-CABG had a significantly lower percentage of postoperative stroke (2.4% vs. 3.9%; P<.001) and a trend toward lower combined stroke and death rates (6.9% vs. 8.6%; P=.1) compared with patients undergoing CEA-CABG, although in-hospital death rates were similar (5.2% vs. 5.4%, respectively). Univariate analysis revealed that CEA-CABG patients had a 65% increased risk of postoperative stroke compared with patients undergoing CAS-CABG (OR, 1.65; 95% CI, 1.1-2.6; P=.02). However, no differences in the risk of combined stroke and death were observed (OR, 1.26; 95% CI, 0.9-1.6; P=NS).

Stratified analyses according to symptomatic status and type of carotid revascularization revealed that among 973 patients with symptomatic carotid stenosis, the vast majority (96.4%) underwent CEA-CABG. Postoperative stroke occurred in 14.2% of these patients. Only 25 patients with symptomatic carotid stenosis in this series underwent CAS-CABG. Postoperative stroke occurred in 11 of these 25 patients (44%). Symptomatic patients undergoing CAS-CABG, therefore, had a fivefold increased risk of postoperative stroke compared with those undergoing CEA-CABG (OR, 4.7; 95% CI, 2.1-10.6; P<.001).

According to multivariate logistic regression analysis, CEA-CABG was associated with a 66% increased risk of postoperative stroke compared with CAS-CABG after adjusting for age, gender, symptomatic status, and comorbidities (OR, 1.66; 95% CI,

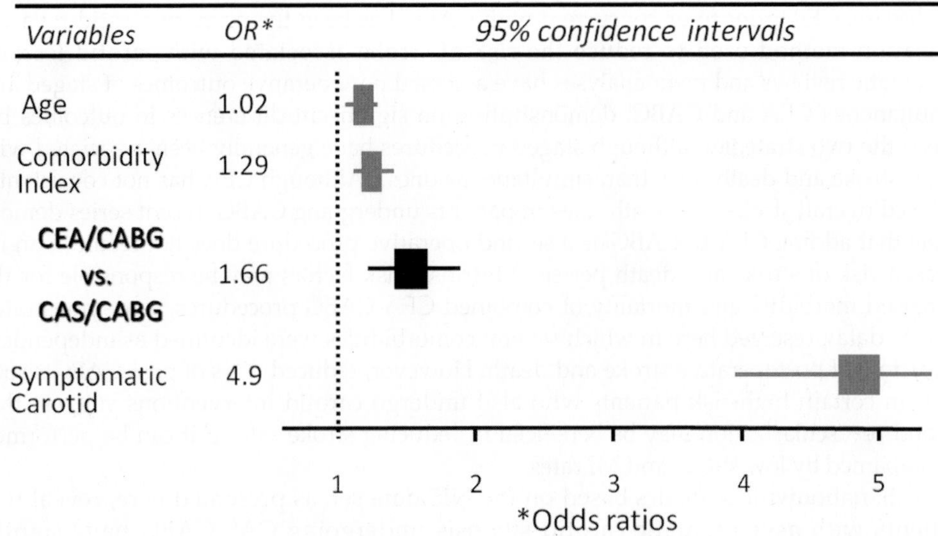

Figure 1-2. Multivariate logistic regression identified CEA-CABG (compared with CAS-CABG), increasing age, symptomatic carotid stenosis, and Charlson comorbidity index (CCI) as independent predictors for postoperative stroke.

1.12-2.7; P=.015). Other independent predictors for postoperative stroke included age, symptomatic carotid stenosis, and CCI (Fig. 1–2). Stratified logistic regression models revealed that octogenarians had a 25% increased risk of postoperative stroke compared with patients younger than 80 years (OR, 1.25; 95% CI, 1.06-1.5; P=.011), whereas high-risk patients (CCI>1) had a 70% increased risk of postoperative stroke compared with low-risk patients (CCI≤1; OR, 1.7; 95% CI, 1.5-1.94; P<.001).

Age, female sex, acute MI, renal failure, and elective hospital admission were identified as independent predictors of in-hospital mortality by stepwise logistic regression (see Figure 1–2). By separate analysis in which age was substituted for octogenarian status in the logistic regression model, octogenarians were found to have a threefold increase risk of in-hospital mortality (OR, 2.9; 95% CI, 2.6-3.3; P<.001).

IMPLICATIONS OF OUTCOMES OF CAS VERSUS CEA PRIOR TO OR CONCURRENT WITH CORONARY BYPASS

The risk of stroke associated with CABG is reported to be less than 2% in patients with no significant carotid disease and 3% in patients with asymptomatic severe carotid stenosis. These figures, however, increase to 5% in those with bilateral carotid stenosis and to 7 to 11% in patients with carotid occlusion.[2] Stroke remains, therefore, the major noncardiac complication following CABG. Optimal treatment of patients with concurrent carotid and coronary artery disease, however, remains unresolved despite over 110 publications during the last 30 years reporting results in over 9000 patients.[1–2,21] Although only 40 to 50% of strokes after CABG are ipsilateral to an existing carotid lesion, carotid revascularization could potentially reduce postoperative stroke and death in patients with combined vascular disease. CEA prior to or concurrent with CABG has been the primary carotid revascularization method used to reduce the risk of stroke associated with carotid lesions. Systematic reviews and meta-analyses have assessed perioperative outcomes of staged and simultaneous CEA and CABG, demonstrating no significant differences in outcomes between the two strategies, although staged procedures have generally been associated with lower stroke and death rates than simultaneous ones.[2] Although CEA has not consistently reduced overall stroke and death rates in patients undergoing CABG, recent series demonstrate that adding CEA to CABG as a second operative procedure does not result in an increased risk of stroke and death per se.[3,6] Intrinsic risk factors may be responsible for the increased morbidity and mortality of combined CEA-CABG procedures, as demonstrated by U.S. data presented here in which several comorbidities were identified as independent predictors of postoperative stroke and death. However, reduced rates of post-CABG stroke rates in certain high-risk patients who also undergo carotid interventions suggest that carotid revascularization may be beneficial in reducing stroke rates if it can be performed accompanied by low stroke and MI rates.

U.S. nationwide statistics based on the NIS data set, as presented here, reveal that patients with asymptomatic carotid stenosis undergoing CAS-CABG have significantly decreased stroke rates than those undergoing CEA-CABG but similar in-hospital mortality. CAS is, however, performed infrequently in patients who require concurrent treatment of carotid artery lesions and CABG. On the basis of these stroke and death figures, CAS-CABG could be explored as an alternative combined revascularization strategy in high-risk asymptomatic patients who require CABG. Further improvements are still necessary to reduce in-hospital mortality, irrespective of the carotid revascularization technique, in patients who require concurrent carotid intervention and CABG. The role of CAS-CABG in symptomatic patients remains undefined because, according to these data, it is very rarely performed.

In the United States, carotid stenting under cerebral embolic protection is currently approved for the treatment of high-risk patients, particularly those with unstable CAD.[8,22] Current evidence indicates that CAS can be used in such patients with acceptable morbidity and mortality rates, particularly when patients are neurologically asymptomatic.[22,24] More recently, the results of staged CAS prior to CABG have been reported with low periprocedural major adverse events and complication rates.[10-13,25–26] In a few instances, however, CAS and CEA prior to or concomitant with CABG have been compared. Early results tend to favor CAS. The long-term results of staged CAS followed by CABG in asymptomatic patients have been recently reported. Not only low periprocedural morbidity and mortality but also long-term durable results (4.8% death and stroke rates at 30 days and 71.4% 5-year freedom from all stroke and death) were seen.[25] U.S. data confirm the safety and efficacy of staged CAS and CABG in terms of perioperative complications among asymptomatic patients and suggest that staged CAS-CABG may be a useful if not preferable alternative to CEA-CABG.

The role of CAS prior to CABG in patients with symptomatic carotid stenosis deserves further investigation. The increased risk of symptomatic patients after carotid interventions appears to be disproportionably higher after CAS compared with after CEA.[27] In the NIS series, CAS-CABG was disturbingly associated with a fivefold increased risk of postoperative stroke compared with CEA-CABG among symptomatic patients. This finding, however, needs to be interpreted with caution given the small number of symptomatic patients undergoing CAS-CABG in this series. The performance of CAS and CABG during the same hospitalization could have been carried out only with aspirin and heparin therapy, which may have resulted in adverse outcomes owing to stent thrombosis and embolization. Clopidogrel is frequently avoided in order to prevent its associated intrinsic increased risk of bleeding in patients undergoing CABG and is only started once mediastinal bleeding has been excluded. Although the reported experience with this approach is limited and has been restricted primarily to asymptomatic patients in whom no postoperative neurologic adverse events have occurred,[13,28] its utility in symptomatic patients has not been determined. The data presented here suggest that if combined carotid and coronary interventions are required in patients with symptomatic carotid stenosis, CEA-CABG is probably the best option.

CAS-induced hemodynamic depression is a well-known complication that results from mechanical stimulation of the carotid sinus baroreceptors and may induce major adverse cardiac events.[29] It is unknown to what extent CAS may result in major adverse cardiac events in patients requiring CABG. Although postprocedural MI data are not available in the NIS data set, major postoperative cardiac complications were not reported after either CAS-CABG or CEA-CABG, and in-hospital death rates were similar, thereby suggesting a similar incidence of major cardiac adverse events for both carotid revascularization techniques in patients requiring CABG. The potential advantage of CAS over CEA related to its theoretical reduced invasiveness that may prevent cardiac events in patients with significant and unstable coronary artery disease has, therefore, not been proven.

Unfortunately, combined CAS or CEA and CABG included in the NIS data set are performed during the same hospitalization, because unique subject identifiers within the data set prevent the identification of multiple admissions for the same patient. The importance of including only patients undergoing combined carotid and coronary procedures during the same hospitalization, however, is based on the inclusion of patients with such severe carotid and coronary artery disease that requires immediate treatment, which constitutes the heart of the controversy regarding the best management of patients with combined vascular disease. In fact, the vast majority of patients with combined carotid and coronary artery stenosis have varying degrees of severity of their vascular diseases that allow them to safely undergo carotid interventions or CABG in different hospitalizations according to clinical priority. In practice, therefore, only a small minority of patients have such severe combined disease that a staged or simultaneous revascularization is required.[2] The current series focuses on such patients, that is, those with severe combined disease who are more likely to undergo their combined reconstructions during the same hospitalization.

The best treatment strategy of patients who require combined carotid and coronary revascularization procedures should ideally be determined by a multicenter randomized clinical trial, the design and implementation of which have, unfortunately, been shown to be impractical and unfeasible. The heterogeneity of patients with varying degrees of coronary and carotid artery disease and the preference of carotid intervention are the main limitations for such a trial. Current evidence should, therefore, focus on the outcomes of those patients with severe combined disease who required simultaneous or staged urgent procedures.

Several limitations of this report should be acknowledged regarding the outcomes of CAS-CABG and CEA-CABG procedures in the United States. First, miscoding and missing data may occur in large administrative data sets such as the NIS. HCUP quality routine control procedures verify to some extent that NIS data values are valid, consistent, and reliable.[20] Second, the NIS data set does not distinguish among the severity of comorbidities, which prevents an accurate risk stratification of patients. In the current series, however, only high-risk patients with unstable CAD were included. Third, only in-hospital stroke and death rates are reported in the NIS data set, which may erroneously be considered too low when compared with the usually reported 30-day rates of MAEs after carotid interventions. Moreover, the inability to include postprocedural MI rates, which are not reported in this series, as part of the primary endpoint would also suggest an apparently lower combined major adverse event rate in this series. Fourth, the inability to perform an intention-to-treat analysis in patients undergoing staged procedures may bias the results against patients undergoing simultaneous CEA-CABG, because patients who suffer a major complication or death associated with the carotid revascularization are unlikely to undergo subsequent CABG. Finally, anatomic, procedural, and other patient characteristics that could be explored as possible predictors of adverse outcomes are not available in the NIS data set. Future studies assessing their effects on the outcomes of combined procedures as well as the influence of the severity and stability of both carotid and coronary conditions will probably alter the strategy and type of procedures used for the treatment of patients requiring concurrent carotid and coronary interventions. The effects of the degree of carotid stenosis and the presence of bilateral critical carotid stenosis in asymptomatic patients also need further investigation, as most patients undergoing combined carotid and coronary interventions in the United States have asymptomatic carotid disease.

In conclusion, CAS is infrequently used in patients who require concurrent carotid and coronary interventions in the United States. Patients with asymptomatic carotid stenosis undergoing CAS-CABG have significantly lower stroke rates than those undergoing CEA-CABG but have similar in-hospital mortality. CAS may be a safer carotid revascularization option for patients with asymptomatic carotid stenosis requiring CABG in terms of postoperative stroke prevention, but further improvements in in-hospital mortality are necessary. Conversely, in patients with symptomatic carotid stenosis, CEA-CABG is probably a better option. The best treatment approach for patients requiring combined carotid and coronary interventions is, however, still undefined and should be established comparing the two strategies in the setting of a well-powered randomized clinical trial.

REFERENCES

1. Naylor AR, Mehta Z, Rothwell PM, Bell PR. Carotid artery disease and stroke during coronary artery bypass: a critical review of the literature. Eur J Vasc Endovasc Surg 2002;23:283–94.
2. Naylor AR, Cuffe RL, Rothwell PM, Bell PR. A systematic review of outcomes following staged and synchronous carotid endarterectomy and coronary artery bypass. Eur J Vasc Endovasc Surg 2003;25:380–9.
3. Ricotta JJ, Wall LP, Blackstone E. The influence of concurrent carotid endarterectomy on coronary bypass: a case-controlled study. J Vasc Surg 2005;41:397–401.
4. Myers SI, Valentine RJ, Estrera A, Clagett GP. The intra-aortic balloon pump, a novel addition to staged repair of combined symptomatic cerebrovascular and coronary artery disease. Ann Vasc Surg 1993;7:239–42.

5. Hertzer NR, Mascha EJ. A personal experience with coronary artery bypass grafting, carotid patching, and other factors influencing the outcome of carotid endarterectomy. J Vasc Surg 2006;43:959–68.
6. Ricotta JJ, Char DJ, Cuadra SA, et al. Modeling stroke risk after coronary artery bypass and combined coronary artery bypass and carotid endarterectomy. Stroke 2003;34:1212–7.
7. Brown KR, Kresowik TF, Chin MH, et al. Multistate population-based outcomes of combined carotid endarterectomy and coronary artery bypass. J Vasc Surg 2003;37:32–9.
8. Veith FJ, Amor M, Ohki T, et al. Current status of carotid bifurcation angioplasty and stenting based on a consensus of opinion leaders. J Vasc Surg 2001;33:S111–S116.
9. Ohki T, Timaran CH, Yadav JS. Technique of carotid angioplasty and stenting. In: Moore WS, ed. Vascular and Endovascular Surgery: A Comprehensive Review. 7th ed. Philadelphia: Saunders Elsevier; 2006, pp. 355–82.
10. Ziada KM, Yadav JS, Mukherjee D, et al. Comparison of results of carotid stenting followed by open heart surgery versus combined carotid endarterectomy and open heart surgery (coronary bypass with or without another procedure). Am J Cardiol 2005;96:519–23.
11. Kovacic JC, Roy PR, Baron DW, Muller DW. Staged carotid artery stenting and coronary artery bypass graft surgery: initial results from a single center. Catheter Cardiovasc Interv 2006;67:142–8.
12. Randall MS, McKevitt FM, Cleveland TJ, et al. Is there any benefit from staged carotid and coronary revascularization using carotid stents? A single-center experience highlights the need for a randomized controlled trial. Stroke 2006;37:435–9.
13. Mendiz O, Fava C, Valdivieso L, et al. Synchronous carotid stenting and cardiac surgery: an initial single-center experience. Catheter Cardiovasc Interv 2006;68:424–8.
14. Overview of the Nationwide Inpatient Sample (NIS) of the Healthcare Cost and Utilization Project (HCUP). http://www.hcup-us.ahrq.gov/nisoverview.jsp Accessed January 4, 2008.
15. Nowygrod R, Egorova N, Greco G, et al. Trends, complications, and mortality in peripheral vascular surgery. J Vasc Surg 2006;43:205–16.
16. McPhee JT, Hill JS, Ciocca RG, et al. Carotid endarterectomy was performed with lower stroke and death rates than carotid artery stenting in the United States in 2003 and 2004. J Vasc Surg 2007;46:1112–8.
17. Healthcare Cost and Utilization Project (HCUP) Clinical Classifications Software (CCS). http://www.hcup-us.ahrq.gov/toolssoftware/ccs/ccs.jsp Accessed January 4, 2008.
18. Deyo RA, Cherkin DC, Ciol MA. Adapting a clinical comorbidity index for use with ICD-9-CM administrative databases. J Clin Epidemiol 1992;45:613–9.
19. Karp HR, Flanders WD, Shipp CC, et al. Carotid endarterectomy among medicare beneficiaries: A statewide evaluation of appropriateness and outcome. Stroke 1998;29:46–52.
20. Healthcare Cost and Utilization Project (HCUP) Quality Control Procedures. http://www.hcup-us.ahrq.gov/db/quality.jsp Accessed January 2, 2008.
21. Eagle KA, Guyton RA, Davidoff R, et al. ACC/AHA guidelines for coronary artery bypass graft surgery: executive summary and recommendations: A report of the American College of Cardiology/American Heart Association Task Force on Practice Guidelines (Committee to revise the 1991 guidelines for coronary artery bypass graft surgery). Circulation 1999; 100:1464–80.
22. Yadav JS, Wholey MH, Kuntz RE, et al. Protected carotid-artery stenting versus endarterectomy in high-risk patients. N Engl J Med 2004;351:1493–501.
23. Gray WA, Hopkins LN, Yadav S, et al. Protected carotid stenting in high-surgical-risk patients: the ARCHeR results. J Vasc Surg 2006;44:258–68.
24. Fairman R, Gray WA, Scicli AP, et al. The CAPTURE registry: analysis of strokes resulting from carotid artery stenting in the post approval setting: timing, location, severity, and type. Ann Surg 2007;246:551–6.
25. Van der HJ, Suttorp MJ, Bal ET, et al. Staged carotid angioplasty and stenting followed by cardiac surgery in patients with severe asymptomatic carotid artery stenosis: early and long-term results. Circulation 2007;116:2036–42.

26. Kramer J, Abraham J, Jones PA. Carotid artery stenting before CABG: a better alternative to treat concomitant coronary and carotid artery disease. Stroke 2006;37:1359.
27. Mas JL, Chatellier G, Beyssen B, et al. Endarterectomy versus stenting in patients with symptomatic severe carotid stenosis. N Engl J Med 2006;355:1660–71.
28. Chiariello L, Tomai F, Zeitani J, Versaci F. Simultaneous hybrid revascularization by carotid stenting and coronary artery bypass grafting. Ann Thorac Surg 2006;81:1883–5.
29. Gupta R, bou-Chebl A, Bajzer CT, et al. Rate, predictors, and consequences of hemodynamic depression after carotid artery stenting. J Am Coll Cardiol 2006;47:1538–43.

2

Interventional Approaches to Acute Stroke

Omar M. Arnaout, B.A., Anitha Nimmagadda, M.D., Joseph Adel, M.D., Guilherme Dabus, M.D., and Bernard R. Bendok, M.D.

INTRODUCTION

Stroke continues to be the third leading cause of death in the United States, with an approximate incidence of 800,000 people annually. Eighty-five percent of strokes are ischemic in nature, with an associated mortality between 53% and 92%.[1-4] Over the past two decades, several studies have shown that the effectiveness of interventional therapy for stroke is time-dependent.[5] Furthermore, successful recanalization of a previously occluded vessel correlates with improvement in clinical outcomes.[2,6–7] As a result, the current focus of treatment for acute stroke is the delivery of prompt therapy that effectively restores flow to the occluded vascular territory.

In assessing the time frame available to salvage brain tissue, studies have suggested that tissue may continue to be at risk up to 24 hours after stroke onset; however, the clinical significance of this extended window is unclear.[8–9] While intravenous tissue plasminogen activator (IV tPA) administration has shown benefit up to 3 hours from stroke onset, extension of the window to 6 hours has failed to show benefit.[10–11] On the other hand, recent combined analysis of several studies has suggested that the benefit of IV tPA may extend to 4.5 hours after stroke onset.[5,12–13] More recently, European Cooperative Acute Stroke Study (ECASS) 3 demonstrated that intravenous alteplase administered 3 to 4.5 hours after the onset of symptoms improved clinical outcomes in patients with acute ischemic stroke.[13] However, patients with severe ischemic strokes were excluded from the trial. This raises a concern regarding the applicability of these data to patients with large intracranial vessel occlusions. The limited time window for IV tPA infusion and the multitude of contraindications to full dose IV tPA have spawned interest in infusion of local tPA at lower doses and/or mechanical approaches to revascularizing acutely occluded intracranial vessels. Additionally, a number of trials have investigated the use of intra-arterial (IA) infusion of thrombolytics at the location of the thrombus within 6 hours of stroke onset.[14-17]

For patients presenting outside the window for tPA and for those in whom tPA is contraindicated, mechanical interventional devices including the MERCI clot retrieval system (Concentric Medical, Mountain View, CA) and the Penumbra system (Penumbra, Inc., Alameda, CA), have recently been approved for up to 8 hours after stroke onset.[19-21]

TABLE 2-1. SUMMARY OF RECENT LANDMARK TRIALS IN THE TREATMENT OF ACUTE STROKE

						Window			
Study	**Year**	**#**	**Study Type**	**Population**	**Median NIHSS**	**Goal**	**Median**	**Drug Infusion**	**Dose/Hour**
PROACT I	1998	46	Multicenter, prospective, randomized, double-blind, controlled	Symptomatic M1/M2	17 (19 placebo)	6 hours	5.4 hours (5.7 hours placebo)	Pro-UK	6 mg/hr
PROACT II	1999	180	Multicenter, prospective, randomized, open-label, controlled	Symptomatic M1/M2	17 (17 control)	6 hours	5.3 hours	Pro-UK	9 mg/hr
IMS	2006	80	Multicenter, prospective, nonrandomized, single arm	ICA, MCA, ACA, PCA, BA	18	3 hours	2.3 hours	re-tPA	0.6 mg/kg IV, plus up to 22 mg IA @ 9 mg/hr
IMS II	2007	81	Multicenter, prospective, nonrandomized, single arm	Same as IMS I	19	3 hours	2.4 hours	re-tPA	0.6 mg/kg IV, plus up to 22 mg IA @ 9 mg/hr
MERCI	2005	151	Multicenter, prospective, nonrandomized, single arm	VA, BA, ICA, M1, M2	20	8 hours	4.3 hours (mean)	None	N/A
Multi MERCI	2008	164	Multicenter, international, prospective, nonrandomized, single arm	VA, BA, ICA, M1, M2	19	8 hours	4.3 hours	IV tPA	N/A
Penumbra	2009	125	Multicenter, prospective, nonrandomized, single arm	"large intracranial vessels"	17	8 hours	4.3 hours (mean)	None	N/A
SARIS	2009	20	Prospective pilot, single arm, single center	Intracranial artery <14 mm	13	8 hours	4.9 hours	60% of patients: eptifibatide, reteplase	13 mg, 6 mg respectively

This chapter summarizes recent landmark studies related to the treatment of acute ischemic stroke, ongoing promising trials, and potential future directions and concludes with case illustrations. Table 2–1 and Figure 2–1 provide a summary of the landmark studies discussed below.

Pharmacologic Agent							
IV Heparin	**Device**	**mRS≤2 @ 90 days**	**Recannalization Rate (TIMI 2 or 3)**	**Asymptomatic Hemorrhage**	**Symptomatic Hemorrhagic Conversion**	**Procedural Complications**	**All-Cause Mortality @ 90 days**
Yes, high dose initially, low dose later.	None	30.8% (21.4% placebo)* mRS≤1	57.7% (14.3% placebo)	42.3% (7.1% placebo)	15.4% (vs. 7.1% placebo)	N/A	26.9% (42.9% placebo)
Yes, low dose	None	40% (25% control)	66% (18% control)	35% (13% control)	10% (vs. 2% control)	9% (7% control)	25% (vs. 27% control)
Yes	None	43%	56%	43%	6.30%	10%	16%
Yes	EKOS micro-infusion catheter	46%	60%	32.10%	9.90%	3.70%	16%
Yes	Merci Retrieval System (X5,X6)	22.60%	48.0%	27.7%	7.80%	13.00%	43.5%
Yes	Merci Retrieval System (L5)	36%	55.0%	N/A	9.80%	9.80%	34.0%
Yes, no standard dose	Penumbra System	25%	81.60%	28%	11.20%	12.80%	32.80%
Yes	Wingspan SES, Enterprise SES	45%* mRS≤1	100%	10%	5%	N/A	25% (1 month)

PROACT: Prolyse in Acute Cerebral Thromboembolism
IMS: Interventional Management of Stroke
MERCI: Mechanical Embolus Removal in Cerebral Ischemia
SARIS: Stent-Assisted Recanalization in Acute Ischemic Stroke
pro-UK: pro-urokinase
tPA: tissue plasminogen activator
ICA: internal carotid artery
MCA: middle cerebral artery
ACA: anterior cerebral artery
PCA: posterior cerebral artery
BA: basilar artery
VA: vertebral artery
M1: horizontal segment of MCA
M2: insular segment of MCA

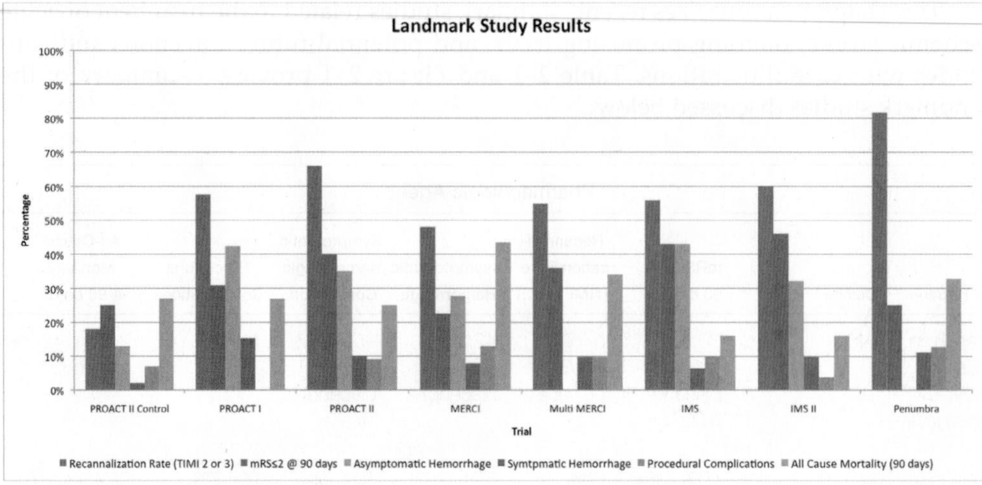

Figure 2-1. Summary of recent landmark trials in the treatment of acute stroke. MERCI: Mechanical Embolus Removal in Cerebral Ischemia, SES: self-expanding stent

LANDMARK STUDIES

PROACT I (1998, N=46)[16]

The Prolyse in Acute Cerebral Thromboembolism (PROACT) trial was a multicenter, prospective, randomized control trial that compared the efficacy of direct IA infusion of pro-urokinase (pro-UK) versus placebo for the treatment of symptomatic middle cerebral artery (MCA) occlusion within 6 hours of stroke onset. The investigators chose to include only stroke patients with acute MCA occlusions (M1 and M2 branches) to increase the homogeneity of the patient population. Pro-UK is a proenzyme that is locally converted to urokinase by fibrin-associated plasmin at the thrombus surface and whose effects are augmented by the presence of heparin. In this study, the recanalization of an occluded vessel, evidenced by achieving a Thrombolysis in Myocardial Infarction (TIMI) score of 2 or 3, was significantly more likely in the pro-UK group than the placebo group (57.7% vs. 14.3%, respectively). There was also a 9.4% improvement in clinical outcome (assessed by a modified Rankin score [mRS] of 0 or 1) and a 16% reduction in mortality at 90 days, although neither change was statistically significant. The overall risk of intracranial hemorrhage (ICH) was elevated in the pro-UK group to 42.3% (compared with 7.1% in the placebo group), although only 15.4% of hemorrhages were symptomatic (defined as a decline in neurologic status).

Notably, the rate of developing ICH postprocedurally decreased to 20% from 72.7% after the investigators reduced the dose of heparin being used. Concurrently, there was a reduction in the rate of recanalization from 81.8 to 40%.

PROACT II (1999, N=180)[17]

The PROACT II study, which was enrolling at the time the results of PROACT were published, was a multicenter, prospective, randomized control trial that primarily aimed at assessing the neurologic outcome of the use of IA pro-UK in the treatment of MCA strokes. Unlike the original PROACT trial, the investigators used a control group in which no IA infusion was performed in place of a placebo infusion. Although the investigators used the lower heparin dose from the latter part of the original trial, they increased the dose of IA pro-UK to 9 mg/hr from 6 mg/hr.

The recanalization rate in the pro-UK group was 66%, representing a statistically significant 15% absolute increase over the control group, which was attributed to the higher pro-UK dose. Although the rate of ICH was 35% (compared with 13% in the control group), the rate of symptomatic hemorrhage was 10% (compared with 2% in the control group). Although mortality at 90 days was not significantly improved (25% vs. 27% in the control group), neurologic outcomes (mRS≤2) were significantly better in the pro-UK group (40% vs. 25% in the control group).

IMS I (2006, N=80)[14]

The Interventional Management of Stroke (IMS) study was a multicenter, prospective, single-arm study aimed at assessing the feasibility and safety of combined IV and IA tPA administered within 3 hours of stroke onset. The investigators used historical controls from the National Institute of Neurological Disorders and Stroke (NINDS) trial of IV tPA alone[10] and built upon earlier data from the Emergency Management of Stroke (EMS) Study.[18]

The investigators found that neurologic outcome at 90 days (43%) and mortality at 90 days (16%) were significantly improved when compared with the placebo arm of the NINDS trial (28% and 24%, respectively). There was no difference in the rate of symptomatic hemorrhage comparable to the IV tPA arm of the NINDS study (6.3% vs. 6.6%, respectively). Although there was no significant improvement in neurologic outcome or mortality rates compared with the IV tPA arm of NINDS, the IMS study included patients with a higher median NIHSS score (18 vs. 14) and more patients with atrial fibrillation (increasing their risk for larger emboli). As such, the results were considered promising for potential benefit over IV tPA alone and as warranting further investigation.

Notably, there was a trend toward significance for improvement in neurologic outcome at 90 days in the subgroup of patients treated within the first 3 to 4 hours of onset compared with those treated more than 4 hours later, affirming the association between earlier revascularization and outcome.

IMS II (2007, N=81)[15]

The second IMS trial employed an identical protocol to IMS I, with the addition of an investigational EKOS microinfusion catheter. The catheter combines a traditional targeted drug infusion mechanism with a low-energy ultrasound in order to facilitate penetration of tPA into the thrombus and theoretically enhance thrombolysis. Of the 81 enrolled patients, ultrasound was activated for use in 33 patients (40.7%). The investigators also aimed to further demonstrate the results of IMS I while plans for a phase III trial were ongoing.

Whereas there was an increase in the incidence of ICH in IMS II compared with IMS I patients (9.9% vs. 6.3%, respectively), the results were not significantly different for hemorrhage, neurologic outcome, revascularization rate, or mortality. However, again demonstrated was a significant improvement over the placebo arm of the NINDS trial, supporting direct comparison between a combined IA/IV approach and IV alone.

MERCI (2005 N=151, 2008 N=164)[19,20]

The Mechanical Embolus Removal in Cerebral Ischemia (MERCI) trial evaluated the efficacy and safety of a mechanical endovascular device (which consists of a Nitinol core wire with shaped loops at the distal end designed to engage the thrombus) in the revascularization of an occluded large cerebral vessel within 8 hours of stroke onset. The original study was subsequently updated by the Multi MERCI trial incorporating a newer generation of the device.[20] The population of patients included in both studies were those ineligible to receive IV tPA (either arriving too late or having a contraindication for its use). The MERCI trial was a multicenter, prospective, single-arm trial that referred to the control arm of the PROACT II trial as the historical control.

Although the therapeutic window was 8 hours, the median time from onset to treatment was 4.3 hours in both studies. The recanalization rate was significantly higher than that in the control arm of PROACT II (48% vs. 18%), but lower than that in the IA tPA group (66%). The proportion of patients achieving mRS≤2 at 90 days was comparable with that in the control arm of PROACT II (22.6% vs. 25%). On the other hand, the mortality rate was significantly higher than that reported in most prospective studies of the treatment of acute stroke, at 43.5%. The investigators attributed this elevated mortality to a higher baseline NIHSS score (median 18), and a higher proportion of basilar artery and internal carotid artery terminus occlusions. The introduction of a new generation of the device in the Multi MERCI trial resulted in a significantly higher recanalization rate (55%) and an improvement in the mortality or neurologic outcome at 90 days, although it was not statistically significant.

Penumbra (2009, N=125)[21]

The Penumbra device was introduced in the United States in 2008 after results from a European safety trial were published. The system consists of a thrombus debulking and aspiration component as well as a direct thrombus extraction component. The safety and efficacy of the device were reported in a multicenter, prospective single-arm trial.

Although the revascularization rate using the Penumbra device was the highest of the prospective trials at 81.6% (compared with 55% in the Multi MERCI trial and 66% in the PROACT II trial), the neurologic outcome was comparable or lower (25% with mRS≤2, vs. 36% in the Multi MERCI trial and 40% in the PROACT II trial). The investigators attribute this disparity to the lack of sufficient power and higher baseline NIHSS score.[17,19–20] Further studies are under way to better define outcomes with this promising device.

SARIS (2009, N=20)[23]

The use of endovascular stents has been recently advocated in the setting of acute stroke.[23] Based on retrospective data regarding the use of intracranial stents as a salvage technique in acute stroke, the SARIS trial (Stent-Assisted Recanalization in Acute Ischemic Stroke) aimed to evaluate the safety of stent deployment as a primary therapeutic intervention for acute stroke using a prospective, single-arm study design. The investigators used the Wingspan (Boston Scientific, Natick, MA) and the Enterprise (Cordis. Bridgewater, NJ) intracranial self-expanding stents.

All 20 cases included in the trial were successfully revascularized, although 60% of the patients required the use of an adjuvant intraprocedural pharmacologic infusion (eptifibatide or tPA) or angioplasty. The risk of subsequent asymptomatic and symptomatic hemorrhage was 10% and 5%, respectively, and no procedure-related complications were reported. With regards to neurologic outcomes, 45% of patients achieved an mRS score of 1 or less at 1-month follow-up. The results of the SARIS trial are difficult to directly compare with the large, randomized prospective trials, because it included a small number of patients with a relatively low median NIHSS score (13 vs. 19 in IMS II and 17 in PROACT II), was nonrandomized, and included only a short follow-up; nonetheless, the results represent an encouraging foundation for further investigation into the role of stenting for stroke treatment.

CASE EXAMPLES

Case 1: Left M1 Occlusion – angioplasty

The patient is an 80-year-old right-handed female with a history of hypertension and hypercholesterolemia who awoke with acute onset of aphasia and right-sided weakness. She was brought to the emergency room, admitted to the neurology service, and started on antiplatelet agents. An MRI of the brain 24 hours after admission showed left basal ganglia stroke and a left M1 occlusion (Figures 2–2 and 2–3). The patient's right motor function became pressure-dependent and therefore mechanical endovascular intervention was requested to open the left M1. An M1 angioplasty was performed with successful recanalization of the vessel (Figures 2–4 and 2–5). Her exam improved significantly after angioplasty. She was discharged home after return to her baseline neurologic condition.

Case 2: Left M1 Occlusion: Thrombolysis and Thrombectomy – MERCI

The patient is a 76-year-old female who developed aphasia and right-sided weakness after endovascular repair of a thoracic aortic aneurysm. An MRI of the brain showed restricted diffusion of the left caudate and lentiform nuclei (Figure 2–6). She was taken to the angiography suite within 8 hours of the onset of her symptoms for cerebral angiography with possible intervention. A cerebral angiogram demonstrated left M1 occlusion (Figures 2–7 and 2–8). Left M1 thrombolysis and thrombectomy were performed with the MERCI device (Figure 2–9). The cerebral angiogram after thrombolysis and thrombectomy demonstrated

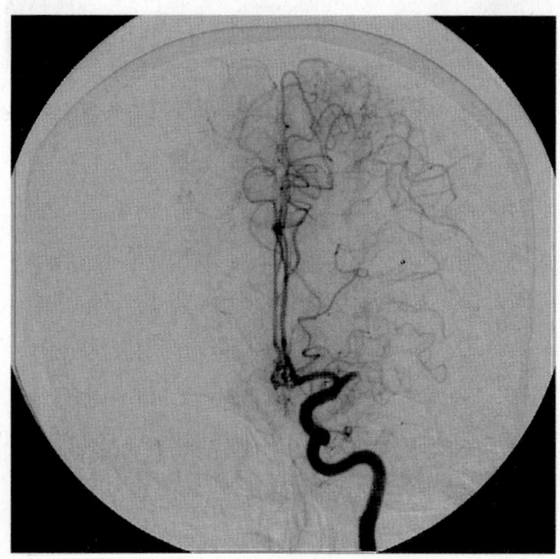

Figure 2-2. Cerebral angiogram. AP view demonstrating left M1 occlusion.

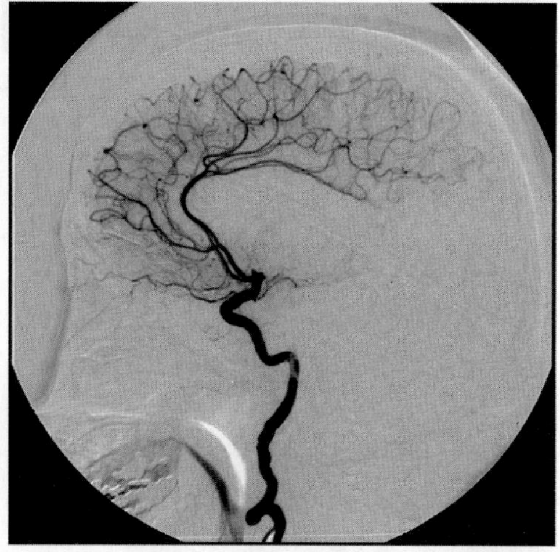

Figure 2-3. Cerebral angiogram. LICA injection - Lateral view demonstrating left M1 occlusion.

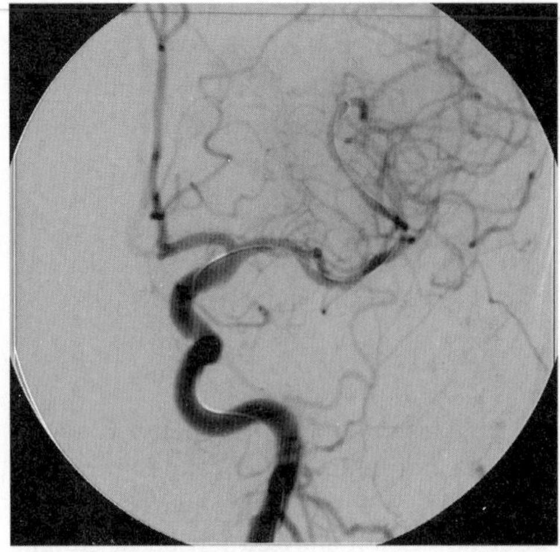

Figure 2-4. Cerebral angiogram. LICA injection - AP view during left M1 angioplasty.

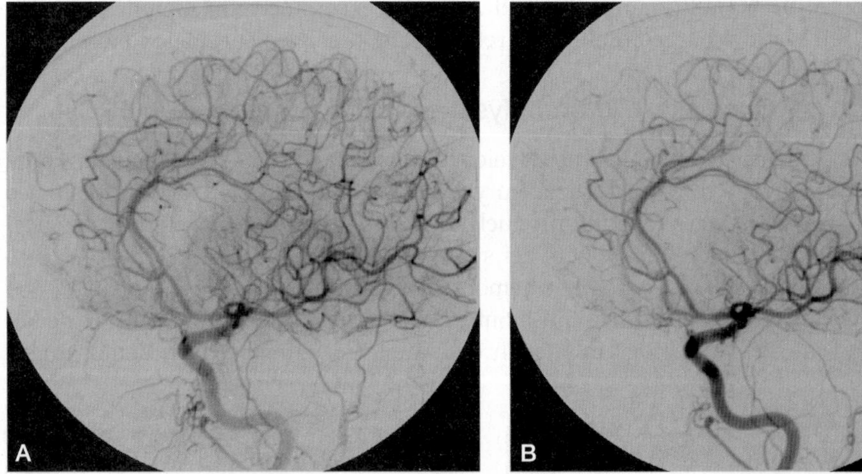

Figure 2-5. Cerebral angiogram. LICA injection - Lateral views post successful left M1 angioplasty demonstrating restored flow.

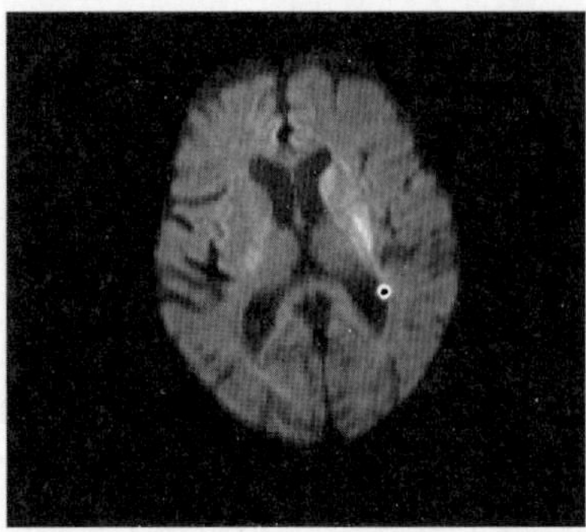

Figure 2-6. MRI brain diffusion weighted imaging (DWI) sequence showing restricted diffusion of left caudate and lentiform nuclei.

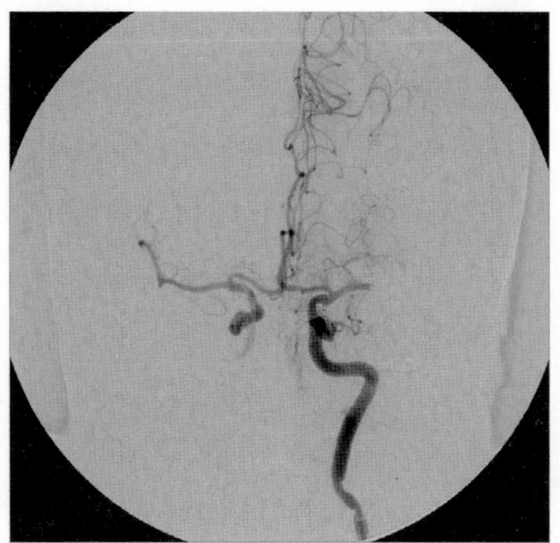

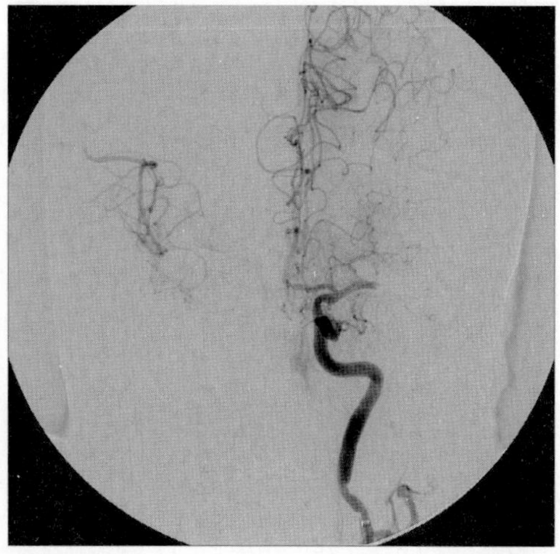

Figure 2-7. Cerebral angiogram. LICA injection - AP views demonstrating left M1 occlusion.

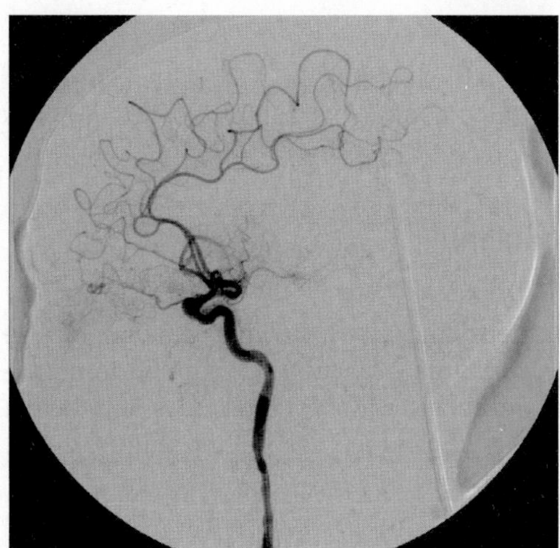

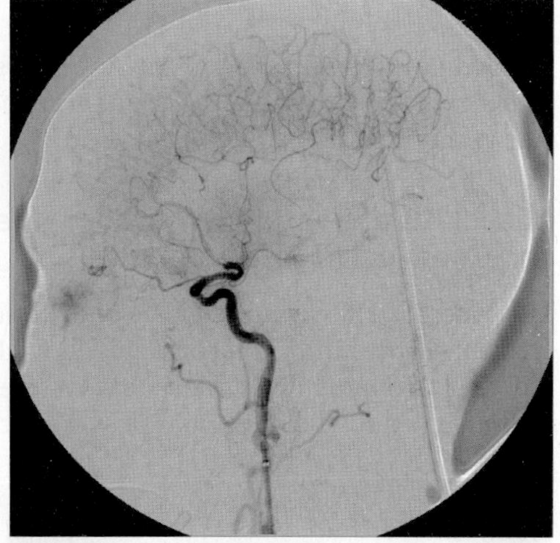

Figure 2-8. Cerebral angiogram. LICA injection lateral views demonstrating left M1 occlusion.

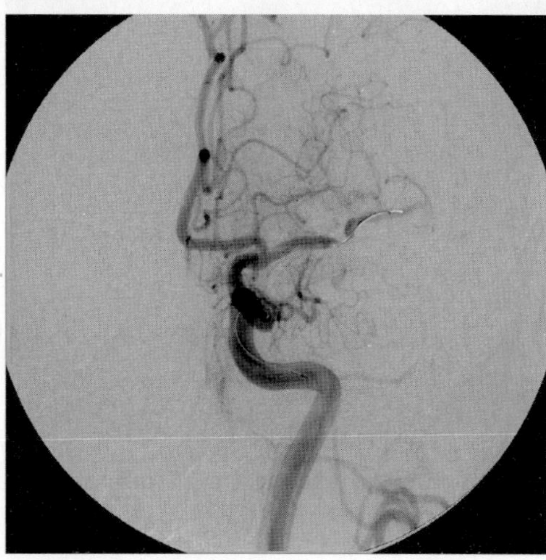

Figure 2-9. Cerebral angiogram. LICA injection AP view during mechanical thrombolysis.

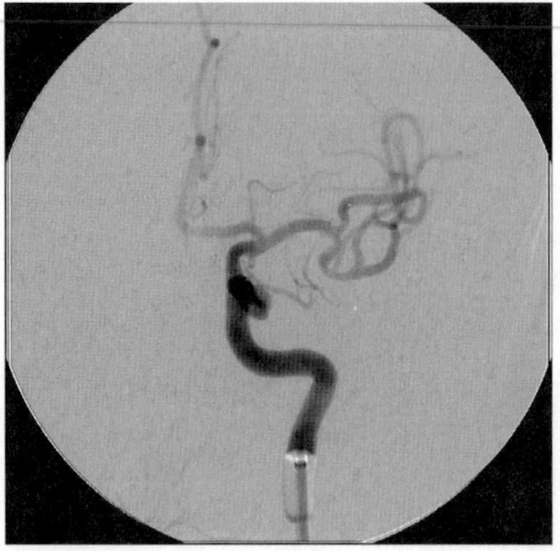
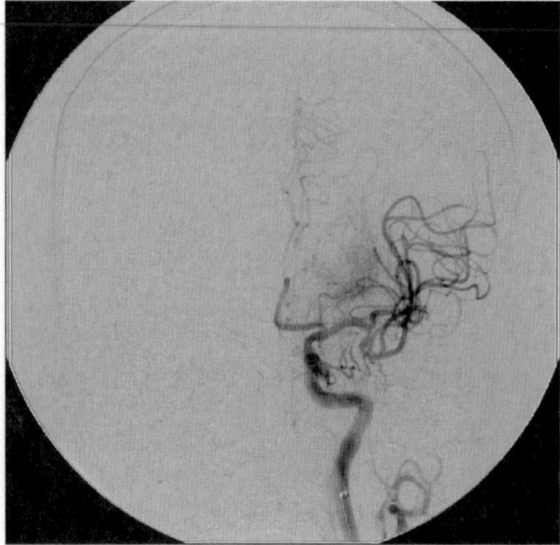

Figure 2-10. Cerebral angiogram. LICA injection AP views post mechanical thrombolysis demonstrating restored flow and successful left M1 thrombolysis.

restored flow in the distal left MCA (Figures 2–10 and 2–11). Postprocedurally, she recovered significant strength in her right arm and leg and showed significant improvement of her speech.

Case 3: Basilar Artery Occlusion – Mechanical and Chemical (tPA) Thrombolysis

The patient is a 43-year-old female who declined neurologically 1 day after a motor vehicle accident that resulted in a comminuted C1 left lateral mass fracture. Computed tomography (CT) angiography revealed a basilar artery thrombosis. MRI revealed areas of ischemia and infarction in the pons, right posterior occipital lobe, and left cerebellum (Figure 2–12).

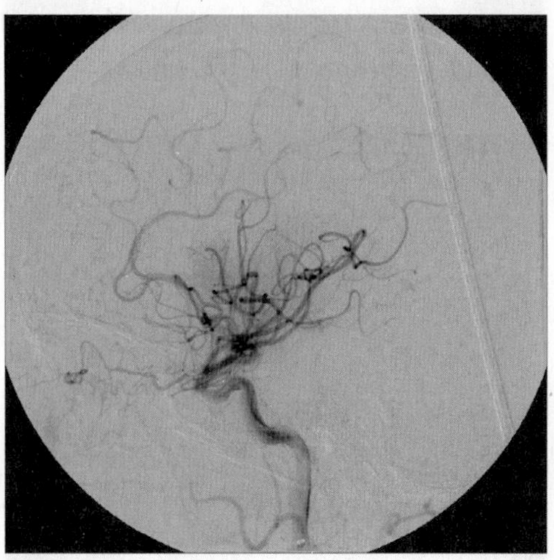
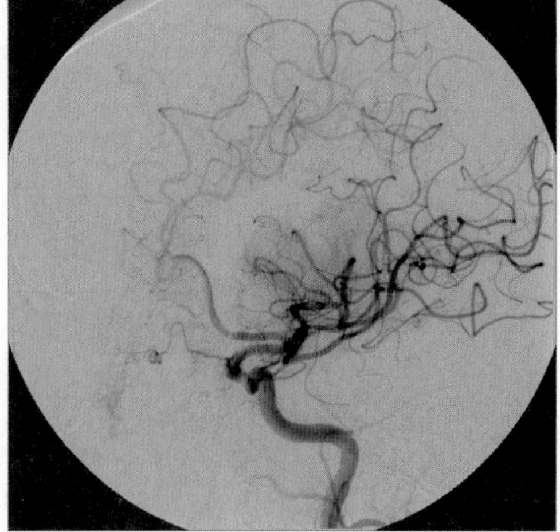

Figure 2-11. Cerebral angiogram. LICA injection lateral views demonstrating restored flow after successful left M1 thrombolysis.

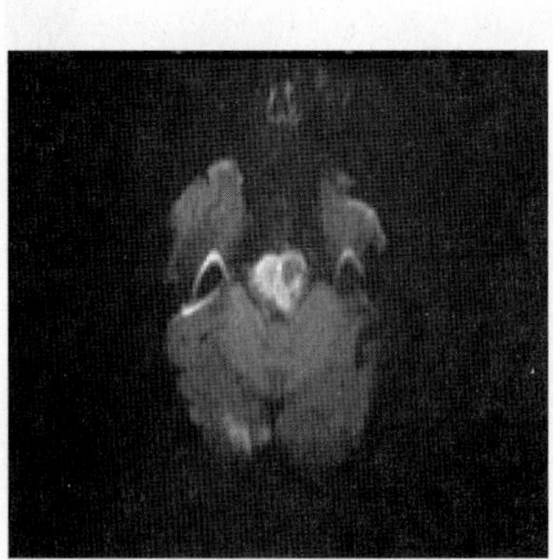

Figure 2-12. MR DWI sequence demonstrating areas of restricted diffusion consistent with infarction in the pons and right occipital lobe.

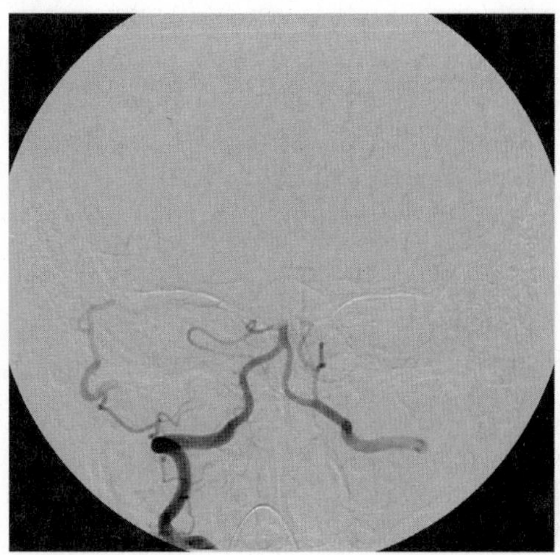

Figure 2-13. Cerebral angiogram. RVA injection AP view demonstrating basilar artery occlusion.

The patient was transferred to our institution for intervention. At the time of transfer, she had significant weakness of all extremities, right third nerve palsy, and left sixth nerve palsy. Cerebral angiogram demonstrated basilar artery occlusion (Figures 2–13 and 2–14). Chemical and mechanical thrombolysis of the basilar artery was performed with the Merci device. Cerebral angiography performed after thrombolysis showed restored flow in the basilar artery (Figures 2–15 through 2–17). At 1-year follow-up, the patient was independent with an excellent neurologic exam.

Case 4: Right Supraclinoid ICA Occlusion – Stent Placement

The patient is a 47-year-old female who presented with mild left-sided weakness. Three days after admission she developed increasing left-sided weakness and lethargy. An MRI showed

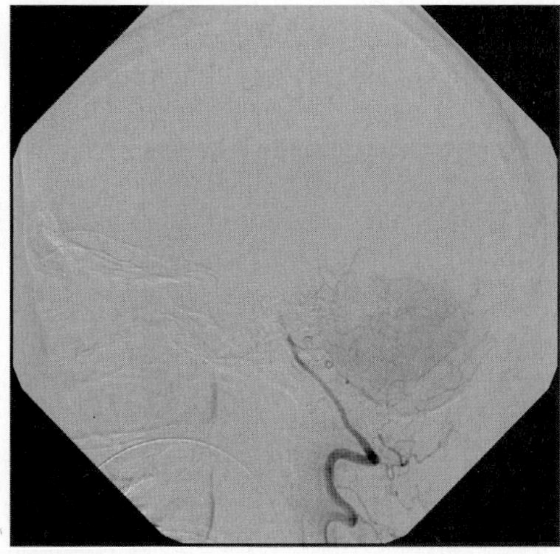

Figure 2-14. Cerebral angiogram. RVA injection AP view demonstrating basilar artery occlusion.

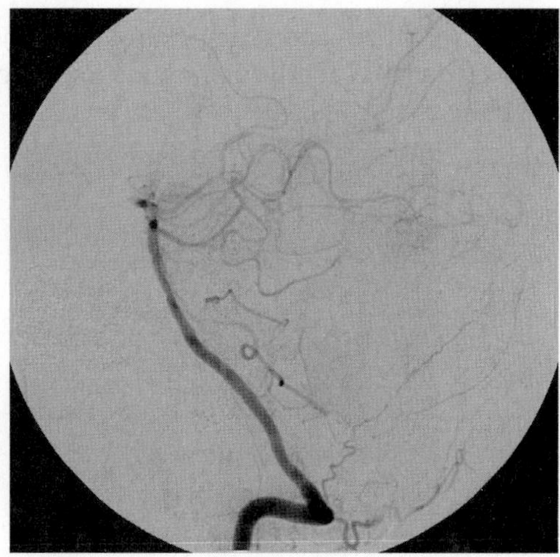

Figure 2-15. Cerebral angiogram. RVA injection lateral view post mechanical thromobolysis.

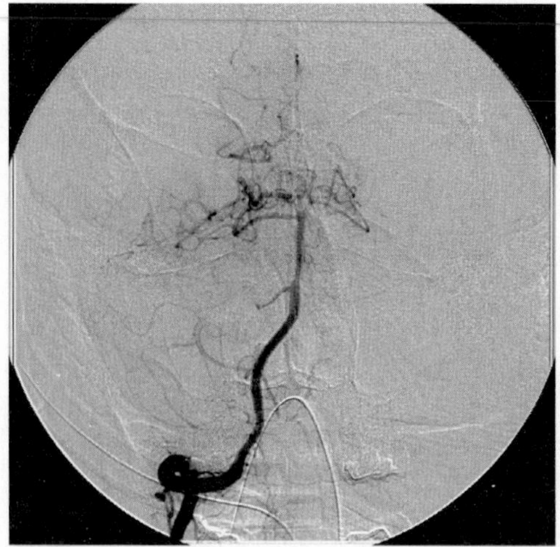

Figure 2-16. Cerebral angiogram. RVA injection AP view post mechanical and chemical thromoblysis demonstrating restored basilar artery flow.

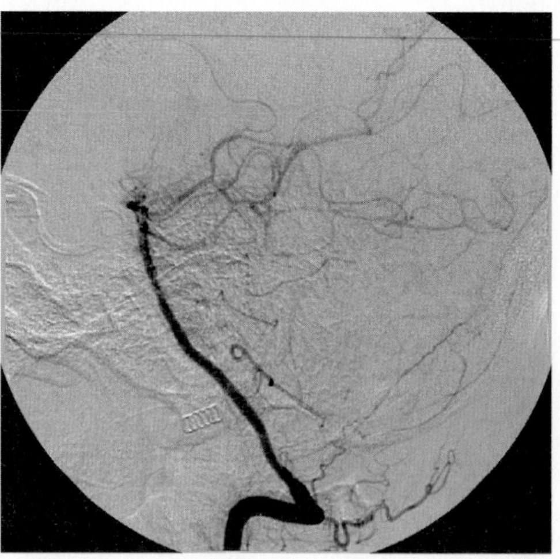

Figure 2-17. Cerebral angiogram. RVA injection lateral view post mechanical and chemical thrombolysis demonstrating restored flow in the basilar artery.

new right hemisphere infarction (Figure 2–18). A perfusion study showed severe hypoperfusion of the hemisphere (beyond areas of acute infarction, i.e., a large perfusion- diffusion mismatch). Cerebral angiography showed significant narrowing of the supraclinoid right internal carotid artery (ICA) (Figure 2–19). The patient was taken to the angiography suite and underwent stenting of the supraclinoid ICA (Figures 2–20 and 2–21). Cerebral angiography post-stenting demonstrated restored flow of the supraclinoid ICA (Figure 2–22). Repeat cerebral angiography 6 months post-stenting demonstrated patency of the supraclinoid right ICA without in-stent thrombosis or stenosis (Figures 2–23 and 2–24).

FUTURE DIRECTIONS

Despite recent advances, acute stroke continues to be a source of considerable morbidity, mortality, and disability. Continued improvement in outcomes will require improved and

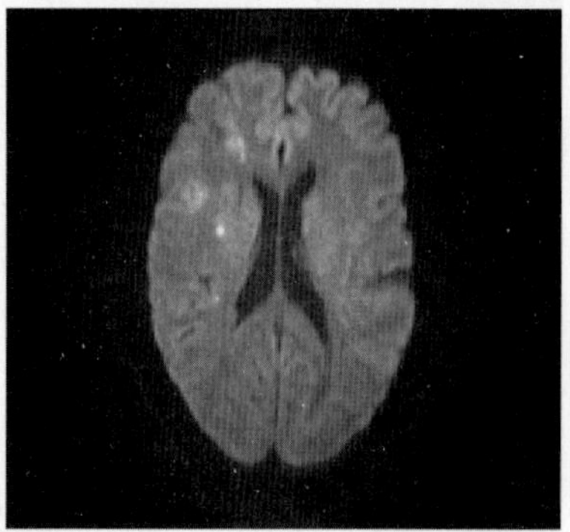

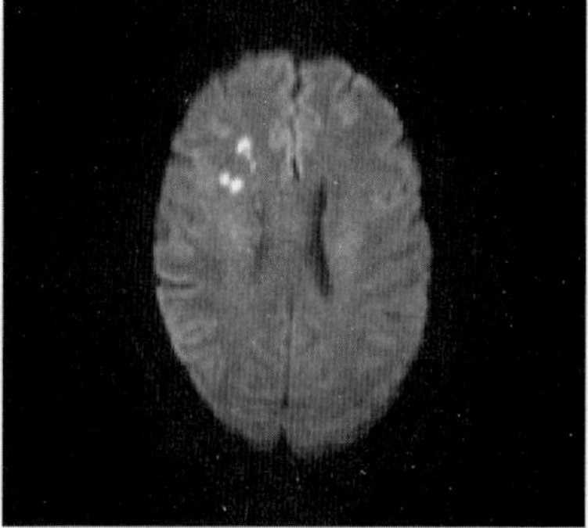

Figure 2-18. MRI brain. B1000 sequence. Acute infarcts in anterior division R MCA distribution in right frontal lobe white matter.

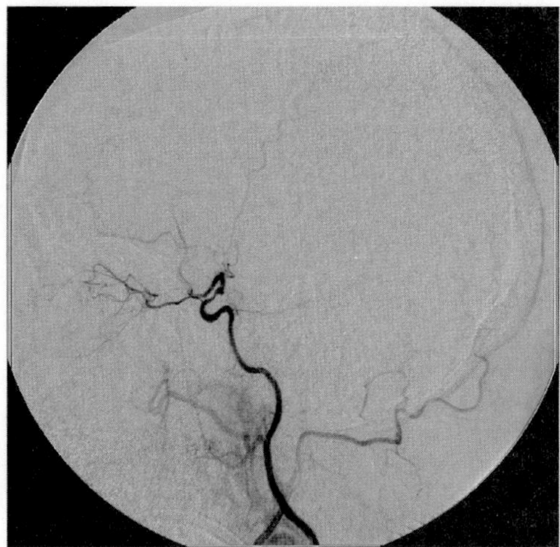

Figure 2-19. Cerebral angiogram. RICA injection lateral view demonstrating right supraclinoid ICA high grade narrowing secondary to dissection.

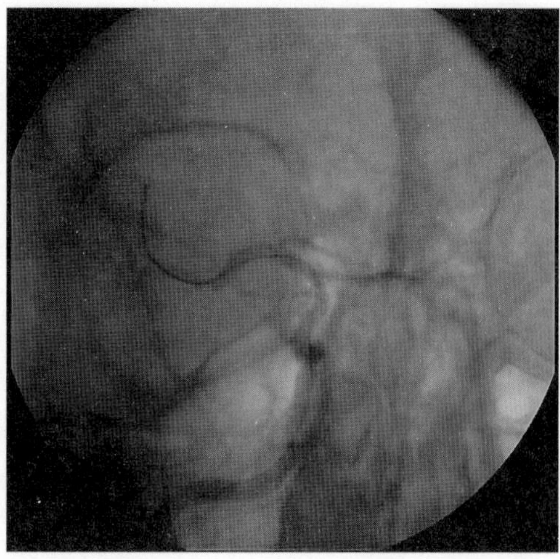

Figure 2-20. Cerebral angiogram. RICA injection AP view during stent deployment.

timely access of patients to treatment as well as refined patient selection for treatment. Furthermore, the multiplicity of available strategies requires investigation into their potential combinations. Interestingly, recent studies have suggested that a majority of patients presenting with stroke are unable to receive IV tPA, most frequently because they do not arrive soon enough.[22] This emphasizes the importance of improving currently available strategies in order to extend the therapeutic window.

With regard to imaging, computed tomography (CT) is most commonly used to evaluate acute stroke patients for both ischemia and hemorrhage. However, more recent studies suggest that gradient recall echo magnetic resonance imaging (GRE MRI)

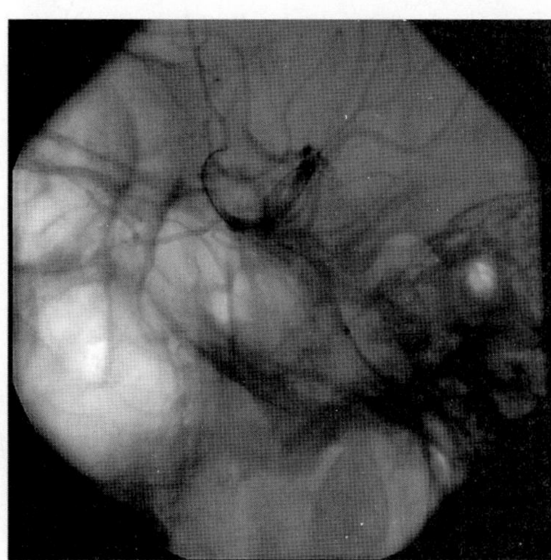

Figure 2-21. Cerebral angiogram. RICA injection lateral view during stent deployment.

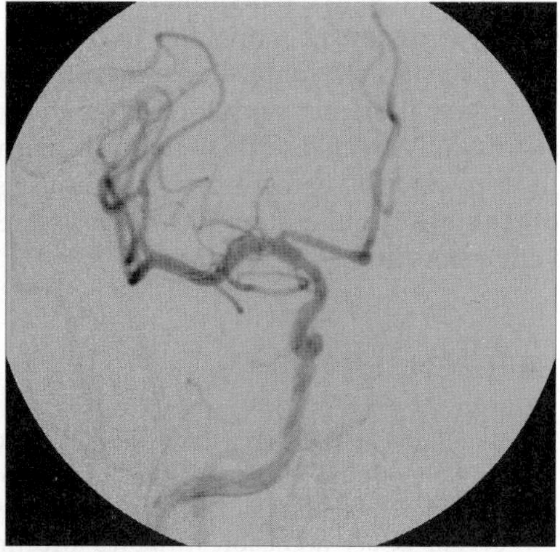

Figure 2-22. Cerebral angiogram. RICA injection AP view immediately post stent deployment demonstrating restored flow of supraclinoid ICA.

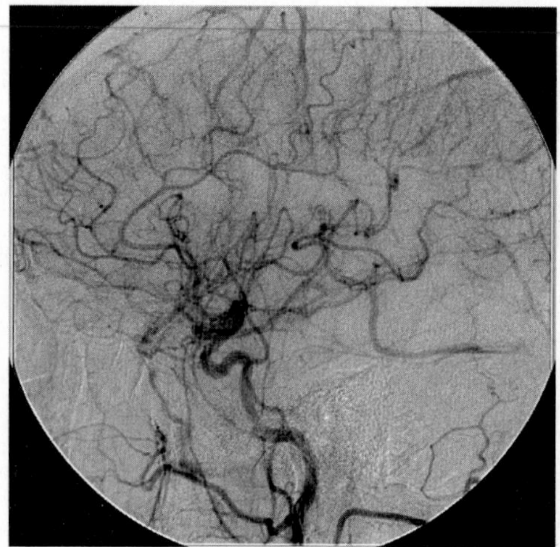

Figure 2-23. Cerebral angiogram 6 months post stent deployment. RICA injection lateral view demonstrating patency of stented supraclinoid ICA.

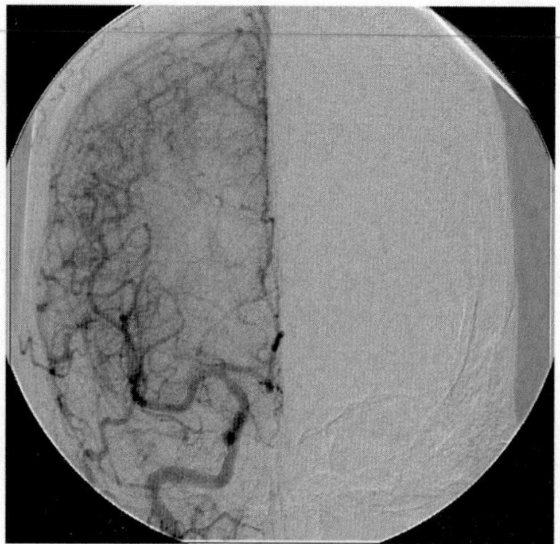

Figure 2-24. Cerebral angiogram 6 months post stent deployment. RICA injection AP view demonstrating patency of stented supraclinoid ICA.

may be a more specific modality for the detection of acute hemorrhage.[23] Incorporation of improved imaging techniques in future studies may provide a more accurate assessment of the risk of hemorrhage and hemorrhagic conversion following reperfusion, especially for patients with early hemorrhage who may be at risk by receiving thrombolytics.

The currently enrolling IMS III trial is a large, international, multicenter, prospective randomized control trial (Phase III) that will enroll a projected 900 subjects within 3 hours of stroke onset. The trial aims to compare combined IV/IA approaches with IV tPA alone. The highly anticipated results of this trial will provide sound scientific evidence allowing direct comparison between a combined approach and the standard IV approach.

In addition to the treatment of acute stroke, there has been recent interest in applying these treatment modalities to the treatment of subacute stroke (>8 hours of window). We recently published a report of two cases of subacute vascular occlusion with persistent ischemic symptoms referable to the affected ischemic territory that were successfully treated with angioplasty with no residual neurologic deficits.[24] The benefit of restoration of vessel patency in the setting of subacute occlusion and the use of other endovascular strategies such as mechanical thrombectomy may be interesting venues for future investigation.

REFERENCES

1. Bruckmann H, Ferbert A, Del Zoppo G, et al. Acute vertebral-basilar thrombosis. Angiologic-clinical comparison and therapeutic implications. Acta Radio Suppl 1986;369:38.
2. Brandt T, von Kummer R, Muller-Kuppers M, Hacke W. Thrombolytic therapy of acute basilar artery occlusion variables affecting recanalization and outcome. Stroke 1996;27: 875–81.
3. Hacke W, Schwab S, Horn M, et al. 'Malignant' middle cerebral artery territory infarction: clinical course and prognostic signs. Archiv Neurol 1996;53:309–15.

4. Jansen O, Von Kummer R, Forsting M, et al. Thrombolytic therapy in acute occlusion of the intracranial internal carotid artery bifurcation. AJNR Am J Neuroradiol 1995;16:1977–86.
5. Hacke W, Donnan G, Fieschi C, et al. Association of outcome with early stroke treatment: pooled analysis of ATLANTIS, ECASS, and NINDS rt-PA stroke trials. Lancet 2004;363:768.
6. Hacke W, Zeumer H, Ferbert A, et al. Intra-arterial thrombolytic therapy improves outcome in patients with acute vertebrobasilar occlusive disease. Stroke 1988;19:1216–22.
7. Suarez J, Sunshine J, Tarr R, et al. Predictors of clinical improvement, angiographic recanalization, and intracranial hemorrhage after intra-arterial thrombolysis for acute ischemic stroke. Stroke 1999;30:2094–100.
8. Fisher M, Prichard J, Warach S. New magnetic resonance techniques for acute ischemic stroke. JAMA 1995;274:908-11.
9. Staroselskaya I, Chaves C, Silver B, Linfante I, Edelman R, Caplan L, Warach S, Baird A. Relationship between magnetic resource arterial patency and perfussion-diffusion mismatch in acute ischemic stroke and its potential clinical use. Arch Neurol 2001;58:1069.
10. Tissue plasminogen activator for acute ischemic stroke. The national institute of neurological disorders and stroke rt-pa stroke study group. N Engl J Med 1995;333:1581–7.
11. Yamaguchi T, Hayakawa T, Kiuchi H. Intravenous tissue plasminogen activator ameliorates the outcome of hyperacute embolic stroke. Cerebrovasc Dis 1993;3:269–72.
12. Kidwell C, Wintermark M. Imaging of intracranial haemorrhage. Lancet Neurol 2008;7: 256–67.
13. Hacke W, Kaste M, Bluhmki E, et al. Thrombolysis with Alteplase 3 to 4.5 hours after acute ischemic stroke. N Engl J Med 2008;359:1317–28.
14. Combined intravenous and intra-arterial recanalization for acute ischemic stroke: The Interventional Management of Stroke Study. Stroke 2004;35:904–11.
15. The interventional management of stroke (IMS) II study. Stroke 2007;38:2127–35.
16. del Zoppo GJ, Higashida RT, Furlan AJ, et al. A phase II randomized trial of recombinant pro-urokinase by direct arterial delivery in acute middle cerebral artery stroke. PROACT investigators. Prolyse in acute cerebral thromboembolism. Stroke 1998;29:4–11.
17. Furlan A, Higashida R, Wechsler L, et al. Intra-arterial prourokinase for acute ischemic stroke. The PROACT II study: A randomized controlled trial. Prolyse in acute cerebral thromboembolism. JAMA 1999;282:2003–11.
18. Lewandowski C, Frankel M, Tomsick T, et al. Combined intravenous and intra-arterial r-tPA versus intra-arterial therapy of acute ischemic stroke emergency management of stroke (EMS) bridging trial. Am Heart Assoc 1999;30:2598–2605.
19. Smith W, Sung G, Starkman S, et al. Safety and efficacy of mechanical embolectomy in acute ischemic stroke results of the MERCI trial. Am Heart Assoc 2005;36:1432–8.
20. Smith W, Sung G, Saver J, et al. Mechanical thrombectomy for acute ischemic stroke: final results of the multi MERCI trial. Stroke 2008;39:1205.
21. The penumbra pivotal stroke trial. Safety and effectiveness of a new generation of mechanical devices for clot removal in intracranial large vessel occlusive disease. Stroke 2009;40: 2761–8.
22. Barber P, Zhang J, Demchuk A, et al. Why are stroke patients excluded from tPA therapy? An analysis of patient eligibility. Neurology 2001;56:1015–20.
23. Levy E, Siddiqui A, Crumlish A, et al. First Food and Drug Administration-Approved Prospective Trial of Primary Intracranial Stenting for Acute Stroke. SARIS (Stent-Assisted Recanalization in Acute Ischemic Stroke). Stroke 2009.
24. Gross B, Hurley M, Bernstein R, et al. Endovascular recanalization for subacute symptomatic intracranial arterial occlusion: a report of two cases. Clin Neurol Neurosurg 2008; 110:1058–63.

3

High Risk — What Does It Mean?

Tamara N. Fitzgerald, M.D., Ph.D. and
Alan Dardik, M.D., Ph.D.

SYSTEMIC ILLNESS AND THE "HIGH-RISK" STATE

It is a common belief within the medical and surgical communities that patients with vascular disease tend to be more ill than patients with nonvascular diseases. Vascular patients, more often than not, have multiple comorbid conditions and are of advanced age. Furthermore, they tend to have a similar constellation of risk factors, and their numerous comorbid conditions are often related to the same risk factors that predict outcome. Age, diabetes, cigarette smoking, hyperlipidemia, and obesity have all been identified as contributors to the atherosclerotic process and play a role in other systemic problems such as impaired cardiovascular, pulmonary, and renal function. As such, are all patients undergoing vascular procedures at "high risk" for developing some sort of complication? Are all patients that vascular surgeons care for "high risk"?

Vascular risk factors influence both perioperative and long-term outcome, with increasing numbers of risk factors subsequently increasing the risk of early and late complications.[1] Diabetes in particular affords patients a larger surgical risk, with recent reports of decreased primary patency rates after interventions for lower extremity occlusive disease.[2] Perioperative cardiac risk level and early cardiac complications have been shown to predict patient longevity.[3] "High-risk" patients may have a serious postoperative complication after abdominal aortic aneurysm (AAA) repair, the most common of which is a cardiac event. In addition to cardiovascular risk factors, chronic kidney disease independently predicts long-term mortality.[4]

The most convincing evidence of the relationship between vascular disease and other illness relates to the ankle-brachial index (ABI). The ABI is a simple and noninvasive marker of vascular disease, with values of less than 0.9 being diagnostic of disease. Reduced ABI has been shown to be predictive of functional impairment, congestive heart failure, major coronary events, cardiac mortality,[5] renal failure, vascular dialysis access failure, peritoneal dialysis failure,[6] stroke, and dementia,[7] all of which cause mortality. Therefore, it is not surprising that patients undergoing vascular procedures are likely to have multiple comorbid medical conditions.

DEFINING "HIGH RISK"

With the introduction of endovascular techniques, the "high-risk" vascular patient has become a controversial area of research. Before the endovascular era, it was well known that vascular patients were often at increased risk for complications of surgery, and that the natural course of vascular disease and patient risk factors would lead to serious and disabling consequences, including stroke, limb loss, and death without additional therapy. Therefore, the large benefit of surgery in ameliorating the vascular problem typically outweighed the risk of periprocedural complications; other than some extremely ill patients for whom surgery would not be offered, most patients accepted surgical therapy as necessary for their condition and less risky than the inherent risks of the natural course of their disease. However, when endovascular therapy came into existence, proponents hoped for faster recovery times, decreased hospital stays, and decreased morbidity and mortality when compared with the corresponding open procedure. In particular, it was hoped that endovascular therapy, with its potential for the decreased risk of complications inherent in minimally invasive procedures, would expand the patient pool to which therapy could be offered. Several clinical trials have been completed and others are under way to investigate the outcomes between open and endovascular interventions. Some of these trials have even specifically defined and focused on "high-risk" patients.

Despite the overwhelming interest in patients with complex vascular problems, current risk stratification paradigms are not well established. For example, Weiss et al.[8] compared the "high-risk" inclusion criteria for carotid artery stenting (CAS) with carotid endarterectomy (CEA) trials and found that there was great variation in the physiologic parameters used between trials. Parameters included the presence of advanced age, congestive heart failure, recent coronary artery bypass grafting (CABG), angina, a positive cardiac stress test, recent myocardial infarction (MI), ejection fraction, degree of chronic obstructive pulmonary disease (COPD), creatinine levels, and recent stroke or transient ischemic attacks (TIAs). Of the seven studies that were compared, no two used the same set of parameters, and different threshold values were used for each parameter from study to study. Studies also varied in the percentage of patients who met the "high- risk" criteria (17-50%). [8]

Therefore, the term "high risk" must be defined. We believe that the concept of high risk should be divided into distinct categories of medical high-risk and surgical high risk. **Medical high risk** is related to the presence of multiple preexisting risk factors and comorbidities that impact the patient's long-term survival and ultimately the risk-benefit ratio of treatment of the patient's vascular disease. Medical high-risk criteria must be distinguished from those of surgical high risk. **Surgical high risk** implies the increased likelihood that a patient will develop a complication in the perioperative period from the nature of the procedure itself. Examples of surgical high risk include extended supraceliac clamp time predisposing to development of a perioperative MI, redo CEA predisposing to an increased risk of cranial nerve injury, ligation of the inferior mesenteric artery in a patient with concomitant visceral artery stenosis predisposing to ischemic colitis, or administration of dye to a patient predisposing or leading to renal failure. Thus, surgical high risk is the likelihood of developing perioperative complications as determined by surgical parameters such as the procedure length, major vessel clamp time, blood loss, fluid resuscitation, type of anesthesia, physiologic stress, organ ischemia, the extent of postoperative healing required, or simply whether the procedure is an open or an endovascular repair. A patient's medical risk status has the potential to affect the surgical risk; administration of intravenous contrast medium to a patient carries an increased risk of renal failure in those with preexisting renal insufficiency. Because different vascular procedures create different risks or complications, patients may have very different risks for different procedures. For example, a patient at high risk for complications after an AAA repair may be at very low risk for complications after CEA. Overall high-risk status should be determined by both the health of the patient and the stress of the procedure.

Several classification schemes can be used to assess the medical risk status of the patient. Three commonly used classification systems are the American Society of Anesthesiologists (ASA) Score, the Modified Goldman-Detsky Cardiac Risk Index, and the Eagle Criteria for Cardiac Risk Stratification (Table 3–1). The ASA classification is a well-known scheme, and although subjective, it uses simple clinical findings to rank the overall physiologic state of a patient before surgery. The Modified Goldman-Detsky Cardiac Risk Index stratifies patients undergoing noncardiac surgery into four categories based on their cardiac status. It has been shown to be predictive of cardiac morbidity and mortality.[9] The Eagle Criteria can be used to stratify patients into major,

TABLE 3-1. MEDICAL RISK STRATIFICATION SCHEMES

ASA Classification

I	Normal, healthy patient with good exercise tolerance
II	Controlled medical conditions without significant systemic effects
III	Medical conditions with systemic effects; functional compromise
IV	Medical condition with significant dysfunction; potential threat to life
V	Critical medical condition; little chance of survival with or without surgery
VI	Brain death; anesthesia performed for organ donation

Modified Goldman-Detsky Cardiac Risk Index

Risk Factor	Points
MI within 6 months	10
MI more than 6 months	5
Canadian CV Society angina class	
Class III	10
Class IV	20
Unstable angina within 6 months	10
Alveolar pulmonary edema	
Within 1 week	10
Ever	5
Suspected critical aortic stenosis	20
Rhythm other than sinus	5
>5 PVCs	5
Poor general medical status	5
Age >70	5
Emergency operation	10

Risk Class (points)	Cardiac Morbidity[9]
Class I (0-5)	1%
Class II (6-12)	4%
Class III (13-25)	15%
Class IV (>25)	56%

(Continued)

TABLE 3-1. MEDICAL RISK STRATIFICATION SCHEMES (*Continued*)

Eagle Criteria	
Major Criteria	Minor Criteria
Unstable angina	Advanced Age
Recent MI	Abnormal ECG
Decompensated CHF	Rhythm other than sinus
Significant arrhythmias	Poor functional capacity
Severe valvular disease	History of stroke
	Hypertension
Intermediate Criteria	
Mild angina	
Prior MI by history or ECG	
Prior congestive heart failure	
Diabetes mellitus	
Renal insufficiency	

MI, myocardial infarction; CV, cardiovascular; PVCs, premature ventricular contractions; CHF, congestive heart failure; ECG, electrocardiogram.

intermediate, or minor cardiac risk. The presence of major predictors may necessitate coronary angiography if surgery is deemed necessary or justify cancellation of the proposed procedure. The presence of intermediate predictors warrants careful consideration of whether preoperative cardiac testing is necessary. Patients with minor predictors usually do not warrant further cardiac testing.

These classification schemes address the physiologic state of the patient and medical high-risk status but do not take into account the surgical risk status. Unfortunately, objective predictors and classification schemes for the surgical risk of a procedure are not commonly used. The Physiologic and Operative Severity Score for Enumeration of Mortality and Morbidity (POSSUM) uses a wide range of physiologic parameters but also classifies surgery as moderate, major, or major plus.[10] Peripheral vascular procedures and amputations are considered major surgery and any aortic procedure is considered major plus. The POSSUM score then calculates a predicted morbidity and mortality rate.

The ASA Relative Value Guide uses basic units to assign a complexity level to operative cases. However, it has mainly been used for the purposes of anesthesia billing, operating room scheduling, and to monitor trends in case complexity.[11] It was not designed to predict surgical risk and has not been used in this way.

NOT ALL VASCULAR SURGERY AFFORDS THE SAME RISK

In many classification schemes, surgical procedures are often grouped as vascular versus nonvascular, with a higher risk profile associated with the vascular grouping. These grouping strategies do not take into account the details of the procedure – the surgical risk – and thus the actual risk to the patient. For example, CEA generally entails a much smaller risk of perioperative complications than open AAA repair but both are considered vascular procedures.

Figure 3–1 shows complication rates published in randomized trials that have compared open versus endovascular procedures for AAA, peripheral occlusive disease, and carotid stenosis.[12-17] Death is a more common complication after AAA repair

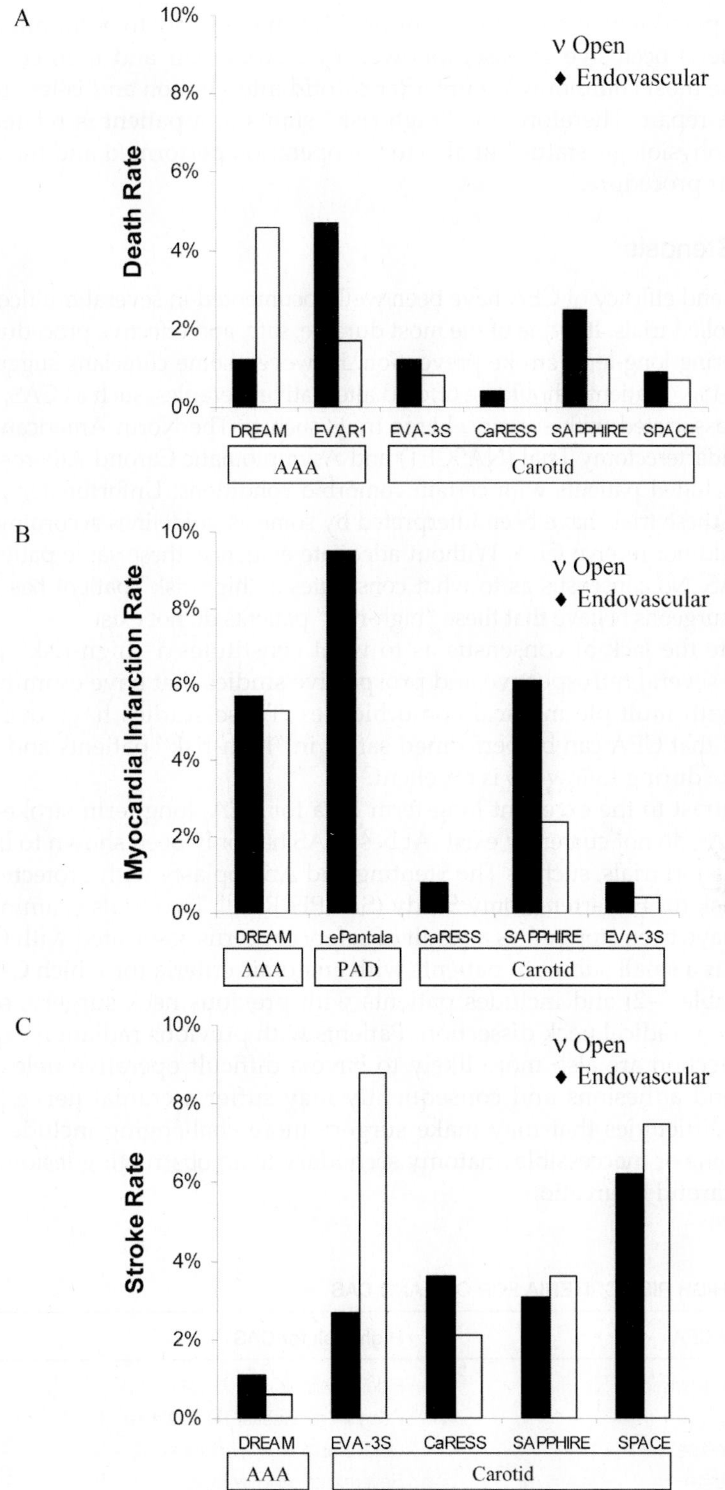

Figure 3-1. Postoperative (<30 days) complication rates for death, myocardial infarction, and stroke. Data as published in randomized, controlled trials comparing open versus endovascular intervention for aortic aneurysm (AAA), peripheral arterial disease (PAD), and carotid stenosis. Open bars, open surgical rate. Shaded bars, endovascular rate.

when compared with carotid intervention. MI is more likely to occur after intervention for peripheral occlusive disease, followed by AAA repair and then carotid intervention. Stroke most commonly occurs after carotid intervention and is less likely to occur after AAA repair. Therefore, the "high-risk" status of a patient is related not only to his or her physiologic status but also to the operation performed and the risk profile of a particular procedure.

Carotid Stenosis

The safety and efficacy of CEA have been well documented in several multicenter, randomized, controlled trials. It is one of the most durable, safe, and effective procedures performed today, offering long-term stroke prevention. However, some clinicians suggest that "medically high-risk" patients should be offered alternative therapies, such as CAS, to avoid complications associated with surgery. Large trials such as The North American Symptomatic Carotid Endarterectomy Trial (NASCET) and Asymptomatic Carotid Atherosclerosis Study (ACAS) excluded patients with certain comorbid conditions. Unfortunately, the exclusion criteria for these trials have been interpreted by some as guidelines according to which patients should not receive CEA. Without adequate evidence, these same patients have been offered CAS. No consensus as to what constitutes a "high-risk" patient has been reached, and some surgeons believe that these "high-risk" patients do not exist.

Despite the lack of consensus as to what constitutes a "high-risk" patient, there have been several retrospective and prospective studies that have examined cohorts of patients with multiple medical comorbidities. These studies have overwhelmingly concluded that CEA can be performed safely in "high-risk" patients and that freedom from stroke during follow-up is excellent.

In contrast to the excellent long-term data for CEA, long-term stroke-free survival data for CAS do not currently exist. At best CAS has only been shown to be noninferior to CEA in short trials, such as The Stenting and Angioplasty with Protection in Patients at High Risk for Endarterectomy Study (SAPPHIRE).[18] Two trials examining CAS versus CEA have been stopped as a result of safety concerns associated with CAS.

There is a small subset of patients with anatomic criteria for which CAS has a clear benefit (Table 3–2) and includes patients with previous neck surgery, such as a tracheostomy or radical neck dissection. Patients with previous radiation exposure or extensive infection are also more likely to have a difficult operative field secondary to scarring and adhesions and consequently may suffer a cranial nerve injury. Other anatomic difficulties that may make surgery more challenging include an immobile cervical spine or inaccessible anatomy secondary to an obstructing lesion or an unusually high carotid bifurcation.

TABLE 3-2. HIGH RISK CRITERIA FOR CEA AND CAS

High Risk for CEA	High Risk for CAS
Previous neck dissection	Elderly patients
Tracheostomy	Recent (<2 weeks) TIA or stroke
Radiation exposure	Unfavorable arterial anatomy
Extensive infection	Severely calcified lesions
Neck immobility	"String-sign" stenoses

CEA, carotid endarterectomy; CAS, carotid artery angioplasty and stenting; TIA, transient ischemic attack.

Likewise, there is also a group of patients at high risk for CAS (see Table 3–2). Elderly patients are likely to have a worse outcome with CAS. Analysis of the NASCET data has demonstrated that patients 75 years or older derive a substantially improved outcome after CEA, especially those with severe stenosis. In patients with 70 to 99% stenosis, the absolute risk reduction of ipsilateral stroke at 2 years is 28.9%, suggesting that these patients have much to gain from CEA. Studies on the outcomes of stenting in elderly high-risk patients continue to show unacceptably high rates of perioperative stroke in the range of 8 to 19.2%. The Carotid Revascularization Endarterectomy vs. Stent Trial (CREST) revealed that rates of periprocedural stroke or death were significantly higher for older patients than they were for younger patients (12.1% vs. 4.0%).[19]

In addition to elderly patients, symptomatic patients may not be ideal candidates for CAS. Patients with recent (<2 weeks) symptoms of ipsilateral carotid-territory ischemia and those with extensively calcified lesions or "string-sign" stenoses are probably best served by CEA. Unfavorable arch anatomy (type C arch) and severely angulated common or internal carotid anatomy also make access and distal-filter deployment problematic.

In the case of combined carotid and coronary disease, where intervention is needed for two different vascular territories, it is still an area of debate as to whether CAS is preferred to CEA. One potential advantage of CAS over CEA is a reduced rate of myocardial events in patients who need CABG because CAS is less invasive than CEA. However, the need for dual antiplatelet therapy and the potential adverse hemodynamic depression associated with CAS may limit its utility in patients with unstable coronary artery disease (CAD).

Also, it should be noted that the Centers for Medicare and Medicaid Services continue to support reimbursement for CEA. Current policies support CAS only for high-risk, symptomatic patients with severe stenosis. This policy is problematic, as "high-risk" is once again not well defined, and several reports have shown that symptomatic patients and those with severe stenosis do not do as well after CAS compared with CEA. Additionally, CAS offers no financial advantage over CEA as a result of high materials cost.

Therefore, patients who are at "medical high risk" for CEA may include a very small subset of extremely ill patients with such limited life expectancy that they will not derive benefit from stroke-risk reduction. Patients at "surgical high risk" for CEA include those patients with previous neck surgery, radiation exposure, extensive infection, or severe neck immobility. Patients at "medical high risk" for CAS include the elderly and those with recent TIA or stroke. Patients with severely calcified lesions and "string-sign" stenoses are at higher risk for complications related to the CAS procedure, that is, at "surgical high risk" for CAS.

Peripheral Arterial Occlusive Disease

Peripheral arterial disease (PAD) presents a complex relationship between the medical and the surgical high-risk states. Most surgery for peripheral disease does not involve entering the abdomen and therefore spares the patient massive fluid shifts, aggressive resuscitative efforts, and a prolonged postoperative ileus leading to malnourishment. In fact, many procedures for peripheral occlusive disease can be conducted under local or spinal anesthesia, negating the need for general anesthesia and intubation. Therefore, it might be presumed that surgery for PAD would be surgically low risk.

However, these patients often have complications following surgery. Patients with PAD tend to be very ill, with multiple medical comorbidities such as CAD, hypertension, hyperlipidemia, and chronic renal disease. They have a three- to sixfold increased risk of coronary artery disease (CAD) and stroke and a three- to fivefold increased risk of death caused by cardiovascular disease compared with patients without PAD. Patients with multivessel PAD have a particularly poor long-term prognosis, with a 15-fold increased risk of cardiovascular mortality over 10 years. They experience the highest fatality rates due to stroke, MI, or other vascular causes.[20] Patients with PAD and metabolic syndrome are more likely to experience a cardiovascular event such as MI, stroke, or death from a peripheral vascular event than are patients without metabolic syndrome.[21]

Peripheral bypass with vein graft is considered the gold standard for revascularization of the lower extremities in patients with critical limb ischemia. However, in medically high-risk patients, angioplasty and stenting have been considered less invasive revascularization alternatives. Few studies have examined the outcome in "high-risk" PAD patients; one recent study investigated the outcome of angioplasty and stenting in patients with ASA >3 and severe symptomatic disease confined to the superficial femoral artery. Perioperative mortality was 0%, and limb salvage rate was 92%. There were no severe complications, hematomas, pseudoaneurysms, dissections, or emboli. The 2-year primary and primary-assisted patency were 68% and 90%, respectively, which is lower than that of femoropopliteal bypass surgery with vein grafts (81%) but similar to that of polytetrafluoroethylene (PTFE) grafts (69%). Although the combination of ASA >3 with severe symptomatic presentation is not a validated measure of risk, nevertheless it may be clinically useful.[22]

Therefore, the "medical high-risk" status for peripheral interventions, both open and endovascular, may be increased by the presence of CAD, cerebrovascular disease, renal disease, metabolic syndrome, or an increased ASA classification status. MI rates are higher after peripheral bypass than AAA repair or CEA. Therefore, peripheral bypass likely exerts a "surgical high-risk" status for MI; it is not clear what increased surgical risk aortic procedures impart above and beyond the risk of infrainguinal arterial reconstruction, although intuitively aortic procedures have a higher risk. Other complications that are associated with peripheral arterial surgical intervention include renal failure, infection, and amputation. As additional information is learned regarding the mechanical forces present in the superficial femoral and popliteal arteries and how these forces exert effects on endovascular treatments, it is likely that surgical high risk for infrainguinal endovascular procedures is due to the anatomic location of the intervention. For example, superficial femoral artery and popliteal artery motion may increase the risk of complications after stent placement, whereas the small diameter of the tibial and peroneal arteries may increase the risk of early restenosis.

Abdominal Aortic Aneurysm

Open AAA repair is an extensive and invasive procedure, and patients must be carefully evaluated before a decision for operation or endovascular intervention is reached. Endovascular aneurysm repair (EVAR) has become popular for "high-risk" patients, but again the term "high risk" has not been universally defined. Infected AAA, cardiac disease, ASA score, and age have been shown to be positive predictors of perioperative mortality after AAA repair and increase a patient's "medical high-risk" status. Other factors that may impart a "medical high-risk" status include pulmonary and renal disease.

Infected AAA carries a high rate of morbidity and is almost always fatal without undergoing aortic resection. Common pathogens include *Salmonella* and *Staphylococcus aureus*. Therefore, a patient with an infected aneurysm is at medical high risk, regardless of the presence or absence of other medical comorbidities. In patients considered high risk for surgery, medical treatment can be attempted but offers disappointing results. EVAR is controversial due to its propensity for graft infection, with an in-hospital mortality of 10 to 20%. In patients treated nonoperatively, the hospital mortality rate is approximately 50%, and of those who survive, half will die of aneurysm-related causes after leaving the hospital. Therefore, traditional surgical excision of infected aortic aneurysms with revascularization should be attempted, even in medically high-risk patients. EVAR may be used as a bridge to surgical repair in select cases.

The most common complications after AAA repair are cardiac in nature, and MI is the leading cause of postoperative morbidity and mortality. Not only is CAD a risk factor for complications after AAA repair, but AAA is also a risk factor for adverse outcome after CABG. In a study of 32 patients with CAD in at least three vessels and AAA >6 cm, 13% of patients undergoing CABG died in the perioperative period from a ruptured AAA, and mortality for patients undergoing concomitant CABG and AAA repair was 10%.[23]

A history of erectile dysfunction and low ABI, both of which reflect the overall vascular disease state, has been shown to be predictive of death after AAA repair. Similarly, a history of heart valve replacement is also predictive of complications after repair. The Society for Vascular Surgery's pulmonary risk score has been shown to be predictive of death after AAA repair. Factors that may lead to pulmonary complications after open AAA repair include perioperative fluid shifts and aggressive fluid resuscitation, long operative time, and prolonged postoperative intubation. Tracheostomy is associated with a high incidence of in-hospital mortality. The preoperative diagnosis of COPD is associated with improved survival, whereas postoperative sepsis is associated with increased mortality. Therefore, it is important to identify patients with impaired pulmonary function, CAD, decreased ABI, and renal insufficiency preoperatively, as these patients may be at "medical high risk."

Perioperative mortality, length of hospital admission, and respiratory complications have been shown to be similar after EVAR in patients with and without COPD. Also, the presence of pulmonary disease is not associated with higher rates of aortic neck dilatation or type I endoleak.

Finally, the coexistence of AAA and lung cancer is a challenging paradigm. The prognosis is generally poor and largely determined by the lung cancer stage. In patients with potentially curable cancer, AAA repair should be considered. Repair rarely is justified in patients with advanced disease unless the AAA is symptomatic.

Chronic renal failure with preoperative serum creatinine levels equal to or greater than 1.5 mg/dL is a strong predictor of late mortality after AAA repair, and patients with normal preoperative renal function recover more quickly. Renal insufficiency after open repair is associated with increased mesenteric ischemic time, supraceliac clamping, left renal vein division, and renal artery bypass, but renal artery reimplantation and endarterectomy do not appear to contribute to postoperative renal failure.

Both open repair and EVAR can lead to renal injury. During open repair, hypotension, suprarenal aortic clamping, and nephrotoxic agents can lead to renal insufficiency and in some cases to new-onset dialysis. EVAR can incur renal injury via contrast dye nephropathy or stent migration, leading to renal artery occlusion. Contrast dye nephropathy is of particular concern, as EVAR patients require periodic CT scans to evaluate stent position and the presence of endoleaks. Therefore, open AAA repair carries an immediate "surgical high risk" of renal injury but is relatively free of late risk. EVAR carries a cumulative renal risk that increases each year with subsequent CT scanning.

In elderly patients, PAD is often asymptomatic. However, an abnormal ABI is still associated with an increased mortality risk.[24] Therefore, elderly patients at high risk may be more difficult to identify. Octogenarians undergoing AAA repair more frequently have cardiac disease, impaired renal function, pulmonary disease, and larger aneurysm diameter. Device-related complications, systemic complications, and incidence of hematoma are all more common in octogenarians, but the rate of aneurysm rupture is not significantly different.[25] In most studies, advanced age alone does not constitute a risk factor for perioperative death. Most octogenarians (>75%) are able to maintain their previous lifestyles with the independent activities of everyday life after open repair. Differences in morbidity and mortality in EVAR versus open repair have not been demonstrated in the elderly population.

Does EVAR Decrease Risk?

The EVAR 1 and 2 and Dutch Randomized Endovascular Aneurysm Management (DREAM) trials addressed management of AAAs larger than 5.5 cm in diameter. Both the DREAM and the EVAR 1 trials showed a 3% lower initial mortality for EVAR but no difference in overall late survival. EVAR was found to be associated with significantly higher intervention rates and higher hospital costs. Similarly, the EVAR 2 trial found that EVAR did not demonstrate a survival benefit compared with open repair but was associated with a higher rate of subsequent interventions and higher costs. It did demonstrate a brief quality of life benefit for EVAR. As expected, patient survival was much worse in patients enrolled in EVAR 2 compared with those enrolled in EVAR 1.

In one recent study, "high-risk" patients were randomized into open repair versus EVAR. High risk was defined as age >60 years plus at least one cardiac, pulmonary, or renal comorbidity. The investigators did not find any significant difference in perioperative mortality or aneurysm rupture at 4 years, but the endoleak rate for EVAR was 19% at 4 years.[26] In another European study, for patients with at least three cardiac risk factors, EVAR was associated with improved cardiac event-free survival but not overall survival when compared with open repair. Statin therapy was associated with both cardiac event-free survival and overall survival in both the open and the EVAR groups.[27] In a study of Veteran's Affairs patients, those who were classified as high risk underwent elective EVAR with significantly lower 30-day and 1-year mortality than patients having open repair, and the risk of perioperative complications was significantly lower.[28]

Therefore, when considering EVAR versus open repair in patients with multiple medical comorbidities, both the short- and the long-term outcomes must be examined. If EVAR does impart a perioperative improvement in quality of life and some protection from cardiac complications, the long-term outcome must also be considered. The durability of EVAR is not yet known, whereas open repair is known to result in good long-term freedom from aneurysm rupture. Also, EVAR requires surveillance for endoleak, with many institutions continuing to use serial CT scans. Many patients with vascular disease have concurrent renal disease; therefore, repeated contrast loads can be nephrotoxic and may lead to renal failure.

Many patients initially seeking consultation for aneurysm repair specifically request performance of EVAR, possibly because of the novelty of minimally invasive procedures, fear of surgery, media perception, and advertising. However, a careful conversation must be initiated with patients so that an informed decision can be made. Recent data show that patients undergoing both EVAR and open repair did not appreciate the scope of their options, were not adequately informed prior to making a decision, and were influenced by their trust in the surgeon.[29]

The process of informed consent first requires that clinicians be informed so as to pass on this knowledge to their patients. Therefore, the term "high risk" must be better defined as it relates to the patient with AAA. The risk that is conferred by cardiac, pulmonary, and renal disease and advanced age must be further investigated and quantified. At present, most studies focusing on "high-risk" patients have grouped individuals with varying degrees of comorbidities into a single "high-risk" group. However, diseases affecting different organ systems likely incur different risk profiles that have yet to be established. Whether this risk is reduced by open repair or EVAR must also be decided. At present, the durability of EVAR is unknown. Surgical risk of open repair includes the risk of aortic clamping, such as renal emboli, as well as risk to surrounding structures such as the bowel and ureters. The surgical risk of EVAR includes risk of embolization of a thrombus or calcium into the renal arteries from wire or catheter manipulation, covering the renal arteries with the endograft, and femoral artery trauma, including pseudoaneurysm formation and distal embolization.

MINIMIZING RISK

Primary and Secondary Prevention of Medical Risk

Risk to the vascular patient may be minimized by proper medical management and careful surgical planning. Primary prevention of vascular disease should be emphasized in the primary care setting and in public health education and initiatives, as atherosclerosis is a disease process that begins in early life. Dyslipidemia, hypertension, and smoking are modifiable medical high-risk factors that are increasingly prevalent in the youth of today. The incidence of metabolic syndrome is high, and rates of obesity and diabetes continue to climb. This problem is expected to become worse with increasing industrialization and those with a sedentary lifestyle. More education and treatment efforts should be focused on women because, despite the presence of multiple vascular risk factors, women tend to have low levels of knowledge and awareness about vascular diseases.[30]

For most patients presenting to the vascular surgeon, the opportunity for primary prevention has been lost and secondary prevention must be achieved. The role of the vascular surgeon is expanding, and comprehensive vascular care should include review and modification of a patient's pharmacotherapy according to the best medical practice. However, recent data suggest that many vascular surgeons are not aware of the target values for cholesterol, blood pressure, and blood glucose control, and risk factor screening in the surgical setting is suboptimal. Because of the chronic nature of vascular disease, the vascular surgeon is likely to care for a patient over several years.

Therefore, the surgeon has an opportunity to positively intervene in risk factor modification.

Patients with vascular disease benefit from a medical regimen of antiplatelet therapy, 3-hydroxy-3-methylglutaryl-coenzyme A (HMG-CoA) reductase inhibitors ("statins"), beta blockers, and angiotensin-converting enzyme (ACE) inhibitors. Previous studies have shown that lipid-lowering therapy with HMG-CoA reductase inhibitors is associated with a reduction in stroke, cardiovascular mortality, and overall mortality, but patients with PAD remain undertreated. The American Heart Association has recommended strict modification of atherosclerotic risk factors, including a low-density lipoprotein (LDL) goal of <100 mg/dL. The National Cholesterol Education Program recommends that for "high-risk" patients (patients with CAD, noncoronary atherosclerotic disease, diabetes, or multiple cardiovascular risk factors), an LDL goal of <70 mg/dL is a therapeutic option. Clinicians should also focus on modifying other medical high-risk factors such as smoking, hypertension, and sedentary lifestyle. Weight loss and glycemic control are also instrumental in preventing vascular events.

Perioperative Medical Risk Management

Every patient undergoing elective vascular surgery should have a preoperative assessment that includes a thorough history and physical examination, blood analysis, electrocardiogram (ECG), and a chest x-ray. Severe anemia and electrolyte abnormalities should be corrected prior to surgery, as deficiencies can impact cardiac status. Glucose levels should be tightly controlled before, during, and after surgical intervention. Endocrine consultation may be obtained for patients with challenging diabetic control. For those patients taking warfarin or other anticoagulants, an appropriate anticoagulation scheme should be decided upon prior to surgery. Blood typing should be performed and appropriate blood products placed on reserve. Optimizing the coagulation status and having appropriate blood products available may decrease the surgical risk status of some procedures.

In patients with a cardiac history or troublesome cardiac findings, preoperative cardiac clearance should be obtained and perioperative beta blockade should be initiated. Patients should also receive a statin when appropriate. In select patients, more advanced testing may be required, such as a dobutamine stress echocardiogram. Pulmonary function tests should be obtained in patients with a history of COPD or questionable lung capacity. A preoperative FEV1<60% should alert the surgeon to potential postoperative respiratory problems. Teaching in incentive spirometry should begin in the preoperative period, and aggressive pulmonary toilet should be implemented after surgery.

In all patients, a baseline creatinine concentration should be obtained to identify problems with renal clearance and to establish baseline renal function in the event that renal compromise occurs. If the patient receives dialysis, then it should be performed before surgery and arrangements for postoperative dialysis should be made.

Patients undergoing vascular surgery have high rates of malnutrition, and therefore, the nutritional status of the patient should be assessed, as malnutrition may also place patients in a "medical high-risk" category. For elective surgery, nutrition should be optimized preoperatively via increased oral intake of appropriate foods. A consult to a nutritionist may be helpful for some patients. If patients are unable to maintain appropriate oral intake, enteral nutrition should be considered. In the postoperative period, feeding should begin as soon as possible. In patients with prolonged postoperative ileus, total parenteral nutrition should be considered.

Nicotine dependence should be evaluated. Patients who currently smoke have a twofold increased risk of postoperative complications, with the highest risk in patients who have smoked within the last 2 months. Patients who have quit smoking more than 6 months ago have a risk similar to those who do not smoke. The beneficial effects of smoking cessation, including improvement in ciliary function and a decrease in sputum production, occur gradually over several weeks. The abrupt absence of the irritant effect of cigarette smoke in the postoperative period inhibits coughing and leads to retention of secretions and small airway obstruction. For elective surgery, patients should be instructed to abstain from smoking at least 8 weeks before surgery. For patients who continue to smoke, nicotine replacement therapy should be initiated in the perioperative period.

Patients should also be screened for alcohol abuse. The rate of morbidity and mortality due to infections, cardiopulmonary insufficiency, or bleeding disorders is two to four times greater in chronic alcoholics. When alcohol dependence is suspected, delirium tremens prophylaxis should be initiated with intermittent benzodiazepine therapy.

Surgical Risk Management

It is intuitive that the surgical risks of open and endovascular procedures must be accepted and taken when the procedure is performed. Yet, risk can be minimized. For example, it is possible that renal injury may be minimized during suprarenal aortic clamping by administration of mannitol; carotid thrombosis and distal emboli after CEA may be minimized by postoperative administration of dextran. Performance of procedures by surgeons who carry out the surgery — often "high-volume surgeons" — is thought to be an important factor in preventing complications, even in the presence of medical high-risk factors.[31] Similarly, performance of procedures by board-certified vascular surgeons may be a similar surrogate marker of quality control processes in place to reduce risk to patients.[32–33] For example, meticulous attention to operative details as well as clear communication between the surgeon and the nursing and anesthesia teams improves outcomes.[34] Last, as technology evolves and procedures change, it is likely that surgical risks will be reduced accordingly.

CONCLUSIONS

Vascular patients often have a complex constellation of risk factors and comorbid conditions that place them at high risk for complications after surgical and endovascular interventions. However, the term "high risk" is still not well defined. Risk includes both a medical component relating the physiologic status of the patient and a surgical component that is inherent in the risks of a particular procedure. The decision to treat medically, surgically, or with endovascular means must be carefully considered in light of the limited data currently available, especially regarding the differential impact of medical and surgical risks. When an intervention has been decided upon, risk can be minimized with careful preoperative work-up and treatment of underlying comorbid disease.

REFERENCES

1. Bonardelli S, Parrinello G, De Lucia M, et al. Risk factors for immediate results and long-term survival following elective open surgery for AAA. Statistical analysis of 1111 consecutively-treated patients. Ann Ital Chir 2007;78:265–76.
2. Derubertis BG, Pierce M, Ryer EJ, et al. Reduced primary patency rate in diabetic patients after percutaneous intervention: results from more frequent presentation with limb-threatening ischemia. J Vasc Surg 2008;47:101–8.
3. Back MR, Leo F, Cuthbertson D, et al. Long-term survival after vascular surgery: specific influence of cardiac factors and implications for preoperative evaluation. J Vasc Surg 2004;40:752–60.
4. Pasqualini L, Schillaci G, Pirro M, et al. Renal dysfunction predicts long-term mortality in patients with lower extremity arterial disease. J Intern Med 2007;262:668–77.
5. Fowkes FG, Murray GD, Butcher I, et al. Ankle brachial index combined with Framingham risk score to predict cardiovascular events and mortality: a meta-analysis. JAMA 2008; 300:197–208.
6. Liu JH, Lin HH, Yang YF, et al. Subclinical peripheral artery disease in patients undergoing peritoneal dialysis: risk factors and outcome. Perit Dial Int 2009; 29:64–71.
7. Laurin D, Masaki KH, White LR, Launer LJ. Ankle-to-brachial index and dementia: the Honolulu-Asia aging study. Circulation 2007;116:2269–74.
8. Weiss JS, Dumas P, Cha C, et al., Safety of carotid endarterectomy in a high-risk population: lessons from the VA and Connecticut. J Am Coll Surg 2006;203:277–82.
9. Bronson DL, Halperin AK, Marwick TH. Evaluating cardiac risk in noncardiac surgery patients. Cleve Clin J Med 1995;62:391–400.
10. Copeland GP, Jones D, Walters M. POSSUM: a scoring system for surgical audit. Br J Surg 1991;78:355–60.
11. Dexter F, Thompson E. Relative value guide basic units in operating room scheduling to ensure compliance with anesthesia group policies for surgical procedures performed at each anesthetizing location. AANA J 2001;69:120–3.
12. Carotid revascularization using endarterectomy or stenting systems (CARESS) phase I clinical trial: 1-year results. J Vasc Surg, 2005;42:213–9.
13. Endovascular aneurysm repair versus open repair in patients with abdominal aortic aneurysm (EVAR trial 1): randomised controlled trial. Lancet 2005;365:2179–86.
14. Lepantalo M, Laurila K, Roth WD, et al. PTFE bypass or thrupass for superficial femoral artery occlusion? A randomised controlled trial. Eur J Vasc Endovasc Surg 2009;37:578–84.
15. Mas JL, Chatellier G, Beyssen B, et al. Endarterectomy versus stenting in patients with symptomatic severe carotid stenosis. N Engl J Med 2006;355:1660–71.
16. Prinssen M, Verhoeven EL, Buth J, et al. A randomized trial comparing conventional and endovascular repair of abdominal aortic aneurysms. N Engl J Med 2004;351:1607–18.
17. Ringleb PA, Allenberg J, Bruckmann H, et al. 30 day results from the space trial of stent-protected angioplasty versus carotid endarterectomy in symptomatic patients: a randomised non-inferiority trial. Lancet 2006; 368:1239–47.
18. Yadav JS, Wholey MH, Kuntz RE, et al. Protected carotid-artery stenting versus endarterectomy in high-risk patients. N Engl J Med 2004;351:1493–501.
19. Hobson RW 2nd, Howard VJ, Roubin GS, et al. Carotid artery stenting is associated with increased complications in octogenarians: 30-day stroke and death rates in the CREST lead-in phase. J Vasc Surg 2004;40:1106–11.
20. Cotter G, Cannon CP, McCabe CH, et al. Prior peripheral arterial disease and cerebrovascular disease are independent predictors of adverse outcome in patients with acute coronary syndromes: Are we doing enough? Results from the orbofiban in patients with unstable coronary syndromes-thrombolysis in myocardial infarction (OPUS-TIMI) 16 study. Am Heart J 2003;145:622–7.

21. Vlek AL, van der Graaf Y, Sluman MA, et al. Metabolic syndrome and vascular risk in patients with peripheral arterial occlusive disease: a 5.5-year follow-up study. J Vasc Surg 2009;50:61–9.
22. Nishibe T, Kondo Y, Nishibe M, et al. Stent placement for superficial femoral arterial occlusive disease in high-risk patients: preliminary results. Surg Today 2009;39:21–6.
23. Ruddy JM, Yarbrough W, Brothers T, et al. Abdominal aortic aneurysm and significant coronary artery disease: strategies and options. South Med J 2008;101:1113–6.
24. Suominen V, Rantanen T, Heikkinen E, et al. Peripheral arterial disease and its clinical significance in nonagenarians. Aging Clin Exp Res 2008;20: 211–5.
25. Lange C, Leurs LJ, Buth J, Myhre HO. Endovascular repair of abdominal aortic aneurysm in octogenarians: An analysis based on eurostar data. J Vasc Surg 2005;42:624–30; discussion 630.
26. Sicard GA, Zwolak RM, Sidawy AN, et al. Endovascular abdominal aortic aneurysm repair: long-term outcome measures in patients at high-risk for open surgery. J Vasc Surg 2006; 44:229–36.
27. Schouten O, Lever TM, Welten GM, et al. Long-term cardiac outcome in high-risk patients undergoing elective endovascular or open infrarenal abdominal aortic aneurysm repair. Eur J Vasc Endovasc Surg 2008;36:646–52.
28. Bush RL, Johnson ML, Hedayati N, et al. Performance of endovascular aortic aneurysm repair in high-risk patients: results from the Veterans Affairs national surgical quality improvement program. J Vasc Surg 2007;45:227–233; discussion 233–5.
29. Berman L, Dardik A, Bradley EH, et al. Informed consent for abdominal aortic aneurysm repair: assessing variations in surgeon opinion through a national survey. J Vasc Surg 2008; 7:287–5.
30. Bush RL, Kallen MA, Liles DR, et al. Knowledge and awareness of peripheral vascular disease are poor among women at risk for cardiovascular disease. J Surg Res 2008;145:313–9.
31. Dardik A., Bowman HM, Gordon TA., et al. Impact of race on the outcome of carotid endarterectomy: a population-based analysis of 9,842 recent elective procedures. Ann Surg 2000;232:704–9.
32. Teso D, Edwards RE, Antezana JN, et al. Do vascular surgeons improve the outcome of carotid endarterectomy? An analysis of 12,618 elective cases in the state of Connecticut. Vascular 2004;3:1–11.
33. Teso D, Frattini JC, Dardik A., Carotid endarterectomy: the critical role of vascular surgeons. Semin Vasc Surg 2004;17:214–8.
34. Barkhordarian S, Dardik A. Preoperative assessment and management to prevent complications during high-risk vascular surgery. Crit Care Med 2004;32(Suppl 4):S174–85.

4

Carotid Stents and Embolic Protection Devices

Mark K. Eskandari, M.D.

INTRODUCTION

Although it is well known that early outcomes of carotid artery stenting (CAS) can be influenced by the skills of the interventionalist, symptomatic status of the patient, and characteristics of the target lesion, what many treating physicians want to know is the impact of the type of stent used in conjunction with the efficacy of cerebral protection employed. Approved carotid stents are all self-expanding but vary in architecture and metal composition, which may impact early and late outcomes of CAS. Three categories of embolic protection devices (EPDs) are recognized; however, currently only the distal filter devices are readily available in the United States. The design characteristics of each of these systems may influence the periprocedural events associated with CAS. This chapter will review the currently approved carotid stent systems and approved mechanical EPDs.

CAROTID STENTS

To date, there are a number of stent designs indicated for use in CAS: Wallstent (Boston Scientific, Natick, MA), Acculink (Abbott Vascular, Santa Rosa, CA), X-act (Abbott Vascular), Precise (Cordis, a Johnson and Johnson Company, Miami, FL) and Protégé (ev3 Inc., Plymouth, MN). All are self-expanding stents, yet their metal alloys, architecture, and configurations differ. Any or all of these properties may have a clinical impact on the early and long-term success of CAS.

Stent Alloys

There exist two primary materials by which most self-expanding carotid stents are created: elgiloy and nitinol. Elgiloy, also known as conichrome, is a biomedical grade cobalt-chromium-iron-nickel-molybdenum alloy which is then braided into a tubular mesh configuration creating what is best recognized as the carotid Wallstent. This particular stent is stainless steel and designed with a closed cell configuration. The second major self-expanding stent alloy is made of nickel and titanium and is commonly referred to as nitinol. Stents constructed of this alloy include Precise, X-act, Acculink, and Protégé. Most of these stents are constructed from a nitinol tube that is laser-cut during production to create a meshed device with thermal expansion properties. At room temperature, the stent exists in a compact shape and can be placed within a delivery sheath. Once exposed to body temperature, the stent conveniently expands as the sheath is withdrawn based upon a predetermined shape. These stents can be of either open or closed cell design and can be configured into a straight tubular or tapered design.

Theoretically, one of the biggest differences between elgiloy and nitinol stents occurs with respect to their behavior in the deployed state. The woven mesh structure of elgiloy allows it to adapt its diameter to the width of a vessel lumen, thereby allowing for more optimal vessel conformability versus the behavior of nitinol stents, which are completely determined by their thermal memory. A downside of the adaptation process of elgiloy stents is that the implanted stent length is highly dependent on the vessel diameter. Thus, excessive oversizing of the stent relative to the true vessel luminal diameter can result in significant variations in overall length of the implanted device. However, in contrast to nitinol stents, the Wallstent is reconstrainable, meaning that after partial deployment, if positioning is not appropriate, the device can be recaptured, repositioned, and deployed once more. Last, the chronic outward radial force of the Wallstent is significantly less than the available nitinol stents, which may contribute to plaque protusion after implantation.[1] Although no prospective, randomized data are yet available to compare the results of these two alloys, the lack of radial force may have implications for late embolic events as a result of plaque protusion and unstable plaque trapping.

Stent Architecture

Scaffolding of the carotid bifurcation lesion is achieved after placement of the self-expanding stent across the atherosclerotic lesion. Approved carotid stents are either open cell or closed cell systems. However, newer stents in clinical trials have been developed that are a hybrid—mixing areas of open cell design with a closed cell structure. Cell structure and geometry of a stent are critical determinants of stent flexibility. In general, open cell stents tend to be more conformable and flexible as compared with closed cell designs because of fewer connections between individual hooped cells. Unfortunately, increases in flexibility tend to compromise strength and "therefore" make these stents more susceptible to compression and elongation once implanted. Additionally, increased flexibility leads to lower scaffolding, which allows for stent strut protrusion into the lumen at points of curvature of the vessel or excessive irregularity of a rigid plaque and subsequent particle protrusions. Clinically, the reduction in particle trapping may increase the risk of delayed embolic events.

Based on these concepts, some believe that closed cell stents may be best suited for CAS, because the design would improve chronic outward radial force, increase scaffolding, and reduce free cell area. One notable restrospective study by Bosiers et al., examined the clinical impact of cell design on CAS outcomes.[2] The investigators found that closed cell stents were superior in reducing postprocedural neurologic events in symptomatic patients but not in asymptomatic patients. Despite this data, open cell stents should not be excluded from our arsenal because they are clearly more advantageous in tortuous vessels due to their improved conformability.

Stent Configurations

Cell structure, extent of scaffolding and composition of the stents are part of the equation, and yet changes from a straight to a tapered stent to accommodate the anatomic carotid bifurcation might also have clinical consequences. This becomes important because in the majority of cases, stent placement crosses the external carotid artery (ECA) orifice and needs to be well apposed to both the common carotid artery (CCA) and the internal carotid artery (ICA) lumina. The natural size mismatch between the ICA and CCA leads to more stent oversizing in the ICA. Additionally, "self-tapering" of straight stents may not allow for good wall apposition along the entire length of the treated segment. The impact of these two circumstances are excessive oversizing in the ICA, increased chronic outward radial force in the ICA, decreased free cell area in the ICA, and poor or no scaffolding along portions of the atherosclerotic plaque.

Two primary configurations of tapered stents have been developed:

1. conical represented by Acculink and X-act, and
2. shouldered represented by Protégé. In the conical tapered stents, there is a gradual decrease in the diameter of the stent from proximal to distal, whereas in the shouldered tapered stents, there exists a short transition point in the mid-segment of the stent. When considering the carotid vasculature, a significant diameter reduction occurs at the bifurcation, thus theoretically making conical tapered stents more favorable. The primary concern of too much oversizing in the ICA to accommodate to the diameter of the CCA is the risk of restenosis from either excessive metal coverage or undue chronic outward radial force.

Unfortunately, few data exist at this point to allow for a direct comparison of tapered versus nontapered stents. Our institution recently published results from a single-center retrospective review of 308 cases of CAS treated with EPDs and either tapered or nontapered self-expanding nitinol stents.[3] A total of 156 tapered stents were evaluated as well as 152 nontapered stents. The study revealed no statistical difference between the 30-day ipsilateral stroke/transient ischemic attack (TIA) rates in tapered (3.2%) and nontapered stents (1.3%, P=0.5). However, at mid-term follow-up, restenosis (≥ 80%) or asymptomatic stent occlusion was detected in 2.3% of cases in arteries treated with nontapered stents as compared with 0% in the tapered stent group. This analysis is underpowered, but the observed trend was that tapered stents had a lower incidence of restenosis or asymptomatic occlusion. Larger studies are needed to confirm these results.

EMBOLIC PROTECTION DEVICE

Three general categories of mechanical EPDs have been developed to guard against distal cerebral embolization during CAS: (1) distal balloon occlusion, (2) distal filtration, and (3) proximal balloon occlusion.

Distal Balloon Occlusion

Distal balloon occlusion systems are most commonly represented by the PercuSurge GuardWire (Medtronic Vascular, Santa Rosa, CA) in which the balloon blocks flow within the ICA and emboli are aspirated before balloon deflation and catheter removal.

Advantages of this approach tend to include a lower crossing profile as well as the ability of the balloon to capture particles of all sizes. Disadvantages include theoretical local injury to the ICA by balloon overnflation, possible embolization via ECA branches, intolerance of total ICA occlusion by the patient, "suction shadowing," and of most concern, the possibility of embolization during initial lesion crossing prior to inflation of the balloon.[4–5] "Suction shadow" was reported by Tuber et al. in which a 5.2% periprocedural adverse neurologic event rate was noted despite use of balloon occlusion. It is theorized that this effect occurs when suction catheters fail to aspirate all emboli because some emboli may be too large or the blood column adjacent to the balloon device may not be effectively aspirated.[6] The TriActiv FX (Kensey Nash), a more recently introduced distal balloon occlusion system, helps reduce "suction shadow" through the introduction of an active flush system that allows for aggressive particle removal from vessel walls and areas adjacent to the inflated balloon. An additional complication reported with distal balloon occlusion EPDs is the risk of neurologic intolerance during balloon occlusion.[5] This can manifest with a variety of symptoms ranging from mild confusion to seizures. Fortunately, the majority of instances are transient and resolve after re-establishing antegrade flow by deflating the occlusion balloon.

Distal Filters

Distal filters tend to be the most commonly employed cerebral protection devices in most centers. This form of protection allows for continued antegrade cerebral flow through the device while emboli are captured. At the end of the procedure, the filter element is reconstrained and removed with the captured particulate debris. Advantages include the ability to perform angiograms throughout the procedure as well as maintenance of flow, thereby reducing the likelihood of cerebral hypoperfusion. Disadvantages include a larger crossing profile, thereby making it difficult to cross some more tortuous, possibility of incomplete apposition of the filter to the arterial wall, concern for filter thrombosis, filter pore size limitations, and risk of embolization during the initial lesion crossing prior to positioning and deployment of the filter. A review of the current literature evaluating the outcomes of 2263 CAS procedures using various filter devices—Spider Embolic Protection Device (ev3), AngioGuard XP (Cordis), FilterWire EZ (Boston Scientific), AccuNet (Abbott Vascular), and Emboshield (Abbott Vascular)—demonstrated a periprocedural stroke rate of roughly 2%.[7-19]

Proximal Balloon Occlusion

The third and final category of EPD used for carotid interventions is the proximal balloon occlusion devices. These are represented by the NPS (Neuroprotection system, formerly known as PAES—Parodi Anti-Emboli System—W.L. Gore & Associates, Flagstaff, AZ) and the Mo.Ma device (Invatec, Roncadelle, Italy). Both utilize the concepts of carotid occlusion that are used to measure carotid stump pressures during carotid endarterectomy procedures. Instead of clamping the CCA and ECA, each vessel is controlled with balloon occlusion. The balloon for the CCA is mounted on a working sheath placed in the distal CCA, which provides a platform to proceed with CAS after flow reversal is instituted. The NPS device uses both passive and active flow reversal through a sumping mechanism created by an external arteriovenous shunt created between the femoral artery and the femoral vein.[11,20] The Mo.Ma device utilizes flow stagnation as a mechanism to provide for cerebral protection—this is achieved by occlusion of the ECA as well as ICA by two independently inflated low-pressure compliant balloons.[21] This allows for intermittent collection of debris between steps of the procedure and of aspiration of debris at the conclusion of the procedure through a separate working channel. Taken together, advantages of these devices include complete protection of both the ICA as well as the ECA. Protection starts prior to crossing the lesion, there is greater freedom for wire choices, and the device is capable of capturing particles of all sizes. Disadvantages include the need for a larger groin sheet, typically 9-10 Fr, potential arterial injury at balloon inflation sites, and most importantly, total arrest of antegrade flow on the protected side. The largest series of reports using these devices has shown a periprocedural stroke rate of approximately 1 to 2%.[13,15,20,22–23] Notably transient neurologic intolerance, which resolved at the conclusion of the flow reversal, occurred in roughly 10 to 12% of cases. One additional study by Criado et al. showed that cerebral venous oxygen saturation, as measured in the internal jugular vein, was significantly lower during ICA occlusion than during ICA flow reversal.[24] Presumably, this is due to enhancement of collateral flow via the circle of Willis during periods of passive or active flow reversal.

A primary advantage of the proximal occlusion devices is the ability to capture particulate debris of all sizes. In one ex vivo study,[25] a filter device captured only 88% of embolized particles as indicated by transcranial Doppler monitoring. Interestingly, Angelini et al.[8] have shown through histopathologic analysis that microscopic emboli captured in distal filters during CAS have a mean particle size of 289.5 ± 512 micrometers in the major axis and a mean of 119.7 ± 186.7 μ in the minor axis. Prior data have shown that cerebral microcirculation is composed of numerous vessels with diameters less than 300 microns: arterioles tend to have a diameter of between 12 and 100 microns, and capillaries a diameter of approximately 12 microns. Current distal filter devices use membranes with wide-ranging pore sizes (80-500 μ).[10] Thus it is possible that small microemboli may escape the pores of the filter devices and create short-term effects such as stroke or long-term problems including dementia or cognitive failure. According to recent studies, small microemboli showers can potentially trigger platelet aggregation and may cause microvascular obstruction with concomitant prolonged vessel vasospasm and subsequent cerebral infarction.[16,26]

Although the use of EPDs during CAS has not been validated in randomized trials, data from registries and observational studies support their routine use and most interventionalists consider them to be the standard of care. Advocates of performing CAS without the uses of EPDs argue that the larger proportion of strokes occurs postprocedurally, and indeed this seems to be the case. Four studies were identified that distinguished between intraprocedural stroke and postprocedural stroke as identified by clinical findings and/or diffusion-weighted MRI. A total of 368 cases identified were done without the use of EPDs and closed cell stent types, in which there was a 2.5% cumulative incidence of all intraprocedural stroke. Postprocedure, a 5.2% incidence of all stroke was noted.[27-29] In addition, in two other studies, 1069 cases were performed with the use of distal filters EPDs and primarily closed cell stents, in which there was a 1.6% and 1.9% cumulative incidence of intraprocedural stroke and postprocedure stroke, respectively.[27,29] When both subsets of data were combined a total of 65 strokes, both major and minor were identified, of which 60% occurred in the postprocedural period. Indeed, a larger proportion of strokes do occur postprocedure; however, it remains that the incidence of intraprocedural stroke with the use of EPDs is lower than without their use.

SUMMARY

The outcomes of CAS with EPDs have improved markedly over the last decade. This can be attributed to advances in technology, training, and patient selection. While we await results from randomized trials on symptomatic and asymptomatic standard-risk patients treated with CEA or CAS to guide us on the role of these two modalities, it is crucial that we remain committed to understanding potential areas of improvement with regards to the equipment at our disposal. More data on the early and long-term effects of stent design are needed as well as more comprehensive data on the limitations of EPDs.

REFERENCES

1. Muller-Hulsbeck S, Schafer PJ, Charalambous N, et al. Comparison of carotid stents: an in-vitro experiment focusing on stent design. J Endovasc Ther 2009;16:168–77.
2. Bosiers M, de Donato G, Deloose K, et al. Does free cell area influence the outcome in carotid artery stenting? Eur J Vasc Endovasc Surg Feb 2007;33:135–41; discussion 142–3.
3. Brown KE, Usman A, Kibbe MR, et al. Carotid stenting using tapered and nontapered stents: associated neurological complications and restenosis rates. Ann Vasc Surg Jul-Aug 2009;23:439–45.
4. Eskandari MK. Design and development of mechanical embolic protection devices. Expert Rev Med Devices May 2006;3:387–93.
5. Eskandari MK, Najjar SF, Matsumura JS, et al. Technical limitations of carotid filter embolic protection devices. Ann Vasc Surg Jul 2007;21:403–7.
6. Tubler T, Schluter M, Dirsch O, et al. Balloon-protected carotid artery stenting: relationship of periprocedural neurological complications with the size of particulate debris. Circulation Dec 4 2001;104:2791–6.
7. Al-Mubarak N, Colombo A, Gaines PA, et al. Multicenter evaluation of carotid artery stenting with a filter protection system. J Am Coll Cardiol Mar 6 2002;39:841–6.
8. Angelini A, Reimers B, Della Barbera M, et al. Cerebral protection during carotid artery stenting: collection and histopathologic analysis of embolized debris. Stroke Feb 2002;33: 456–61.
9. Castellan L, Causin F, Danieli D, Perini S. Carotid stenting with filter protection. Correlation of ACT values with angiographic and histopathologic findings. J Neuroradiol Mar 2003;30:103–8.
10. Fanelli F, Bezzi M, Boatta E, Passariello R. Techniques in cerebral protection. Eur J Radiol Oct 2006;60:26–36.
11. Green DW, Sanchez LA, Parodi JC, et al. Acute thromboembolic events during carotid artery angioplasty and stenting: etiology and a technique of neurorescue. J Endovasc Ther Jun 2005;12:360–5.
12. Hart JP, Peeters P, Verbist J, et al. Do device characteristics impact outcome in carotid artery stenting? J Vasc Surg Oct 2006;44:725–30; discussion 730–21.
13. Henry M, Polydorou A, Henry I, et al. Carotid angioplasty and stenting under protection. Techniques, results and limitations. J Cardiovasc Surg (Torino) Oct 2006;47:519–46.
14. Kasirajan K, Schneider PA, Kent KC. Filter devices for cerebral protection during carotid angioplasty and stenting. J Endovasc Ther Dec 2003;10:1039–45.
15. Rabe K, Sugita J, Godel H, Sievert H. Flow-reversal device for cerebral protection during carotid artery stenting—acute and long-term results. J Interv Cardiol Feb 2006;19:55–62.
16. Reimers B, Corvaja N, Moshiri S, et al. Cerebral protection with filter devices during carotid artery stenting. Circulation Jul 3 2001;104:12–5.

17. Reimers B, Tubler T, de Donato G, et al. Endovascular treatment of in-stent restenosis after carotid artery stenting: immediate and midterm results. J Endovasc Ther Aug 2006;13: 429–35.
18. Rubartelli P, Brusa G, Arrigo A, et al. Transcranial Doppler monitoring during stenting of the carotid bifurcation: evaluation of two different distal protection devices in preventing embolization. J Endovasc Ther Aug 2006;13:436–42.
19. White CJ, Iyer SS, Hopkins LN, et al. Carotid stenting with distal protection in high surgical risk patients: the BEACH trial 30 day results. Catheter Cardiovasc Interv Apr 2006;67: 503–12.
20. Adami CA, Scuro A, Spinamano L, et al. Use of the Parodi anti-embolism system in carotid stenting: Italian trial results. J Endovasc Ther Apr 2002;9:147–54.
21. Scheinert D, Scheinert S, Sax J, et al. Prevalence and clinical impact of stent fractures after femoropopliteal stenting. J Am Coll Cardiol Jan 18 2005;45:312–5.
22. Reimers B, Schluter M, Castriota F, et al. Routine use of cerebral protection during carotid artery stenting: results of a multicenter registry of 753 patients. Am J Med Feb 15 2004; 116:217–22.
23. Reimers B, Sievert H, Schuler GC, et al. Proximal endovascular flow blockage for cerebral protection during carotid artery stenting: results from a prospective multicenter registry. J Endovasc Ther Apr 2005;12:156–65.
24. Criado E, Doblas M, Fontcuberta J, et al. Carotid angioplasty with internal carotid artery flow reversal is well tolerated in the awake patient. J Vasc Surg Jul 2004;40:92–7.
25. Ohki T, Roubin GS, Veith FJ, et al. Efficacy of a filter device in the prevention of embolic events during carotid angioplasty and stenting: an ex vivo analysis. J Vasc Surg Dec 1999; 30:1034–44.
26. Williams DO. Carotid filters: new additions to the interventionist's toolbox. Circulation Jul 3 2001;104:2–3.
27. Alexandrescu V, Ngongang C, Proumen J, et al. Filter-protected carotid stenting via a minimal cervical access with transitory aspirated reversed flow during initial passage of the target lesion. J Endovasc Ther Apr 2006;13:196–204.
28. Davila-Roman VG, Murphy SF, Nickerson NJ, et al. Atherosclerosis of the ascending aorta is an independent predictor of long-term neurologic events and mortality. J Am Coll Cardiol Apr 1999;33:1308–16.
29. Verzini F, Cao P, De Rango P, et al. Appropriateness of learning curve for carotid artery stenting: an analysis of periprocedural complications. J Vasc Surg Dec 2006;44:1205–11; discussion 1201–02.

SECTION II

Upper Extremity

5

Treatment Options for Hand Ischemia

Gregory A. Dumanian, M.D., F.A.C.S.

Hand ischemia is rendered difficult by what it is not: It is not pure vascular surgery, it is not pure hand surgery and it is not common. The anatomy is relatively unfamiliar. The physiology of hand blood flow is generally not well understood. The disease entities causing hand ischemia are in some instances unique to the hand in comparison with the rest of the body. The surgical adjuncts of microscopes and tourniquets are not used in most surgical practices but are often used in hand surgery. Finally, the postoperative splints, rehabilitation protocols, nerve issues, and prostheses in cases of failed salvage are all the domain of hand surgery rather than vascular surgery. The goal of this chapter is to give an overview of the treatment of a patient with hand ischemia.

HAND BLOOD FLOW ANATOMY AND PHYSIOLOGY

The parallel blood supply to the hand from the radial and ulnar arteries has been extensively studied in the dissection laboratory. Coleman and Anson, in their landmark studies, demonstrated an anatomic connection in 80% of hands.[1] A "complete palmar arch" was defined as when the superficial palmar arch was in continuity or "completed" by a branch from the deep palmar arch, the radial artery itself, or a persistent median artery. The ulnar artery, being the supplier to the superficial palmar arch, was considered the major blood vessel to the hand. For hands with a Coleman and Anson incomplete arch, damage to the radial artery at the wrist should theoretically cause decreased blood flow to the thumb.

Blood flow physiology is significantly different from blood vessel anatomy. Differences between radial and ulnar artery contributions to hand blood flow were documented from following soldiers in World War II with arterial ligations in the forearm. Surprisingly, soldiers with radial artery ligations had five times the rate of hand tissue loss than soldiers who underwent ulnar artery ligation for trauma. More recently, the advent of use of the radial artery in coronary artery bypass grafting has led to studies

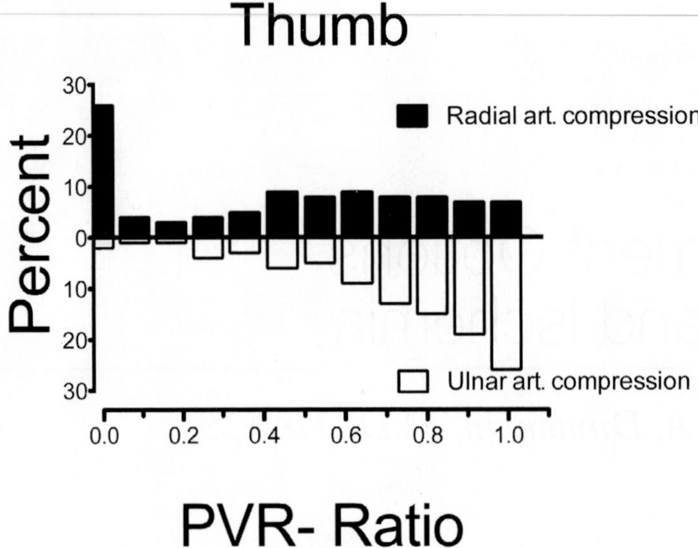

Figure 5-1. Percent reduction in surface area under PVR tracing for the thumb with either radial or ulnar artery compression at the wrist; 294 hands. Twenty-five percent of thumbs lose pulsatile flow with compression of the radial artery at the wrist, whereas 3% of thumbs lose pulsatile flow with ulnar artery compression. A PVR tracing =1 shows no change in blood flow with compression of the artery, whereas a PVR tracing = 0 shows a complete loss of pulsatile flow.

testing the importance of the radial artery for digital pulsatile blood flow.[2] Manual compression of the radial artery at the wrist caused the loss of pulsatile flow seen on pulse volume recordings (PVRs) of the thumb and fifth fingers in approximately 20% of hands, while compression of the ulnar artery caused similar flat line PVR tracings in only 4% of hands (Figures 5–1 and 5–2). This supports the World War II data of the radial artery's being critical to hand blood flow five times as often as the ulnar artery.

What is most surprising from these data is that for hands that lose pulsatile blood flow to the thumb with radial artery compression at the wrist, fully 70% of the fifth fingers will also lose pulsatile blood flow. In only 1% of all tested hands was there blood flow maintained in the fifth finger despite a loss of pulsatile blood flow in the thumb with compression of the radial artery at the wrist (Figure 5–3). For the majority of hands, the physiology is that the hand acts as a single vascular bed supplied by two different arteries. A drop in pressure with the loss of one blood vessel affects the entire hand rather than the loss of perfusion of just the radial or just the ulnar side of the hand. Anatomy is different from physiology. Coleman and Anson predict that fully 20% of hands should act as two separate beds and that the ulnar artery is the dominant vessel for blood flow. Instead, the hand acts as a single vascular bed in 99% of hands tested. In the overwhelming majority of hands, the fingers act more similarly than dissimilarly from drops in perfusion pressure. Images of ischemic hands demonstrate digits affected simultaneously on the radial and ulnar sides of the hand (Figures 5–4 and 5–5). This concept that the hand acts more as a single vascular bed is critical when bypass grafting of the hand is considered. Rather than needing to revascularize multiple arteries, increased inflow to the hand at one site will improve its overall condition.

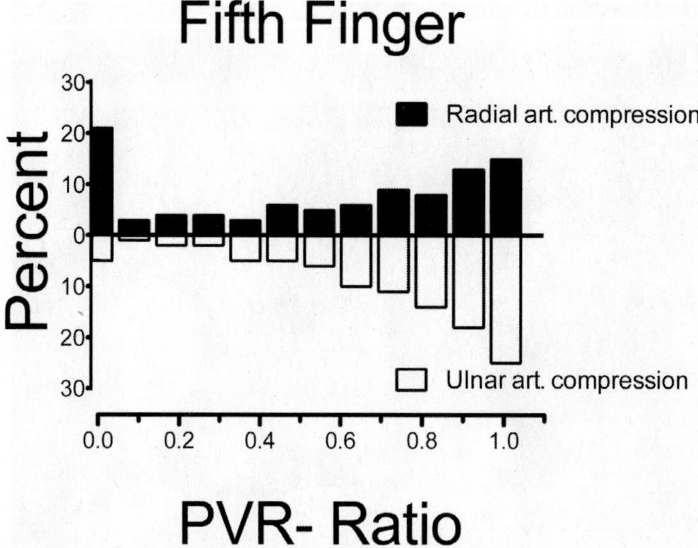

Figure 5-2. Percent reduction in surface area under PVR tracing for fifth finger with either radial or ulnar artery compression at the wrist; 578 hands. Twenty-one percent of fifth fingers lose pulsatile flow with compression of the radial artery at the wrist, whereas 5% of fifth fingers lose pulsatile flow with ulnar artery compression. A PVR tracing = 1 shows no change in blood flow with compression of the artery, whereas a PVR tracing = 0 shows a complete loss of pulsatile flow.

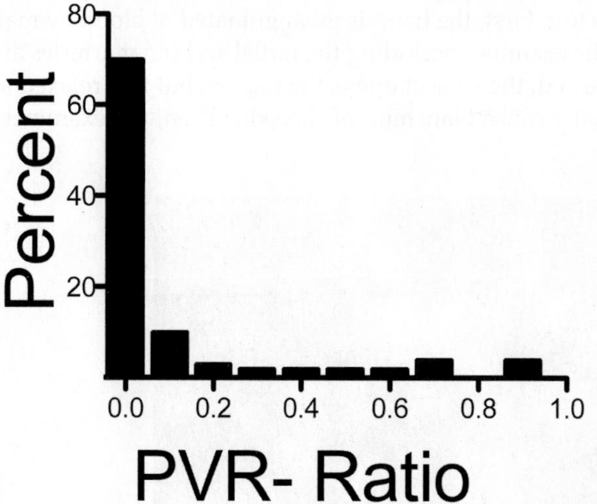

Figure 5-3. Percent reduction in fifth finger PVR tracings in the 86 hands that lost thumb blood flow with radial artery compression at the wrist. Seventy percent of fifth fingers also lost pulsatile flow, demonstrating that the fifth finger and the thumb act similarly. On the right, 4% of these 86 hands maintained normal blood flow to the fifth finger despite losing pulsatile flow to the thumb with radial artery compression. This minority of test hands has two distinct vascular beds.

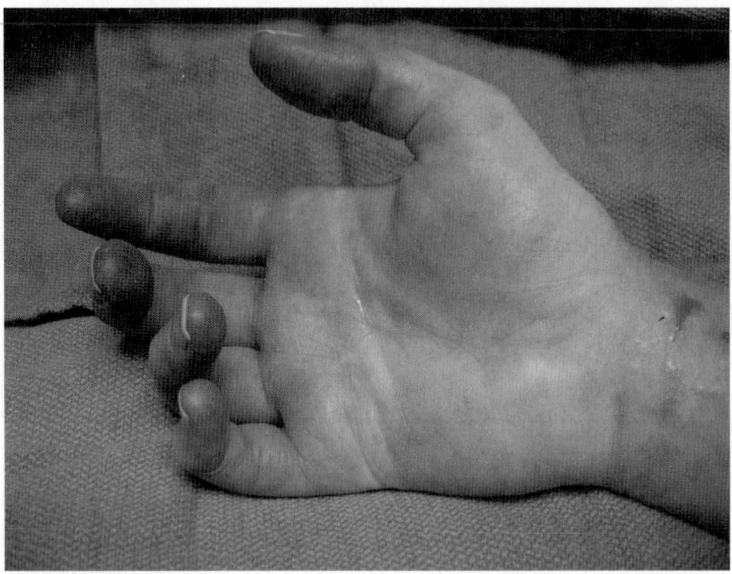

Figure 5-4. Global hand ischemia in a critically ill patient on vasopressors.

Physical and Vascular Examinations

Palpation of the brachial and radial artery pulses is mandatory in the initial evaluation of the blood flow in the hand. The radial artery pulse can also be palpated in the anatomic snuffbox on the dorsal radial aspect of the hand. The ulnar artery is typically difficult to palpate because of the stout flexor carpi ulnaris tendon overlying the vessel. To better evaluate the radial and ulnar artery contributions to hand blood flow, Allen, a medical student, devised the Allen's test. First, the hand is exsanguinated of blood by making a fist, opening and closing, with the examiner occluding the radial and ulnar arteries at the wrist. With the arteries still compressed, the subject opens the fingers, but in a relaxed and normal cascade so as not to artificially cause blanching of the skin. Then, the examiner releases either the

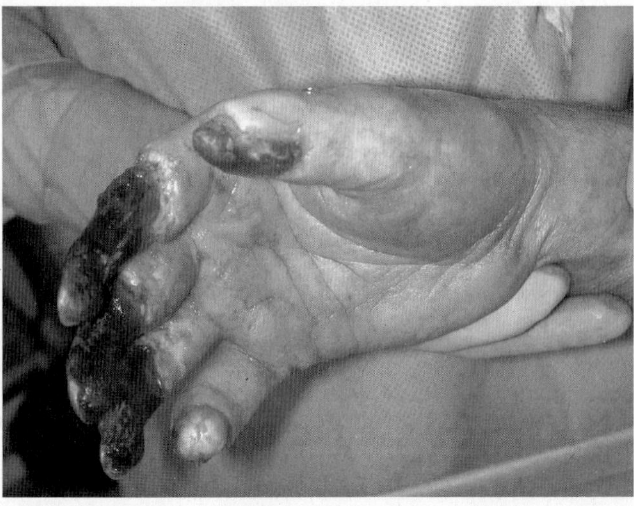

Figure 5-5. Multiple necrotic digits demonstrating the hand acting as a single vascular bed.

radial or the ulnar artery in order to assess the reperfusion of the hand from that vessel. The fingers should appear pink within 5 seconds. Digits that remain white demonstrate either a lack of patency of the artery at the wrist or poor flow of the vessel into the hand. This test is especially important for testing the patency of the radial artery before arterial catheter placement.

The vascular laboratory and radiologic tests are also helpful in the treatment of patients with hand ischemia. PVRs, digital pressures, and Doppler waveforms can adequately assess pulsatile flow and are useful for postoperative evaluation of therapies. MRA, CT angiography, and arteriograms are often necessary to plan surgical procedures.

ACUTE HAND ISCHEMIA

A thorough history and physical examination must be obtained upon the presentation of an individual with a cool, mottled, and painful hand. Patient age, handedness, smoking history, occupation, heart history, trauma, athletic history, recent upper extremity surgery or catheter placement, and a history of a hypercoagulable state must be obtained. Establishment of the presence or absence of a sinus rhythm, evidence of endocarditis or septic emboli, pulses at the level of the humerus and wrist, an Allen's test, and the presence of Doppler signals in the palm and fingers are mandatory. Full anticoagulation is usually the first step. along with pain control in the emergency room. After admission, the patient needs an echocardiogram to look for mural thrombi and any valvular disease (Figures 5–6 and 5–7). A chest x-ray and a chest CT may show evidence of a subclavian aneurysm from hypermobility of shoulder movements or compression of the artery from thoracic outlet syndrome.[3] Along with these tests, an arteriogram that includes the take-off of the subclavian artery from the aorta is typically required to complete the work-up of a proximal source of emboli to the arm and hand.

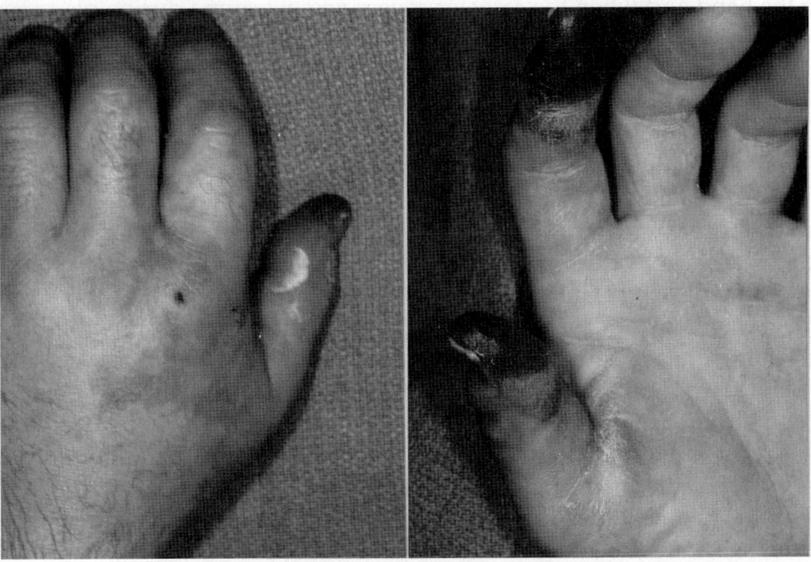

Figure 5-6. Volar and dorsal views of a patient with acute hand ischemia, presenting 1 full week after the beginning of severe pain. He was treated for thumb and index finger paronychias initially.

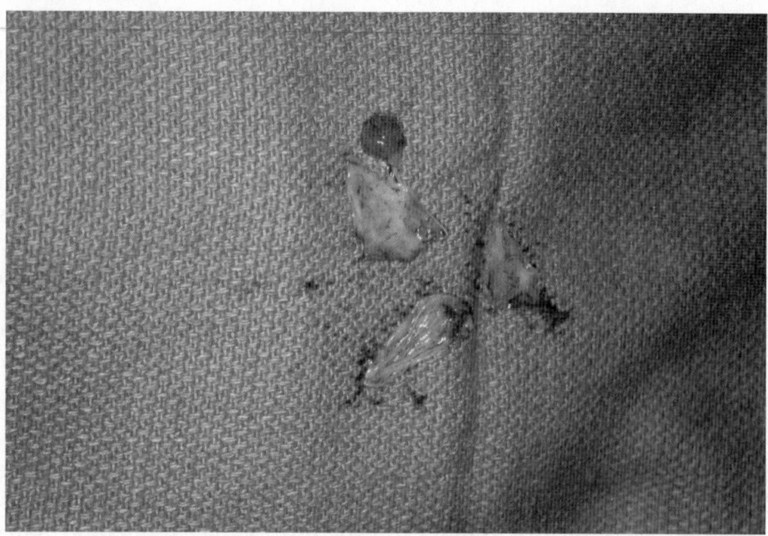

Figure 5-7. Nonseptic degenerative lesion excised from the patient's aortic leaflets at the time of aortic valve replacement.

Hand ischemia caused by a more distal process is typically understandable on physical examination and may or may not need an arteriogram for evaluation. In children, supracondylar fractures are associated with acute limb ischemia. This can be due to an intimal stretch injury at the time of a bony injury to the artery, or being associated with a newly reduced fracture that was reduced and pinned. Also at the level of the brachial artery, distal embolizations from inadvertent intra-arterial injections in drug abusers can cause profound ischemia. In the forearm, trauma to either the radial or the ulnar arteries would be apparent on physical examination. Radial arterial catheters can produce hand ischemia when the radial artery is the dominant source of blood to the hand and when the catheter causes vessel trauma during placement.

The management of patients with acute hand ischemia is rendered difficult by several factors. First, due to its relative rarity, many patients present late, with tissue loss that is unrecoverable. Embolic disease from aneurysms often occurs in subacute fashion over a prolonged period of time, with the "acute" final event occurring after many of the vessels have already been chronically occluded. This is the pathophysiology from both subclavian artery and ulnar artery aneurysmal disease. When emboli do occur, they are difficult to retrieve because of the small vessel size that is unreachable with Fogarty catheters.

The treatment of proximal causes of hand ischemia is beyond the scope of this chapter. At the elbow, supracondylar fractures with ischemia must be brought urgently to the operating room. After reduction by the orthopedic service, the hand is evaluated for a wrist pulse and capillary refill. The quality of blood flow that is considered acceptable after reduction of the fracture remains controversial. My opinion is that a palpable pulse at the wrist is mandatory before leaving the operating room to ensure normal growth of the maturing arm. If the blood flow is considered inadequate, the brachial artery should be explored. If the artery is within the fracture line, the pins must be removed and the artery restored to its normal position. If the artery is in a normal position but there is still no pulsatile flow after adventitial stripping, then an intimal injury must be suspected. Excision of the damaged artery and possible repair with a vein graft are necessary to reestablish a pulse at the wrist. This often requires microsurgery and consideration of a postrevascularization fasciotomy. In the forearm, repair of a single vessel in the arm at the time of forearm trauma when the hand is pink and has pulsatile flow also is controversial. Repair of single-vessel arterial injuries in the forearm perhaps decreases the rate of cold intolerance, although this may also be related to associated nerve injuries. Radial artery catheter–induced hand ischemias should be treated with immediate catheter removal. If this does not improve the hand, then an immediate exploration is required to repair the injured radial artery. After removal of large emboli from the vascular tree and repair of the radial artery injury, there still may be ischemia of the hand due to distal microemboli. Embolectomy catheter retrieval of these emboli is generally not feasible owing to the small size of these vessels. In these instances, intra-arterial infusions of thrombolytic agents are often helpful. A tourniquet is placed on the arm, and an intra-arterial injection of 10% of the systemic dose of tissue plasminogen activator (tPA) mixed in 30 cc of volume is administered through the radial artery into the vascular tree (Figures 5–8 and 5–9). The tourniquet allows the tPA to remain in the limb to improve its efficacy while still at a dose that would not cause systemic fibrinolysis. After 20 minutes, the tourniquet is let down, and much of the tPA is already degraded due to its short half-life. Alternatively, the tPA can be administered over time using a superselective catheter threaded from the groin adjacent to the occluded vessel. Carpal tunnel and intrinsic muscle fasciotomies are necessary for hands that have had a prolonged ischemic event.

Vasopressor-associated hand hypoperfusion and ischemia occur in critically ill patients in intensive care unit settings. Treatment of hand ischemia is typically not feasible in these patients other than removal of any arterial blood pressure catheters in line with the extremity. Conservative treatment is typically in order rather than aggressive amputations in which suture lines tend to suffer from marginal ischemia and necrosis. If the patient recovers, the tissue loss tends to be less marked than would otherwise be expected on initial presentation, although motion and function are poor.

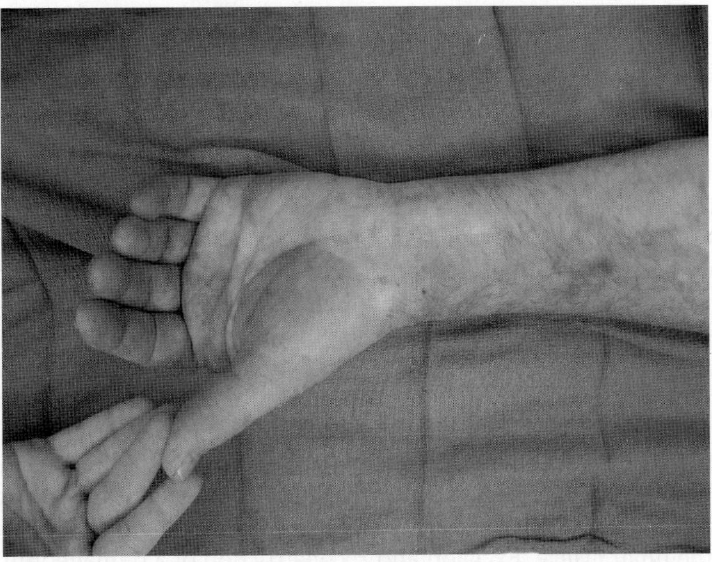

Figure 5-8. Hand ischemia due to a radial arterial line placement.

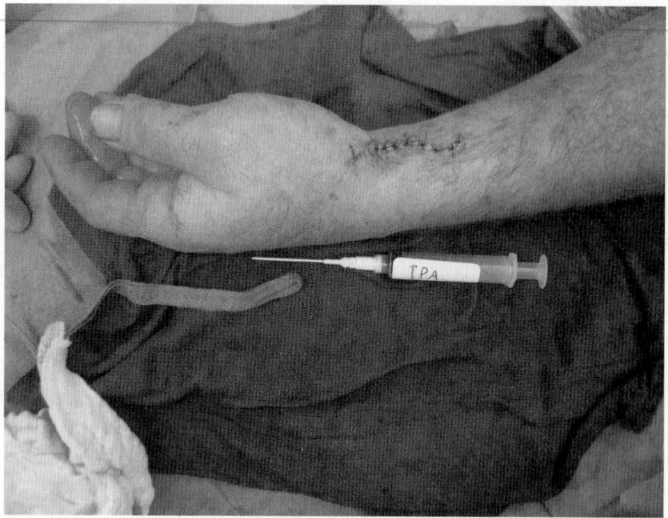

Figure 5-9. Resolution of hand ischemia with repair of the radial artery, carpal tunnel release for a fasciotomy, and infusion of tPA under a tourniquet.

Chronic Hand Ischemia

Patients with chronic hand ischemia present with painful digital ulcers and cold intolerance. The two main etiologies that exist for chronic hand ischemia are divided into the causes of repeated embolization and the causes of multiple-vessel thrombosis. In terms of embolization, the subclavian artery and the ulnar artery both can cause repeated distal embolization. Patients with proximal vessel injury with repeated distal embolization initially present with "acute" hand ischemia, with the most recent embolization upon an already damaged vascular tree tipping the hand into the ischemic zone. Some patients with chronic ischemia become symptomatic only on "stress" tests of increased activity or with challenges of a cold environment. It is only by obtaining an arteriogram that the multiple shower of emboli are seen filling the vascular tree. Arteriograms should begin at the aortic arch to rule out emboli coming from a subclavian ostial lesion. Aneurysms are tip-offs for the site of repeated distal embolization. Emboli-induced ischemia should be treated initially with anticoagulation and then with prevention of further emboli. Subclavian artery injury from atherosclerosis, excess mobility, or brachial plexus compression is managed with combinations of endovascular techniques, brachial plexus decompression, and subclavian artery resection and replacement. This is beyond the scope of this chapter.

The ulnar artery is another source of multiple emboli to the ulnar digits. In so-called hypothenar hammer syndrome, the ulnar side of the hand is used to strike objects such as paint cans or tire hubcaps, traumatizing the ulnar artery against the hook of the hamate bone. After the diagnosis is made, treatment is controversial. Excision of the ulnar artery aneurysm and ligation prevent new emboli from occurring. If the collateral flow to the digits is acceptable, tissue loss will not occur. However, patients still tend to complain of cold intolerance after the procedure. Cold intolerance is a complex subject and may be due to nerve injury from the chronic emboli as opposed to decreased digital pressures. However, to optimize all components of the hand, I tend to reconstruct the ulnar artery. Excision and reconstruction of a damaged ulnar artery require the use of an operating microscope and a vascular conduit. I prefer to use a tourniquet for the bloodless field and a reversed lesser saphenous vein graft for a vascular conduit for its size and handling characteristics.[4] Extensile palmar incisions to perform adventitectomies of the superficial palmar arch and common digital vessels, such as are done for patients with scleroderma, are often necessary as adjuncts to ulnar artery replacement.

Thrombotic causes of hand ischemia are generally caused by collagen vascular diseases such as scleroderma. The radial artery tends to have a palpable pulse at the wrist, and the ulnar artery also tends to have inflow. Between the wrist and the fingers, the vessels have a constricting periadventitial fibrosis that causes them to look small on an arteriogram (Figure 5–10). The superficial palmar arch is often thrombosed, although the deep arch is often patent. Thromoboses tend to occur at the level of PIP joints. Medical treatment for these patients includes cessation of smoking, avoidance of cold, anticoagulation with antiplatelet agents, and vasodilating agents such as calcium channel blockers. A relatively new and poorly understood agent for treatment of chronic hand ischemia is the injection of botulinum toxin A into the skin of the palm.[5–6] Initially injected into the hand for treatment of hyperhidrosis, botulinum toxin A was found to be successful for the amelioration of ischemia symptoms of Raynaud's phenomenon. Treatment with 50 to 100 units of this agent divided into 15 to 20 injections has been shown to help a percentage of patients in terms of wound healing, pain, and digital blood flow. It is unclear how often these agents need to be reinjected. It is also unclear if patients with vaso-occlusion will do as well as patients with a vasospastic etiology of their ischemia.

Surgical treatment of chronic ischemia of the hand due to scleroderma is generally done either with a digital sympathectomy or with microscope-assisted bypass grafting. Indications for surgery include nonhealing tip ulcers and pain that are refractory to medical treatment.[7] There also must be something to save, because frank digital ischemia with tissue loss up to the DIP joint is probably best served by amputation. Digital sympathectomy is somewhat of a misnomer because the procedure is more

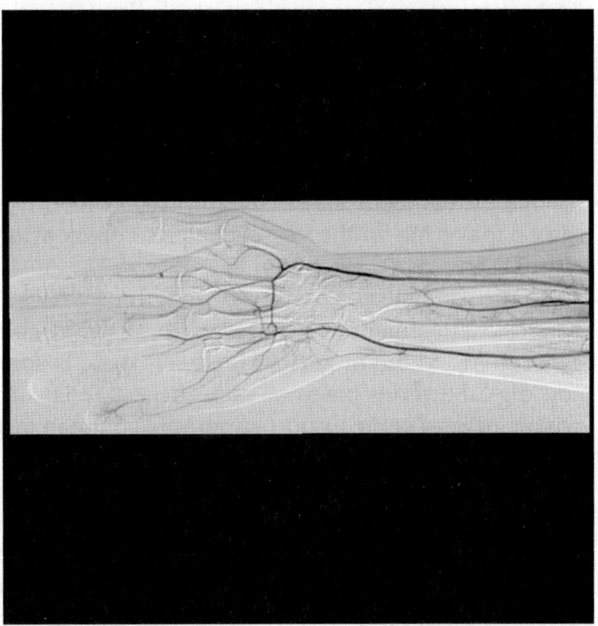

Figure 5-10. Arteriogram of a patient with digital ulcerations due to scleroderma.

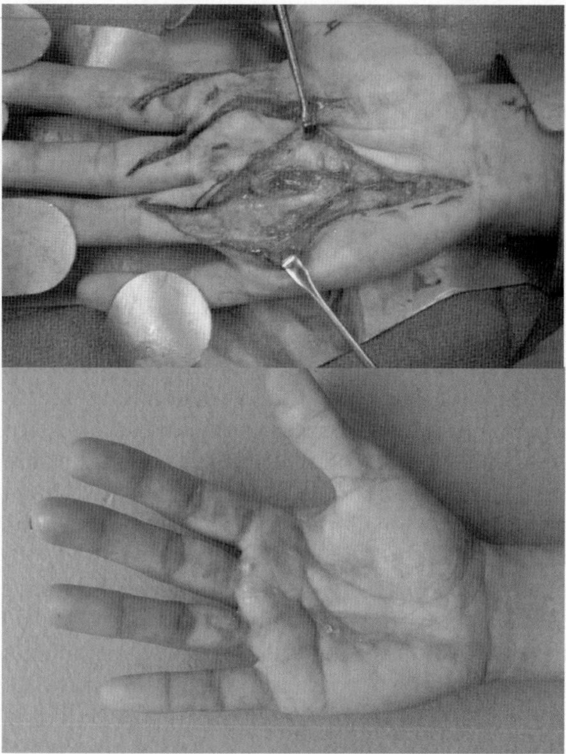

Figure 5-11. Intraoperative and postoperative views of digital sympathectomy/radical adventiectomy for the arteriogram seen in Figure 5-10.

directed at periadventitial stripping of fibrotic tissue than it is a sympathectomy. The digital sympathetics leave the common digital nerves at right angles to reach the digital arteries over a 2- to 3-cm area proximal to the PIP joints. In a classic digital sympathectomy under microscopic control, Bruner incisions are used to expose both the radial and the ulnar digital arteries from the palmar arch to the PIP joint (Figures 5–11 through 5–14). Circumferential adventitial stripping opens the vessels, removes any sympathetics, alleviates extrinsic vasoconstriction, and permits vasodilatation. It is important not to damage any connections between the deep and the superficial palmar arches, as these collaterals are occasionally the only blood supply to the digits. A brachial plexus block anesthetic improves blood flow in the postoperative period, and using papaverine on the vessels helps to break arterial spasm induced during the procedure.

Controversy exists over what length of vessel the stripping should be performed. Classically, treatment of a 2-cm length of vessel up to the PIP joint divides the sympathetics going to the fingerip. However, there is some rationale for following the common digital arteries onto the superficial palmar arch, and even onto the palm to the wrist if necessary to divide superficial palmar fascial bands compressing the ulnar artery.

Also controversial is the need to perform bypass grafting of the hand. Bypass grafts have typically been considered surgical challenges, with diagrams demonstrating multiple arterial microanastomoses with reimplantation of each of the common digital arteries end-to-side off the bypass graft.[8] A critical issue in deciding whether to perform a long vessel adventiectomy or a hand bypass is the issue of the presence or

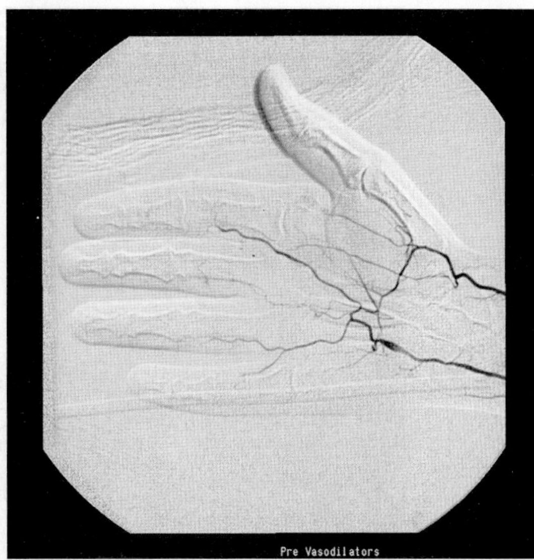

Figure 5-12. Patient with scleroderma and a proximal compression of the ulnar artery in Guyon's canal.

absence of "in-line" flow. Narrowed arteries that are in continuity between the forearm up to the PIP joints would be treated with a digital sympathectomy, whereas digits with critical ischemia supplied via collaterals from the deep palmar arch would potentially be candidates for a hand bypass procedure. Bypasses are done in a unique manner for hand ischemia.[9] First, a tourniquet is used so as to be able to work in a bloodless environment. The tourniquet perhaps provides a privileged environment that does not allow any blood to clot in the operative field while it is elevated. However, surgeries then must be performed within the customary 2-hour window that the tourniquet can be safely elevated. Second, the superficial palmar arch or a

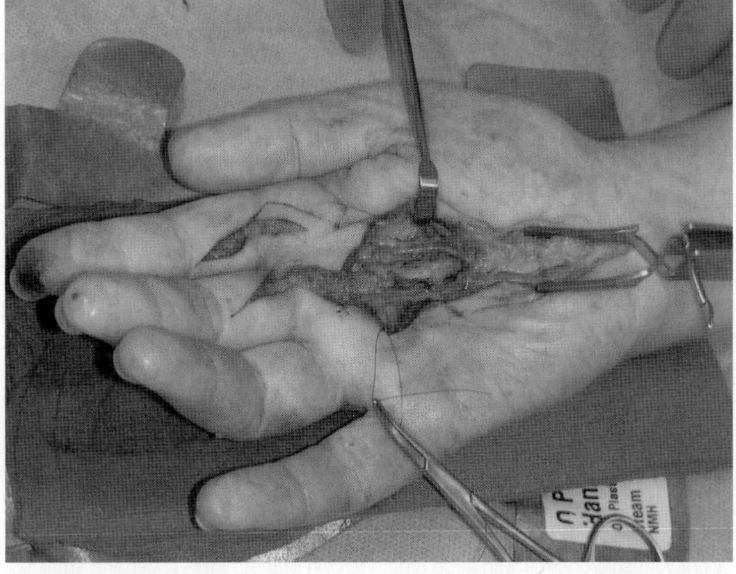

Figure 5-13. Digital sympathectomy/radical adventitiectomies for the patient in Figure 5-12.

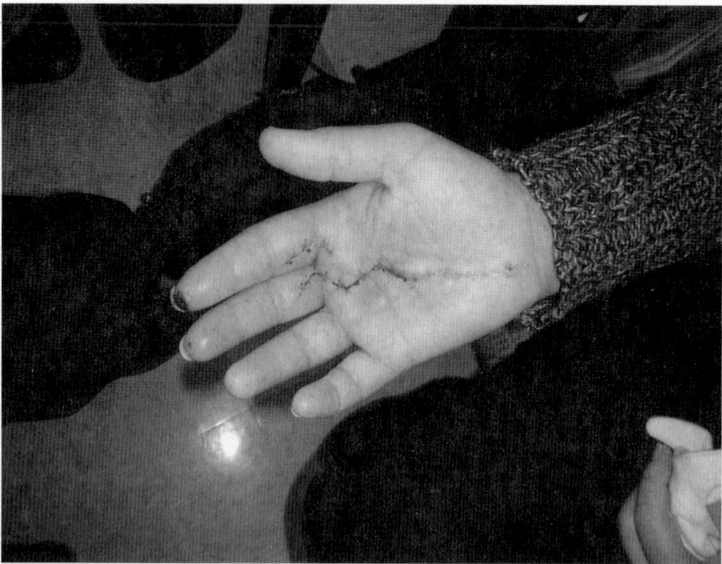

Figure 5-14. Postoperative view of patient in Figure 5-12.

common digital artery is the distal target as the sole outflow anastomosis (Figures 5–15 through 5–18). The hand acts as a single vascular bed, and therefore one outflow vessel can revascularize the entire hand. This decreases operative times and allows the procedure to be done within one tourniquet run. Third, the tunneling of the graft within the tight confines of the skin of the hand can be difficult. My preferred tech-

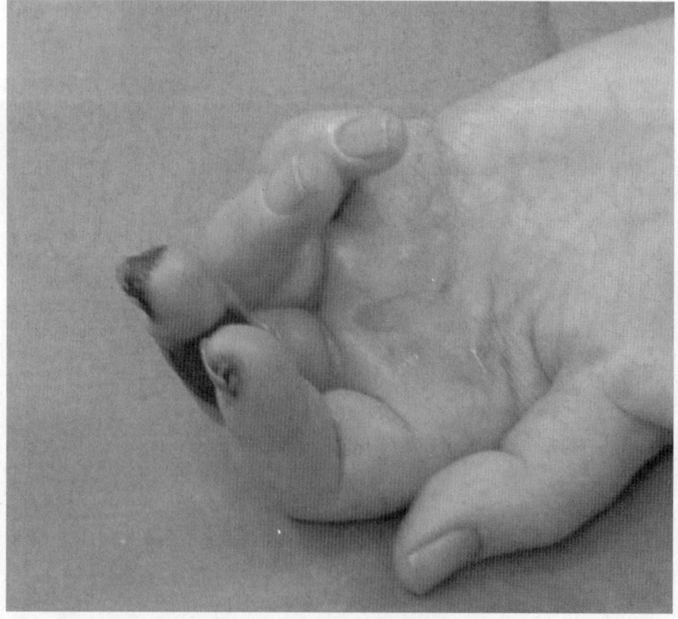

Figure 5-15. Patient with scleroderma with large area necrosis of the middle finger and small tip necrosis of the index finger. She has a radial artery pulse at the wrist.

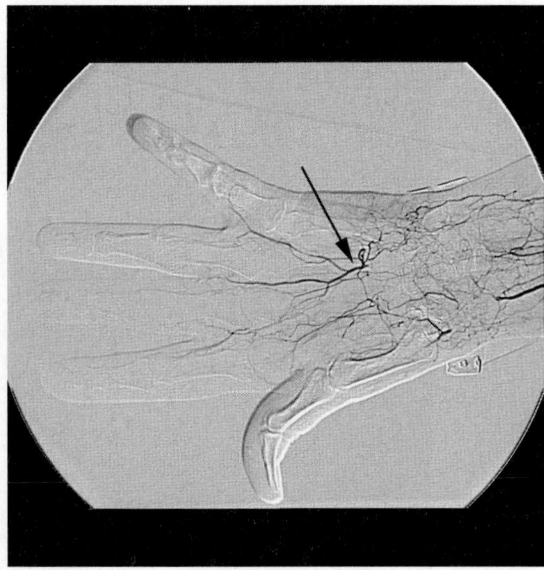

Figure 5-16. Arteriogram of patient in Figure 5-15. The arrow demonstrates a patent superficial arch.

nique is to perform the proximal anastomosis of a reversed lesser saphenous vein graft to either the radial or the ulnar artery and to tunnel the graft through the carpal canal enlarged with the help of an endoscopic carpal tunnel release. The graft is allowed to fill with nonclotting blood while still under the tourniquet to ensure proper length of the construct. The distal anastomosis is done to a vessel selected with the help of a preoperative arteriogram, either end-to-end or end-to-side, depending of whether or not there is a proximal occlusion. The tourniquet is then let down, and hemostasis in the newly revascularized hand takes some additional time to achieve.

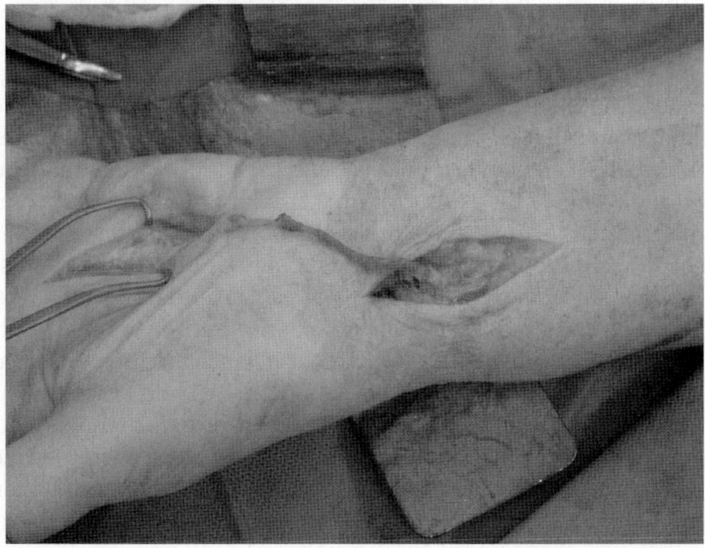

Figure 5-17. Bypass from the radial artery through the carpal canal end-to-end to the superficial palmar arch using the thoracodorsal artery for conduit.

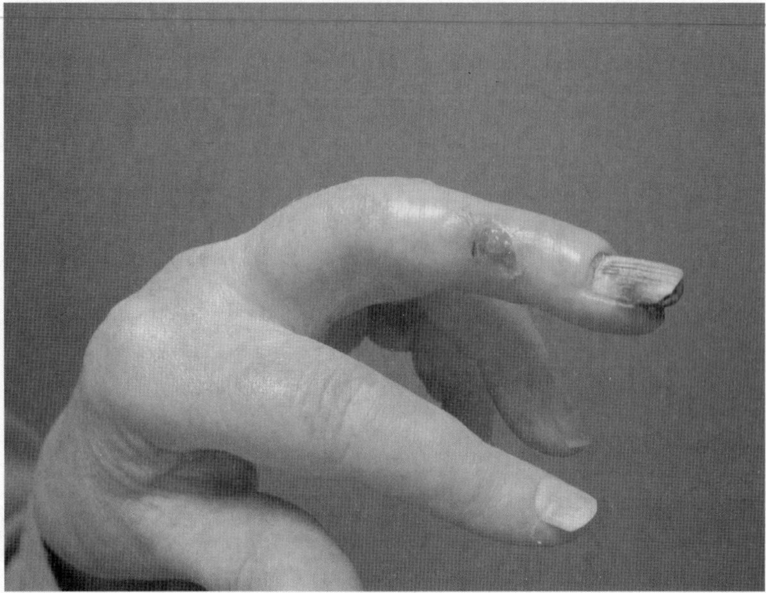

Figure 5-18. Healed fingers and a patent graft.

AMPUTATIONS

Performance of amputations is one of the necessary adjuncts to the care of the ischemic hand patient. The goal of surgery is a mobile pain-free digit, whereas digital length is only secondary. Persistently ischemic tissue generating pain in a stiff finger is not as good an outcome as a well-healed incision with good soft tissues covering the digital nerve amputations. Under local anesthesia and without stopping anticoagulation, digital amputations can be done without too much difficulty. Fish-mouth incisions with dog-ears taken out in the midlateral lines tend to do well. There should be absolutely no tension on the skin flaps, and so the bone should be divided a bit more proximally than thought necessary. The skin edges tend to die back a bit due to decreased skin blood flow caused by the sutures. In general, the amputations across the midportion of the middle phalanx do not heal reliably for a patient with a necrotic digital tip, and the PIP joint does not tend to maintain its motion. Amputations across the proximal phalanx tend to heal completely, and metacarpophalangeal movement tends to be maintained. The bone end should be contoured so as not to look bulbous. Nerves found on either side of the tendon sheath should be placed on traction and divided as proximally as possible to decrease the chance of a symptomatic neuroma found under the skin. Similarly, traction should be placed on both flexor tendons before a proximal division to decrease the chance of an infected tendon end festering in the mid-palm. The flexor tendons specifically should not be sewn to the extensor tendon mechanism for added bone coverage. The profundus tendon placed and fixed on unusual tension in that manner is a cause of "quadrigia" and decreased motion of adjacent fingers. Digital prostheses are available for the patient with amputations. Although they do not improve function, custom-made digits made out of latex materials can assist patients in camouflaging the sequelae of their vascular injuries.

POSTOPERATIVE CARE

Digital tip ulcers are treated with gentle wound care, very conservative removal of necrotic tissue, and a topical antimicrobial with a silver-containing compound. If bypass surgery is performed, prevention of occlusion of the graft from wrist flexion or pressure on the graft can be achieved with a volar well-padded splint placed in the operating room with the metacarpophalangeal joints extended and the PIP joints flexed slightly. Splints help to immobilize the soft tissues to achieve early postoperative healing and they also help with postoperative pain. Patency of the bypass graft is followed in the postoperative period by an arterial saturation monitor placed on a finger. Early digit motion and nighttime splints in full extension help to prevent PIP flexion contractures that develop in these patients who are prone to develop thick scars. If a graft is done, a well-padded wrist splint with the fingers free worn for 3 to 4 weeks will help to prevent occlusion of the graft from wrist flexion or direct compression.

CONCLUSIONS

The complete treatment of a patient with hand ischemia requires a working knowledge of vascular surgery, hand surgery, and reconstructive microsurgery. Lasting improvements in patient function are achievable using the principles presented in this chapter.

REFERENCES

1. Coleman SS, Anson BJ. Arterial patterns in the hand based upon a study of 650 specimens. Surg Gyncol Obstet 1961;113:409.
2. Dumanian GA, Segalman K, Beuhner JW, et al. Analysis of digital pulse-volume recordings with radial and ulnar artery compression. Plast Reconstr Surg 1998;102:1993–8.
3. Durham JR, Yao JST, Pearce WH, et al. Arterial injuries in the thoracic outlet syndrome. J Vasc Surg 1995;21:57.
4. Dumanian GA, Chen A. Microsurgery in a bloodless field. Microsurgery 2000;20:221–4.
5. Van Beek AL, Lim PK, Gear AJ, Pritzker MR. Management of vasospastic disorders with botulinum toxin A. Plast Reconstr Surg 2007;119:217.
6. Fregene A, Ditmars D, Siddiqui A. Botulium toxin type A: a treatment option for digital ischemia in patients with Raynaud's phenomenon. J Hand Surg 2009;34A:446–52.
7. Wilgis EF. Evaluation and treatment of chronic digital ischemia. Ann Surg 1981;193:693–8.
8. Jones NF. Ischemia of the hand in systemic disease. The potential role of microsurgical revascularization and digital sympathectomy. Clin Plast Surg 1989;16:547–56.
9. Kryger ZB, Rawlani V, Dumanian GA. Treatment of chronic digital ischemia with direct microsurgical revascularization. J Hand Surg 2007;32A:1466–70.

6

Subclavian Artery Aneurysms

Audrey Rosinberg, M.D. and William H. Pearce, M.D.

Subclavian artery aneurysms (SAAs) are an uncommon clinical entity. Clinical reviews by Hobson, Pairolero, and Dougherty provide an excellent overview of the world's literature.[1–3] Because of the rarity of these lesions, it is difficult to predict their behavior with any accuracy, since most reports were written prior to the era of CT and MR imaging, making natural history studies difficult. Except for the smallest of aneurysms, the majority of SAAs are repaired because of their propensity for distal embolization with digital ischemia. This chapter reviews the etiology, diagnosis, and management of SAAs. With the advent of endoluminal treatment for vascular disease, the treatment paradigm for SAA has changed. However, open surgery remains the primary treatment for SAAs associated with the thoracic outlet syndrome.

ETIOLOGY

In Hobson's report, atherosclerosis was the most common cause of subclavian aneurysm.[1] However, in our own experience, atherosclerosis is a rare cause of SAA and subclavian aneurysms are most likely to be associated with abnormalities of the thoracic outlet.[4] Table 6–1 reviews the various etiologies associated with SAAs. Unlike aneurysms of the lower extremity, there are a wide variety of potential etiologies for SAAs. Upper extremity arteries are particularly prone to large-vessel vasculitis. These diseases include giant cell arteritis, Behçet's disease, Wegener's granulomatosis, sarcoidosis, and Takayasu's disease.[5–9] In addition, there are a number of infectious diseases that have been associated with SAAs, including syphilis, HIV, and Kawasaki's disease.[10] The thoracic outlet syndrome with associated cervical ribs, direct trauma, or iatrogenic trauma is perhaps the most common cause of SAAs.[11–13] In addition to these etiologies, inherited connective tissue diseases such as Marfan's disease, Ehlers-Danlos syndrome, and neurofibromatosis have been reported as causes of SAAs.[14–18] Perhaps what is most unusual about SAAs is their congenital etiology. It is rare to find congenital causes for aneurysms elsewhere in the body, but this is not un-

TABLE 6-1. ETIOLOGIES ASSOCIATED WITH SAAs

Atherosclerotic	Infectious
Inflammation	Syphilis
Giant cell	Human Immunodeficiency Virus
Wegener's	Kawasaki's disease
Sarcoidosis	Thoracic outlet
Behçet's	Trauma
Takayasu's	Congenital
Connective tissue disease	Atherosclerotic
Marfan's	
Ehlers-Danlos syndrome	
Neurofibromatosis	

common in the upper extremity. The most common congenital abnormality associated with SAAs is an aberrant right subclavian artery with associated aneurysm formation.[19–20] SAAs are also associated with coarctation, ipsilateral congenital absence of the internal carotid artery, and bilateral SAA.[21] Aneurysms of the subclavian artery have also been associated with the Blalock-Taussig operation with aneurysm formation following coarctation repair and congenital heart repair.[22] Finally, fibromuscular dysplasia has been reported to be associated with an unusual grape cluster aneurysm of the SA.[23]

SYMPTOMS

Nearly one third of patients with SAAs are asymptomatic. Aneurysms tend to occur more frequently on the right than the left side and are more frequent (2:1) in males than females. Mean age of onset is 49 to 61 and between 33% and 47% of patients have multiple aneurysms.[3] This high frequency of associated aneurysms reflects the underlying connective tissue disease or inflammatory process. The symptoms associated with SAAs are related to rupture, compression, or distal embolization. Compressive symptoms include brachial plexopathy, ipsilateral Horner's syndrome, and dysphagia lusoria. Rupture presents with death from hemothorax or massive hematemesis or hemoptysis. Distal embolization is manifested by acute arterial ischemia, digital gangrene, unilateral Reynaud's phenomenon, and splinter hemorrhages. Fifty percent of subclavian aneurysms are intrathoracic in location, which probably reflects the high incidence of SAAs associated with an aberrant right subclavian artery.

DIAGNOSIS

The diagnosis of extrathoracic SAA is made on physical examination. The supraclavicular pulsatile mass is easily identified. However, a long cervical rib will cause the subclavian artery to pass more cephalad, mimicking an SAA. A close examination of the hand is important to detect digital emboli or splinter hemorrhages in the nail bed. For SAAs not associated with thoracic outlet abnormalities, computed tomographic angiography (CTA) is

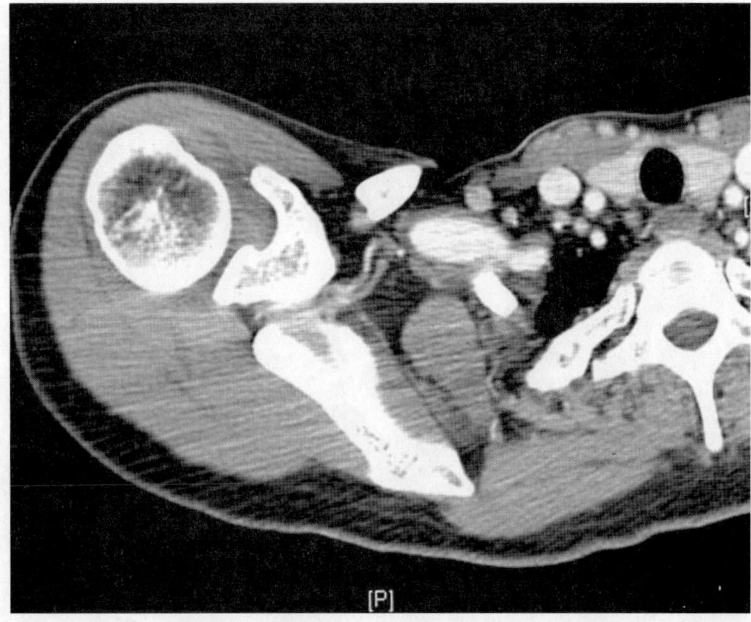

Figure 6-1. Transaxial CT image demonstrating the cervical rib in relationship to the SAA.

sufficient (Figures 6–1, through 6–3). However, in patients with thoracic outlet syndrome (TOS), angiography is important to identify distal emboli, which may alter the surgical procedure (distal revascularization). In patients with an associated vasculitis or connective tissue disease, multiple aneurysms may be present in other locations. In these cases, total body CTA or MRA should be performed.

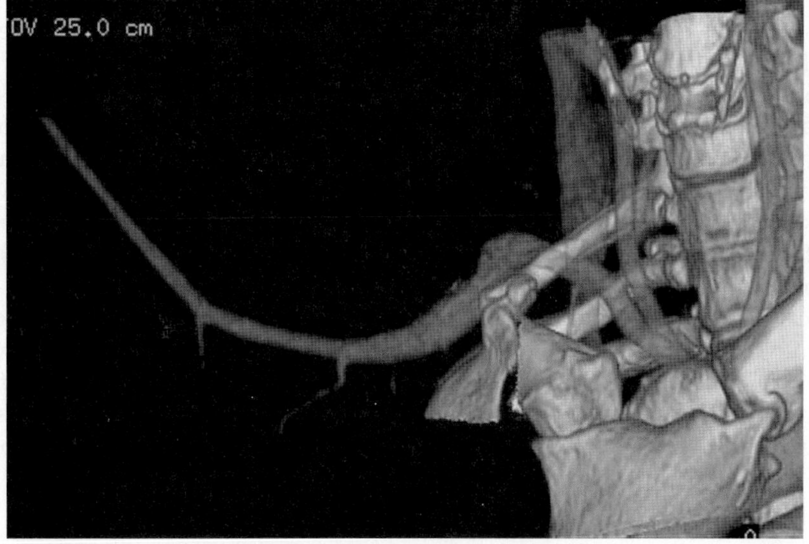

Figure 6-2. Three-dimensional reconstruction of the CT shown in Figure 6-1 illustrating the relationship in three dimensions. Note the SAA distal to the cervical rib.

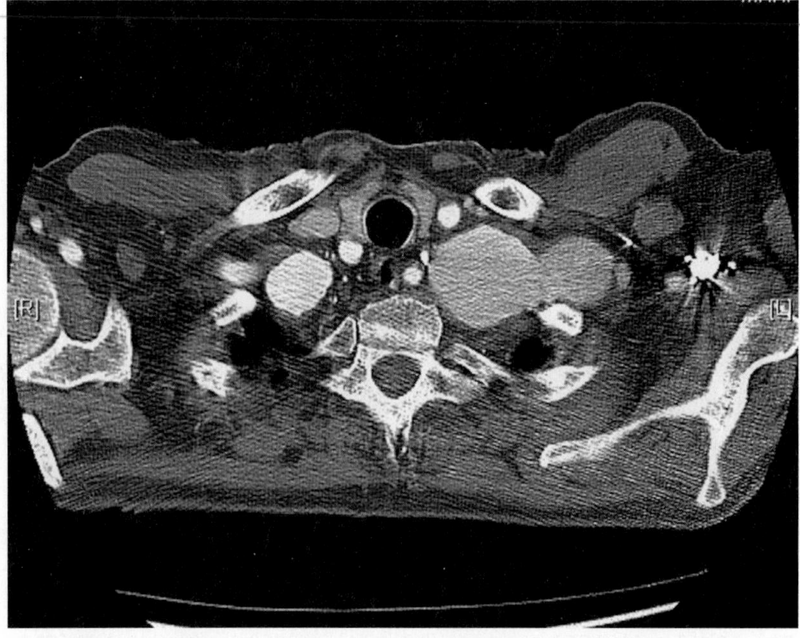

Figure 6-3. Left atherosclerotic SAA.

TREATMENT

For asymptomatic aneurysms, it is not clear as to the size at which they should be repaired. Several authors have suggested 4 cm, although there is no clear evidence as to the appropriate size for intervention. Because of the rarity of these lesions, the decision to intervene is based on a wide variety of factors, including associated diseases, presence or absence of symptoms, and patient age. Endovascular stent grafts provide a wider array of treatment options and have reduced perioperative morbidity. However, it is unclear whether endoluminal therapy has changed the indications for intervention.

For patients with extrathoracic SAAs, there is no clear answer as to the most appropriate treatment. A stent graft may be placed across the thoracic outlet. However, it is unknown whether these grafts will function well in an environment in which there is repeated trauma (from the clavicle and first rib). The literature contains several case reports of patients treated effectively with stent grafts, probably representing an older, less active population.[24–26]

However, in patients in whom there is bony compression of the thoracic outlet by a cervical rib or an anomalous first rib, surgery should be performed. The surgical procedure involves removing the compressive elements and reconstructing the damaged artery.[27–28] The compressive elements may be cervical ribs, abnormalities of the first ribs, or complications associated with clavicular fracture. Furthermore, these patients are young and the long-term durability of an intraluminal stent graft is unknown.

Open Repair

The surgical repair of a SAA with cervical rib involves both a supraclavicular and an infraclavicular incision (Figure 6–4a–d). In the supraclavicular incision, the subclavian artery is identified behind the anterior scalene muscle. The anterior scalene muscle is resected, taking care not to injure the phrenic nerve, which passes from the lateral side of the muscle to the medial side over the anterior surface. The subclavian artery often takes an unusual course in the presence of a cervical rib, and this may be associated with abnormalities of the brachial plexus and may involve a very elongated proximal or first part of the subclavian artery. Once proximal control of the subclavian artery has been obtained, the infraclavicular incision is made, the pectoralis muscles are divided, and the axillary artery is identified. The axillary artery is encircled by the brachial plexus and the subclavian vein. Working from above and below the clavicle, the neurovascular structures are freed in the costoclavicular space. Once there is full mobility of all of the structures in the infraclavicular and supraclavicular spaces, the subclavian and axillary arteries are clamped. The supreme thoracic and small branches of the subclavian artery may be patent, which requires careful dissection under the clavicle to identify them and ligate them with surgical clips. Once these branches have been clipped, it is possible to pass the subclavian artery beneath the clavicle into the supraclavicular space (Figure 6–4b). Within this location, it is easy to resect the remaining portion of the subclavian artery and to reconstruct the artery with a saphenous vein graft (Figure 6–4c–d). Potential complications include injury to the phrenic nerve and to the brachial plexus. The procedure is well tolerated and appears to be

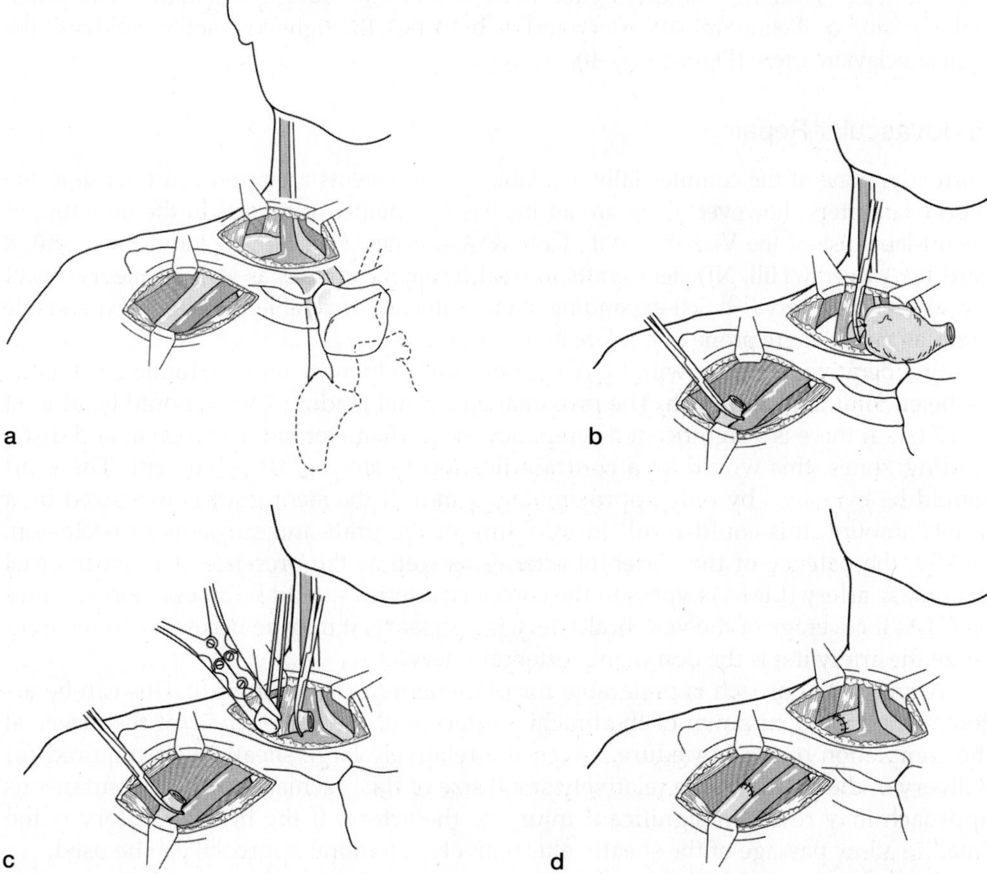

Figure 6-4. a. Supraclavicular incision for the exposure of the subclavian artery and an infraclavicular incision to expose the axillary artery. **b.** The transected subclavian artery is pulled back into the supraclavicular incision. **c.** The cervical rib is removed. **d.** Autogenous reconstruction with the saphenous vein. With the SAA removed, there is adequate space for the reconstruction.

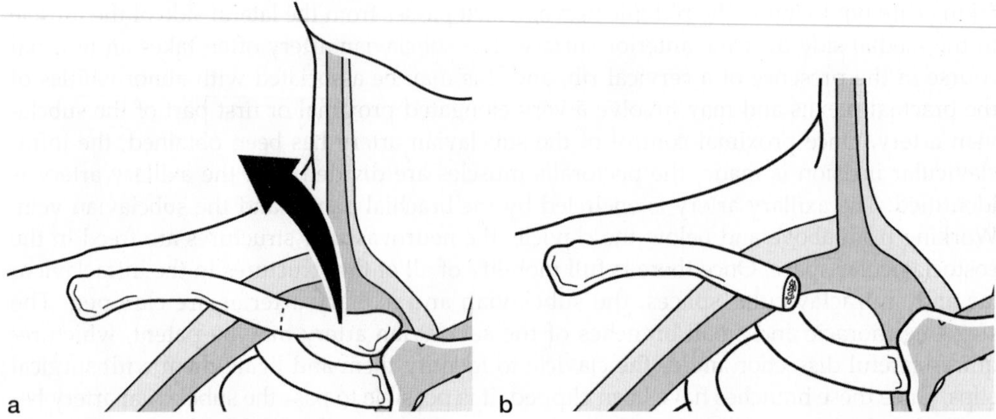

Figure 6-5. a. Removing the head of the clavicle on the right side provides excellent exposure of the innominate artery bifurcation. **b.** The innominate artery and proximal subclavian artery lie behind the left internal jugular vein and innominate vein.

very durable. On the right side, resection of the head of the clavicle will allow more proximal exposure of the innominate artery and its branches, the right common carotid and the right subclavian artery (Figure 6–5a–b).

Endovascular Repair

Currently, none of the commercially available covered stents are approved for use in the subclavian artery; however, there are an increasing number of reports in the literature of the off-label use of the Viabahn (W.L. Gore & Associates, Flagstaff, AZ) and Fluency (CR Bard Inc., Murray Hill, NJ) stent grafts to treat traumatic injuries as well as aneurysms of the subclavian artery.[11,24] Self-expanding stent grafts are preferable to balloon-expandable grafts as the latter are prone to fracture in this location.

Preoperative planning with CTA is important to identify any anatomic limitations to the endoluminal approach. The proximal and distal landing zones should be at least 2 to 3 cm. If there is a significant discrepancy in the diameter of the proximal and distal landing zones, this would be a contraindication to stent graft placement. The graft should be oversized by only approximately 1 mm. If the stent graft is oversized by a larger amount, this could result in infolding of the graft and subsequent occlusion. Finally, the patency of the vertebral arteries as well as the presence of a left internal mammary artery (LIMA) bypass to the coronary arteries should be assessed in advance on CTA. If coverage of the vertebral artery is necessary, it may be necessary to revascularize the artery if it is the dominant vertebral artery.

A brachial approach is preferable for placement of the stent graft. This can be accomplished via a cutdown of the brachial artery with primary repair of the artery at the completion of the procedure. Given the relatively large sheath sizes required for delivery of the graft and the relatively small size of the brachial artery, a percutaneous approach may result in significant injury to the artery. If the brachial artery is too small to allow passage of the sheath, alternatively, a femoral approach can be used.

A 6F sheath is initially placed over a wire. A glidewire (Terumo Medical Corp., Somerset, NJ) and a glide catheter (Terumo Medical Corp., Somerset, NJ) can be used to maneuver through the aneurysm and into the aorta. A straight marked angio-

TABLE 6-2. STENT GRAFT/SHEATH SIZE CHART

Viabahn Diameter	Required Sheath Size
7 mm	8F
8 mm	8F
9 mm	11F
10 mm	11F
11 mm	12F
13 mm	12F
Fluency Diameter	**Required Sheath Size**
7 mm	8F
8 mm	9F
9 mm	9F
10 mm	9F

graphic catheter is then placed over the wire, and angiography is performed to confirm the length of stent graft required. A stiff Amplatz (Boston Scientific, Natick, MA) is placed into the aorta, and the angiographic catheter is removed. A long sheath of the appropriate diameter (Table 6–2) is then advanced over the wire through the aneurysm. Ideally, the stent graft should not be advanced bare through the artery. Placement can be confirmed again with an angiogram through the sheath prior to deployment (Figures 6–6 and 6–7).

The sheath is then pulled back to uncover the stent graft, and the stent graft is deployed. A balloon is then advanced over the wire, and the stent graft is dilated to ensure complete expansion and good wall apposition at the landing zones. Completion

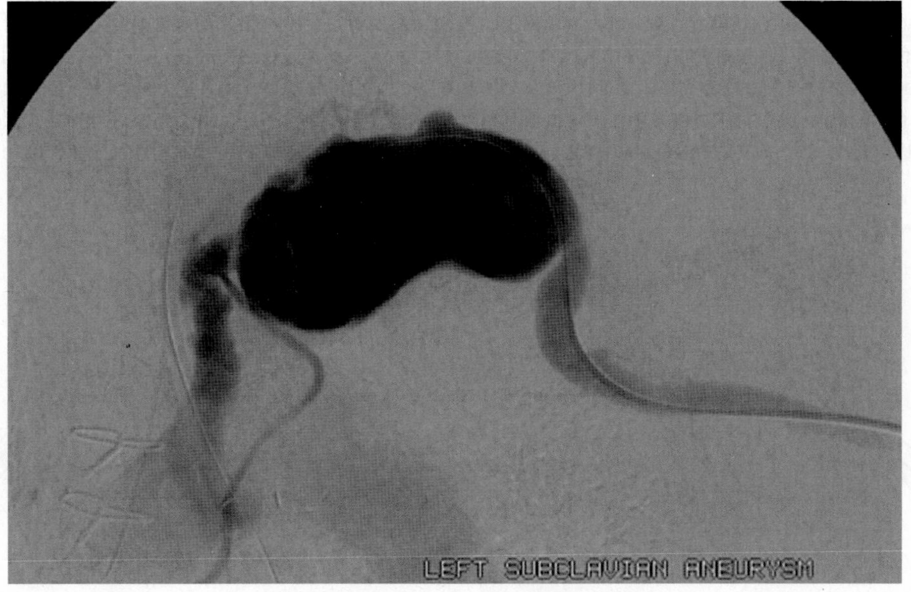

Figure 6-6. Atherosclerotic subclavian artery aneurysm (SAA).

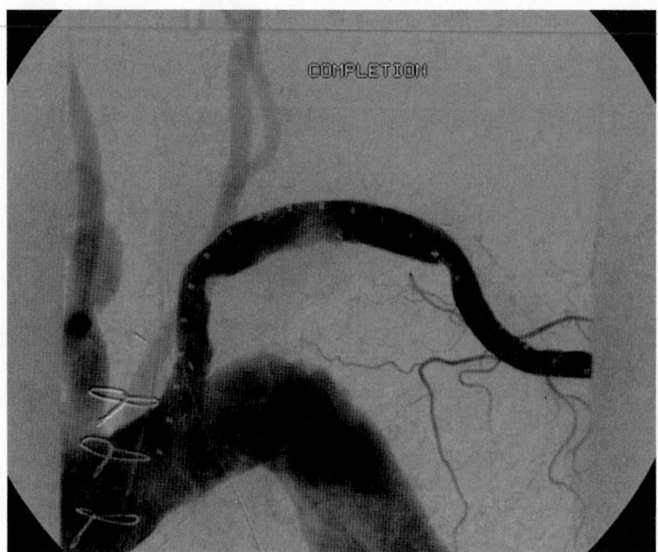

Figure 6-7. Stent graft placement.

angiography should then be performed to evaluate for an endoleak as well as the patency of any critical branches.

ANEURYSMS OF AN ABERRANT RIGHT SUBCLAVIAN ARTERY

Aneurysmal degeneration of the aorta and proximal subclavian artery occurs with aberrant right subclavian artery[17,29] (Figure 6–8a, b). It is uncertain why this lesion occurs, and it may be related to congenital abnormalities of the architecture of the blood vessel or flow characteristics. These aneurysms have been associated with dysphagia lusoria as well as exsanguinating hemorrhage via the esophagus or trachea. When identified, the lesions in the past have been treated utilizing a left thoracotomy and plagetting, suturing the takeoff of the aberrant subclavian or aortic replacement[30] (Figure 6–9). This is difficult because the

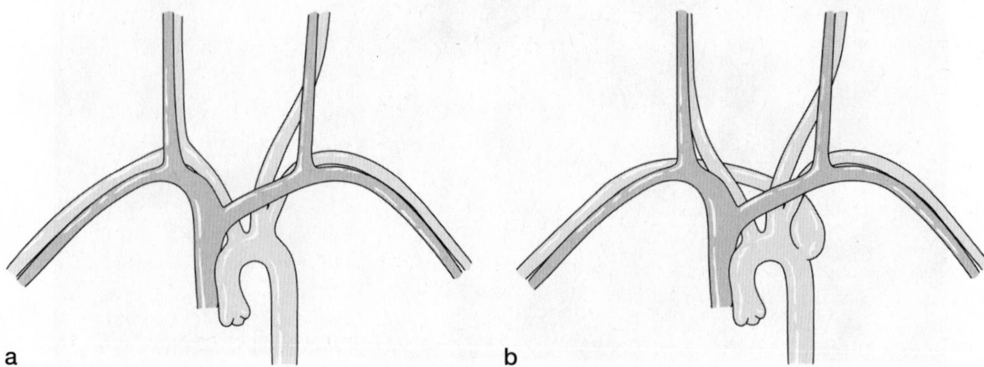

Figure 6-8 a. Normal aortic arch anatomy. **b.** Aberrant right subclavian artery with proximal aneurysm.

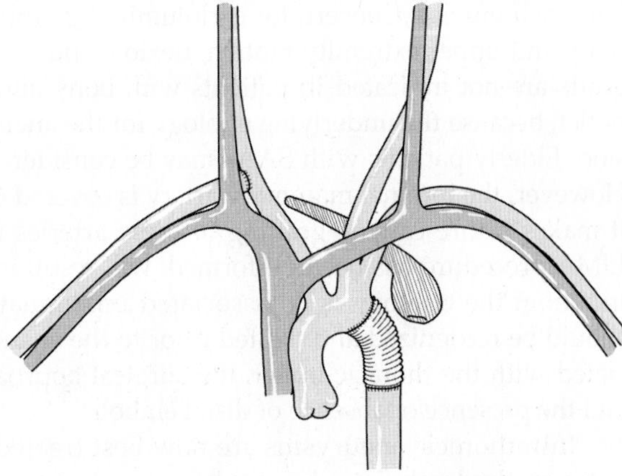

Figure 6-9. Aortic replacement with right subclavian artery to right carotid artery transposition.

aorta may be aneurysmal and degenerative at this location. The use of thoracic endovascular aneurysm repair (TEVAR) has dramatically changed our approach to these aneurysms.[31] They may be treated with extracavitary bypass (a right subclavian-carotid transposition) and placement of an endovascular stent graft (Figure 6–10). The technology developed by TEVAR allows the use of large-diameter grafts. The selection of appropriate landing zones and sizing plays an important role. The operation may be performed simultaneously or staged. The right subclavian artery transposition is performed with a supraclavicular incision. The subclavian artery is sometimes difficult to locate because of its aberrant course. However, it does lie in front of the brachial plexus and can be palpated. Once the sufficient length has been identified, either a carotid-subclavian bypass or a subclavian transposition may be performed. If a bypass is performed, the SAA is ligated proximally to prevent retrograde flow into the aneurysm. Long-term follow-up of these patients has shown gradual shrinking of the aneurysm sac and resolution of symptoms.

COMMENT

SAAs occur infrequently. Extrathoracic aneurysms are best treated by direct surgical repair unless there are significant comorbidities or anatomic considerations that make this

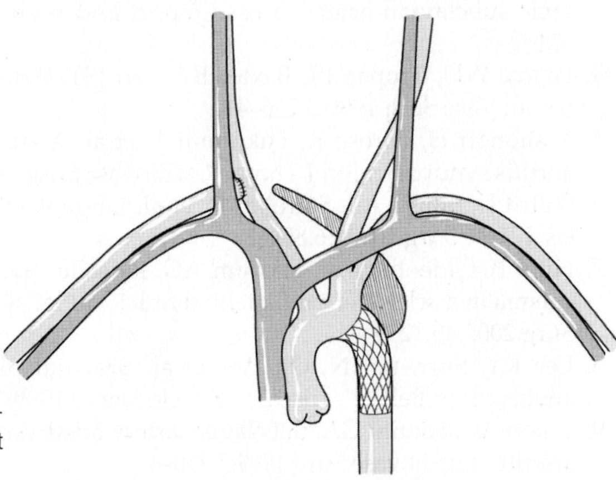

Figure 6-10. Right subclavian to carotid transposition is performed followed by the placement of a TEVAR.

approach unwise. Concern for endoluminal grafting in this location is the long-term durability and upper extremity motion, flexion, abduction, and external rotation. Endovascular grafts are not indicated in patients with bony abnormalities associated with the thoracic outlet, because the underlying etiology for the aneurysm formation is mechanical compression. Elderly patients with SAAs may be considered candidates for endovascular therapy. However, the internal mammary artery is covered during this procedure. If this is the case, it makes future cardiac grafting of these arteries impossible and, in patients in whom a LIMA procedure has been performed, will result in catastrophic consequences. In patients in whom the etiology is an associated inflammatory condition, the underlying disease should be recognized and treated prior to the aneurysm repair. In patients with SAA associated with the thoracic outlet, the surgical approach is tailored to the patient's anatomy and the presence or absence of distal emboli.

Intrathoracic aneurysms are now best treated by endovascular methods. Endovascular methods obviate the need for a thoracotomy and attendant complications with this incision. Endovascular stent grafts are placed via the groin into suitable candidates. Careful attention must be paid as to whether the patients have undergone coronary artery bypass surgery using the ipsilateral internal mammary artery. In patients with aberrant right subclavian artery aneurysms, endovascular methods have greatly changed the operative approach and the comorbidities associated with the open procedure. Several reports have described the successful treatment of these aneurysms using a carotid-subclavian bypass on the right side followed by or in conjunction with endovascular coverage of the subclavian aneurysm and, in one case, the use of an Amplatz or even a clamshell device to cover the orifice of the subclavian. The use of a covered aortic stent graft seems to be a better solution than simple coiling or the use of clamshells in the cases of dislodgement and continued perfusion of the subclavian aneurysm.

REFERENCES

1. Hobson RW, Sarkaria J, O'Donnell J, Neville W. Atherosclerotic aneurysms of the subclavian artery. Surgery 1979;85:368–71.
2. Pairolero PC, Walls JT, Payne WS, et al. Subclavian-axillary artery aneurysms. Surgery 1981;90:757–63.
3. Dougherty MJ, Calligaro KD, Savarese RP, et al. Atherosclerotic aneurysm of the intrathoracic subclavian artery: a case report and review of the literature. J Vasc Surg 1995;21:521–9.
4. Pearce WH, Tropea BI, Baxter BT, Yao JST. Arterial complications in the thoracic outlet. Semin Vasc Surg 1990;3:236–41.
5. Nishimori H, Hirose K, Fukutomi T, et al. A subclavian artery aneurysm associated with aortitis syndrome. Jpn J Thorac Cardiovasc Surg 1999;47:621–4.
6. Shitrit D, Shitrit AB, Starobin D, et al. Large vessel aneurysms in Wegener's granulomatosis. J Vasc Surg 2002;36:856–8.
7. Hugl B, Oldenburg A, Hakaim AG, Persellin ST. Unusual etiology of upper extremity ischemia in a scleroderma patient: thoracic outlet syndrome with arterial embolization. J Vasc Surg 2007;45:1259–61.
8. Lee KY, Sunwoo IN, Oh WS, et al. Brachial plexopathy caused by subclavian artery aneurysm in Behçet's disease. Muscle Nerve 1999;22:1721–3.
9. Chiou AC, Fantini GA. Subclavian artery aneurysm: an unusual manifestation of Takayasu's arteritis. Cardiovasc Surg 1999;7:310–4.

10. Muzaffer MA, Al-Mayouf SM. Pattern of clinical features of Kawasaki disease. Saudi Med J 2002;23:409–12.
11. du Toit DF, Lambrechts AV, Stark H, et al. Long-term results of stent graft treatment of subclavian artery injuries: management of choice for stable patients? J Vasc Surg 2008;47: 739–43.
12. Hood DB, Kuehn J, Yellin AE, Weaver FA. Vascular complications of thoracic outlet syndrome. Am Surg 1997;63:913–7.
13. Nehler MR, Taylor LM Jr, Moneta GL, Porter JM. Upper extremity ischemia from subclavian artery aneurysm caused by bony abnormalities of the thoracic outlet. Arch Surg 1997;132:527–32.
14. Tassiopoulos AK, Nadalin BA, Labropoulos N, et al. Endovascular repair of a symptomatic subclavian artery aneurysm in a patient with Marfan syndrome: a case report. Vasc Endovasc Surg 2006;40:409–13.
15. Gonzalez JMD, Garcia BA, Lebrun JM, Docampo MM. Combined surgery for the treatment of bilateral subclavian artery aneurysm in Marfan syndrome. J Vasc Surg 2007;45:180–2.
16. Seow VK, Chong CF, Wang TL, et al. Ruptured left subclavian artery aneurysm presenting as upper airway obstruction in von Recklinghausen's disease. Resuscitation 2007;74:563–6.
17. Jebara VA, Arnaud-Crozat E, Angel F, et al. Aberrant right subclavian artery aneurysm: report of a case review of the literature. Ann Vasc Surg 1989;3:68–73.
18. Schievink WI, Piepgras DG. Cervical vertebral artery aneurysms and arteriovenous fistulae in neurofibromatosis Type 1: case reports. Neurosurgery 1991;29:760–5.
19. Myers JL, Gomes MN. Management of aberrant subclavian artery aneurysms. J Cardiovasc Surg 2000;41:607–12.
20. Hiller N, Verstanding A, Simanovsky N. Coarctation of the aorta associated with aneurysm of the left subclavian artery. Br J Radiol 2004;77:335–7.
21. Lin PC, Jacobowitz GR, Rockman CB. Subclavian artery aneurysm in association with congenital absence of ipsilateral internal carotid artery. J Vasc Surg 2004;39:682–5.
22. McGahan JP, Bogren HG, Foerster JM, Mason DT. Subclavian artery aneurysm: Unique late complication of Blalock-Taussig anastomosis. AJR AM JRoentgenol 1978;130:1181–3.
23. Steinmetz EF, Berry P, Shames ML, et al. "Grape cluster" aneurysm of the right subclavian artery: an unusual manifestation of fibromuscular dysplasia. Ann Vasc Surg 2003;17:296–301.
24. Chambers CM, Curci JA. Treatment of nonaortic aneurysms in the endograft era: aneurysms of the innominate and subclavian arteries. Semin Vasc Surg 2005;28:184–90.
25. MacSweeney ST, Holden A, Harltley D, Lawrence-Brown M. Endovascular repair of subclavian artery aneurysm. J Vasc Surg 1996;24:304–5.
26. May J, White G, Waugh R, et al. Transluminal placement of a prosthetic graft-stent device for treatment of subclavian artery aneurysm. J Vasc Surg 1993;18:1056–9.
27. Keiffer E. Arterial complications of the thoracic outlet syndrome. In Bergan JJ, Yao JST, eds. Evaluation and Treatment of Upper and Lower Extremity Circulatory Disorders. New York: Grune & Stratton; 1984, pp. 249–75.
28. Scher LA, Veith FJ, Samson RH, et al. Vascular complications of thoracic outlet syndrome. J Vasc Surg 1986;3:565–8.
29. Pifarre R, Dieter RA Jr, Niedballa RG. Definitive surgical treatment of the aberrant retroesophageal right subclavian artery in the adult. J Thorac Cardiovasc Surg. 1971;61:154–9.
30. Smythe WR, Reznik SI. Optimal exposure of thoracic inlet vascular structures: transmanubrial approach. Semin Vasc Surg 2008;21:21–4.
31. Davidian M, Kee ST, Kato N, et al. Aneurysm of an aberrant right subclavian artery: treatment with PTFE covered stent-graft. J Vasc Surg 1988;28:335–9.

7

Raynaud's: Update on Diagnosis and Treatment

Thom W. Rooke, M.D. and Cindy Felty, C-ANP

INTRODUCTION

Some medical students are more productive than others. In 1862, Maurice Raynaud (1834-1881) defended his medical school thesis; in the process, he described the constellation of symptoms that now bears his name.[1] Classic *Raynaud's phenomenon*[1]* (or *"Raynauds"*) consists of intermittent attacks of blanching or cyanosis involving one or more digits or extremities. These episodes are typically precipitated by exposure to cold, although other factors (e.g., stress, tobacco, hormones) may also trigger attacks.[2] Raynauds is common; epidemiologic studies estimate its incidence at 5 to 10% or more of the general population, with women being affected more often than men.[3] Most cases are due to primary Raynauds, in which the large, small, and microvessels are patent and attacks are caused by intermittent episodes of exaggerated vasospasm. Primary (vasospastic) Raynauds is usually benign, rarely causes significant damage to the digits, and typically enjoys a good long-term prognosis. Secondary Raynauds, caused by "fixed" obstruction of the large or small vessels (upon which attacks of intermittent vasospasm may be superimposed), tends to be more serious. It can be associated with infarction of the digits and, by definition, occurs because of underlying illnesses or abnormalities. In general, patients with secondary Raynauds have a less optimistic prognosis than those with the primary condition.[4]

The diagnosis of Raynauds can usually be made from the history and physical examination. However, it is not sufficient to simply make a clinical diagnosis. The treatment – and prognostic implications – of the condition are linked to its etiology and mechanism, and it is therefore important for the physician to determine whether

* I am using the term "Raynaud's phenomenon" to describe the typical color and temperature changes that occur during an attack. Raynaud's phenomenon may be a primary condition (often called *"Raynaud's disease, Raynaud's syndrome, or primary Raynaud's*), or it can occur secondary to other disorders (*secondary Raynaud's*). In this chapter, I refer to both the phenomenon and the disease or syndrome as simply "Raynauds."

the condition is primary (i.e., vasospastic, easier to treat, good prognosis) or secondary (i.e., obstructive, more difficult to treat, often serious). Unfortunately, most physicians are far better at diagnosing the presence of Raynauds than they are at figuring out whether it is primary or secondary in origin.

DIAGNOSIS

As noted above, the diagnosis of Raynauds can usually be made on the basis of history and physical examination. The clinical assessment may also help to distinguish between primary and secondary causes of Raynauds. Historical elements such as tobacco use, clotting abnormalities, and a previous diagnosis of connective tissue disease suggest secondary causes; similarly, examination findings such as ulceration, digital telangiectasias, subcutaneous calcium, and sclerodactyly are consistent with secondary causes such as scleroderma. In addition to inspection of the limbs, hands, digits, and skin, all extremity pulses should be palpated. If the upper extremity is involved, the Allen's test[5] may provide useful information about the patency of the ulnar artery (occult ulnar artery occlusion may predispose to or aggravate Raynauds).

In some situations, it may not be possible to determine the presence or severity of arterial occlusion based upon the history and physical examination alone. Fortunately, there are a variety of simple, noninvasive, widely available tests that can help to identify the presence of "fixed" vascular obstruction. These include tests such as pulse volume recordings, photoplethysmography, and digital pressure measurements obtained using small pneumatic occlusion cuffs and various digital blood flow detectors. In many cases, these tests (as opposed to imaging studies) are all that is necessary to identify and characterize the presence of arterial obstruction associated with "secondary" Raynauds.

In patients without evidence of "fixed" arterial obstruction, the key question is "does the patient have inducible vasospasm?" The traditional method for identifying inducible vasospasm is the *ice water immersion test*. Ice water immersion testing is generally performed when there is (1) no demonstrable "fixed" arterial obstruction, and (2) normal resting digital temperatures (typically greater than or equal to 30 degrees centigrade after the patient has been seated for 10 to 20 minutes in a comfortable room.)

The test is conceptually simple. After baseline temperatures of all digits are measured, the hands are cooled by immersion in ice water for 30 seconds. In most individuals, this reduces the fingertip skin temperature to 20 degrees centigrade or less. Upon re-exposure to room temperature, patients with normal blood flow rewarm quickly (most digits return to normal temperature within 10 to 15 minutes or less). However, if ice water immersion triggers vasospasm, digital blood flow decreases or stops and the rewarming time is prolonged (typically to 15 to 20 minutes or more.) Patients with normal arterial studies and normal baseline digital temperatures are assumed to have "inducible vasospasm" if their post–ice water immersion rewarming times are delayed.

A dilemma arises in patients who have normal upper extremity and digital arteries by objective testing (plethysmography and/or digital pressure measurements) but who have reduced digital temperatures under baseline conditions (fingertip skin temperatures less than 30 degrees centigrade). Ice water immersion is rarely valuable in these patients, because virtually all of them will have delayed rewarming (the low initial skin temperatures reflect the fact that baseline cutaneous/digital blood flow is

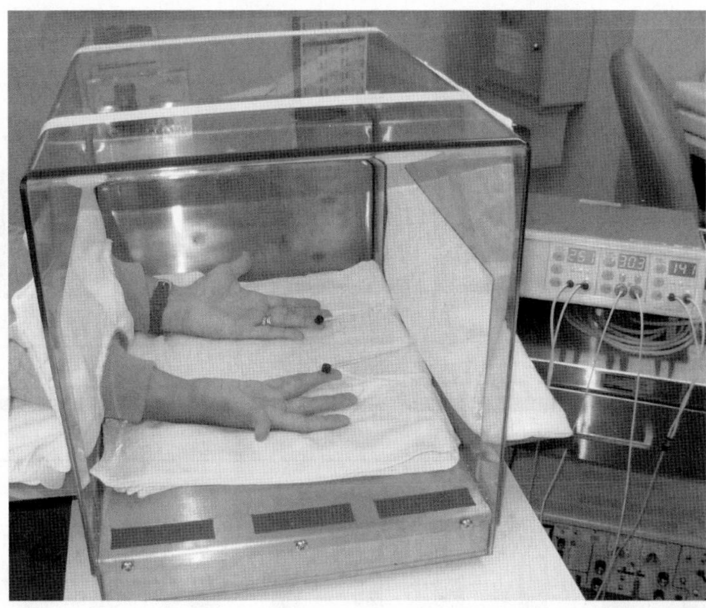

Figure 7-1. "Hot box." This device (heated internally to 45 degrees centigrade) gently and uniformly warms the hands, which produces maximal cutaneous vasodilation in the digits. Laser Doppler probes are used to measure the changes in fingertip skin blood flow produced by ambient warming.

already reduced). In these patients, it is important to ascertain why the baseline digital cutaneous blood flow and temperatures are reduced. Is continuous vasospasm present (suggesting that the Raynauds is likely primary)? Is there "fixed" obstructive disease of the larger arteries or, more likely, the microvasculature (consistent with a secondary cause for the Raynauds)? It is now possible to distinguish between these possibilities by using various cutaneous blood flow sensing techniques such as laser Doppler flowmetry to assess profusion changes produced by ambient warming (which is a potent cutaneous vasodilator). In our laboratory, we have developed a "hot box" for the purpose of warming the hands and digits (Figure 7–1). Briefly, patients with objectively normal upper extremity and digital arteries — but abnormally cold baseline digital temperatures — have laser Doppler measurements obtained at the distal tip of each finger. The values obtained are invariably reduced in comparison to values from normal digits. The hands are then placed inside the hot box (which is maintained at a constant temperature of 45 degrees centigrade) for a period of 15 minutes. Digital skin temperature generally increases to 35 degrees centigrade or higher during the ambient warming period. Laser Doppler measurements are subsequently repeated on the warmed fingertips. Normal subjects (Figure 7–2 A), or patients with baseline vasospasm (Figure 7–2 B) demonstrate a marked increase in laser Doppler flow following ambient warming. Digits with "fixed" large or small vessel obstruction do not demonstrate the expected increase in flow (Figure 7–2 C), or may even show a decrease in flow (due to vasodilation-induced shunting and stealing of cutaneous blood flow). The "hot box" technique has proved extremely useful at detecting vascular obstruction that is not evident by physical examination or conventional noninvasive testing modalities (especially obstruction in the small or microvessels).

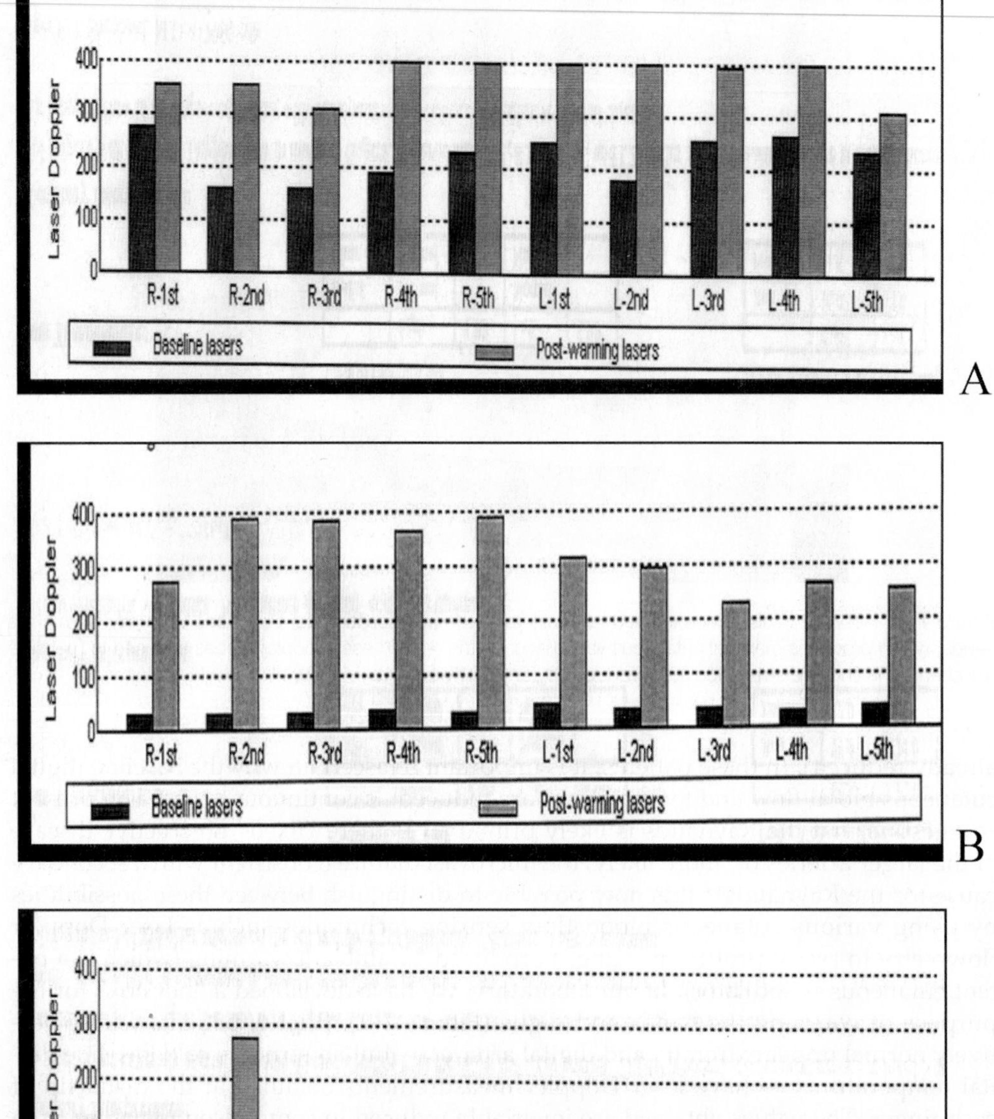

A. Normal. Baseline laser Doppler (LD) flux is greater than 100; peak (post-warming) flux is greater than 200.

B. Vasospasm. Baseline LD flux is less than 100; peak flux is greater than 200.

C. "Fixed" obstruction. Baseline LD flux is less than 100; peak flux is less than 200.

Figure 7-2. A-C. Laser Doppler response to ambient warming.

TREATMENT

The initial treatment of Raynauds is identical for both the primary and the secondary forms. One of the simplest and most effective ways to treat Raynauds is by avoiding the things that precipitate it. By far the most important of these is *exposure to cold*. Staying indoors during cold weather when possible or dressing warmly when outside or otherwise exposed to low temperatures is essential.[6] The use of hats, gloves, or mittens, boots, and other garments may be all that is necessary to avoid symptoms with either form of Raynauds. In extreme cases, patients have benefited by moving to a warmer climate.[2†]

It is also important to avoid other stimuli that can trigger Raynauds attacks. These include tobacco use, stress, certain medications or substances that may cause vasoconstriction (such as beta blockers and caffeine) and other potential insults.[7]

Traditional pharmacologic treatments for Raynauds include calcium blockers (e.g., nifedipine, nimodipine),[8] alpha-one receptor blockers (prazosin, doxazosin, terazosin),[9] and other vasodilators (ACE inhibitors). Novel pharmacologic approaches include topical vasodilators such as nitroglycerin ointment[10–11] and drugs with vasodilating side-effects such as sildenafil.[12]

Although both primary and secondary forms of Raynauds have inducible vasospasm as a component of their pathophysiology, it is the "fixed" small vessel (and occasionally larger vessel) obstruction seen in the secondary form that is most problematic. Small vessel arterial obstruction can lead to trophic skin changes, skin breakdown, ulcerations, gangrene, and eventually digital loss. Scleroderma is probably the most common underlying etiology for severe secondary Raynauds, but other connective tissue or vascular obstructive diseases (e.g., thromboangiitis obliterans, microemboli) may cause ischemic tissue damage. These conditions have traditionally proven extremely difficult to manage; for many, there is no pharmacologic treatment. If obstruction affects the small vessels, bypass or other revascularization techniques are not feasible. A variety of hemorheologic agents, lytic agents, and potent vasodilators have been tried — especially in connective tissue disorders — with minimal if any success.

One form of adjuvant therapy that may be useful in secondary forms of Raynauds is *intermittent pneumatic compression*.[13] This approach is widely used to treat severe ischemia of the lower extremities (usually caused by atherosclerosis or other obstructive diseases).[14–15] In recent years, it has been adapted for treatment of the upper extremities in situations in which "fixed" untreatable obstruction is present. The concept is simple: intermittent pneumatic compression (usually 1 to 3 seconds of transient rapid cuff compression to 60 mm Hg or more, administered at three cycles per minute) is applied over the forearms using a commercially available pneumatic impulse pump (Figure 7–3). This action enhances venous return and pushes arterial blood through or around obstructed vessels. The effect of arm pumping on blood flow can be demonstrated by measuring laser Doppler flow in the (ischemic) fingertips during pneumatic pumping; this forms the basis of a provocative test to predict whether pumping will be effective for a given individual.

Patients are typically asked to pump multiple times per day; these sessions last anywhere from 15 minutes to an hour or more (sessions are typically 30 to 45 minutes in duration, although many patients will pump more-or-less continuously). Preliminary work confirms the efficacy of this form of treatment in patients for whom no other

† Medicare or other insurance does not usually cover this expense, even with a prescription.

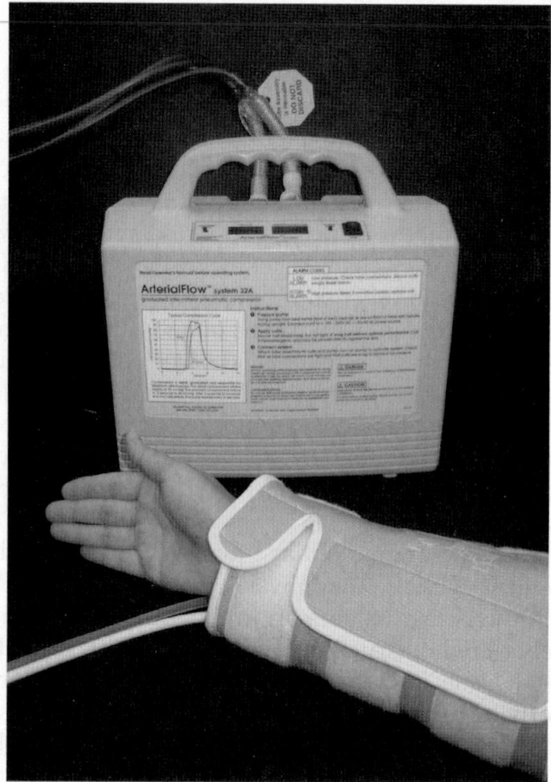

Figure 7-3. Intermittent pneumatic compression pump.

therapy is available. Pumping might be combined in the future with other modalities, such as hyperbaric oxygen, to further enhance the beneficial effects of treatment.

SUMMARY

When evaluating patients with Raynauds, it is important to determine whether the condition is primary or secondary in etiology. After the history and physical are obtained, appropriate measurements of upper extremity and/or digital pressures, arterial wave forms, and skin temperatures should be made. If the arteries appear to be patent and the baseline temperatures are normal, ice water immersion can be used to test for inducible vasospasm. If arterial waveforms or pressures are abnormal, or if baseline temperatures are reduced, the effect of ambient warming on laser Doppler flow measurements can be used to determine whether there is pre-existing vasospasm versus "fixed" occlusive disease.

Regardless of whether Raynauds is primary or secondary in etiology, treatment consists of initial conservative measures such as *avoidance of cold* and *elimination of factors* that can precipitate vasospastic attacks. If significant vasospasm (either intermittent or constant) is confirmed, specific vasodilating drugs may be of value. If "fixed" small (or larger) vessel obstruction is present (i.e., secondary Raynauds), intermittent pneumatic compression pumping may be useful, particularly when severe sequelae occur.

REFERENCES

1. Raynaud M, De I'asphyxie locale et de la gangrène symétrique des extrémities (Local asphyxia and symmetrical gangrene of the extremities), PhD thesis, February 25, 1862, Paris, Rignoux, 1867;15–20. English translation by Thomas Barlow. In Selected Monographs, London: New Sydenham Society; 1888:1–199.
2. Brown KM, Middaugh SJ, Haythornthwaite JA, Bielory L. The effects of stress, anxiety, and outdoor temperature on the frequency and severity of Raynaud's attacks: the Raynaud's treatment study. J Behav Med 2001;24:137–53.
3. Silman A, Holligan S, Brennan P, Maddison P. Prevalence of symptoms of Raynaud's phenomenon in general practice. BMJ 1990;301:590–2.
4. Spencer-Green G. Outcomes in primary Raynaud's phenomenon: a meta-analysis of the frequency, rates, and predictors of transition to secondary disease. Arch Intern Med 1988;158: 595–600.
5. Greenwood NJ, Della-Siega AJ, Fretz EB, et al. Vascular communication of the hand in patients being considered for transradial coronary angiography: is the Allen's test accurate? J Am Coll Cardiol 2005;46;2013–7.
6. Goodfield MJ, Hume A, Rowell NR. The acute effects of cigarette smoking on cutaneous blood flow in smoking and non-smoking subjects with and without Raynaud's phenomenon. Br J Rheumatol 1990;29:89–91.
7. Palesch YY, Valter I, Carpentier PH, Maricq HR. Association between cigarette and alcohol consumption and Raynaud's phenomenon. J Clin Epidemiol 1999;52:321–8.
8. Thompson SE, Shea B, Welch V, et al. Calcium-channel blockers for Raynaud's phenomenon in systemic sclerosis. Arthritis Rheum 2001;44:1841–7.
9. Pope JE, Fenlon D, Thompson A, et al. Prazosin for Raynaud's phenomenon in progressive systemic sclerosis. Cochrane Database Syst Rev 2000;2:CD000956.
10. Denton CP, Fiorentino D, Herrick A, et al. A multicenter crossover study of MQX-503, a topical formulation of nitroglycerin, in patients with Raynaud's phenomenon. Presented at: American College of Rheumatology Meeting; November 7–11, 2007; Boston, MA. Presentation L12.
11. Peterson LL, Vorhies C. Raynaud's syndrome: treatment with sublingual administration of nitroglycerin, swinging arm maneuver, and biofeedback training. Arch Dermatol 1983; 119:396–9.
12. Fries R, Shariat K, Wilmowsky HV, Bohm M. Sildenafil in the treatment of Raynaud's phenomenon resistant to vasodilator therapy. Circulation 2005;112:2980–5.
13. Pfizenmaier DH 2nd, Kavros SJ, Liedl DA, Cooper LT. Use of intermittent pneumatic compression for treatment of upper extremity vascular ulcers. Angiology 2005;56:417–22.
14. Montori VM, Kavros SJ, Walsh EE, Rooke TW. Intermittent compression pump for nonhealing wounds in patients with limb ischemia. The Mayo Clinic experience (1998-2000). 2002; 21:360–6.
15. Kavros SJ, Delis KT, Turner NS, et al. Improving limb salvage in critical ischemia with intermittent pneumatic compression: a controlled study with 18-month follow-up. J Vasc Surg 2008;47:543–9.

SECTION III

Thoracic Outlet Syndrome

8

Imaging for Thoracic Outlet Syndrome

John W. Hallett, M.D., F.A.C.S.

Thoracic outlet syndrome (TOS) is a *dynamic* physical impairment of the upper extremity. The symptoms (Table 8–1) generally occur when the upper extremity is engaged in some action, for example, overhead activity or in an awkward position while sleeping with the arm and hand behind the head. The *dynamic or positional* nature of TOS makes diagnosis difficult (Figure 8–1). There is simply no single diagnostic test or imaging modality that unequivocally confirms the diagnosis.[1–2] In addition, one must sort through several other common causes of complex regional pain syndrome.

This chapter reviews and reflects on how we can "image" the patient with suspected TOS.[1-11] The author sets imaging choices for TOS in the total context of how one approaches making an accurate diagnosis and selecting the optimal treatment plan. Four key concepts are emphasized:

First, the most important imaging modality remains the physician's eyes and ears.[1–2] The evaluating physician must create a dynamic image in his or her mind of what activities or positions precipitate the upper limb symptoms. This preliminary picture will help select the appropriate imaging modalities to confirm or refute the initial clinical impression. There are many choices, and therefore, careful selection is paramount in making a diagnosis at the best cost.[4]

Second, basic radiographs and ultrasound provide the essential images at the initial evaluation.[1,4] They reveal most of the critical anatomic information to supplement the thorough history and physical examination.

Third, magnetic resonance imaging (MRI) may be the best single imaging modality for TOS.[7] MRI and MRA provide multidimensional views of all the potential compressive components of TOS: the bones, muscles, nerves, arteries, veins, and abnormalities of any or all of these anatomic structures.[9] MRI is also invaluable in evaluating the cervical spine and shoulder for pathology in these areas.

Fourth, standard venography or arteriography remains essential in the diagnosis and treatment of vascular complications of TOS.[10–11] Venography with thrombolysis is key in the initial relief of effort subclavian vein thrombosis (Paget-Schroetter syndrome). Arteriography of the entire aortic arch with downstream views of all upper

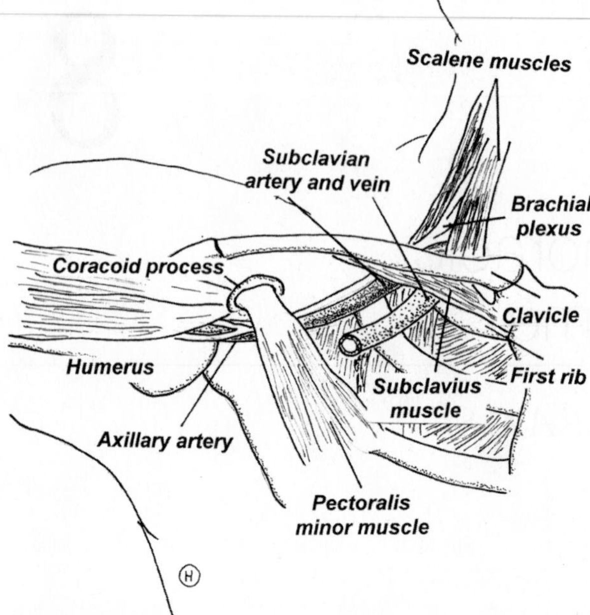

Figure 8-1. Normal thoracic outlet anatomy.

extremity arteries, including the hand and digits, is critical in evaluating arterial thromboembolism related to subclavian artery aneurysms that are often associated with cervical ribs.

THE INITIAL LOOK AT THE PATIENT

Set aside all the sophisticated imaging technology options at first. Simply take a careful history and do a comprehensive physical examination. The vast majority of critical "imaging"

TABLE 8-1 COMMON SYMPTOMS OF THORACIC OUTLET SYNDROME (TOS)

Neurogenic TOS
Upper plexus symptoms (C5, C6, C7): neck and occipital pain radiating to rhomboid region, pectoral area, or lateral upper arm
Lower plexus symptoms (C8 and T1): anterior or posterior shoulder pain radiating down the arm classically with tingling of ring and fifth fingers with frequent autonomic features of vasomotor disturbance (Raynaud's syndrome)
Venous TOS
Chronic intermittent swelling and cyanosis of hand with some painful discomfort and heaviness of the arm with exercise or work
Acute onset of diffuse upper limb swelling, cyanosis and pain associated frequently with strenuous upper limb exercise or work (Paget-Schroetter syndrome)
Arterial TOS
Chronic upper limb tiring and heaviness with exercise (upper limb equivalent of lower limb claudication)
Repetitive painful, blue fingertips suggesting thromboembolism
Acute arterial ischemia with pain, pallor, paresthesia, and paresis of upper extremity

occurs with the initial history and examination. They guide the selection of more high-tech modalities such as MRI or computed tomography (CT). A few points deserve emphasis.

History

TOS, whether acute or chronic, is related to certain activities or positions of the upper extremity. The evaluating physician must not only record this history but also form an image in his or her mind of what activities cause the patient's symptoms.

Begin with simply asking When did the symptoms first appear? Were they acute or insidious? Auto accidents with whiplash are a common story of acute onset. Onset and progression of symptoms with a new job are also typical of a more chronic history, for example, packing and lifting boxes at a busy outlet store. Are the symptoms worse with certain activities at home or at work, for example, changing a ceiling light bulb? Patterns of symptom development become clear.

In addition to certain activities, are symptoms worse in certain positions, such as sleeping with the arm and hand over the head? It is remarkable how many patients with severe TOS awaken at night with a "dead arm." Just as remarkable is how easily symptoms occur with simple elevation of the arms while driving a car or typing on a computer.

Finally, listen closely for any symptoms of arterial compression (Raynaud's syndrome) or venous compression (arm swelling). Hand pallor and coolness on elevated activity are common in TOS. If the patient has experienced acute, painful blue fingertips, microemboli from a suspected subclavian artery aneurysm mandates imaging the arteries. Likewise, chronic intermittent arm swelling with overhead activity (e.g., painting) suggests venous compression or stenosis. At the other extreme, sudden upper limb pain, swelling, and cyanosis are classic symptoms of acute subclavian vein thrombosis (effort vein thrombosis or Paget-Schroetter syndrome).

When the initial history and physical examination are completed, the physician can then design an imaging plan that is most likely to assist with the diagnosis. Subsequent imaging should be performed in positions that are usually related to the patient's symptoms. Otherwise, the imaging may miss the anatomic signs of vascular or neurologic compression in that particular patient. For example, a baseball pitcher may only develop progressive hand swelling with a certain windup pattern of his throwing arm. Venous ultrasound should be performed in that exaggerated position of abduction and external rotation of the upper limb.

Physical Examination

When all else fails, examine the patient! This time-honored clinical principle is very important for deciding how to image a patient with possible TOS. Certain physical findings reveal so much about where the neurovascular compression may be and what is causing the symptoms. A few findings are essential in every patient.[1–2,11]

First, simply look at the patient's general emotional affect and shoulder-girdle posture. An affect of chronic depression should not go unnoticed. There is often considerable psychological overlay to any chronic upper extremity pain syndrome, whether it is due to TOS or some other pathology. Likewise, downward sloping shoulders and poor posture can exacerbate TOS. Look at the clavicles for deformity from a previous fracture (Figure 8–2) or natural concavity that pushes the clavicle posterior and inferior toward the first rib, tightening the thoracic outlet across the first rib. Is the neck

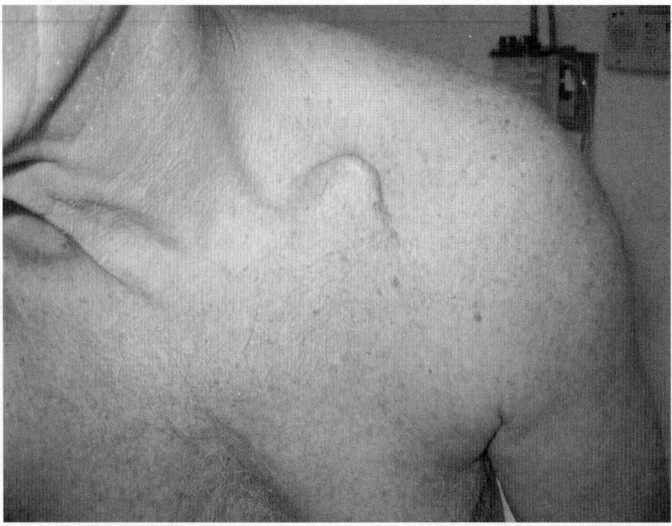

Figure 8-2. Chronic malunion and deformity of left clavicular fracture from bicycle accident in 68-year-old white male presenting with Raynaud's syndrome of left hand and absent left radial pulse. The patient had extensive chronic thrombosis of the left subclavian and proximal axillary arteries.

elongated ("giraffe neck")? The scalene triangle may be elongated and compressed in such patients, who are usually young athletic women. Finally, is the upper extremity swollen or are there any signs of arterial emboli in the fingertips?

Next, assess the full range of motion of the upper limbs, both overhead and behind the back. Internal shoulder problems, for example, torn rotator cuff, may cause painful limitation of range of motion, which is uncommon with TOS.

Palpation plays a key role in the examination as well. Palpate the supraclavicular area first. TOS patients may have a tight and tender anterior scalene muscle. A cervical rib should be suspected if the subclavian pulse is prominent and a firmness lies beneath it (i.e., the cervical rib). Occasionally, a palpable supraclavicular mass may be lymphadenopathy from regional or gastrointestinal cancer, especially if it is present on the left side where the thoracic duct courses.

Palpation with auscultation of the upper limb arteries is another essential step in the examination. I like to palpate the radial pulse *and* listen to the infraclavicular subclavian artery with my stethoscope as I move the arm from the position of rest to elevation and external rotation (Figure 8–3). If arterial compression is present in the thoracic outlet, an infraclavicular bruit is often heard before the radial pulse obliterates.

The physical examination should culminate in the Elevated Activity Stress Test (EAST).[2] This test is designed to reproduce the patient's symptoms with the arms elevated over the head and exercising. It is best to ask the patient to simply describe the onset and nature of any symptoms. Avoid leading questions. Patients with TOS frequently develop neck or shoulder discomfort with arm heaviness and hand tingling in less than a minute of overhead activity. If arterial compression is severe, the hand may show pallor. When the patient relaxes the upper limb and hand to the neutral position of rest, he or she often describes a "rush of blood" back into the hand.

At the end of the initial history and examination, the physician should have an impression of whether TOS is present. Other causes of chronic upper extremity pain may

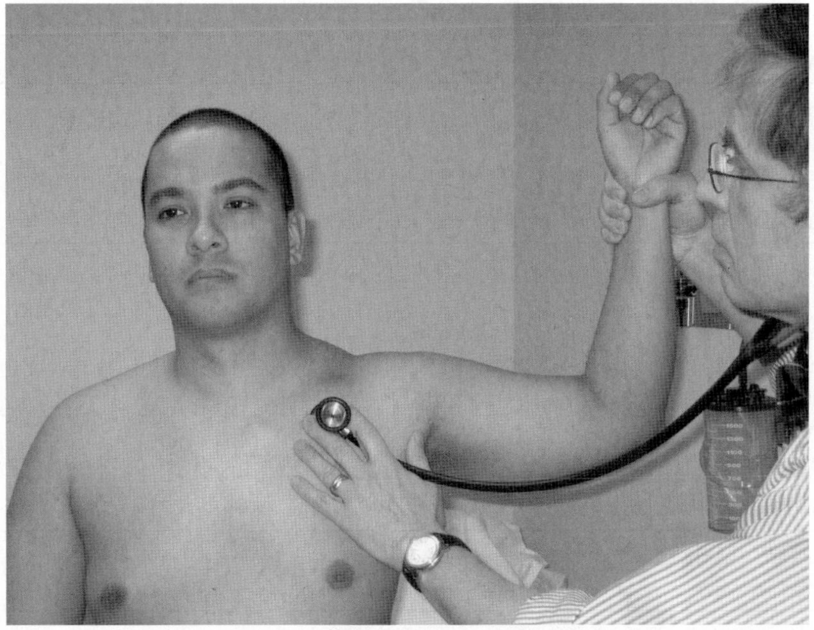

Figure 8-3. Auscultation of left subclavian artery for bruit secondary to compression of subclavian artery in thoracic outlet with abduction and external rotation of the arm.

also be evident and not previously evaluated, for example, cervical disk disease, rotator cuff tear, carpel tunnel syndrome, or brachial plexus trauma. These initial impressions set in motion a series of diagnostic and imaging tests to confirm or refute the clinical surmises.

THE COMPRESSIVE ZONES

The compression of blood vessels or nerves generally occurs at one of three *compressive zones* along the course of the thoracic outlet from the neck to the outer limit of the pectoralis minor muscle. Imaging modalities can often help to identify where the most important compression is occurring (Figure 8–4, Table 8–2).

BASIC IMAGING TESTS

Several basic tests should be done as part of the initial evaluation of every patient suspected of having TOS. A chest x-ray is mandatory. It shows the configuration of the first rib and may reveal a complete or partial cervical rib. A separate cervical rib series is also helpful (Figure 8–5). The chest x-ray also reveals any pulmonary pathology that may be impinging on the brachial plexus, for example, a Pancoast lung tumor (Figure 8–6).

The vascular laboratory may assist in diagnosing TOS in several ways. First, basic digital Photoplethysmographies (PPGs) or arm pulse volume recordings (PVRs)

TABLE 8-2 PRINCIPAL CAUSES OF THORACIC OUTLET SYNDROME[4]

Skeletal Abnormalities
Cervical rib
Elongated C7 transverse process
Exostosis or tumor of the first rib or clavicle
Soft Tissue Abnormalities
Fibrous band*
Congenital muscle abnormalities
Supernumerary muscles (e.g., scalenus minimus/intermedius)
Muscles insertion variations
Acquired fibrotic problems
Post-traumatic fibrous scars+
Postoperative scarring
Posture and Predisposing Morphotype
Poor posture and weak muscular support of shoulder girdle
Hypertrophied neck and scalene muscles in athletes

* With or without an associated cervical rib or elongated C7 transverse process.
+ Due to direct trauma or work-related repetitive microstress on scalene muscles.

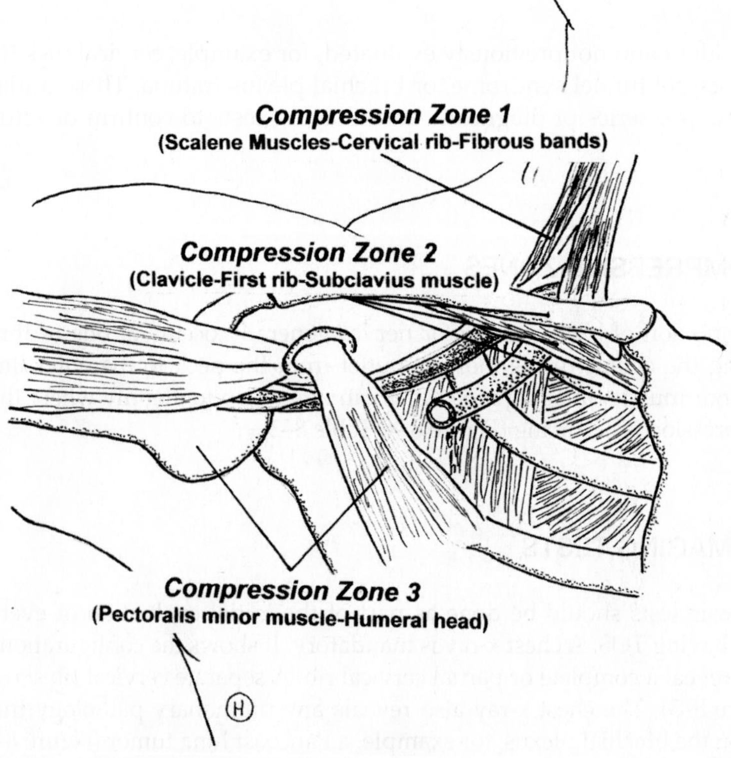

Figure 8-4. Compressive zones of the thoracic outlet. Patients may experience compression of the nerves or blood vessels at one of more of these anatomic points.

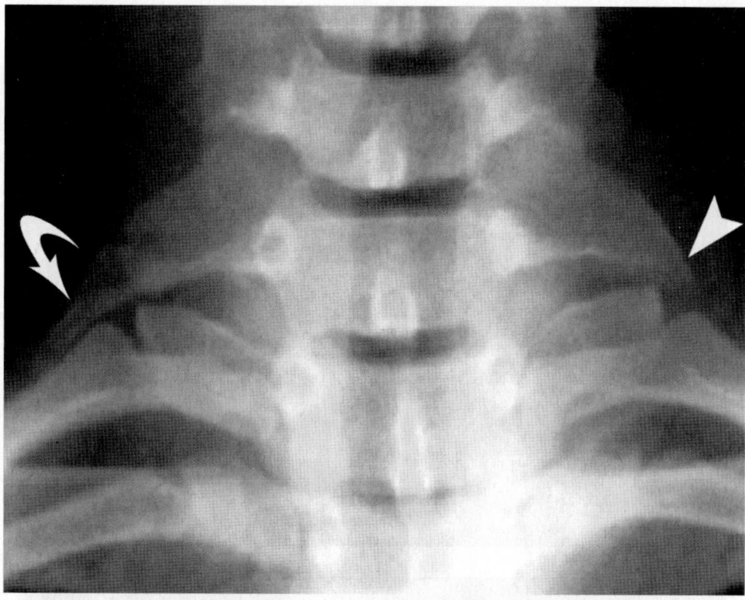

Figure 8-5. Cervical ribs. Cervical ribs may be either complete with extension to the first rib (right side in this x-ray) or partial with a fibrous or cartilaginous band to the first rib (left side).

taken at various positions of rest, military brace, and hyperabduction with external rotation may confirm arterial compression (Figure 8–7). Second, ultrasound allows views of arterial and venous flow in various arm positions. The clavicle may partially obstruct clear visualization of the vessels, but generally a significant portion of the artery and vein can be revealed. Acute venous thrombus is usually easy to see. When arterial microembolization from a subclavian aneurysm is evident, digital pulse waveforms will confirm markedly diminished perfusion.

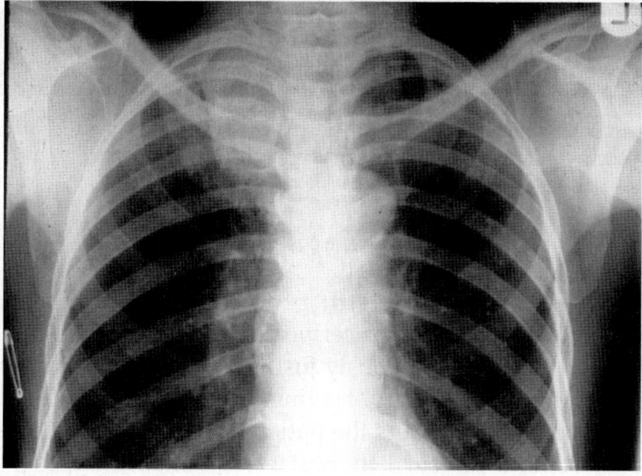

Figure 8-6. Pancoast tumor of the lung that may present with brachial plexus symptoms of chronic regional pain syndrome of the upper extremity.

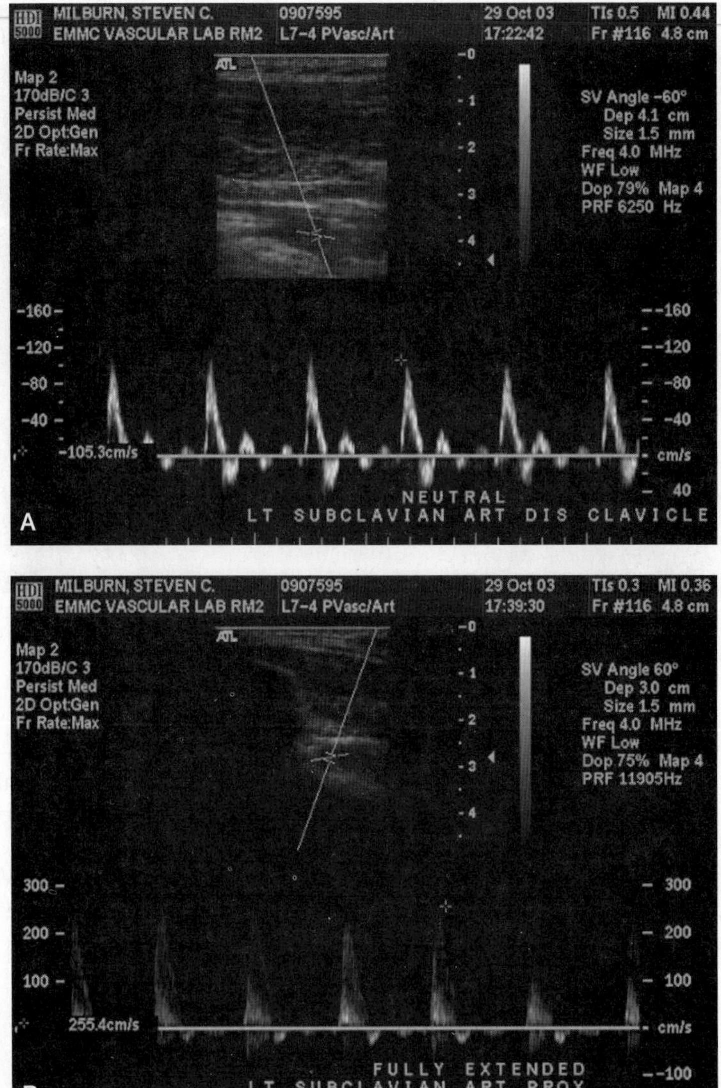

Figure 8-7. Ultrasound of the arterial waveform in a 40-year-old male with neurogenic thoracic outlet syndrome and associated Raynaud's syndrome. With abduction and external rotation of the affected limb, the arterial flow and waveform are diminished significantly compared with the normal resting position.

When orthopedic (e.g., rotator cuff problems) or neurologic (carpal tunnel syndrome, ulnar nerve entrapment, or cervical radiculopathy) issues are suspected, a consult with these specialists is obviously justified. They can decide what imaging or electrophysiologic testing is necessary. Having a neurologist evaluate a patient before any thoracic outlet surgery also offers the patient at least two opinions before any surgical intervention. Also, a physical therapist and rehabilitation/pain management physician are key to managing any complex upper extremity pain syndrome. They are especially helpful in cases of post-traumatic TOS.

THREE-DIMENSIONAL IMAGING

Ideally, one would like to view the thoracic outlet in three dimensions and in dynamic positions that cause symptoms. Three modalities provide this type of imaging: (1) ultrasound, (2) CT, and (3) MRI and MRA (Figure 8–8).[4-8]

Ultrasound

Ultrasound with both continuous waveforms and B-mode imaging can provide physiologic and anatomic information with the arm in various TOS positions.[5] Generally, subclavian-axillary venous thrombosis can be visualized easily. Although the clavicle may obstruct the view, an axillary aneurysm may be seen in cases of severe arterial compressive damage from a cervical rib. These are static images with the arm in a neutral position.

We also find ultrasound useful in visualizing what happens to arterial and venous flow in various TOS positions, for example, military brace and various abduction/external rotations. The best window to flow patterns can be via the axilla. This axillary approach allows the sonographer to look at the downstream impact on arterial or venous flow, especially when the arm is abducted to 180 degrees.

If venous thrombosis is identified with ultrasound, venography with intent for thombolysis is the next step. If impairment of arterial flow or signs of aneurysmal degeneration are identified, selective digital angiography of the entire upper extremity is usually the best method to get details of the thoracic outlet and any distal emboli. Fast CT scanning or MRA are other reasonable choices, depending on their availability and the expertise of the radiologist.

Computed Tomography

Fast CT angiography with the arm alongside the body and then with the upper limb elevated can demonstrate arterial compression (see Figure 8–8).[4,6] To enhance visualization of the arteries without venous artifacts, some experts suggest injecting the contrast medium into a vein in the contralateral extremity. One recommended method is beginning the scan 15 to 20 seconds after the start of a monophasic injection of approximately 90 mL of contrast material at a rate of 4 mL/sec. Volume-rendered images before and after postural maneuvers also provide images of the bony relationships with any vascular abnormalities. In addition, CT is also an excellent method to image the upper lung for any tumors impinging on the brachial plexus.

However, CT scanning has three potential disadvantages. If the patient is large, arm abduction and elevation cannot fit into the CT tube. In addition, contrast toxicity may be problematic for patients with chronic renal disease. Finally, the radiation dose is substantial, making repetitive examinations of concern for future cancer risk in younger patients.

Magnetic Resonance Imaging

MRI of the soft and bony structures with MRA may be preferable if arterial symptoms or signs exist.[4,7–8] A noninvasive and nonionizing technique, MRI scanning in a phased-array body coil provides three-dimensional, accurate images of all the anatomic components of the thoracic outlet (see Figure 8–8). Sagittal T1-weighted sequences can depict the vascular and nerve compressions in the anterioposterior and craniocaudal direction. Coronal views provide important images of the brachial plexus and any abnormal fibrous bands. It

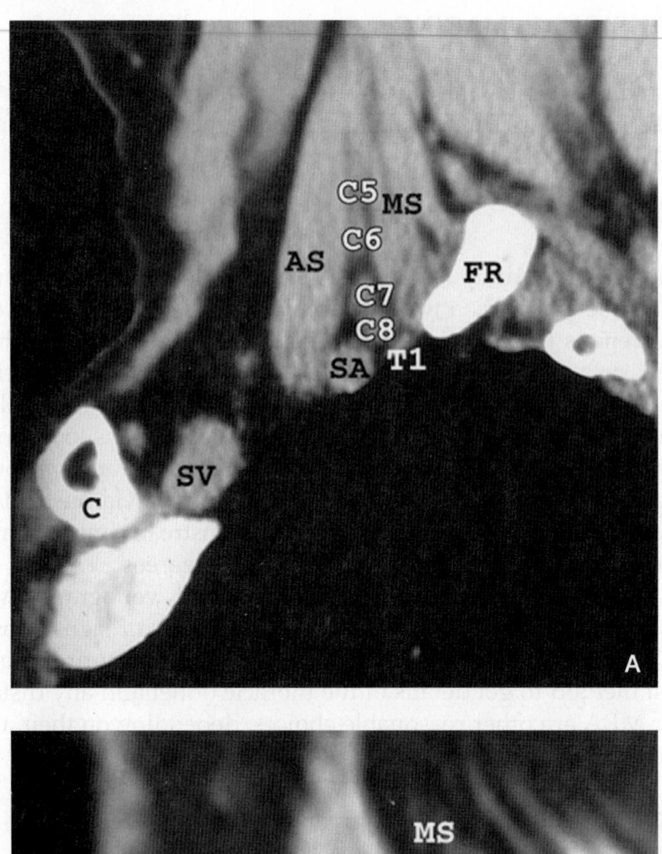

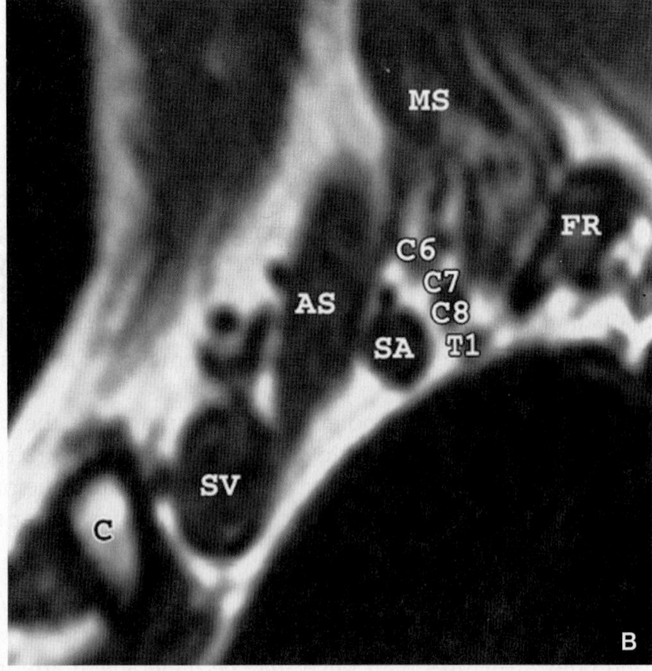

Figure 8-8. Computed tomographic (A) and magnetic resonance T1-weighted (B) images of sagittal anatomy of thoracic outlet showing anterior scalene muscle (AS), middle scalene (MS), clavicle (C), first rib (FR), subclavian artery (SA), subclavian vein (SV), and cervical and thoracic nerve roots (C5-8 and T1). (With permission from Demondion X, Vidal C, Herbinet P, et al. Ultrasonographic assessment of arterial cross-sectional area in the thoracic outlet on postural maneuvers measured with power Doppler ultrasonography in both asymptomatic and symptomatic populations. J Ultrasound Med 2006;25:217–48.)

is essential that images be taken with the arm elevated, because most symptoms from neurovascular compression occur in this position.

Arterial and venous compressions may be seen by comparing cross-sectional images of the vessels with the arm at the side and then elevated. Vessel caliber will decrease with compression. In addition, neurologic compression of the brachial plexus is manifested by disappearance of the fat surrounding the plexus and close contact with the adjacent osseous structures. Finally, MRI can reveal muscular hypertrophy (scalene, subclavius, or pectoralis minor muscles), fibrous bands, and supernumerary muscles (e.g., scalenus minimus or intermedius).

MRI also faces limitations similar to those of CT: (1) fitting the extended upper extremity into the tube, (2) chronic renal insufficiency in which gadolinium may cause nephrogenic fibrotic syndrome, and (3) inaccuracy in very thin patients in whom adipose tissue is too sparse to delineate compressive changes.

VENOGRAPHY

Patients with symptoms and signs of subclavian venous stenosis or occlusion require standard digital venography.[10–11] The precise site and extent of venous pathology are clarified. If acute venous thrombosis is present, catheter-directed thrombolysis is used if the symptoms have occurred recently, that is, in the past 7 to 10 days. The best results are achieved when the thrombus is less than 3 days' duration.

Once the vein is recannalized, a venous stenosis at the first rib is common (Figure 8–9). Although such a stenosis may be dilated gently immediately after thrombolysis, angioplasty generally does not help much at this point. The next therapeutic step is first rib resection. Stents should be avoided before the rib has been resected and generally do not work well even after thoracic decompression. Surgical venoplasty may be necessary for significant residual venous stenosis after rib resection.[10]

ARTERIOGRAPHY

Patients with symptoms and signs of subclavian artery stenosis or aneurysm generally benefit from digital angiography.[11] The study should survey the upper limb from the origin of the aortic arch to the fingertips. Although MRA or CT angiography may obtain this information, digital arteriography usually provides clearer images for therapeutic planning. Although some authors have reported catheter-directed arterial thrombolysis for distal forearm and hand emboli, these thrombi are often more chronic and not generally amenable to thorough thrombolysis. Again, arteriography should be performed with the arm at the side and then elevated (Figure 8–10).

FINAL WORDS OF CAUTION

TOS is a conundrum in many patients. The wrong diagnosis with unnecessary or poorly performed thoracic outlet surgery is a common cause of both disability for the patients and also litigation for the surgeon. Physicians and surgeons who evaluate and manage patients with complex upper extremity pain syndromes should create collaborative teams. These teams often include a vascular surgeon, a neurologist, an orthopedist, a neurosurgeon, and

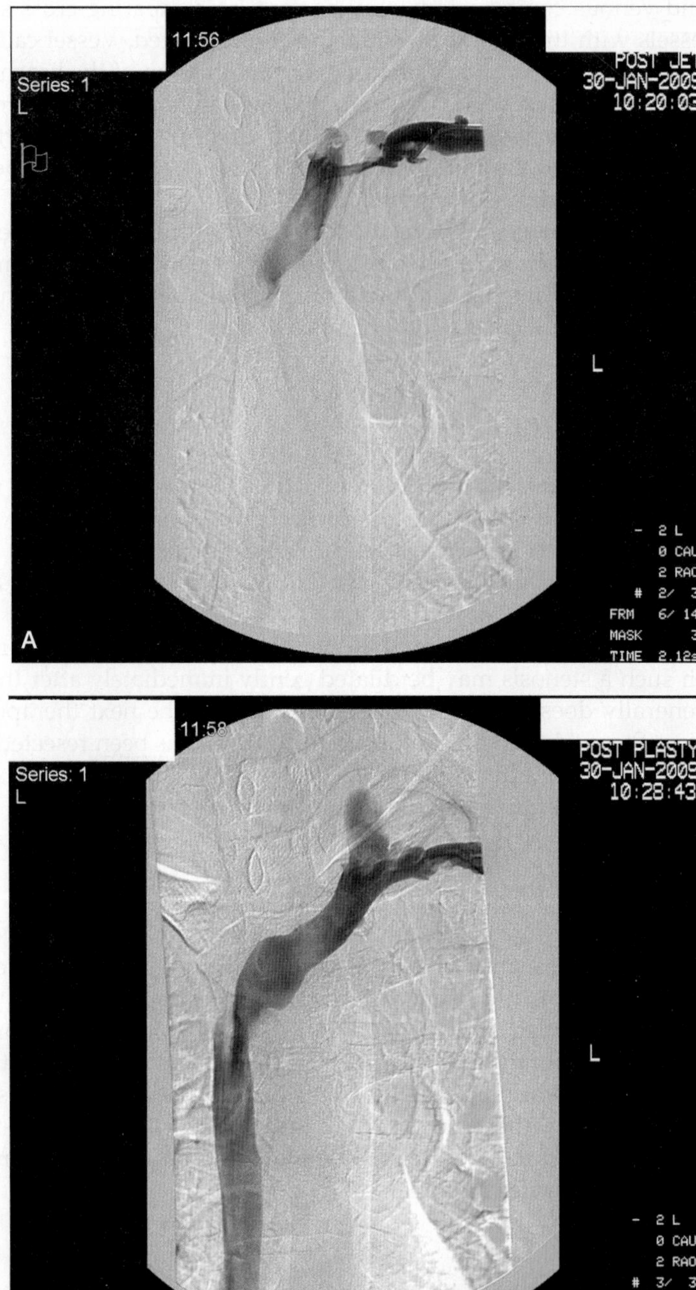

Figure 8-9. Venogram of patient presenting with Paget-Schroetter syndrome (A). After thrombolysis of the subclavian vein thrombus, a residual venous stenosis (B) from thoracic outlet compression is obvious.

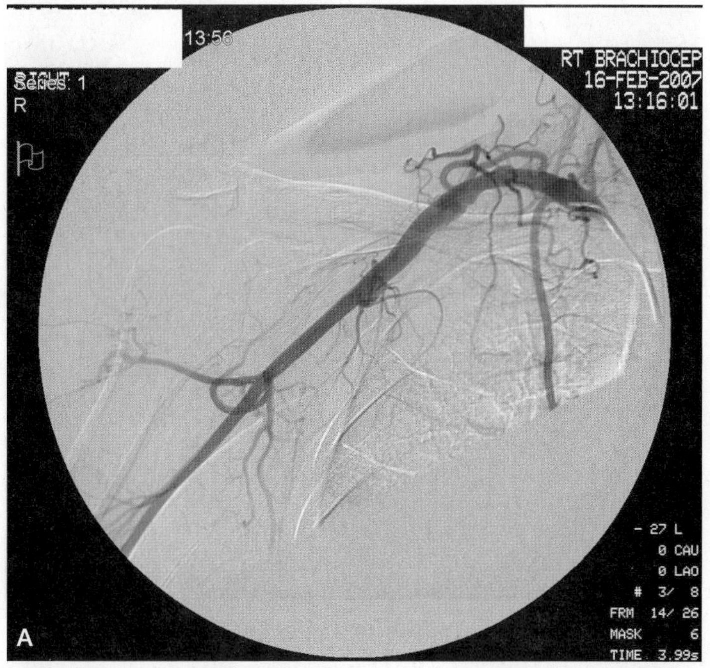

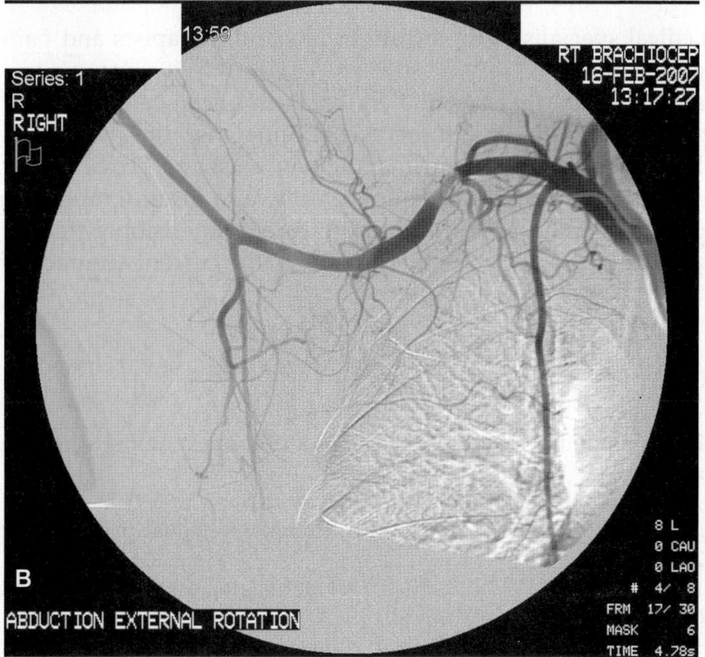

Figure 8-10. Arteriogram of right subclavian artery in a 45-year-old woman presenting with microemboli to fingertips. Note mild irregularity and early aneurysmal degeneration of subclavian artery at rest (A) with marked stenosis and abduction and external rotation of the upper extremity (B) and digital artery occlusions in the fingers (C). *(Continued)*

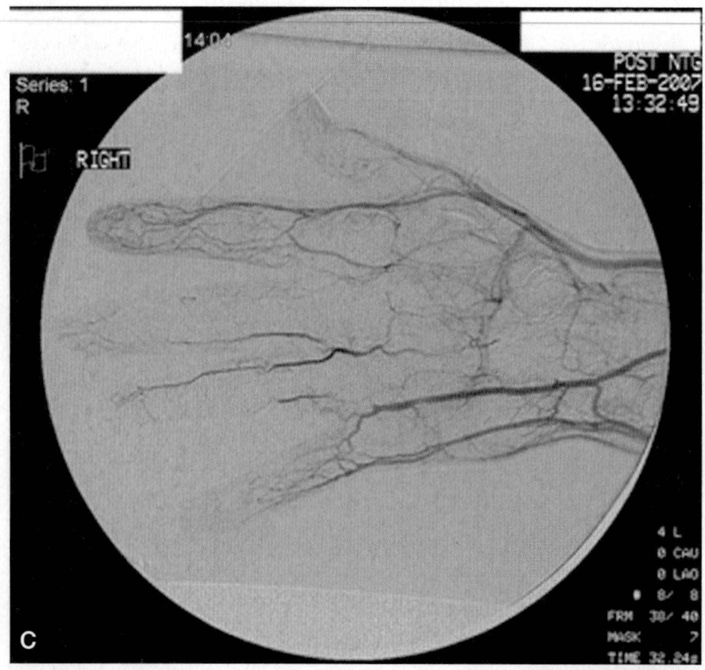

Figure 8-10. *(Continued)*

a physical medical specialist with a team of physical therapists and pain-management anesthesiologists.

This chapter has emphasized the enduring importance of a careful history and physical examination as the initial method of "imaging" the thoracic outlet. In addition, multiple methods of radiologic imaging now exist and provide important options for both diagnosis and management. Venography and arteriography remain essential in both diagnosis and therapy. In addition, three-dimensional imaging with ultrasound, CT, and MRI have added immeasurably to the current accuracy of diagnosis.

REFERENCES

1. Sander RJ, Hammond SL, Rao NM. Diagnosis of thoracic outlet syndrome. J Vasc Surg 2007;46:601–4
2. Roos DB, Owens JC. thoracic outlet syndrome. Arch Surg 1966;93:71–4.
3. Rho RH, Brewer RP, Jamer TJ, Wilson PR. Complex regional pain syndrome. Mayo Clin Proc 2002;77:174–80.
4. Demondion X, Herhinet P, Van Sint Jan S, et al. Imaging assessment of thoracic outlet syndrome. RadioGraphics 2006;26:1735–50.
5. Demondion X, Vidal C, Herbinet P, et al. Ultrasonographic assessment of arterial cross-sectional area in the thoracic outlet on postural maneuvers measured with power Doppler ultrasonography in both asymptomatic and symptomatic populations. J Ultrasound Med 2006;25:217–24.
6. Matsumura JS, Rilling WS, Pearce SH, et al. Helical computed tomography of the normal thoracic outlet. J Vasc Surg 1997;26:776–83.

7. Demondion X, Bacqueville E, Paul C, et al. Thoracic outlet: assessment with MR imaging in asymptomatic and symptomatic populations. Radiology 2003;227:461–8.
8. Charon JP, Milne W, Sheppard JG. et al. Evaluation of MR angiographic technique in the assessment of thoracic outlet syndrome. Clin Radiol 2004;59:588–95.
9. Makhoul RG, Machleder HI. Developmental anomalies at the thoracic outlet: an analysis of 200 consecutive cases. J Vasc Surg 1992;16:534–45.
10. Melby SJ, Vedantham S, Thompson RW. et al. Comprehensive surgical management of the competitive athlete with effort thrombosis of the subclavian vein (Paget-Schroetter syndrome). J Vasc Surg 2008;47:809–20.
11. Frieischlag J, Rigberg DA. thoracic outlet syndrome. In: Hallett JW, Mills JL, Earnshaw JJ, et al, eds. Comprehensive Vascular and Endovascular Surgery. Edinburgh: Mosby (Elsevier); 2009, pp.318–35.

9

Thoracic Outlet Syndrome: Too Many Operations Or Too Few?

Kaj H. Johansen, M.D., Ph.D.

INTRODUCTION

Thoracic outlet syndrome (TOS) is a term signifying a variety of neurovascular compressive states at the thoracic outlet – where the brachial plexus, the subclavian and axillary arteries, and the axillosubclavian vein pass from the base of the neck and the upper mediastinum into the upper extremity. Along their course, these elements of the upper extremity neurovascular bundle may potentially be compressed by one or another of a series of musculotendinous, osseous. or other structures.

When prolonged or unduly significant, such compression may result in arterial, venous, or neurogenic syndromes, each with its characteristic presentation, natural history, diagnosis, and treatment. To varying degrees, the indications for and means of operative intervention for these thoracic outlet compression syndromes remain topics of lively discussion and even dispute. Whether these various syndromes are being recognized and managed appropriately is timely and is the topic of this discussion.

GENERAL ASSESSMENT

Whether a particular medical condition is being treated adequately would seem to be straightforward. Indeed, when the natural history of such a condition is well understood and an effective, safe, and durable treatment has been established, little debate attends the utilization of that treatment; subsequent discussion is reserved for such issues as the sensitivity and specificity of various diagnostic evaluations or the utility of various new treatment technologies and modalities.

For example, the natural history of appendicitis is well-established, and so is its operative treatment: what remains debatable are collateral issues such as whether physical examination suffices or routine emergency department CT scans are indicated,[1] or whether a laparoscopic approach is any better than a standard open operation.[2]

In considering TOS, the extent to which indications for and conduct of surgical therapy are in dispute depends upon what is understood about the natural history of each of the three forms of TOS. As we shall see, little uncertainty accompanies the natural history of *arterial* TOS, and the primary issue for this condition revolves around identifying individuals at risk and intervening before limb-threatening manifestations of the condition develop. *Venous* TOS, a condition currently presumed generally to be optimally managed operatively, is undergoing a fresh evaluation in light of new studies suggesting that the natural history of the condition may be relatively benign and self-limited. And for *neurogenic* TOS, whereas we are likely past the point at which the very validity of the diagnosis is questioned (if not ridiculed), the questions of whether patients appropriate for intervention are being selected, whether patients with similar but non-TOS conditions are being ruled out, and whether the operative therapy currently identified to treat this most common of the three forms of TOS is safe, durable, and efficacious remain vigorously debated.

ARTERIAL THORACIC OUTLET SYNDROME

The subclavian artery is at risk for extrinsic compression during its course through the thoracic outlet – from the root of the neck all the way out into the axilla beneath the pectoralis minor tendon. Consequently, either direct trauma to the artery along this course or, alternatively, chronic extrinsic compression and torsion (most commonly when the subclavian artery is tented over a cervical rib, as in Figure 9–1) can result in various arterial derangements with locoregional implications (e.g., poststenotic or false aneurysms or arterial thrombosis) and/or peripheral implications (arterial embolization into the hand or wrist arteries).

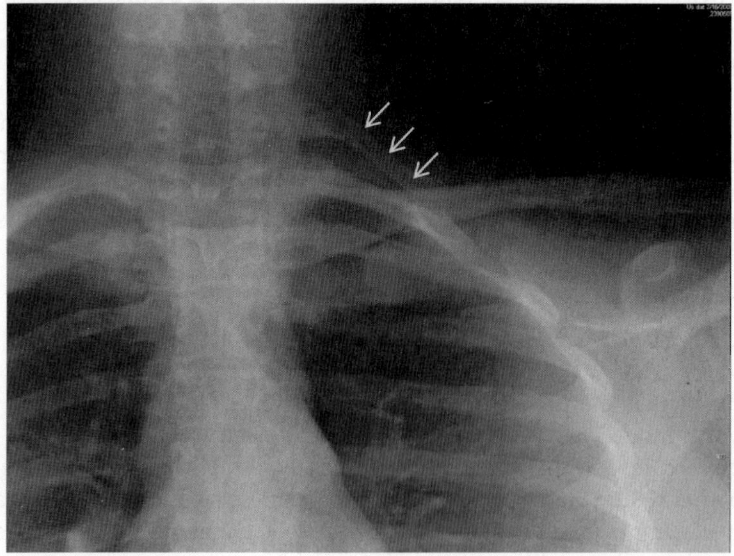

Figure 9-1. A pseudoaneurysm of the left subclavian artery developed where the vessel was draped over this 18 year old woman's large left cervical rib (arrows).

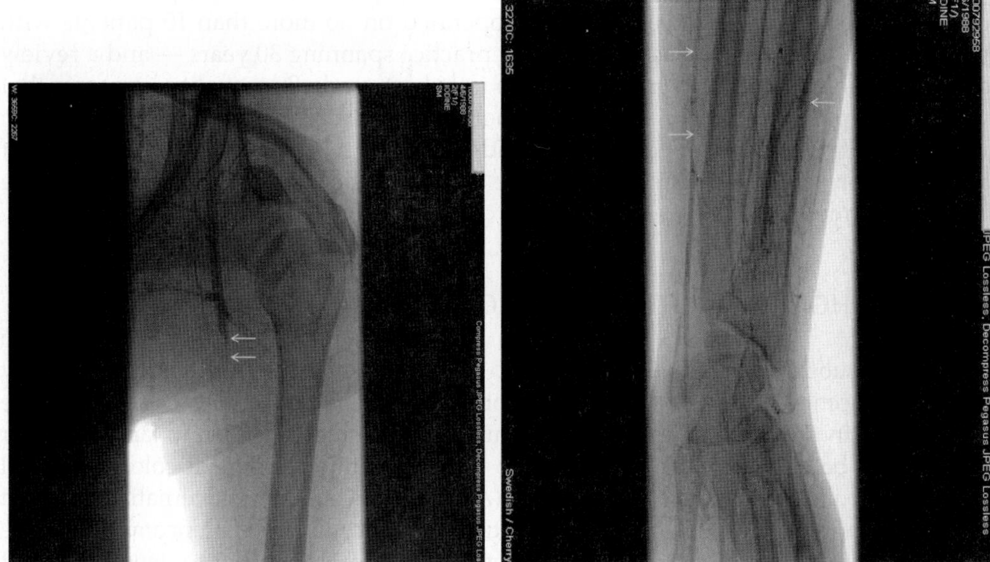

Figure 9-2. Emboli from left subclavian artery pseudoaneurysm (Figure 1) into the proximal brachial artery (arrows, left panel) and, in the forearm to the ulnar and radial arteries (right panel).

Arterial TOS is very rare, constituting only about 1% of all patients with symptomatic TOS. The largest contemporary series of patients with arterial TOS rarely number more than a few dozen, even from major referral centers reviewing a decade or more of their cumulative practices.[3-6]

A majority of patients with arterial TOS are initially identified after development of ischemic symptoms in the limb peripheral to the site of arterial thoracic outlet involvement. Most commonly, patients present with finger or hand ischemia and upon arteriographic evaluation are discovered to have evidence of diffuse chronic thromboembolization into the finger, hand, and wrist arteries (Figure 9–2). These emboli have generally resulted from a pseudoaneurysm, or less commonly, an ulcerative plaque, in the ipsilateral subclavian artery, commonly just distal to a previously undiagnosed cervical rib.

Not infrequently, the ischemic symptoms of the distal upper extremity have been dismissed as Raynaud's syndrome, and only in belated fashion is the diagnosis confirmed of a proximal arterial site causing chronic embolization into the outflow arterial circulation. In this context, the findings are similar to the natural history of popliteal artery aneurysms and their chronic embolization into the distal arteries of the lower extremities.[7]

Patients who have an embolic source identified in the subclavian artery (or those who for some unrelated reason have identification of such an arterial problem prior to distal ischemic symptoms) are generally managed in a straightforward fashion — either with a vascular graft interposition following resection of the offending arterial segment or by means of a bypass, commonly from the ipsilateral common carotid artery to the axillary artery.[3-6] Excision of the cervical rib is carried out simultaneously: performance of a complete thoracic outlet decompression (scalenectomy, first rib resection) is reserved for the very occasional patient with demonstrable concurrent neurogenic TOS.

Is the appropriate number of operations being performed for arterial TOS? The clinical scenario is rare — the author has operated on no more than 10 patients with true arterial TOS during a vascular surgery practice spanning 30 years — and a review of the available literature,[3-6] most of which is at best grade B in quality, suggests that virtually all patients with *arterial* TOS sooner or later undergo operation. However, in view of the fact that fingers and even hands continue to be lost as a consequence of this condition,[8] it is reasonable to conclude that a number of these operations may be being performed too late.

VENOUS THORACIC OUTLET SYNDROME

Because the subclavian vein passes anterior to the anterior scalene muscle, it does not truly traverse the central aspects of the thoracic outlet: this vein can, however, potentially be compressed in the costoclavicular space. Thus, several times a year, any large vascular practice will be confronted by a patient who presents with a swollen, discolored, painful arm due to axillosubclavian vein thrombosis (ASVT). This condition is alternatively known as "effort" thrombosis (based on the observation that such subjects not uncommonly have engaged in strenuous or unaccustomed upper extremity exertion prior to development of their ASVT): classically, it has been known as Paget-Schroetter syndrome.

Patients with ASVT generally are symptomatic as a result of arm swelling, pain, and discoloration. They thus commonly seek medical attention relatively soon — generally within days — after the onset of symptoms. The diagnosis of upper extremity deep venous thrombosis (DVT) is readily confirmed by noninvasive vascular laboratory examination,[9] and anticoagulation is generally begun.[10] This is given additional impetus by the fact that pulmonary embolization has been reported following upper extremity DVT.[11]

In contemporary practice, transcatheter lysis of axillosubclavian DVT is commonly attempted.[10,12] Because many patients with ASVT present soon after onset of their symptoms, such lytic therapy is predictably successful in completely or at least partially clearing the axillosubclavian venous thrombus burden. Residual thrombus or a stricture may be amenable to balloon angioplasty[13]; whether this is useful or durable is debatable. Stenting is not indicated because these devices commonly fracture due to extrinsic compression.[14]

Studies published in the 1960-1990 era appeared to suggest that the natural history of venous TOS is that of chronic arm swelling, pain, and dysfunction, that is, the post-thrombotic syndrome (PTS).[15-17] This assertion led to the recommendation in many centers that surgical decompression of the involved vein[18-21] should be the norm. This approach, sometimes combined with reconstruction of the damaged axillosubclavian vein itself,[20-23] has become commonplace, and reviews of outcomes suggest that 80 to 90% of such patients have restitution of relatively normal venous and upper extremity function.

However, more recent natural history studies have suggested that the natural history of venous TOS may not be nearly as morbid as previously thought. Older studies, upon which subsequent enthusiasm for aggressive axillosubclavian venous decompressive/reconstructive surgery had been based, only irregularly utilized thrombolysis or even anticoagulation for the initial treatment of ASVT.[15-17] However, *all* contemporary studies have included at least 3 months of anticoagulation as well as an aggressive initial effort at lytic recanalization of the involved axillosubclavian vein. These more recent studies appear to document that a substantial majority — 80 to 90% — of such ASVT patients who are observed rather than operated on continue to do well, with little or no arm swelling or other manifestations of PTS.[24-29] Interestingly, these results pertain even when the axillosubclavian vein is partially or completely occluded.[28,29]

An explanation for this apparently benign natural history for ASVT may arise from the following observations. In comparison with the lower extremities (where DVT is commonly associated with later PTS symptoms), the upper extremities have a significantly lower total limb blood flow and a shorter distance across which venous collaterals need to develop. Further, most individuals are relatively sedentary, which results in an asymptomatic limb following upper extremity venous thrombosis, not only at rest but even after upper extremity exercise. And, unlike the lower extremities, gravity plays a significantly less significant role in producing venous stasis in the upper extremities.

Accordingly, if 80 to 90% of individuals who have suffered upper extremity DVT are asymptomatic *whether or not* they undergo venous decompression and/or reconstruction, the necessity for (and certainly what some believe to be the virtually obligatory role of) aggressive operative therapy for this condition becomes controversial. There is a very real possibility that those who champion the beneficial effects of axillosubclavian venous decompression/reconstruction following upper extremity DVT take advantage of the fact that such patients were going to do well anyway!

The author has recently presented data suggesting that 90% of patients with ASVT treated with initial thrombolysis and anticoagulation followed by observation alone did well without surgical intervention.[29] This reflects the results of other series raising questions about the validity of routine operative therapy for ASVT.[27–28] I believe that more of these venous decompression/reconstructive operations are performed than may be warranted by contemporary ASVT natural history data. Although conceding that there may be subgroups of individuals with effort thrombosis in whom upper extremity venous decompression/reconstruction is justified (e.g., elite athletes[30]), I believe even that assertion is speculative. At the current time, I believe that venous TOS is generally a benign condition and aggressive surgical reconstruction offers risk without predictable functional benefit in most such patients for whom operation is recommended.

Because venous TOS patients often present in the early stages of the condition in stereotypic fashion, the clinical scenario seems well-suited for a multicenter randomized controlled trial of observational therapy versus aggressive surgical reconstruction for ASVT.

NEUROGENIC THORACIC OUTLET SYNDROME

The vast majority of individuals with TOS — more than 95% of them — present with complaints of upper extremity and neck pain, weakness, numbness and tingling, and limitation of motion at the shoulder and arm. These symptoms arise from compression of trunks of the brachial plexus at one of three sites along the thoracic outlet: (1) between the anterior and the middle scalene muscles, (2) within the costoclavicular space, and (3) beneath the pectoralis minor tendon near its attachment to the coracoid process.

In contrast to arterial or venous TOS, in which the clinical manifestations of the problem often are obvious and imaging studies accurately confirm the presence of an arterial or venous abnormality, symptoms associated with neurogenic TOS are diffuse, particularly in that they wax and wane relative to neck and upper extremity posture.

Further, objective diagnostic modalities are sparse, disputed, and incompletely validated.

It has thus been easy for skeptics and provocateurs[31] to question whether the condition really exists at all. To be sure, such critics concede that the identical syndrome, when the consequence of a cervical rib, is indeed a real clinical phenomenon that can be mitigated by an appropriate operation.[6] Even so, identifying patients who truly do have brachial plexus compression across the thoracic outlet and excluding those who have other conditions (cervical spine or shoulder abnormalities, peripheral nerve compression) but a similar clinical presentation remains challenging. How to carry out a safe, effective, and durable decompression of the brachial plexus remains a topic of vigorous discussion. Few really credible long-term analyses of outcomes following decompressive surgery for neurogenic TOS are available.[32–33] In addition, the operation may be attended by significant complications.[34–35]

Making the diagnosis of neurogenic TOS remains problematic. Although the presence of an appropriate trauma history, a worsening of symptoms with the arms outfront or overhead, an ulnar predominance of neuritic radiation out the affected arm, and a negative work-up for cervical spine, shoulder, and peripheral nerve problems can help confirm the diagnosis, in substantial numbers of patients, false-positive and false-negative diagnostic assessments continue to be made. In our view, the pioneering work of Jordan and his colleagues at UCLA[36–37] in validating the use of chemodenervation of the scalene muscles has made objective diagnosis of the problem (as well as the primacy of the scalene muscles in the pathophysiology of the condition) vastly more objective.

Further, the choice of surgery to treat neurogenic TOS is controversial. Transaxillary,[38] supraclavicular,[39] and posterior[40] approaches each have their adherents, and removing the first rib, although commonplace,[38] remains unproven.[41] Sanders promotes the relevance of pectoralis minor compression of the brachial plexus as a component of this syndrome.[42] At least 5 to 10% of individuals will have recurrent symptoms: did they have an inadequate operation[43] or did they not have neurogenic TOS at all?

Operative techniques to treat neurogenic TOS are not performed or taught in vascular residencies on a consistent basis, nor are such procedures commonly performed by other specialists such as neurosurgeons or orthopedists. The combination of a lack of familiarity with both the condition and the operation and the well-documented litigation risk associated with the complications of this operation[44] has thus limited performance of this operation to a few high-volume centers throughout North America.

Restriction of this operation to regional "centers of excellence" has both positive and negative implications. Favorable aspects include relatively high volumes of patients being operated upon at each of these centers, such that the well-established relationship between operative volumes and their outcomes likely means that when patients are operated upon at these sites, adverse outcomes (e.g., due to lack of familiarity with the anatomy or the basic rules of the operative procedure) are likely minimized. On the other hand, restriction of performance of this operation to a few isolated centers, free of any substantive outside critique or influence, may promote continuation of outmoded or incorrect theories or practices regarding the identification and the management of this constellation of problems.

Are too many or two few operations being performed for neurogenic TOS in the United States? It is impossible to tell. Because of a lack of recognition or understanding of the condition among primary care practitioners, a substantial number of such patients may end up undergoing therapy for other conditions — cervical spine disease, shoulder dysfunction, fibromyalgia — because the proper diagnosis has not been made. Such patients predictably continue to suffer pain and disability and their physicians may then ultimately assign them a chronic pain diagnosis. It is assuredly true that such patients injured on the job and ensnared in a worker's compensation system may frequently be denied timely and appropriate care because of obsolete and/or frankly invalid criteria for the condition.[45]

CONCLUSION

Whether the proper number of operations are being performed for the various forms of TOS remains unclear. For *arterial* TOS, because the condition's problems are exclusively related to peripheral embolization (or the subclavian arterial aneurysms or intimal plaques that result in embolization), it is likely that an appropriate number of operations are being performed, but some of them too late. Just as for popliteal artery aneurysms in the lower extremities, the damage resulting from arterial TOS often results in a diffuse obliteration of all distal upper extremity arteries, eventuating in chronic digital and hand ischemia that may be difficult to resolve.

Over the past 25 years, an increasingly aggressive operative approach, based on historical studies suggesting the morbid natural history of *venous* TOS, has been promoted in such patients. However, more recent observational studies, following up on patients treated with anticoagulation after aggressive lytic recanalization of their thrombosed axillosubclavian veins, suggest that robust collateralization occurs in patients with partial or complete venous occlusion, rendering most of them normal or only minimally symptomatic even after upper extremity exertion. It seems likely that a number of venous TOS patients are being subjected to operation who in fact do not really need such an aggressive intervention.

Patients with *neurogenic* TOS are victimized by the fact that diagnostic tests with appropriate sensitivities and specificities for the condition are inadequately validated or understood, operative techniques remain disputed, and outcomes are poorly documented. Many such individuals ultimately become identified as chronic pain patients and fail to undergo the operative therapy that might significantly improve their chronic pain and disability. A more objective diagnostic assessment of the condition, a more widespread education of primary care providers about the quite stereotypic presentation of the condition, and broader education of surgeons in the conduct of surgical therapy of neurogenic TOS would be timely.

REFERENCES

1. Andre JB, Sebastian BA, Ruchman RM, Saad SA. CT and appendicitis: evaluation of correlation between CT diagnosis and pathological diagnosis. Postgrad Med J 2008;84:321–4.
2. Sporn E, Petroski GF, Mancini GJ, et al. Laparoscopic appendectomy – is it worth the cost? Trend analysis in the US from 2000 to 2005. J Am Coll Surg 2009;208:179–85.
3. Davidovic LB, Koncar IB, Pajkic SD, Kuzmanovic IB. Arterial complications of thoracic outlet syndrome. Ann Surg 2009;75:235–9.
4. Cormier JM, Amrane M, Ward A, et al. Arterial complications of the thoracic outlet syndrome: fifty-five operative cases. J Vasc Surg 1989;9:778–87.

5. Durham JR, Yao JS, Pearce WH, et al. Arterial injuries in the thoracic outlet syndrome. J Vasc Surg 1995;21:57–69.
6. Nehler MR, Taylor LM Jr, Moneta GL, Porter JM. Upper extremity ischemia from subclavian artery aneurysm caused by bony abnormalities of the thoracic outlet. Arch Surg 1997;132:527–32.
7. Gouny P, Bertrand P, Duedal V, et al. Limb salvage and popliteal aneurysms: advantages of preventive surgery. Eur J Vasc Endovasc Surg 2000;19:496–500.
8. Bucek RA, Schnurer G, Ahmadi A, et al. A severe case of vascular thoracic outlet syndrome. Wien Klin Wochenschr 2000;112:973–7.
9. Weber TM, Lockhart ME, Robbin ML. Upper extremity venous Doppler ultrasound. Radiol Clin N Am 2007;45:513.
10. Thomas IH, Zierler BK. An integrative review of outcomes in patients with acute primary upper extremity deep venous thrombosis following no treatment or treatment with anticoagulation, thrombolysis or surgical algorithms. Vasc Endovasc Surg 2005;39:163–74.
11. Monreal M, Lafoz E, Ruiz J, et al. Upper-extremity deep venous thrombosis and pulmonary embolism. Chest 1991;99:280–3.
12. Sabeti S, Schillinger M, Miekusch W, et al. Treatment of subclavian-axillary vein thrombosis: longterm outcome of anticoagulation versus systemic thrombolysis. Thromb Res 2002; 108:279–85.
13. Glanz S, Gordon DH, Lipkowitz GS, et al. Axillary and subclavian vein stenosis: percutaneous angioplasty. Radiology 1988;168:371–3.
14. Bjarnason H, Hunter DW, Crain MR, et al. Collapse of a Palmaz stent in the subclavian vein. AJR Am J Roentgenol 1993;160:1123–4.
15. Tilney NL, Griffiths HJG, Edwards E.: Natural history of major venous thrombosis of the upper extremity. Arch Surg 1970;101:792–6.
16. Gloviczki P, Kazmier FS, Hollier LH: Axillary-subclavian venous occlusion: the morbidity of a non-lethal disease. J Vasc Surg 1986;4:333–7.
17. Kunkel JM, Machleder HI: Treatment of Paget-Schroetter syndrome. Arch Surg 1989;124: 1153–8.
18. Taylor LM, McAllister WR, Dennis DL, et al. Thrombolytic therapy followed by first rib resection for spontaneous ("effort") subclavian vein thrombosis. Am J Surg 1985;149:644–7.
19. Rutherford RB, Hurlbert SN: Primary subclavian-axillary vein thrombosis: consensus and commentary. Cardiovasc Surg 1996;4:420–3.
20. Thompson RW, Schneider PA, Nelken NA, et al. Circumferential venolysis and paraclavicular thoracic outlet decompression for "effort thrombosis" of the subclavian vein. J Vasc Surg 1992;16:723–32.
21. Lee MC, Grassi CJ, Belkin M, et al. Early operative intervention after thrombolytic therapy for primary subclavian vein thrombosis: an effective treatment approach. J Vasc Surg 1998:27:1101–8.
22. Sanders RJ, Cooper MA: Surgical management of subclavian vein obstruction, including six cases of subclavian vein bypass. Surgery 1995;118:856–63.
23. Adelman MA, Stone DH, Riles TS, et al. A multidisciplinary approach to the treatment of Paget-Schroetter syndrome. Ann Vasc Surg 1997;11:149–54.
24. Hingorani A, Ascher E, Lorenson E, et al. Upper extremity deep venous thrombosis and its impact on morbidity and mortality rates in a hospital-based population. J Vasc Surg 1997;26:853–60.
25. Heron E, Lozinguez O, Emmerich J, et al. Long-term sequelae of spontaneous axillary-subclavian venous thrombosis. Ann Intern Med 1999;131:510–3.
26. Martinelli I, Battoglioli T, Bucciarelli P, et al. Risk factors and recurrence rate of primary deep vein thrombosis of the upper extremities. Circulation 2004;110:566–70.
27. Lee WA, Hill BB, Harris JJ, et al. Surgical intervention is not required for all patients with subclavian vein thrombosis. J Vasc Surg 2000;32:57–67.
28. Lokanathan R, Salvian AJ, Chen JC, et al. Outcome after thrombolysis and selective thoracic outlet decompression for primary axillary vein thrombosis. J Vasc Surg 2001;33:783–8.

29. Johansen K. Does axillosubclavian vein ("effort") thrombosis oblige first rib resection? Arch Surg In press.
30. Melby SJ, Vedantham S, Narra VR, et al. Comprehensive surgical management of the competitive athlete with effort thrombosis of the subclavian vein (Paget-Schroetter syndrome). J Vasc Surg 2008;47:809–20.
31. Wilbourn AJ, Porter JM. Neurogenic thoracic outlet syndrome: surgical versus conservative therapy. J Vasc Surg 1992;15:880–2.
32. Degeorges R, Reynaud C, Becquemin JP. Thoracic outlet syndrome surgery: long-term functional results. Ann Vasc Surg 2004;18:558–65.
33. Axelrod DA, Proctor MC, Geisser ME, et al. Outcomes after surgery for thoracic outlet syndrome. J Vasc Surg 2001;33:1220–5.
34. Melliere D, Becquemin JP, Etienne G, Lecheviller B. Severe injuries resulting from operations for thoracic outlet syndrome: can they be avoided? J Cardiovasc Surg (Torino) 1991;32:599–603.
35. Chang DC, Lidor AO, Matsen SL, Freischlag JA. Reported in-hospital complications following rib resections for neurogenic thoracic outlet syndrome. Ann Vasc Surg 2007;21:564–70.
36. Jordan SE, Machleder HI. Diagnosis of thoracic outlet syndrome using electrophysiologically guided anterior scalene blocks. Ann Vasc Surg 1998;12:260–4.
37. Jordan SE, Ahn SS, Gelabert HA. Combining ultrasonography and EMG for botulinum chemodenervation treatment of thoracic outlet syndrome. Comparison with fluoroscopy and EMG guidance. Pain Physician 2007;10:441–52.
38. Roos DB. Transaxillary approach for first rib resection to relieve thoracic outlet syndrome. Ann Surg 1996;163:344–58.
39. Sanders R, Raymar S. The supraclavicular approach to scalenectomy and first rib resection: description of technique. J Vasc Surg 1985;2:751–6.
40. Tender GC, Kline DE: Posterior subscapular approach to the brachial plexus. Neurosurgery 2005;57(4 suppl 2):377–381.
41. Cheng SW, Reilly LM, Nelken NA, et al. Neurogenic chronic outlet decompression rationales for sparing the first rib. Cardiovasc Surg 1995;3:617–23.
42. Sanders RJ. The forgotten pectoralis minor syndrome: report of 100 operations. J Vasc Surg, in press.
43. Ambrad-Chalela E, Thomas GI, Johansen KH. Recurrent neurogenic thoracic outlet syndrome. Am J Surg 2004;187:505–10.
44. Dale WA. Thoracic outlet compression syndrome. Critique in 1982. Arch Surg 1982;17: 1437–45.
45. Wickizer TM, Franklin G, Gluck JV, Fulton-Kehoe D. Improving quality through identifying inappropriate care: the use of guideline-based utilization review protocols in the Washington State Workers' Compensation System. J Occup Environ Med 2004;46:198–204.

10

Long-Term Outcomes for Upper Extremity Deep Vein Thrombosis

R. Eugene Zierler, M.D. and
Michael T. Caps, M.D., M.P.H.

There has been a common perception that upper extremity deep vein thrombosis (DVT) is a "benign" process with a low risk for pulmonary embolism and other complications. However, reported experience suggests that this is not true. For example, pulmonary embolism (PE) is present in up to 36% of patients with upper extremity DVT.[1] Mortality associated with this condition is in the range of 12 to 34% and is based on the severity of underlying systemic illness. The rising prevalence of upper extremity DVT can be directly attributed to the increasing use of both cardiac pacemakers and central venous catheters for chemotherapy, hemodialysis, and parenteral nutrition. Thrombosis of the subclavian, axillary, or brachial veins accounts for between 4% and 10% of all venous thromboses.[2] However, this may be an underestimation, because it is likely that many upper extremity venous thromboses are not symptomatic and therefore not documented. Upper extremity DVT can be considered as either *primary* or *secondary* based on the presumed etiology.

CLASSIFICATION OF UPPER EXTREMITY DVT

Primary Thrombosis

Primary upper extremity DVT is a relatively rare disorder, affecting approximately 2 in 100,000 persons per year.[3] This category includes idiopathic thrombosis, effort thrombosis, and venous thoracic outlet syndrome.

Idiopathic Venous Thrombosis. Patients with idiopathic upper extremity DVT have no known or apparent underlying disease that could be considered as the cause of the thrombotic episode at the time that they present. However, many of these patients — up to 25% in one study — are subsequently found to have occult cancer.[4] Hypercoagulable states are another cause of idiopathic upper extremity venous thrombosis and are particularly likely in patients with a family history of venous thromboembolism. Inherited hypercoagulable states include factor V Leiden and the prothrombin gene mutation.

Effort Thrombosis (Paget-Schroetter Syndrome). Patients who present with axillary-subclavian vein thrombosis following vigorous arm activity (usually in the dominant arm) are considered to have *effort thrombosis*. This condition was first described by Paget and von Schroetter in the late 1800s and subsequently named the Paget-Schroetter syndrome. Typical activities associated with this condition involve strenuous arm movements such as swimming, rowing, volleyball, or baseball pitching (Figure 10–1). Effort thrombosis

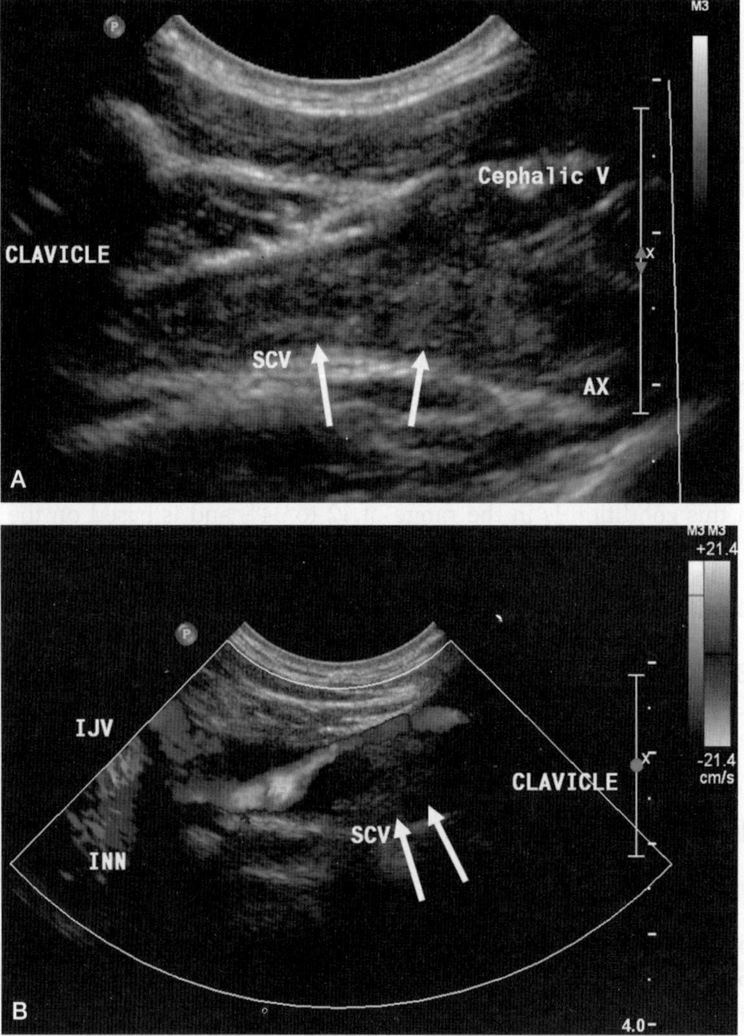

Figure 10-1. Effort thrombosis in a 19-year-old female on the university crew team who presented with a "heavy" and swollen left arm. A. B-mode image shows acute-appearing thrombus (white arrows) in the distal left subclavian vein (SCV) extending into the cephalic and axillary (AX) veins. B. Color Doppler image showing flow in the left internal jugular (IJV) and innominate (INN) veins but minimal flow with thrombus (white arrows) in the proximal subclavian vein (SJV).

is uncommon, accounting for only 1 to 2% of upper extremity DVTs. The patients are generally young and otherwise healthy. If there is mechanical compression of the involved veins at the thoracic outlet, this condition overlaps with venous thoracic outlet syndrome. In these patients, it is assumed that thrombosis is preceded by many years of intermittent compression and repetitive trauma to the venous segments, with eventual accumulation of scar tissue.

Venous Thoracic Outlet Syndrome. Thoracic outlet syndrome refers to compression of the neurovascular structures as they pass out of the thoracic cavity into the arm. The venous variety typically involves the subclavian vein as it passes under the clavicle and over the first rib. Some patients with this syndrome are athletes and can be considered to have a form of effort thrombosis. Cervical ribs and other bony abnormalities can also predispose to compression of the subclavian vein in this location.

Secondary Thrombosis

Secondary upper extremity venous thrombosis accounts for about 70% of upper extremity DVT cases and develops in patients with a central venous catheter (CVC), cardiac pacemaker, or known cancer.[2]

Central Venous Catheters. Upper extremity venous thrombosis occurs most often in response to the presence of a foreign object in the lumen of the vein. In the hospital setting, this typically involves various types of CVCs (Figure 10–2). Peripheral venous catheters cause superficial thrombophlebitis, a painful but generally minor complication. The consequences of DVT associated with CVCs are more serious and include arm, neck, and head swelling, pain, malfunction of the catheter (which interferes with drug therapy, hemodialysis, or parenteral nutrition), and PE. Central catheters can be inserted peripherally through the basilic or cephalic veins (peripherally inserted central catheters or PICC lines) or directly into the internal jugular or subclavian veins (Hickman catheters). These lines can be tunneled under the skin to provide more secure fixation and some protection against infection. Some CVCs contain implanted ports that remain entirely subcutaneous, and medications are injected through the skin into the port. For all types of CVCs, the central end of the catheter is usually positioned in the superior vena cava (SVC) or the right atrium.

Pacemakers. Whereas a pacemaker is placed beneath the skin of the upper chest and presents no direct risk to the vasculature, the lead wires are inserted through the subclavian and innominate veins and the SVC into the heart. As with CVCs, these lead wires are a foreign object in the lumen of the vein and therefore increase the risk for thrombosis. Pacer wires tend to be left in place chronically, exposing the patient to a long-term risk of venous complications.

Known Cancer. Active cancer is often associated with a hypercoagulable state that increases the overall risk of venous thrombosis. In addition, cancer patients frequently require CVCs for treatment, further increasing their risk for DVT in the upper extremities. Chemotherapeutic drugs can be very irritating to the venous endothelium and contribute to sclerosis of the central veins. This combination of a hypercoagulable state, venous intimal injury, and a foreign object within the vessel lumen results in a very high risk for upper extremity venous thrombosis.

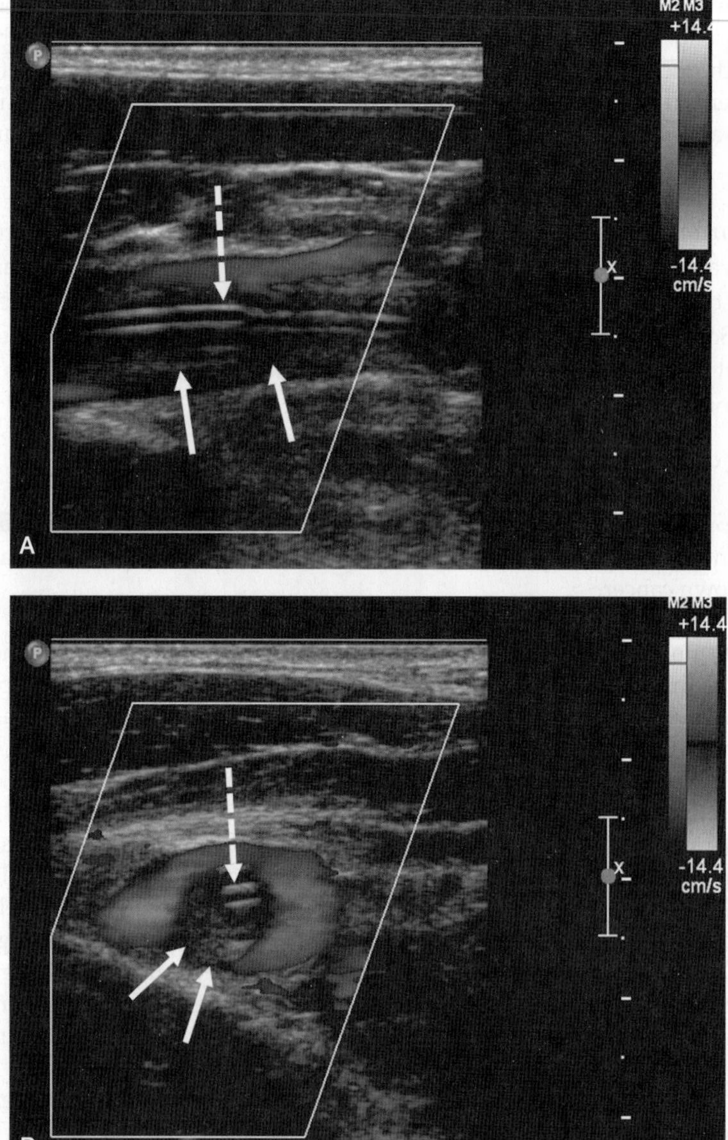

Figure 10-2. Catheter-associated thrombus in a 35-year-old male with a history of liver transplant and a peripherally inserted central line on the left side. He presents with swelling and pain in the left arm and poor function of the catheter. A. Longitudinal duplex image shows the catheter (dashed arrow) with associated thrombus (white arrows) in the left subclavian vein. B. Transverse duplex image shows the catheter (dashed arrow) and thrombus (white arrows) with some flow in the subclavian vein on color Doppler.

CLINICAL PRESENTATION

The clinical presentation of a patient with primary upper extremity DVT typically involves a young, athletic individual with unilateral swelling of the upper arm, forearm, and hand. Pain is a frequent symptom and is usually described as "tightness" or "heaviness" that may be exacerbated by dependency and partially relieved by elevation of the arm. Because these patients have venous hypertension in the affected extremity, the veins of the arm and hand are distended, although this may not be readily apparent because the venous distention is often masked by edema. Although they are not necessarily present in the acute phase, enlarged venous collaterals may be visible around the shoulder. The relative severity of these signs and symptoms depends on the duration and extent of the occlusive process in the upper extremity veins and the capacity of the collateral circulation to compensate for impaired venous drainage.

The symptoms and signs in patients with secondary or CVC-associated upper extremity DVT are similar to those described above, but they can be more subtle than the presentation of primary or effort thrombosis.[5] Thrombus associated with CVCs often develops slowly, allowing more time for development of venous collateral circulation, and typically involves a shorter venous segment than the primary type. In addition, patients with secondary upper extremity DVT are usually hospitalized and have multiple medical comorbidities such as cancer, heart failure, or end-stage renal disease that increase their overall risk for venous thrombosis. Malfunctioning of the CVC may indicate occlusion of the vein at the central end of the catheter. In the extreme case of SVC occlusion (SVC syndrome), facial edema, blurred vision, and dyspnea may occur.

DIAGNOSIS

The most commonly used diagnostic tests for upper extremity DVT are duplex ultrasound and catheter contrast venography, although magnetic resonance venography (MRV) and computed tomographic venography (CTV) may also play a role, depending on local expertise and availability. Duplex scanning is usually the preferred initial imaging test because it is less expensive than the other methods and does not require the use of contrast agents or ionizing radiation (see Figures 10–1 and 10–2). Table 10–1 summarizes the studies in which the accuracy of duplex scanning for the diagnosis of axillary-subclavian DVT has been quantified using catheter contrast venography as the reference or "gold standard."[6-12] However, venography is not a perfect standard in this setting, and there is considerable disagreement when two "blinded" radiologists interpret the same venograms.[13]

The accuracy of duplex scanning for upper extremity DVT has not been as extensively studied as for DVT in the lower extremities. Published studies (see Table 10–1) have shown considerable variability in methodology, including the proportion of patients with CVC-associated DVT. Sensitivities range from 56 to 100%, with a weighted average of 86%. Specificities range from 82 to 100%, with a slightly higher weighted average of 90%. Some of this variability is related to the fact that duplex scanning is operator-dependent and relies heavily on the skill of the examiner and interpreting physician.

TREATMENT

Anticoagulation is indicated for treatment of most patients with DVT involving the axillary, subclavian, or more proximal upper extremity veins.[14] This can consist of initial treatment with unfractionated heparin, low molecular weight heparin, or fondaparinux. Long-term anticoagulation with Coumadin is recommended for at least 3 months, and the guidelines for overall duration of anticoagulation are similar to those for lower extremity

TABLE 10-1. SUMMARY OF STUDIES IN WHICH THE RESULTS OF DUPLEX SCANNING FOR AXILLARY-SUBCLAVIAN VEIN THROMBOSIS WERE VALIDATED USING VENOGRAPHY AS THE "GOLD STANDARD"

Authors	Year	Number of Patients	% Catheter-Related	Sensitivity	Specificity
Faulk and Smith[6]	1987	14	64	88%	100%
Knudson et al.[7]	1990	20	48	78%	92%
Haire et al.[8]	1991	43	91	56%	100%
Baxter et al.[9]	1991	19	74	100%	100%
Koksoy et al.[10]	1995	94	100	94%	88%
Prandoni et al.[11]	1997	58	14	100%	93%
Baarslag et al.[12]	2002	99	41	82%	82%

DVT. Limb elevation may be beneficial to relieve swelling in the acute phase, and a compression sleeve can be used to control swelling over the long term.

Catheter-directed thrombolysis is indicated in selected patients with primary upper extremity DVT. The rationale for thrombolyis is based on the observation that a significant proportion of patients with primary upper extremity DVT who are treated with anticoagulation alone have persistent and often severe post-thrombotic symptoms in the involved extremity.[15] These patients are typically young and active, and they complain of persistent arm swelling and pain exacerbated by upper extremity exercise. Because these patients are usually healthy, there are rarely any contraindications to the use of thrombolytic agents. Thrombolytic therapy is more likely to be successful when the thrombus is relatively fresh, preferably less than 1 week old.[16] In addition to thrombolysis, suction catheter thrombectomy, balloon angioplasty, stenting, and surgical thrombectomy may be useful in some cases. Thoracic outlet decompression should be considered in those patients with bony or other anatomic abnormalities that cause direct compression of veins.

Thrombolytic therapy is generally not indicated for the majority of patients with secondary or CVC-associated upper extremity DVT. If the inciting catheter can be removed, it should be, preferably after anticoagulation has been started. When a catheter has already been removed, some have advocated no anticoagulation at all; however, most clinicians would favor a short course of anticoagulation (4 to 6 weeks) following catheter removal, although there are no reliable data to guide decision-making. For those with secondary upper extremity DVT due to a nonreversible risk factor such as malignancy or a catheter or pacemaker that cannot be removed, a longer course of anticoagulation may be indicated.

CLINICAL OUTCOME

The main complications of upper extremity DVT include PE, right-sided heart thromboembolism, recurrent thrombosis, post-thrombotic syndrome, and death. The mortality in patients with a diagnosis of upper extremity DVT is in the range of 12 to 48%.[1,17-20] It is noteworthy that most of these deaths are not associated with PE but rather with CVCs in the setting of cancer, multisystem organ failure, and infection. Therefore, the relatively high mortality rates associated with secondary upper extremity DVTs can be attributed to the severity of the underlying illness.

Pulmonary Embolism

Reported series of upper extremity DVT vary considerably with regard to the proportion of primary and secondary cases, treatment strategies, and other characteristics. This has given rise to a prevalence of associated PE that ranges from 0 to 25%.[20-23] Because the majority of emboli associated with upper extremity DVT may be asymptomatic, the frequency of detected PE will depend on how aggressively the diagnosis is sought. In a review of 430 patients with lower extremity DVT and 52 patients with upper extremity DVT, PE was documented by ventilation-perfusion scan in 33 (8%) with lower extremity DVT and 9 (17%) with upper extremity DVT.[20] In addition, 6-month mortality in the lower extremity DVT group was 13% compared with 48% in the upper extremity DVT group. In a prospective study of 86 patients with CVC-associated upper extremity DVT, all of whom were anticoagulated and had ventilation-perfusion scans, PE was found in 13 patients (15%).[22] Among these 13 patients, 11 were asymptomatic, whereas 2 had symptomatic and fatal PE.

In a comprehensive literature review of patients with primary upper extremity DVT, the reported incidence of PE was 12% among those managed without anticoagulation (rest, heat, and elevation of the limb) versus 7% for those who were anticoagulated.[23] Although the data are incomplete, the prevalence of PE appears to be similar for patients with primary and secondary upper extremity DVT. Studies on jugular vein thrombosis are also sparse, but the available reports suggest a similar risk of PE compared with that of axillary-subclavian DVT.[24–25] It is generally believed that DVT occurring distal to the shoulder (i.e., in the brachial or forearm veins), as well as superficial venous thrombosis involving the cephalic and basilic veins, are both associated with a very low risk of PE. However, in a clinical review of patients with axillary-subclavian, isolated internal jugular, and isolated brachial DVT, no significant differences were noted among the three groups for mortality or the incidence of PE.[1] It is noteworthy that of 52 patients with isolated brachial DVT, PE was documented in 11.5%.

Right-Sided Heart Thromboembolism

The increased use of transesophageal echocardiography in patients with suspected PE has resulted in the more frequent detection of right-sided heart thromboembolism (RHTE).[26] This includes nonmobile and mobile thrombi located within the right atrium or right ventricle as well as thrombi on foreign bodies such as catheters and pacemaker wires. Highly mobile right-sided heart thrombi are more likely to be associated with PE and death than thrombi that are adherent to the atrial or ventricular walls. The overall mortality of RHTE is approximately 30%.[27–28] The presence of RHTE in association with PE appears to carry a higher mortality than PE alone. Treatment options for RHTE include direct surgical removal and thrombolysis; anticoagulation alone does not appear to be effective.

Recurrent Thrombosis

Patients with a first episode of upper extremity DVT are at risk for recurrent thrombosis. In a follow-up study of 224 patients with a first upper extremity DVT, the cumulative incidence of recurrence after 2 years was 8%.[29] Women had a twofold higher risk of recurrence than men. There was also a higher risk of recurrent thrombosis among patients with a BMI ≥25 kg/m^2. A decreased risk of recurrence was found for patients whose first upper extremity DVT was in the subclavian vein or related to a CVC. As in many of the other reported series of patients with upper extremity DVT, mortality was high and most often related to malignancy. The overall mortality rate was 25% (55 of 224 patients). The presence

TABLE 10-2. SYMPTOMS AND SIGNS IN THE AFFECTED ARM ASSOCIATED WITH POST-THROMBOTIC SYNDROME (PTS) OF THE UPPER EXTREMITY

Symptoms	Signs
Pain	Edema
Swelling	Tenderness
Heaviness	Skin induration
Paresthesia	Dilation of superficial veins
Pruritus	Hyperpigmentation
Functional limitation	Ulceration

of thrombophilia (factor V Leiden, prothrombin G20210A, and protein C, protein S, and antithrombin deficiency) also increases the risk of recurrent symptomatic upper extremity DVT.[30]

Post-Thrombotic Syndrome

The post-thrombotic syndrome (PTS) is best known as a complication of lower extremity DVT that results in chronic, debilitating symptoms of limb pain, heaviness, swelling, varicose veins, and in severe cases, skin hyperpigmentation and ulceration. This syndrome is caused by venous hypertension secondary to persistent venous outflow obstruction and valvular dysfunction. Manifestations of the PTS develop in 20 to 50% of patients after lower extremity DVT.[31] There is currently no standard definition for PTS in the upper extremity. The symptoms and signs that have been attributed to this condition are listed in Table 10–2. In a systematic review of seven clinical studies, the frequency of PTS after upper extremity DVT ranged from 7 to 46%, with a weighted average of 15%.[32] The presence of residual thrombus on ultrasound evaluation after upper extremity DVT was associated with a fourfold increase in risk for PTS.[18] Patients with thrombosis of the axillary and subclavian veins are 2.9 times more likely to develop PTS than those with upper extremity DVT at other sites. The PTS may be less frequent after CVC-associated upper extremity DVT than after other types of upper extremity DVT.

The effect of treatment with thrombolytic agents or anticoagulants on the incidence of PTS after upper extremity DVT is not known. Based on experience with lower extremity PTS, elastic bandages or compression sleeves have been used to control symptoms of pain and swelling in the involved arm, similar to the measures used for lymphedema.[3] One study has examined function and quality of life in patients with PTS of the upper extremity.[33] Twenty-five limbs in 24 patients were followed for a median of 13 months after the diagnosis of upper extremity DVT. Based on a standard clinical scale, 11 of 25 patients (46%) developed PTS. Patients with PTS had significantly more functional disability and poorer quality of life compared with those without PTS, according to both generic and disease-specific questionnaires. These measures showed an even greater impact when the PTS involved the dominant arm.

CONCLUSIONS

Primary and secondary upper extremity DVT are associated with significant complications that include PE, RHTE, recurrent thrombosis, and PTS. Patients with primary upper extremity DVT are typically young and relatively healthy, and they present with acute, severe signs and symptoms. Secondary upper extremity DVT is usually less symptomatic, but it is often associated with a severe underlying illness that is responsible for the high mortality rate.

Because venous thromboembolism can be regarded as a systemic disease with local manifestations, it is not surprising that upper and lower extremity DVT can coexist in the same patient. Among 211 patients with upper extremity DVT who also had lower extremity venous duplex examinations, 45 (21%) were found to have lower extremity DVT, and 8 of the remaining 166 patients with initially negative duplex scans developed a lower extremity DVT at a later date.[34] These data emphasize that patients with upper extremity DVT are also at high risk for DVT in the lower extremity.

REFERENCES

1. Hingorani A, Ascher E, Marks N, et al. Morbidity and mortality associated with brachial vein thrombosis. Ann Vasc Surg 2006;20:297–300.
2. Flinterman LE, Van der Meer FJM, Rosendahl FR, et al. Current perspective of venous thrombosis in the upper extremity. J Thromb Haemost 2008;6:1262–6.
3. Joffe HV, Goldhaber SZ. Upper-extremity deep vein thrombosis. Circulation 2002;106: 1874–80.
4. Girolami A, Prandoni P, Zanon E, et al. Venous thromboses of upper limbs are more frequently associated with occult cancer as compared with those of lower limbs. Blood Coagul Fibrinolysis 1999;8:455–7.
5. Lindblad B, Tengborn L, Bergqvist D. Deep vein thrombosis of the axillary-subclavian veins: epidemiologic data, effects of different types of treatment and late sequelae. Eur J Vasc Surg 1988;2:161–5.
6. Falk RL, Smith DF. Thrombosis of upper extremity thoracic inlet veins: diagnosis with duplex Doppler sonography. AJR Am J Roentgenol 1987;149:677–82.
7. Knudson GJ, Wiedmeyer DA, Erickson SJ, et al. Color Doppler sonographic imaging in the assessment of upper-extremity deep venous thrombosis. AJR Am J Roentgenol 1990;154: 399–403.
8. Haire WD, Lynch TG, Lieberman RP, et al. Utility of duplex ultrasound in the diagnosis of asymptomatic catheter-induced subclavian vein thrombosis. J Ultrasound Med 1991;10: 493–6.
9. Baxter GM, Kincaid W, Jeffrey RF et al. Comparison of colour Doppler ultrasound with venography in the diagnosis of axillary and subclavian vein thrombosis. Br J Radiol 1991; 64:777–81.
10. Koksoy C, Kuzu A, Kutlay J, et al. The diagnostic value of colour Doppler ultrasound in central venous catheter related thrombosis. Clin Radiol 1995;50:687–9.
11. Prandoni P, Polistena P, Bernardi E, et al. Upper-extremity deep vein thrombosis. Risk factors, diagnosis, and complications. Arch Intern Med 1997;157:57–62.
12. Baarslag HJ, van Beek EJ, Koopman MM, et al. Prospective study of color duplex ultrasonography compared with contrast venography in patients suspected of having deep venous thrombosis of the upper extremities. Ann Intern Med 2002;136:865–72.
13. Baarslag HJ, van Beek EJ, Tijssen JG, et al. Deep vein thrombosis of the upper extremity: intra- and interobserver study of digital subtraction venography. Eur Radiol 2003;13:251–5.
14. Kearon C, Kahn SR, Agnelli G, et al. Antithrombotic therapy for venous thromboembolic disease: American College of Chest Physicians Evidence-Based Clinical Practice Guidelines (8th Edition). Chest 2008;133:454–545.
15. Donayre CE, White GH, Mehringer SM, et al. Pathogenesis determines late morbidity of axillosubclavian vein thrombosis. Am J Surg 1986;152:179–84.

16. Wilson JJ, Zahn CA, Newman H. Fibrinolytic therapy for idiopathic subclavian-axillary vein thrombosis. Am J Surg 1990;159:208–10.
17. Marinella MA, Kathula SK, Markert RJ. Spectrum of upper-extremity deep venous thrombosis in a community teaching hospital. Heart Lung 2000;29:113–7.
18. Prandoni P, Bernardi E, Marchiori A, et al. The long term clinical course of acute deep vein thrombosis of the arm: prospective cohort study. BMJ 2004;329:484–5.
19. Hingorani A, Ascher E, Markevich N, et al. Risk factors for mortality in patients with upper extremity and internal jugular deep venous thrombosis. J Vasc Surg 2005;41:476–8.
20. Hingorani A, Ascher E, Hanson J, et al. Upper extremity versus lower extremity deep vein thrombosis. Am J Surg 1997;174:214–7.
21. Ascher E, Salles-Cunha S, Hingorani A. Morbidity and mortality associated with internal jugular vein thromboses. Vasc Endovascular Surg 2005;39:335–9.
22. Monreal M, Raventos A, Lerma R, et al. Pulmonary embolism in patients with upper extremity DVT associated to venous central lines—a prospective study. Thromb Haemost 1994;72:548–50.
23. Thomas IH, Zierler BK. An integrative review of outcomes in patients with acute primary upper extremity deep venous thrombosis following no treatment or treatment with anticoagulation, thrombolysis, or surgical algorithms. Vasc Endovascular Surg 2005;39:163–74.
24. Sheikh MA, Topoulos AP, Deitcher SR. Isolated internal jugular vein thrombosis: risk factors and natural history. Vasc Med 2002;7:177–9.
25. Major KM, Bulic S, Rowe VL, et al. Internal jugular, subclavian, and axillary deep venous thrombosis and the risk of pulmonary embolism. Vascular 2008;16:73–9.
26. Burns KEA, McLaren A. A critical review of thromboembolic complications associated with central venous catheters. Can J Anesth 2008;55:532–41.
27. Kinney EL, Wright RJ. Efficacy of treatment of patients with echocardiographically detected right-sided heart thrombi: a meta-analysis. Am Heart J 1989;118:569–73.
28. Rose PS, Punjabi NM, Pearsse DB. Tretament of right heart thromboemboli. Chest 2002; 121:806–14.
29. Flinterman LE, van Hylckama Vlieg A, Rosendaal FR, et al. Recurrent thrombosis and survival after a first venous thrombosis of the upper extremity. Circulation 2008;118:1366–72.
30. Martinelli I, Battaglioli T, Buciarelli P, et al. Risk factors and recurrence rate of primary deep vein thrombosis of the upper extremities. Circulation 2004;110:566–70.
31. Kahn SR, Ginsberg JS. The post-thrombotic syndrome: current knowledge, controversies, and directions for future research. Blood Rev 2002;16:155–65.
32. Elman EE, Kahn SR. The post-thrombotic syndrome after upper extremity deep venous thrombosis in adults: a systematic review. Thromb Res 2006;117:609–14.
33. Kahn SR, Elman EE, Bornais C, et al. Post-thrombotic syndrome, functional disability and quality of life after upper extremity deep venous thrombosis in adults. Thromb Haemost 2005;93:499–502.
34. Hingorani A, Ascher E, Markevich N, et al. Prospective evaluation of combined upper and lower extremity DVT. Vasc Endovasc Surg 2006;40:131–4.

11

Diagnosis of Neurogenic Thoracic Outlet Syndrome

Valerie B. Emery, R.N., Rahul Rastogi, M.D., Matt R. Driskill, M.S.P.T., and Robert W. Thompson, M.D.

INTRODUCTION

Thoracic outlet syndromes (TOSs) are rare conditions caused by compression of neurovascular structures within the anatomic space posterior to the clavicle and above the first rib (Figure 11–1). The most frequent of these conditions is *neurogenic thoracic outlet syndrome* (NTOS), representing 85 to 95% of all patients. NTOS is due to brachial plexus nerve root compression caused by a combination of congenital *variations in anatomy* (such as a cervical rib, anomalous scalene musculature, and/or aberrant fibrofascial bands) coupled with a history of *neck or upper extremity injury* that has resulted in scalene muscle spasm, fibrosis, and other pathologic changes.[1-4] Acquired changes in posture, abnormalities in neck and shoulder muscle mechanics, and excessive perineural fibrosis contribute to nerve compression in the scalene triangle.[5] An additional location of nerve compression in NTOS may occur just beyond the first rib, underneath the pectoralis minor muscle, producing the "hyperabduction" syndrome.[6-8] In some cases, NTOS may be combined with additional peripheral nerve compression disorders (e.g., carpal tunnel, cubital tunnel, and/or radial canal syndromes) or with cervical spine radiculopathy to produce what has been termed the "double-crush" phenomenon.[9-12]

In the presence of a congenital cervical rib, some patients with NTOS present with weakness, overt electrophysiologic abnormalities, and thenar or hypothenar muscle atrophy (Gilliatt-Sumner hand).[13–14] Although this clinical presentation has been termed "true" NTOS, these findings may simply represent a particularly advanced form of NTOS with long-standing and possibly irretrievable nerve injury. In contrast, most patients with NTOS exhibit varying degrees of *sensory symptoms* with no hand muscle weakness or atrophy and have normal or nonspecific findings on conventional electrophysiologic testing and/or imaging studies. These individuals are identified primarily through comprehensive clinical diagnosis and the exclusion of other conditions. Because there remain no validated objective tests by which to definitively estab-

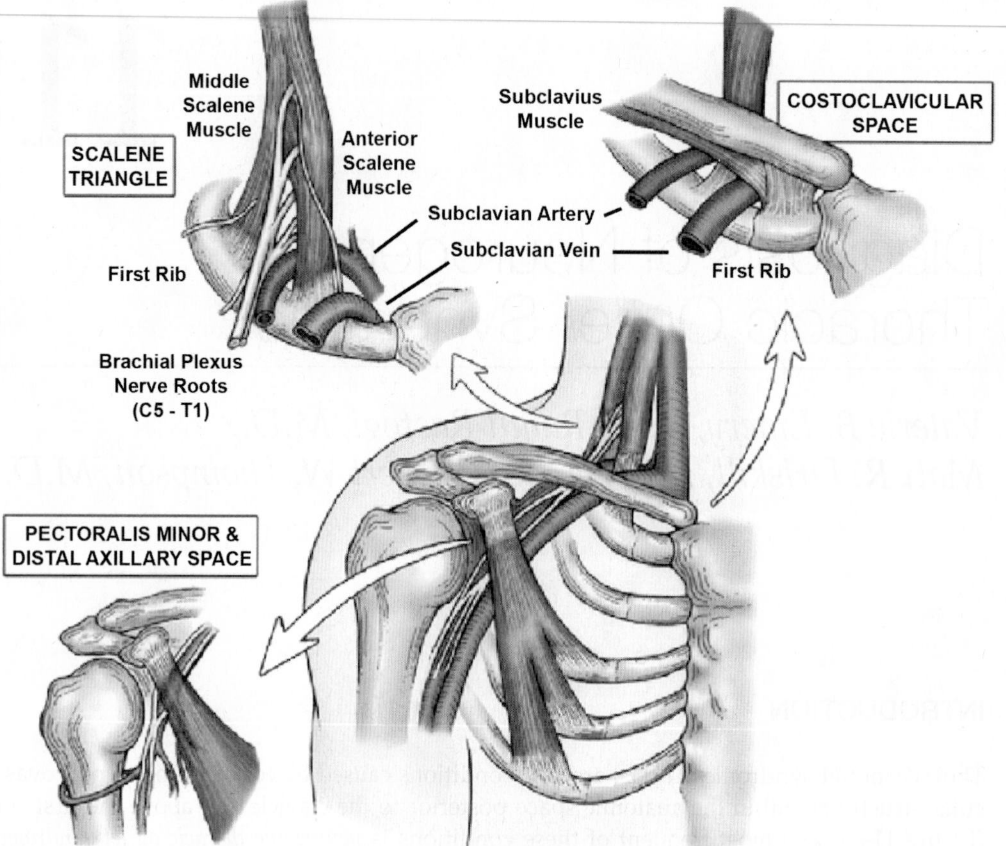

Figure 11-1. Anatomy of the Thoracic Outlet. Standard anatomic relationships between the neurovascular structures and the musculoskeletal components of the thoracic outlet. Brachial plexus compression resulting in NTOS may occur at one or more of three levels: the scalene triangle, the costoclavicular space, or the subpectoralis space.

lish the diagnosis of brachial plexus compression in such patients, these individuals are often considered to have "nonspecific" or "disputed" NTOS. Such modifying terms for NTOS have not been found to be particularly helpful, either in understanding the condition or in clinical evaluation and management, and they have been largely discarded.

NTOS is clinically important because when it goes unrecognized and/or is inadequately treated, it can cause chronic pain syndromes and/or long-term restriction in use of the upper extremities and because it produces substantial disability in relatively young, active, and otherwise healthy individuals in the prime of their working lives. Accurate diagnosis of NTOS remains a significant challenge in clinical practice; yet properly identified patients can respond quite well to treatment. At present, NTOS is initially treated with physical therapy and occupational rehabilitation approaches to relieve scalene/pectoralis muscle spasm, improve relevant postural disturbances, enhance functional limb mobility, strengthen associated shoulder girdle musculature, and diminish repetitive strain exposure or overuse in the workplace.[5,15-21] Pharmacologic management typically includes nonsteroidal anti-inflammatory agents, muscle relaxants, and analgesics as needed. In some cases, localized injection of botulinum toxin is utilized to produce chemodenervation of muscles thought to be responsible for brachial plexus nerve root compression, particularly the anterior and middle scalene and/or pectoralis minor.[22-24] Surgical treatment is considered in patients with substantial disability in whom conservative measures have failed to produce sufficient clinical improvement. Operative treatment is based on removing one or more of the structures considered responsible for brachial plexus nerve root compression, including the anterior and middle scalene muscles, any additional scalene muscle anomalies or fibrofascial bands that may be encountered, the first rib (and cervical rib if present), and fibrous scar tissue that may have accumulated around the brachial plexus nerve roots; in some patients, pectoralis minor tenotomy may also be performed, either as an isolated procedure or in combination with supraclavicular or transaxillary decompression.[1,3,25-46]

NTOS can be readily differentiated from venous TOS, which produces marked arm swelling, cyanotic discoloration, and distention of subcutaneous veins around the shoulder and chest wall; it also often presents with the axillosubclavian vein "effort thrombosis" syndrome. NTOS is also distinguished from arterial TOS, which causes fixed subclavian obstruction resulting in cramping muscular fatigue with arm use similar to what occurs with intermittent claudication or poststenotic subclavian artery aneurysm formation that can cause thromboembolism, hand ischemia, rest pain, and/or digital ulceration and necrosis. The symptoms, diagnosis, and management of NTOS often overlap with other upper extremity neurologic and musculoskeletal disorders, producing a particularly broad differential diagnosis (Table 11–1). Many of the unresolved issues surrounding NTOS revolve around defining the most accurate criteria to differentiate this condition from other cervical-brachial syndromes and the optimal means to select patients for different forms of treatment. Thus, long-standing effort has been exerted to establish testing procedures that can better predict outcomes

TABLE 11-1. DIFFERENTIAL DIAGNOSIS OF NTOS

Condition	Differentiating Features
Carpal tunnel syndrome	Hand pain and paresthesia in median nerve distribution; positive findings on nerve conduction studies; treatment with physical/occupational therapy or surgical decompression.
Cubital canal syndrome	Hand pain and paresthesia in ulnar nerve distribution; positive findings on nerve conduction studies; treatment with physical/occupational therapy or surgical mobilization.
Rotator cuff tendinitis	Localized pain and tenderness over biceps tendon and shoulder pain on abduction; positive findings on MRI; relief from NSAIDs, local steroid injections or arthroscopic surgery.
Cervical spine strain	Post-traumatic neck pain and stiffness localized posteriorly along cervical spine; paraspinal tenderness; relief with conservative measures over weeks to months.
Cervical disk disease	Neck pain and stiffness, arm weakness, and paresthesia involving thumb and index finger (C5-6 disk); symptom improvement with arm elevation; positive findings on CT or MRI.
Cervical arthritis	Neck pain and stiffness; arm or hand paresthesia infrequent; degenerative rather than post-traumatic; positive findings on spine radiographs.
Fibromyositis	Post-traumatic inflammation of trapezius and parascapular muscles; tenderness, spasm and palpable nodules over affected muscles; may coexist with TOS and persist after surgery.

(Continued)

TABLE 11-1. DIFFERENTIAL DIAGNOSIS OF NTOS *(Continued)*

Condition	Differentiating Features
Brachial plexus injury	Caused by direct injury or stretch; arm pain and weakness, hand paresthesias; symptoms constant not intermittent or positional; positive findings on neurophysiologic studies.
Acromioclavicular joint	Localized pain and tenderness over AC joint; arthritis/bursitis on MRI; responds to NSAIDs, local steroid injections, or distal claviculectomy.
Fibromyalgia	Pain and tenderness in multiple (>10) muscle sites; responds to trigger point injections.
Vasculitis	Digital ischemia or arm claudication; diagnosis by arteriography and serologic tests; treatment with systemic steroids; arterial bypass of proximal occlusive lesions once quiescent.
Atheroembolism	Digital ischemia with localized fixed skin changes/mottling in the presence of radial/ulnar pulses, proximal atherosclerotic arterial source detected by CT/MR/contrast arteriography, often follows intravascular catheterization, surgical manipulation, or Coumadin treatment; treatment by removal of proximal source, oral vasodilators, or intra-arterial vasodilator infusion; consider sympathetic blocks/sympathectomy; digital amputation when necessary.
Raynaud's syndrome	Episodic digital vasospasm, often cold- or activity-induced; absence of serologic/rheumatologic findings; treatment with oral vasodilators and avoidance of cold exposure; cervical sympathetic blocks or sympathectomy only for nonhealing lesions with threatened tissue loss.
Scleroderma	Sustained digital vasospasm with ischemic ulceration; systemic manifestations, elevated ESR and serologic tests; conservative management of digital lesions with oral vasodilators; consider sympathetic blocks/sympathectomy; digital amputation when necessary.
CRPS/RSD	Chronic pain syndrome with digital vasospasm and allodynia in extremity/neck, usually following relatively minor trauma; diagnosis by response to sympathetic blockade; comprehensive pain management with serial cervical sympathetic blocks or cervical sympathectomy.
Cervical dystonia	Severe, spontaneous, repetitive neck muscle spasm; responds to Botox injections.
Lymphedema	Nonpitting arm edema in absence of venous obstruction; responds to compression and massage.
Psychogenic syndrome	Debilitating symptoms, often chronic pain, with no definable pathophysiologic abnormality; counseling, psychiatric consultation, and comprehensive pain management required.
Parsonage-Turner syndrome	Spontaneous brachial neuritis resolving within 3 weeks; no specific treatment.
Nerve sheath neoplasm	Neck or axillary mass and neurologic deficit; well detected by MRI; treatment by resection.
Pancoast tumor	Apical lung neoplasm; brachial plexus, sympathetic chain, or subclavian vessel involvement; detected by CT/MRI; treatment by resection with/without radiation/chemotherapy.
Catheter-induced thrombosis	Central venous access or pacemaker; initial treatment by catheter removal; anticoagulation.
Primary thrombosis	Hypercoagulable disorder with spontaneous thrombosis at multiple sites or times; defined by laboratory coagulation studies; treatment with anticoagulant and/or antiplatelet medications.
Arterial embolism	Digital ischemia with a defined proximal source of thromboembolism, possibly with acute ischemia and/or tissue loss; detected by CT/MR/contrast angiography; treatment by exclusion of proximal artery source, anticoagulation, oral vasodilators; consider arterial vasodilator infusion or cervical sympathectomy.

of treatment, including various forms of soft tissue imaging,[47-52] improvements in electrophysiologic testing,[53-56] the application of selective scalene and pectoralis muscle blocks,[24] and ongoing refinement of clinical criteria.

PATIENT POPULATION

NTOS is most frequently seen between the ages of 20 and 40 years and over 50% of those affected are women. There are no known disease conditions that specifically predispose to NTOS, and most patients have been otherwise healthy and physically active prior to the onset of symptoms. NTOS often occurs in individuals engaged in occupational or recreational activities that involve repetitive overhead use of the arms and/or heavy lifting, and it may develop following various types of injury to the head, neck, or upper extremity (e.g., motor vehicle collisions or falls upon the outstretched arm). The presence of a cervical rib is often cited as a predisposing factor in the development of NTOS. However, few patients with NTOS actually exhibit a definable cervical rib or first rib anomaly, and the development of symptoms of NTOS is rare, even in patients with known cervical ribs in the absence of additional injury. NTOS may also develop in patients with no apparent predisposition, due to either anatomic variations or a history of trauma. Although the incidence and overall prevalence of NTOS are unknown, data from the Nationwide Inpatient Sample suggest that there are approximately 1900 operations performed for this condition each year in the United States.[57] Because surgical treatment is required in fewer than 10% of patients with NTOS, these findings indicate that approximately 20,000 new patients undergo treatment each year. The actual prevalence of NTOS is probably substantially higher, as patients are often symptomatic for long periods of time prior to diagnosis and are frequently treated for years with nonsurgical approaches.

PRESENTING SYMPTOMS

The principal symptoms of NTOS are pain, numbness, and tingling (paresthesias) in the arm and hand. These symptoms may be accompanied by a perception of weakness in using the arm or hand, particularly in elevated positions, although actual muscle weakness or visible muscle atrophy is rare. The symptoms of NTOS are typically present throughout the affected arm or hand without specific localization to a single peripheral nerve or cervical nerve root distribution, and they often involve different areas of the entire upper extremity. Thus, symptoms in the hand may involve all fingers, thereby extending beyond the typical sensory distribution of either the median or the ulnar nerves. Symptoms that might otherwise appear to be related to the median or ulnar nerve distributions often extend above the level of the wrist or elbow, respectively, implying a more proximal site of nerve compression than the carpal tunnel or cubital canal. Some have attempted to differentiate symptomatic presentations of NTOS based on the brachial plexus nerve roots that appear to be principally involved, with "upper plexus" disorders (nerve roots C5, C6, C7) dominated by symptoms in the distribution of the radial and musculocutaneous nerves, and "lower plexus" disorders (nerve roots C7, C8, T1) most commonly involving the median and ulnar nerves. In many cases, it is not possible to draw these distinctions because of a wider distribution of symptoms; indeed, it is not uncommon for patients to describe an extension of symptoms from the hand to include the shoulder, neck, and upper back, and in many the neck or upper back symptoms are perceived to be the most functionally disabling. Most patients with NTOS have symptoms affecting just one upper extremity; however, bilateral symptoms are not uncommon. Although the dominant extremity is often more symptomatic at first presentation, the opposite extremity may become involved over time, perhaps as a result of compensatory overuse in protecting the affected extremity.

An important aspect of NTOS is that almost all patients describe reproducible exacerbation of symptoms with arm elevation or sustained overhead use of the arms or hands. Such activities include reaching for objects or lifting with the outstretched arm, throwing or catching, prolonged typing or work at computer consoles, driving a motor vehicle, holding a phone, and combing, brushing, or drying the hair. Positional complaints consistent with NTOS may even be brought on while lying supine, especially when the arms are positioned overhead, resulting in pain, numbness, tingling, and difficulty sleeping.

Headaches are a common but often overlooked symptom of NTOS.[58] This is most frequently exhibited as a result of referred pain to the back of the neck and head, due to secondary spasm within the trapezius and paraspinous muscles. Headaches associated with NTOS are typically occipital in nature, whereas frontal headaches are not specifically associated with brachial plexus compression. Although many patients with NTOS also have migraine headaches, there is no clear pathophysiologic association between these two conditions.

Prolonged peripheral nerve compression can result in muscle weakness and atrophy, but such findings are actually rare in patients with NTOS. This is probably due to the intermittent nature of brachial plexus nerve compression in NTOS, which produces pain and other sensory symptoms but prevents permanent motor nerve dysfunction. The presence of objective muscle weakness or atrophy may therefore indicate particularly severe and long-standing compression of the brachial plexus nerve roots, due to either NTOS or another condition. Because hand or arm pain with use of the affected extremity may lead to the perception of weakness in patients with NTOS, these symptoms should be clearly distinguished from objective muscle weakness or detectable atrophy to help identify other neuromuscular conditions that may be present.

The majority of individuals with NTOS have only positional upper extremity complaints and are affected to a mild and tolerable degree. These symptoms are usually due to transient irritation of the brachial plexus in certain positions or activities of the arm, and to some extent they are frequent in the normal population. There is little risk of progressive injury in these situations and most will improve with conservative management, not requiring more specific interventions. In contrast, there remains a smaller subset of patients with clinically significant NTOS who exhibit progressively disabling symptoms that effectively prevent them from working or carrying out simple daily activities. These patients often describe progressive disability, a long history of specialist physician consultations, and multiple partial or ineffective treatments. They may have been prevented from working for long periods of time prior to consultation or may have attempted to persist in work-related activities despite ongoing neurogenic symptoms. An important part of the initial assessment is concerned with evaluating the extent of the patient's disability and expectations for continuing or returning to work. It is particularly helpful to obtain a detailed description from the patient of activities that exacerbate symptoms associated with NTOS as well as those activities normally required in the workplace. Documentation of this assessment is often required if relief from work is necessary in initial management and in guiding later decisions about surgical treatment.

Upper extremity vascular symptoms should be specifically sought in the history of patients with suspected NTOS, and descriptions of cold sensations or intermittent discoloration in the hands and fingers are not uncommon in those with long-standing or severe symptoms. This type of vasomotor disturbance is thought to result from associated sympathetic overactivity. In some situations, the symptoms of NTOS may have progressed to resemble those of complex regional pain syndrome (CRPS; formerly known as causalgia or reflex sympathetic dystrophy), with persistent vasospasm, disuse edema, and extreme hypersensitivity (allodynia). The acuity of these symptoms often leads to avoidance and withdrawal from even a light touch of the affected extremity. In most cases, the diagnosis of associated CRPS can be made on clinical grounds but may be supported by vascular laboratory studies (revealing abnormal vasoconstrictive responses in the cold-pressor test), imaging studies of the hand (assessing microcirculation and osseous changes), and cervical sympathetic (stellate) ganglion blocks. The identification of coexisting CRPS is quite important in patients with NTOS because it may require different considerations for operative treatment, such as concomitant use of cervical sympathectomy.

In the presence of a history suggesting arterial insufficiency or thromboembolism, vascular laboratory studies and contrast-enhanced arteriographic imaging are necessary to exclude the presence of subclavian artery stenosis or aneurysm. Conversely, a history of arm swelling, cyanotic discoloration, and distended subcutaneous collaterals may indicate venous TOS due to obstruction of the subclavian vein, which requires contrast venography for full evaluation. At present we find contrast-enhanced magnetic resonance angiography (MRA), with the arms at rest and in an overhead position, to be the most useful noninvasive approach to vascular forms of TOS. Identification of associated vascular conditions is vital in patients with NTOS, because the coexistence of neurogenic and vascular forms of TOS will have a substantial impact on decisions and planning for surgical treatment.

PHYSICAL EXAMINATION

Physical examination is initially directed toward identifying particular factors that exacerbate painful hand and arm complaints and determining the degree of neurogenic disability. The resting posture is assessed while the patient is sitting comfortably, often revealing the "slumped-forward" position of the head and neck that commonly accompanies NTOS. The patient is initially asked to describe any symptoms present at rest and to clarify their distribution. The presence of any swelling, edema, discoloration, or distention of subcutaneous veins in the upper extremities is noted, and arterial perfusion of the hands is evaluated with assessment of color, capillary refill, digital vasospasm, emboli, ulcerations, and palpation of the radial, ulnar, and brachial artery pulses. The hands are evaluated for evidence of thenar or hypothenar muscle atrophy and weakness of hand-grip strength. Weakness of the fifth finger is often present in NTOS, which can be assessed by having the patient press the tips of the fifth finger and thumb together and evaluating resistance while the examiner attempts to pull them apart. Thorough examination of the peripheral nerves by palpation and assessment for Tinel's sign is performed to determine if there is evidence of median nerve compression at the carpal tunnel, ulnar nerve entrapment at the cubital canal, or radial nerve compression in the extensor forearm. The range of motion of the upper extremities is then assessed under both passive and active conditions, with the patient asked to identify any exacerbation of pain, numbness, or tingling along with their specific distribution. Evidence of scapular winging is sought with the arms outstretched in front of the patient and placed through a range of motion.

The effects of arm elevation on the strength of the radial pulse or visible changes in perfusion of the hand are evaluated during the Adson maneuver. When the patient describes an increase in neurogenic symptoms during arm elevation, it is specifically noted whether there is a concomitant decrease in the radial pulse. It is notable that many patients with NTOS exhibit a pale color in the affected hand during elevation, sometimes referred to as the "white hand sign." Careful examination often reveals that this is due to sympathetic vasoconstriction rather than detectable changes in the pulse caused by subclavian artery compression, although the two findings may coexist. It is important to recognize that a positive Adson sign is also quite common in the asymptomatic general population. This maneuver may therefore serve to support but not prove the diagnosis of NTOS, and it is equally important to recognize that negative findings of subclavian artery compression do not exclude a diagnosis of NTOS. Thus, many physicians with experience in the management of NTOS find the Adson test of little diagnostic value.

Range of motion of the neck is evaluated with respect to both lateral turning and flexion toward the shoulder (head-tilt), with the symptoms of NTOS elicited on the opposite side, and Spurling's sign and the axial compression test are used to identify symptoms associated with the cervical spine. The clavicle and sternoclavicular joint are examined to identify any focal tenderness or palpable deformity that might be associated with a previous fracture or dislocation. Pain and tenderness over the shoulder joint are evaluated as potentially related to rotator cuff tears, biceps tendinitis, or degenerative conditions of the acromioclavicular joint. Palpation over the sternocleidomastoid, trapezius, parascapular, and paraspinous muscles is used to localize specific areas that reproduce symptoms of pain. The presence of multiple muscular "trigger points" is a characteristic feature of fibromyalgia, another condition that can overlap with NTOS.

A critical aspect of the physical examination is palpation of the supraclavicular space to determine the presence of scalene muscle spasm, localized tenderness, and reproduction of upper extremity symptoms. Almost all patients with NTOS exhibit both tenderness over the scalene triangle and exacerbation of pain and numbness and tingling in the arm and/or hand upon supraclavicular palpation, whereas these findings are infrequent in patients with other cervicobrachial syndromes. Palpable spasm in the anterior scalene muscle is not uncommon in NTOS, and a firm supraclavicular mass may also be palpable in patients with a complete cervical rib anomaly.

Palpation over the infraclavicular space is used to help identify those with symptoms related to brachial plexus compression at the level of the pectoralis minor muscle, which occurs in 30 to 50% of patients with NTOS. The pectoralis minor can usually be identified by palpation over the lateral infraclavicular space just below the coracoid process, medial to the deltopectoral groove. Mild pressure over the muscle is often accompanied by reproduction of upper extremity symptoms that are not present with palpation over the medial infraclavicular area. Relief of symptoms while having the patient simultaneously contract the superimposed pectoralis major muscle, which prevents transfer of digital pressure to the underlying pectoralis minor during this maneuver, helps distinguish the pectoralis minor syndrome from more generalized muscle tenderness.

Provocative positional maneuvers remain one of the most important components of the examination for NTOS, because the symptoms of brachial plexus compression are usually specifically exacerbated by elevated arm positioning. The "upper limb tension test" (ULTT) is performed by having the patient place both arms at 90 degrees of abduction from the trunk with the elbows extended and the palms flat. Reproduction of arm or hand symptoms during wrist extension, with some degree of relief during wrist flexion, is a frequent finding in those with NTOS. Perhaps the most widely used and informative provocative maneuver is the "elevated arm stress test" (EAST), in which the patient is positioned with the arms elevated in a 90/90 degree "surrender" position and asked to repetitively open and close the hands for up to 3 minutes. Patients are asked to describe all changes in the nature and distribution of symptoms in the neck and upper extremity and are instructed to lower the arms if unable to continue due to pain. Most patients with NTOS report the rapid onset of typical upper extremity symptoms within 20 to 30 seconds of initiating the EAST and are often unable to continue the exercise beyond 60 seconds. Indeed, the diagnosis of NTOS is suspect when there is no difficulty performing the EAST for 3 minutes, and an alternative explanation for the symptoms should be considered.

IMAGING STUDIES

NTOS is considered to be caused by functionally significant anatomic compression of the brachial plexus nerve roots within and adjacent to the scalene triangle. A number of structures and anatomic variations have been described in the thoracic outlet region based on observations during surgical operations and in cadaver studies.[47-52,59-68] In addition to congenital cervical ribs and first rib anomalies, which are present in <1% of the population,[41] there are a variety of soft tissue abnormalities that can affect the brachial plexus.[26] It has been considered for many years that radiographic imaging might be applied to help define these anatomic features in the assessment of patients with a clinical diagnosis of NTOS.

Plain radiographs of the neck are helpful in determining if an osseous cervical rib or abnormally wide transverse process of the seventh cervical vertebra is present. Although each of these findings may solidify a diagnostic impression of NTOS, neither of them is essential and in most patients the results are negative. Additional imaging studies, such as computed tomography (CT) and magnetic resonance imaging (MRI), may be important to exclude other conditions that could be responsible for upper extremity symptoms, including degenerative cervical disk or spine disease, shoulder joint pathology, and various forms of intracranial pathology.

The results of CT and MRI of the brachial plexus are usually negative in patients with NTOS, because the anatomy leading to intermittent or positional nerve compression is usually beyond the resolution of these studies. Even in situations in which an apparent imaging abnormality exists in the region of the scalene triangle, it is difficult to prove the functional importance of such abnormalities with respect to specific upper extremity complaints. More recent approaches using contrast-enhanced MRI "neurography" have the capacity to provide far greater anatomic detail of the thoracic outlet than previously available, and several investigators have described successful use of MRI in patients with NTOS.[50-52,62] Unfortunately, anatomic variations in the thoracic outlet region are relatively frequent and it has not yet been firmly established whether the detection of specific findings will be helpful in diagnosis or prediction of treatment outcomes. At present, the presence of radiographic abnormalities cannot be considered either necessary or sufficient for the existence of clinically apparent NTOS until correlations between imaging findings and clinical assessment have been evaluated with sufficient rigor to guide treatment.

ELECTROPHYSIOLOGIC TESTING

Nerve conduction (NC) and electromyographic (EMG) studies are usually performed during the initial evaluation of patients suspected of having NTOS. These studies are particularly useful when positive electrophysiologic results can confirm another specific condition that must be evaluated further, such as cervical radiculopathy, peripheral nerve syndromes or a general myopathy. However, the results of conventional NC/EMG studies are usually negative in NTOS, because nerve root compression occurs in an extremely proximal location and because nerve root compression in NTOS is intermittent and not usually associated with permanent changes in motor nerve function.[69] Indeed, positive NC/EMG findings in patients with NTOS may be considered a relatively poor prognostic finding (in the absence of an alternative explanation), potentially indicating an advanced stage of neural damage unlikely to resolve even with adequate thoracic outlet decompression.

Several studies have suggested that NC studies of the medial antebrachial cutaneous (MAC) nerve may provide a more sensitive and specific test for NTOS.[53-55,70-77] As illustrated in Figure 11–2 A, the MAC nerve is derived from the C8 and T1 nerve roots and it arises from the medial cord of the brachial plexus, immediately proximal to the origin of the ulnar nerve. It passes along the medial aspect of the upper arm and emerges from the deep fascia, along with the basilic vein, just proximal to the antecubital space. The sensory distribution of the MAC nerve encompasses the medial forearm to the wrist. The proximal origin of the MAC nerve within and just distal to the scalene triangle and the correspondence of its distribution to a pattern of sensory symptoms frequently observed in patients with NTOS has suggested a useful target for diagnostic studies. Seror first reported the use of MAC studies in 16 patients with NTOS in whom conventional NC/EMG studies were normal.[73] The utility of MAC NC studies was further supported by Machanic and Sanders in evaluating patients with a clinical diagnosis of NTOS in comparison to asymptomatic healthy volunteers as well as in patients in whom MAC NC studies were repeated 3 months after thoracic outlet decompression (Figure 11–2 B-C).[56] The high sensitivity and specificity observed in this study suggest that MAC NC studies may provide a novel and reliable electrophysiologic test by which to help confirm the clinical diagnosis of NTOS.

SCALENE/PECTORALIS MUSCLE BLOCKS

Infiltration of local anesthetics into the anterior scalene muscle (ASM) was introduced over 10 years ago by Jordan et al. as a means to improve the diagnosis of NTOS and to help predict outcomes of treatment.[78] This approach was based on the recognition that reversible muscle relaxation during ASM block can temporarily decompress neural elements passing through the thoracic outlet. This occurs through relief of compression exerted directly by ASM spasm as well as through indirect effects to decrease narrowing of the costoclavicular space. Successful ASM blocks are associated with prompt improvement in symptoms of numbness, tingling, pain, and fatigability of the affected limb in patients with NTOS and

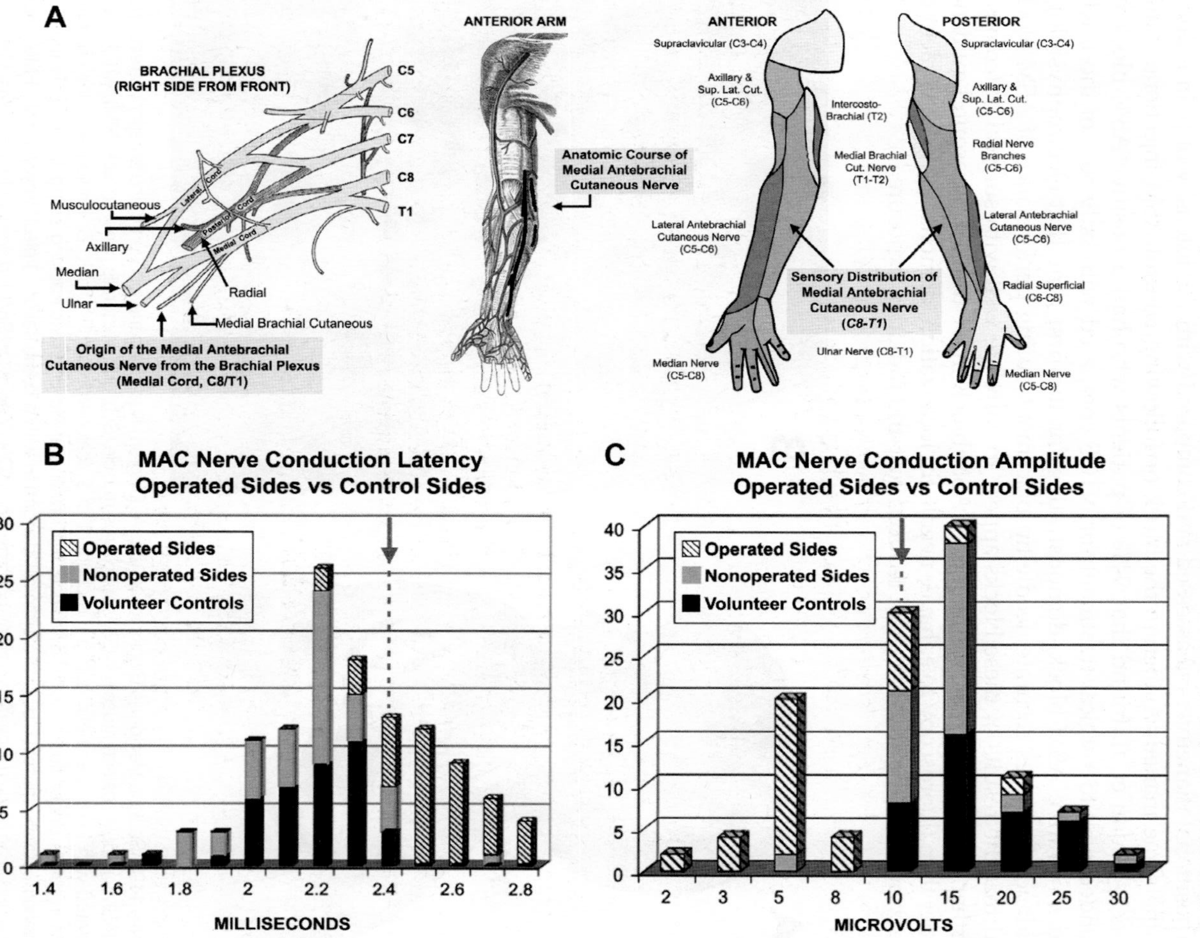

Figure 11-2. Nerve Conduction Studies of the Median Antebrachial Cutaneous Nerve. **A:** Anatomy of the median antebrachial cutaneous (MAC) nerve. **B** and **C:** MAC nerve conduction studies were performed prior to surgery in 41 patients with NTOS (operated and nonoperated sides, n = 41 each) and in 19 healthy volunteers (n = 38 sides). MAC nerve conduction latency values above or below a threshold of 2.4 msec had a specificity of 99% and a sensitivity of 73% in the diagnosis of NTOS (P<.001) (B), while MAC amplitude values above or below a threshold of 10 uV had a specificity of 97% and a sensitivity of 68% (P<.001) (C). (Data adapted from Machanic and Sanders).[56]

are thereby thought to strongly confirm the diagnosis otherwise based on clinical criteria. Sanders and others have reported a strong correlation between the relief of symptoms following scalene muscle block and the success of surgical decompression.[78-80]

Techniques for ASM block initially used surface landmarks. However, spread of anesthetic into surrounding tissues results in inadvertent somatic and/or sympathetic blockade, which can impair interpretation of the results. Increasingly rigorous testing protocols have been developed to improve the sensitivity and specificity of this technique (Figure 11–3).[22,78] To help improve needle tip localization, percutaneous insertion of an insulated hypodermic needle into the ASM is guided by EMG monitoring from the needle tip, with stimulation used to verify that the needle tip is not in the brachial plexus. After instillation of local anesthetic into the ASM, the intensity of pain induced by positional maneuvers is assessed and compared with the intensity of pain induced by the same maneuvers before the block or following control ASM injections (saline alone). Jordan et al. found that 94% of patients who had a positive ASM block responded well to surgical treatment for NTOS compared with only 50% of those who had a negative ASM block, demonstrating for the first time that electrophysiologic guidance facilitates accurate needle tip placement during performance of ASM blocks and that the results of these blocks appear to correlate well with surgical outcomes.[22] Further refinements in the technique for ASM blocks have utilized ultrasound guidance rather than fluoroscopy to enhance needle tip localization, demonstrating equivalent efficacy but with the advantages of reduced cost and radiation exposure.[23]

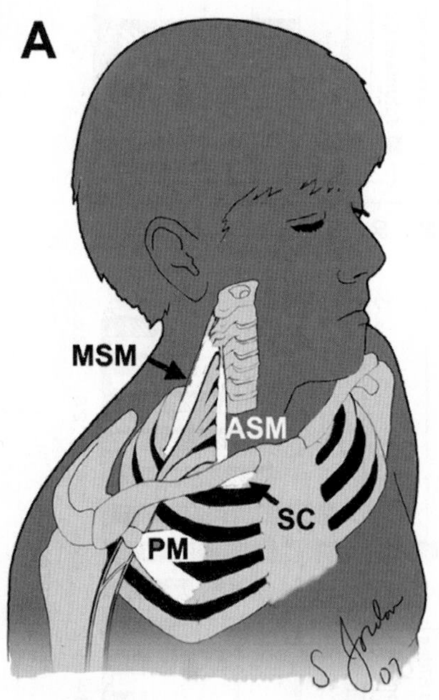

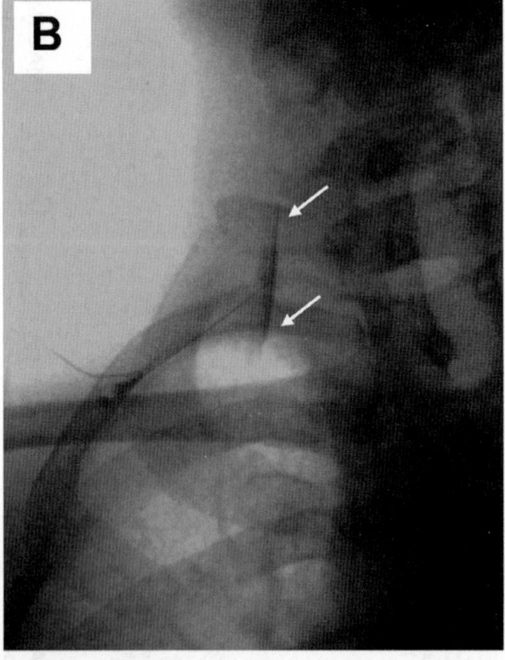

Figure 11-3. Scalene/Pectoralis Blocks for NTOS. **A:** Diagram illustrating the location of the anterior scalene muscle (ASM), middle scalene muscle (MSM), subclavius muscle (SC), and pectoralis minor muscle (PM), which are all infiltrated with local anesthetic during the conduct of a scalene/pectoralis block. **B:** Radiograph demonstrating ASM injection under fluoroscopic guidance, with radiographic contrast tracking along the muscle (arrows). Scalene/pectoralis muscle blocks are optimally performed with a combination of electromyographic (EMG) monitoring and imaging guidance (fluoroscopy or ultrasound). (Courtesy of Dr. Sheldon Jordan, Los Angeles, CA.)

CLINICAL PREDICTORS OF RESPONSE TO TREATMENT

Beyond the use of scalene blocks, there are currently few criteria that have been thoroughly evaluated by which to predict responses to treatment for NTOS. In one recent investigation, Axelrod et al. evaluated associations between psychological and socioeconomic characteristics and the long-term outcomes of operative treatment.[40] They examined 170 patients with an average follow-up of 47 months after thoracic outlet decompression, with 65% reporting improved symptoms and 64% being satisfied with their operative outcome; however, 35% of patients remained on medication and 18% were disabled. Based on multivariate logistic regression models, three independent preoperative risk factors were identified to have a significant association with persistent postoperative disability: major depression, unmarried status, and low educational attainment (less than high school).

To acquire further understanding of preoperative factors that influence outcome in NTOS, Jordan et al. examined a variety of clinical features and the results of a patient self-assessment survey they developed for this purpose: the Cervical-Brachial Symptom Questionnaire (CBSQ).[24] The CBSQ was initially validated in a group of 50 patients, with a test-retest reliability of 0.87 and an internal consistency of 0.93 (Cronbach's alpha). In 140 patients, the correlation between CBSQ and the Brief Pain Inventory (BPI) was 0.70, and the responsiveness to change, when comparing patients before and after treatment, was excellent. A prospective series of 85 patients were then evaluated for at least 6 months after treatment for NTOS. As shown in Table 11-2, a positive scalene block was significantly associated with a treatment-responsive condition. Significant predictors of treatment-resistant NTOS included (1) a coexisting widespread pain syndrome, (2) past surgery for a cervical-brachial condition other than NTOS, (3) widespread sensory

TABLE 11-2. CLINICAL FEATURES AND RESPONSIVENESS TO TREATMENT FOR NTOS

	Treatment-Responsive	Treatment-Resistant	Difference
Patients studied	n = 59	n = 26	
Disability status	49%	69%	NS*
Ongoing worker's compensation claim	46%	27%	NS*
Positive scalene block	100%	38%	P<.01*
Ultrasound abnormalities in neck	80%	65%	NS*
Decreased arterial flow in hyperabduction	34%	34%	NS*
Comorbid widespread pain syndrome	12%	81%	P<.01*
Past surgery for other than TOS	17%	50%	P=.01*
Wide sensory symptoms upper arm/face	10%	42%	P=.01*
Weakness extending beyond lower trunk	12%	29%	P=.01*
Presence of depression	10%	35%	P<.01*
BPI rating (combined pain + interference)	78.5 ± 25	79.2 ± 16	NS†
CBSQ Rating	78.5 ± 25	94.1 ± 17	P=0.039†

BPI = Brief Pain Inventory.
CBSQ = Cervical-Brachial Symptom Questionare.
NS = Not Significant.
*Fisher's exact test, 2-tailed.
†Mann-Whitney U test.
Data from Jordan et al.[24]

symptoms involving the upper arm and/or face, (4) weakness extending beyond the lower trunk dermatomes, and (5) the presence of depression. In addition, 92% of treatment-resistant patients had the combination of either a negative scalene block or a coexisting widespread pain syndrome as compared with 12% of the treatment-responsive patients, and pretreatment CBSQ scores were significantly higher in the treatment-resistant patients as compared with the treatment-responsive group.

CONSENSUS-BASED DIAGNOSTIC CRITERIA

Factors limiting efforts to compare outcomes of treatment for NTOS include the diverse diagnostic criteria that are used in various studies and a corresponding lack of uniformity in patient populations. To help address this issue, we and others recently began a multidisciplinary effort to facilitate comparative-effectiveness research, the Consortium for Outcomes Research and Education on Thoracic Outlet Syndrome (CORE-TOS). One of the first tasks of the CORE-TOS planning group was to undertake a consensus-building process to establish a defined set of diagnostic criteria for NTOS. This was achieved utilizing a Delphi process approach, a group-consensus strategy that has been widely utilized in other specialties of medicine.[81-83]

The CORE-TOS planning group first identified a broad list of 223 clinical features considered to be potentially important in establishing a diagnosis of NTOS, including features related to (a) history, (b) symptoms, (c) physical examination, and (d) tests and studies. These data elements also included clinical features associated with poor clinical outcomes of treatment in patients with NTOS in previous studies, including signs and symptoms of depression, fibromyalgia, CRPS, peripheral nerve compression syndromes, and coexisting musculoskeletal disorders.[24,40] A panel of experienced clinicians with expertise in the care of patients with NTOS participated in the survey process. In the first round of the Delphi survey, 162 of the initial 223 features were considered to be of potential diagnostic value by >50% of the evaluators. These features were then modified and/or consolidated, and additional features were added for more specificity. In a second round of evaluation, the consensus panel evaluated 242 features of which 183 were considered to be of potential value by >50% of evaluators. In the third and subsequent rounds, panel members were asked to score each feature with respect to (1) the "proportion of patients with a cervical-brachial syndrome attributed to NTOS that would be expected to exhibit that feature" (diagnostic sensitivity) and (2) the "proportion of patients with a cervical-brachial syndrome not attributed to NTOS that would be expected to exhibit that feature" (reverse diagnostic specificity). Following analysis of the results and additional surveys, the list of features was consolidated to 62 that appeared to exhibit the greatest estimated diagnostic sensitivity, specificity, and accuracy (Table 11–3). Although this is still a "work-in-progress," these features will provide a basis for further evaluation and modification by a wider group of clinical specialists. It is anticipated that this type of standardized process will help establish a set of sound consensus-based criteria for the clinical diagnosis of NTOS, which can be subsequently used in clinical outcomes research, comparative-effectiveness studies, and clinical practice.

TABLE 11-3. CONSENSUS-BASED DIAGNOSTIC CRITERIA FOR NTOS

	SENS	SPEC
No. Type and Description of Feature	**+ NTOS**	**− NTOS**
Clinical History		
1 Symptoms not explained by other condition	100	1
2 Symptoms worsened by work	90	60
3 History of neck/arm injury (all types)	80	50
4 Repetitive strain injury	78	25
5 Age 15-35 years	70	60
6 Symptoms worse/minimally improved with conservative treatment	58	37
7 Substantial improvement with conservative treatment specific for TOS	15	5
8 History of cervical rib	10	1
9 Performance music or sports, arm overhead/weights	10	5
10 History of peripheral nerve surgery (median, ulnar)	8	6
11 History of previous treatment or surgery for TOS	5	3
12 History of clavicle or first rib fracture	4	2
Symptoms		
13 Paresthesias in digits 4 and 5	90	12
14 Complaint of hand/digit numbness	90	25
15 Symptom exacerbation with daily activities or work	90	60
16 Symptom exacerbation with arm use, especially overhead	88	35
17 Pain interferes with sleep	85	37
18 Paresthesias radiate in ulnar distribution	83	20
19 Pain in neck, upper back, shoulder, and/or arm	83	70
20 Complaint of weakness in arm or hand	72	25
21 Paresthesias radiate from supraclavicular space	70	5
22 Headache occipital	60	20
23 Pain in hand/digits, especially with arm use	50	23
24 Complaint of hand/digit swelling or coldness	50	22
25 Paresthesias in hand and/or all digits	43	15
26 Complaint of neck swelling	20	10
Physical Examination		
27 Tenderness/pain on palpation scalene triangle	95	5
28 Upper limb tension test reproduces symptoms	95	20
29 Tenderness/pain on palpation >1 areas	90	30
30 Hand/digit paresthesias on passive arm elevation	90	10
31 Head tilt/neck rotation reproduces symptoms contralateral only	83	22
32 Palpable muscle spasm scalene triangle	80	5
33 Hand/digit paresthesias on palpation scalene triangle	80	5
34 Positive Tinel's supraclavicular	80	15
35 Head tilt/neck rotation reproduces symptoms, ipsilateral only	80	30
36 Postural abnormalities (e.g., slumped head forward)	68	20
37 Tenderness/pain on palpation of pectoralis minor	60	10

(Continued)

TABLE 11-3. CONSENSUS-BASED DIAGNOSTIC CRITERIA FOR NTOS *(Continued)*

No.	Type and Description of Feature	SENS + NTOS	SPEC − NTOS
Physical Examination			
38	3-minute EAST unable to complete or moderate symptoms	60	17
39	1-minute EAST unable to complete	55	5
40	Radial pulse ablated or diminished on arm elevation	55	17
41	Palpable muscle spasm pectoralis and/or trapezius	50	20
42	Pale hand upon arm elevation	50	10
43	Diminished sensation in hand/digits especially digits 4/5	49	12
44	Hand/digit paresthesias on palpation pectoralis minor	45	7
45	Weakness of handgrip, intrinsic muscles, or digit 5	44	18
46	Pain-limited ROM neck, shoulder, or arm	33	33
47	Tenderness/pain SCM, anterior chest, rhomboid, or trap	29	21
48	Visible arm swelling, cyanosis, distended subcutaneous veins	9	4
49	Hyperalgesia/allodynia neck	8	5
50	Palpable supraclavicular mass	5	2
51	Digital ischemia, ulceration, emboli, or Raynaud's phenomenon	4	2
52	Thenar or hypothenar atrophy	4	5
53	Radial, brachial, or axillary pulse not palpable at rest	2	1
54	Indwelling subclavian vein access, past or present	1	3
Tests and Studies			
55	Cervical imaging: normal C-spine	80	50
56	Scalene muscle block moderate or dramatic improvement	79	3
57	Vascular lab: diminished arterial pressures arm elevation	72	21
58	Venogram: Subclavian vein stenosis and/or thrombosis	34	15
59	Cervical imaging: cervical rib or wide C7 affected side	13	1
60	Abnormal EMG/NC studies: brachial plexus	8	5
61	Arteriogram: Subclavian artery aneurysm and/or stenosis	5	1
62	Vascular lab: Axillary-subclavian vein thrombosis	5	0

Unpublished data from the Consortium for Outcomes Research and Education on Thoracic Outlet Syndrome (CORE-TOS), based on Delphi process evaluation of diagnostic criteria for NTOS. SENS (+NTOS) = diagnostic sensitivity based on the estimated percentage of patients *with NTOS* who will exhibit the feature listed (mean of expert panel evaluators). SPEC (−NTOS) = diagnostic specificity based on the estimated percentage of patients *without NTOS* who will exhibit the feature listed (mean of expert panel evaluators).

SUMMARY

The diagnosis of NTOS depends upon both clinical suspicion and pattern-recognition as well as exclusion of more common conditions that have overlapping features. Diagnostic suspicion is raised by the clinical history and description of symptoms, with provisional diagnosis supplemented by physical examination. In most patients, a diagnosis of NTOS can be made or excluded on this basis. A limited number of diagnostic studies may be of value, both in excluding other conditions and in supporting the suspected diagnosis, but with the exception of scalene/pectoralis muscle blocks, no single diagnostic test is entirely specific for NTOS. In the end, a satisfactory response to treatment targeted to NTOS, particularly when other treatments have failed, remains the most convincing means to confirm the cause of the underlying condition. Careful follow-up studies using standardized assessment instruments, particularly through consortium efforts involving a larger number of patients than available at any single center, will provide further insight into the most accurate diagnostic and prognostic criteria for NTOS.

REFERENCES

1. Sanders RJ. Thoracic Outlet Syndrome: A Common Sequelae of Neck Injuries. Philadelphia: J. B. Lippincott Company; 1991.
2. Mackinnon SE, Novak CB. Thoracic outlet syndrome. Curr Probl Surg 2002;39:1070–145.
3. Thompson RW, Bartoli MA. Neurogenic thoracic outlet syndrome. In: Rutherford RB, ed. Vascular Surgery, 6th Edition. Philadelphia: Elsevier Saunders; 2005;1347–65.
4. Sanders RJ, Hammond SL, Rao NM. Diagnosis of thoracic outlet syndrome. J Vasc Surg 2007;46:601–4.
5. Novak CB. Thoracic outlet syndrome. Clin Plast Surg 2003;30:175–88.
6. Lord JWJ, Stone PW. Pectoralis minor tenotomy and anterior scalenotomy with special reference to the hyperabduction syndrome and effort thrombosis of the subclavian vein. Circulation 1956;13:537–42.
7. McIntyre DI. Subcoracoid neurovascular entrapment. Clin Orthop Relat Res 1975;108: 27–30.
8. Ambrad-Chalela E, Thomas GI, Johansen KH. Recurrent neurogenic thoracic outlet syndrome. Am J Surg 2004;187:505–10.
9. Upton AR, McComas AJ. The double crush in nerve entrapment syndromes. Lancet 1973;2:359–62.
10. Osterman AL. The double crush syndrome. Orthop Clin North Am 1988;19:147–55.
11. Dellon AL, Mackinnon SE. Chronic nerve compression model for the double crush hypothesis. Ann Plast Surg 1991;26:259–64.
12. Schenardi C. Whiplash injury: TOS and double crush syndrome, forensic medical aspects. Acta Neurochir Suppl 2005;92:25–7.
13. Gilliatt RW, Le Quesne PM, Logue V, et al. Wasting of the hand associated with a cervical rib or band. J Neurol Neurosurg Psychiatry 1970;33:615–24.
14. Tender GC, Thomas AJ, Thomas N, et al. Gilliatt-Sumner hand revisited: a 25-year experience. Neurosurgery 2004;55:883–90.
15. Totten PA, Hunter JM. Therapeutic techniques to enhance nerve gliding in thoracic outlet syndrome and carpal tunnel syndrome. Hand Clin 1991;7:505–20.
16. Aligne C, Barral X. Rehabilitation of patients with thoracic outlet syndrome. Ann Vasc Surg 1992;6:381–9.
17. Novak CB. Conservative management of thoracic outlet syndrome. Semin Thorac Cardiovasc Surg 1996;8:201–7.
18. Edgelow P. Neurovascular consequences of cumulative trauma disorders affecting the thoracic outlet: a patient centered treatment approach. In: Donatelli R, ed. Physical Therapy of the Shoulder. New York: Churchill Livingstone; 2004, pp. 205–38.
19. Wehbe MA, Schlegel JM. Nerve gliding exercises for thoracic outlet syndrome. Hand Clin 2004;20:51–5.
20. Crosby CA, Wehbe MA. Conservative treatment for thoracic outlet syndrome. Hand Clin 2004;20:43–9.
21. Vanti C, Natalini L, Romeo A, et al. Conservative treatment of thoracic outlet syndrome: a review of the literature. Eura Medicophys 2007;43:55–70.
22. Jordan SE, Ahn SS, Freischlag JA, et al. Selective botulinum chemodenervation of the scalene muscles for treatment of neurogenic thoracic outlet syndrome. Ann Vasc Surg 2000;14: 365–9.

23. Jordan SE, Ahn SS, Gelabert HA. Combining ultrasonography and electromyography for botulinum chemodenervation treatment of thoracic outlet syndrome: comparison with fluoroscopy and electromyography guidance. Pain Physician 2007;10:541–6.
24. Jordan SE, Ahn SS, Gelabert HA. Differentiation of thoracic outlet syndrome from treatment-resistant cervical brachial pain syndromes: development and utilization of a questionnaire, clinical examination and ultrasound evaluation. Pain Physician 2007;10:441–52.
25. Roos DB. Transaxillary approach for first rib resection to relieve thoracic outlet syndrome. Ann Surg 1966;163:354–8.
26. Roos DB. Congenital anomalies associated with thoracic outlet syndrome. Am J Surg 1976; 132:771–8.
27. Sanders RJ, Monsour JW, Gerber WJ. Recurrent thoracic outlet syndrome following first rib resection. Vasc Surg 1979;13:325–30.
28. Hempel GK, Rusher AH Jr. Wheeler CG, et al. Supraclavicular resection of the first rib for thoracic outlet syndrome. Am J Surg 1981;141:213–5.
29. Sanders RJ, Raymer S. The supraclavicular approach to scalenectomy and first rib resection: description of technique. J Vasc Surg 1985;2:751–6.
30. Sanders RJ, Pearce WH. The treatment of thoracic outlet syndrome: a comparison of different operations. J Vasc Surg 1989;10:626–34.
31. Machleder HI. The treatment of thoracic outlet syndrome: a comparison of different operations. J Vasc Surg 1990;12:220–1.
32. Machleder HI. Thoracic outlet syndromes: new concepts from a century of discovery. Cardiovasc Surg 1994;2:137–45.
33. Cheng SW, Stoney RJ. Supraclavicular reoperation for neurogenic thoracic outlet syndrome. J Vasc Surg 1994;19:565–72.
34. Cheng SW, Reilly LM, Nelken NA, et al. Neurogenic thoracic outlet decompression: rationale for sparing the first rib. Cardiovasc Surg 1995;3:617–23.
35. Hempel GK, Shutze WP, Anderson JF, et al. 770 consecutive supraclavicular first rib resections for thoracic outlet syndrome. Ann Vasc Surg 1996;10:456–63.
36. Thompson RW, Petrinec D. Surgical treatment of thoracic outlet compression syndromes. I. Diagnostic considerations and transaxillary first rib resection. Ann Vasc Surg 1997;11: 315–23.
37. Thompson RW, Petrinec D, Toursarkissian B. Surgical treatment of thoracic outlet compression syndromes. II. Supraclavicular exploration and vascular reconstruction. Ann Vasc Surg 1997;11:442–51.
38. Kashyap VS, Ahn SS, Machleder HI. Thoracic outlet neurovascular compression: approaches to anatomic decompression and their limitations. Semin Vasc Surg 1998;11:116–22.
39. Urschel HC Jr. Razzuk MA. Neurovascular compression in the thoracic outlet: changing management over 50 years. Ann Surg 1998;228:609–17.
40. Axelrod DA, Proctor MC, Geisser ME, et al. Outcomes after surgery for thoracic outlet syndrome. J Vasc Surg 2001;33:1220–5.
41. Sanders RJ, Hammond SL. Management of cervical ribs and anomalous first ribs causing neurogenic thoracic outlet syndrome. J Vasc Surg 2002;36:51–6.
42. Huang JH, Zager EL. Thoracic outlet syndrome. Neurosurgery 2004;55:897–902.
43. Atasoy E. Combined surgical treatment of thoracic outlet syndrome: transaxillary first rib resection and transcervical scalenectomy. Hand Clin 2004;20:71–82.
44. Sanders RJ, Hammond SL. Supraclavicular first rib resection and total scalenectomy: technique and results. Hand Clin 2004;20:61–70.
45. Sheth RN, Campbell JN. Surgical treatment of thoracic outlet syndrome: a randomized trial comparing two operations. Neurosurg Spine 2005;3:355–63.
46. Sanders RJ, Hammond SL, Rao NM. Observations on the use of seprafilm on the brachial plexus in 249 operations for neurogenic thoracic outlet syndrome. Hand 2007;2:179–83.
47. Collins JD, Disher AC, Miller TQ. The anatomy of the brachial plexus as displayed by magnetic resonance imaging: technique and application. J Natl Med Assoc 1995;87:489–98.

48. Saxton EH, Miller TQ, Collins JD. Migraine complicated by brachial plexopathy as displayed by MRI and MRA: aberrant subclavian artery and cervical ribs. J Natl Med Assoc 1999;91:333–41.
49. van Es HW. MRI of the brachial plexus. Eur Radiol 2001;11:325–36.
50. Demondion X, Bacqueville E, Paul C, et al. Thoracic outlet: assessment with MR imaging in asymptomatic and symptomatic populations. Radiology 2003;227:461–8.
51. Demondion X, Herbinet P, Van Sint Jan S, et al. Imaging assessment of thoracic outlet syndrome. Radiographics 2006;26:1735–50.
52. Demirbag D, Unlu E, Ozdemir F, et al. The relationship between magnetic resonance imaging findings and postural maneuver and physical examination tests in patients with thoracic outlet syndrome: results of a double-blind, controlled study. Arch Phys Med Rehabil 2007;88:844–51.
53. Rubin M, Lange DJ. Sensory nerve abnormalities in brachial plexopathy. Eur Neurol 1992;32:245–7.
54. Nishida T, Price SJ, Minieka MM. Medial antebrachial cutaneous nerve conduction in true neurogenic thoracic outlet syndrome. Electromyogr Clin Neurophysiol 1993;33:285–8.
55. Cruz-Martinez A, Arpa J. Electrophysiological assessment in neurogenic thoracic outlet syndrome. Electromyogr Clin Neurophysiol 2001;41:253–6.
56. Machanic BI, Sanders RJ. Medial antebrachial cutaneous nerve measurements to diagnose neurogenic thoracic outlet syndrome. Ann Vasc Surg 2008;22:248–54.
57. Chang DC, Lidor AO, Matsen SL, et al. Reported in-hospital complications following rib resections for neurogenic thoracic outlet syndrome. Ann Vasc Surg 2007;21:564–70.
58. Raskin NH, Howard MW, Ehrenfeld WK. Headache as the leading symptom of the thoracic outlet syndrome. Headache 1985;25:208–10.
59. Estilaei SK, Byl NN. An evidence-based review of magnetic resonance angiography for diagnosing arterial thoracic outlet syndrome. J Hand Ther 2006;19:410–9.
60. Charon JP, Milne W, Sheppard DG, et al. Evaluation of MR angiographic technique in the assessment of thoracic outlet syndrome. Clin Radiol 2004;59:588–95.
61. Yanaka K, Asakawa H, Matsumaru Y, et al. Diagnosis of vascular compression at the thoracic outlet using magnetic resonance angiography. Eur Neurol 2004;51:122–3.
62. Demondion X, Boutry N, Drizenko A, et al. Thoracic outlet: anatomic correlation with MR imaging. AJR Am J Roentgenol 2000;175:417–22.
63. Cherington M, Wilbourn AJ, Schils J, et al. Thoracic outlet syndromes and MRI. Brain 1995;118:819–21.
64. Panegyres PK, Moore N, Gibson R, et al. Thoracic outlet syndromes and magnetic resonance imaging. Brain 1993;116:823–41.
65. Ohkawa Y, Isoda H, Hasegawa S, et al. MR angiography of thoracic outlet syndrome. J Comput Assist Tomogr 1992;16:475–7.
66. Sullivan JM, Wszolek ZK, Lund G, Pfeiffer RF. Magnetic resonance imaging in thoracic outlet syndrome. Nebr Med J 1988;73:70–2.
67. Filler AG, Kliot M, Howe FA, et al. Application of magnetic resonance neurography in the evaluation of patients with peripheral nerve pathology. J Neurosurg 1996;85:299–309.
68. Filler AG, Maravilla KR, Tsuruda JS. MR neurography and muscle MR imaging for image diagnosis of disorders affecting the peripheral nerves and musculature. Neurol Clin 2004;22:643–82.
69. Komanetsky RM, Novak CB, Mackinnon SE, et al. Somatosensory evoked potentials fail to diagnose thoracic outlet syndrome. J Hand Surg [Am] 1996;21:662–6.
70. Chiu YN, Huang YL, Chang CW. Medial antebrachial cutaneous neuropathy: a case report. Electromyogr Clin Neurophysiol 2008;48:125–7.
71. Seror P. Symptoms of thoracic outlet syndrome in women with carpal tunnel syndrome. Clin Neurophysiol 2005;116:2324–9.

72. Seror P. Frequency of neurogenic thoracic outlet syndrome in patients with definite carpal tunnel syndrome: an electrophysiological evaluation in 100 women. Clin Neurophysiol 2005;116:259–63.
73. Seror P. Medial antebrachial cutaneous nerve conduction study, a new tool to demonstrate mild lower brachial plexus lesions: a report of 16 cases. Clin Neurophysiol 2004;115: 2316–22.
74. Seror P. The medial antebrachial cutaneous nerve: antidromic and orthodromic conduction studies. Muscle Nerve 2002;26:421–3.
75. Seror P. Brachial plexus neoplastic lesions assessed by conduction study of medial antebrachial cutaneous nerve. Muscle Nerve 2001;24:1068–70.
76. Tavana B, Moghaddam FR, Pajhouh RR. Medial brachial cutaneous nerve conduction study. Electromyogr Clin Neurophysiol 2000;40:393–6.
77. Ferrante MA, Wilbourn AJ. The utility of various sensory nerve conduction responses in assessing brachial plexopathies. Muscle Nerve 1995;18:879–89.
78. Jordan SE, Machleder HI. Diagnosis of thoracic outlet syndrome using electrophysiologically guided anterior scalene blocks. Ann Vasc Surg 1998;12:260–4.
79. Gage M. Scalenus anticus syndrome: a diagnostic and confirmatory test. Surgery 1939;5: 599–601.
80. Sanders RJ, Monsour JW, Gerber FG, et al. Scalenectomy versus first rib resection for treatment of the thoracic outlet syndrome. Surgery 1979;85:109–21.
81. Holey EA, Feeley JL, Dixon J, et al. An exploration of the use of simple statistics to measure consensus and stability in Delphi studies. BMC Med Res Methodol 2007;7:52.
82. Kellum JA, Mehta RL, Levin A, et al. Development of a clinical research agenda for acute kidney injury using an international, interdisciplinary, three-step modified Delphi process. Clin J Am Soc Nephrol 2008;3:887–94.
83. Dahmen R, van der Wilden GJ, Lankhorst GJ, et al. Delphi process yielded consensus on terminology and research agenda for therapeutic footwear for neuropathic foot. J Clin Epidemiol 2008; 61:819–26.

12

Pectoralis Minor Syndrome

Richard J. Sanders, M.D.

INTRODUCTION

Although pectoralis minor syndrome (PMS) was described more than 60 years ago, it has received little attention. Although the pectoralis minor space is usually included in general descriptions of thoracic outlet syndrome (TOS), recognition of PMS as a separate entity has escaped our attention. Stimulated by Dr. George Thomas of Seattle to look more closely at PMS, in 2005 we began to evaluate all patients with TOS symptoms for PMS as well as TOS. The surprising finding was that at least 75% of "TOS patients" had positive findings of PMS. Some patients had only PMS, whereas others had both TOS and PMS. This chapter describes the features of PMS, how closely the clinical picture is to TOS, and how to differentiate and treat the two conditions.

HISTORY

PMS was first described by Wright in 1945 and called the hyperabduction syndrome.[1] It was described as symptoms of paresthesia in the hands when sleeping with the arms overhead. Wright attributed the symptoms to compression of the axillary neurovascular bundle by the pectoralis minor (PM) tendon. This was treated by teaching patients to sleep with their arms at their sides. It was also recognized that in patients with more extensive symptoms, surgery might be indicated.

Wright observed that when elevating the arms 180 degrees overhead, the radial pulse was occluded in over 80% of 150 asymptomatic volunteers. He concluded that pulse obliteration in this position was a normal phenomenon

The first pectoralis minor tenotomy (PMT) for symptoms of pectoralis minor compression was a report of five cases by Lord and Stone in 1956. Their patients had both venous and neurogenic symptoms.[2]

The next report of this condition was 19 years later when McIntyre reported the condition as "subcoracoid neurovascular entrapment."[3] In this report of 22 limbs in 19 patients, half responded to conservative therapy and the other half underwent PMT with complete relief in 80% and partial relief in 20%.

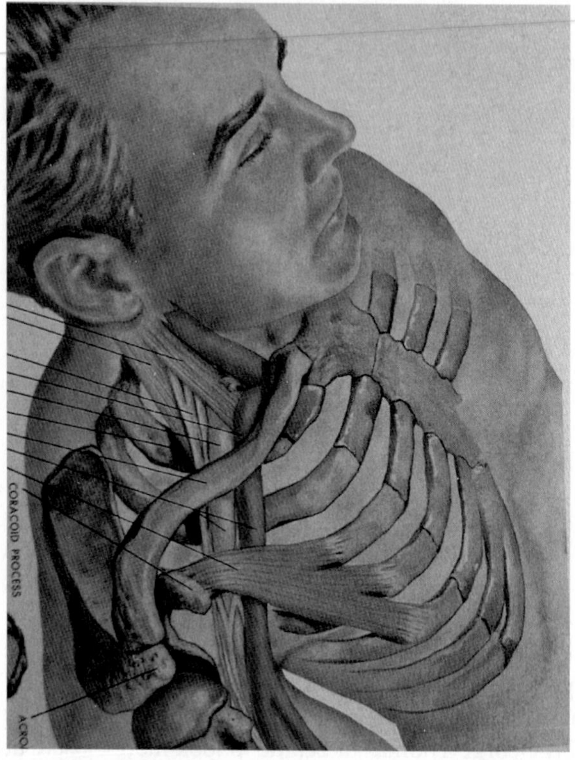

Figure 12-1. Anatomy of the pectoralis minor space below the clavicle and thoracic outlet area above the clavicle. (From Lord JWJr, Rosati LM. Thoracic outlet syndromes. Ciba Symposium 1971;23:1–13.)

In 1977, Stallworth pointed out that symptoms of neurogenic TOS (NTOS) could be relieved by cutting soft tissues and that routine first rib resection was unnecessary. His later report in 1984 noted that PMT was performed in 156 of a total of 194 operations for relief of NTOS symptoms.[4] PMT was combined with other muscle releases in 63 (anterior scalene or subclavius), but in 93 patients, PMT was the only procedure. He reported over a 90% success rate.

Recurrent NTOS treated by combined thoracic outlet decompression plus PM release was reported in 2004.[5] All 20 patients in this study had good improvement from surgery, with 13 patients receiving PMT.

ANATOMY

The PM muscle lies below the clavicle. It originates from ribs 3, 4, and 5 and inserts on the coracoid process of the scapula. Below the PM muscle is the PM space, which contains the axillary neurovascular bundle consisting of axillary artery, axillary vein, and branches of the brachial plexus (Figure 12–1).

The thoracic outlet area lies above the clavicle. It contains a similar neurovascular bundle consisting of the subclavian artery, subclavian vein, and nerve roots of the brachial plexus.

The fact that the composition of the neurovascular bundle is the same above and below the clavicle explains why the symptoms of brachial plexus compression are similar regardless of where the site of compression lies. Although the brachial plexus has progressed from cords above the clavicle to branches under the PM, the nerve fasciculi are the same, just rearranged.

Under the PM muscle, the artery usually lies cephalad to the vein, and the nerve branches lie in a variety of patterns but usually are more superficial so that the nerves are the closest structures to the PM muscle. This probably explains why nerve compression is much more common than vascular compression.

THREE TYPES OF PMS

Like thoracic outlet compression, PM compression can involve any of the three structures in the axillary neurovascular bundle: nerve, vein, or artery. And similar to TOS, the neurogenic PMS (NPMS) is the form seen in over 90% of patients with PMS.

Axillary vein compression by PM is much less common. It presents with arm swelling and cyanosis and can be differentiated from subclavian vein obstruction only by venography.[6] Venous PMS is usually nonthrombotic venous obstruction. All of the patients we have seen with axillary vein thrombosis had developed this condition as an extension of subclavian vein thrombosis. We have not seen a single case of just axillary vein thrombosis.

Axillary artery compression is the least common form of PM compression. Only a handful of patients have been reported and the majority were athletes, some with thrombosis, most without.[7-9]

ETIOLOGY

Trauma to the neck and/or shoulder girdle was the etiology in 80% of the patients seen with NPMS. The same was true of patients with NTOS. Whiplash injuries experienced in motor vehicle accidents were the most common type of trauma. Other causes were falls on floors, ice, or stairs, repetitive stress injuries at keyboards, and quite a few athletic injuries. The sports associated with NPMS were those that involved hyperabduction of the shoulder, which stretches PM. The common sports were swimming, gymnastics, baseball pitching, and weight-lifting. Athletic injuries were more common among NPMS patients than NTOS patients.

SYMPTOMS

The symptoms of NPMS are similar to those of NTOS. The triad of nerve compression symptoms is present in both conditions: pain, paresthesia, and weakness in the upper extremity. In NPMS, pain or tenderness is almost always present in the anterior chest wall and/or the axilla. Pain is also frequent in the trapezius, arm, and forearm. Pain may occur in the neck and supraclavicular area but occipital headaches, which frequently occur with NTOS, are seen much less often with NPMS.

Paresthesia is present in about 90% of NPMS patients. Involvement of all five fingers is the most common distribution, with fourth and fifth fingers next most common.

Weakness is present in about half the NPMS patients but is usually less severe than is seen in NTOS patients.

Patients with NTOS tend to have more intense pain, paresthesia, and weakness compared with those with NPMS. NTOS patients have a higher incidence of neck pain and occipital headaches, which are more intense than those in NPMS patients.

PHYSICAL EXAMINATION

Physical examination for PMS is the same as for TOS plus checking for tenderness over the PM tendon and axilla. Complete physical examination should also include evaluation for nerve compression at the elbow and forearm.

Tenderness

Areas of tenderness to check include the anterior scalene muscle, PM tendon just below the clavicle, axilla, shoulder, trapezius, and rhomboid muscles. Areas of tenderness below the upper arm include the ulnar nerve at the elbow, supinator tunnel, and pronator tunnel.

Tinel's Sign

Finger tapping over the course of nerves is performed over the brachial plexus above the clavicle, over the ulnar nerve at the elbow, and over the supinator and pronator tunnels. Positive responses at the elbow and forearm may indicate compression in the respective area, compression on the brachial plexus higher up, or both could coexist—a double-crush phenomenon.[10]

Provocative Maneuvers

Four provocative maneuvers are helpful in eliciting symptoms or in aggravating symptoms that are already present. Each maneuver applies stress and stretching on the brachial plexus both above and below the clavicle. The single most helpful maneuver is the modified Upper Limb Tension Test (ULTT) originally described by Elvey[11] (Figure 12–2).

Other provocative maneuvers are the Elevated Arm Stress Test[12–13] (Figure 12–3), neck rotation (Figure 12–4), and head tilt (Figure 12–5). A positive response to neck rotation and head tilt elicits radiating symptoms of pain and paresthesia into the contralateral arm and hand within 60 seconds and often within 30 seconds.

Positive responses to provocative maneuvers may be absent or minimal in NPMS patients, whereas they are usually stronger and most or all are present in NTOS patients.

DIAGNOSTIC TESTS

Muscle blocks and electrodiagnostic tests are the two tests of greatest value in the diagnosis of NPMS. The most helpful test is a PM muscle block. Also helpful in these patients is a scalene muscle block.

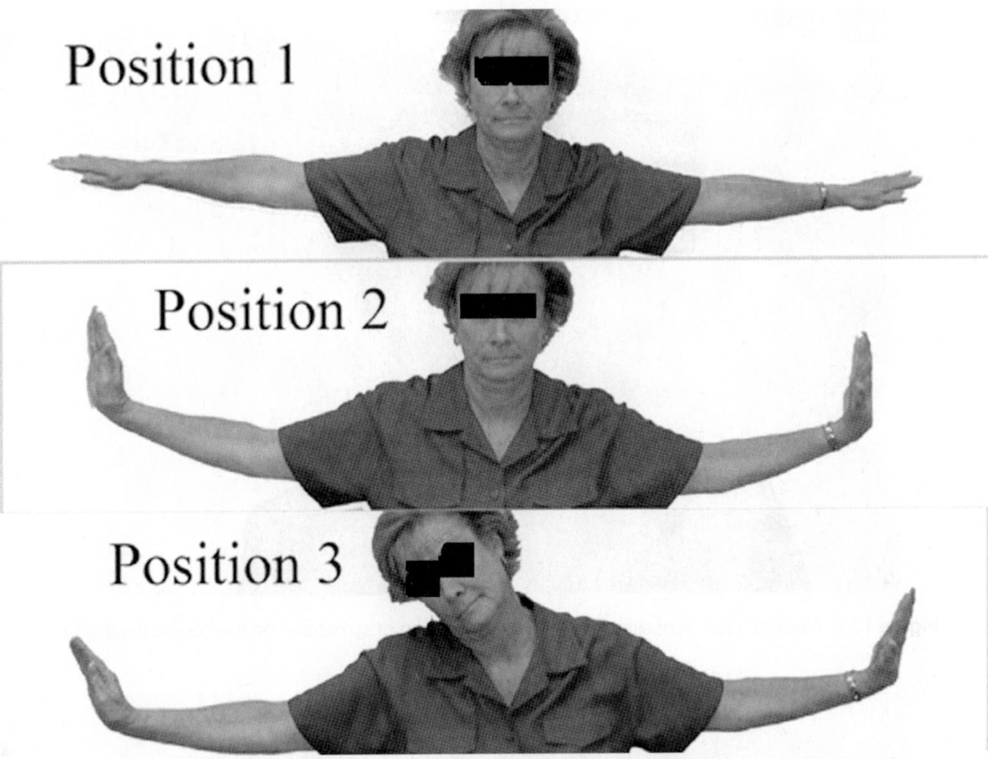

Figure 12-2. Upper limb tension test. Position one: Arms at 90°, elbows extended; Position two: Wrists dorsiflexed; Position three: Head tilted to contralateral side. A positive response is symptoms of pain and paresthesia in arm and hand. The earlier it occurs, the stronger the response.

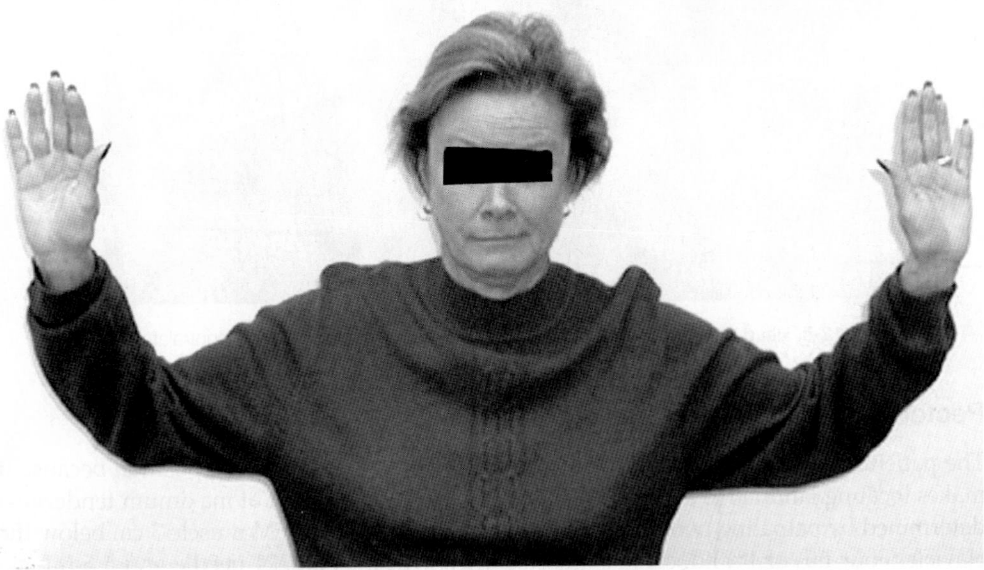

Figure 12-3. Arms abducted to 90 degrees. The elevated arm stress position. A positive response is duplication of symptoms in less than 60 seconds.

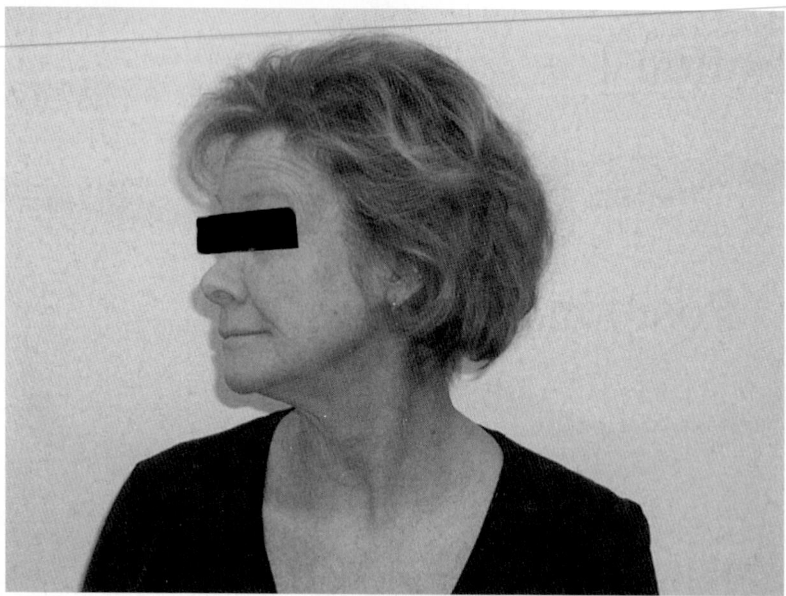

Figure 12-4. Neck rotation. A positive response is duplication of symptoms on the contralateral side.

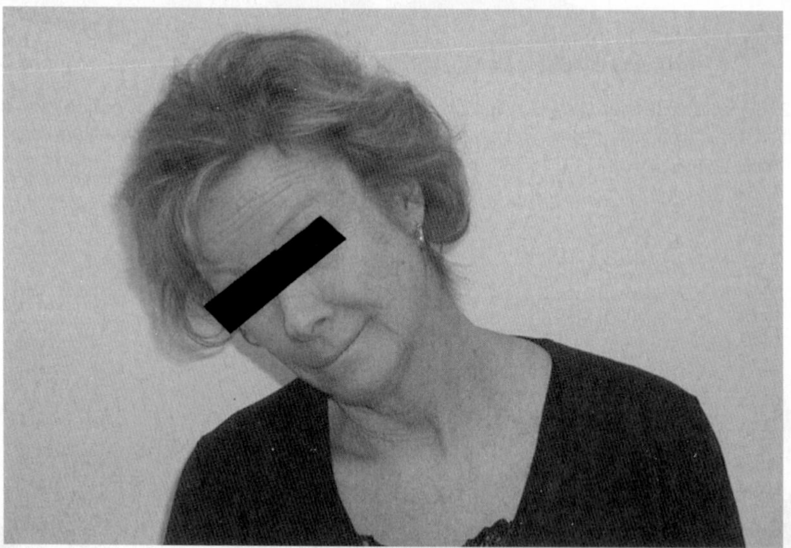

Figure 12-5. Head tilt: A positive response is duplication of symptoms on the contralateral side.

Pectoralis Minor Muscle Block

The patient may be sitting or lying down. Our preference is the sitting position because it makes locating landmarks easier. The spot of injection is the point of maximum tenderness determined by palpating two or three spots over the area of the PM muscle 3 cm below the clavicle. Four mL of 1% lidocaine is injected with a 1½-inch No. 21 needle and a 5-mL syringe. The needle is aimed upward toward the coracoid process at a 45-degree angle to avoid entering the pleura. No attempt is made to feel the coracoid process. The needle is moved frequently to spread the 4 mL over a wide area. The needle is aspirated each time it is moved to avoid injecting into the axillary artery or vein. If a vessel is entered, the needle is pulled back a few millimeters, repositioned, and the injection continued. A good response is improvement in symptoms at rest (if there were any at rest) and improvement on repeat physical examination, emphasizing the provocative maneuvers and points of tenderness.

Scalene Muscle Block

This can be performed sitting or reclining. The spot to introduce the needle is the point of maximum tenderness over the anterior scalene muscle, 2 to 3 cm above the clavicle. Four mL of 1% lidocaine is injected with a one and 1½-inch No. 21 needle and 5-mL syringe. The needle is aimed upward into the muscle at a 45-degree angle to avoid entering the pleura. The needle is moved frequently to spread the 4 mL over a wide area. Just as in the PM block, the needle is aspirated each time it is moved to avoid injecting it into subclavian artery or vein. If a vessel is entered, the needle is pulled back a few millimeters, repositioned, and the injection continued. A good response is improvement in symptoms at rest and improvement on repeat physical examination, emphasizing the provocative maneuvers and points of tenderness.[14]

Electrodiagnostic Studies (Edx)

Most electromyography (EMG) and nerve conduction velocity (NCV) studies are normal or show nonspecific changes. However, a more specific variation of NCV measurement is of the medial antebrachial cutaneous nerve (MAC). We have found the MAC test to be the most reliable measurement of brachial plexus compression.[15] Normal ranges of latency and amplitude should be established for each EMG laboratory. In patients with unilateral symptoms, the uninvolved arm can serve as the control. In patients with bilateral symptoms, the established normal range for each laboratory must be used.

DIFFERENTIATING NTOS FROM NPMS

History and physical examination can usually differentiate NTOS and NPMS. NPMS is recognized by a history of pain or tenderness in the anterior chest wall and/or the axilla. Tenderness on palpation supports the diagnosis and a good response to the PM muscle block confirms it. NPMS also has the same extremity symptoms as NTOS and may also have neck pain and headache. However, many NPMS patients have no headache or neck pain, or if they do, it is a minor symptom. Physical examination, other than the tenderness over the PM and axilla, usually finds that responses to the provocative maneuvers are minimal or absent in NPMS patients. Most patients with NPMS alone are still gainfully employed.

In contrast, NTOS patients usually have stronger positive symptoms of neck pain and headache plus stronger responses to all four of the provocative maneuvers. If a patient is tender over the PM and scalenes and has strong responses to all the provocative maneuvers, a diagnosis of both NTOS and NPMS is suspected. A good response to the PM muscle block, which is always performed first, and more improvement with the scalene muscle block confirm the diagnosis of both NPMS and NTOS, a double-crush syndrome.[10]

TREATMENT

Conservative Treatment: Stretching is the specific treatment for NPMS. The stretch is a corner stretch or the door jamb stretch. With each hand on the jambs of an open door, the body drops forward into the open doorway. This brings the two scapulae toward each other and stretches the PM muscle. The same stretch can be achieved by standing in the corner of a room or by sitting in a chair and assuming a military position. The position should be held for 15 to 30 seconds. After resting 30 seconds, this should be repeated three to five times, three times a day. This should be given a trial of 2 to 3 months. If it fails, the options are to continue to live with the symptoms or consider surgery.

Surgery

PMT with partial myomectomy will decompress the PM space. There are three surgical approaches to the pectoralis minor tendon: Through an infraclavicular incision, splitting the pectoralis major muscle parallel to its fibers; and through a vertical incision over the lateral edge of the pectoralis major muscle, which must be retracted to reach the coracoid process; or through a transverse incision in the axilla. Our preference is for the transaxillary approach, as it provides better exposure and the scar is hidden in the axilla.

Anesthesia

The operation is usually performed on an outpatient basis under local anesthesia with an anesthesiologist providing heavy sedation. A frequent combination of drugs used is Propythal, Fentanyl, and Versed. One percent lidocaine is infiltrated into the skin of the incision. Additional lidocaine is injected as needed into the deeper tissues, but in the majority of patients, little additional local anesthetic is needed.

Technique

The skin incision for the transaxillary approach is 5 to 7 cm long and is made 1 cm above the bottom of the hairline. The incision is placed in the anterior part of the axilla and begins within 1 cm of the anterior axillary fold. Placing the incision here can usually avoid the second intercostal brachial cutaneous nerve, although not always. Placing the incision here also makes is easier to identify the lateral edge of the pectoralis major, which is the first landmark. Once subcutaneous fat has been divided, the lateral edge of pectoralis major is identified. The pectoralis major is retracted medially and the coracoid process is identified by finger palpation. The PM can often be palpated and its medial edge isolated by finger dissection, even before the PM has been visualized. If the PM is not easily palpated, exposure is obtained with a retractor and the muscle identified.

In some patients, PM is fused to the pectoralis major. When PM does not readily appear as a distinct muscle inserting into the coracoid, fusion to pectoralis major should be suspected. In such cases, the coracoid process is exposed and the muscle fibers inserting into the coracoid are separated from the fibers just above the coracoid with a spreading instrument, such as the back of a scissors. This will usually lead into an avascular plane separating the two muscles. If the plane is not avascular, another nearby plane should be sought until the avascular one is identified.

The PM tendon is divided against the coracoid with a cautery. The end of the muscle is grasped with a heavy clamp and 2 to 3 cm of muscle isolated with another heavy clamp. This portion of the PM muscle is then excised to prevent it from scarring to the axillary neurovascular bundle in the future and causing recurrent symptoms. Care should be observed to make sure that the pectoral nerve to the pectoralis major is not injured when excising the 2 to 3 cm of PM.

The axillary neurovascular bundle is inspected, and tight bands of clavipectoral fascia are divided. Occasionally, a thick band of fascia is found crossing the neurovascular bundle, which we observed in one patient. This has been described previously and labeled Langer's arch.[16] Prior to closing, the deep wound is inspected and any small bleeders meticulously cauterized with a bipolar bovie. The wound is closed with subutaneous and subcuticular absorbable sutures.

RESULTS OF SURGERY

PMT as Solo Operation

Between 2005 and 2007, PMT was performed as a primary operation and also as a secondary operation for patients with recurrent NTOS. As a solo operation, PMT was carried out in three groups of patients: those with a diagnosis of NPMS alone; those with both NPMS and NTOS; and patients with recurrent NTOS. In these three groups, a total of 164 PMT operations were carried out and their results are shown in Table 12–1. PMT in patients with NPMS alone had a failure rate of only 8% compared with PMT in patients with combined NPMS and NTOS whose failure rate was 46%. Most of the patients with poor results had thoracic outlet decompression at a later date. This significant difference emphasizes the importance of thorough history and physical examination in order to recognize the difference between the two conditions and be aware of the frequency of their coexistence.

PMT Accompanying TOS Operations

PM decompression along with thoracic outlet decompression was performed for both primary and recurrent NTOS.[5] PMT accompanied a total of 121 TOS operations, 91 being primary procedures and 30 for recurrence (Table 12–2). Failure rates were 18% and 14%, respectively, and fair results were 14% and 33%, respectively. Thus, good improvement was noted in 68% and 53%. Note that for recurrent NTOS, although the failure rate is low, the

TABLE 12-1. RESULTS OF SURGERY

Pectoralis minor tenotomy as only operation				
Indication	#Ops	Good	Fair	Failed
NPMS only	52	(44) 84%	(4) 8%	(4) 8%
NPMS+NTOS	48	(17) 35%	(9) 19%	(22) 46%
Recurrent NTOS	64	(45) 70%	(7) 11%	(12) 19%
Total ops	164	(106) 65%	(22) 13%	(36) 22%

Time: 2005-2007
Follow up: 1-3 years
NPMS= neurogenic PMS
NTOS = neurogenic thoracic outlet syndrome
#Ops = number of operations
Good = improvement in most symptoms
Fair = improvement in a few symptoms but some major symptoms remain
Failed = not enough improvement to have made operation worthwhile

TABLE 12-2. RESULTS OF SURGERY

Combined PMT and TOS operations				
Operation	**#Ops**	**Good**	**Fair**	**Failed**
PMT + TOS op	91	(62) 68%	(13) 14%	(16) 18%
PMT + TOS Reop	30	(16) 53%	(10) 33%	(4) 14%
Total ops	121	(78) 64%	(23) 19%	(20) 17%

Time: 2005-2007
Follow up: 1-3 years
Good = improvement in most symptoms
Fair = improvement in a few symptoms but some major symptoms remain
Failed = not enough improvement to have made operation worthwhile
PMT= pectoralis minor tenotomy
TOS = thoracic outlet syndrome
#Ops = number of operations

good results are also low. The number of patients with a fair result, 33%, is quite high. indicating that failure rate alone is not the only criterion of a good result. The addition of PMT with TOS operations has reduced the failure rates a few percentage points compared with TOS operations without PMS (failure at 1 to 2 years for primary operations was 22% and reoperations 28%[17]). The differences were not statistically significant but did suggest a trend.

Impact of Pectoralis Minor on Operations Performed

Between 2005 and 2008, 413 operations for NTOS and NPMS were performed. PMT only was the operation in 220 of these, and combined PMT with a TOS operation was performed in the other 193. Over all, PM decompression was performed in 82% of all operations (Table 12–3).

Complications of PMT

Complications have been minor and temporary. There were five wound infections in 413 PMTs. Four of the five occurred before we began using prophylactic antibiotics. Injury to the second intercostal antebrachial cutaneous nerve occurred 10% of the time. Even by placing the incision as far anterior in the axilla as possible, this nerve was still encountered. If the nerve is cut, numbness under the arm occurs and is not a problem. However, if the nerve is stretched or bruised, burning pain and hyperesthesia may occur in this area. This usually will subside in a few weeks. If it does not, the wound can be explored and the nerve divided to convert the pain to numbness, which is well tolerated.

The only other complications noted are aching and tenderness in the chest wall over the end of the divided PM muscle. This can occur a few weeks to several months postoperatively. It is treated by steroid injection into the tender area. The incidence of this has been 1%.

Time of Failure

Following TOS operations, failures in the first 3 months are usually the result of a wrong diagnosis, an error in technique, or an associated diagnosis. Failures that occur between 6 and 24 months are the result of scar tissue formation around the nerve roots and account for at least half of the failures following TOS operations. Following PMT alone, almost all failures are seen within the first 3 months. However, failures more than three months after

TABLE 12-3. IMPACT OF PMS ON TREATMENT OF TOS

	Primary Operations		
	No. Ops	With PMT	Without PMT
PMT Alone	153	153	0
Scalenectomy	82	44	38
Scalenectomy and 1st Rib Resect	40	26	14
Cerv Rib Resect w/wo 1st rib	25	11	14
Total Primary Ops	300	234 (78%)	66 (22%)
	Reoperations		
	No. Ops	With PMT	Without PMT
Neurolysis Brachial Plexus	46	37	9
PMT Alone	67	67	0
Total Ops for Recurrence	113	104 (92%)	9 (8%)
Total All Operations	413	338 (82%)	75 (18%)

Time: 2005-2008
PMT = pectoralis minor tenotomy

PMT as a solo operation are rare. The explanation for this is that the nature of the two operations is different. In both transaxillary and supraclavicular operations for TOS, the nerves of the plexus are cleaned of bands and scar tissue. This encourages postoperative scar tissue formation and adherence of scar tissue to the nerve roots. which is the explanation for the late failures. In contrast, PMT is performed by lifting the PM muscle off the axillary neurovascular bundle. Bands of clavipectoral fascia are also removed, but the fat covering the nerves is left undisturbed, and the nerves are usually not touched. Thus postoperative scarring does not occur around the axillary nerves and late failures are avoided.

CONCLUSION

The high incidence of PM involvement should lead physicians who see patients with arm pain and hand paresthesia to think first of brachial plexus compression and then determine if compression is above the clavicle, below the clavicle, or both. PMS commonly accompanies NTOS and frequently exists alone. Recognition is important, because many patients with suspected NTOS can be treated successfully with a simple, essentially risk-free PMT. Should this fail, thoracic outlet decompression can always be performed at a later date.

REFERENCES

1. Wright IS. The neurovascular syndrome produced by hyperabduction of the arms: the immediate changes produced in 150 normal controls, and the effects on same persons of prolonged hyperabduction of the arms, as in sleeping, and in certain occupations. Am Heart J 1945;29:1–19.

2. Lord JW Jr, Stone PW. Pectoralis minor tenotomy and anterior scalenotomy with special reference to the hyperabduction syndrome and effort thrombosis of the subclavian vein. Circulation 1956;13:537–42.
3. McIntyre DI. Subcoracoid neurovascular entrapment. Clin Orthop Rel Res 1975;108:27–30.
4. Stallworth JM, Horne JB. Diagnosis and management of thoracic outlet syndrome. Arch Surg 1984;119:1149–51.
5. Ambrad-Chalela E, Thomas GI, Johansen KH. Recurrent thoracic outlet syndrome. Am J Surg 2004;187:505–10.
6. Sanders RJ, Rao NM. Pectoralis minor obstruction of the axillary vein: report of six patients. J Vasc Surg 2007;45:1206–11.
7. Finkelstein JA, Johnston KW. Thrombosis of the axillary artery secondary to compression by pectoralis minor muscle. Ann Vasc Surg 1993;7:287–90.
8. McCarthy WJ, Yao JST, Schafer MF, et al. Upper extremity arterial injuries in athletes. J Vasc Surg 1989;9:317–27.
9. Tullos HS, Erwin WD, Woods W, et al. Unusual lesions of the pitching arm. Clin Orthop 1972;88:169–82.
10. Upton ARM, McComas AJ: The double crush in nerve-entrapment syndromes. Lancet 1973; 2:359–62.
11. Sanders RJ, Hammond SL. Diagnosis of thoracic outlet syndrome. J Vasc Surg 2007;46: 601–4.
12. Gilroy J, Meyer JS: Compression of the subclavian artery as a cause of ischemic brachial neuropathy. Brain 1963;86:733–45.
13. Roos DB, Owens JC: Thoracic outlet syndrome. Arch Surg 1966;93:71–4.
14. Sanders RJ, Haug CE: Thoracic outlet syndrome: a common sequela of neck injuries. Philadelphia: Lipppincott; 1991, p. 91.
15. Machanic BI, Sanders RJ. Medial antebrachial cutaneous nerve measurements to diagnose neurogenic thoracic outlet syndrome. Ann Vasc Surg 2008;22:248–54.
16. Sachatello CR. The axillopectoral muscle (Langer's axillary arch): a cause of axillary vein obstruction. Surgery 1977;5:610–2.
17. Sanders RJ, Haug CE: Thoracic outlet syndrome: a common sequela of neck injuries. Philadelphia: Lipppincott; 1991; pp. 183, 204.

13

Thoracic Outlet Syndrome – Which Way To Go?

Eitan S. Barbalat, M.S.-2 and William H. Pearce, M.D.

The thoracic outlet syndrome (TOS) is a broad description of any condition in which there is neurovascular compression in the thoracic outlet. Because the shoulder is dynamic, neurovascular compression may not be present with the arm in the neutral position but may be present and aggravated when the arm is abducted and externally rotated. Symptoms related to TOS have been recognized since the early part of the 18th century.[1-2] However, despite a large body of literature, there is no consensus as to the diagnosis and treatment of this disease. Much of the problem revolves around the lack of objective testing and the nature of the pathologic process leading to the patient's symptoms. Traditionally, the TOS has been divided into arterial, venous, and neurogenic (true and disputed). In addition, some patients may manifest combinations of neurovascular compression. In our practice, neurogenic thoracic outlet syndrome (NTOS) is commonly associated with venous thoracic outlet syndrome (VTOS). With the diversity of structures that can be compressed in the thoracic outlet, there are also a variety of anatomic elements that may produce the compression. Therefore, it is important to understand the anatomy of the thoracic outlet and how symptoms may arise.

The anterior and middle scalene muscles arise from the upper portions of the cervical vertebrae and insert in either the first or the second rib. The anterior scalene muscle inserts primarily on the scalene tubercle of the first rib, and the middle scalene inserts on the first and second ribs. There is a great deal of variability in the scalene triangle, with interdigitation between the two muscles, which is particularly prominent when there is a cervical rib.[3] Scalene muscles can be considered as an extension of the intercostal muscles with penetration of this muscle layer by the brachial plexus. These interdigitations of muscles and fibers may produce symptoms in and by themselves. These fibrous bands have been well described by Roos[4] and are thought to be the source of symptoms in patients with NTOS. With this anatomic variability, various trunks of the brachial plexus may be irritated. Another location in which the neurovascular bundle can be compressed is in the costoclavicular space. The costoclavicular space is a tight space that is bordered by the clavicle, subclavius muscles, first rib, and anterior scalene muscle and contains the subclavian vein. From an anatomic viewpoint, it can be seen that any one of these structures can be the pathologic process leading to obstruction of the subclavian vein and venous thrombosis. Finally, the venous and arterial structures may be compressed more distally beneath either the pectoralis minor muscle or the head of the humerus. An understanding of the varieties of neurovascular compression and the various elements leading to this compression underscores why there is such difficulty in making the diagnosis, tailoring the treatment, and understanding the results associated with its treatment. This chapter reviews the various forms of TOS and provide some insights into the appropriate surgical approach and expected results. In addition, this chapter reviews the various diagnostic modalities available and the pitfalls in interpreting results associated with this diagnosis.

ARTERIAL THORACIC OUTLET SYNDROME

Arterial injuries of the thoracic outlet occur as the result of bony abnormalities of either an abnormal first rib, the presence of a cervical rib, or injury to the clavicle.[5-10] These bony abnormalities produce intima ulceration at the location of the abnormality with and without a distal aneurysm.[10] These aneurysms are very prone to distal embolization, and symptoms are most commonly related to the peripheral emboli rather than to the proximal stenotic lesion. On very rare occasions, occlusion of the artery occurs with retrograde thrombosis into cerebral vessels, producing stroke.[11] Branches of the subclavian artery have been reported to thrombose as the result of muscle hypertrophy, particularly subclavian muscle, leading also to distal embolization.[9]

The evaluation and planning of the surgical procedure for ATOS with subclavian artery aneurysms (SAA) has been discussed in Chapter 6). The treatment of ATOS without SAA is similar. The only nuance in this situation is the presence of ulcerative lesions in arteries of relatively normal diameter. It may be difficult to image these lesions without intravascular ultrasound. However, in patients with bony abnormalities in the thoracic outlet and evidence of peripheral embolization, the intimal ulcer should be suspected. The reported risk of injury to nerves is 3 to 5% for the phrenic or the long thoracic and 1% for the brachial plexus (temporary and permanent). The most common complication is a pneumo- or hemothorax as a result of manipulation of the first or cervical ribs, resulting in pleural injury.

The preoperative evaluation of patients with ATOS requires computed tomographic angiography (CTA) imaging with the arm in a neutral position and with abduction and external rotation or position of use. Bony three-dimensional reconstructions and arteriography have been most useful in our practice (Figure 13–1). In this case, a 17-year-old female swimmer presented with arm fatigue and digital ischemia. The CT demonstrated a long transverse process of C7 and compression of the subclavian vein by fibrous band. The three-dimensional reconstruction of the thoracic outlet provides a clear anatomic depiction of the bony abnormalities and where the resection of bone should occur. The CTA is also performed in the abducted and externally rotated position. The dynamic nature of the thoracic outlet mandates dynamic imaging because the anatomic structures shift as the shoulder is moved. Even though the CTA may provide important information, it is not as accurate as standard arteriography. We have at least one example in our practice of a young baseball pitcher who could not obtain maximal abduction and external rotation within the CT scanner but could duplicate his pitching movement in the angiography suite, eliciting the dynamic compression of the subclavian artery (Figure 13–2A–D).

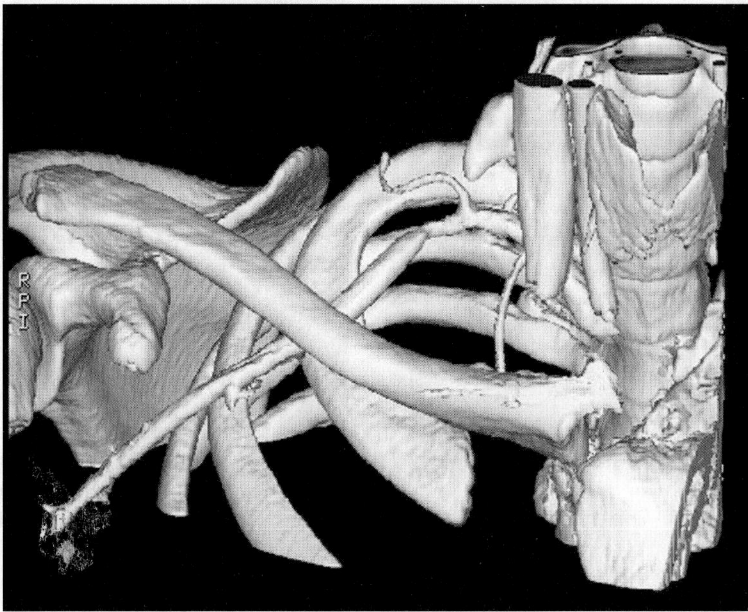

Figure 13-1. Long transverse process of C7 with fibrous band narrowing of the subclavian artery.

Selection of an appropriate surgical approach is based on the patient's anatomy and the surgeon's experience. For example, in the patient with no bony or arterial abnormality in whom compression occurs only in extreme positions, resection of the first rib seems most appropriate without arterial reconstruction. In the patient demonstrated in Figure 13–2, the posterior rib appeared to be the compressive element. Therefore, every effort was made to remove as much of the posterior rib as could be performed safely from the transaxillary approach. However, in patients who require arterial reconstruction, the supra- and infraclavicular approaches are more appropriate (see discussion in Chapter 6 on subclavian artery aneurysms). This approach allows for maximal exposure and control of the subclavian and axillary arteries.

VENOUS THORACIC OUTLET SYNDROME

There is a broad spectrum of viewpoints in treating patients with effort vein thrombosis. The approaches vary from anticoagulation only, to thrombolysis and first rib removal, to first rib removal and venous reconstruction with distal arteriovenous (AV) fistula and clavectomy.[12-15] Generally, although most surgeons have agreed with the aggressive approach to young patients' effort vein thrombosis, both Olcott and Johansson have suggested a more conservative approach in selective individuals.[16-17] Freischlag has reviewed the variety of surgical algorithms used for the treatment of VTOS and has concluded that no one approach is applicable to all.[12] In our own practice, we have used first rib decompression with or without postoperative venoplasty. We have had two serious complications with hemothorax when there was concomitant use of venoplasty along with anticoagulation. We no longer recommend the use of perioperative anticoagulation when venoplasty is being considered.

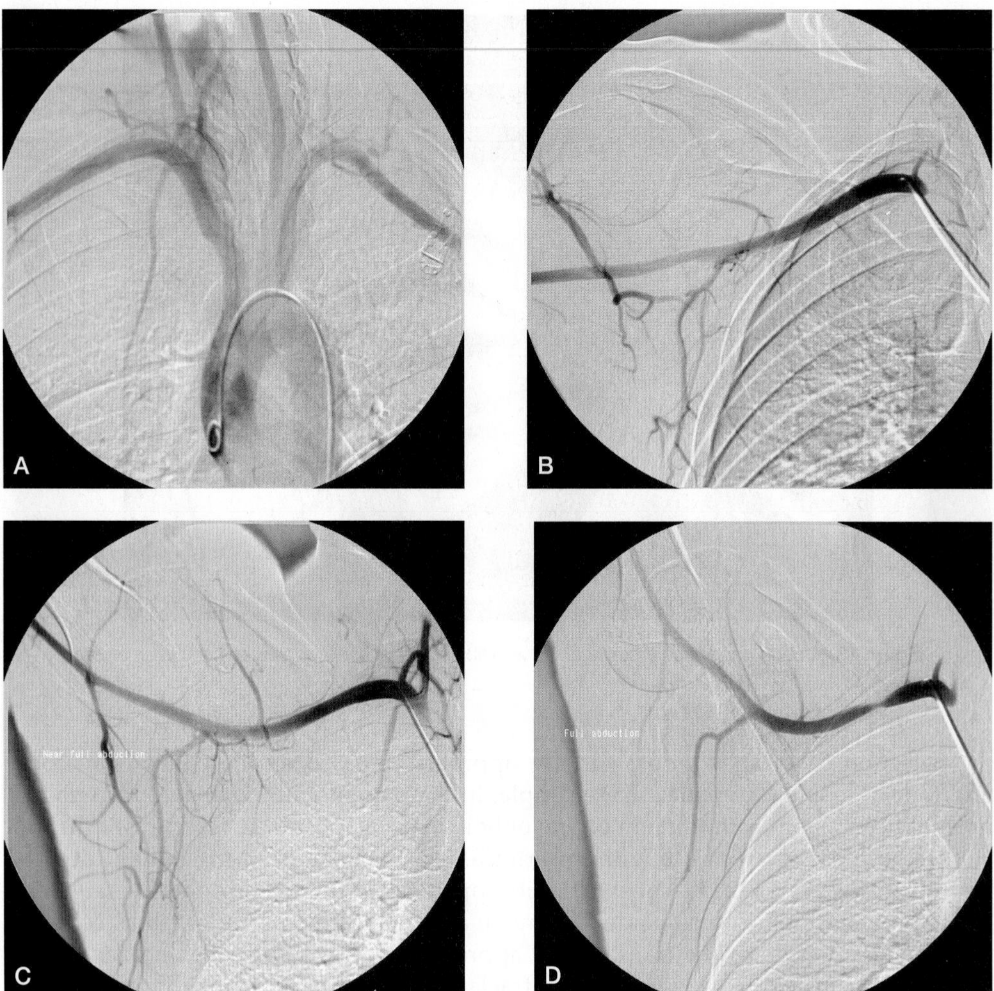

Figure 13-2. Subclavian artery of 19-year-old baseball player with ischemic finger and splinter hemorrhages.
A. Arm in neutral position.
B. Arm partially abducted.
C. Arm in near full abduction.
D. Arm in full abduction and in position of pitching.

The underlying surgical principle for decompressing patients with VTOS is to remove the obstructive elements. Here the obstructive elements may represent the clavicle, subclavius muscle, first rib, or scalene muscle hypertrophy. A transaxillary rib resection removes much of the floor of the scalene triangle as well as the scalene muscle. The transaxillary approach affords the best view of the inferior border of the subclavian vein and allows an adequate resection of this bony structure. A supraclavicular approach affords a view of only the first rib a few centimeters distal to the insertion of the scalene muscle. Retraction of the subclavian vein may provide an additional few millimeters to resect the rib directly underneath the vein. The approach advocated by Thompson et al., using a second incision below the clavicle, is most appropriate in muscular patients and where it is very difficult to see the rib underneath the subclavian vein.[18] With this incision, there is a clear view of the margins of resection below the vein. Thompson has reported excellent results using this approach with surgical venoplasty and the creation of a distal AV fistula.[19] There are rare reports of axillary vein occlusion due to pectoralis minor hypertrophy.[20] In these instances, resection of the pectoralis muscles relieves the compression.

NEUROGENIC THORACIC OUTLET SYNDROME

NTOS is by far the most common presentation of neurovascular compression. True NTOS is rare and is manifested by hypothenar wasting and a mixed picture of motor function loss in the median nerve distribution and sensory loss in the ulnar distribution. This lesion is localized to the lowest trunk of the thoracic outlet. In such instances, resection of the first rib is mandatory and can be accomplished from either above or below the clavicle. In our experience, complete neurologic recovery is unusual. Chronic compression of the nerve often accounts for the permanency of the injury.

In patients with a disputed form of TOS (the most common form), the surgical approach is much more variable. The variety of approaches and reported outcomes are the result of the lack of consensus on the diagnosis of NTOS and the measures of success. Sanders, in Table 13–1, reported a variety of symptoms associated with TOS.[21] As one can see, none is either specific or sensitive to the disease process and can be produced by a variety of other conditions. The most suggestive symptoms of NTOS include numbness and paresthesia in the ulnar distribution and difficulty with the use of the arms above the head. Similarly, positive physical findings are variable and, indeed, may not be specific or sensitive, given the selected patient population (Table 13–2). The most reliable sign is that at 90 degrees of abduction and external rotation, symptoms should occur within 60 seconds (East/Roos test). Electrodiagnostic tests, nerve conductive velocity (NCV), and electromyography (EMG) have been used primarily to rule out other neurologic conditions, including carpal tunnel syndrome, cubital tunnel

TABLE 13-1. INCIDENCE OF SPECIFIC SYMPTOMS IN LAST 50 PATIENTS

Symptoms	50 patients (%)
Neck pain	88
Trapezius pain	92
Supraclavicular pain	76
Chest pain	72
Shoulder pain	88
Arm pain	88
Occipital headache	76
Paresthesia:	98
All 5 fingers	58
4th and 5th fingers	26
1st to 3rd fingers	14
No paresthesia	2

This table was published in Journal of Vascular Surgery, Vol. 46, Sanders RJ, Hammond SL, Rao NM. Diagnosis of thoracic outlet syndrome, 601–604. Copyright 2007 by The Society for Vascular Surgery.

TABLE 13-2. POSITIVE PHYSICAL FINDINGS IN 50 PATIENTS

Positive Physical Findings	50 Patients (%)
Upper Limb Tension Test (ULTT)[22]	98
90-degree abduction in external rotation	100
Scalene muscle tenderness	94
Scalene pressure yields radiating symptoms	92
Neck rotation to opposite side	90
Head tilt to opposite side	90
Sensation to light touch	68

syndrome, or cervical radiculopathy. Recently, it has been reported that the median antebrachial cutaneous nerve (MAC) is a sensitive test to detect changes in sensory nerve transmission. It is not routinely used but may be one of few tests that are specific to the TOS. A scalene block is commonly used to confirm the diagnosis. Although it may be performed blindly, we recommend the use of ultrasound to ensure direct injection of the scalene muscle. A positive test, that is, relief of symptoms, has a high predictive value for good outcome following surgery.

Surgeons have also divided neurologic symptoms of the TOS into upper plexus symptoms versus lower plexus symptoms or combinations. Because of the variability of the anatomy of the scalene muscles, it is possible that multiple nerve trunks are being irritated simultaneously. Therefore, what is the best surgical approach to relieve symptoms in these patients? Surgical treatment of thoracic outlet has generally been to remove either the scalene muscles or the first rib or both. The first rib may be removed by a variety of techniques, including a posterior approach, a transaxillary approach, or a supraclavicular approach. The transaxillary approach was popularized by Roos, who performed detailed studies of the scalene anatomy and its relationship to symptoms.[4] The transaxillary approach is cosmetic and avoids the large operative procedure involved with the posterior approach. The transaxillary approach also provides a clearer exposure of the neurovascular bundle and the pectoralis minor muscle. However, it is a difficult operation, particularly in muscular patients, with poor lighting and visibility. As a result, injuries could occur to any of the neurovascular structures, at times resulting in disastrous consequences.[23] Other surgeons believe that when upper brachial plexus symptoms are present, a supraclavicular approach is more appropriate. The supraclavicular approach provides a clear exposure of all the brachial plexus and possible interdigitations of the scalene muscles. Removal of the anterior scalene muscle, either in total or in part, has been employed along with partial resection of the middle scalene muscle. The supraclavicular approach provides the clearest view of the potential pathologic process. In addition, surgeons have used combinations of the two approaches using the transaxillary approach as a first procedure followed by a supraclavicular scalenectomy should recurrence occur or if the patient's symptoms are unresolved following the first procedure.

In this discussion, the focus has been on making an accurate diagnosis of TOS and then tailoring the operative procedure to address those concerns. Because of the variabilities in the definition of TOS and the potential compressive elements, there has been a wide selection of approaches. This problem is compounded by the fact that, because there are no diagnostic criteria prior to the procedure, improvement is similarly subjective. The outcomes of these many surgical options fall into several categories (Table 13–3). The most reliable category is the rate of perioperative neurologic and the pulmonary complication rate. Overall, the total supraclavicular complication rates ranged from 8 to 72% (small series). Other complications of this approach included pneumothorax (0 to 5%) and neurologic (0 to 5%). For the transaxillary approach, overall complication rates ranged from 10 to 45%, pneumothorax (7-15%), and neurologic (0-31%). Complication rates for simultaneous axillary-supraclavicular procedures were 2% neurologic and <10% pneumothorax. Chang et al. from Johns Hopkins, using a national database, evaluated 2016 TOS operations.[24] The majority of these patients were treated at teaching hospitals and, overall, there was a 0.6% brachial plexus injury rate and 1.74% for vascular injuries. The complications rates were lower at teaching hospitals than at community hospitals. However, the determination of long-term outcome is much more complicated. Many authors have simply used either telephone or mail surveys to ask the patients whether their symptoms have improved, remained unchanged, or worsened since the operative procedure. Numerous problems exist with these small surveys, particularly when a telephone survey is made by the operating surgeon or his/her office. The number of patients considering an excellent-to-good response varies between 50 and 100%. This seems to be true whether the approach is transaxillary, supraclavicular, or a combination. In addition, the general trend is that, as follow-up is extended, good and excellent outcomes tend to diminish.

Some investigators have increased the spectrum of endpoints, using pain scales of 5 or 10 to discriminate the pain symptoms, and others have used return to work and functional outcome studies such as the SF-36 and SF-12 as the endpoints. Axelrod and his colleagues at the University of Michigan reported on the results of the supraclavicular approach with an average follow-up of 40 months. In this study, 65% of patients reported improved outcomes. However, 35% of patients remained on medication and 18% were disabled. Perioperative factors that were associated with persistent disability and failure to improve included depression and having less than a high school education.[25] The TOS program at the University of Maryland is staffed not only by physical therapists but also by psychiatrists who perform preoperative psychological evaluations. Chang et al. from Johns Hopkins reported a more recent study of 105 patients undergoing transaxillary rib resection for NTOS.[24] These patients were evaluated by a disabilities of the arm, shoulder, and hand (DASH) survey and SF-12 quality of life survey. The DASH survey is specific to the upper extremity for orthopedic problems. Half of the neurogenic patients returned to full-time work or activity by 5 months. These patients had SF-12 physical component scores similar to patients with chronic heart failure, which did improve by 0.2 points following surgery. The DASH scores were similar to those of patients with rotator cuff tears and improved with surgery (0.85 point). Secondary interventions were common in patients with NTOS, including the requirement for additional physical therapy, Botox injections, muscle relaxation, and pain management referrals. In the only randomized controlled study of patients with NTOS, Sheth et al. randomized patients between supraclavicular and neuroplasty of the brachial plexus and transaxillary first rib resections.[26] Fifty-five patients were randomized in this study. The preoperative signs that were consistent with TOS included onset of symptoms with provocative positioning and tenderness in the supraclavicular space. With a median follow-up of 37 months, the group that underwent transaxillary first rib resection had better outcomes than those undergoing supraclavicular scalenectomy. Patients undergoing transaxillary first rib resections re-

(Text continues on page 175)

TABLE 13-3. NEUROGENIC THORACIC OUTLET SYNDROME

Supraclavicular Approach

Series	Number of Procedures	Method	Outcome Metric	Results	Mean Follow-Up	Complications (Nerve, Pneumothorax, Total)
Axelrod et al. (2001)[25]	170	Questionnaires	Short term - Patients were questioned about their overall satisfaction, their activity and work status, and the amount of pain and paresthesia. Wound healing, range of motion, and muscle/joint dysfunction were evaluated, and an overall assessment of the patients' progress was reported.	Short-term, pain improved 80%, paresthesia improved 81%, range of motion improved 82%, Moderately or highly satisfied- 86%, full activity (self-reported) 55%, full employment 80%, restricted work 30%, taking medication 29%, taking narcotics 9%, taking nonsteroidal anti-inflammatory drugs 20%, Progress (good/average 67%).	Short term: 10.4 months	18/170 (10.6%) had complications 9/170 pneumothorax requiring chest tube placement 6/170 pleural entry not requiring a chest tube 1/170 - transient phrenic nerve injury
			Long term - Questionnaire to assess patients' perceptions of their current status and level of satisfaction; asked to grade their symptoms of pain; also reported their activity level and overall satisfaction with the operation	Long term, still have symptoms 65%, taking medication 35%, symptoms improved with surgery 66%, satisfied 64%, would have operation again 69%, 75% employed/homemaker, prolonged disability 18%.	Long term: 47 months	
McCarthy et al. (1999)[27]	37 total (33 with neurogenic symptoms)	Questionnaire	Patients categorized themselves: 1) asymptomatic/cured, 2) significantly improved, 3) minimal improvement or the same as their preoperative symptoms, 4) symptoms had been made worse	18/33 (55%) were asymptomatic/cured 7/33 (21%) had significantly improved symptoms 8/33 (24%) had minimal or no improvement 0/33 (0%) had worse symptoms postoperatively	12 months	3/37 (8%) had complications. 0/37 had pneumothorax 1/37 had nerve injury (Horner's syndrome; resolved after 2 months)
Sheth and Campbell (2005)[26]	25	Questionnaire and telephone interview	Percentage of pain relief: Pain level status VAS (100 mm-line) Categorical assessment of pain relief postoperatively (excellent, good, fair, or poor) Average pain level (9-point affective scale (0 = no pain, 8 = very intolerable pain)	30 ± 8% pain relief. preoperative VAS score = 82 ± 3, and postoperative VAS score = 61 ± 7 48% reported good or excellent pain relief. Patients went from 6.5 ± 0.2 preoperatively to 5.1 ± 0.5 postoperatively.	37 months	No complications

			Were symptoms better or same during the arm-raise maneuver strategy? Numbness Would they undergo surgery again for same results?	Lowest pain experienced postoperatively = 49 ± 7. Greatest amount of pain felt during the day was 67 ± 8 48% felt improvement postoperatively compared with preoperative symptoms when raising their arm. Preoperatively 5.5 ± 0.5 areas were numb, whereas postoperatively 4.6 ± 0.6 areas were numb. 56% said they would undergo this surgery again for the same results.		
Urschel (1999)[28]	336	Questionnaire		Early results = 310/336 improvement 5-yr improvement 150/336 20-yr improvement = 31/336 still improved	Not stated	Not stated
Sanders and Pearce (1989)[29]	278	Questionnaire	Asked for patients' subjective evaluation postoperatively at different time points. Improved = total of excellent, good, and fair responses.	92% improved at 1-3 mo, 79% improved at 1-2 yr, 72% improved at 3-5 yr, 72% improved at 5-10 yr.	N/A	13/278 (4.7%) neurologic 7/278 (2.5%) pneumothorax requiring tap 59/278 (21.2%) total complications
Reilly and Stoney (1988)[30]	39		Used a subjective grading system	59% Good 33% Fair 8% Failed	Length of follow-up = 1-30 mo	
Thompson and Hernandez (1979)[18]	15		Used a subjective grading system	87% Good 0% Fair 13% Failed	Not stated	
Colli et al. (2006)[31]	22		Subjective comparison between preoperative and postoperative sensory and motor symptoms. Outcome was evaluated based on overall working capacity after treatment = normal when patient returned to previous job without limitations; working limitation when patient returned to the same job with some limitation, unchanged - no improvement of symptoms, or worsened.	16/20 (80%) of patients became normal/marked improvement of their pain/paresthesias. 4/11 (36.4%) of patients had improvement in sensory function of their limb postoperatively. 11/18 (61.1%) returned to their same work with no or slight limitation postoperatively.	137 months	10/22 (45.5%) neurologic complications 1/22 (4.5%) pneumothorax 16/22 (72.7%) total complications

(Continued)

TABLE 13-3. NEUROGENIC THORACIC OUTLET SYNDROME *(Continued)*

Transaxillary Approach

Series	Number of Procedures	Method	Outcome Metric	Results	Mean Follow-Up	Complications (Nerve, Pneumothorax, Total)
Leffert and Perlmutter (1999)[32]	282	Telephone interview	Completely asymptomatic, substantially improved, improved, no relief from operation, worse pain after operation.	Completely asymptomatic - 98/282 (34.75%) Substantially improved: requiring no analgesics - 97/282 (34.04%) Improved but using occasional non-narcotic analgesics - 45/282 (15.96%) No relief from operation - 39/282 (13.8%) Worse pain after operation - 3/282 (1.06%)	55 months	127/282 (45%) had complications; 89/282 (31%) = intraoperative pneumothorax - no permanent residua; 2/282 (0.7%) - pneumothorax postoperatively; 89/282 (31%) - nerve injury - 43 complete recovery within 6 weeks, - 36 the recovery took longer; 10 patients had permanent numbness
		Also objectively compared swelling, motor loss, and sensory loss preoperatively and postoperatively	Objective determination if the problem existed preoperatively and postoperatively	Swelling - 67 preoperatively, 2 postoperatively Motor loss - 138 preoperatively, 17 postoperatively Sensory loss - 136 preoperatively, 14 postoperatively		
Sheth and Campbell (2005)[26]	24	Questionnaire and telephone survey	Percentage of pain relief Pain level status represented by a score on a VAS (100 mm-line) Categorical assessment of pain relief postoperatively (excellent, good, fair, or poor) Average pain level (on a 9-point affective scale (0 = no pain, 8 = very intolerable pain) Pain level at its worst and best.	Patients said they had 52 ± 8% pain relief. Preoperative VAS score = 77 ± 3, and postoperative VAS score = 39 ± 7 75% reported good or excellent pain relief Patients went from 6.5 ± 0.2 preoperatively to 3.7 ± 0.4 postoperatively.	37 months	No complications

			Were symptoms better or same during the arm-raise maneuver strategy.	Least pain experienced postoperatively = 30 ± 6. Greatest amount of pain felt during the day in the postoperative period was 47 ± 8	
			Numbness	72% felt improvement postoperatively compared with preoperative symptoms when raising their arm. Preoperatively 5.2 ± 0.61 areas were numb, and postoperatively 2.8 ± 0.6 areas were numb.	
			Would they undergo surgery again for same results?	79% said they would undergo this surgery again for the same results.	
Fulford et al. (2001)[33]	83	Questionnaire and telephone survey	Postoperative outcome was retrospectively graded into the following categories: 1) completely better, 2) partially better, 3) no change, 4) worse. Also, in order to assess functional recovery, patients were asked if their symptoms had prevented them from performing activities at work or at home and if there had been any improvement in this regard subsequent to surgery. Patients were also asked if there had been a short-term symptomatic benefit following surgery, and finally, if they felt the operation had been beneficial.		Short-term median follow-up (6 months) Long-term median follow-up (4 years)
Altobelli et al. (2005)[34]	254	Patients were asked to judge their symptomatic improvement	Success = greater than or equal to 50% improvement on the operation side, the patient returning to preoperational work status without the need for an additional ipsilateral procedure, or both.	118/254 (46%) successful	25 months

(Continued)

TABLE 13-3. NEUROGENIC THORACIC OUTLET SYNDROME *(Continued)*

Transaxillary Approach

Series	Number of Procedures	Method	Outcome Metric	Results	Mean Follow-Up	Complications (Nerve, Pneumothorax, Total)
Urschel (1997)[35]	2210 (250 for upper plexus compression only; 452 for combined upper and lower plexus compression; 1508 for lower plexus compressions.	Looked at symptom relief postoperatively	Percentage of symptom relief for each type of plexus compression	96% patients had relief of symptoms of the upper plexus; 95% had relief of symptoms for combined upper and lower plexus; 95% had relief of symptoms for lower plexus compression.		
Chang et al. (2009)[36]	44	Administered Quality of Life Surveys to patients	Short-Form 12 (SF-12) and Disability of Arm, Hand and Shoulder (DASH) given preoperatively and then again at 3, 6, 12, 18, and 24 months. These are Quality of Life Instruments. Determined rate of recovery, and used Kaplan-Meier method to analyze time to return to work.	Neurogenic had SF-12 of 33.8 on Physical Component Score (PCS), and 44.5 on Mental Component Score (MCS). PCS improved by 0.24 points and MCS scores improved 0.15 points per month. Initial DASH score was 50.2, and that improved by 0.85 points per month postoperatively. 15/44 (34.1%) patients were unemployed or disabled upon presentation, but 22/44 (50%) patients eventually returned to full-time work or activity during the study follow-up period, half of them doing so by 4 months and 75% by 5 months. Median time to recovery of normal quality of life was 23 months for physical function and 12 months for mental function.	24 months of follow up	Pneumothorax = 7/44 (15.9%) Nerve injury = 0/44 (0%) Total = 10/44 (22.7%)

Sanders and Pearce (1989)[29]	111	Survey: Subjective grading of excellent, good, and fair.		91% improved at 1-3 mo, 76% improved at 1-2 yr, 73% improved at 3-5 yr, 69% improved at 5-10 yr, 64% improved at 10-15 yr	N/A	4/111 (3.6%) neurologic complications 10/111 (9.0%) pneumothorax requiring tap 50/111 (45%) total complications
Roos (1982)[37]	1315	Questionnaire	Used a subjective grading system	92% Good 0% Fair 8% Failed	3-180 months	

Axillary-Supraclavicular Sequentially Approach

Series	N	Outcome Metric		Results	Mean Follow-Up	Complications (Nerve, Pneumothorax, Total)
Altobelli et al. (2005)[34]	80	Patients were asked to judge their symptomatic improvement	Success = greater than or equal to 50% improvement on the operation side, the patient returning to preoperational work status without the need for an additional ipsilateral procedure, or both.	45/80 (56.3%) successful	25 months	

Axillary-Supraclavicular Simultaneously Approach

Series	Number of Operations	Method	Outcome Metric	Results	Mean Follow-Up	Complications (Nerve, Pneumothorax, Total)
Atasoy (2004)[38]	532 total surgeries, 102 respondents to questionnaire	Gave patients a questionnaire regarding the outcome of their surgery.	Excellent (70-100% improvement) Good (50-70% improvement) Better (30-50 percent improvement) Fair (10-30% improvement) Very Poor (less than 10% improvement)	36/102 (35.2%) 24/102 (23.5%) 26/102 (25.5%) 9/102 (8.8%) 5/102 (4.9%)		Pneumothorax = less than 10% Nerve = several patients had temporary phrenic nerve palsy caused by surgical manipulation and traction; 12-14 other complications occurred.

(Continued)

TABLE 13-3. NEUROGENIC THORACIC OUTLET SYNDROME *(Continued)*

Other

Series	Number of Operations	Method	Outcome Metric	Results	Mean Follow-Up	Complications (Nerve, Pneumothorax, Total)
Sanders and Pearce (1989)[29]	279	Asked for patients' subjective evaluation postoperatively at different time points. Improved = total of excellent, good, and fair responses.	Excellent (relief of all symptoms); good (relief of the major symptoms with some residual pain or paresthesias); fair (improvement in some symptoms, but persistence in major ones, but the patient felt the operation was worthwhile in spite of limited relief); poor/failure (no significant improvement)	93% improved at 1-3 mo, 77% improved at 1-2 yr, 70% improved at 3-5 yr, 69% improved at 5-10 yr, and 65% improved at 10-15 yr	NA	17/279 (6%) temporary phrenic palsy; 1 /279 (0.4%) pneumothorax requiring tap; 23/279 (8.2%) total complications
Sharp et al. (2001)[39]	36 total (27 with neurogenic symptoms)	Contacted patients for a phone interview postoperatively, where patients rated their relief of symptoms and satisfaction with the operation.	Excellent = relief of all symptoms Good = relief of most major symptoms Fair = relief of some symptoms Poor = no improvement or worsening of symptoms. Would they undergo procedure again for same results? (Measure of Patient Satisfaction)	5/27 (18%) = Excellent result 13/27 (48%) = Good result 1/27 (4%) = Fair result 1/27 (4%) = Poor result 7/27 (26%) lost to follow-up 14/16 (88%) of patients would have the same surgery again for relief of thoracic outlet syndrome.	4 years	Transaxillary approach = 1/28 procedures (3.5%) (neurologic); supraclavicular approach = 3/8 procedures (37.5%) (neurologic) 0/36 (0%); pneumothorax 4/36 (11%) total complications (all neurologic)

ported significantly less pain and a greater percentage of pain relief as compared with those undergoing scalenectomies.

From Table 13–3, there is a broad spectrum in reported results whether one uses functional outcomes, neurologic evaluations, subjective improvement, or SF-12 surveys, reflecting the lack of sensitivity and specificity in the diagnosis of NTOS and outcome measures used.[25-39]

The role of physical therapy in nonoperative treatment of TOS has been poorly studied. There is no standardized recommended physical therapy program for NTOS, and it varies dramatically from center to center. Retraining of cervical and scapular muscles is important to realign posture and location of the clavicle. There is only one indirect study that looks at the question of nonoperative therapy versus surgical therapy. Landry evaluated patients who were seen for independent medical evaluations for work-related injuries. The patients were studied using a standardized telephone interview or patient questionnaire.[40] The patient's ability to return to work and assessment of their current level of symptoms were accessed. This was performed preoperatively and in follow-up. Nineteen percent of all patients underwent first rib resections and the remainder were treated nonoperatively. Sixty percent of patients who underwent first rib resection returned to work compared with 78% who did not have a surgical procedure. Patients' estimate of severity of symptoms preoperatively was not different between the two groups. In late follow-up, in the operated group there was complete resolution of symptoms in 7%, marked improvement in 27%, minimal improvement in 40%, no improvement in 13%, and feeling worse in 13%. In the nonoperated group, the change with physical therapy was not different from the operative group: 2% resolution, 30% marked improvement, 22% minimal improvement, 31% no improvement, and 16% worse. The authors concluded that there may not be a significant benefit from surgical intervention.

COMMENT

There is little debate over the operative approach in treatment of patients with ATOS. Limb salvage and prevention of embolus has been demonstrated consistently in the literature. In patients with axillary-subclavian vein thrombosis, the literature predominantly supports an aggressive approach with immediate thrombolysis followed by thoracic outlet decompression. However, this treatment paradigm recently has been challenged by several authors, suggesting that long-term outcomes may be just as good using a nonoperative approach. However, long-term symptoms (postphlebitic syndrome) may be substantial.[41] It is reasonable to use thoracic outlet decompression in conjunction with thrombolytic therapy in young active individuals in whom the long-term outcome remains debatable. In older less active patients and in those patients who have developed substantial collateral venous outflow, surgery may not be necessary.

The most difficult problem that faces clinicians is the disputed form of NTOS. In these patients, it is often difficult to make the diagnosis, and one relies on clinical experience and many subjective factors. The rapid reproduction of symptoms with the arms abducted and externally rotated and tenderness over the scalene muscle seem to be the most consistent presenting symptoms. A good response to a scalene muscle block is also predictive of a good clinical outcome. However, in the literature reviewed, this outcome may be no different than those receiving physical therapy alone.

Because of the many discrepancies and controversies surrounding NTOS, Robert Thompson from Washington University established a core study group in an attempt to standardize the diagnosis, nomenclature, and evaluation of patients with TOS. In addition, because nonoperative therapy has also been poorly defined, further biomechanical investigations in shoulder function and the particular physiologic abnormalities associated with TOS must be pursued. It is clearly the time to put TOS under scientific scrutiny to understand its pathogenesis and its optimal treatment.

REFERENCES

1. Cooper A. On exostosis. In: Cooper A, Travers B, eds. Surgical Essays, 3rd ed. London: Cox & Son; 1820, p. 128.
2. Sanders RJ. History. In: Sanders RJ, Haug CE, eds. Thoracic Outlet Syndrome: A Common Sequela of Neck Injuries. Philadelphia: J.B. Lippincott Company; 1991, pp. 11–20.
3. Kirgis HD, Reed AF. Significant anatomic relations in the syndrome of the scalene muscle. Ann Surg 1948;127:1182–201.
4. Roos DB. Congenital anomalies associated with thoracic outlet syndrome. Anatomy, symptoms, diagnosis, and treatment. Am J Surg 1976;132:771–8.
5. Keiffer E. Arterial complications of the thoracic outlet syndrome. In: Bergan JJ, Yao JST, eds. Evaluation and Treatment of Upper and Lower Extremity Circulatory Disorders. New York: Grune & Stratton; 1984, pp. 249–75.
6. Scher LA, Veith FJ, Samson RH, et al. Vascular complications of thoracic outlet syndrome. J Vasc Surg 1986;3:565–8.
7. Short DW. The subclavian artery in 16 patients with complete cervical ribs. J Cardiovasc Surg 1975;16:135–41.
8. Eden KC. The vascular complications of cervical ribs and first thoracic rib abnormalities. Br J Surg 1939;27:111–39.
9. Abouljoud MS, Obeid FN, Horst HM, et al. Arterial injuries of the thoracic outlet: a ten-year experience. Am Surg 1993;59:590–5.
10. Durham JR, Yao JS, Pearce WH, et al. Arterial injuries in the thoracic outlet syndrome. J Vasc Surg 1995;21:57–69.
11. Yamaguchi R, Kohga H, Kurosaki M, et al. Acute basilar artery occlusion in a patient with left subclavian artery occlusion due to first rib anomaly: case report. Neurol Med Chir (Tokyo) 2008;48:355–8.
12. deLeon RA, Chang DC, Hassoun HT, et al. Multiple treatment algorithms for successful outcomes in venous thoracic outlet syndrome. Surgery 2009;145:500–7.
13. Molina JE. Approach to the confluence of the subclavian and internal jugular veins without claviculectomy. Semin Vasc Surg 2000;13:10–9.
14. Green RM, Waldman D, Ouriel K, et al. Claviculectomy for subclavian venous repair: long-term functional results. J Vasc Surg 2000;32:315–21.
15. Doyle A, Wolford HY, Davies MG, et al. Management of effort thrombosis of the subclavian vein: Today's treatment. Ann Vasc Surg 2007;21:723–9.
16. Lee WA, Hill BB, Harris EJ Jr, et al. Surgical intervention is not required for all patients with subclavian vein thrombosis. J Vasc Surg 2000;32:57–67.
17. Johansen KH. Does axillosubclavian vein thrombosis oblige first rib resection? Presented at Western Surgical Association 116th Scientific Session, Santa Fe, NM, November 9–12, 2008.
18. Thompson JB, Hernandez IA. The thoracic outlet syndrome: a second look. Am J Surg 1979;138:251–3.
19. Thompson RW, Schneider PA, Nelken NA, et al. Circumferential venolysis and paraclavicular thoracic outlet decompression for "effort thrombosis" of the subclavian vein. J Vasc Surg 1992;16:723–32.

20. Sanders RJ, Rao NM. Pectoralis minor obstruction of the axillary vein: report of six patients. J Vasc Surg 2007;45:1206–11.
21. Sanders RJ, Hammond SL, Rao NM. Diagnosis of thoracic outlet syndrome. J Vasc Surg 2007;46:601–4.
22. Gilroy J, Meyer JS. Compression of the subclavian artery as a cause of ischemic brachial neuropathy. Brain 1963;86:733–45.
23. Cherington M, Happer I, Machanic B, Parry L. Surgery for thoracic outlet syndrome may be hazardous to your health. Muscle Nerve 1986;9:632–4.
24. Chang DC, Lidor AO, Matsen LS, Freischlag JA. Reported in-hospital complications following rib resections for neurogenic thoracic outlet syndrome. Ann Vasc Surg 2007;21:564–70.
25. Axelrod DA, Proctor MC, Geisser ME, et al. Outcomes after surgery for thoracic outlet syndrome. J Vasc Surg 2001;33:1220–5.
26. Sheth RN, Campbell JN. Surgical treatment of thoracic outlet syndrome: a randomized trial comparing two operations. J Neurosurg: Spine 2005;3:355–63.
27. McCarthy MJ, Varty K, London NJ, Bell PR. Experience of supraclavicular exploration and decompression for treatment of thoracic outlet syndrome. Ann Vasc Surg 1999;13:268–74.
28. Urschel HC Jr. Neurovascular compression in the thoracic outlet: changing management over 50 years. Adv Surg 1999;33:95–111.
29. Sanders RJ, Pearce WH. The treatment of thoracic outlet syndrome: a comparison of different operations. J Vasc Surg 1989;10:626–34.
30. Reilly LM, Stoney RJ. Supraclavicular approach for thoracic outlet decompression. J Vasc Surg 1988;8:329–34.
31. Colli BO, Carlotti CG Jr, Assirati JA Jr, Marques W Jr. Neurogenic thoracic outlet syndromes: a comparison of true and nonspecific syndromes after surgical treatment. Surg Neurol 2006;65:262–71.
32. Leffert RD, Perlmutter GS. Thoracic outlet syndrome. Results of 282 transaxillary first rib resections. Clin Orthop 1999;368:66–79.
33. Fulford PE, Batuneid MS, Ibrahim MR, et al. Outcome of transaxillary rib resection for thoracic outlet syndrome—a 10 year experience. Cardiovasc Surg 2001;9:620–4.
34. Altobelli GG, Kudo T, Haas BT, et al. Thoracic outlet syndrome: pattern of clinical success after operative decompression. J Vasc Surg 2005;42:122–8.
35. Urschel HC Jr, Razzuk MA. Upper plexus thoracic outlet syndrome: optimal therapy. Ann Thorac Surg 1997;63:935–9.
36. Chang DC, Rotellini-Coltvet LA, Mukherjee D, et al. Surgical intervention for thoracic outlet syndrome improves patient's quality of life. J Vasc Surg. 2009;49:630–7.
37. Roos DB. The place for scalenectomy and first-rib resection in thoracic outlet syndrome. Surgery 1982;92:1077–85.
38. Atasoy E. Combined surgical treatment of thoracic outlet syndrome: transaxillary first rib resection and transcervical scalenectomy. Hand Clin 2004;20:71–82.
39. Sharp WJ, Nowak LR, Zamani T, et al. Long-term follow-up and patients' satisfaction after surgery for thoracic outlet syndrome. Ann Vasc Surg 2001;15:32–6.
40. Landry GJ, Moneta GL, Taylor LM Jr, et al. Long-term functional outcome of neurogenic thoracic outlet syndrome in surgically and conservatively treated patients. J Vasc Surg 2001;33:312–9.
41. Zierler RE, Caps MT. Long-term outcomes for upper extremity deep vein thrombosis. In: Pearce WB, Yao JST, Eskandari MK, Morasch MD, eds. Vascular Surgery – A Manual for Survival. Shelton, CT: PMPH USA, Ltd.; 2009.

14

Quality of Life Research in Thoracic Outlet Syndrome

Hayley B. Osen, B.A., David C. Chang, Ph.D., M.P.H., M.B.A., and Julie Freischlag, M.D.

INTRODUCTION

Quality of life research provides a conceptual framework to judge patient outcomes, health status, and the effectiveness of specific treatments. Quality of life research also has extensive applications: in descriptive research, it is used to characterize the burdens of disease and injury; in clinical research, it is used to test the efficacy of treatments; and for clinicians, it can be used to monitor outcomes and evaluate performance. Quality of life research is especially important for analyzing the outcomes of surgery, particularly as modern medicine has evolved and the emphasis has shifted from mortality to perceived health status, wellness, and patient preference. Quality of life measurements can therefore help clinicians and researchers identify determinants of health and investigate illness.

Quality of life measurement is especially important in thoracic outlet syndrome (TOS) patients. Whereas venous TOS may be confirmed by ultrasound or venogram, no definitive diagnostic tests have been validated for neurogenic TOS. Thus, the diagnosis of TOS remains largely a clinical diagnosis, with patients often being seen by multiple physicians and labeled as either disabled or malingering. The same uncertainty carries forward to the evaluation of patient outcomes postoperatively, and to date, many were based on unstructured subjective assessment. A structured, validated assessment of the quality of life and functional outcomes of TOS patients is necessary to advance the state of the clinical science in this field.

QUALITY OF LIFE DATA IN THORACIC OUTLET SYNDROME

TOS represents a constellation of signs and symptoms of the upper limb caused by compression of the neurovascular plexus passing through the "thoracic outlet," the anatomic space posterior to the clavicle and overlying the first rib. Clinical features of TOS differ between the neurogenic and the venous forms of the syndrome, which represent 95% and 2% of all TOS cases, respectively.[1-2] Both forms of TOS tend to manifest during active, working years of life (20-50 years of age).[3-5] Neurogenic TOS commonly presents in patients with a history of neck trauma and with symptoms including neck pain and occipital headaches as well as pain, paresthesia, and weakness of the upper extremity. In contrast, venous TOS commonly presents in patients who have a history of excessive activity of the upper extremity and with symptoms including pain, cyanosis, and swelling of the arm with secondary paresthesia.

To date, there are limited data in the literature on the quality of life and functional outcome of these patients, and many were based on unstructured subjective assessments. We thus decided to undertake a study to quantify the degree and characteristics of TOS patient disability using structured and validated patient-reported quality of life instruments and to assess their long-term quality of life outcomes following transaxillary first rib resection and scalenectomy.[6-10]

PATIENTS AND METHODS

With Institutional Review Board (IRB) approval, patients ages 18 and older presenting to a TOS clinic at an academic medical center between February 2005 and March 2008 were asked to participate. Informed consent was obtained by the attending surgeon or the physician assistant in the clinic. These patients had failed physical therapy prior to their referrals.

All patients then underwent transaxillary first rib resection at our center. Preoperative treatments for the venous population included venography with clot lysis and placement on anticoagulation if necessary. Postoperative treatment for all patients included physical therapy for 2 months. All venous TOS patients also underwent venogram and dilatation 2 weeks following surgery, and anticoagulation was administered if necessary. Secondary intervention for recurrent symptoms during the follow-up period included additional physical therapy, botulinum toxin injections for chemodenervation, and muscle relaxation in the residual scalene anticus muscle, pectoralis major, trapezius, or the rhomboids, and/or pain management referral.

For the study, preoperative patient demographics and postoperative clinical outcomes, including time to return to work, were abstracted from clinical records. Quality of life data were gathered using two surveys: the Disability of the Arm, Shoulder and Hand (DASH), and the Short-Form 12 (SF-12). DASH was selected for its disease-specific focus. DASH was developed by the American Academy of Orthopaedic Surgeons as an outcomes tool to evaluate "upper extremity-related symptoms and measure functional status at the level of disability."[11-12] Concepts covered by DASH include symptoms (pain, weakness, stiffness, and tingling/numbness), physical function (daily activities, house/yard chores, shopping, errands, recreational activities, self-care, dressing, eating, sexual activities, sleep, and sport/performing arts), social function (family care occupation, socializing with friends/family), and psychological function (self-image). To complement the DASH, the SF-12 was selected as an adjunctive instrument to measure the overall health status of our patients. The SF-12 is a condensed version of the popular SF-36 that was developed from the Medical Outcomes Study in the early 1990s.[13] The SF-12 was chosen instead of SF-36 to decrease patient response burden; because its purpose was to serve as an adjunctive instrument to the DASH, we believe it would be unnecessarily burdensome to include the longer SF-36 version. Understandability and acceptability of the questionnaire instruments were assessed by open discussion with the first five patients.

The patient surveys were created with Optical Mark Reader technology (Figure 14–1).[14] These computer-readable forms can be answered with any writing instruments and do not require the "bubbles" to be completely filled; instead they can be marked with simple check marks. The software system generates the database automatically after scanning, without need for manual data entry. These surveys were administered preoperatively and then again at 3, 6, 12, 18, and 24 months after surgery.

In analysis, the Physical Component Score (PCS) and Mental Component Score (MCS) on the SF-12 scale were standardized and normalized to population data (mean 50, standard deviation [SD] 10). Means were compared with population norms with one-sample t tests. Reliability of the survey package was assessed by internal consistency, by calculation of Cronbach's alpha of the SF-12 subscales. Validity of the survey package was assessed by convergent validity via simple regression to determine association between SF scores and DASH. The rate of recovery was determined with population-averaged models using generalized estimating equations (GEE) method. The Kaplan-Meier method was used to analyze time to return to work. Patients with bilateral TOS who had had previous rib resection were excluded from this analysis in order to avoid confounding of the second surgery with long-term outcomes analysis.

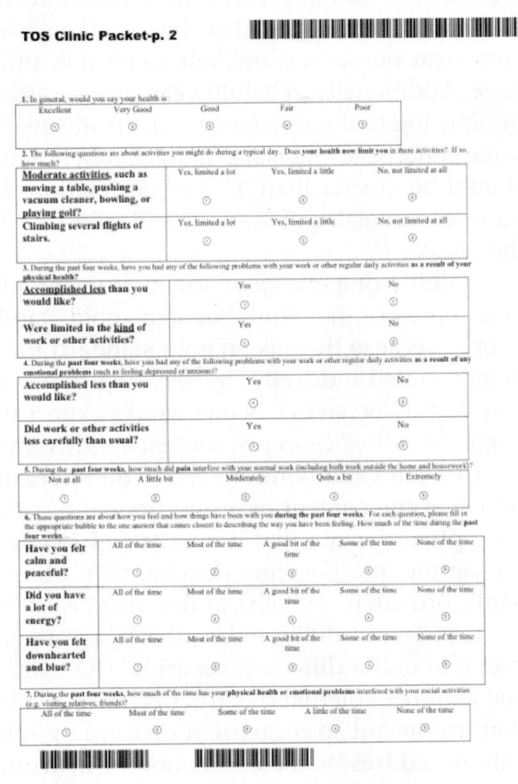

TOS Clinic Packet-p. 2

1. In general, would you say your health is:

Excellent	Very Good	Good	Fair	Poor

2. The following questions are about activities you might do during a typical day. Does **your health now limit you** in these activities? If so, how much?

Moderate activities, such as moving a table, pushing a vacuum cleaner, bowling, or playing golf?	Yes, limited a lot	Yes, limited a little	No, not limited at all
Climbing several flights of stairs.	Yes, limited a lot	Yes, limited a little	No, not limited at all

3. During the past four weeks, have you had any of the following problems with your week or other regular daily activities **as a result of your physical health?**

Accomplished less than you would like?	Yes	No
Were limited in the kind of work or other activities?	Yes	No

4. During the **past four weeks**, have you had any of the following problems with your work or other regular daily activities **as a result of any emotional problems** (such as feeling depressed or anxious)?

Accomplished less than you would like?	Yes	No
Did work or other activities less carefully than usual?	Yes	No

5. During the **past four weeks**, how much did **pain** interfere with your normal work (including both work outside the home and housework)?

Not at all	A little bit	Moderately	Quite a bit	Extremely

6. These questions are about how you feel and how things have been with you **during the past four weeks**. For each question, please fill in the appropriate bubble to the one answer that comes closest to describing the way you have been feeling. How much of the time during the **past four weeks**...

Have you felt calm and peaceful?	All of the time	Most of the time	A good bit of the time	Some of the time	None of the time
Did you have a lot of energy?	All of the time	Most of the time	A good bit of the time	Some of the time	None of the time
Have you felt downhearted and blue?	All of the time	Most of the time	A good bit of the time	Some of the time	None of the time

7. During the **past four weeks**, how much of the time has your **physical health or emotional problems** interfered with your social activities (e.g. visiting relatives, friends)?

All of the time	Most of the time	Some of the time	A little of the time	None of the time

Figure 14-1. Portion of the survey package generated with Optical Mark Reader (OMR) technology, which can be read by computers to automatically generate a database without manual data entry.

THEORIES OF QUALITY OF LIFE RESEARCH

There are three fundamental principles of any form of survey research, including quality of life research: acceptability, reliability, and validity.

Questions on a survey should be acceptable to the target population. This is assessed with focus groups in order to determine the appropriateness and understandability of the wording to the target population in terms of language, culture, and educational level. In analysis, acceptability of the survey can be assessed with data completeness and score distributions. Ideally, there should be less than 5% missing data for summary scores that are to be generated. Higher prevalence of missing data may suggest that respondents have difficulty in understanding the questions. And there should be an even distribution of frequencies across response categories, with less than 10% floor/ceiling effects—that is, no more than 10% of responses clustered at the low end (floor effect) or high end of the spectrum of response categories. The presence of ceiling/floor effect would suggest that the questions may not be meaningful.

The concept of reliability is demonstrated by Figure 14–2. This is usually demonstrated with a test-retest reliability protocol, which involves administering the same survey on two different occasions and then examining the correlation in scores between the two administrations. The correlation should ideally be greater than 0.80. The time interval should be short enough to ensure that no clinically meaningful change is likely to occur (e.g., both surveys should be preoperative, or both should be postoperative, but one administration cannot be preoperative while the second administration is postoperative); however, the interval should be long enough to ensure that the subjects do not recall their answers during the first assessment. Problems with reliability may suggest that the questions are unclear and vague in their wording; a very clear question is unlikely to elicit a different response each time from a respondent. Additionally, reliability can also be assessed during the analysis phase by determining internal consistency, which means that items on a scale are measuring the same concept. Cronbach's alpha can be calculated for summary scores, which ideally should be greater than 0.70; or correlations between individual items and summary score can be calculated, which ideally should have a correlation coefficient greater than 0.20.

Validity of a questionnaire instrument addresses the concept that it should somehow represent the "truth" or some gold standard. This is difficult in quality of life research, because there is no gold standard for quality of life measures. Validity is thus demonstrated indirectly, by showing that a questionnaire instrument "makes sense" and that it "behaves" as one would expect it to in different scenarios. There are two major "validity" concepts: content validity and construct validity.

Content validity means that a questionnaire "makes sense." It represents the concept that the content of a questionnaire instrument should be representative of the conceptual domain that it is intended to cover. This is usually assessed qualitatively during the questionnaire development phase or through the focus groups (with patients, providers, or both), as described earlier in acceptability study.

Construct validity means that a questionnaire should "behave" as one would expect it to under different scenarios. There are two forms of construct validity: internal and external. Internal construct validity relates to the concept that questionnaire items that are meant to measure a concept should correlate with one another. External validity addresses the correlation of instruments or concepts outside of the current questionnaire. There are three possible methods to demonstrate external validity:

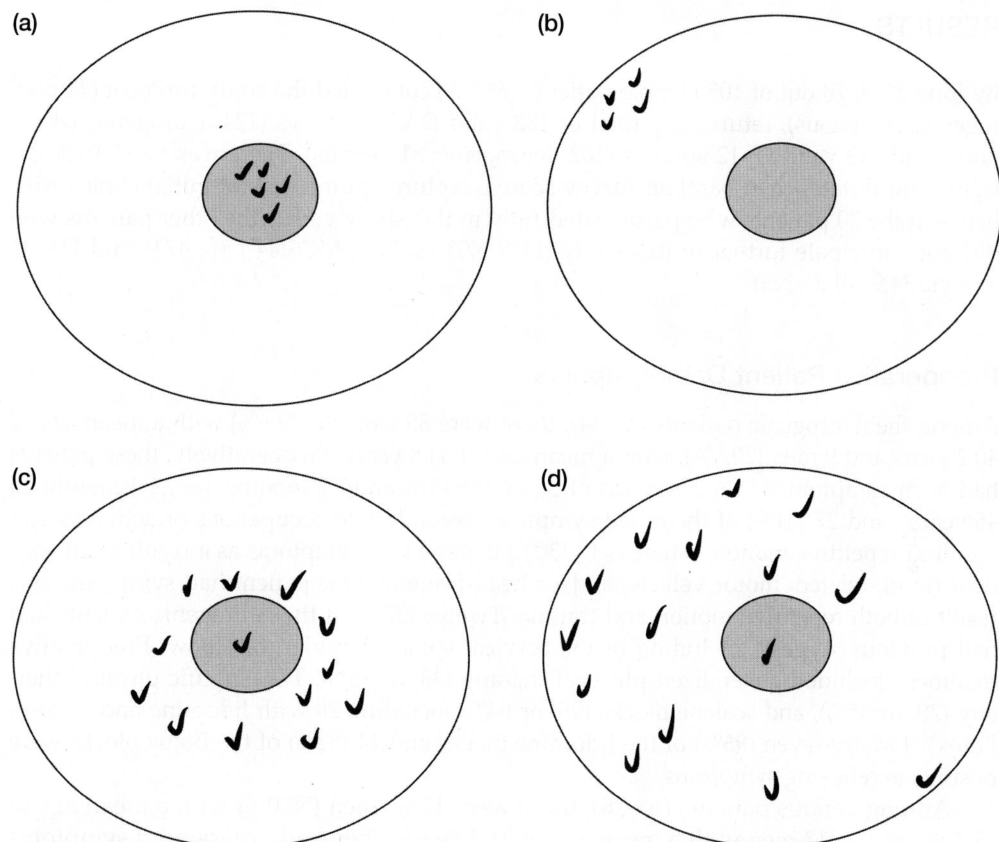

Figure 14-2. Demonstration of the concepts of reliability versus validity. Assuming that the red circle represents "truth," then the pattern of checkmarks in (a) would be valid, "hitting the truth," and reliable. Pattern (b) would be reliable but not valid. Pattern (c) would probably be valid but not reliable. And pattern (d) would not be valid nor reliable.

(1) Convergent validity: An instrument is said to have convergent validity if it is correlated with another instrument that is meant to measure a similar construct. The degrees of correlation are expected to vary according to the similarity of the concepts being measured by each instrument; for example, because DASH and SF-36 differ in being disease-specific versus generic, correlations are expected to be in moderate range; and because DASH items are meant to capture more physical than mental issues, higher correlations are expected between DASH and the PCS of the SF-36 than the MCS. (2) Discriminant validity: In contrast to the concept of convergent validity, a questionnaire is said to demonstrate discriminant validity if it is not correlated with another instrument that is meant to measure a different concept. For example, the DASH, because it is meant to measure disability and not general health status, should not correlate with age and gender in healthy subjects. (3) Known-group differentiation validity: A questionnaire is said to have known-group differentiation validity if it can differentiate between patients who are known to be different. For example, DASH scores should increase (i.e., denoting more frequent symptoms) with increasing severity of TOS.

RESULTS

By June 2008, 70 out of 105 eligible patients (66.7%) completed the study protocol (44 neurogenic; 26 venous), returning a total of 188 valid DASH surveys (124 neurogenic; 64 venous) and 243 valid SF-12 surveys (162 neurogenic; 81 venous). There was no statistically significant difference in baseline survey scores, captured at the time of initial clinic visits, between the 70 patients who participated fully in this study versus the other patients who did not participate further in this study (PCS 37.3 vs. 37.9, MCS 44.1 vs. 47.9, and DASH 41.9 vs. 34.9, all P=NS).

Preoperative Patient Demographics

Among the neurogenic patients (n=44), there were 35 women (79.5%) with a mean age of 40.2 years and 9 men (20.5%), with a mean age of 34.8 years. Preoperatively, these patients had been symptomatic for a median of 36 months (mean 67.7 months; range 4 months to 45 years), and 27 (61%) of them had symptoms secondary to occupations or activities that required repetitive motion, whereas 13 (30%) experienced symptoms as a result of an accident (work-related, motor vehicle, and/or head trauma). One patient had symptoms as a result of both repetitive motion and trauma. Twelve (27%) of the neurogenic patients had had previous surgery, including of the cervical spine, shoulder, or elbow. Preoperative treatment included generalized physical therapy (33, or 75%), TOS-specific physical therapy (20, or 45%), and scalene blocks (28, or 64%, including 28 with lidocaine and 17 with Botox). Twenty-seven (96%) of the lidocaine blocks and 14 (82%) of the Botox blocks were positive in relieving symptoms.

Among venous patients (n=26), there were 13 women (50.0%) with a mean age of 37.1 years and 13 men with a mean age of 31.2 years. They had experienced symptoms for a median of 4.5 months (mean 10.4 months; range 0-72 months) prior to consultation. Ten (38%), attributed their condition to chronic repetitive motion; their occupations included painting, carpentry, mechanics, and music composition or performance. Acute effort thromboses (2, or 8%) were common among the athlete population. These patients were active as quarterbacks, pitchers, swimmers, and runners. Few (3, or 12%) had trauma to or surgery on the affected arm, a significantly lower rate than the neurogenic patients.

Return to Work

Although 15/44 (34%) of neurogenic patients and 2/26 (8%) of venous patients were disabled or unemployed upon presentation, 22 (50%) neurogenic patients and 20 (77%) venous patients eventually returned to full-time work or activity at some time during the study follow-up period. Additionally, there were 2 neurogenic patients and 2 venous patients who returned to part-time activity. For the purpose of this study, we considered full-time activity to be equivalent to employment to account for patients who were not formally employed at baseline such as athletes, college students, musicians, and homemakers. This included 3 of the 15 neurogenic patients and 1 of the 2 venous patients.

The time course of returning to full-time work or activity is presented in Figure 14–3. Half of the patients had returned to full-time work or activity by 4 months and more than 75% had returned by 5 months. There was no statistically significant difference in this rate of return to work between neurogenic and venous patients.

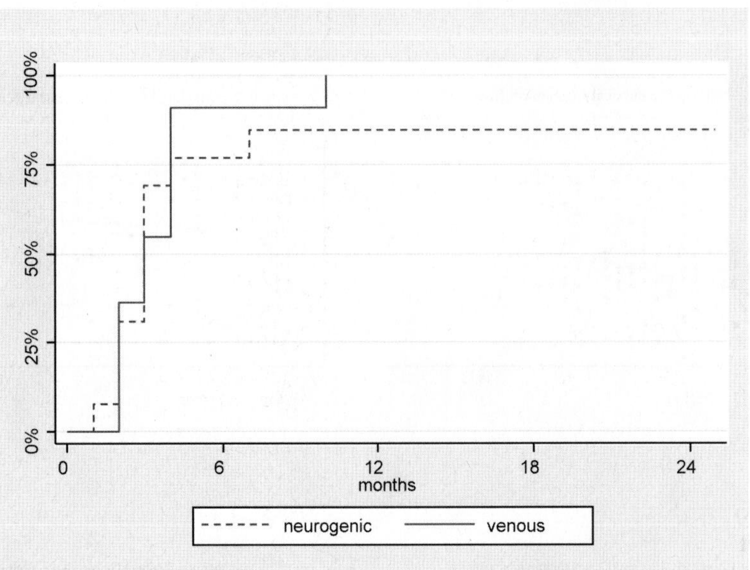

Figure 14-3. Proportion of patients returning to full-time work or activity over time.

Quality of Life Outcome

Separating neurogenic and venous TOS patient data on baseline, it was found that neurogenic TOS patients had significantly worse PCS values than venous TOS patients (33.8 vs. 43.6, $P<.001$). In contrast, there was no significant difference between their MCS scores (44.5 vs. 43.5, P=NS). The DASH scores were also significantly worse among neurogenic TOS patients than venous TOS patients (50.2 vs. 25.0, $P<.001$).

In follow-up, PCS scores for neurogenic patients improved 0.24 points ($P<.001$) and MCS scores improved 0.15 points per month on average ($P=.01$) (Figure 14–4 a). PCS scores for venous patients improved 0.40 points ($P=.004$) and MCS scores improved 0.55 points per month ($P<.001$) on average (Figure 14–4 b). DASH scores also improved 0.85 points ($P<.001$) for neurogenic patients and 0.81 points ($P<.001$) for venous patients per month on average.

Additionally, it was determined that the median time to recovery of normal quality of life for neurogenic patients was 23 months for physical function and 12 months for mental function. In contrast, for venous TOS patients, the median time to recovery of normal quality of life was 11 months for physical function and 8 months for mental function. Note that these quality of life recovery times were significantly longer than the time it took for the patients to return to full-time work or activity.

DISCUSSION

Although some risk factors for persistent postoperative disability in TOS have been identified, measurement of long-term postoperative mental and physical functional outcomes has been lacking.[15-17] Because surgical intervention for TOS has demonstrated low rates of complication, analysis of long-term functional outcomes in TOS patients may provide

(a)

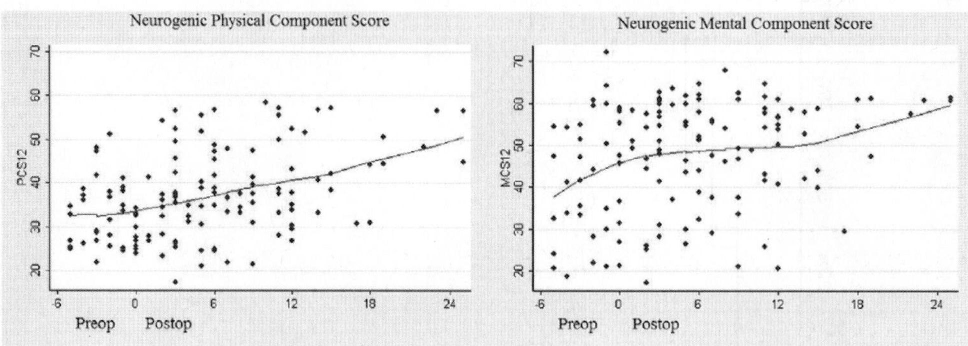

(b)

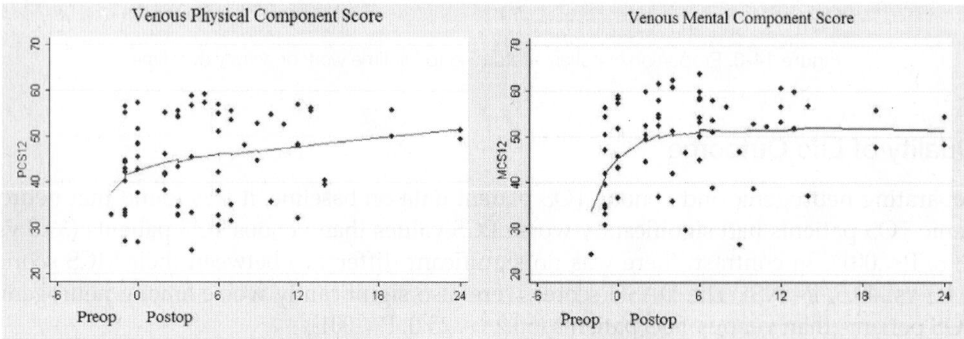

Figure 14-4. Quality of life outcome of: (a) neurogenic TOS patients and (b) venous TOS patients.

useful additional insight into the postoperative course of patients.[18-19] Although there have been some attempts to assess long-term outcomes, these efforts have primarily focused on diffuse measures of patient satisfaction using unvalidated tools.[20-23] A recent report by Cordobes-Gual et al. presented some functional data using the validated DASH instrument on 23 patients, but they included only a single follow-up at approximately 4 to 6 months after surgery.[24]

In contrast to the limited studies in the literature, our current study presents functional data on a larger group of patients (n=70) followed over a longer period of time (up to 2 years) using objective and well-established quality of life instruments. The findings of this study suggest that despite the seemingly nebulous nature of their complaints, these patients suffer striking physical morbidity from TOS. The mean PCS of 37.5 on baseline was approximately 1.3 SDs below the population norm. This score was much worse than the mean score of 46.4 that has been reported for chronic prostatitis patients, 46.5 for hypertension patients, or 44.8 for diabetes patients, and was actually similar to the mean score of 34.0 that has been reported for chronic heart failure patients.[25-27] Similarly, the mean DASH score of 41.4 was similar to the mean value of 43.7 that has been reported for patients with chronic rotator cuff tears.[27] The validity of

TOS patients' physical complaints was further supported by their MCS being within 1 SD of the population norm. Of note, the reported MCS on the SF-12 were also similar between baseline TOS patients in this study (43.7) versus chronic heart failure patients (48.2).[27]

We observed significant differences between recovery to full-time work or activity versus recovery to normal quality of life scores. Half of patients were able to return to full-time work or activity by 3 months and 75% were able to do so by 6 months in contrast to the 1 to 2 years of recovery time until normal quality of life is achieved. This observation suggests that patients can return to full-time work or activity while they continue to recover. This is an important point to convey during patient counseling on their expected recovery course.

In conclusion, neurogenic TOS patients who are refractory to physical therapy and venous TOS patients present with significant physical disability. Their quality of life profile in general is similar to that of patients with chronic heart failure, and, more specifically in relation to upper extremity functions, similar to that of patients with chronic rotator cuff tears. Following first rib resection, venous TOS patients typically improved both physical and mental quality of life in shorter periods of time than their neurogenic counterparts. Additionally, neurogenic and venous TOS patients returned to full-time work/activity within the same length of time postoperatively; however, neurogenic patients required more secondary interventions. Therefore, in appropriately selected patients with either neurogenic or venous TOS, surgical intervention can improve their quality of life over time.

FUTURE DIRECTIONS

Although quality of life instruments are structured and have undergone extensive validation testing, the verbal nature of these reports still presents a concern for some investigators, especially considering the difficulty of making the diagnosis in these patients. A biomechanical validation of the quality of life reports will be valuable not only to further objectively confirm patient recovery following surgery but also as a possible new tool to assist in making an objective diagnosis.

One such tool would be an accelerometer. An accelerometer is a device that measures changes in angular position over time. The most basic form of accelerometer is the pedometer, which measures the number of steps taken. Accelerometers have been used in biomedical research. For example, an ankle version of the device has been used to measure ambulation among stroke patients.[28]

However, the functional use of the upper extremity, as would be affected by TOS, has different characteristics than ambulation. The swinging motion of the arm, as captured by the acceleration measurement, is not important; rather, the ability to raise the arm to a certain angle and hold it there would be more indicative of arm function. Therefore, we would need to track both the angular data and the time data to determine the total length of time that the arm is being used.

An ideal accelerometer should measure tilt in three planes simultaneously, allowing capture of abduction/adduction and flexion/extension of the arm in the same device. It should record data in standard comma-delimited format onto standard digital camera-type flash cards and include a USB connection that can be easily connected to any computer for data downloading. A patient could wear such a device just above the elbow in order to maximize its distance from the shoulder so that angular motion about the shoulder can be measured easily, but it should not to be worn below the elbow in order to prevent it from measuring motion around the elbow joint. A patient should also wear two of these devices, one on each arm, so that data can be collected from both arms to adjust for personal activity level and arm dominance.

The functional use of the arm, as captured by the angular tracing (with some exclusions based on angle of elevation and minimum time thresholds in order to eliminate noise from random arm swings), should then serve as an external validation of the quality of life data obtained in TOS patients. This can enhance the objectivity of outcomes measurement and further advance the state of the clinical science in this field. We are in the process of evaluating the use of such a device to compare normal volunteers versus TOS patients to determine baseline differences and then to compare TOS patients before and after surgical interventions.

REFERENCES

1. Podlaha J. Thoracic outlet syndrome—24 years of experience. Bratisl Lek Listy 2007;108: 429–32.
2. Sanders RJ, Hammond SL, Rao NM. Diagnosis of thoracic outlet syndrome. J Vasc Surg 2007;46:601–4.
3. Leffert RD. Thoracic outlet syndrome. J Am Acad Orthop Surg 1994;2:317–25.
4. Leffert RD, Perlmutter GS. Thoracic outlet syndrome: results of 282 transaxillary first rib resections. Clin Orthop Relat Res 1999;368:66–79.
5. Köknel Talu G. Thoracic outlet syndrome. Agri 2005;17:5–9.
6. Howard M, Lee C, Dellon AL. Documentation of brachial plexus compression (in the thoracic inlet) utilizing provocative neurosensory and muscular testing. J Reconstr Microsurg 2003;19:303–12.
7. Lee GW, Massry DR, Kupfer DM, Abrams R. Documentation of brachial plexus compression in the thoracic inlet with quantitative sensory testing. J Reconstr Microsurg 2000;16: 15–20.
8. Novak CB, Mackinnon SE, Patterson GA. Evaluation of patients with thoracic outlet syndrome. J Hand Surg 1993;18:292–9.
9. Parziale JR, Akelman E, Weiss AP, Green A. Thoracic outlet syndrome. Am J Orthop 2000;29:353–60.
10. Chang DC, Rotellini-Coltvet LA, Mukherjee D, et al. Surgical intervention for thoracic outlet syndrome improves patient's quality of life. J Vasc Surg 2009;49:630–5.
11. Hudak PL, Amadio PC, Bombardier C. Development of an upper extremity outcome measure: the DASH (Disabilities of the Arm, Shoulder and Hand) [corrected]. The Upper Extremity Collaborative Group (UECG). Am J Ind Med 1996;29:602–8.
12. Kirkley A, Griffin S, Dainty K. Scoring systems for the functional assessment of the shoulder. Arthroscopy 2003;19:1109–20.
13. Ware J Jr, Kosinski M, Keller SD. A 12-Item Short-Form Health Survey: construction of scales and preliminary tests of reliability and validity. Med Care 1996;34:220–33.
14. Bergeron BP. Optical mark recognition. Tallying information from filled-in "bubbles." Postgrad Med 1998;104:23–5.
15. Gockel M, Lindholm H, Vastamäki M, et al. Cardiovascular functional disorder and distress among patients with thoracic outlet syndrome. J Hand Surg [Br] 1995;20:29–33.
16. Yavuzer S, Atinkaya C, Tokat O. Clinical predictors of surgical outcome in patients with thoracic outlet syndrome operated on via transaxillary approach. Eur J Cardiothorac Surg 2004;25:173–8.

17. Axelrod DA, Proctor MC, Geisser ME, et al. Outcomes after surgery for thoracic outlet syndrome. J Vasc Surg 2001;33:1220–5.
18. Divi V, Proctor MC, Axelrod DA, Greenfield LJ. Thoracic outlet decompression for subclavian vein thrombosis: experience in 71 patients. Arch Surg 2005;140:54–7.
19. Chang DC, Lidor AO, Matsen SL, Freischlag JA. Reported in-hospital complications following rib resections for neurogenic thoracic outlet syndrome. Ann Vasc Surg 2007;21: 564–70.
20. Sharp WJ, Nowak LR, Zamani T, et al. Long-term follow-up and patient satisfaction after surgery for thoracic outlet syndrome. Ann Vasc Surg 2001;15:32–6.
21. Bhattacharya V, Hansrani M, Wyatt MG, et al. Outcome following surgery for thoracic outlet syndrome. Eur J Vasc Endovasc Surg 2003;26:170–5.
22. Degeorges R, Reynaud C, Becquemin JP. Thoracic outlet syndrome surgery: long-term functional results. Ann Vasc Surg 2004;18:558–65.
23. Rochkind S, Shemesh M, Patish H, et al. Thoracic outlet syndrome: a multidisciplinary problem with a perspective for microsurgical management without rib resection. Acta Neurochir Suppl 2007;100:145–7.
24. Cordobes-Gual J, Lozano-Vilardell P, Torreguitart-Mirada N, et al. Prospective study of the functional recovery after surgery for thoracic outlet syndrome. Eur J Vasc Endovasc Surg 2008;79–83. Epub 2007 Oct 4.
25. McNaughton-Collins M, Pontari MA, O'Leary MP, et al. Quality of life is impaired in men with chronic prostatitis: the Chronic Prostatitis Collaborative Research Network. J Gen Intern Med 2001;16:656–62.
26. Baker DW, Brown J, Chan KS, et al. A telephone survey to measure communication, self-management, and health status for patients with heart failure: the Improving Chronic Illness Care Evaluation (ICICE). J Card Fail 2005;11:36–42.
27. Tashjian RZ, Henn RF, Kang L, Green A. The effect of comorbidity on self-assessed function in patients with a chronic rotator cuff tear. J Bone Joint Surg Am 2004;86:355–62.
28. Busse ME, Pearson OR, Van Deursen R, Wiles CM. Quantified measurement of activity provides insight into motor function and recovery in neurological disease. J Neurol Neurosurg Psychiatry 2004;75:884–8.

SECTION IV

Trauma

15

Civilian Experience With Temporary Arterial Shunts

John Blebea, M.D. and Rashad Choudry, M.D.

INTRODUCTION

Successful clinical management of penetrating vascular trauma in the urban environment, especially in the context of high-velocity and multiple gunshot wounds, requires utilization of the entire breadth of contemporary vascular surgical techniques. Whereas the emphasis within the past decade has focused on innovative endovascular diagnostic and therapeutic options, extensive extremity injuries will occasionally require the ability to employ less commonly used techniques for vascular control and repair for limb salvage.

One such method that should be a part of the armamentarium of all vascular surgeons involved in the management of trauma patients is the use of intra-arterial shunting (IAS). The technique itself is commonplace and routinely used by many surgeons during the performance of carotid endarterectomy. For trauma, it was described as early as 1919 by Makins as a way of maintaining blood flow after gunshot injuries to blood vessels during World War I.[1] This technical option was reintroduced for use in civilian trauma in the 1970s but is likely underutilized in most surgical practices and not well described or taught to vascular trainees.[2]

A critical evaluation of the use of intra-arterial shunts in civilian extremity trauma remains limited, mostly because of the small numbers of patients in whom these devices have been used and the absence of long-term follow-up in young, often transient, trauma patients.[3-9] Recent reports from vascular and trauma surgeons participating in the wars in Iraq and Afghanistan have brought a renewed interest in the use of IASs for peripheral extremity trauma.[10] The more liberal use of IASs in military hospitals by combat surgeons has provided additional clinical data and made possible some recommendations for possible application in civilian trauma patients.[11]

INTRA-ARTERIAL SHUNTS

Effectively any tube of sufficient diameter and acceptable handling characteristics can be utilized as a vascular shunt. The majority of research and design of vascular shunts has been for elective intraoperative use in the carotid artery (Figure 15–1). They all are rather similar, and most perform adequately for their intended short-term duration for preservation of end-organ blood flow. However, intraluminal diameter, length, and tapered configurations may all contribute to discrepancies in the volume of blood flow delivered. A limited but important group of studies has been published regarding the hemodynamic function of shunts. Although in vivo data are limited, bench-top analysis has provided valuable information regarding the different commercially available shunts.[12] Verkerke et al. described a considerable difference in blood flow among shunts.[13] Javid shunts (Bard; Tempe, AZ) were shown to have the highest blood flow in their model as compared with the Pruitt-Inahara type (LeMaitre Vascular; Burlington, MA). As would be expected, the larger-diameter, straight shunts performed better than their smaller counterparts. Within the smaller-diameter group, the tapered shunts offered improved flow rates. Overall, higher shunt flow rates produce higher distal perfusion pressure.[14] At the molecular level, animal research, which has focused on the cellular effects of shunt use in the coronary circulation, has demonstrated a beneficial preservation of cellular architecture, including endothelial function.[15]

At present, there is no commercially available shunt specific for use in traumatic vascular injury. Likely reasons for this include an overall low clinical demand for such a specialized product and a lack of compelling research data to support any specific type of shunt. Available arterial shunts have been fabricated for application only in the cerebrovascular circulation and other use is off-label. Nonetheless, these have been the ones most employed for injured peripheral vessels due to their ready availability, surgeon familiarity, and reasonable size approximation to the arteries in the extremities.

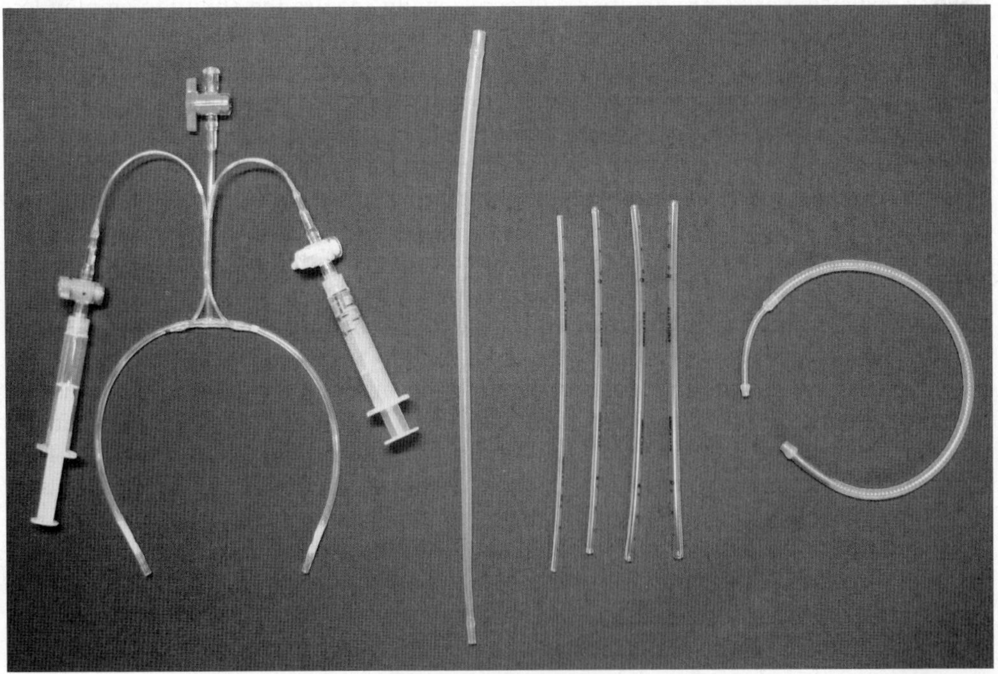

Figure 15-1. Examples of commonly available carotid shunts. Left to right: the Pruitt-Inahara, Javid, Argyle, and Sundt shunts.

The most commonly used IASs in the contemporary literature for traumatic peripheral vascular injuries is the Argyle shunt (Covidien; Mansfield, MA).[16] It is a polyvinyl chloride (PVC) tube available in sizes 8, 10, 12, and 14 French combined in a standard kit. Both 6-inch straight and 11-inch looped varieties are available, but the straight version is most frequently available in operating rooms. The Sundt shunt (Integra; Plainsboro, NJ) is similar but is tapered to a smaller diameter distally, varying from 3.0 to 5.0 mm. It is constructed of a soft silicone elastomer with cone-shaped bulb ends that the manufacturer claims are less traumatic to the vessel intima, allow for easier extraluminal clamp or tourniquet to hold the shunt in place, and may have a more hemostatic seal when properly sized. Additional features of the Sundt shunt include stainless steel wire reinforcement to prevent kink formation as well as availability in both internal (10 cm) and external (30 cm) loop placement configurations. The Javid shunt shares a similar tapered design; however, it may require cutting for in-line internal placement given the greater lengths which are commercially available.

The Pruitt-Inahara shunt is a unique shunt system with particular technical aspects that some operators may find helpful in trauma situations (Figure 15–2). The shunt (8 to 10 French; inlying, 15 cm; outlying, 25 to 31 cm length) is color-coded for luminal orientation and each end has an inflatable balloon for proximal (14 mm diameter at full expansion) and distal (8 mm) fixation, with a safety sleeve to prevent overdistention of the distal balloon. No external fixation is required, making extensive dissection unnecessary, particularly in situations of anatomically high vascular injuries in which clamp or tourniquet placement is not possible. Additionally, a special side port allows for flushing of debris, blood sampling, or measurement of arterial pressure. This side port also provides access for infusion of vasodilators, anticoagulants, or dye contrast should distal arterial evaluation be needed postoperatively.

In situations in which commercially available shunts may not be optimal, because of either their length or, more frequently, their small diameter that either may limit flow or would be a size mismatch with native vessels, alternative devices can be modified and used. As reported by military surgeons in Operation Iraqi Freedom, several

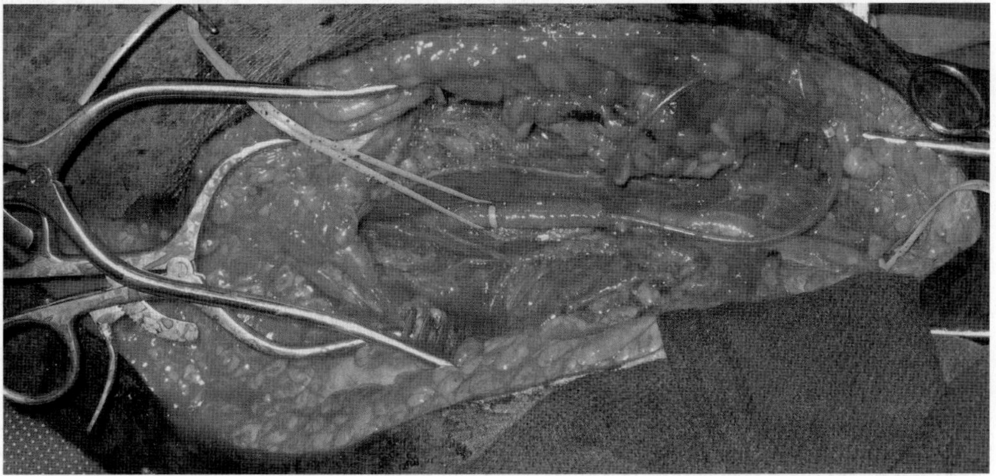

Figure 15-2. Example of an intra-arterial shunt (Pruitt-Inahara) during an arterial reconstruction of the mid-superficial femoral artery.

routinely available luminal devices may be used as temporary vascular conduits. These include large-diameter angiocatheters, pediatric feeding tubes, small-caliber chest tubes, and even endotracheal tubes. As with other shunts, these devices are not specifically designed for use in this capacity and may be subject to malfunction because of kinking, dislodgement, or thrombosis.

Certain types of traumatic wounds may prove challenging for straight or looped shunts. Arterial bifurcation injuries may be best treated by shunt placement into both branch vessels. In the authors' experience with such injuries, we found successful shunting of both the superficial femoral and the profunda femoris arteries using a double-lumen hemodialysis access catheter (Mahurkar MAXID 14.5 French; Covidien, Mansfield, MA) customized to the patients' femoral anatomy and secured with silk suture.[17] This custom-made shunt allowed for peripheral shunting for 2 full days prior to definitive vascular reconstruction. Similar shunts can be constructed from other hemodialysis access catheters (Figure 15–3). Another consideration for IAS in proximal extremity lesions, in which ligation of inflow may be required, is temporary external shunting from the contralateral extremity.[18]

Innovative technologies that may provide utility when IASs are used include the real-time monitoring of volume flow and blood pressure through the shunt and into the distal extremity or end organ. Temporary hand-held Doppler assessment in the operating room is useful only for immediate evaluation of shunt patency. Postoperative monitoring may be necessary if the IAS is to remain for longer than during the initial intraoperative time period. In such cases, flow monitoring can be difficult, particularly with inlying straight shunts, which can be neither visualized nor directly transonated due to the need to maintain sterility of the vascular wound. Outlying shunts, if a portion is left exposed through the wound, could be intermittently examined with a Doppler probe to confirm continued flow. For continuous monitoring, a

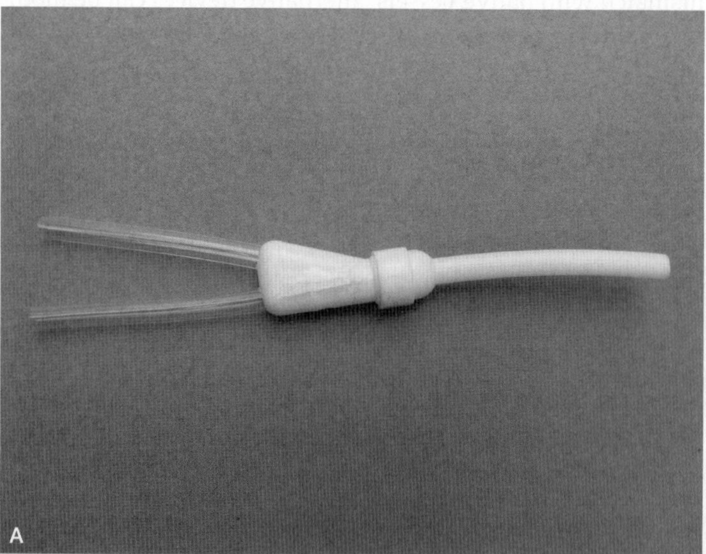

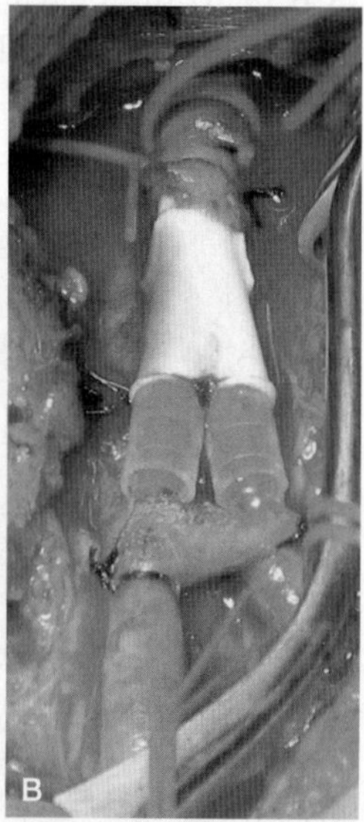

Figure 15-3. **A.** A modified dual-lumen hemodialysis catheter that has been cut so that it may be used in a reversed fashion at a vascular bifurcation. **B.** Another dual-lumen hemodialysis catheter that has been inserted into the left common femoral artery (top) and the superficial (medial) and profunda (lateral) femoral arteries prior to vascular reconstruction.

Pruitt-Inahara type of shunt could have the aspiration channel connected to an arterial pressure monitor that would be an indirect confirmation of continued function. The same type of shunt, with a built-in Doppler probe, would be a better direct indicator of continuing blood flow through the shunt. For larger vessels such as the iliac or common femoral arteries, however, larger-diameter tubing may be required beyond what is available with the Pruitt-Inahara shunts. In such circumstances, with larger tubes serving this role, a flow sensor placed around the catheter itself can measure flow when a prolonged period of patient resuscitation is required prior to definitive vascular reconstruction. Such devices are available and have been used in experimental research for many years to measure liquid flow through any type of sterile tubing (Bypass Flowmeter; Transonic Systems Inc., Ithaca, NY).[19] Using transit-time ultrasound technology composed of two transducers and an acoustic reflector, accurate volume flow measurements may be obtained across any IAS. Sterile packaging and reusability make it highly attractive for temporary surgical implantation. However, these systems are not customarily available in the operating room and pose a potential infectious risk because the wiring would be maintaining a track through the wound. The authors are examining the efficacy of implantable wireless flow-sensors, but such a device is not yet commercially available (DVX, Princeton, NJ).

Although publications have thus far emphasized the potential usefulness of IASs, complications of shunting are likely under-reported. A key tenet to the safe placement of an IAS is visualization of the distal vessel to evaluate and confirm that no dissection flap has been caused by placement of the shunt, which can lead to lack of flow through the shunt and distal vessel thrombosis. In the trauma patient, injury to the intima as a result of hurried or inappropriate shunt placement can complicate vascular reconstruction, may require additional operative time for vessel dissection in circumstances in which time is of the essence, and may lead to avoidable morbidity and limb loss. Choosing the appropriately sized shunt to fit both the inflow and the outflow vessels is important. Unless the shunt is placed into a segment of the same vessel or into vessels of similar diameters, a tapered shunt may be most appropriate. A variety of sizes are typically available for straight shunts and many manufacturers distribute them as a part of a kit. Although one should avoid inserting a shunt that is too large for the recipient vessel, the largest appropriate diameter should be used to maximize flow to the extremity. In situations in which size measurement is difficult and distal vessel control is not easily achieved, a shunt with balloon-inflatable ends may be advantageous.

Once in place, subsequent shunt dislodgement and associated arterial bleeding can be a significant challenge, especially if the shunt is to stay in place for more than a few hours and the patient will be undergoing multiple transfers. Military surgeons involved in the transfer of soldiers with in-line shunts have recommended the placement of shunts well into the native vessel both proximally and distally with adequate external fixation using sutures to prevent accidental and potentially catastrophic bleeding complications.[20]

Shunt thrombosis remains a very real concern when used for more than a limited period of time during the index operation. It is plausible, although not proven, that longer shunts, particularly those that are also angled with external loops, are more likely to experience this problem. Shunts that extend across joints may be prone to kink formation, and extremity splinting may be helpful in preventing this problem.[20] Shunts utilized during planned elective procedures in stable patients, such as tumor resections involving critical vessels, may benefit from receiving systemic heparinization prior to shunt insertion. Multiple-trauma civilian patients with vascular injuries requiring shunt placement, similar to casualties seen in the military, are typically coagulopathic and systemic anticoagulation may be both unnecessary and contraindicated.[20-22] By the time that normal hemodynamic and hematologic functions are restored, the vascular injury can typically be repaired in controlled situations in which anticoagulation may be administered either locally or systemically. The potential benefit of a heparin-coated shunt for trauma patients has theoretical appeal to maintain shunt patency, but no such product is commercially available. The overall low incidence of shunt thrombosis during carotid surgery has not encouraged the development of such a product.

Often referred to as "dwell time," the length of time that a shunt can be left in situ before removal is unknown. This time period is most frequently determined by the patient's overall clinical status and cardiopulmonary stability. From the vascular perspective, in order to prevent shunt thrombosis or vessel and wound infection, the shunt should be removed and definitive vascular repair performed as soon as possible. When a patient's resuscitative phase is protracted and cardiovascular stability is not quickly attained, shunt dwell time becomes more critical. In our experience, a temporary IAS functioned appropriately and remained patent by duplex ultrasound for 2 full days prior to reconstruction despite massive fluid resuscitation and on-going hypotension. Granchi reported shunt patency for 52 hours without anticoagulation.[5] The longest reported shunt patency in the literature is 72 hours.[16] With such extended periods of shunt use, if clinically possible, systemic anticoagulation even at low doses should be considered.

CONTEMPORARY CLINICAL USE

The largest reported number of patients in the modern era with the use of IASs is from experiences during the Iraqi war. Woodward et al. reported vascular shunt use in 40% of femoral and popliteal segment injuries.[10] Although the data retrieved from these studies are important and helpful in the evaluation of shunt use, they should be analyzed carefully to exclude variables that are not relevant to civilian vascular injuries. Of these, the most important are demographics and prehospital care. Injured soldiers are almost always young with normal vasculature, are in excellent physical condition, and rarely have associated medical comorbidities. In addition, modern battlefield injuries are treated by medical personnel trained and experienced in dealing with such injuries on the scene with rapid transfer times to hospitals and short extremity ischemia time. Excellent limb salvage rates have been reported by military surgeons in this war.[10,23] In another reported series of 18 patients with 26 IASs, an early shunt patency of 96% was reported with 100% limb salvage after vascular reconstruction.[23] These authors commented that their observed shunt patency was based on technical factors, including optimum short intraluminal shunt length, which may reduce stasis and thrombus formation, and the use of in-line (internal) shunting with appropriate extremity positioning to avoid kink formation.

Location of vessel injury and required shunting may be an important variable. Rasmussen et al. also reported on the use of IASs during contemporary wartime conditions.[21] In their analysis of 126 vascular injuries, they found that two thirds of traumatic vascular injuries occurred in the lower extremities, with the remainder involving the upper extremity. This pattern is similar to that seen in civilian injuries of the extremities.[16] Of 30 shunted vessels (26 arterial, 4 venous), 22 were placed in proximal vessels, with the remainder in more distal vasculature below the elbow or knee. Impressively, 100% of venous shunts, 86% of proximal arterial, but only 12% of those shunts below the knee were patent at vessel exploration, although 28 of 30 shunted patients achieved limb viability at discharge.[21] Some have suggested that distal vascular injuries should not be routinely shunted given this high thrombosis rate and advocate vessel ligation or amputation, depending on the viability of the distal extremity.[23]

Injury to major veins in the same extremity can also negatively affect the success of arterial shunts. Chambers and associates reported on 27 shunts in 20 patients, of whom 12 had combined arterial and venous injuries. Two arterial shunts thrombosed when proximal venous ligation was performed.[20] This experience reconfirmed the importance of venous outflow restoration whenever possible, and as early as possible, to augment shunt patency and reduce extremity ischemia-reperfusion injury.[24] This may be particularly valuable in instances of extensive soft tissue destruction in which important venous collaterals are lost. Concomitant intravenous shunting, when expeditious repair cannot be performed, can also be useful in the absence of life-threatening hemorrhage.

As in military combat injuries, the femoral artery is the most commonly injured vessel and also the most frequent to be shunted.[10,16] The mechanism of vessel injury in the military has characteristically been high-velocity bullets or blast injuries with resultant massive soft tissue destruction, which makes treatment much more challenging. Increasingly, however, injuries with multiple gunshots and higher-velocity weapons are being seen in the civilian population in large urban areas. In such circumstances, injury patterns and clinical results in the civilian population will be similar to those seen among the military.[25] Extensive débridement of injured soft tissue and associated damaged vasculature are a must. Under such circumstances, temporary vascular shunting can be a necessary rather than merely an adjunctive maneuver. Similarly, blunt injuries with extensive soft tissue damage and associated multisystem trauma can benefit from shunting as part of the prioritization of treatment and improve the survivability of such patients. Regardless of mechanism of injury, if revascularization is not successful, amputation is more likely to result.[26] Subramanian et al. have recently reported the largest series of civilian patients who incurred a traumatic vascular injury and had a vascular shunt employed (67 patients, 101 shunts, 72 arterial, 29 venous).[16] The most common reason (44%) for shunt placement was as part of "damage control" surgery en route to postoperative resuscitation and later definitive vascular repair. A large majority (81%) of this group had extremity injuries, with the remainder having shunts placed for abdominal visceral arterial injuries. The second most common reason for IASs, in 42% of patients, was in the treatment of complex Gustilo IIIc open tibial extremity fractures. Similar to the military experience, temporary shunt patency was excellent at 91%. Of the three thromboses, two were of shunts placed in the visceral circulation (superior mesenteric artery). Despite liberal shunt application in both arteries and veins, below the knee popliteal injuries resulting from either blunt or penetrating trauma did not ultimately show improved amputation rates. However, in a smaller retrospective series of seven civilian patients in whom shunts were used for blunt popliteal injuries, Hosnny reported favorable outcomes with shortened total ischemia time, fewer fasciotomies and wound infections, and a reduced length of hospital stay.[27] Overall, however, the limited published data on the use of IASs for popliteal injuries bring into question the clinical efficacy of shunts when used in this location.

A number of other reports in the literature have evaluated the role of IASs in traumatic vascular extremity injury in combination with complex orthopedic fractures. An age-old dilemma has been which injury to correct first and whether bone fracture stabilization should precede revascularization. Generally speaking, an ischemic extremity makes vascular repair the top priority, whether by direct revascularization or temporary IAS to allow for fracture stabilization followed by definitive vascular repair. Vascular bypass graft disruption or shunt dislodgement during orthopedic reconstruction remains a largely theoretical risk but is often cited by orthopedic surgeons as a concern during their portion of the surgery.[28] In the authors' respective institutions, vascular repair is almost always possible prior to bony stabilization. It is our policy to have both surgical specialists available in-house during the surgery. External fixation of flail limbs may be accomplished in under 30 minutes when experienced orthopedic surgeons are available and work in concert with both trauma and vascular surgical specialists. Internal fixation, including intramedullary rod placement, is not routinely employed, particularly in patients with multisystem injuries.

McHenry et al. reported on 27 patients with complex vascular and orthopedic extremity injuries. Of these, 22 initially underwent revascularization, with 59% of them having IAS followed by fracture repair and subsequent vascular reconstruction. Neither bypass graft nor shunt dislodgement during orthopedic repair was observed.[29]

Similarly, Huynh et al. have strongly advocated that vascular repair be performed first. In their report of 36 patients who underwent both vascular and orthopedic repairs, two thirds had bone fixation after revascularization.[30] There were no vascular graft injuries when revascularization preceded fixation.

In the authors' unpublished experience of 71 patients at two different urban Level I trauma centers over 4 years, we have found IASs to be unnecessary in the majority of patients with only 2 (3%) requiring IASs en route to definitive revascularization, consistent with the experience of others.[31] In both cases, a concomitant venous injury was present and required repair. In one case, a damage control approach was initiated for multisystem injuries.[17] The second patient was transferred to us several hours after the injury and required reestablishment of blood flow as soon as possible. We have found that the majority of civilian arterial injuries are recognized quickly at Level 1 trauma centers and expeditious repair of injured extremity vessels by qualified vascular specialists can make the need for IAS infrequent. Low-velocity gunshot wounds or sharp penetrating injuries, without associated multiorgan trauma, require infrequent use of IAS. Multiple gunshots wounds and/or severe multitrauma patients with complex vascular and orthopedic injuries are the settings in which temporary arterial shunts can be limb- or life-saving techniques.

RECOMMENDATIONS

In the context of an elective community vascular surgical practice, noncarotid temporary IASs are unlikely to be needed. However, for vascular or trauma surgeons participating at a Level 1 trauma center, an IAS is a useful technique to have available. It can be of value in patients with multiple gunshot wounds, high-velocity injuries, or complex combined vascular/orthopedic/multiorgan trauma. In patients with combined arterial and venous injury, massive soft tissue destruction, or multisystem injuries that mandate a damage control operative conduct, an IAS may be used for limb salvage or life preservation. A variety of devices are commercially available for surgeons as well as the preparation of custom-designed shunts modified for patient needs. In general, the same principles of application should be used as for the carotid artery. The largest-diameter and shortest-length shunt should be used based on the size and distance of the injured vessel. In-lying shunts most often best fulfill this requirement. Shunts that will be used for more than just the intraoperative time period will need to be monitored for flow status. In this circumstance, a shunt with an incorporated Doppler flow sensor or a side-branch through which arterial pressure may be continuously monitored may be of additional benefit. When the common femoral artery is disrupted at its bifurcation, a reversed hemodialysis catheter can provide perfusion to both the superficial and the profunda femoral arteries.

REFERENCES

1. Makins GH. On Injuries to the Blood Vessels, Founded on Experience Gained in France During the Great War, 1914-1918. Bristol: John Wright and Sons; 1919, pp. 109–11.
2. Eger M, Goleman L, Goldstein A, et al. The use of a temporary vascular shunt in the management of arterial vascular injuries. Surg Gynecol Obstet 1971;132:67–70.
3. Sriussadaporn S, Pak-art R. Temporary intravascular shunt in complex extremity vascular injuries. J Trauma 2002;52:1129–33.
4. Reber PU, Patel AG, Ris HB, et al. Selective use of temporary intravascular shunts in coincident vascular and orthopedic upper and lower limb trauma. J Trauma 1999;47:72–6.
5. Granchi T, Schmitting Z, Vasquez J, et al. Prolonged use of intraluminal arterial shunts without systemic anticoagulation. Am J Surg 2000;180:493–7.
6. Husain AK, Khandeparker JM, Tendolkar AG, et al. Temporary intravascular shunts for peripheral vascular trauma. J Postgrad Med 1992;38:68–9.
7. Khalil IM, Livingston DH. Intravascular shunts in complex lower limb trauma. J Vasc Surg 1986;4:582–7.
8. Nichols JG, Svoboda JA, Parks SN. Use of temporary intraluminal shunts in selected peripheral arterial injuries. J Trauma 1986;26:1094–6.
9. Johansen K, Bandyk D, Thiele B, et al. Temporary intraluminal shunts: resolution of a management dilemma in complex vascular injuries. J Trauma 1982;22:395–402.
10. Woodward EB, Couse WD, Eliason JL, et al. Penetrating femoropopliteal injury during modern warfare: experience of the Blad Vascular Registry. J Vasc Surg 2008;47:1259–65.
11. Starnes BW, Beekley AC, Sebesta JA, et al. Extremity vascular injuries on the battlefield: tips for surgeons deployed to war. J Trauma 2006;60:432–42.
12. Grossi EA, Giangola G, Parish G, et al. Differences in carotid shunt flow rates and implications for cerebral blood flow. Ann Vasc Surg 1993;7:605–6.
13. Verkerke GJ, van den Dungen JJ, Meyer T, et al. Flow analysis in vascular shunts that bypass the carotid artery. Int J Artif Organs 2001;24:636–41.
14. Aufiero TX, Thiele BL, Rossi JA, et al. Hemodynamic performance of carotid artery shunts. Am J Surg 1989;158:95–9.
15. Wipperman J, Albes JM, Bruhin R, et al. Chronic ultrastructural effects of temporary intraluminal shunts in a porcine off-pump model. Ann Thorac Surg 2008;78:543–8.
16. Subramanian A, Vercruysse G, Dente C, et al. A decade's experience with temporary intravascular shunts at a civilian Level I trauma center. J Trauma 2008;65:316–26.
17. Choudry R, Schmieder F, Blebea J, et al. Temporary femoral artery bifurcation shunting following penetrating trauma. J Vasc Surg 2009;49:779–81.
18. Lee YC, Lee JW. Cross-limb vascular shunting for major limb replantation. Ann Plast Surg 2009;62:139–43.

19. Drost, CJ, "Vessel Diameter-Independent Volume Flow Measurements Using Ultrasound," Proceedings of the San Diego Biomedical Symposium, 1978;17, pp. 299–302.
20. Chambers LW, Green DJ, Sample K, et al. Tactical surgical intervention with temporary shunting of peripheral vascular trauma sustained during operation Iraqi Freedom: one unit's experience. J Trauma 2006;61:824–30.
21. Rasmusen TE, Clouse WD, Jenkins DH, et al. The use of temporary vascular shunts as a damage control adjunct in the management of wartime vascular injury. J Trauma 2006; 61:8–15.
22. Dawson DL, Putnam AT, Light JT, et al. Temporary arterial shunts to maintain limb perfusion after arterial injury: an animal study. J Trauma 1999;47:64–71.
23. Taller J, Kamdar JP, Greene JA, et al. Temporary vascular shunts as initial treatment of proximal extremity vascular injuries during combat operations: the new standard of care at Echelon II facilities? J Trauma 2008;65:595–603.
24. Harkin DW, D'Sa AA, Yassin MM, et al. Reperfusion injury is greater with delayed restoration of venous outflow in concurrent arterial and venous limb injury. Br J Surg 2002;89:245.
25. Peck M, Clouse WD, Cox MW, et al. The complete management of extremity vascular injury in a local population: a wartime report from the 332nd Expeditionary Medical Group/Air Force Theatre Hospital, Balad Air Base, Iraq. J Vasc Surg 2007;45:1197–205.
26. Hafez H, Woolgar J, Robbs J. Lower extremity arterial injury: results of 550 cases and review of risk factors associated with limb loss. J Vasc Surg 2001;33:1212–9.
27. Hossny A. Blunt popliteal artery injury with complete lower limb ischemia: is routine use of temporary intraluminal arterial shunt justified? J Vasc Surg 2004;40:61–6.
28. Ashworth EM, Dalsing MC, Glover JL, et al. Lower extremity vascular trauma: a comprehensive, aggressive approach. J Trauma 1988;28:329–36.
29. McHenry TP, Holcomb JB, Aoki N, et al. Fractures with major vascular injuries from gunshot wounds: implications of surgical sequence. J Trauma 2002;53:717–21.
30. Huynh TT, Pham M, Griffin LW, et al. Management of distal femoral and popliteal arterial injuries: an update. Am J Surg 2006;192:773–8.
31. Hussain MI, Zahid M, Khan AW, et al. Extremity vascular trauma—a 7 year experience in Lahore, Pakistan. Saudi Med J 2009;30:50–5.

16

Fasciotomies

Neha D. Shah, M.D. and Joseph R. Durham, M.D., F.A.C.S.

INTRODUCTION

A properly timed, expertly performed fasciotomy procedure is an invaluable tool to have in the surgeon's armamentarium. Knowledge of the appropriate indications as well as the anatomy involved will lead to decreased patient morbidity and enhanced functional outcomes. Fasciotomies are performed to treat existing or developing compartment syndromes, and the most common anatomic sites are the leg and forearm. This is because of the well-defined, rigid fascial boundaries of these locations and the frequency of injury to the distal extremities. Other less common sites for fasciotomy include the arm and the thigh.[1] Compartment syndromes involving the hand,[2] foot,[3,5] shoulder, abdomen, lumbar paraspinous muscles, and spinal cord also exist but are not addressed here.

INDICATIONS FOR FASCIOTOMY

The presence of an existing or a developing acute compartment syndrome is the typical indication for a fasciotomy procedure. Another indication is a clinical situation in which the incipient development of a significant compartment syndrome is very likely, such as prolonged extremity ischemia or combined extremity arterial and venous injuries (especially the popliteal vessels and ligation of the popliteal vein). Other clinical situations that may result in an acute compartment syndrome include severe burns and prolonged limb compression following loss of consciousness from a drug overdose or a stroke. Delayed development of a compartment syndrome is common and may be very difficult to document, especially in the patient with altered mental status or the trauma patient with multiple injuries. Discussion of fasciotomy for chronic compartment syndrome is well recognized but is beyond the scope of this chapter.[6-7]

The most common cause for the development of increased compartmental pressures is a bony fracture, especially of the tibia. Consequently, these are managed by the orthopedic surgery service in most institutions. Arterial bleeding into rigid, fixed compartments, reperfusion following prolonged extremity ischemia due to arterial injury (traumatic or iatrogenic), embolic disease, popliteal aneurysm thrombosis, or failure of an existing bypass often result in compartment syndromes. Not surprisingly, compartment syndrome following penetrating trauma is due to direct vascular injury with resultant ischemia and reperfusion injury. Blunt trauma typically results in compartment syndrome from musculoskeletal injury or direct tissue damage. These are the patients we routinely encounter at the John H. Stroger, Jr. Hospital of Cook County (formerly the Cook County Hospital). Development of a clinically relevant compartment syndrome following elective extremity revascularization for chronic extremity ischemia may occur but is distinctly uncommon.

The diagnosis of a compartment syndrome is based upon clinical suspicion, the mechanism and location of the injury, physical examination findings, and objective compartment pressure measurements. Physical examination findings suggestive of an acute compartment syndrome may include rigidity and tenderness of muscles in the involved compartment, loss of arterial pulses, or neurologic deficits. Severe pain (often out of proportion to the physical findings) or severe tenderness and pain on passive stretching are suggestive of an existing compartment syndrome. Possible neurologic findings are hypesthesia, paresthesia, or decreased motor function (e.g., peroneal nerve involvement and decreased foot dorsiflexion). Diminished sensation in the distribution of relevant nerves within the compartment in question may be an early finding due to ischemia of the nerves. Muscle weakness or paralysis follows if the compartment is not promptly released. These findings are often straightforward and readily evident in the awake and alert patient. Diagnosis is much more challenging in the patient with an altered mental state or neurologic deficit due to alcohol or drug influence, general or regional anesthesia, spinal cord injury, or unconsciousness. Loss of arterial pulses may be a late sign or could be due to an arterial injury itself rather than resulting from a compartment syndrome. An elevated serum creatine phosphokinase level is an ominous finding signifying late diagnosis and established myonecrosis. Myoglobinuria and renal failure add to the morbidity and mortality of this disorder (Figure 16–1).

Unfortunately, these findings are all nonspecific and none is diagnostic for an established, significant compartment syndrome. Noninvasive assays exist to assist in the determination of an acute compartment syndrome but are still in the development stage and not widely used; these tend to have a high specificity but low sensitivity for reliable diagnosis. Our preference is to proceed with direct pressure measurements of the involved compartments using the Stryker intracompartmental pressure monitoring system (Stryker Surgical, Kalamazoo, MI). This direct approach allows serial measurements at multiple sites and has been very easy, quick, reasonably reliable, and reproducible. A surgical culture that melds a high index of clinical suspicion, serial surveillance, and measurement of compartment pressures will yield excellent clinical outcomes.

Normal compartment tissue pressures range from 0 to 10 mm Hg. Concern for a compartment syndrome and the consideration of a fasciotomy intervention occur when the compartmental pressure reaches 30 mm Hg or greater. The degree of tissue perfusion has been shown to correlate with diastolic blood pressure; when the compartment pressure exceeds the diastolic blood pressure, perfusion ceases. Consequently, some clinicians rely upon the comparison of the compartment pressure to the diastolic blood pressure. When the compartment pressure rises to within 30 mm Hg of the diastolic

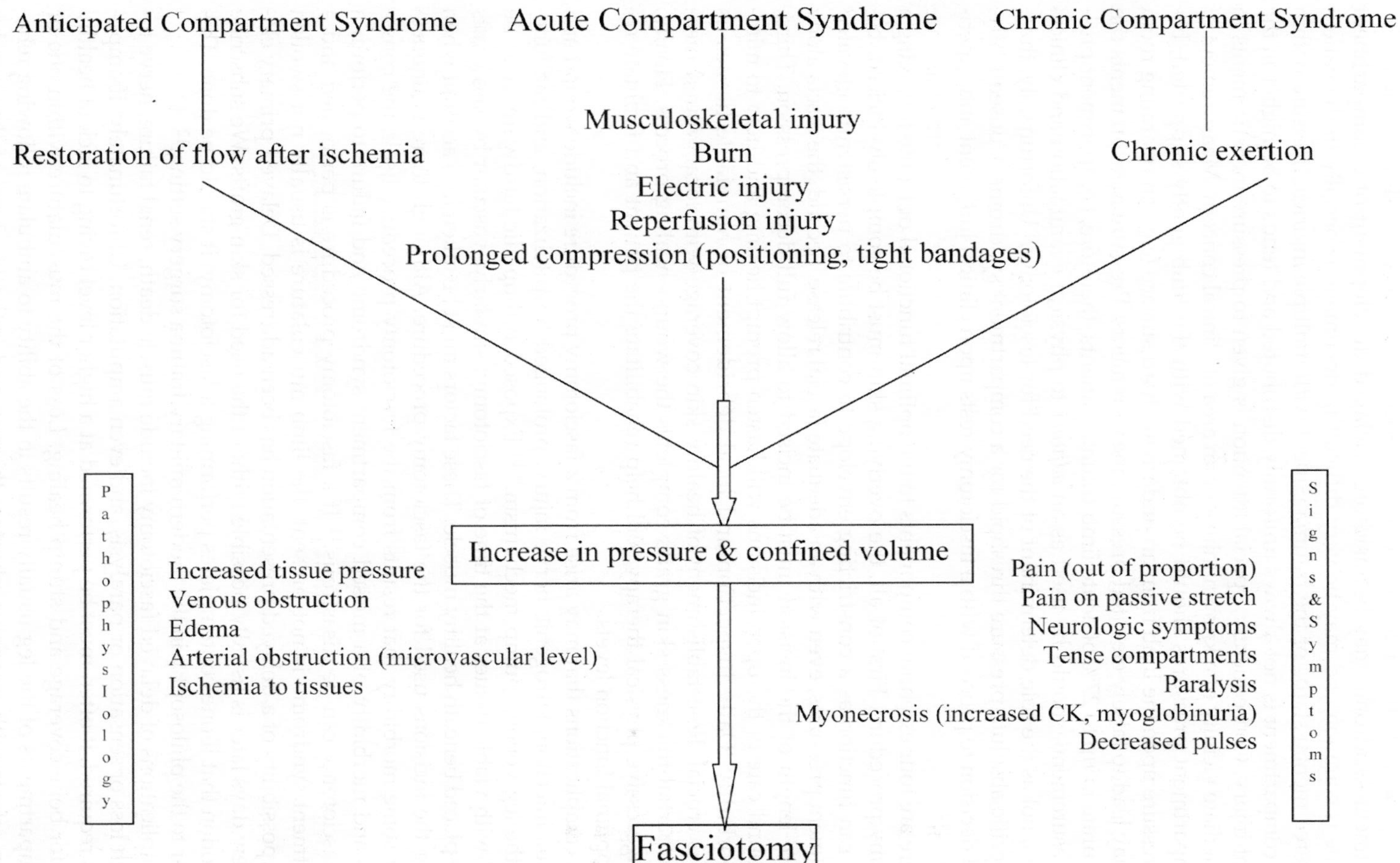

Figure 16-1. The causes of impending compartment syndrome, acute compartment syndrome, and chronic compartment syndrome are reviewed. All of these lead to a common pathophysiologic process, initiated by increased pressure in a confined space. The listed signs and symptoms (in order from early to late) will lead one to the diagnosis. The suspicion of compartment syndrome should prompt the surgeon toward fasciotomy. CK: creatine kinase.

blood pressure, serious consideration should be given to performing a prompt fasciotomy. Serial pressure measurements are essential, because the development of a compartment syndrome may be insidious. Delayed development of a compartment syndrome is common and may be very difficult to document, especially in the patient with altered mental status or the trauma patient with multiple injuries. Pressure within a given compartment is not always uniformly distributed and tends to be higher in the region of injury. Consequently, special attention is given to pressure measurements in the immediate vicinity of a known injury or an area of clinical concern. Measurement of the compartment pressures should be obtained with the limb gently supported, because pressure upon the limb from an underlying hard surface (e.g., an operating room table) may lead to falsely elevated pressure measurements. Pressure measurements can be inaccurate in up to 27% of acute limb trauma patients; therefore, compartment pressure measurements should be used as an *adjunct* to physical examination and clinical suspicion, not as the sole determinant of the need for fasciotomy.[8] Unfortunately, there is no specific absolute pressure threshold for a compartment syndrome. Consequently, the final decision to proceed with a fasciotomy rests upon clinical judgment and experience.

There are four essential components to the optimal functional outcome following a fasciotomy procedure. First of all, the overlying skin must be completely incised, because it can function as a constricting envelope to contribute to persistently elevated compartment pressures, even with an adequate fascial release. Second, the fascia along the entire length of the incision must be incised to allow full decompression. Third, local wound care of the open incisions will hasten prompt healing and help to minimize morbidity. Daily inspection and local débridement of nonviable tissues as needed is crucial. Re-establishment of healthy skin coverage with local wound measures or partial-thickness skin grafts completes the wound healing process. Finally, timely aggressive physical therapy will help rehabilitate the patient and facilitate return to optimal function levels.

The complications that may arise from a fasciotomy procedure include wound and soft tissue infection, iatrogenic nerve injury, prolonged hospitalization, and malfunction of the leg venous pump mechanism.[9-10] Exposed orthopedic hardware must be covered with viable tissues at the time of fasciotomy; similarly, vascular bypass grafts must be placed beneath healthy muscle. These factors must be taken into account when planning the incisions used for the fasciotomy procedure. Although there is unquestionably some morbidity that results from the fasciotomy procedure itself, the consequences and morbidity of a missed compartment syndrome and failure to perform a timely fasciotomy can be disastrous.[11] If a fasciotomy procedure is performed and a compartment syndrome is not present, the limb musculature is usually not swollen and the possibility of a delayed presentation has been addressed. Delayed primary closure a few days later is usually possible without the need for skin grafts. We subscribe to the notion that if one contemplates performing a fasciotomy, it should be done. This is similar to the philosophy in the modern military trauma surgery setting.[12]

Complications of delayed fasciotomy include muscle death, renal failure, nerve injury with loss of sensation or paralysis, and even amputation. Unfortunately, if amputation is required, it often must be performed at a higher level owing to lack of healthy muscle for bone coverage and stump healing. Loss of the musculature within one or two compartments of the leg usually results in the ability to ambulate following rehabilitation efforts with intensive physical therapy and orthotics. Loss of the muscles with three or more leg compartments almost always results in a functionless limb; in this setting, an early amputation at a level sure to heal followed by aggressive prosthetic rehabilitation may yield independent ambulation.[13]

ANATOMY AND SURGICAL TECHNIQUES

The Leg

The leg has four compartments: anterior, lateral, superficial posterior, and deep posterior. Each of these four compartments has a significant nerve coursing through it: the anterior compartment (deep peroneal nerve), the lateral compartment (superficial peroneal nerve), the posterior compartment (sural nerve), and the deep posterior compartment (posterior tibial nerve) (Figure 16–2). Whereas the anterior compartment is the compartment most commonly involved, more significant damage tends to occur from involvement of the deep posterior compartment.

Certain types of clinical situations may predispose to the development of a leg compartment syndrome. Injuries to the proximal half of the below-knee arterial segment are the most common cause for development of compartment syndrome from penetrating trauma of the lower extremity.[14-18] Shock also predisposes to compartment syndrome.[16]

Three distinct surgical techniques are available for complete decompression of all four leg compartments. The most commonly employed is the dual-incision technique, which involves separate medial and lateral leg incisions. Two other approaches permit

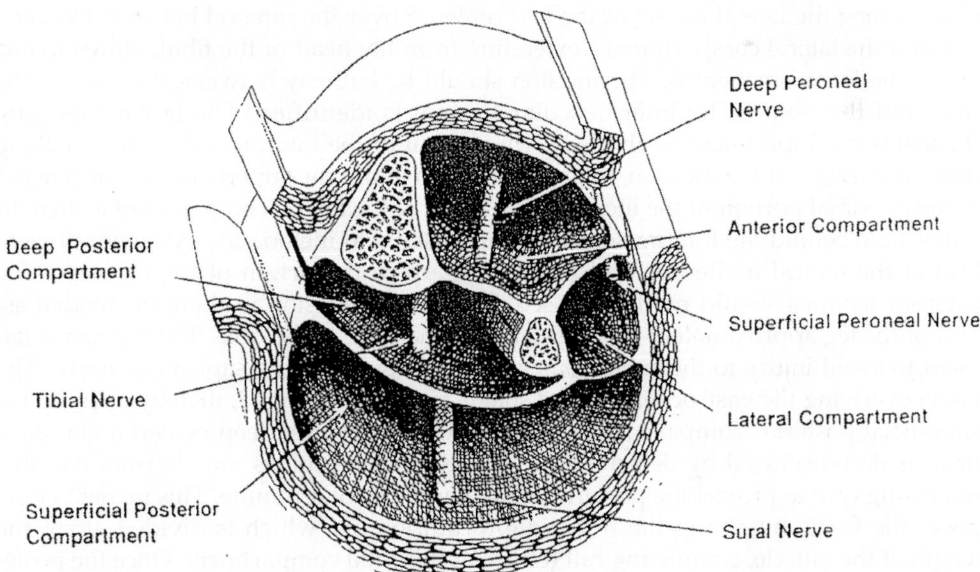

Figure 16-2. The four compartments of the leg are shown with the respective nerves running through them. The deep peroneal nerve in the anterior compartment, the superficial peroneal nerve in the lateral compartment, the sural nerve in the superficial posterior compartment, and the tibial nerve in the deep posterior compartment. Access to each compartment via two incisions is demonstrated in cross-section. (Reprinted with permission from Ernst CB, Stanley JC. Fasciotomy in vascular trauma and compartment syndrome. In: Mills JL, ed. Current Therapy in Vascular Surgery. Philadelphia: Mosby Elsevier; 1995, Figure 2.)

decompression through a single lateral incision. One involves actual resection of the fibula and is probably of historical interest only. The other is a perifibular technique. These single lateral incision approaches may have some utility if preservation of the integrity of the skin of the medial leg is essential, such as with the presence of a comminuted tibia fracture. A medial leg incision in this setting could convert a closed fracture to an open fracture with attendant risk of infection. However, in most vascular surgery settings, we believe that the dual-incision approach is safer, faster, and more effective than the single-incision methods.

The single lateral incision four-compartment leg fasciotomy is accomplished through a long incision in line with the fibula that extends from just distal to the head of the fibula down to several centimeters proximal to the lateral malleolus (Figure 16–3). If performed too far posteriorly, the anterior compartment may not be identified properly and not decompressed adequately. The skin and subcutaneous tissues are undermined anteriorly with care taken not to injure the superficial peroneal nerve in the proximal aspect of the incision. The intermuscular septum is identified, and a longitudinal fasciotomy of each of the anterior and lateral compartments is performed for the entire length of the incision. The skin and subcutaneous tissues are then undermined posteriorly to gain access to the superficial posterior compartment, which is released. Then, the interval between the lateral and the superficial posterior compartments is defined and separated. This exposes the flexor hallucis longus muscle, which is dissected off the fibula and retracted posteromedially, along with the peroneal vessels. Finally, the fascial attachment of the posterior tibial muscle to the fibula is cut longitudinally to allow decompression of the deep posterior compartment.[7]

The dual-incision technique is accomplished through two vertical skin incisions that are separated by a bridge of skin at least 8 cm wide (Figure 16–4). The first incision is along the lateral aspect of the leg, centered over the interval between the anterior and the lateral compartments, extending from the head of the fibula down to just above the lateral malleolus. The incision should be halfway between the crest of the tibia and the fibula. The intermuscular septum is identified. The fascia overlying the anterior compartment is divided 1 cm in front of the intermuscular septum along the entire length of the incision, taking care not to injure the superficial peroneal nerve in the proximal portion of the incision. The fascia of the lateral compartment is then divided 1 cm behind the intermuscular septum distally to include the extensor retinaculum at the lateral malleolus and proximally up to the origin of the muscles. The extensor tendons should not be exposed. The second incision is along the medial aspect of the leg approximately 2 cm posterior to the edge of the tibia. The incision is tailored to avoid injury to the saphenous vein and accompanying saphenous nerve. The fascia overlying the gastrocnemius and soleus muscles is divided, thereby opening the superficial posterior compartment. Using electrocautery, the deep posterior compartment is decompressed by detaching the insertion of the soleus muscle from the tibia but taking care to protect the posterior tibial neurovascular bundle. This maneuver exposes the fascia overlying the flexor digitorum longus, which is divided along the length of the muscle, completing full release of this vital compartment. Once the posterior aspect of the tibia is visualized directly, one knows that the deep posterior compartment has been fully decompressed.

The Thigh and Buttocks

The thigh has three compartments: anterior, medial, and posterior. Most thigh compartment syndromes involve the anterior and posterior compartments, each of which has a

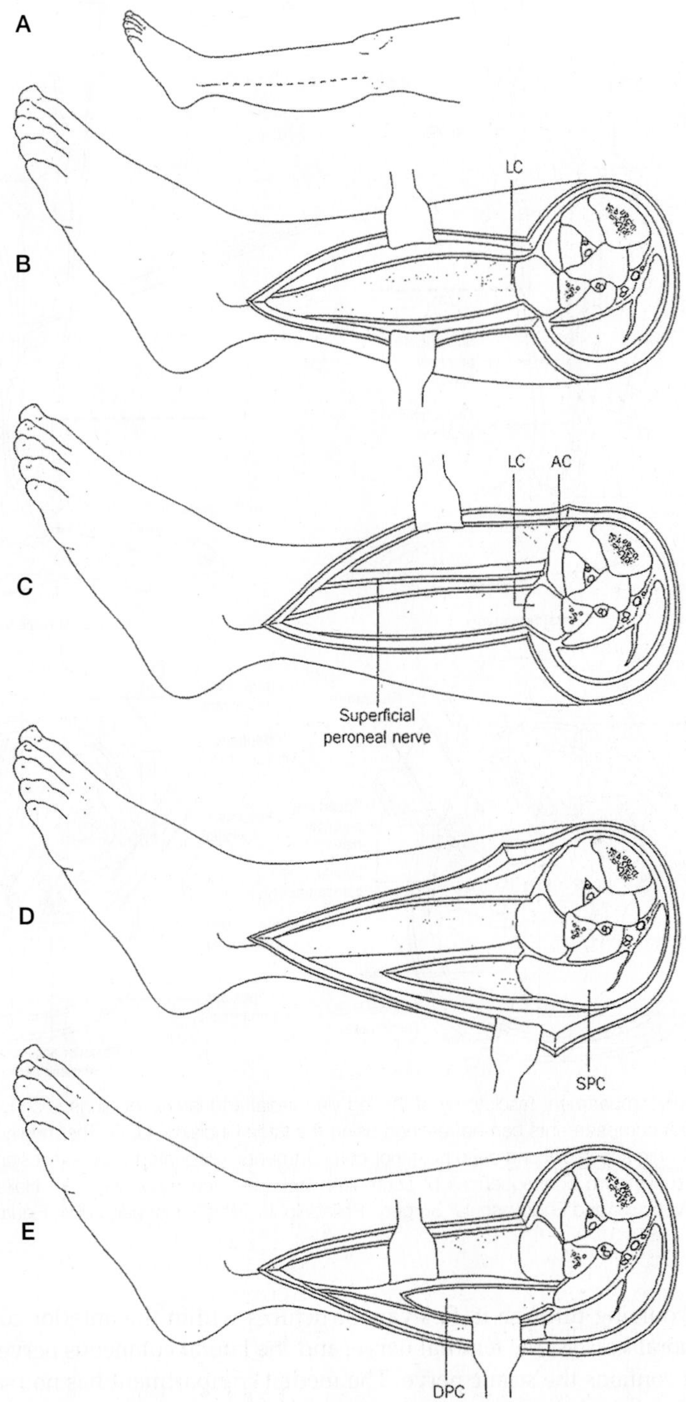

Figure 16-3. A. The leg fasciotomy via single incision is shown here. **B.** The decompression of the lateral compartment (LC). **C.** The decompression of the anterior compartment (AC). **D.** The decompression of the superficial posterior compartment (SPC). **E.** The decompression of the deep posterior compartment (DPC). (Reprinted with permission from Varma S, et al. Metabolic and systemic consequences of acute limb ischemia and reperfusion. In: Hallett JW, et al, eds. Comprehensive Vascular and Endovascular Surgery. Philadelphia: Mosby Elsevier; 2004, Figure 18–6.)

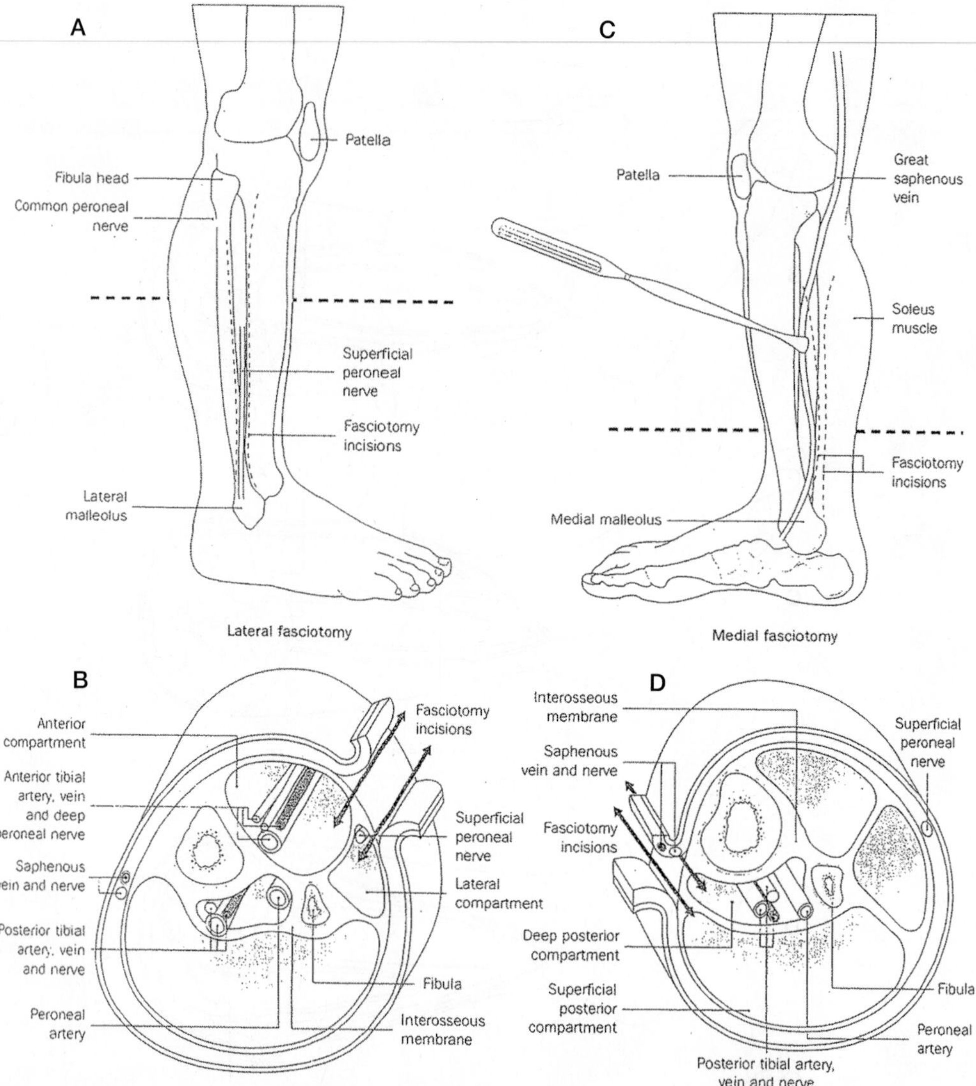

Figure 16-4. Four compartment fasciotomy of the leg via medial and lateral incisions is shown here. **A, B:** The anterior and lateral compartments can be reached using the lateral incision. **C, D:** The medial incision allows for decompression of the superficial and deep posterior compartments. (Reprinted with permission from Varma S, et al. Metabolic and systemic consequences of acute limb ischemia and reperfusion. In: Hallett JW, et al, eds. Comprehensive Vascular and Endovascular Surgery. Philadelphia: Mosby Elsevier; 2004, Figure 18–5.)

major nerve coursing through it. Relevant structures within the anterior compartment include the femoral vessels, the femoral nerve, and the lateral cutaneous nerve. The posterior compartment contains the sciatic nerve. The medial compartment has no major neurologic structure within it and does not usually require decompression. Most thigh compartment syndromes are the result of femur fractures or arterial injuries.[19-20] The gluteal muscle group of the buttocks is enclosed by the fascia lata, defining another compartment vulnerable to increased pressures and involvement of the sciatic nerve as well as the muscles themselves.[21]

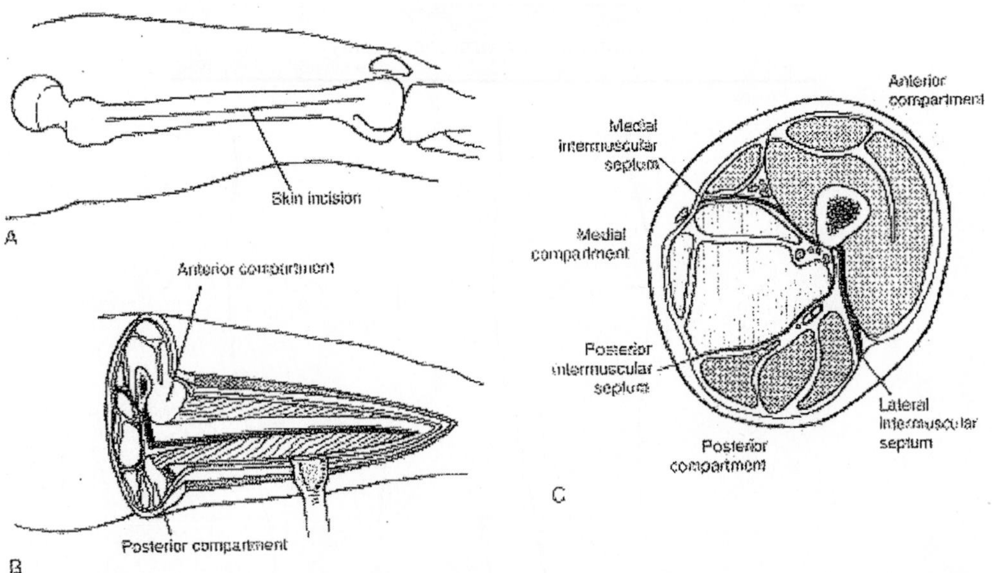

Figure 16-5. A. Thigh fasciotomy incision. **B.** Decompression of anterior compartment by incising fascia lata and exposing lateral compartment by medial retraction of vastus lateralis, and incision of intermuscular septum for decompression of the posterior compartment. **C.** Cross-sectional view. (Reprinted with permission from Canale ST, Beaty JH. Traumatic Disorders from Canale and Beaty: Campbell's Operative Orthopaedics. Philadelphia: Mosby Elsevier, 2007, Figure 46–5.)

Decompression of the anterior and posterior thigh compartments is readily accomplished using a full-length lateral thigh incision extending from the intertrochanteric line down to the lateral femoral epicondyle (Figure 16–5). The anterior compartment is opened by incising the underlying fascia lata. The posterior compartment is decompressed by retracting the vastus lateralis muscle medially to expose the lateral intermuscular septum, which is then opened. Following decompression of the anterior and posterior compartments, a pressure measurement of the medial compartment may be obtained. If necessary, the medial compartment is decompressed with the same medial incision used to expose the superficial femoral artery beneath the sartorius muscle; anterior extension of this approach will also allow decompression of the anterior compartment.[19] Decompression of the gluteal musculature of the buttocks is performed using longitudinal incisions through the skin with additional incisions of the underlying individual epimysial envelopes as needed.[22]

The Forearm

The forearm has three compartments: the volar, the dorsal, and the mobile wad. The volar compartment contains the radial and ulnar arteries plus the median and ulnar nerves. The radial nerve runs through the mobile wad compartment, which is closely associated with the dorsal compartment. The dorsal compartment contains the extensor musculature but no major arteries or nerves.[23] The forearm muscles that are at increased risk for injury are in the volar compartment. The upper extremity compartment most often requiring decompression is the volar compartment of the forearm.

A wide variety of both blunt and penetrating traumatic mechanisms can lead to the development of a compartment syndrome in the upper extremity.[24] The diagnosis

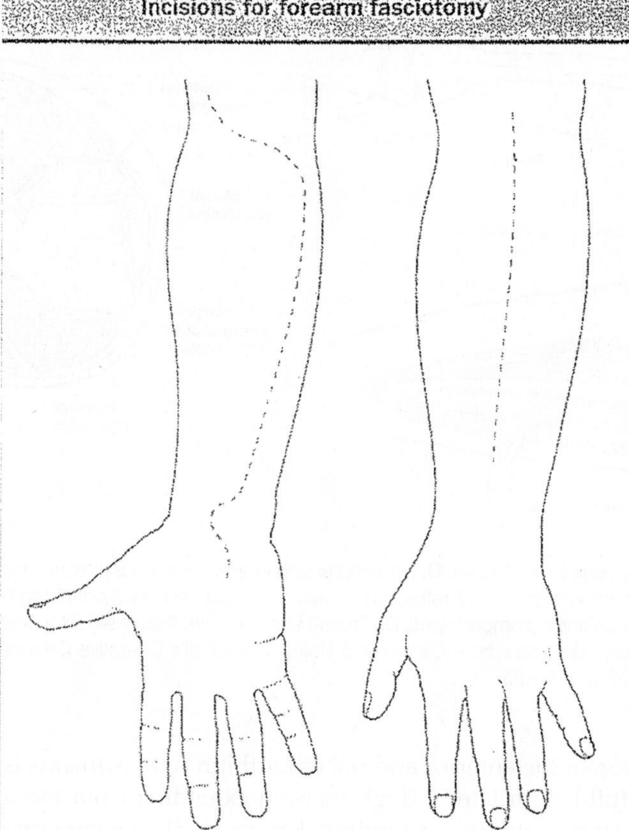

Figure 16-6. Ventral and dorsal incisions for forearm fasciotomy. (Reprinted with permission from Varma S, et al. Metabolic and systemic consequences of acute limb ischemia and reperfusion. In: Hallett JW, et al., eds. Comprehensive Vascular and Endovascular Surgery. Philadelphia: Mosby Elsevier; 2004, Figure 18–7.)

should be suspected in children following supracondylar fracture of the humerus, the mechanism of injury leading to the original description of Volkmann's contracture of the forearm.[25] Other clinical situations possibly leading to a forearm compartment syndrome include high-energy injuries with fractures of the forearm, iatrogenic or traumatic arterial injury, subfascial intravenous fluid infiltration, crush injury, and reimplantation of the hand or forearm.[22,26]

Surgical intervention with fasciotomy is the mainstay of treatment. Complete fasciotomy of the forearm is performed using volar and dorsal incisions. Most forearm compartment syndromes are successfully decompressed with a volar incision only. A curvilinear volar incision allows release of the flexor muscle compartment (Figure 16–6). The course of the incision may be tailored to accommodate pre-existing traumatic wounds and tissue loss.[22] The need for the additional dorsal fasciotomy incision may be determined by intraoperative pressure measurements of the dorsal compartment following release of the volar compartment. A longitudinal incision along the posterior aspect of the forearm releases the dorsal compartment and its extensor musculature. In severe cases, the deep intramuscular fascia enveloping the flexor digitorum superficialis, the flexor digitorum profundus, and the flexor pollicis longus may also require decompression[22] (Figure 16–7).

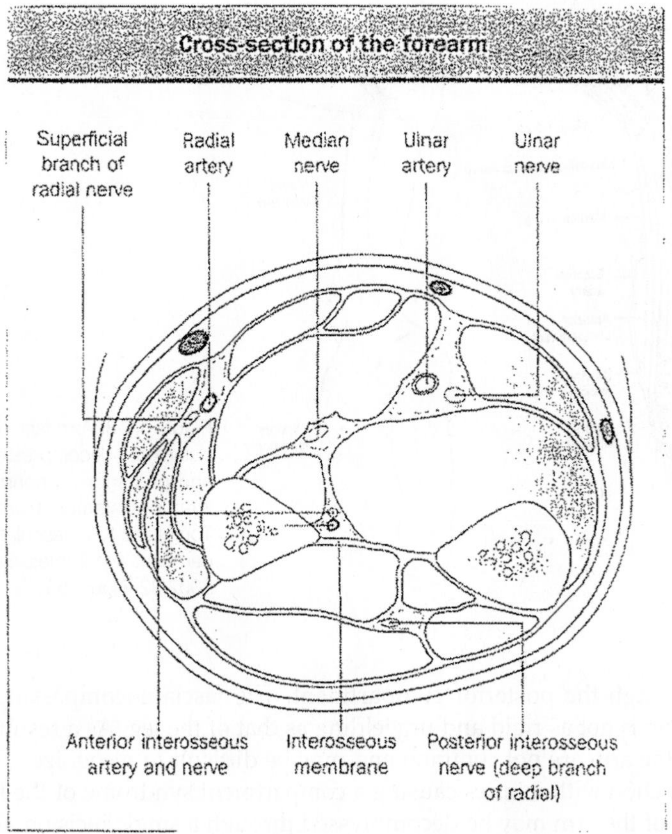

Figure 16-7. Cross-sectional forearm anatomy. (Reprinted with permission from Varma S, et al. Metabolic and systemic consequences of acute limb ischemia and reperfusion. In: Hallett JW, et al, eds. Comprehensive Vascular and Endovascular Surgery. Philadelphia: Mosby Elsevier; 2004, Figure 18–8.)

An alternative incision for fasciotomy of the volar compartment is available. This approach allows exposure of the brachial artery and decompression of the mobile wad compartment, if needed. This volar incision should extend from the distal arm down to the carpal tunnel. The incision is begun medially just proximal to the antecubital crease and is an S-shaped incision that begins medial to the biceps tendon and extends across the antecubital fossa down the lateral (radial) aspect of the forearm. The incision may be extended across the wrist out onto the hand to divide the transcarpal ligament to decompress the carpal tunnel as needed. This maneuver decompresses the median, ulnar, and radial nerves as well as the flexor/pronator musculature and the extrinsic muscles of the fingers and thumb. Proximally at the antecubital fossa, the lacertus fibrosus should be divided to release pressure on the median nerve. The resultant skin flap is designed to maintain coverage of the median nerve and the flexor tendons. Postoperatively, the open incisions are loosely dressed with moist saline gauze and the limb is maintained in a functional position.

The Arm

The arm has two compartments: anterior and posterior. The anterior compartment contains the brachial vessels plus the median, ulnar, and musculocutaneous nerves. The radial

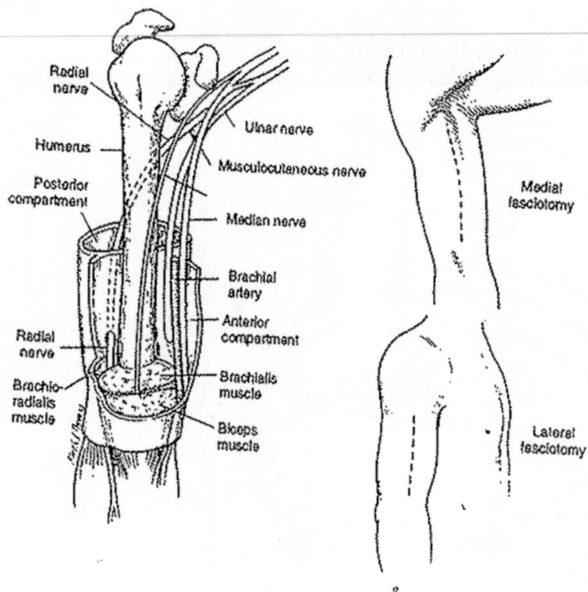

Figure 16-8. Arm fasciotomy, with two incisions for decompression of the anterior and posterior compartment. (Reprinted with permission from Velmahos GS, Toutouzas KG. Vascular trauma and compartment syndromes. Surg Clin North Am 2002;82, Figure 5.)

nerve runs through the posterior compartment. The fascia encompassing the compartments of the arm is not as rigid and unyielding as that of the leg. As a result, compartment syndromes of the arm are not common and may be difficult to recognize. They most often occur in conjunction with injuries causing a compartment syndrome of the forearm.[27] Both compartments of the arm may be decompressed through a single incision along the lateral border of the biceps muscle. This incision releases the anterior compartment. If the posterior compartment requires decompression, it is opened by dividing the intermuscular septum of the arm deep to the biceps muscle. For more extensive injuries with severe swelling, fasciotomy of the arm may be performed using the two incisions depicted in Figure 16–8.

THE AFTERMATH: POSTOPERATIVE CARE AND WOUND CLOSURE

Discussion regarding fasciotomy is usually focused on its appropriate indications and proper technique. Although less glorious than the urgent fasciotomy, its aftermath is equally important. The postoperative care and closure of the wound should not be overlooked. The patient may require support for rhabdomyolysis and renal failure in the acute postoperative phase. Once the patient is clinically stabilized and the acute illness or injury has been overcome, the challenge of closing a large soft tissue defect must be addressed.

Traditionally, wounds have been managed with moist dressings until they are eventually covered with skin grafts or closed primarily. A newer wound management strategy is the Wound Vac device, which employs negative pressure wound therapy (V.A.C. System, KCI Medical, San Antonio, TX); this method is used in place of standard moist gauze dressings, with reports of a higher rate of primary closure[28] (Figure 16–9). For final closure of the wound, several techniques of delayed primary closure have been described for improvement of cosmetic outcome and ease of closure (Figure 16–10).

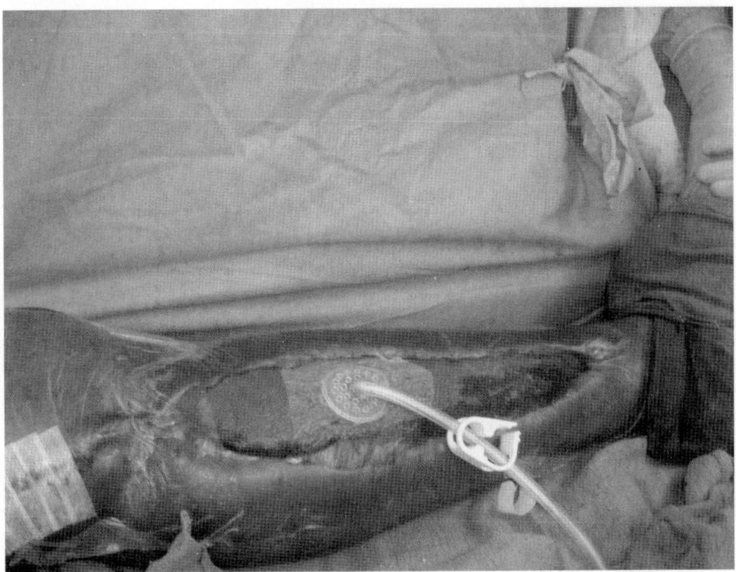

Figure 16-9. Wound management with vacuum suction device.

The most commonly described technique of delayed primary closure is the shoelace technique. A large polypropylene suture can be placed, at the time of fasciotomy, in a crossing, shoelace pattern. This suture is gradually tightened as the swelling decreases (Figure 16–11). It is essential to note that the closure process should not be initiated until the acute compartment syndrome has resolved. Some surgeons have covered the suture with pieces of large drain tubing to protect the tissue in contact with the muscle. Another variant of the shoelace technique utilizes vessel loops or

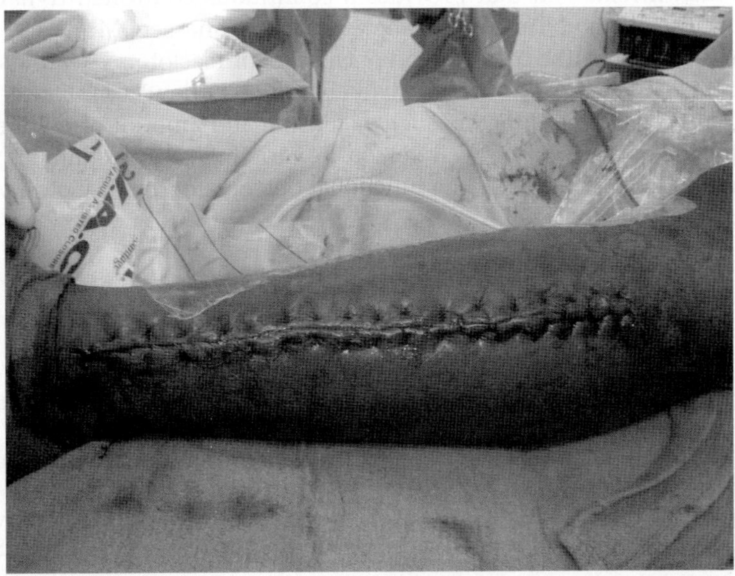

Figure 16-10. Fasciotomy wound with closure sutures following management with vacuum suction device.

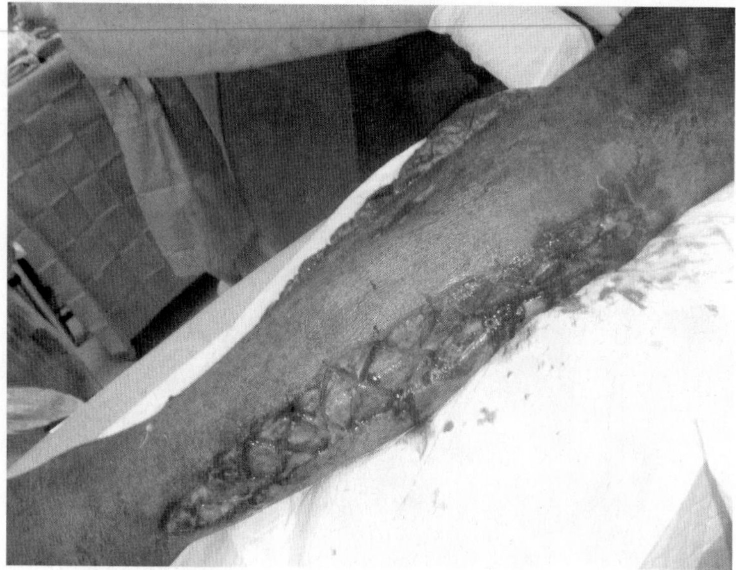

Figure 16-11. Fasciotomy wounds with shoelace closure technique.

rubber bands in the place of suture in order to minimize trauma to the muscle tissue.[29] The vessel loops are stapled to the wound edges of the fasciotomy and gradually tightened in the same manner. Daily advancement of Steri-Strips has also been described.[30] Recently, there have been innovations to achieve the same goal of delayed primary closure. The concept of dermatotraction utilizes the elastic properties of skin to maximize the surgeon's ability to primarily close a fasciotomy wound.[31] More recently, a device using stainless steel skin anchors and a nylon line provides an elegant means of applying a defined, calibrated degree of traction to reapproximate the wound margins; there is a clutch mechanism that provides a continuous controlled dynamic pulling force (Dermaclose, Wound Care Technologies, Inc., Chanhassen, MN).

It is unclear which is the best method of closure for fasciotomy wounds. Certainly, the method of closure must be individualized based on patient compliance, equipment availability, cost, and wound factors such as tension and amount of myonecrosis. It is important for the surgeon to be well versed in varied closure techniques so that the particular method used optimizes the functional outcome of the fasciotomy procedure for that individual patient.

REFERENCES

1. Boland MR, Heck C. Acute exercise-induced bilateral thigh compartment syndrome. Orthopedics 2009;32:218.
2. Spinner M, Aiache A, Silver L, Barsky A. Impending ischemic contracture of the hand. Plast Reconstr Surg 1972;50:341.
3. Ascer E, Strauch B, Calligaro KD, et al. Ankle and foot fasciotomy: an adjunctive technique to optimize limb salvage after revascularization for acute ischemia. J Vasc Surg 1989;9: 594–7.

4. Manoli A II. Compartment releases of the foot. In: Johnson KA, ed. Master Techniques in Orthopaedic Surgery: The Foot and Ankle. New York: Raven Press; 1994, pp. 257–67.
5. Maurel B, Brilhault J, Martinez R, Lermusiaux P. Compartment syndrome with foot ischemia after inversion injury of the ankle. J Vasc Surg 2007;46:369–71.
6. Turnipseed WD. Surgical management of atypical claudication associated with overuse injury. In: Pearce WH, Matsumura JS, Yao JST, eds. Trends in Vascular Surgery 2003. Chicago: Precept Press; 2003, pp. 427–34.
7. Davey JR, Rorabeck CH, Fowler PJ. The tibialis posterior muscle compartment: an unrecognized cause of exertional compartment syndrome. Am J Sports Med 1984;12:391–7.
8. Azar FM. Traumatic disorders. In: Canale ST, Beatty JH, eds. Campbell's Operative Orthopaedics. 11th ed. St. Louis: Mosby; 2008, pp. 2737–88.
9. Nypaver TJ. Fasciotomy in vascular trauma and compartment cyndrome. In: Ernst CB, Stanley JC, eds. Current Therapy in Vascular Surgery. 4th ed. St Louis: Mosby; 2001, pp. 624–8.
10. Bermudez K, Knudson MM, Morabito D, et al. Fasciotomy, chronic venous insufficiency, and the calf muscle pump. Arch Surg 1998;133:1356–61.
11. Ritenour AE, Dorlac WC, Fang R, et al. Complications after fasciotomy revision and delayed compartment release in combat patients. J Trauma 2008;64(2 Suppl):S153–62.
12. Beekley AC, Starnes BW, Sebesta JA. Lessons learned from modern military surgery. Surg Clin North Am 2007;87:157–84.
13. Watson JC, Johansen KH. Compartment syndrome: pathophysiology, recognition, and management. In: Rutherford RB, ed. Vascular Surgery. 6th ed. Philadelphia: Elsevier Saunders; 2005, pp. 1058–65.
14. Gonzalez RP, Scott W, Wright A, et al. Anatomic location of penetrating lower-extremity trauma predicts compartment syndrome development. Am J Surg 2009;197:371–5.
15. Grossman MD, Reilly P, McMahan D, et al. Gunshot wounds below the popliteal fossa: a contemporary review. Am Surg 1999;65:360–5.
16. Asensio JA, Kuncir EJ, Garcia-Nunez LM, Petrone P. Femoral vessel injuries: analysis of factors predictive of outcomes. J Am Coll Surg 2006;203:512–20.
17. Huynh TTT, Pham M, Griffin LW, et al. Management of distal femoral and popliteal arterial injuries: an update. Am J Surg 2006;192:773–8.
18. Woodman G, Croce MA, Fabian TC. Iliac artery ischemia: analysis of risks for ischemic complications. Am Surg 1998;64:833–7.
19. Tarlow, SD, Achterman CA, Hayhurst J, Ovadia DN. Acute compartment syndrome in the thigh complicating fracture of the femur: a report of three cases. J Bone Joint Surg 1986;68A: 1439–43.
20. Hill SL, Bianchi J. The gluteal compartment syndrome. Am Surg 1997;9:823–6.
21. Schwartz JT Jr, Brumback RJ, Lakatos R, et al. Acute compartment syndrome of the thigh, a spectrum of injury. J Bone Joint Surg 1989;71A:392–400.
22. Varma S, Padberg F Jr, Hobson R II, Duran WN. Metabolic and systemic consequences of acute limb ischemia and reperfusion. In: Hallett JW, Mills JL, Earnshaw JJ, Reekers JA, eds. Comprehensive Vascular and Endovascular Surgery. St. Louis: Mosby; 2004, pp. 235–46.
23. Doyle J. Anatomy of the upper extremity muscle compartments. Hand Clin 1998;14:343–64.
24. Morin RJ, Swan KG, Tan V. Acute forearm compartment syndrome secondary to local arterial injury after penetrating trauma. J Trauma 2009;66:989–93.
25. Mubarak SJ, Hargens AR. Compartment Syndromes and Volkmann's Contracture, Philadelphia: W.B. Saunders; 1981, pp. 106–21.
26. Friedrich JB, Shin AY. Management of forearm compartment syndrome. Hand Clin 2007; 23:245–54.
27. Dente CJ, Feliciano DV, Rozycki GS, et al. A review of upper extremity fasciotomies in a Level I trauma center. Am Surg 2004;70:1088–93.
28. Zannis J, Angobaldo J, Marks M, et al. Comparison of fasciotomy wound closures using traditional dressing changes and the vacuum-assisted closure device. Ann Plast Surg 2009;62: 407–9.

29. Suliman MT, Aizaz S. Closing fasciotomy wounds using plastic bands: an alternative simple and cheap method. Ann Vasc Surg 2008;22:697–700.
30. Harrah J, Gates R, Carl J, Harrah JD. A simpler, less expensive technique for delayed primary closure of fasciotomies. Am J Surg 2000;180:55–7.
31. Taylor RC, Reitsma BJ, Sarazin S, Bell MG. Early results using a dynamic method for delayed primary closure of fasciotomy wounds. J Am Coll Surg 2003;197:872–8.

17

Vascular Injury During Anterior Exposure of the Spine

Frank Pomposelli, M.D.

INTRODUCTION

During the past 15 years, the number of anterior lumbar interbody fusions (ALIFs) alone or in combination with posterior spinal instrumentation has increased significantly. Procedures are most commonly performed for degenerative disk disease, although other indications include scoliosis, spondylolisthesis, and spinal instability due to infection, trauma, or malignancy.[1] In the past, spinal fusion surgery was relatively uncommon and the occasional anterior procedure was usually done through a large left flank incision analogous to that used for renal transplantation or retroperitoneal exposure of the left iliac vessels. The relatively recent development of stand-alone metal alloy cages placed in the disk spaces after lumbar disk excision,[2] along with the development of the artificial implantable lumbar disk,[3] required a different approach because the devices are oriented on the anterior midline of the vertebral column. Proper placement of these devices necessitated the direct exposure and access to the anterior surface of the vertebral bodies. The tremendous growth in volume of ALIF procedures has proved to be a source of new business for vascular surgeons. Because of the proximity of the lower lumbar spine to the aorta, inferior vena cava, and iliac vessels, the anterior approach to the lumbar spine is usually performed by vascular surgeons who function as "exposure surgeons" for the spine surgeon. Several authors have described a variety of complications with this approach, including injury to the bowel and the ureter, infection, lymphocele/seroma, and erectile dysfunction.[4-6] Injury to the adjacent vascular structures is the most common complication, ranging from minor injuries requiring simple suture repair to severe life-threatening hemorrhage from major venous or arterial injuries.[1,4-9] Recognition of the potential for injury with the exposure of the spine places a unique burden on the exposure surgeon, who must minimize the chances of a complication with the approach that might compromise the chance for a successful result with the fusion, which is the ultimate goal of the operation. Vascular surgeons are uniquely suited for this role because of their familiarity with the retroperitoneal structures in this area, their comfort and expertise with vascular dissection and mobilization, and most importantly, their ability to rapidly deal with vascular injury should it occur during the conduct of the procedure.[10]

Although the technology employed for ALIF includes a vast array of metal cages, implants, and insertion devices, the fundamental tenets of the exposure procedure are nearly always the same. Understanding how to expose the spine and mobilize the vessels out of harm's way is the most important measure to prevent vascular injury. Owing to the frequency with which these procedures are now performed, spine exposure should be in the skill set of all vascular surgeons. The following is the author's personal approach and experience developed from a personal experience of over 15 years involving nearly 1500 operations and an analysis of the rate of vascular injury and the factors associated with their occurrence.

TO STAY OR NOT TO STAY

In most ALIFs, the vascular surgical team will open and expose the spine, after which the spine surgical team will perform the spinal fusion portion of the procedure. Closure of the incision can be accomplished by either the vascular surgical or the spine surgical team. Because of time constraints and busy schedules, it is common for one team to function separately from the other, especially in centers where both services are very busy. Although some surgeons are proponents of both teams always being in attendance for the entire procedure,[10] the realities of busy clinical practice make this impractical or impossible for many surgeons. It has been my practice to leave after completing the exposure but to have the good fortune to work in a center where the spine and/or vascular fellows will close the incision. My spine specialists feel no need to have me in attendance once my job is done, and I feel comfortable that they will rarely if ever cause a vascular injury during the fusion. This relationship developed over time from working together frequently and admittedly may not be applicable in different circumstances. Undoubtedly, performing a good exposure and knowing the abilities of your spine surgeon are critical to making this arrangement possible and cannot nor should not be expected unless both of these tenets are met. Vascular surgeons at other busy centers have a similar approach and rarely if ever have problems, which has been our experience.

So when is it advisable as an exposure surgeon to remain for the fusion? Working together throughout an ALIF is strongly advised when the spine and vascular surgeon first start working together and in circumstances in which procedures are performed very infrequently. For vascular surgeons new to the ALIF exposure, working with the spine surgeon during the fusion portion, learning the anatomy of the spine and its relationship to the overlying vascular structures, along with having a working knowledge of how the implants are inserted and when and where the vessels are at risk for injury, are critical for learning how to give the spine specialist adequate exposure. In assisting the vascular surgeon, the spine surgeon gains an appreciation of how to safely retract the iliac vessels and protect them from inadvertent injury. Perhaps most importantly, each learns how skilled and experienced his or her counterpart is and whether a level of comfort and trust can be developed to work independently. In my own early experience, I learned the exposure technique from a senior spine surgeon and assisted him through his portion of the procedure many times. This gave me a good understanding of the procedure and a familiarity with spine anatomy and the devices used. As an experienced exposure surgeon working with a spine surgeon for the first time, I stay beyond the exposure until I feel comfortable with his or her ability to work safely in close proximity to the iliac vessels. Regardless of the level of experience and familiarity, it is important to recognize that certain high-risk cases such as extremely obese patients, redo procedures, and those done for malignancy or infection may require the vascular surgeon's assistance for an extended period beyond the exposure and occasionally for the entire procedure. Moreover, in every case, if the vascular surgeon chooses to leave, he or she must be readily available to return should a problem develop. If the exposure has been done correctly and the spine surgeon is extremely careful, this should happen rarely if ever. However, as with all things in surgery, good judgment and experience are critical and when in doubt, *stay!*

TECHNIQUE

The patient should be positioned supine with a small roll under the lumbar spine that serves to distract the lumbar vertebrae. Having the patient in a slight Trendelenburg position is helpful. A Foley catheter is routinely inserted. Arterial lines and central venous pressure (CVP) lines are generally reserved for older, sicker patients. Although vascular injuries are infrequent, prudence dictates that vascular instruments should be on the field and vascular sutures readily available. Blood loss from ALIF is usually limited; therefore, type and screen are usually adequate for most patients with the exception of those having a concomitant, bloodier, posterior procedure; they should have 2 to 4 units of blood available. Heparin prophylaxis and pneumatic boots are always used. Some spine surgeons use spinal monitoring, usually evoked motor potentials. Working in the pelvis requires good lighting and magnification. The author routinely employs the use of headlights and loupes during these procedures.

The lumbar spine is most readily approached from the left retroperitoneal space. The left iliac vessels are retracted to the right to expose the underlying spine from the level of L3 to the sacrum. Exposure of more proximal levels requires leftward retraction of the distal infrarenal aorta (Figure 17–1). Although vascular surgeons have been traditionally taught to expose the aorta and left renal vessels from an oblique left flank incision, this approach is undesirable for spine exposure because most devices are designed to be inserted on the midline axis of the vertebral column (Figure 17–2), mandating a midline orientation of their delivery instrumentation, which is difficult or impossible to achieve from that incision. Moreover, the lowest lumbar disk, L5-S1, is difficult to expose from the flank. The spine can be exposed from a traditional midline intra-abdominal incision; however, it requires more dissection, increases the risk of ureteral and bowel injury, increases the rate of retrograde ejaculation in males, and may result in increased rates of ileus.

Consequently, most exposure surgeons prefer a modified retroperitoneal approach from a midline or left paramedian incision. The author prefers a midline skin incision with a paramedian incision in the left rectus muscle for the simple reason that midline incisions look better when they heal, especially in obese patients. The length of the incision is dependent of the number and level of disk spaces required for exposure. Exposing the two lowest and most commonly treated levels, L4-5 and L5-S1, can almost always be accomplished with an infraumbilical incision. More proximal levels will require extension lateral to or above the umbilicus. A much preferred alternative for exposure of the L5-S1 disk space alone, especially in women, is a standard

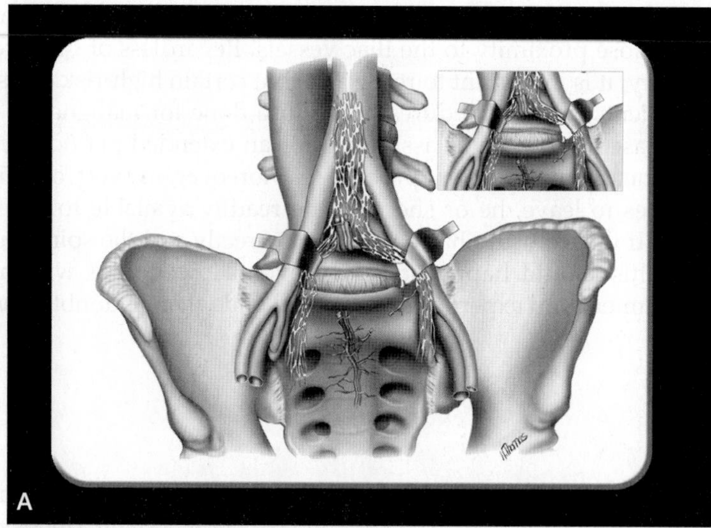

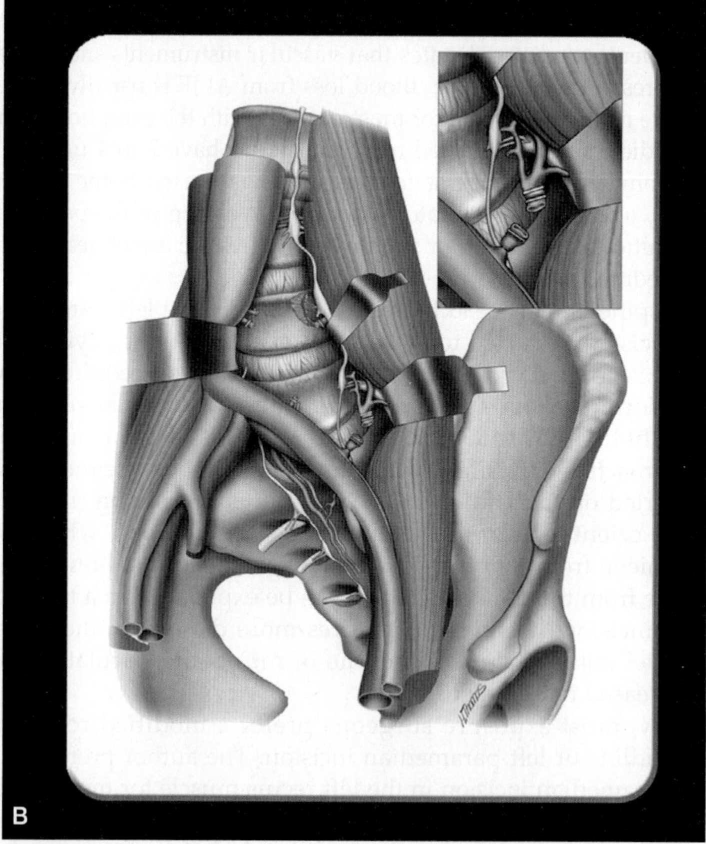

Figure 17-1. Relationship of the aorta, vena cava, and iliac vessels to the lumbar spine. Most spine procedures involve the spine from L4 to S1. The L5-S1 disk can be exposed in the crotch of the bifurcation at the sacral prominence with division of the middle sacral artery and vein (A), while exposure of L4-5 and the more proximal levels will require division of the iliolumbar vein and lumbar segmental vessels to permit rightward retraction of the left common iliac artery and vein (B). (Courtesy of Depuy Spine.)

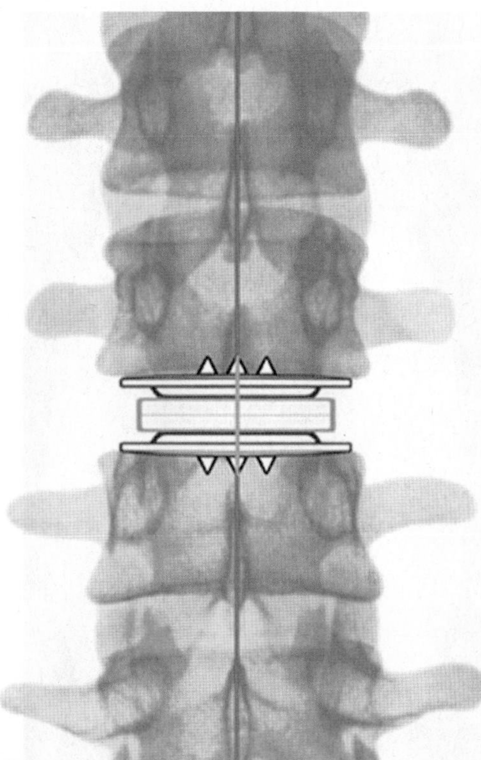

Figure 17-2. Current spinal fusion hardware such as the Charite artificial disk requires placement in the midline axis of the vertebral bodies, which is best accomplished from a midline approach with the patient supine. (Courtesy of Depuy Spine.)

Pfannenstiel incision (Figure 17–3). The incision is deepened to the level of the rectus fascia and then a flap of skin and subcutaneous tissue is raised superiorly to the level of the umbilicus, exposing the left rectus sheath, which can be incised longitudinally. Once the rectus sheath has been opened, the belly of the left rectus muscle is reflected laterally, exposing the transversalis fascia and the lower edge of the posterior rectus sheath at the linea semilunaris. The transversalis fascia and posterior rectus sheath are incised longitudinally without entering the peritoneal cavity (Figure 17–4). Using a combination of sharp and blunt dissection, the peritoneum and its contents can then be mobilized in the preperitoneal space out of the left iliac fossa and reflected to the right, a maneuver that takes some finesse and practice to avoid entering the peritoneal cavity (Figure 17–5). The dissection should extend over the iliac vessels to a point slightly right of the midline. The ureter will usually elevate with the peritoneum during this dissection. In men, the dissection is commenced superior and lateral to the left spermatic cord, which must be mobilized but not skeletonized to facilitate retraction of the peritoneum to the right and exposure of the lower lumbar spine. In women, the round ligament is encountered and can be divided with impunity. Once the peritoneum has been adequately mobilized, a self-retaining abdominal wall retractor is placed. The author prefers the Bookwalter retractor with a small round ring. The left common iliac artery and vein are the first vascular structures encountered. Palpation of the L5-S1 disk is accomplished just proximal to the sacral prominence. Usually, this disk space will be seen to be situated in the crotch created by the bifurcation of the aorta into the left and right common iliac vessels. The middle sacral artery and vein can be seen to vertically cross over the anterior surface of the L5-S1 disk. This disk space is the easiest to expose, because the only vessels crossing over it are the middle

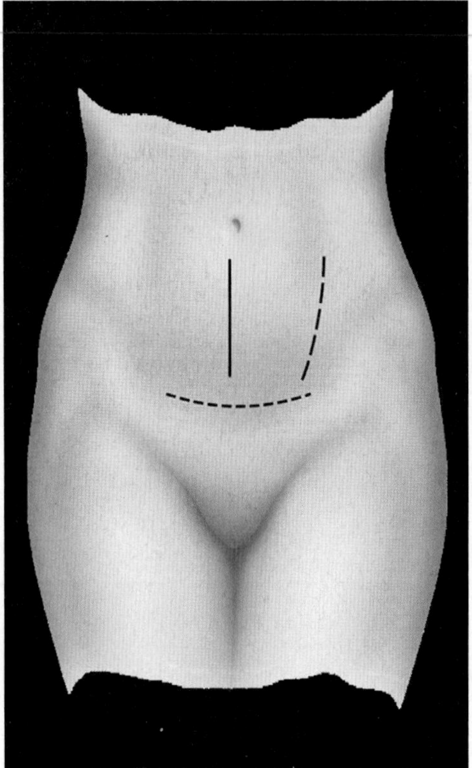

Figure 17-3. Incisions for the anterior approach include infraumbilical midline or paramedian incisions, although the Pfannenstiel incision is well suited for exposing L5-S1. The author prefers a midline or Pfannenstiel skin incision. (Courtesy of Depuy Spine.)

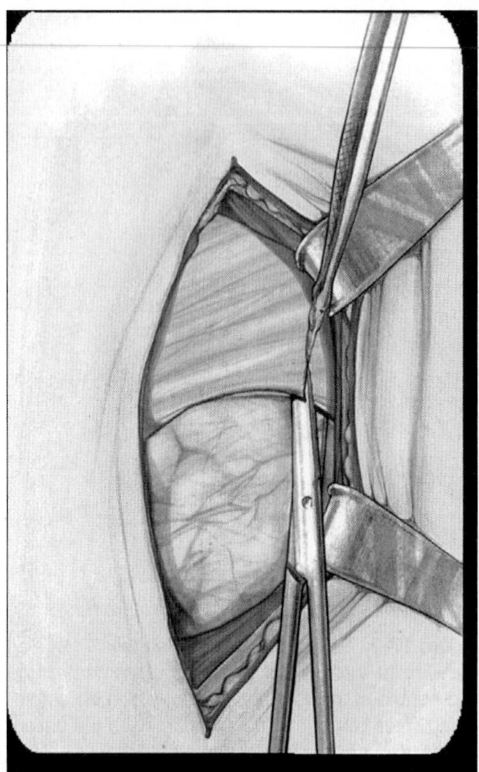

Figure 17-4. After retraction of the left rectus muscle, the transversalis fascia and distal edge of the posterior rectus sheath at the linea semilunaris are seen. Incision of the transversalis fascia and the posterior rectus sheath facilitates entry into the preperitoneal space without tearing the peritoneum. (Courtesy of Depuy Spine.)

sacral vessels. Exposure requires division of these vessels. Frequently, the inferior edge of the left common iliac vein crosses over the left side of the L5-S1 disk and is readily swept off its surface using a peanut sponge without much difficulty. On the right side of the L5-S1 disk, the peritoneum is often encountered and, much less frequently, the right common iliac vein. The distal dissection should not extend beyond the edge of the sacrum to avoid troublesome bleeding by injury of the sacral veins more distally. Proximally, the vessels can be mobilized off the anterior surface of the L5 vertebral body if necessary. In general, extensive mobilization of the left iliac vessels is not necessary for exposure of the L5-S1 disk.

Exposure of the L4-5 disk requires far more extensive mobilization of the left common iliac artery and vein. In most patients, these vessels cross directly over the anterior surface of the L4-5 disk, and they must be retracted medially to expose the disk space. This is best accomplished by sharply and bluntly mobilizing the vessels free from the anterior surface of the lumbar spine along the lateral edge of the left common iliac artery, avoiding the common iliac vein, which tends to be more medial and slightly inferior to the artery. Because the goal is to mobilize the left common iliac vessels so that they can be retracted to the right, the lumbar segmental branches and left

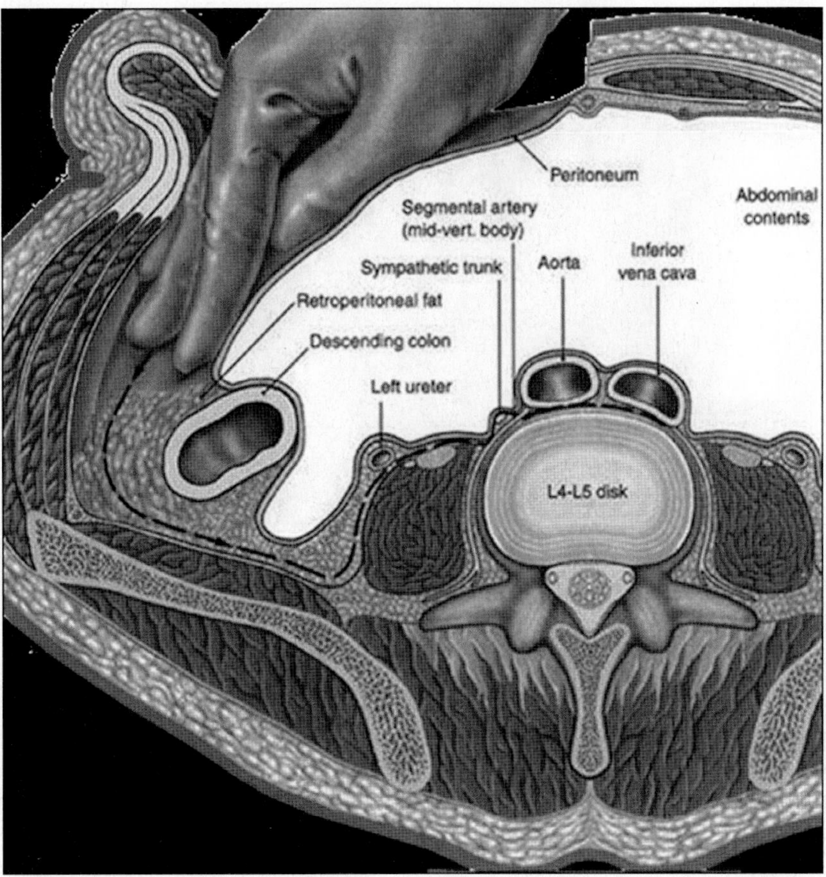

Figure 17-5. Mobilization of the peritoneal cavity and its contents must include its posterior surface over the iliac vessels to obtain adequate exposure. This maneuver requires some finesse and practice to avoid entry into the peritoneal cavity. (Courtesy of Depuy Spine.)

iliolumbar vein must be divided. As a general rule, the lumbar segmental vessels course laterally over the surface of the lumbar vertebrae. The iliolumbar vein courses under the left common iliac artery at the distal end of the L4-5 disk. It is occasionally bifurcated and may be adherent to the disk if it is inflamed. This vein is almost always present and must always be divided when exposing the L4-5 disk (Figure 17–6). If it is left intact, it will be torn when reflecting the iliac vessels to the right, causing severe bleeding. This vein must be carefully ligated. The author has had the unpleasant experience of the tie becoming dislodged when the vessel is being retracted during the fusion portion of the operation. Division of the lumbar segmental vessels is straightforward but important for the same reason. If they are torn during retraction, they can be difficult to control, especially at more proximal levels. As a general rule, it is advisable to divide the lumbar segmental vessels one level above the disk being excised. In addition to the iliolumbar vein and segmental vessels, numerous small, unnamed branches of the common iliac vessels are encountered that tether the posterior surface of the iliac vessels to the spine. These must also be divided. Many can be controlled with electrocautery. In general, most spine surgeons will only use bipolar cautery around the spine to avoid inadvertent conduction thermal injury to the vessels and

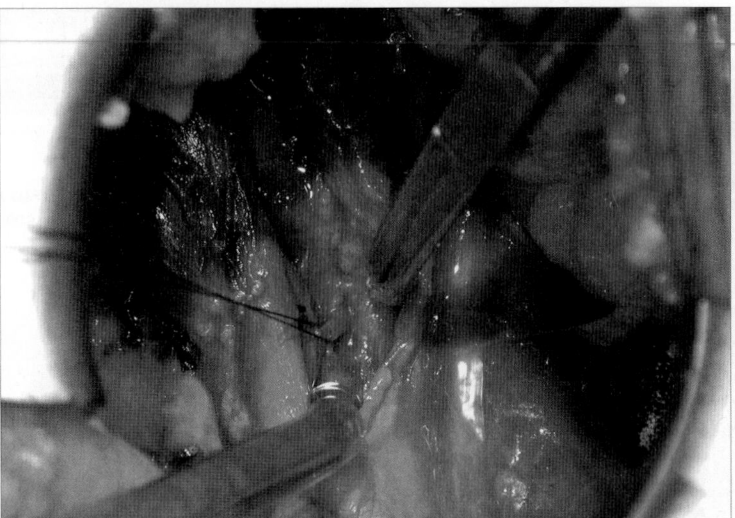

Figure 17-6. Operative view of the iliolumbar vein is a constant structure that must be identified and divided during mobilization of the left iliac vein to allow retraction to the right. Failure to do so will result in its avulsion from the common iliac vein, leading to serious bleeding.

nerves. Some studies have noted a lower incidence of retrograde ejaculation in males with bipolar cautery. Limiting retrograde ejaculation requires preservation of the sympathetic and parasympathetic nerve branches crossing over the left iliac vessels. In most cases, the majority are seen crossing over the external iliac artery, which rarely needs to be mobilized for spine exposure. The exposure of more proximal levels requires more proximal dissection and mobilization of the aortic bifurcation and infrarenal aorta. Lumbar segmental arteries and veins at these levels tend to be larger and will bleed significantly if torn or injured. Gaining exposure proximal to L3 may require mobilization of the lower pole of the kidney and can be exceedingly difficult, especially in obese patients. The author has occasionally extended this exposure to the first lumbar vertebra, although as a rule, exposures proximal to L2 require a lateral approach through the left flank. Exposure is easiest in multiparous women owing to their having a wider pelvis and more lax abdominal tissues and most difficult in obese young males. The likelihood of vascular injury increases with increasing difficulty of exposure and in those cases with inflammatory reaction of the disk spaces, where the iliac vessels and their branches can be densely adhered to the spine, making safe mobilization difficult or even impossible.

Once the vessels have been fully exposed, the spine surgery team will remove the disks and insert metallic implants filled with bone graft and/or bone morphogenic protein,[11] which will ultimately fuse the vertebrae together, eliminating instability, the cause of the pain. Removal of the disks and insertion of the implants requires the use of heavy sharp-edged instruments that can easily injure the adjacent blood vessels if they are not continuously retracted out of the way (Figure 17–7). Although there are fixed vascular retractors that can be attached to the self-retaining retractor, their use is ill-advised because they may occlude blood flow for an extended period, risking venous and arterial thrombosis. A useful retractor for the artery and vein is the hand-held version of the Wylie renal vein retractor with a 7-inch blade (Pilling Surgical

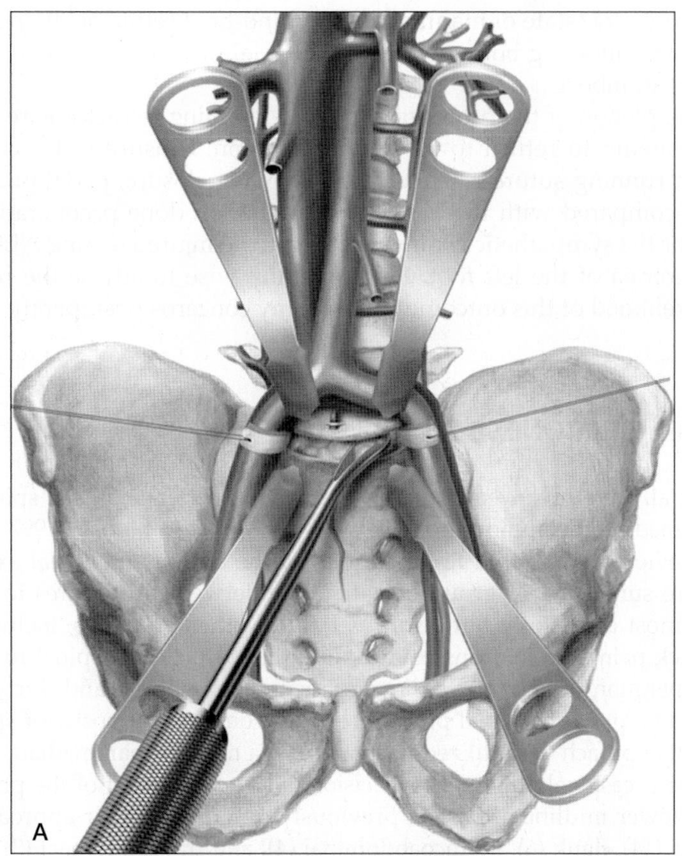

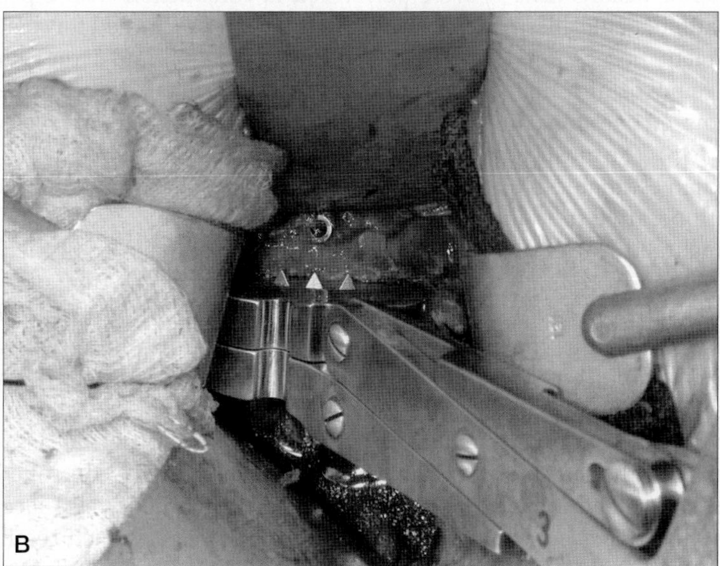

Figure 17-7. Disk excision (A) and hardware insertion (B) involve large sharp-edged instruments that can easily injure the iliac vein and artery if they have been inadequately mobilized to allow retraction out of harm's way. (Courtesy of Depuy Spine.)

Instrument Corp city/state of manufacturer). Hand-held retractors by necessity are relaxed frequently, allowing both venous and arterial flow to continue and minimizing the chance of thrombosis.

At the completion of the procedure, the self-retaining retractor is removed, allowing the peritoneum to return to its normal location. Closure of the anterior rectus sheath with a running suture is preferred. Following closure, pedal pulses should be checked and compared with the vascular examination done preoperatively. It is not uncommon for the sympathetic chain on the left to be injured during ALIF procedures, causing hyperemia of the left foot. It is generally wise to advise the recovery room staff of the likelihood of this outcome to avoid any concerns postoperatively.

BETH ISRAEL DEACONESS RESULTS

The author et al. have reviewed and reported their experience on 482 spine procedures, mostly performed by the author at one spine center between January 1997 and December 2002.[12] This review represented less than half of the author's personal experience with spine exposure surgery. This group of patients underwent procedures for degenerative joint disease most commonly but also a variety of other problems, including scoliosis, diskogenic back pain, and joint instability due to failed previous spinal fusions. The median age at operation was 42 and 55% were men. One hundred and thirty-nine patients (28.8%) had had a previous spinal procedure, most commonly a posterior spinal fusion. A retroperitoneal approach was utilized in 456 cases via midline, paramedian, and transverse Pfannenstiel or occasional oblique skin incision. Fifty-two percent of the procedures were done via the lower midline approach previously described. Other approaches included thoracolumbar (14), flank (6), thoracoabdominal (4), and transperitoneal (3). One hundred eighteen anterior fusions (24.4%) were performed in conjunction with a posterior spinal procedure with the same anesthetic. Seven exposures were performed for the Charité artificial disk implantation as part of the IDE investigational trial and 1 procedure was performed for removal of a dislodged artificial anterior lumbar disk. Forty-two percent (202/482) required one spinal level exposed and the average number of levels exposed was 1.78 (range 1 to 8). The most common levels exposed were L5-S1 and L4-5.

The median estimated blood loss for exposure was approximately 150 cc, and there were no perioperative mortalities. A vascular injury occurred in 11% (54/480) of patients; this included 2 arterial and 52 venous injuries. The majority of the injuries were minor (45/54) and were treated with simple suture repair at the time of exposure. The most common site of injury was the left common iliac vein (Table 17–1). Nine vascular injuries were classified as major, defined as any injury requiring transfusion, vascular reconstruction, or blood loss greater than 300 cc. Seven of these injuries were treated with simple suture repair and did not require any reconstruction. Of these, 2 were arterial injuries and 7 others were venous. One arterial injury occurred as a result of an avulsed branch of the left internal iliac artery, which was easily controlled with surgical clips and suture ligation. The other arterial injury sustained was a laceration of the left common iliac artery secondary to the orthopedic implant, which required a vascular reconstruction using a Dacron graft. Three major injuries to the left common iliac vein and 3 major injuries to the left internal iliac vein were directly repaired with suture. One major injury occurred secondary to a tie that became dislodged from a previously divided iliolumbar vein, and this was repaired with suture ligation. One patient

TABLE 17-1. LOCATION OF VASCULAR INJURY

Location	n	%
Left common iliac vein	44	81.5
Left internal iliac vein	3	5.6
Right common iliac vein	2	3.7
Iliolumbar vein	2	3.7
Inferior vena cava	1	1.9
Left internal iliac artery	1	1.9
Left common iliac artery	1	1.9

From Hamdan AD, Malek JY, Schermerhorn ML, et al. Vascular injury during anterior exposure of the spine. J Vasc Surg 2008; 48:650–4.

sustained an avulsed branch of the left internal iliac vein. This bled sufficiently to require transfusion of 1 unit of Cell Saver blood as well as placement of intra-abdominal packs to control hemorrhage, which were then removed 24 hours later. The patient underwent successful spinal fusion at that juncture. One patient sustained an avulsed branch of the right common iliac vein that was repaired with a suture but required a transfusion of a unit of packed red blood cells. The average estimated blood loss from major vascular injuries was 520 cc. Although not explicitly evaluated in the study, no arterial or deep vein thrombosis, pulmonary emboli, or long-term vascular sequelae were noted from any of these injuries.

In the 318 patients who had exposure of L4-5, 44 patients experienced the vascular some injury (13.8%), whereas in the remaining 162 patients, only 9 experienced any vascular injury (5.6%). Statistical analysis revealed that exposure of L4-5 was associated with an increased rate of injury with an odds ratio of 2.73 (P=.05 for all injuries). A significantly lower risk of injury was seen with isolated L5-S1 exposures (6/23 patients versus 47/358 patients who had exposure of other levels) with an odds ratio equal to 0.34 (P=.01). Multilevel exposures as an independent factor did not predict vascular injury, nor did a history of previous spinal surgery, although the vast majority of these were posterior spinal fusions. No independent variable predicted risk of major vascular injury and no mortalities were noted.

DISCUSSION

The anterior approach for lumbar surgery was first described by Ito for the treatment of Potts disease in 1934.[13] Since its introduction and modification, the anterior approach has been popularized as an acceptable method for exposure of the anterior spine. Up until about 15 years ago, however, this approach was infrequently used. As spinal technology has advanced, principally due to the introduction of new implantable cages for the disk spaces to fuse the lower lumbar vertebrae, this approach has become widely utilized, and vascular surgeons are commonly asked by their spine surgeon colleagues to perform these exposures for them.[2] The use of a multidisciplinary team, including the vascular and spine surgeon, reduces the likelihood of catastrophic vascular injury. With the popularity of these procedures at an all-time high, it is incumbent that all vascular surgeons become familiar with the tenets of anterior spinal exposure.

The overall complication rate for open anterior lumbar exposure has been estimated to be as high as 30 to 40%.[5] Such complications include but are not limited to vascular injury, bleeding, thrombosis, damage to nervous or genitourinary structures, postoperative infection, seroma formation, bowel injury, hernia, and ileus.

The most prevalent and feared complication is due to vascular injury,[14] which has an overall published rate of incidence ranging from 1.9 to 15.6%.[7] When restricted to examining intraoperative vascular injury using the definitions outlined, results of our study indicated that some vascular injury occurred in 11% of patients, although most of these were minor. Our incidence is similar to rates reported by others.[5,7,10] That a majority of these injuries were avulsed branches of the left common iliac vein is not surprising because this vein is most commonly mobilized during exposure of the lower lumbar spine. Careful exposure, dissection, and mobility of the left common iliac vein can avoid many of these injuries and allow for rapid and relatively easy repair when injuries do occur.

Arterial injuries have proven to be relatively rare, occurring in 0.45 to 1.5% of cases[8,15] and only twice in this series of nearly 500 procedures. Most of these have proven to be either thrombosis or vasospasm, although arterial lacerations and avulsions can occur, as was reported in our series. Proper management of arterial injuries is important to avoid postoperative ischemic complications. Like venous injuries, lacerations of the iliac artery are generally immediately apparent and can often be repaired with simple suture. In our own study, one arterial injury was treated with direct surgical repair and the other required a Dacron interposition graft.

Perhaps the most important measure that can be taken to avoid injury to the left common iliac vein is exposure and division of the lumbar branch of the left iliac vein. This vein is almost always encountered during exposure of the lower lumbar spine and must be divided to allow adequate medial retraction of the vessels when exposing the L4-5 intralumbar disk. Proper ligation of this vessel is important to avoid dislodgement of the tie during retraction of the vessels during the orthopedic portion of the procedure. In the author's experience, minor vascular injuries generally occur as a result of injury to the vessels during dissection, and it is usually a simple manner to repair them. More serious vascular injuries generally occur as a result of inadequate mobilization and exposure of the vessels, which leads to injury during excision of the anterior lumbar disk or during the implantation of cages, which often have sharp-edged introducer devices; these may catch the wall of the vein during their insertion into the disk space.

This study, as others,[6,8,10,15] has demonstrated that when venous lacerations are encountered, they usually are typically associated with exposure of the L4-5 inter-lumbar disk. In our series, 85% of patients sustaining vascular injuries had exposure higher than the L5-S1 level and exposure of the L4-5 level was found to be an independent predictor of vascular injury. Given the fact that the L4-5 disk level is frequently exposed and that the left common iliac vein crosses directly over the anterior surface of the disk space, this is not surprising. This study, as others,[6] has shown that exposure of the L5-S1 disk is associated with the lower risk of injury compared with that of the L4-5 disk level.

Other authors[16] have also failed to show a relationship between prior spinal surgeries and increased risk of vascular injury. This may seem counterintuitive but is probably explained by the fact that most prior spinal surgeries are posterior spinal fusions where the peritoneal cavity or retroperitoneal space has not been entered. In the author's experience and that of others,[17] redo anterior spinal exposure and procedures done for infection or malignancy are technically far more difficult and increase the likelihood of vascular injury. Indeed, the one arterial reconstruction that was required occurred as a result of a redo procedure to remove a dislodged artificial disk. It may be advisable when re-exposing the anterior surface of the lower lumbar spine to avoid adhesions by approaching the anterior surface from the right retroperitoneal space; however, this must be weighed against the additional technical difficulties of right-sided exposure, especially for levels proximal to L4 where the inferior vena cava is often encountered. Alternatively, the spine surgeon can elect to avoid the anterior spine altogether in favor of the lateral or posterior approach. Vascular surgeons must allow more time for these cases, be prepared for more significant blood loss due to the higher likelihood of vascular injury, and plan on assisting for most if not all of the procedure.

CONCLUSION

Anterior lumbar surgery has become an increasingly attractive and popular alternative to posterior spinal fusion surgery with the development of new spinal fusion technology. Because of the close prominence of major vascular structures to the anterior surface of the lower lumbar spine, vascular surgeons are often required to perform exposure for their spine surgeon colleagues. It is incumbent upon all vascular surgeons to become familiar with these techniques. The results of the current study and others demonstrate that a skilled vascular surgeon can obtain adequate exposure of the spine to minimize the likelihood of serious vascular injury.

REFERENCES

1. Oskouian RJ Jr, Johnson JP. Vascular complications in anterior thoracolumbar spinal reconstruction. J Neurosurg 2002;96:1–5.
2. Blumenthal SL, Ohnmeiss DD. Intervertebral cages for degenerative spinal diseases. Spine J 2003;3:301–9.
3. Guyer RD, McAfee PC, Banco RJ, et al. Prospective, randomized, multicenter Food and Drug Administration investigational device exemption study of lumbar total disc replacement with the CHARITE artificial disc versus lumbar fusion: five-year follow-up. Spine J 2009;9:374–86.
4. Gumbs AA, Shah RV, Yue JJ, Sumpio B. The open anterior paramedian retroperitoneal approach for spine procedures. Arch Surg 2005;140:339–43.
5. Rajaraman V, Vingan R, Roth P, et al. Visceral and vascular complications resulting from anterior lumbar interbody fusion. J Neurosurg 1999;91:60–4.
6. Sasso RC, Best NM, Mummaneni PV, et al. Analysis of operative complications in a series of 471 anterior lumbar interbody fusion procedures. Spine 2005;30:670–4.
7. Baker JK, Reardon PR, Reardon MJ, Heggeness MH. Vascular injury in anterior lumbar surgery. Spine 1993;18:2227–30.
8. Brau SA, Delamarter RB, Schiffman ML, et al. Vascular injury during anterior lumbar surgery. Spine J 2004;4:409–12.
9. Staehli LM, Zehnder T, Schwarzenbach O, et al. Venous injury in lumbar anterior spine surgery. Swiss Med Wkly 2006;136:670–1.
10. Chiriano J, Abou-Zamzam AM Jr, Urayeneza O, et al. The role of the vascular surgeon in anterior retroperitoneal spine exposure: preservation of open surgical training. J Vasc Surg 2009;50:148–51.
11. Burkus JK. Bone morphogenetic proteins in anterior lumbar interbody fusion: old techniques and new technologies. Invited submission from the Joint Section Meeting on Disorders of the Spine and Peripheral Nerves, March 2004. J Neurosurg Spine 2004;1:254–60.

12. Hamdan AD, Malek JY, Schermerhorn ML, et al. Vascular injury during anterior exposure of the spine. J Vasc Surg 2008;48:650–4.
13. Ito H TJ, Asami G. A new radical operation for Pott's disease. J Bone Joint Surg 1934;16: 499–515.
14. Ikard RW. Methods and complications of anterior exposure of the thoracic and lumbar spine. Arch Surg 2006;141:1025–34.
15. Kulkarni SS, Lowery GL, Ross RE, et al. Arterial complications following anterior lumbar interbody fusion: report of eight cases. Eur Spine J 2003;12:48–54.
16. Bianchi C, Ballard JL, Abou-Zamzam AM, et al. Anterior retroperitoneal lumbosacral spine exposure: operative technique and results. Ann Vasc Surg 2003;17:137–42.
17. Stulik J, Vyskocil T, Bodlak P, et al. [Injury to major blood vessels in anterior thoracic and lumbar spinal surgery]. Acta Chir Orthop Traumatol Cech 2006;73:92–8.

18

Vascular Trauma in a Rural Environment

Joshua P. Froman, M.D. and
Thomas H. Cogbill, M.D., F.A.C.S.

The management of vascular trauma in a rural setting is challenging because of unique mechanisms of injury, difficulties posed by an attenuated prehospital care system, and a wide variety of arterial and venous injuries. Although the epidemiology of vascular injuries has been less well studied in rural areas than in urban centers, several differences have been identified. The incidence of blunt vascular injuries is greater and affected patients are older in rural areas.[1-3] Extremity vascular injuries predominated in studies of two rural states.[2,4] In North Carolina, rural patients with vascular trauma were transported by helicopter more often, and 78% were treated in local community hospitals before transfer to a tertiary care center.[2] Humphrey and associates observed that helicopter transport of patients with vascular trauma was responsible for a decrease in the time from injury to definitive care from 6 to 4 hours. Although survival rates were unchanged with the advent of helicopter transport, amputation rates after vascular injuries declined.[4] Optimal management of patients with vascular trauma depends upon a well-designed regional trauma system with initial stabilization at small community hospitals and definitive care at a referral trauma center. In this chapter, we focus on the unique aspects of vascular trauma in a rural environment, using the experience of our rural referral trauma center as an example.

GUNDERSEN LUTHERAN MEDICAL CENTER

Gundersen Lutheran Medical Center is a 325-bed hospital and multispecialty group practice of 453 physicians in La Crosse, WI (population 51,840). The main campus is part of a physician-led, fully integrated health care system with 25 regional clinics throughout 19 agricultural counties of southwestern Wisconsin, northeastern Iowa, and southeastern Minnesota. The American College of Surgeons verified Level II trauma center in La Crosse is the regional trauma center for this vast rural area. The trauma service is staffed by five trauma surgeons, ten general surgery residents, and one physician assistant. A helicopter transport service has operated from Gundersen Lutheran since 1992. A full range of consultant services is available, including orthopedic surgery, neurosurgery, plastic surgery, critical care, and physical medicine/rehabilitation. Vascular surgery, including both open and endovascular techniques, is performed by four vascular surgeons and three interventional radiologists. Only patients with severe burns (>20% BSA) or limbs for replantation are transferred to other facilities.

CHALLENGES OF A RURAL TRAUMA SYSTEM

Rural areas in the United States present many challenges to the timely transport of injured patients. Unwitnessed accidents in remote areas may lead to long times prior to discovery. Prolonged extrications from complex machines in hostile settings are often necessary. Long transport distances to a Level I or Level II trauma center highlight the need for an inclusive trauma system with initial resuscitation and stabilization performed at small community hospitals.[5] A committed rural general surgeon in a community hospital is often the key to achieving good outcomes in multiply injured patients.[6] Unlike urban settings in which "scoop and run" transports are often best for vascular injuries, prolonged transport times in rural areas require airway and ventilation management and the initiation of treatment for shock prior to transport. The use of tourniquets or temporary vascular shunting may also be indicated for select vascular injuries in remote areas, paralleling the contemporary military experience.[7-8] Limited resources such as a small or absent blood bank may preclude optimal stabilization prior to transport. Variability in the level of care able to be provided by emergency medical services (EMS) personnel may also be a factor affecting the sophistication of treatment prior to arrival at the trauma center. Long times to discovery, long extrication times, extended transport distances, and the effects of inclement weather all combine to cause delays in definitive care. Prior to the initiation of a helicopter transport service, the average time from injury to trauma center arrival in our area exceeded 3 hours.[9-10] In patients with ischemia or hemorrhage due to vascular injuries, these prolonged transport times may lead to increased mortality and greater need for fasciotomy and limb amputations. Although the advent of helicopter transport based at our trauma center has clearly shortened transport times, this service is not always available due to weather, high volume, or maintenance. For optimal care, both ground and air transport rely upon excellent communication, coordination of care, and preexisting transport protocols.

UNIQUE MECHANISMS OF INJURY

Power Take-Off Units

Power take-offs (PTOs) were developed to transfer power from the drive shaft of a tractor to a piece of trailing farm machinery (Figure 18–1). A PTO consists of a rapidly rotating shaft with a coupling device that rotates from 500 to more than 1000 rpm. Although contemporary PTOs are supplied with a totally shielded shaft, older models in wide use have partially protective shields that are often removed for maintenance (Figures 18–2 and 18–3). Injuries result when an article of loose-fitting or bulky clothing becomes entangled in a poorly shielded shaft.[11] The clothing quickly draws the nearest body part into the machinery, and the victim is violently thrown by the force. Multiple fractures, spine and neck injuries, and blunt thoracic and abdominal trauma are common. A victim can die from

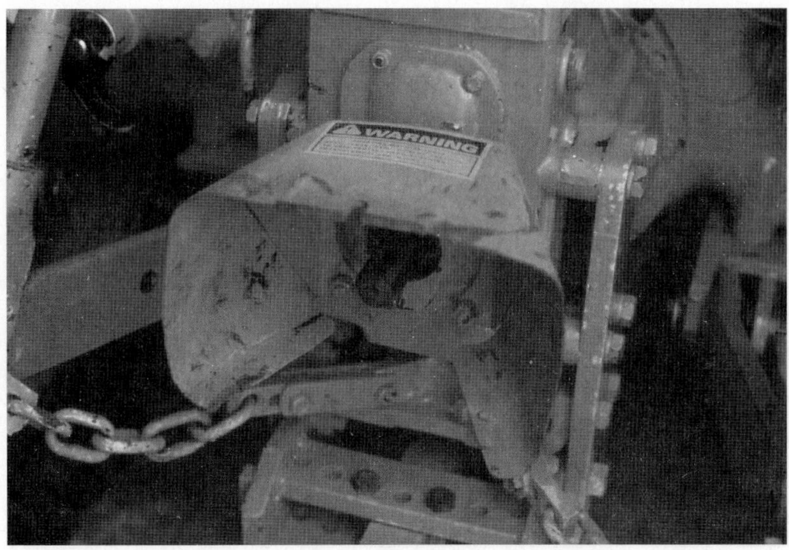

Figure 18-1. Power take-off attaches to tractor drive shaft at back of tractor.

strangulation if upper extremity clothing is entangled. Extremities may be rendered ischemic by arterial disruption or prolonged arterial compression (Figure 18–4).

Corn-Harvesting Equipment

A corn picker is a large combine-like machine designed to separate mature corn cobs from the reminder of the corn plants (Figure 18–5). Plants are drawn into the machine by a series of pulleys, rollers, and chains. Most injuries occur when a farmer attempts to dislodge a

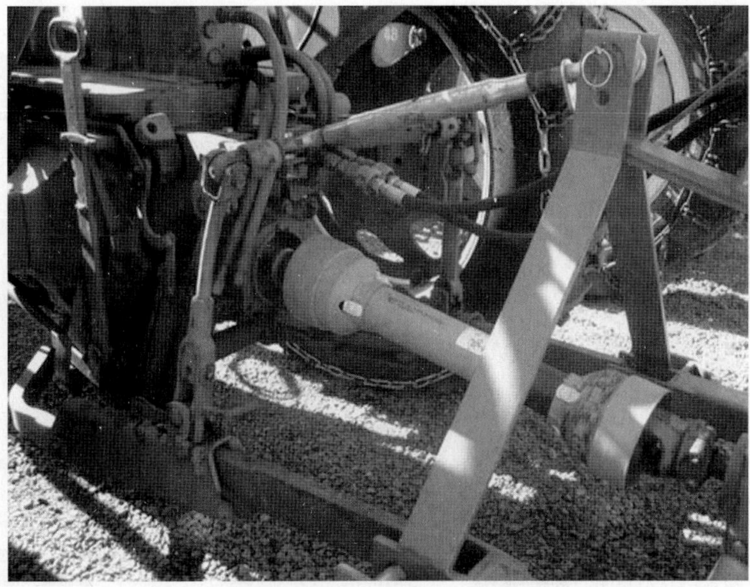

Figure 18-2. Power take-off unit sold today with totally shielded shaft.

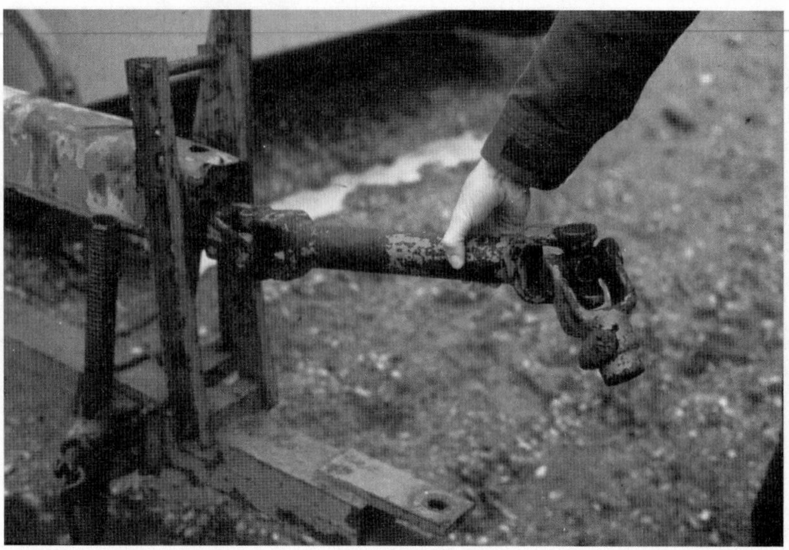

Figure 18-3. Older power take-off shaft with protective shield removed.

bound corn stalk without first turning the machine off.[11] Typical injuries involve the hands or feet, with multiple-level crushing amputations and lacerations with severe contamination (Figure 18–6). Vascular injuries are common with both hemorrhagic and ischemic complications.

Corn augers are long metal troughs with screw-like devices that transport corn from one place to another, as in loading a silo (Figure 18–7). Injuries to the extremities occur when a farmer inadvertently steps into a working auger or attempts to unjam the machine by hand without shutting down the auger first. Typical injuries involve elements of crush and laceration at multiple levels. Vascular injuries are hemorrhagic or ischemic.

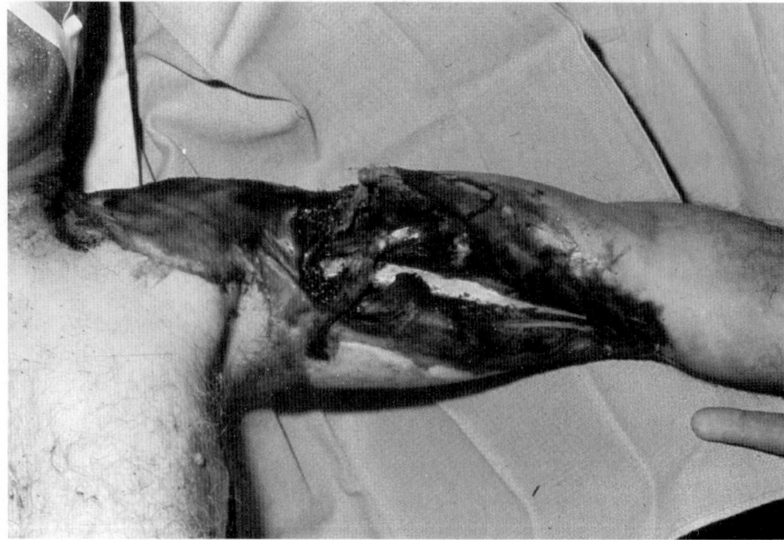

Figure 18-4. Injury from power take-off in which arm was entrapped until the tractor ran out of fuel.

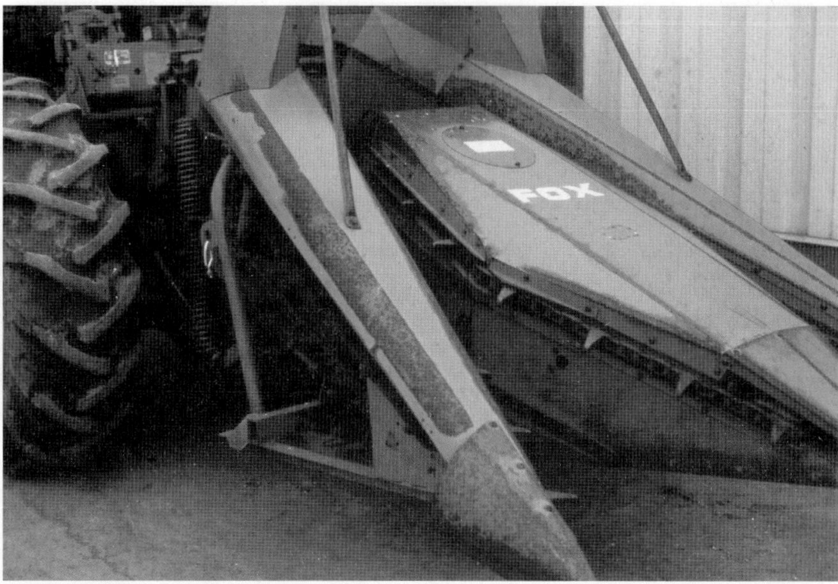

Figure 18-5. Corn picker harvesting machine which separates mature corn cobs from remainder of corn plant.

Farm Tractor Rollovers

Farm tractor rollovers are persistent causes of multiple-system trauma treated at our institution. All 19 counties in our referral area are hilly, with active dairy farms. Contour farming of feed crops is accomplished with tractors operating along an incline. When the ground is soft, these large machines can tip over, thus crushing and/or entrapping the

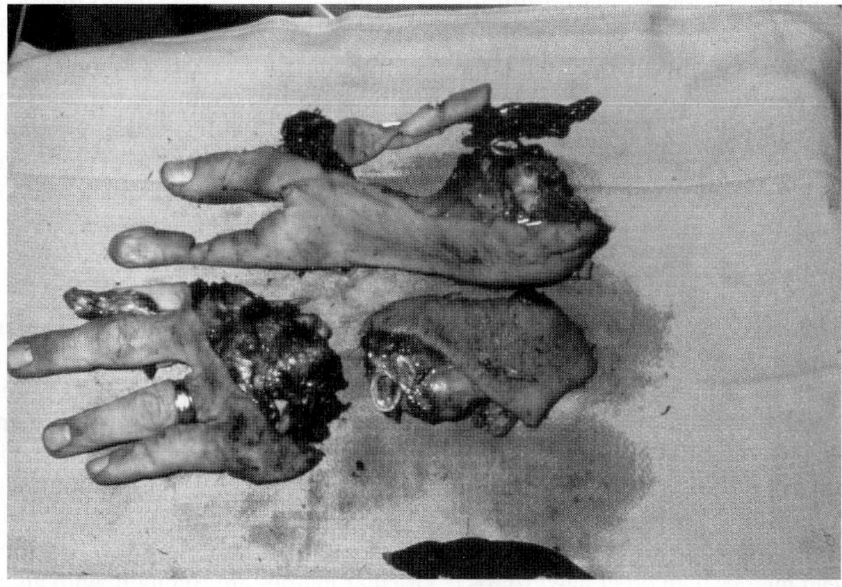

Figure 18-6. Injury from corn picker with multiple levels of amputation and crush injury.

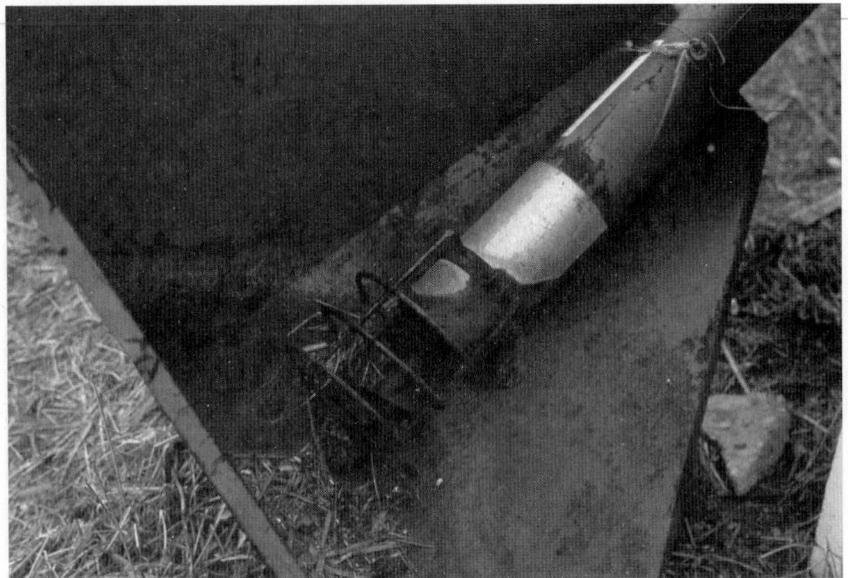

Figure 18-7. Corn auger with screw-like mechanism for moving the corn along a trough.

operators. Tractor rollovers are the most frequent cause of death among agricultural accidents treated at our institution.[11] Thoracoabdominal and spine injuries are common. Two types of vascular injury occur with tractor rollovers: pelvic fractures with arterial and/or venous hemorrhage, and traumatic asphyxia. The source of ongoing arterial bleeding associated with pelvic fractures can be identified by diagnostic arteriography and often controlled with selective embolization.

Traumatic asphyxia is caused by a prolonged thoracic crush by a heavy object such as a farm tractor. Increased intrathoracic pressure against a closed glottis causes a marked increase of blood pressure within the superior vena cava and the valveless veins of the head and neck. Classic stigmata of traumatic asphyxia include craniocervical cyanosis, facial swelling, facial petechiae, and subconjunctival hemorrhages (Figure 18–8). Although victims have a striking moribund appearance, removal of the crushing object and initiation of airway/ventilation management can achieve excellent survival. Neurologic sequelae are rare in patients who survive traumatic asphyxia.[12]

All-Terrain Vehicle Crashes

Since the early 1980s, there has been a proliferation of All-Terrain Vehicks (ATVs) in rural North America. Originally designed for work on ranches and farms, ATVs are now commonly used for recreational purposes. The first models had three wheels and were inherently unstable. Only four-wheeled models are currently sold. Each year, the number of people injured on ATVs increases in the United States.[13] The most frequent mechanisms of injury are loss of vehicle stability, rider thrown from ATV, and ATV collision with stationary object.[14] As with other motor vehicles, alcohol is often a factor in ATV crashes.[13-14] Young adolescents are frequently involved in ATV crashes and sustain more severe trauma and more head injuries than other age groups.[14] Vascular injuries are common, with an increasing number of mangled extremity injuries similar to those seen with motorcycle crashes.[13]

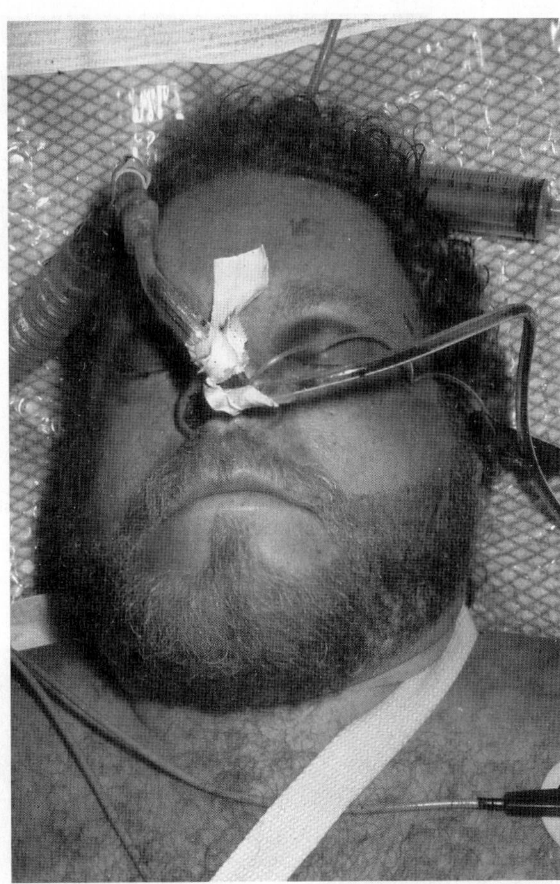

Figure 18-8. Classic physical stigmata of traumatic asphyxia include craniocervical cyanosis, facial swelling, facial petechiae, and subconjunctival hemorrhages.

Scapulothoracic Dissociation

Scapulothoracic dissociation is the result of violent lateral distraction or rotational displacement of the shoulder away from the relatively rigid thorax. The injury is often caused by motorcycle/ATV crashes, motor vehicle crashes, tractor rollovers, and machinery entrapments. Lateral displacement of the scapula on chest radiograph is diagnostic (Figure 18–9). Scapular and clavicular fractures and acromioclavicular and sternoclavicular joint disruptions are frequent. The tremendous forces required to cause these musculoskeletal injuries result in concomitant injuries to the brachial plexus and the subclavian or axillary artery. Vascular injury is suspected based upon physical examination and diagnostic arteriography (Figure 18–10). Functional outcome is primarily based upon the severity of the neurologic injury.[15-16] However, neurologic deficits caused by ischemia may be reversible. Arterial repair should be performed within 4 to 6 hours of injury. In a literature review, brachial plexus injury was complete in 81% of patients with scapulothoracic dissociation and partial in 13%. Vascular injuries included disruption of the subclavian or axillary artery in 88% of patients. However, extensive collateral vessels around the shoulder allow adequate distal perfusion despite occlusion of the subclavian or axillary artery in the majority of patients.[17] Vascular intervention should be limited to cases with limb-threatening ischemia or active hemorrhage.[17] Long-term outcome revealed flail arm in 52%, early amputation in 21%, and death in 10% of patients. Limited functional recovery occurred in only 17% of patients.[15,17]

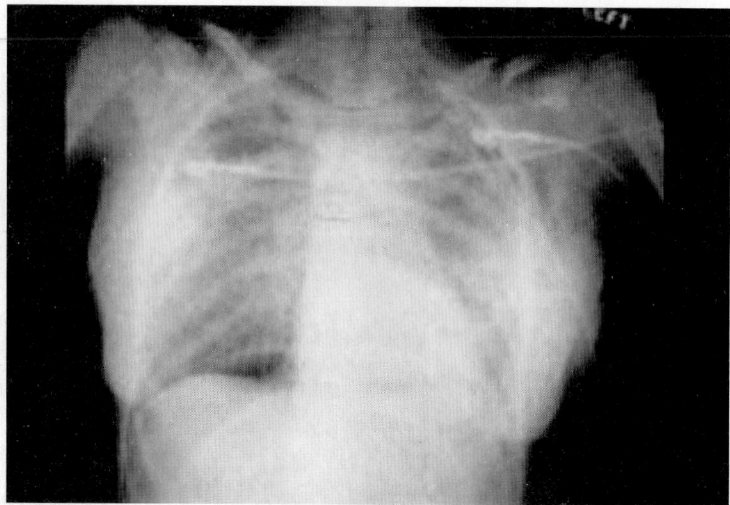

Figure 18-9. Chest radiograph in patient with scapulothoracic dissociation demonstrating left mid-clavicular fracture and lateral displacement of the left scapula.

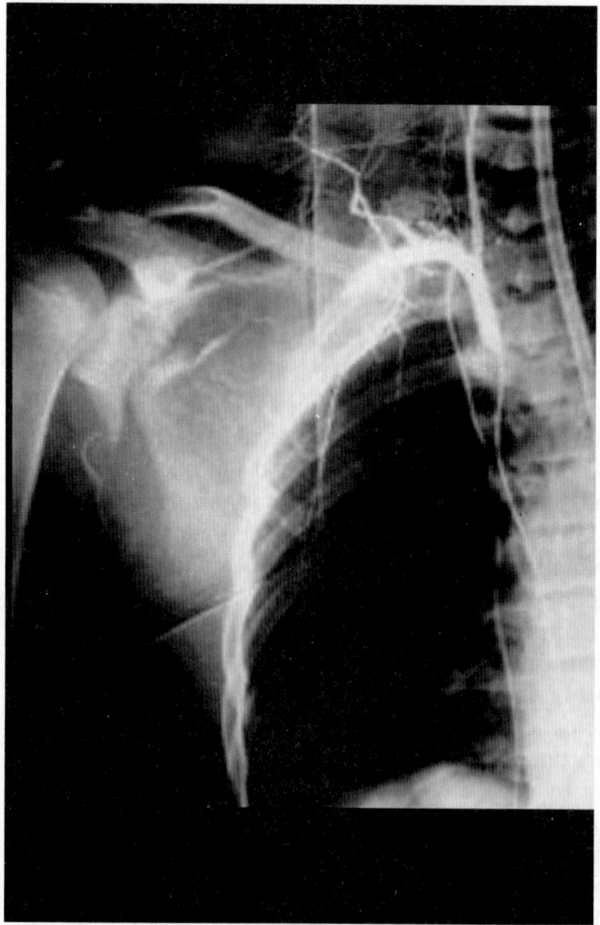

Figure 18-10. Arteriogram of patient with vascular injury associated with scapulothoracic dissociation showing right acromioclavicular joint separation, right scapular fracture, and disruption of the right subclavian artery.

UNUSUAL SOFT TISSUE INFECTIONS

Mutilating injuries from farm accidents frequently involve crushing and multiple lacerations of skin and soft tissues, tissue loss, and ischemia. These wounds are often grossly contaminated with dirt, manure, and plant material. Gram-negative rods have been cultured from 81% of wounds caused by corn-harvesting machinery.[18] The most frequently cultured organisms from these wounds were *Enterobacter* species and *Xeromonas maltophilia*. Broad-spectrum antibiotics with activity against multiple species of both gram-positive bacteria and gram-negative rods are recommended as initial therapy for infections from corn-harvesting wounds.[11,18]

VASCULAR TRAUMA TREATED AT GUNDERSEN LUTHERAN

Vascular injuries were identified from a prospective trauma database from July 1, 2000, to February 28, 2009. Variables available for study in the database included patient demographics, mechanism of injury, injury severity score (ISS), length of stay, functional independence measure (FIM) at discharge, and disposition at discharge. FIM score is calculated at the time of discharge and consists of the sum of three subscores — expression, locomotion, and self-feeding — each ranging from 1 (complete dependence) to 4 (complete independence). Individual chart review was undertaken for exact injury location, specific mechanism of injury, and type of repair.

Over the 8½-year study period, 4933 patients were admitted to the trauma service and 130 (2.6%) patients had a traumatic vascular injury and/or traumatic amputation. The mean age of these patients was 41.2 years (range 7 to 87 years) and 75% were male; 103 (79%) were injured by blunt mechanisms. The majority of these were either motor vehicle or motorcycle crashes. There were also crush injuries, pedestrian versus car, pedestrian versus train, and two blast injuries from explosions. Of those injured from penetrating mechanisms (21%), lacerations were most common, followed by stab wounds and gunshot wounds. Median ISS for the entire group was 11. Sixteen (12.3%) patients died.

Specific Vascular Injuries

Aorta. Sixteen patients sustained traumatic thoracic aortic injuries. Injury mechanisms were motor vehicle crash in 14, motorcycle crash in 1, and pedestrian versus car in 1. These patients were severely injured, with a median ISS of 43. Four (25%) patients died – 1 in the emergency department and 3 in the operating room.

Of the 12 patients who survived, 10 underwent operative repair. Nine patients underwent open repair with synthetic interposition graft. One patient underwent endovascular repair with a stent graft. Endovascular graft placement was attempted in 1 patient, but this was unsuccessful due to unfavorable aortic arch anatomy. This elderly patient was managed by observation alone. The final patient had a partial transection and was treated nonoperatively with anticoagulation and aggressive blood pressure management.

Five (42%) of 12 patients were discharged to their homes. The remaining 7 were discharged either to inpatient rehabilitation (5) or to a skilled nursing facility (2). These patients recovered well, with median FIM score of 10.5.

Carotid Artery. Four patients sustained injuries to the carotid artery: three involved the internal carotid artery and one involved the external carotid artery. Of the internal carotid artery injuries, two were arterial dissections, both resulting from motor vehicle crashes. Both were treated nonoperatively: one was treated with intravenous heparin, and the other was observed because severe head injury precluded anticoagulation. The final internal carotid artery injury was a laceration from a stab wound to the neck. This was repaired primarily. There was one external carotid artery laceration from a motor vehicle crash, which was repaired primarily.

One of these four patients died secondary to a severe head injury. The three remaining patients did well and were discharged home.

Vertebral Artery. Three patients had vertebral artery injuries. All were arterial dissections resulting from motorcycle crashes. All patients were treated nonoperatively. None were anticoagulated because of associated injuries. One of three patients died from severe head injury, one was discharged home, and one was discharged to inpatient rehabilitation. Of the two patients who survived, neither developed a stroke and both had good functional outcomes.

Iliac Artery. Six patients had iliac artery injuries. All were the result of blunt trauma. There were three motor vehicle crashes and three crush injuries. The crush injuries resulted from a logging accident (1), forklift accident (1), and a front-end loader accident (1). All six patients had associated pelvic fractures. One patient had a common iliac artery injury with complete transaction. This was repaired with a common iliac to superficial femoral artery PTFE bypass. The other five patients had avulsed branches of the internal iliac artery, and all were treated with coil embolization. These patients were all severely injured; the median ISS was 37.5. Three (50%) patients died, all secondary to uncontrollable pelvic hemorrhage. Of those who survived, two were discharged to inpatient rehabilitation and one to a skilled nursing facility.

Extremity Arteries. Fifty-one patients had extremity vascular injuries: 29 (57%) were injured from blunt mechanisms. The most common injury mechanisms were motor vehicle or motorcycle crashes, followed by falls, ATV crashes, and crush injuries. Of those injured from penetrating mechanisms, lacerations were most common, followed by stab wounds and gunshot wounds. There were also two impalement injuries and two grain auger injuries.

UPPER EXTREMITY Thirty of 51 patients had injury to upper extremity vessels. Of these 30 patients, 17 had arterial injuries, 7 had venous injuries, and 6 had combined arterial and venous injuries. One patient had two arterial injuries for a total of 18 injured arteries in 17 patients. See Table 18–1 for arterial injury locations and types of repair.

Venous injury to the upper extremity occurred in 13 patients. One patient had two venous injuries, for a total of 14 injuries; all were ligated.

Sixty percent of patients with upper extremity injury were discharged home. There was 1 death in a patient with a severe head injury as well as axillary artery transection. Three patients (10%) underwent secondary amputation after failed attempts at limb salvage. Two of these patients had gunshot wounds to the upper arm with severe bony and soft tissue injury in addition to the vascular injury. The third patient had an insensate, flail arm secondary to complete brachial plexus injury with scapulothoracic dissociation. The remainder of patients did well after repair, with a median FIM score of 12, indicating complete independence with activities of daily living.

TABLE 18-1. UPPER EXTREMITY ARTERIAL INJURIES

Artery	N	Type of repair
Axillary	5	Reversed vein graft - 2 Endoluminal stent - 2 Coil Embolization - 1
Brachial	9	Reversed vein graft - 6 Primary repair - 3
Radial	5	Primary repair - 3 Reversed vein graft - 1 Ligation - 1
Ulnar	5	Ligation - 5

LOWER EXTREMITY Twenty-one of 51 patients had injury to lower extremity vessels. Eight patients had arterial injury alone, 7 had venous injury alone, and 6 patients had both arterial and venous injuries. There was a total of 29 vascular injuries in these patients. Arterial injury location as well as management is listed in Table 18–2.

Venous injury to the lower extremity occurred in 13 patients, with 15 injured veins. Four were common femoral vein injuries – 3 were repaired primarily and 1 was ligated. There was 1 popliteal vein injury, which was ligated. The remaining 10 injuries involved the saphenous vein (7) and the posterior tibial vein (3); all of these were ligated.

Thirteen patients (62%) with lower extremity vascular injury were discharged home. One patient with superficial venous injuries died from a severe head injury. There was 1 secondary amputation (5%) that occurred in a patient with a fracture/dislocation of the knee and complete transection of the popliteal artery and vein. This was repaired with a saphenous vein graft that failed due to venous outflow obstruction. This patient underwent knee disarticulation amputation. In the remaining patients, independent function after repair was excellent, with a median discharge FIM score of 11.

Miscellaneous Arterial Injuries. Eight patients presented with nine arterial injuries not listed in the previous sections (see Table 18–3). Two of these eight patients died. One patient with pulmonary artery injury died in the emergency department. The second death was in a patient with a splenic artery injury as well numerous other injuries. The patients who survived did well, with four out of six (66%) being discharged home. The median discharge FIM score was 12 in these 6 patients.

Miscellaneous Venous Injuries. Nine patients presented with miscellaneous major venous injuries without associated arterial injuries (Table 18–4).

Traumatic Amputations. Twenty-six patients had traumatic amputations. These ranged from partial to complete amputations. Sixteen (62%) patients had finger amputations. The mechanisms of injury were many: table saws (2), rotary lathes (1), snow blowers

TABLE 18-2. LOWER EXTREMITY ARTERIAL INJURIES

Artery	N	Type of Repair
Profunda femoris	1	Ligation
Common femoral	3	Reversed vein graft - 2 Primary repair - 1
Popliteal	5	Primary repair - 3 Reversed vein graft - 1 In situ vein graft - 1
Posterior tibial	5	Reversed vein graft - 1 Ligation - 4

TABLE 18-3. MISCELLANEOUS ARTERIAL INJURIES

Artery	N	Type of Repair
Mesenteric	2	Ligation - 2
Splenic	2	Coil embolization - 1 Splenectomy - 1
Renal	2	Coil embolization - 1 Nephrectomy - 1
Intercostal	1	Ligation - 1
Pulmonary	1	Attempted repair, intra-operative death
Hepatic	1	Endovascular stent

TABLE 18-4. MISCELLANEOUS VENOUS INJURIES

Vein	N	Type of Repair
Superior mesenteric	1	Primary repair
Portal	1	Primary repair
IVC	3	Intra-operative death - 2 primary repair - 1
Internal jugular	2	Primary repair - 2
External jugular	2	Ligation - 2

(1), PTO shafts (1), fireworks (1), tank explosion (1), garage door spring (1), motorcycle crash (2), motor vehicle crash (2), and logging accident (1). Twelve of 16 patients (75%) underwent operation for débridement of the amputation site with either primary or delayed closure. The remainder were transferred to other facilities; 3 of these patients were transferred for replantation. One patient died from major injuries after a tank explosion; the remaining 11 patients were discharged to home.

Eleven patients had major traumatic limb amputations. Nine patients had lower extremity amputation alone, 1 had combined lower extremity/hand amputations, and 1 had combined lower extremity/finger amputations. Motorcycle crash (5) was the most common mechanism, followed by pedestrian versus train (3), grain auger (2), and trash compactor (1) injuries. No patients with major traumatic limb amputations underwent primary closure because all had grossly contaminated wounds at presentation.

The lower extremity amputation site was at the foot/ankle level in 3 patients. All 3 foot/ankle amputations were converted to traditional below-knee amputations. These patients did well: 2 were discharged to inpatient rehabilitation and 1 to home.

Six patients presented with traumatic below-knee (tibia/fibula) amputation. One patient died in the emergency department, and one patient was transferred to another facility prior to operative intervention. Of the four patients treated at our institution, all underwent initial débridement of the amputation site. Two patients went on to heal this site. The other two patients required conversion to above-knee amputation —one during the initial hospitalization due to infection and the other 6 months after injury due to chronic pain and prosthesis fitting problems. The two patients whose below-knee amputation sites healed were discharged to home; the other two were discharged to inpatient rehabilitation.

Two patients presented with traumatic above-knee (femur) amputations. Both of these patients also had concomitant upper extremity traumatic amputations — one had finger amputations and the other had a wrist amputation. The patient with combined above-knee and finger amputations was transferred to another facility prior to operative intervention. The second patient was treated at our institution with débridement of the above-knee and wrist amputation sites. This patient had also sustained scapulothoracic dissociation with complete disruption of the brachial plexus and injury to the axillary artery. Above-elbow amputation was performed for the flail arm.

CONCLUSIONS

1. Prolonged time to treatment due to delayed discovery, difficult extrication, and long distances to regional trauma centers dictate different priorities in rural vascular trauma. Resuscitation and stabilization at local community hospitals are favored over the "scoop and run" concept of prehospital care. Helicopter transport decreases time to definitive care.
2. Unique injury mechanisms occur in rural North America. Knowledge of these mechanisms may improve care and achieve more realistic outcomes.
3. Unique soft-tissue infections are seen with specific rural vascular injuries. Appropriate wounds should be cultured and treated with effective broad-spectrum antibiotics.
4. The management of vascular injuries seen at a rural referral trauma center involves a combination of open and endovascular techniques. Expertise in each of these disciplines is essential for optimal outcomes.
5. Many vascular injuries are associated with significant soft tissue and skeletal trauma. Team management of these patients includes plastic surgeons, orthopedists, and neurosurgeons.
6. Long-term outcome depends on excellent acute care as well as aggressive physical medicine and rehabilitation services.

REFERENCES

1. Caps MT. The epidemiology of vascular trauma. Semin Vasc Surg 1998;11:227–31.
2. Oller DW, Rutledge R, Clancy T, et al. Vascular injuries in a rural state: a review of 978 patients from a state trauma registry. J Trauma 1992;32:740–5.
3. Gupta R, Rao S, Sieunarine K. An epidemiological view of vascular trauma in Western Australia: a 5-year study. Aust N Z J Surg 2001;71:461–6.
4. Humphrey PW, Nichols WK, Silver D. Rural vascular trauma: a twenty-year review. Ann Vasc Surg 1994;8:179–85.
5. Ruby BJ, Cogbill TH, Gardner RS. Role of the rural general surgeon in a statewide trauma system: the Wyoming experience. Bull Am Coll Surg 2006;91:37–40.
6. Bintz M, Cogbill TH, Bacon J. Rural trauma care: role of the general surgeon. J Trauma 1996;41:462–4.
7. Kragh JF Jr, Walters TJ, Baer DG, et al. Practical use of emergency tourniquets to stop bleeding in major limb trauma. J Trauma 2008;64:S38–49.
8. Taller J, Kamdar JP, Greene JA, et al. Temporary vascular shunts as initial treatment of proximal extremity vascular injuries during combat operations: the new standard of care at echelon II facilities? J Trauma 2008;65:595–603.
9. Martin GD, Cogbill TH, Landercasper J, et al. Prospective analysis of rural interhospital transfer of injured patients to a referral trauma center. J Trauma 1990;30:1014–9.
10. Cogbill TH, Busch HM, Jr. The spectrum of agricultural trauma. J Emerg Med 1985;3: 205–10.

11. Cogbill TH, Steenlage ES, Landercasper J, et al. Death and disability from agricultural injuries in Wisconsin: a 12-year experience with 739 patients. J Trauma 1991;31:1632–7.
12. Jongewaard WR, Cogbill TH, Landercasper J. Neurologic consequences of traumatic asphyxia. J Trauma 1992;32:28–31.
13. Bansal V, Fortlage D, Lee J, et al. A 21-year history of all-terrain vehicle injuries: has anything changed? Am J Surg 2008;195:789–92.
14. Smith LM, Pittman MA, Marr AB, et al. Unsafe at any age: a retrospective review of all-terrain vehicle injuries in two level I trauma centers from 1995 to 2003. J Trauma 2005;58: 783–8.
15. Damschen DD, Cogbill TH, Siegel MJ. Scapulothoracic dissociation caused by blunt trauma. J Trauma 1997;42:537–40.
16. Sampson LN, Britton JC, Eldrup-Jorgensen J, et al. The neurovascular outcome of scapulothoracic dissociation. J Vasc Surg 1993;17:1083–8.
17. Riess KP, Cogbill TH, Patel NY, et al. Brachial plexus injury: long-term functional outcome is determined by associated scapulothoracic dissociation. J Trauma 2007;63:1021–5.
18. Agger WA, Cogbill TH, Busch H Jr, et al. Wounds caused by corn-harvesting machines: an unusual source of infection due to gram-negative bacilli. Rev Infect Dis 1986;8:927–31.

19

Endovascular Treatment of Supra-aortic Arterial Trauma

Richard C. Hershberger M.D. and
Bernadette Aulivola M.D., R.V.T.

BACKGROUND

Vascular Trauma

Each year, over 30 million emergency room visits for traumatic injuries are seen, of which up to 4% are associated with vascular injury. Penetrating trauma predominates, with over 90% of vascular injuries related to penetrating and the remainder related to blunt mechanisms. Vascular injury can present with a spectrum of clinical findings, including external hemorrhage, extremity ischemia, internal hemorrhage, and expanding or pulsatile hematoma. Injury to a vascular structure can result in a range of effects on the vessel such as laceration, transection, contusion, arteriovenous fistula, or extrinsic compression. Laceration may allow extravasation of blood flow resulting in a pseudoaneurysm or internal or external hemorrhage. Contusion, laceration, transaction, or compression can result in arterial thrombosis or distal ischemia. Arteriovenous fistula can cause distal ischemia or, in some cases, high-output heart failure.

The clinical presentation of vascular trauma ranges from hemorrhagic shock to limb ischemia. The well-established hard and soft signs of vascular injury aid in guiding work-up and treatment. Hard signs of extremity vascular injury include absent distal pulses, active hemorrhage, ischemia, pulsatile hematoma, and bruit or thrill. Soft signs include decreased distal pulses, proximity of injury to vessels, neurologic deficit, and hypotension or shock. It is well established that routine arteriography for extremity injury in proximity to vascular structures is relatively low yield, and therefore, selective arteriography or exploration is recommended when hard signs of extremity vascular injury are noted.[1] In some cases, operative exploration may be performed unless arteriography is needed to localize or treat the injury.

Endovascular Therapy

Since the concept of endovascular stent grafting for the treatment of abdominal aortic aneurysms was initially described in 1991, this technique has been employed to treat various forms of arterial disease. In addition to aortic aneurysms, endovascular stent grafts have been used to treat arterial occlusive disease, prosthetic and autogenous graft occlusion, peripheral arterial aneurysms, and vascular trauma. Treatment of traumatic vascular injury using endovascular techniques has dramatically evolved as endovascular capabilities have advanced over the past several decades.

Open surgical repair of traumatic arterial injury is often complicated by distorted anatomy secondary to associated hematoma or pseudoaneurysm. The technical aspect of vascular exposure in these cases is often more challenging than in the elective setting. Several endovascular techniques have been employed in the treatment of traumatic arterial injury. These include coil embolization, bare metal stent placement, and covered stent graft placement. Both bare metal stents and covered stent grafts are available in balloon-expandable and self-expanding configurations. Coil embolization is generally reserved for the treatment of small traumatic pseudoaneurysms and arteriovenous fistulas involving nonessential vascular territories. In the treatment of arterial dissection, bare metal stent placement over the dissection entry point serves to reapproximate the intima, media, and adventitia, preventing continued flow into the false vessel lumen and propagation of a dissection flap. Although bare metal stents have proved useful in the repair of intimal flaps, initially described for use in this setting in 1991, they are less well suited for the treatment of arteriovenous fistulas or pseudoaneurysms.[2] Covered stents are more ideally suited for repairing these lesions as well as traumatic arterial transections. Compared with traditional surgical repair, endovascular repair of traumatic arterial injury has several advantages, including a reduction in anesthetic requirement, operative time, blood loss, and perioperative morbidity.[3] Endovascular therapy for traumatic arterial injury has the additional advantages of reduction in ischemia time, limited exposure, and the ability to use a remote access site. In general, endovascular intervention is useful when the morbidity associated with an operative approach is considered prohibitive. Endovascular repair of the aorta and supra-aortic branch vessels has afforded the greatest potential benefit, given that open surgical repair of these arteries often requires thoracotomy or sternotomy. The morbidity of these surgical approaches can be significant, especially in the patient with multiple injuries. In contrast, open surgical repair in most extremity arterial injuries is more straightforward in terms of operative exposure and repair.

This chapter focuses on endovascular repair of traumatic injury to the supra-aortic branches: the carotid, vertebral, and innominate, subclavian, and axillary arteries. Aortic, intra-abdominal, and extremity artery injury are not discussed in depth here.

LITERATURE

Few large-scale published series have evaluated outcomes associated with an endovascular strategy for repair of traumatic arterial injuries. Between January 1995 and December 2007, publications documenting the endovascular treatment of 302 patients with carotid, vertebral, innominate, subclavian, and axillary artery injuries were identified in the literature (Table 19–1). The overall technical success rate for endovascular stenting for repair of arterial injuries was 93.6%. Unsuccessful stent placement, which occurred infrequently, was

TABLE 19-1. SUMMARY OF LITERATURE ON ENDOVASCULAR INTERVENTION FOR ARTERIAL TRAUMA

Artery Injured	n	Mean Follow-up (Months)	Mean Age (Years)	Injury Type n (%)	Technical Success Rate (%)	Periprocedural Morbidity n (%)	Mortality n (%)
Carotid[2-45]	179	10	35	Blunt 137 (76.5%) Penetrating 39 (21.8%) Iatrogenic 7 (3.9%)	91.6%	6 (3.4%)	4 (2.2%)
Vertebral[4,14,41,46-54]	13	7.5	39	Blunt 2 (15.4%) Penetrating 11 (84.6%)	100%	0 (0%)	0 (0%)
Innominate[55-61]	7	5.4	32	Blunt 6 (85.7%) Penetrating 1 (14.3%)	85.7%	0 (0%)	0 (0%)
Subclavian[9,11,18,62-81]	91	17	50	Blunt 14 (15.4%) Penetrating 21 (23.1%) Iatrogenic 26 (28.6%)	96.7%	11 (12.1%)	3 (3.3%)
Axillary[47,66-67,82-86]	11	17	48	Blunt 6 (54.5%) Penetrating 2 (18.2%) Iatrogenic 3 (27.3%)	100%	1 (9.0%)	0 (0%)
Total	301	13.3	40.1	Blunt 165 Penetrating 74 Iatrogenic 36	94.0%	18 (6.0%)	7 (2.3%)

attributed to a variety of reasons, including the inability to traverse the lesion with a guidewire, persistent contrast extravasation after stent placement, or graft migration requiring either placement of coils or conversion to open repair.

Periprocedural morbidity was documented in 18 (6.0%) patients overall. Complications related directly to the endovascular procedure included iatrogenic brachial and femoral artery puncture site injury, in-stent stenosis, stroke, and retroperitoneal hematoma. Average patient follow-up was 13.3 months.

The overall mortality rate was 2.3% (n=7). Deaths were attributable to comorbid conditions associated with polytrauma, including stroke, hemorrhage from a remote site, sepsis, traumatic brain injury, and multisystem organ failure.

Carotid Artery Injury

Blunt carotid artery injury can result from several mechanisms. Hyperextension and lateral flexion of the neck can cause tethering of the internal carotid artery against the transverse process of the axis or lateral aspect of the atlas, resulting in arterial injury.[87] In motor vehicle collision-related carotid injury or forward movement of the patient's trunk while the head remains fixed may be possible mechanisms of injury.[88] Additional mechanisms of blunt carotid injury include intraoral trauma, a direct blow to the neck, strangulation, or injury in association with basilar skull fracture through the foramen lacerum.[89-90] Carotid artery trauma can result in arterial thrombosis, dissection, pseudoaneurysm or dissection, all of which may result in transient ischemic attack or stroke.

Blunt carotid injury accounts for less than 1% of all arterial trauma.[91-92] As many as 94% of cases are associated with a delay in diagnosis because the injury is often asymptomatic or is confounded by intoxication, intracranial injury, extremity or spinal cord injury, or shock.[93-98] The most common signs and symptoms of blunt carotid injury include ipsilateral headache (58-92%), cerebral ischemia (63-90%), Horner's syndrome (9-75%), neck pain (18-46%), and bruit (12-39%).[99] Owing to the delay in detection of this injury and the presence of concomitant injuries, the morbidity rate associated with carotid injury is high. Neurologic morbidity rates of 40 to 80% and mortality rates of 5 to 40% have been described.[92-93,99-100] In an attempt to decrease morbidity and mortality, screening parameters to allow for earlier diagnosis of carotid injury have been developed. Suggested triggers for work-up for carotid artery injury include cervical vertebral body or transverse process fracture, diffuse axonal injury, Horner's syndrome, Le Fort II or III facial fracture, and basilar skull fractures involving the carotid canal.[92,101-102]

Endovascular treatment of blunt carotid injuries can be particularly useful in selected patients. Treatment of carotid artery dissection with systemic anticoagulation alone has been described extensively and is associated with a recanalization rate of 50 to 70% and a 10% incidence of subsequent neurologic events.[103-105] Although the benefits of systemic anticoagulation in the setting of blunt carotid injury have been documented, contraindications to its use may exist in patients with concomitant head or intra-abdominal solid organ injury.[91,105] In this challenging patient population, stent placement may avoid or reduce the need for long-term systemic anticoagulation. Furthermore, endovascular techniques offer potential benefit in cases of distal internal carotid injury, in which surgical exposure is complicated by the need for extensive dissection or mandibular subluxation to gain exposure. Surgical repair of these injuries is associated with a 9% perioperative stroke rate.[10] Surgical repair of blunt carotid artery injury is rarely indicated, however. In one series of carotid injuries, only 1 of 76 patients required surgical repair.[100] Indications for stent placement in the setting of carotid injury include contraindication to anticoagulation, enlarging pseudoaneurysm, progressive dissection, or lesions inaccessible through a high cervical operative approach.

Forty-two publications discussing 179 patients who sustained injuries to the carotid artery are summarized here. Blunt mechanism accounted for 137 (76.5%) of the arterial injuries, whereas 39 (21.8%) occurred due to a penetrating mechanism. There were 7 (3.9%) iatrogenic injuries. The overall technical success rate in these cases was 91.6%. There were 2 technical failures, 1 due to persistent endoleak[4] and 1 attributed to the inability to cross the injury with a guidewire.[5] Eleven patients suffered from carotid artery occlusion after stent placement.[6-9] None of these patients were symptomatic from the acute occlusion. Five patients suffered from a periprocedural stroke.[4,7,10] Four mortalities were reported.

The timing of repair of blunt carotid injury is somewhat controversial. Some interventionalists advocate delay of carotid stenting, thus decreasing the risk of thrombotic or embolic events related to catheter manipulation in the acutely injured vessel. The role of anticoagulation as both treatment for injury and prevention of acute stent thrombosis must be evaluated taking into consideration the patient's other injuries. Maintaining a partial thromboplastin time (PTT) between 40 to 50 seconds is thought to be sufficient anticoagulation in the treatment of blunt carotid artery injury when medical management is utilized.[91,106]

The management of periprocedural anticoagulation in this setting has evolved. This evolution has potential influence on arterial patency as evidenced by long-term patency rates in two of the larger series identified. Cothren and associates[7] placed carotid stents in 23 patients for traumatic dissection. On follow-up, 8 patients were found to have an asymptomatic occlusion of the carotid artery stent. In this setting, carotid occlusion could be attributed to factors such as accelerated neointimal hyperplasia or a hypercoagulable state in the younger trauma patient population, but it is likely also related to the management of systemic anticoagulation. In contrast, Edwards et al.[10] placed carotid stents in 22 patients for traumatic injuries, none of which demonstrated occlusion on follow-up. All of these patients received treatment with clopidogrel for a minimum of 6 weeks after stent placement. Some advocate the use of clopidogrel for at least 2 weeks following stent placement with conversion to lifelong aspirin therapy. Although long-term follow-up is limited, these studies suggest that outcome in patients undergoing carotid stent placement for traumatic lesions is improved with the post-procedural use of antiplatelet agents such as clopidogrel.

Duplex imaging is typically used for surveillance of carotid interventions in the atherosclerotic patient population. This standard of care generally mandates serial duplex scans for the lifetime of the patient. Although the comorbidities of the average trauma patient reduce the risk for the development of stenosis secondary to atherosclerosis, neointimal hyperplasia-related stenosis is possible and must be ruled out on serial imaging studies. Long-term outcomes related to stenting of the carotid artery for the repair of traumatic injuries have not been well established. Routine surveillance should mirror that for carotid stenting for atherosclerotic disease with duplex evaluation at 1, 3, 6, 12, 18, and 24 months and annually thereafter.

Vertebral Artery Injury

Few studies describe the use of endovascular means for treatment of vertebral artery injury. A total of 12 reports were found in the literature, including a description of 13 cases.

Seven of these cases reported arteriovenous fistulas that required intervention. Patients in this group had a mean age of 39 years and a mean follow-up of 7.5 months. No morbidities or mortalities were reported in this group of patients.

The most common presenting symptoms in patients with vertebral artery trauma were tinnitus and pain. These findings are consistent with the open surgical literature, which indicates that the majority of vertebral artery injuries can be managed non-operatively or with embolization. The majority of these lesions are not life-threatening.[107] In the literature, one patient presented with a life-threatening injury. This patient had a sudden and significant decrease in mental status due to a vertebral artery dissection causing basilar artery occlusion. Although rarer, reports of patients presenting in shock due to vertebral artery injury are documented.[108]

Innominate, Subclavian, and Axillary Artery Injury

Seven reports of innominate artery injury and eight reports of 11 patients with axillary artery injury managed with endovascular techniques are available for review. No periprocedural morbidity was noted in the innominate group and 9.0% morbidity was noted in the axillary artery injury group.

Endovascular repair of subclavian artery injury is much more prevalent in the literature, with 23 reports describing 91 patients. Eleven complications occurred in the subclavian artery injury group (12.1%). These included pseudoaneurysms at the access site,[46,62] arm claudication occurring 3 months after stent placement,[11] stent fracture requiring placement of a second stent,[63-64] stent graft thrombosis,[62] and diminished distal pulses occurring 4 months after initial treatment requiring balloon angioplasty. Three deaths were documented in the subclavian artery injury group.[65] The periprocedural death rate was 1.1%, with 1 death occurring less than 30 days after the injury as a result of multisystem organ failure. Two deaths occurred longer than 30 days after the injury.

The choice of endoprosthesis used in treating injury to the innominate, subclavian, and axillary arteries varied by authors. For isolated dissection, the primary treatment method is placement of a bare metal stent.[66] The potential for stent compression, stent fracture, and in-stent stenosis is well documented, especially in arteries subject to strong mechanical forces.[66-68] All documented cases of in-stent stenosis occurred in the setting of covered stent graft placement. In regard to the choice of covered stent type, some advocate the use of Dacron-covered stents.[69] According to their rationale, trauma patients are notoriously noncompliant with follow-up, and therefore, physicians have difficulty ensuring that appropriate antiplatelet therapy is continued. For this reason, the authors support the use of Dacron because the more rapid neointimal response to the material may help to prevent graft thombosis in the patient who is noncompliant with antiplatelet therapy. The limited number of cases available for review makes outcome analysis with respect to specific covered endoprosthesis difficult. Although the mean follow-up in the innominate artery injury group was relatively short at 5.4 months, the mean follow-up for patients in which a stent or stent graft was placed for subclavian or axillary artery injury was 18 months and 13 months, respectively. During the follow-up period, 8 patients (8.8%) had documented stent fracture, stenosis, or occlusion. Three of the 8 patients with stent complications were asymptomatic. Given so few documented cases in the literature on the endovascular treatment of innominate, subclavian, and axillary artery injuries, more information is needed before the long-term durability of these repairs can be assessed.

Despite the above-mentioned limitations, stent grafting within the innominate and subclavian arteries provides short-term advantages. In the hemodynamically unstable patient, stent grafting eliminates the need for thoracotomy, sternotomy, and clavicular resection. In one report, 78% of their patients had either a serious illness or major trauma.[62] Furthermore, endovascular repair does not preclude future open repair and can thus be used as a bridge to definitive therapy in the hemodynamically unstable patient. Finally, concerns regarding stent fracture may be self-limiting when detected early and have the potential to be corrected. Three patients (3.3%) who developed a stent fracture or kink were successfully revised using endovascular devices.[62-64]

CONCLUSION

Endovascular intervention for repair of arterial trauma involving the supra-aortic vessels can be performed safely and effectively. An overall technical success rate upward of 90% and morbidity and mortality rates of 3.0 and 2.3 respectively, demonstrate a potential benefit compared with traditional open surgical repair. The most significant limitation to the evaluation of endovascular stenting for vascular trauma is the lack of long-term data and controlled trials comparing outcomes with those with open surgical repair. Long-term follow-up for stent durability is of particular concern in the trauma population, which tends to comprise younger patients with minimal atherosclerotic disease compared with the typical older patient treated by endovascular means for aneurysmal or occlusive disease. Another concern is the long-term effect of the stent on the vessel wall, with the radial force exerted by the stent having possible adverse effects on the arterial wall, which may already be fragile due to injury. Long-term follow-up of patients treated by endovascular techniques for arterial trauma during the past decade will provide useful information regarding the durability and complications that may result. Routine surveillance imaging for graft migration, kinking, endoleak, delayed rupture, and vascular or neurologic complications related to the stent should be closely monitored in these cases.

Other limitations of endovascular techniques include reliance on the availability of suitably skilled interventionalists and an angiography suite that can also be used as an operating room when endovascular attempts at repair fail and conversion to open repair is required. Positive outcomes also rely on the availability of a variety of stents and stent graft devices, which allow a more precise tailoring to the anatomy of the vessels and the injury. An additional limiting factor in the endovascular treatment of arterial injury is the presence of large pseudoaneurysms that may require open decompression because of impingement of adjacent structures that is unrelieved by endovascular stent graft placement. In these cases, endovascular repair may be used in combination with open hematoma decompression. In summary, the use of endovascular intervention for the treatment of arterial trauma should not be considered a replacement for open surgical repair but rather an adjunct in the armamentarium of the vascular interventionalist who treats arterial traumatic injuries.

REFERENCES

1. Dennis JW, Frykberg ER, Veldenz HC, et al. Validation of nonoperative management of occult vascular injuries and accuracy of physical examination alone in penetrating extremity trauma: 5 to 10-year follow-up. J Trauma 1998;44:243–53.

2. Lyden S, Srivastava SD, Waldman DL, et al. Common iliac artery dissection after blunt trauma: case report of endovascular repair and literature review. J Trauma 2001;50:339–42.
3. Marin ML, Veith FJ, Panetta TF, et al. Transluminally placed endovascular stented graft repair for arterial trauma. J Vasc Surg 1994;20:466–73.
4. Sakat RR, Razavi MK, Sze DY, et al. Stent-graft treatment of extracranial carotid and vertebral arterial lesions, J Vasc Interv Radiol 2004;15:1151–6.
5. Szopinski P, Ciostek P, Kielar M, et al. A series of 15 patients with extracranial carotid artery aneurysms: surgical and endovascular treatment. Eur J Vasc Endovasc Surg 2005; 29:256–61.
6. Archondakis E, Pero G, Valvassori L, et al. Angiographic follow-up of traumatic carotid cavernous fistulas treated with endovascular stent graft placement. AJNR Am J Neuroradiol 2007;28:342–7.
7. Cothren CC, Moore, EE, Ray CE, et al. Carotid artery stents for blunt cerebrovascular injury. Arch Surg 2005;140:480–6.
8. Duane TM, Parker F, Stokes GK, et al. Endovascular carotid stenting after trauma. J Trauma 2002;52:149–53.
9. Parodi JC, Schonholz C, Ferriera LM, Bergan J. Endovascular stent-graft treatment of traumatic arterial lesions. Ann Vasc Surg 1999;13:121–9.
10. Edwards NM, Fabian TC, Claridge JA, et al. Antithrombotic therapy and endovascular stents are effective treatment for blunt carotid injuries: results from longterm followup. J Am Coll Surg 2007;204:1007–15.
11. du Toit DF, Leith JG, Strauss DC, et al. Endovascular management of traumatic cervicothoracic arteriovenous fistula. Br J Surg 2003;90:1516–21.
12. Ahn JY, Chung YS, Lee BH, et al. Stent-graft placement in traumatic internal carotid-internal jugular fistula and pseudoaneurysm. J Clin Neurosci 2004;11:636–9.
13. Akiyam Y, Nakahara I, Tanaka M, et al. Urgent endovascular stent-graft placement for a ruptured traumatic pseudoaneurysm of the extracranial carotid artery. J Trauma 2005;58:624–7.
14. Amar AP, Teitelbaum GP, Giannotta SL, et al. Covered stent-graft repair of the brachiocephalic arteries: technical note. Neurosurgery 2002;51:247–53.
15. Bejjani GK, Monsein LH, Laird JR, et al. Treatment of symptomatic cervical carotid dissections with endovascular stents. Neurosurgery 1999;44:755–61.
16. Bernstein SM, Coldwell DM, Prall JA, Brega KE. Treatment of traumatic carotid pseudoaneurysm with endovascular stent placement. J Vasc Interv Radiol 1997;8:1065–8.
17. Biffl WL, Moore EE, Offner PJ, et al. Blunt carotid arterial injuries: implications of a new grading scale. J Trauma 1999;47:845–53.
18. Brandt M, Kazanjian S, Wahl W. The utility of endovascular stents in the treatment of blunt arterial injuries. J Trauma 2001;51:901–5.
19. Cohen JE, Ben-Hur T, Gomori JM, et al. Stent-assisted arterial reconstruction of traumatic extracranial carotid dissections. Neurol Res 2005;27:S73–8.
20. Coldwell DM, Novak Z, Ryu RK, et al. Treatment of posttraumatic internal carotid arterial pseudoaneurysms with endovascular stents. J Trauma 2000;48:470–2.
21. Diaz-Daza O, Arriaza FJ, Barkley JM, et al. Endovascular therapy of traumatic vascular lesions of the head and neck. Cardiovasc Intervent Radiol 2003;26:213–21.
22. Duncan IC, Rad FF, Fourie PA. Percutaneous management of concomitant post-traumatic high vertebral and caroticojugular fistulas using balloons, coils, and covered stent. J Endovasc Ther 2003;10:882–6.
23. Duke BJ, Ryu RK, Coldwell DM, et al. Treatment of blunt injury to the carotid artery by using endovascular stents. J Neurosurg 1997;87:825–9.
24. Fateri F, Groebli Y, Rufenacht DA, et al. Intraarterial thrombolysis and stent placement in the acute phase of blunt internal carotid artery trauma with subocclusive dissection and thromboembolic complication: case report and review of the literature. Ann Vasc Surg 2005;19:1–4.
25. Feugier P, Vulliez A, Bina N, et al. Urgent endovascular covered-stent treatment of internal carotid artery injury caused by a gunshot. Eur J Vasc Endovasc Surg 2007:34;663–5.

26. Fusonie GE, Edwards JD, Reed AB. Covered stent exclusion of blunt traumatic carotid artery pseudoaneurysm: case report and review of the literature. Ann Vasc Surg 2004;18: 376–9.
27. Joo JY, Ahn JY, Chung YS, et al. Therapeutic endovascular treatments for traumatic carotid artery injuries. J Trauma 2005;58:1159–66.
28. Kerby JD, May AK, Gomez CR, et al. Treatment of bilateral blunt carotid injury using percutaneous angioplasty and stenting: case report and review of the literature. J Trauma 2000;49:784–7.
29. Klein GE, Szolar DH, Raith J, et al. Posttraumatic extracranial aneurysm of the internal carotid artery: combined endovascular treatment with coils and stents. AJNR Am J Neuroradiol 1997;18:1261–4.
30. Kubaska SM, Greenberg RK, Clair D, et al. Internal carotid artery pseudoaneurysms: treatment with the wallgraft endoprosthesis. J Endovasc Ther 2005;10:182–9.
31. Layton KF, Kim YW, Hise JH. Use of covered stent grafts in the extracranial carotid artery: report of three patients with follow-up between 8 and 42 months. AJNR Am J Neuroradiol 2004;25:1760–3.
32. Lee CY, Yim MB, Kim IM, et al. Traumatic aneurysm of the supraclinoid internal carotid artery and an associated carotid-cavernous fistula: vascular reconstruction performed using intravascular implantation of stents and coils. J Neurosurg 2004;100:115–9.
33. Liu AY, Paulsen RD, Marcellus ML, et al. Long-term outcomes after carotid stent placement for treatment of carotid artery dissection. Neurosurgery 1999;45:1368.
34. Malek AM, Higashida RT, Phatouros CC, et al. Endovascular management of extracranial carotid artery dissection achieved using stent angioplasty. AJNR Am J Neuroradiol 2000;21: 1280–92.
35. Marotta TR, Buller C, Taylor D, et al. Autologous vein-covered stent repair of a cervical internal carotid artery pseudoaneurysm: technical case report. Neurosurgery 1998;42: 408–13.
36. Matsuura JH, Rosenthal D, Jerius H, et al. Traumatic carotid artery dissection and pseudoaneurysm treated with endovascular coils and stent. J Endovasc Surg 1997;4:339–43.
37. McNeil JD, Chiou AC, Gunlock MG, et al. Successful endovascular therapy of a penetrating zone III internal carotid injury. J Vasc Surg 2002;36:187–90.
38. Parikh AA, Luchette FA, Valente JF, et al. Blunt carotid artery injuries. J Am Coll Surg 1997;185:80–6.
39. Patel JV, Rossbach MM, Cleveland TJ, et al. Endovascular stent-graft repair of traumatic carotid artery pseudoaneurysm. Clin Radiol 2002;57:308–11.
40. Perez-Cruet MJ, Patwardhan RV, Mawad ME, et al. Treatment of dissecting pseudoaneurysm of the cervical internal carotid artery using a wall stent and detachable coils: case report. Neurosurgery 1997;40:622–6.
41. Redekop G, Weill MT, Treatment of traumatic aneurysms and arteriovenous fistulas of the skull base by using endovascular stents. J Neurosurg 2001;95:412–9.
42. Reiter BP, Marin ML, Teodorescu VJ, Mitty HA. Endoluminal repair of an internal carotid artery pseudoaneurysm. J Vasc Interv Radiol 1998;9:245–8.
43. Scavee V, De Wispelaere JF, Mormont E, et al. Pseudoaneurysm of the internal carotid artery: treatment with a covered stent. Cardiovasc Interv Radiol 2001;24:283–5.
44. Self ML, Mangram A, Jefferson H, et al. Percutaneous stent-graft repair of a traumatic common carotid-internal jugular fistula and pseudoaneurysm in a patient with cervival spine fractures. J Trauma 2004;57:1331–4.
45. Shames ML, Davis JW, Evans AJ. Endoluminal stent placement for the treatment of traumatic carotid artery pseudoaneurysm: case report and review of the literature. J Trauma 1999;46:724–6.
46. Waldmen DL, Barquist E, Poynton FG, Numaguchi Y. Stent graft of a traumatic vertebral artery injury: case report. J Trauma 1998;44:1094–7.
47. Gonzalez A, Mayol A, Gil-Peralta, Gonzalez-Marcos JR. Endovascular stent-graft treatment of an iatrogenic vertebral arteriovenous fistula. Neuroradiology 2001;43:784–6.

48. Horowitz MB, Miller G 3rd, Meyer Y, et al. Use of intravascular stents in the treatment of internal carotid and extracranial vertebral artery pseudoaneurysms. AJNR Am J Neuroradiol 1996;17:693–6.
49. Mourikis D, Chatziioanou A, Doriforou O. Endovascular treatment of a vertebral artery pseudoaneurysm in a drug user. Cardiovasc Intervent Radiol 2006;29:662–4.
50. Price RF, Sellar R, Leung C, O'Sullivan MJ. Traumatic vertebral arterial dissection and vertebrobasilar arterial thrombosis successfully treated with endovascular thrombolysis and stenting. AJNR Am J Neuroradiol 1998;19:1677–80.
51. Priestly R, Bray P, Bray A, Hunter J. Iatrogenic vertebral arteriovenous fistula treated with a hemobahn stent-graft. J Endovasc Ther 2003;10:657–63.
52. Ruckert RI, Rutsch W, Filimonow S, Lehman R. Successful stent-graft repair of a vertebrojugular arteriovenous fistula. J Endovasc Ther 2001;8:495–500.
53. Singer RJ, Dake MD, Norbash A. Covered stent placement for neurovascular disease. AJNR Am J Neuroradiol 1997;18:507–9.
54. Surber R, Werner GS, Cohnert TU, et al. Recurrent vertebral arteriovenous fistula after surgical repair: treatment with a self-expanding stent-graft. J Endovasc Ther 2003;10:49–53.
55. Axisa BM, Loftus IM, Fishwick G, et al. Endovascular repair of an innominate artery false aneurysm following blunt trauma. J Endovasc Ther 2000;7:245–50.
56. Blatman SB, Landis GS, Knight M, et al. Combined endovascular and open repair of a penetrating innominate artery and tracheal injury. Ann Thorac Surg 2002;74:237–9.
57. Chandler TA, Fishwick G, Bell PRF. Endovascular repair of a traumatic innominate artery aneurysm. Eur J Vasc Endovasc Surg 1999;18:80–2.
58. Miles EK, Blake A, Thompson W, et al. Endovascular repair of acute innominate artery injury due to blunt trauma. Am Surg 2003;69:155–9.
59. Reubben A, Merlo M, Verri A, et al. Combined surgical and endovascular treatment of a traumatic pseudoaneurysm of the brachiocephalic trunk with anatomic anomaly. J Cardiovasc Surg 1997;38:173–6.
60. Waldenberger P, Fraedrich G, Mallouhi A, et al. Emergency endovascular treatment of traumatic aortic arch rupture with multiple arch vessel involvement. J Endovasc Ther 2003;10: 728–32.
61. Zoffoli G, Saccani S, Larini P, et al. Endovascular treatment of traumatic aortic dissection and innominate artery pseudoaneurysm. J Trauma 2006;61:447–50.
62. Hilfiker PR, Razavi MK, Kee ST, et al. Stent-graft therapy for subclavian artery aneurysms and fistulas: single-center mid-term results. J Vasc Interv Radiol 2000;11:578–84.
63. Ohki T, Veith FJ, Kraas C, et al. Endovascular therapy for upper extremity injury. Semin Vasc Surg 1998;11:106–15.
64. Patel AV, Marin ML, Veith FJ, et al. Endovascular graft repair of penetrating subclavian artery injuries. J Endovasc Surg 1996;3:382–8.
65. White R, Krajcer Z, Johson M, et al. Results of a multicenter trial for the treatment of traumatic vascular injury with a covered stent. J Trauma 2006;60:1189–96.
66. Castelli P, Caronno R, Piffaretti G, et al. Endovascular repair of traumatic injuries of the subclavian and axillary arteries. Injury 2005;36:778–82.
67. Piffaretti G, Tozzi M, Lomazzi C, et al. Endovascular treatment for traumatic injuries of the peripheral arteries following blunt trauma. Injury 2007;38:1091–7.
68. Schoder M, Cejna M, Holzenbein, et al. Elective and emergent endovascular treatment of subclavian artery aneurysms and injuries. J Endovasc Ther 2003;10:58–65.
69. Bates MC, Campbell J. Emergent stent graft isolation of a knife-related subclavian arterial venous fistula: lessons learned during long-term follow-up. Catheter Cardiovasc Interv 2005; 66:483–6.
70. Babatasi G, Massetti M, Bhoyroo S, et al. Non-penetrating subclavian artery trauma: management by selective transluminally placed stent device. Thorac Cardiovasc Surg 1999;47: 190–3.
71. Criado E, Marston WA, Ligush J, et al. Endovascular repair of peripheral aneurysms, pseudoaneurysms, and arteriovenous fistulas. Ann Vasc Surg 1997;11:256–63.

72. Meyer T, Merkel S, Lang W. Combined operative and endovascular treatment of a post-traumatic embolizing aneurysm of the subclavian artery. J Endovasc Surg 1998;5:52–5.
73. Pfammater T, Kunzli T, Hilfliker PR, et al. Relief of subclavian venous and brachial plexus compression syndrome caused by traumatic subclavian artery aneurysm by means of transluminal stent-grafting. J Trauma 1998;45:972–4.
74. Renger RJ, de Bruijn AJ, Aarts HC, et al. Endovascular treatment for pseudoaneurysm of the subclavian artery. J Trauma 2003;55:969–71.
75. Sanchez LA, Veith FJ, Ohiki T, et al. Early experience with the Corvita endoluminal graft for treatment of arterial injuries. Ann Vasc Surg 1999;13:151–7.
76. Sivamurthy N, Eichler C, Schneider DB. Endovascular eclusion of subclavian artery pseudoaneurysm. Vascular 2006;14:231–5.
77. Stecco K, Meier A, Seiver A, et al. Endovascular stent-graft placement for treatment of traumatic penetrating subclavian artery injury. J Trauma 2000;48:948–50.
78. Stokkeland PJ, Soreide K, Fjetland L. Acute endovascular repair of right subclavian arterial perforation from clavicular fracture after blunt trauma. J Vasc Interv Radiol 2007;18: 689–90.
79. Strauss DC, du Toit DF, Warren BL. Endovascular repair of occluded subclavian arteries following penetrating trauma. J Endovasc Ther 2001;8:529–33.
80. Watelet J, Clavier E, Reiz T, et al. Traumatic subclavian artery pseudoaneurysm: periprocedural salvage of failed stent-graft exclusion using coil embolization. J Endovasc Ther 2001;8:197–201.
81. Ahn SH, Cutry A, Murphy TP, Slaiby JM. Traumatic thoracic aortic rupture: treatment with endovascular graft in the acute setting. J Trauma 2001;50:949–51.
82. Martinez R, Lermusiaux P, Podeur L, et al. Endovascular management of axillary artery trauma. J Cardiovasc Surg 1999;40:413–5.
83. Onal, Baran, Ilgit ET, Kosar S, Akkan K, et al. Endovascular treatment of peripheral vascular lesions with stent-grafts. Diag Interv Radiol 2005;11:170–4.
84. Stahnke M, Duddy MJ, Endovascular repair of a traumatic axillary pseudoaneurysm following anterior shoulder dislocation. Cardiovasc Intervent Radiol 2006;29:298–301.
85. Turner PJ, Turon EP, Kessel D. Post-traumatic axillary artery pseudoaneurysm: treatment with a covered endoluminal stent. J Interv Radiol 1997;12:154–5.
86. Valentin MD, Tulsyan N, James K. Endovascular management of traumatic axillary artery dissection: a case report and review of the literature. Vasc Endovasc Surg 2004;38:473–5.
87. Parikh AA, Luchette FA, Valente JF, et al. Blunt carotid artery injuries. J Am Coll Surg 1997;185:80–6.
88. Perez-Cruet MJ, Patwardhan RV, Mawad ME, et al. Treatment of dissecting pseudoaneurysm of the cervical internal carotid artery using a wall stent and detachable coils: case report. Neurosurgery 1997;40:622–6.
89. Krajewski LP, Hertzer NR. Blunt carotid artery trauma: report of 2 cases and review of the literature. Ann Surg 1980;191:341–6.
90. New PF, Momose KJ. Traumatic dissection of the internal carotid artery at the atlantoaxial level, secondary to nonpenetrating injury. Radiology 1969;93:41–9.
91. Fabian TC, Patton JH Jr, Croce MA, et al. Blunt carotid injury: importance of early diagnosis and anticoagulant therapy. Ann Surg 1996;223:513–25.
92. Davis JW, Holbrook TL, Hoyt DB, et al. Blunt carotid artery dissection: incidence, associated injuries, screening, and treatment. J Trauma 1990;30:1514–7.
93. Cogbill TH, Moore EE, Meissner M, et al. The spectrum of blunt injury to the carotid artery: a multicenter perspective. J Trauma 1994;37:473–9.
94. Kraus RR, Bergstein JM, DeBord JR. Diagnosis, treatment, and outcome of blunt carotid arterial injuries. Am J Surg 1999;178:190–3.
95. Zetterling M, Carlstrom C, Konrad P. Review article: internal carotid artery dissection. Acta Neurol Scand 2000;101:1–7.
96. Mokri B, Houser OW, Sandok BA, et al. Spontaneous dissections of the vertebral arteries. Neurology 1988;38:880–5.

97. Biousse V, D'Angelajan-Chatillon J, Touboul PJ, et al. Time course of symptoms in extracranial carotid artery dissections. A series of 80 patients. Stroke 1995;26:235–9.
98. DiPerna CA, Rowe VL, Terramani TT, et al. Clinical importance of the "seat belt sign" in blunt trauma to the neck. Am Surg 2002;68:441–5.
99. Singh RR, Barry MC, Ireland A, et al. Current diagnosis and management of blunt internal carotid artery injury. Eur J Vasc Endovasc Surg 2004;27:577–84.
100. Biffl WL, Moore EE, Offner PJ, et al. Blunt carotid arterial injuries: implications of a new grading scale. J Trauma 1999;47:845–53.
101. Duke BJ, Ryu RK, Coldwell DM, et al. Treatment of blunt injury to the carotid artery by using endovascular stents. J Neurosurg 1997;87:825–9.
102. Biffl WL, Moore EE, Offner PJ, Burch JM. Blunt carotid and vertebral injuries. World J Surg 2001;25:1036–43.
103. Watridge CB, Muhlbauer MS, Lowery RD. Traumatic carotid artery dissection: diagnosis and treatment. J Neurosurg 1989;71:854–7.
104. Pozzati E, Giuliani G, Acciarri N, Nuzzo G. Long-term follow up of occlusive cervical carotid dissection. Stroke 1990;21:528–31.
105. Wahl WL, Brandt MM, Thompson BG, et al. Antiplatelet therapy: an alternative to heparin for blunt carotid injury. J Trauma 2002;52:896–901.
106. Biffl WL, Moore EE, Ray C, Elliott JP. Emergent stenting of acute blunt carotid artery injuries: a cautionary note. J Trauma 2001;50:969–70.
107. Moore EE, Feliciano DV, Mattox KL, eds. Trauma. 5th ed. New York: McGraw-Hill; 2004.
108. Reid JD, Weigelt JA. Forty-three cases of vertebral artery trauma. J Trauma 1988;28:1007–12.

SECTION V

AV Access

20

Strategies of Hemodialysis Access

Robyn A. Macsata, M.D., F.A.C.S. and
Anton N. Sidawy, M.D., F.A.C.S.

As the population ages and the incidence of diabetes rises, chronic kidney disease (CKD) and end-stage renal disease (ESRD) are becoming increasingly common diagnoses in the United States. In 2005, data from the U.S. Renal Data System (USRDS) showed more than 106,000 new patients began therapy for ESRD while the prevalent dialysis population reached 341,000 and the prevalent transplant population reached 143,693[1] (Figure 20–1). Total Medicare costs for CKD patients neared $42 billion and for ESRD patients neared $20 billion; this accounts for 13% and 6%, respectively, of the total Medicare spending in 2005 (Figure 20–2); not surprisingly, most of these costs come between the transition from CKD to ESRD and are related to hemodialysis access.[2] With these ever-increasing numbers and the cost of care of renal patients, placement of successful long-term arteriovenous (AV) access has become imperative. In response to this need, the Society for Vascular Surgery (SVS) sponsored a multispecialty expert panel to establish clinical practice guidelines for the surgical placement and maintenance of AV access. These guidelines address appropriate timing of referral for ESRD patients to a nephrologist and vascular access surgeon, preoperative evaluation for AV access, configurations, and strategies to optimize autogenous AV access placement, postoperative management, long-term care, and treatment of AV access failure. These guidelines were published in the Journal of Vascular Surgery in November 2008; this chapter is based on that summary document.[3]

TEMPORARY HEMODIALYSIS ACCESS

Short-Term Dialysis Catheters

Short-term dialysis catheters are double-lumen noncuffed nontunneled catheters that can be placed at the bedside without fluoroscopic guidance. These catheters should be placed in patients needing acute dialysis access and used for less than 3 weeks' duration. If

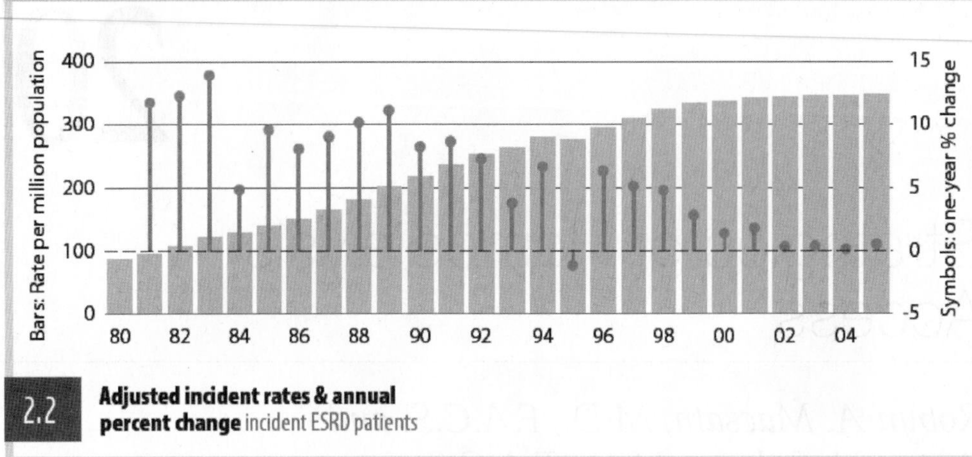

Figure 20-1. Adjusted incident rates and annual percent change of U.S. ESRD patients. (Reproduced from U.S. Renal Data System, USRDS 2007 Annual Report: Atlas of Chronic Kidney Disease and End-Stage Renal Disease in the United States, National Institutes of Health, National Institute of Diabetes and Digestive and Kidney Disease, Bethesda, MD, 2007. http://www.usrds.org)

dialysis is required longer than this time frame, the catheter should be converted to a long-term dialysis catheter. Short-term dialysis catheters may be placed in the internal jugular, subclavian, or femoral veins. With upper extremity catheters, to achieve best flow rates, the distal tip should be placed in the superior vena cava just above the atrial caval junction. The subclavian vein should be avoided if at all possible to prevent central venous stenosis, which may have an impact on future placement of ipsilateral AV access. When femoral ac-

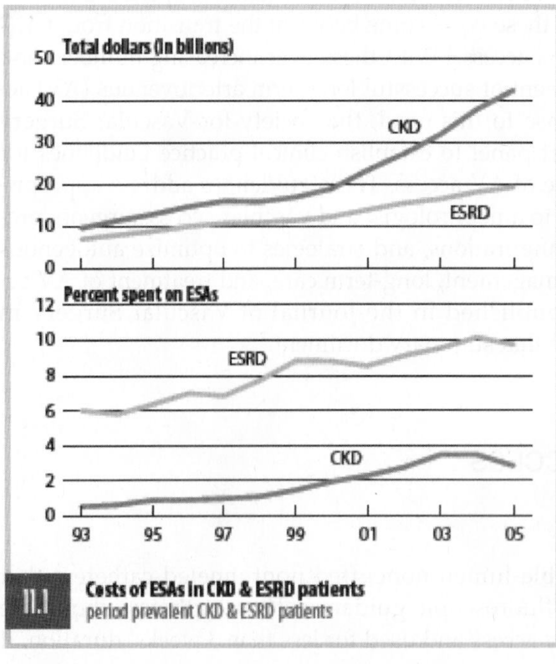

Figure 20-2. Annual Medicare costs for CKD and ESRD patients. (Reproduced from U.S. Renal Data System, USRDS 2007 Annual Report: Atlas of Chronic Kidney Disease and End-Stage Renal Disease in the United States, National Institutes of Health, National Institute of Diabetes and Digestive and Kidney Disease, Bethesda, MD, 2007. http://www.usrds.org)

cess is used, long catheters (24-31 cm) should be placed so the tip can reach the inferior vena cava for best flow rates.[4]

Long-Term Dialysis Catheters

Long-term dialysis catheters are double-lumen cuffed tunneled catheters that are placed with fluoroscopic guidance and are intended to be used over weeks' to months' duration. Because of higher blood flow and lower complication rates, access through the right internal jugular vein with the distal catheter tip in the right atrium is preferred[5-6]; however, left internal jugular and femoral approaches are also suitable. To decrease the risk of central venous stenosis and subsequent venous hypertension, dialysis catheters should be placed contralateral to the side of any maturing or planned permanent AV access and the subclavian vein approach should be avoided if at all possible.[4,7]

Complications of Temporary Dialysis Catheters

The most common indication and main benefit of short- and long-term dialysis catheters is the need for immediate use for dialysis. Other advantages include their universal applicability, their ability to be placed in multiple access sites without hemodynamic compromise, and no need for repeated skin punctures with dialysis sessions. Also, long-term dialysis catheters may be used for months while waiting for permanent AV access to mature. However, less than half of dialysis catheters are removed electively after successful placement of permanent AV access; the remainder are removed as a result of complications. Catheter thrombosis attributable to development of an intraluminal fibrin sheath leads to removal in up to 31% of patients. Catheter infections are another frequent cause for removal, occurring in up to 20% of patients; this is most commonly seen with short-term dialysis catheters placed in the femoral position.[8] Catheter malfunction, including cracked catheters, is cause for removal in 1% of patients.[9] Other disadvantages include the discomfort of an external device and lower blood flow rates leading to longer dialysis times or less effective dialysis.[4] A frequently seen long-term complication of dialysis catheters is subclavian stenosis, which occurs in up to 50% of patients with a subclavian catheter in place for as few as 6 weeks and leads to difficulty with permanent AV access.[7,10-11]

PERMANENT HEMODIALYSIS ACCESSES

Timing of Referral

The National Kidney Foundation-Dialysis Outcomes Quality Initiative (NKF-KDOQI) and the SVS Clinical Practice Guidelines both recommend that patients should be referred to a vascular access surgeon for permanent dialysis access when their creatinine clearance is less than 25 mL/min. Once preoperative evaluation is completed, if the patient is felt to be an adequate candidate for autogenous AV access, the access should be constructed as soon as possible to give adequate time to mature; ideally, this should be longer than 6 months before the anticipated need for dialysis. However, because prosthetic access patency is limited by time of access placement and not by access use, if a patient is felt to require a prosthetic access, the access placement should be delayed until 3 to 6 weeks prior to the initiation of dialysis.[3-4]

Preoperative Evaluation

History and Physical Examination. A thorough patient history should be taken documenting the patient's dominant extremity, recent history of peripheral intravenous lines, site of indwelling or previous central lines including pacemakers and defibrillators, all previous access procedures, any history of trauma or previous nonaccess surgery to the extremity, and all comorbid conditions. On physical examination, the brachial, radial, and ulnar arteries should be evaluated for compressibility and equality bilaterally. An Allen's test should be performed to evaluate palmar arch patency. The superficial venous system should be evaluated with and without a pressure tourniquet in place, examining for distensibility and interruptions. The arm should be examined for prominent venous collaterals and edema, which are signs of central venous stenosis.[4]

Arterial Assessment. If any abnormality is noted on the clinical arterial examination, the patient should be further evaluated with segmental pressures and duplex ultrasound scanning and/or pulse volume recordings (PVRs). For optimal outcome, there should be no pressure gradient noted between the bilateral upper extremities, arterial diameter should be equal to or greater than 2.0 mm throughout the extremity, and a patent palmer arch should be present.[12] Any abnormality noted on noninvasive testing should prompt alternate site selection or be further evaluated with an arteriogram, which gives the surgeon the ability to both identify and possibly treat an arterial inflow stenosis. In patients nearing dialysis, the risk of contrast arteriography should be weighed against the need for access to mature before beginning dialysis. Renal protective agents should be used pre-arteriogram; these include intravenous fluids, N-acetylcysteine, and sodium bicarbonate.[13-16]

Venous Assessment. If superficial veins cannot be visualized with a pressure tourniquet in place or any abnormality is noted on the superficial venous examination, the patient should be further evaluated with superficial venous duplex ultrasound scanning. Using venous duplex imaging, superficial veins should be examined for diameter, distensibility, and continuity. Superficial veins should be of a diameter of 2.5 mm or greater to be used for autogenous AV access.[12] Central venous stenosis should be suspected if there are any prominent venous collaterals or edema, a differential in extremity diameter, any history of previous central venous catheter placement, or multiple previous accesses in the planned extremity to be used for access. If any of these abnormalities is identified, the patient should be examined first with deep venous duplex ultrasound.[4] A venogram should be obtained in patients with either nondiagnostic or abnormal duplex ultrasound imaging for further evaluation and possible treatment.[17] As with the arteriogram, in predialysis patients the risk of contrast venogram needs to be weighed against the need for access to mature in time for dialysis. Patients should be treated prior to the venogram with intravenous fluids, N-acetylcysteine, and/or sodium bicarbonate.[13-16]

Access Location Selection

Table 20–1 lists the various types of autogenous and prosthetic AV access available in the upper extremity. We focus on simple autogenous and prosthetic upper extremity access only; more complex venous translocations, two-stage procedures, lower extremity, and body wall access are beyond the scope of this chapter. When planning upper extremity AV access, a few general principles apply.

1. AV accesses are placed as far distally in the extremity as possible to preserve proximal sites for future accesses.

TABLE 20-1. ARTERIOVENOUS ACCESS CONFIGURATION

Forearm

1. Autogenous
   a. Autogenous posterior radial branch–cephalic wrist direct access (snuff-box fistula)
   b. Autogenous radial–cephalic wrist direct access (Brescia-Cimino-Appel fistula)
   c. Autogenous radial–cephalic forearm transposition
   d. Autogenous brachial (or proximal radial)–cephalic forearm looped transposition
   e. Autogenous radial–basilic forearm transposition
   f. Autogenous ulnar–basilic forearm transposition
   g. Autogenous brachial (or proximal radial)–basilic forearm looped transposition
   h. Autogenous radial–antecubital forearm indirect femoral vein translocation
   i. Autogenous brachial (or proximal radial)–antecubital forearm indirect looped femoral vein translocation
   j. Autogenous radial–antecubital forearm indirect saphenous vein translocation
   k. Autogenous brachial (or proximal radial)–antecubital forearm indirect looped saphenous vein translocation
2. Prosthetic
   a. Prosthetic radial–antecubital forearm straight access
   b. Prosthetic brachial (or proximal radial)–antecubital forearm looped access

Upper Arm

1. Autogenous
   a. Autogenous brachial (or proximal radial)–cephalic upper arm direct access
   b. Autogenous brachial (or proximal radial)–cephalic upper arm transposition
   c. Autogenous brachial (or proximal radial)–basilic upper arm transposition
   d. Autogenous brachial (or proximal radial)–brachial vein upper arm transposition
   e. Autogenous brachial (or proximal radial)–axillary (or brachial) upper arm indirect femoral vein translocation
   f. Autogenous brachial (or proximal radial)–axillary (or brachial) upper arm indirect saphenous vein translocation
2. Prosthetic
   a. Prosthetic brachial (or proximal radial)–axillary (or brachial) upper arm straight access

Adapted from Sidawy AN, et al. Recommended standards for reports dealing with arteriovenous hemodialysis accesses. J Vasc Surg 2002;35:603–10.

2. Given their superior patency rates and lower complication rates, autogenous AV accesses should always be attempted before a prosthetic AV access. These autogenous access configurations should include, in order of preference, direct AV anastomosis, venous transpositions, and venous translocations.
3. Owing to easier accessibility and lower infection rates, upper extremity access sites are used first, with the nondominant arm given preference over the dominant arm.

Forearm Accesses

AUTOGENOUS FOREARM ACCESSES

CEPHALIC VEIN For autogenous forearm access, use of the cephalic vein is preferred to the basilic vein because of its lateral location and the need for only minimal dissection. Possible sites of arterial inflow include the posterior branch of the radial artery, the trunk of the radial artery, the ulnar artery, and the brachial artery. The ulnar artery is usually not the first arterial option because of its distance from the cephalic vein. The access is placed as distally in the arm as possible, where an adequate artery is identified by preoperative evaluation to preserve more proximal sites of inflow for future accesses. Therefore, in

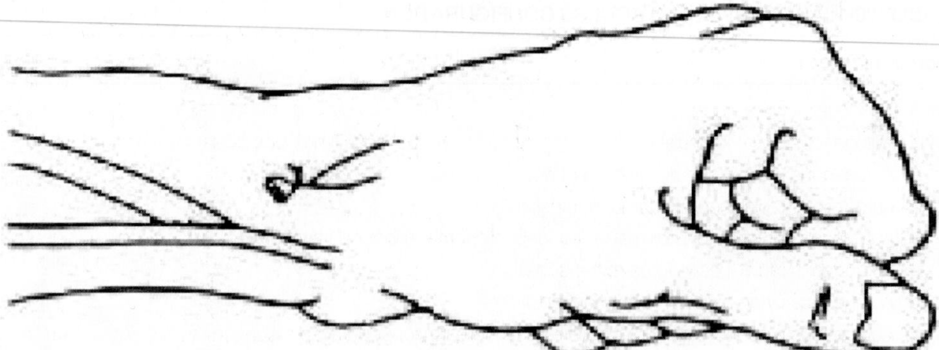

Figure 20-3. Autogenous posterior radial branch-cephalic direct wrist access (snuff-box fistula). (Reproduced with permission from Weiswasser JM, Sidawy AN. Strategies of Arteriovenous Dialysis Access. In: Rutherford R, ed. Vascular Surgery, 6th ed. Philadelphia: Elsevier Saunders; 2005, p. 1672.)

patients with an adequate posterior branch of the radial artery, an autogenous posterior radial branch–cephalic wrist direct access (snuff-box fistula) (Figure 20–3) is performed. In patients with an inadequate posterior branch of the radial artery but an adequate radial artery, an autogenous radial–cephalic wrist direct access (Brescia-Cimino-Appel fistula) (Figure 20–4) is performed. In either of these cases, if the cephalic vein is felt to be too deep, as seen in obese patients, or is not located in close proximity to the radial artery in the wrist, an autogenous radial-cephalic forearm transposition (Figure 20–5) is performed. If the radial artery is inadequate, the ulnar artery may provide an alternative distal inflow site; alternatively, the entire trunk of either the radial or the ulnar artery may provide an arterial source. If the radial and ulnar arteries are inadequate but the brachial or proximal radial arteries are adequate, an autogenous brachial (or proximal radial)–cephalic forearm looped transposition can be performed.

BASILIC VEIN When the cephalic vein is not felt to be adequate for an autogenous AV access, the basilic vein is the preferred alternative. Secondary to its medial location in the forearm, a transposition is always required. Possible sites of arterial inflow include the distal radial artery, the ulnar artery, the proximal radial artery, and the brachial artery. Use of

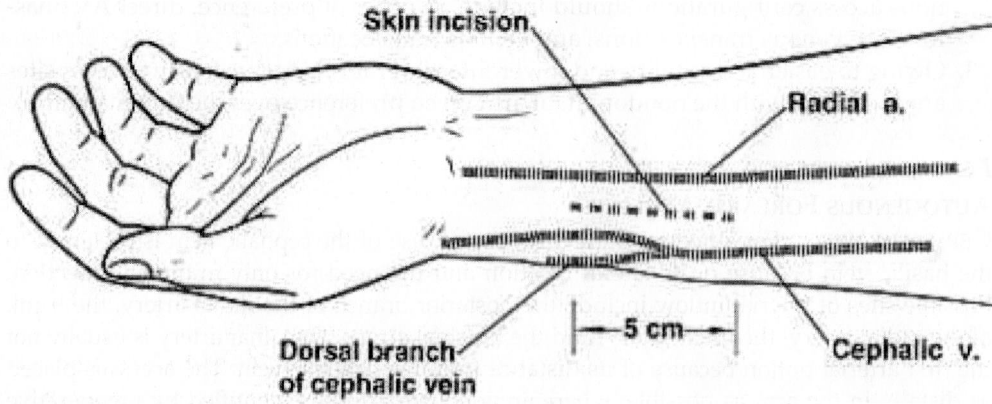

Figure 20-4. Autogenous radial–cephalic direct wrist access (Brescia-Cimino-Appel fistula).

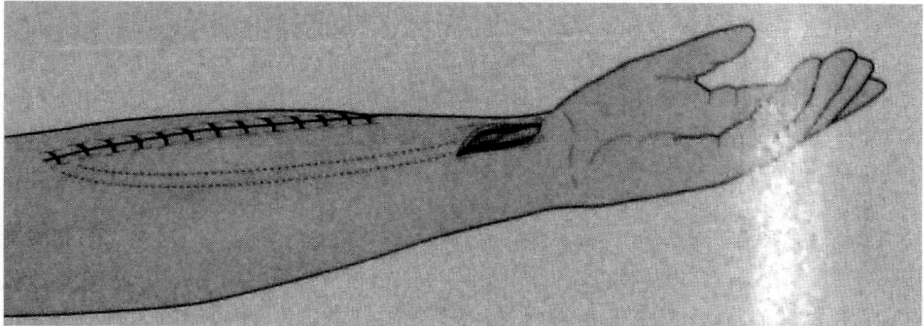

Figure 20-5. Autogenous radial-cephalic forearm transposition. (Reproduced with permission from Weiswasser JM, Sidawy AN. Strategies of arteriovenous dialysis access. In: Rutherford R, ed. Vascular Surgery, 6th ed. Philadelphia: Elsevier Saunders; 2005, p. 1672.)

the posterior branch of the radial artery is usually not possible secondary to the distance from the basilic vein. Similar to the cephalic vein, the AV access is placed as distally in the arm as possible, where an adequate artery is identified by preoperative evaluation to preserve more proximal sites of inflow for future accesses. Therefore, when the radial artery is adequate, an autogenous radial–basilic forearm transposition is performed. If the radial artery is inadequate but the ulnar artery is adequate, an autogenous ulnar–basilic forearm transposition is performed. If the distal radial and ulnar arteries are inadequate, a more proximal segment may be used (autogenous proximal radial–basilic forearm looped transposition). If the radial and ulnar arteries are inadequate throughout but the brachial artery is adequate, an autogenous brachial–basilic forearm looped transposition is performed.

Prosthetic Forearm Accesses

If no vein is available, a prosthetic AV forearm access is performed. Sources of arterial inflow include the distal or proximal radial and brachial arteries. Similar to autogenous access, to preserve more proximal arteries for future accesses, the prosthetic AV access is placed as distally in the arm as possible, where an adequate artery is identified by preoperative evaluation. Therefore, when the distal radial artery is adequate, a prosthetic radial–antecubital forearm straight access is performed. If the radial artery is inadequate but the brachial or proximal radial artery is adequate, a prosthetic brachial (or proximal radial)–antecubital forearm looped access (Figure 20–6) is performed. Patients should be told that this forearm prosthetic access is a "bridge" to an autogenous access. The nephrologists should be told to minimize the number of attempts to salvage the access with endovascular means in order to avoid damaging the venous outflow so it can still be used for an upper arm autogenous access. One of the interesting debates in this area is whether, after exhausting the forearm autogenous options, the surgeon should recommend a forearm prosthetic access before placing an upper arm autogenous access. The SVS AV Access Practice Guidelines recommend that the surgeon discuss these alternatives and their advantages and disadvantages with the patient to arrive at an informed decision.[3]

Upper Arm Access

Autogenous Upper Arm Accesses

Cephalic Vein When use of the forearm has been exhausted, efforts at access are directed to the upper arm. Similar to the forearm, use of the upper arm cephalic vein is preferred to the basilic vein because of its lateral location and need for only minimal

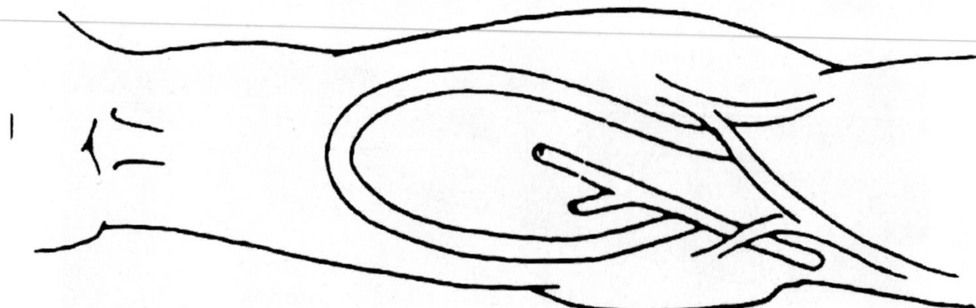

Figure 20-6. Prosthetic brachial (or proximal radial)–antecubital forearm looped access. (Reproduced with permission from Weiswasser JM, Sidawy AN. Strategies of arteriovenous dialysis access. In: Rutherford R, ed. Vascular Surgery, 6th ed. Philadelphia: Elsevier Saunders; 2005, p. 1674.)

dissection. For upper arm access, possible sites of arterial inflow include the proximal radial and brachial arteries. The AV access is placed as distally in the arm as possible, where an adequate artery is identified by preoperative evaluation to lower the risk of arterial steal. Therefore, in patients with an adequate cephalic vein and an adequate proximal radial artery, an autogenous proximal radial–cephalic upper arm direct access is performed. If the proximal radial artery is inadequate and the brachial artery is adequate, an autogenous brachial–cephalic upper arm direct access (Figure 20–7) is performed. If the cephalic vein is felt to be too deep or is located far from the artery, an autogenous brachial (or proximal radial)-cephalic upper arm transposition is performed.

Basilic Vein When the cephalic vein is felt to be inadequate for an autogenous AV access, the upper arm basilic vein is the preferred alternative. Secondary to its medial and deep location, transpositions are required for all accesses using the basilic vein. Similar to upper arm cephalic vein AV accesses, possible sites of arterial inflow include the proximal radial and brachial arteries; the AV access is placed as distally in the arm as possible, where an adequate artery is identified by preoperative evaluation to lower the risk of arterial

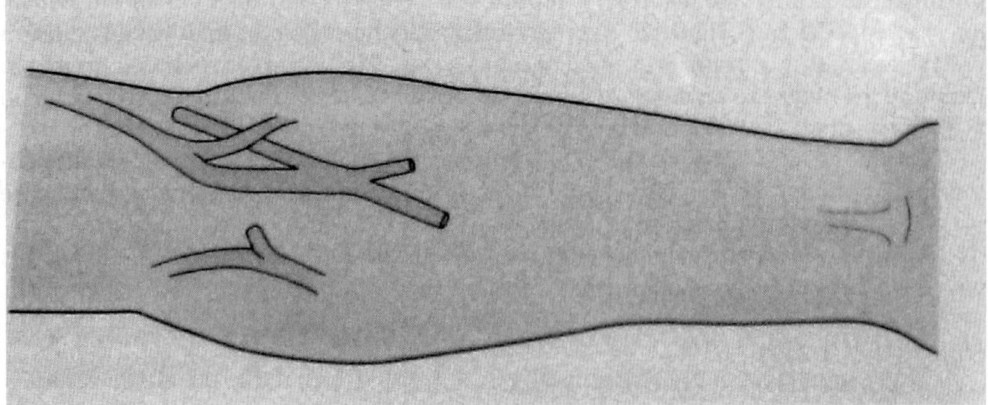

Figure 20-7. Autogenous brachial (or proximal radial)–cephalic upper arm direct access. (Reproduced with permission from Weiswasser JM, Sidawy AN. Strategies of arteriovenous dialysis access. In: Rutherford R, ed. Vascular Surgery, 6th ed. Philadelphia: Elsevier Saunders; 2005, p. 1672.)

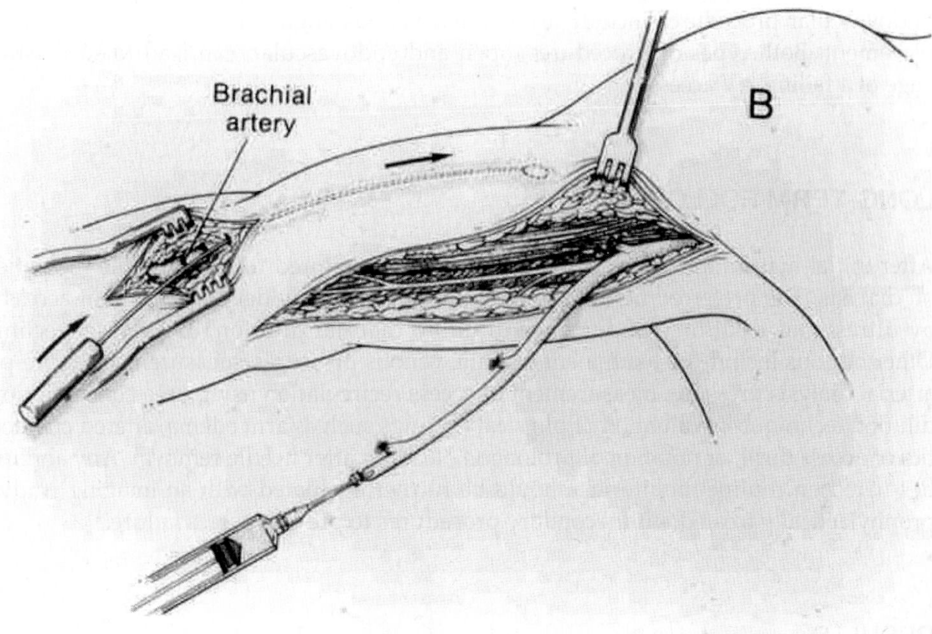

Figure 20-8. Autogenous brachial (or proximal radial)–basilic upper arm transposition.

steal. Therefore, in patients with an adequate basilic vein and an adequate proximal radial artery, an autogenous proximal radial–basilic upper arm transposition (Figure 20–8) is performed. If the proximal radial artery is inadequate and the brachial artery is adequate, an autogenous brachial–basilic upper arm transposition is performed.

Prosthetic Upper Arm Accesses

If no vein is available, an upper arm prosthetic AV access is performed. Similar to upper arm autogenous AV accesses, possible sites of arterial inflow include the proximal radial and brachial arteries. The AV access is placed as distally in the arm as possible, where an adequate artery is identified by preoperative evaluation to lower the risk of arterial steal. Therefore, when the proximal radial artery is adequate, a prosthetic proximal radial–axillary vein (or brachial vein) upper arm straight access is performed. If the proximal radial artery is inadequate and the brachial artery is adequate, a brachial–axillary vein (or brachial vein) upper arm straight access is performed.

POSTOPERATIVE FOLLOW-UP

From the time of the access placement, autogenous AV access should be mature and ready for cannulation by 12 weeks postoperatively and prosthetic AV access should be mature and ready for cannulation by as early as 2 weeks postoperatively. If any access is noted as failing to mature, it should be further examined with access duplex followed by venogram if further information is necessary. Secondary procedures include open surgical or endovascular. Open surgical procedures include vein patches, interposition vein grafts, vein transposition to proximal arteries, branch ligations, and vein superficialization. Endovascular procedures include arterial and venous angioplasties with or without stent placement. Both types of procedures, open and endovascular, can lead to successful salvage of a failing AV access.[18-19]

LONG-TERM FOLLOW-UP

After initial maturation, the AV access should be monitored routinely while the patient is on dialysis. The preferred method of monitoring is monthly determinations of access flow by ultrasound dilution, conductance dilution, thermal dilution, or Doppler technique. Other options include measurement of static venous pressures, measurement of pre-pump arterial dialysis pressure, measurement of access recirculation using urea concentrations or dilution techniques, evaluation of physical findings such as arm edema, altered characteristics of access thrill, or notation of prolonged bleeding after needle removal. Any abnormalities noted on routine monitoring should be further evaluated with an imaging study and prophylactically treated with secondary procedures to prevent access failure.[4]

RESULTS

Autogenous AV access has consistently been shown to have excellent primary and secondary patency rates when compared with prosthetic AV access. One-year primary patency rates of autogenous AV access range from 43 to 85%,[20,27] and 2-year primary patency rates range from 40 to 69%.[21,24,28-29] In comparison, 1-year primary patency rates of prosthetic AV access range from 40 to 54%,[20-21,26-27] and 2-year primary patency rates range from 18 to 30%.[21,28-29] Similarly, secondary patency rates are superior in autogenous access, ranging from 46 to 90%[20-21,24-26] at 1 year and from 62 to 75%[21,28-30] at 2 years; prosthetic access ranges from 59 to 65%[20-21,24] at 1 year and from 40 to 60% at 2 years.[21,28-29] Also of note, in order to maintain these secondary patency rates, prosthetic AV access requires a higher number of interventions than autogenous AV access. These superior patency rates of autogenous access include basilic vein transpositions, which have demonstrated 1-year primary patency rates from 35 to 76%[20,23,25,31-32] and secondary patency rates from 47 to 90%.[20,25,31] A common trade-off for the higher long-term patency rates associated with autogenous AV access is higher primary failure rates due to failure of access maturation or primary thrombosis. Initial success rates leading to a functional AV access range from 55 to 97%.[22-25,28] These poor maturation rates do appear to correspond to the increasing use of small and suboptimal veins for autogenous access.

NONTHROMBOTIC COMPLICATIONS OF AV ACCESS

In addition to its superior patency rate, multiple nonthrombotic AV access complications may be avoided with the use of autogenous access. Venous hypertension occurs irrespective of whether an autogenous or prosthetic access is placed and is due to subclavian vein or outflow stenosis with valvular incompetence; subclavian vein stenosis is seen anatomically in up to 50% of patients; of these, 15 to 20% will become clinically symptomatic.[33-34]

Similarly, arterial steal occurs in both autogenous and prosthetic access and is due to low access track resistance along with arterial occlusive disease; it occurs in up to 10% of all access placed, more so in accesses based on upper arm arteries, and it is commonly asymptomatic.[35] Ischemic monomelic neuropathy is a form of arterial steal that is seen rarely; it affects nerves only and if left untreated may lead to hand paralysis.[36] High-output congestive heart failure is secondary to decreased total peripheral resistance and is seen in 2 to 4% of accesses placed.[37] Access infection is most commonly due to *Staphylococcus aureus* but can be caused by multiple organisms; one of the biggest advantages of autogenous access is average infection rates of 5%, which are clearly superior to infection rates of 20% seen with prosthetic accesses.[8] Pseudoaneurysms are due to repeated punctures of the same access site; they also are seen much more frequently in prosthetic access with an occurrence rate of 5 to 11% compared with an average rate of 3% seen in autogenous access.[38] Seromas occur almost exclusively in prosthetic access (0.5 to 4.0% of patients); they are thought to be due to transudation of serous fluid through porous grafts.[39-40]

REFERENCES

1. Incidence & Prevalence. In: U.S. Renal Data System, USRDS 2007 Annual Report: Atlas of Chronic Kidney Disease and End-Stage Renal Disease in the United States, National Institutes of Health, National Institute of Diabetes and Digestive and Kidney Disease, Bethesda, MD, 2007. www.usrds.org/2007/view/02_incid_prev.asp Accessed 6/18/08.
2. Costs of CKD & ESRD. In: U.S. Renal Data System, USRDS 2007 Annual Report: Atlas of Chronic Kidney Disease and End-Stage Renal Disease in the United States, National Institutes of Health, National Institute of Diabetes and Digestive and Kidney Disease, Bethesda, MD, 2007. www.usrds.org/2007/view/11_econ Accessed 6/18/08.
3. Sidawy AN, Spergel LM, Besarab A, et al. The Society for Vascular Surgery: clinical practice guidelines for the surgical placement and maintenance of arteriovenous hemodialysis access. J Vasc Surg 2008;48:2S–25S.
4. http://www.kidney.org/professionals/KDOQI/guidelines.cfm Accessed 4/25/08.
5. Salgado OJ, Urdaneta B, Colmenares B, et al. Right versus left internal jugular vein catheterization for hemodialysis: complications and impact on ipsilateral access creation. Artif Organs 2004;28:728–33.
6. Moss AH, McLaughlin MM, Lempert KD, Holley JL. Use of a silicone catheter with a Dacron cuff for dialysis short-term vascular access. Am J Kidney Dis 1988;12:49–98.
7. Spinowitz BS, Galler M, Golden RA, et al. Subclavian vein stenosis as a complication of subclavian catheterization for hemodialysis. Arch Intern Med 1987;147:305–7.
8. Saad T. Bacteremia associated with tunneled, cuffed hemodialysis catheters. Am J Kidney Dis 1999;34:1114–24.
9. Jefferys A, Chow J, Suranyi M. Acute vascular access catheters for haemodialysis: complications limiting technique survival. Nephrology 2003;8:16–20.
10. Cimochowski GE, Worley E, Rutherford WE, et al. Superiority of the internal jugular over the subclavian access for temporary dialysis. Nephron 1990;54:154–61.
11. Schillinger F, Schillinger D, Montagnac R, Milcent T. Post catheterisation vein stenosis in haemodialysis: comparative angiographic study of 50 subclavian and 50 internal jugular accesses. Nephrol Dial Transplant 1991;6:722–4.
12. Silva MB, Hobson RW, Pappas PJ, et al. A strategy for increasing use of autogenous hemodialysis access procedures: Impact of preoperative noninvasive evaluation. J Vasc Surg 1998;27:302–7.
13. Kimmel M, Butscheid M, Brenner S, et al. Improved estimation of glomerular filtration rate by serum cystatin C in preventing contrast induced nephropathy by N-acetylcysteine or zinc-preliminary results. Nephrol Dial Transplant 2008;23:124–45.

14. Stenstrom DA, Muldoon LL, Armijo-Medina H, et al. N-Acetylcysteine use to prevent contrast medium-induced nephropathy: premature phase III trials. J Vasc Interv Radiol 2008;19: 309–18.
15. Kelly AM, Kwamena B, Cronin P, et al. Meta-analysis: Effectiveness of drugs for preventing contrast-induced nephropathy. Ann Intern Med 2008;148:284–94.
16. Morcos SK. Prevention of contrast media-induced nephrotoxicity after angiographic procedures. J Vasc Interv Radiol 2005;16:13–23.
17. Passman MA, Criado E, Farber MA, et al. Efficacy of color flow duplex imaging for proximal upper extremity venous outflow obstruction in hemodialysis patients. J Vasc Surg 1998;28:869–75.
18. McLafferty RB, Pryor RW, Johnson CM, et al. Outcome of a comprehensive follow-up program to enhance maturation of autogenous arteriovenous hemodialysis access. J Vasc Surg 2007;45:981–5.
19. Berman SS, Gentile AT. Impact of secondary procedures in autogenous arteriovenous fistula maturation and maintenance. J Vasc Surg 2001;34:866–71.
20. Choe HM, Lal B, Cerveira JJ, et al. Durability and cumulative functional patency of transposed and nontransposed arteriovenous fistulas. J Vasc Surg 2003;38:1206–12.
21. Huber TS, Carter JW, Carter RL, Seeger JM. Patency of autogenous and polytetrafluoroethylene upper extremity arteriovenous hemodialysis accesses: a systematic review. J Vasc Surg 2003;38:1005–11.
22. Silva MB, Hobson RW, Pappas PJ, et al. Vein transposition in the forearm for autogenous hemodialysis access. J Vasc Surg 1997;26:981–6.
23. Obialo CI, Tagoe AT, Martin PC, Asche-Crowe PE. Adequacy and survival of autogenous arteriovenous fistula in African American hemodialysis patients. ASAIO J 2003;49: 435–9.
24. Rooijens PP, Tordoir JH, Stijnen T, et al. Radiocephalic wrist arteriovenous fistula for hemodialysis: meta-analysis indicates a high primary failure rate. Eur J Vasc Endovasc Surg 2004;28:583–9.
25. Keuter XH, van der Sande FM, Kessels AG, et al. Excellent performance of one-stage brachial-basilic arteriovenous fistula. Nephrol Dial Transplant 2005;20:2168–71.
26. Hodges TC, Fillinger MF, Zwolak RM, et al. Longitudinal comparison of dialysis access methods: risk factors for failure. J Vasc Surg 1997;26:1009–19.
27. Ascher E, Gade P, Hingorani A, et al. Changes in the practice of angioaccess surgery: impact of dialysis outcome and quality initiative recommendations. J Vasc Surg 2000;31: 84–92.
28. Gibson KD, Gillen DL, Capt MT, et al. Vascular access survival and incidence of revisions: a comparison of prosthetic grafts, simple autogenous fistulas, and venous transposition fistulas from the United States renal data system dialysis morbidity and mortality study. J Vasc Surg 2001;34:694–700.
29. Kalman, PG, Pope M, Bhola C, et al. A practical approach to vascular access for hemodialysis and predictors of success. J Vasc Surg 1999;30:727–33.
30. Wolford HY, Hsu J, Rhodes JM, et al. Outcome after autogenous brachial-basilic upper arm transpositions in the post-National Kidney Foundation Dialysis Outcomes Quality Initiative era. J Vasc Surg 2005;42:951–6.
31. Rao, RK, Azin GD, Hood D, et al. Basilic vein transposition fistula: a good option for maintaining hemodialysis access site options? J Vasc Surg 2004;39:1043–7.
32. Casey K, Tonnessen BH, Mannava K, et al. Brachial versus basilic vein dialysis fistulas: a comparison of maturation and patency rates. J Vasc Surg 2008;47:402–6.
33. Vanherweghem JL, Yassine T, Goldman M, et al. Subclavian vein thrombosis: a frequent complication of subclavian vein cannulation for hemodialysis. Clin Nephrol 1986;26:235–8.
34. Barrett N, Spencer S, McIvor J, Brown EA. Subclavian stenosis: a major complication of subclavian dialysis catheters. Nephrol Dial Transplant 1988;3:423–5.
35. Murphy GJ, White SA, Nicholson ML. Vascular access for haemodialysis. Br J Surg 2000; 87:1300–15.

36. Wilbourn AJ, Furlan AJ, Hulley W, Ruschhaupt W. Ischemic monomelic neuropathy. Neurology 1983;33:447–51.
37. Taylor SM, Eaves FL, Weatherford DA, et al. Results and complications of arteriovenous access dialysis grafts in the lower extremity: a five year review. Am Surg 1996;62:188–91.
38. Lenz BJ, Veldenz HC, Dennis JW, et al. A three-year follow-up on standard versus thin wall ePTFE grafts for hemodialysis. J Vasc Surg 1998;28:464–70.
39. Ahn SS, Machleder HI, Gupta R. Perigraft seroma: clinical, histologic, and serologic correlates. Am J Surg 1987;154:173–8.
40. Szilagyi DE. In discussion of Kaupp et al. Graft infection or graft rejection? Arch Surg 1979;114:1422.

21

Management of Access-Related Hand Ischemia

Thomas S. Huber, M.D., Ph.D.

Hand ischemia is one of the most troublesome or worrisome adverse outcomes after an upper extremity arteriovenous hemodialysis access. In the most extreme situations, it can result in gangrene and/or a nonfunctional hand requiring amputation. However, it is somewhat debatable whether it represents a true "complication" or, more appropriately, an adverse, hemodynamic outcome within the standard of care. Regardless, it is incumbent upon all access surgeons to be familiar with every aspect of its management, including the preoperative predictors, definitive diagnostic approach, and the various treatment options.

DEFINITIONS AND CLASSIFICATION

A variety of different terms and acronyms have been used to describe access-related hand ischemia including ARI (access-related ischemia), ARHI (access-related hand ischemia), ISS (ischemic steal syndrome), DASS (dialysis-associated steal syndrome), HAIDI (hemodialysis access–induced distal ischemia), and DHIS (distal hypoperfusion ischemic syndrome). The most commonly used descriptive term is simply "steal syndrome." However, this is a misnomer, because there is nothing particularly "illegal" about the phenomenon in that the blood flow (including any "alleged" diversion of flow from the hand) simply follows the pressure gradients and obeys the underlying hemodynamic principles. The reporting standards from the Society for Vascular Surgery define "steal syndrome" among the remote complications after hemodialysis access procedures and classify the severity using a scale ranging from 0-3 (0-none; 1-mild, cool extremity with few symptoms; 2-moderate, intermittent ischemia during dialysis; and 3-severe, ischemic pain at rest/ tissue loss).[1]

PATHOPHYSIOLOGY AND RISK FACTORS

The construction of a direct communication between the artery and vein (i.e., arteriovenous fistula) establishes a low-resistance circuit through which the blood flow is preferentially directed based upon the pressure gradients (Figure 21–1). The blood flow in the arterial segment immediately distal to the fistula can be directed retrograde, antegrade, or "to and fro" based upon the timing of the cardiac cycle, again, as dictated by the pressure gradients. The perfusion of the tissues distal to the fistula (i.e., the hand) is maintained by the recruitment of collateral channels and peripheral vasodilation. Given these mechanisms, it is not surprising that the arterial pressure and blood flow at the wrist and digits (i.e., distal to the fistula) decrease in most cases. Notably, Papasavas and associates[2] reported that the digital/brachial index (DBI) decreased in 80% of patients after an ipsilateral arteriovenous access. This "physiologic steal" syndrome is tolerated in the majority of cases but becomes problematic (or patients develop hand ischemia) when the compensatory changes are inadequate to meet the metabolic needs of the tissue. Within this context, it is easy to see how a

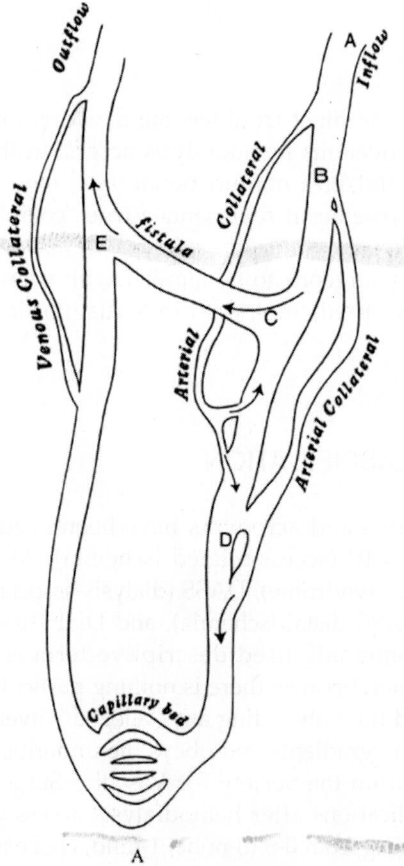

Figure 21-1. A representative diagram of an autogenous arteriovenous hemodialysis access is shown. Note the retrograde blood flow through the anastomosis from the arterial segment immediately distal to the anastomosis. The perfusion of the tissues distal to the anastomosis is supplied predominantly by the arterial collaterals. (Reproduced with permission from Wixon CL, et al. Understanding strategies for the treatment of ischemic steal syndrome after hemodialysis access. J Am Coll Surg 2000;191:301–10.)

significant arterial occlusive lesion in the inflow (i.e., proximal to the fistula) or outflow (i.e., distal to the fistula) vessels could potentially exacerbate the hemodynamic changes. The low-resistance/high-flow fistula can cause an energy loss or pressure drop across an inflow lesion similar to the underlying mechanisms of a peripheral vasodilator challenge (e.g., papaverine) used to interrogate the hemodynamic significance of an aortoiliac stenosis. Significant arterial occlusive disease in the forearm or hand, commonly seen in the diabetic population, can further exacerbate the drop in pressure from the fistula alone and inhibit the compensatory responses.

Some type of ARHI (grades 1-3) can occur in up to 20% of patients after a brachial artery–based arteriovenous access, although the incidence of symptoms (grades 2-3) that merits intervention is roughly half or 10%.[2-9] Indeed, Keuter et al.[3] prospectively documented the incidence of hand ischemia after brachial artery–based procedures using clinical and noninvasive examinations and reported that 28% of the patients developed ischemic symptoms but only 10% required intervention. ARHI can occur after radial artery–based procedures, although the incidence is significantly less and treatment is rarely required.[10-11] The responsible mechanisms in this setting are slightly different and are due predominantly to retrograde perfusion of the fistula from the ulnar artery and palmar arch.

The natural history of ARHI is poorly documented and subject to a certain degree of selection bias, because all patients with grade 3 ischemia (severe) and some of those with grade 2 (moderate) undergo definitive treatment. It has been my anecdotal impression that the mild ischemic symptoms can resolve over time, presumably secondary to arterial remodeling and collateral recruitment. However, the mild symptoms can progress to more advanced grades of ischemia and, therefore, merit close observation. In our series of patients requiring revascularization for ARHI, 44% of the remedial procedures were performed >30 days after the index access procedure as a result of progression of the initial complaints.[12] It has also been my anecdotal impression that the moderate and severe symptoms do not improve without some type of intervention. Notably, Papasavas et al.[2] reported no additional decreases in the DBI after a month despite the significant early drop noted above. Scheltinga and associates[13] performed a systematic review of the literature to identify the relationship between the type of access and the onset of ischemic symptoms and reported that prosthetic accesses were associated with acute symptoms (<24 hr) whereas autogenous accesses were associated with chronic symptoms (>1 mo). Interestingly, van Hoek and associates[14] reported a single case study of a pediatric patient with retarded hand growth presumed secondary to a functional access, a mechanism likely similar to the limb-length discrepancy seen in children after unrepaired femoral artery catheter injuries.

A variety of clinical risk factors have been identified as predictors of ARHI, including advanced age, diabetes mellitus, female gender, peripheral vascular occlusive disease, use of large conduits/veins, multiple prior access procedures, and prior episodes.[6,8,15-18] Indeed, it has been our anecdotal impression that the incidence of hand ischemia is almost 100% in patients with a prior episode. This emphasizes the importance of identifying any potential contributing factors (e.g., subclavian artery stenosis) in this subset of patients and underscores the potential problem with ligating and resiting the access in a patient with hand ischemia (due to the high likelihood that it will occur again in the absence of a contributing factor). Unfortunately, the clinical predictors, even in aggregate, cannot predict when ARHI is inevitable and the procedure should be avoided. However, they can be used to "heighten the awareness" about the potential outcome and the need for vigilance in the perioperative period.

Similar to the clinical predictors, the utility of preoperative noninvasive vascular laboratory studies has been somewhat inconclusive as a tool to identify patients in whom ARHI is inevitable. Valentine et al.[18] prospectively examined patients undergoing brachial artery–based access procedures and reported that there was not an absolute finger pressure or DBI below which hand ischemia was inevitable, although they did report that patients with hand ischemia had lower values. Goff et al.[19] identified a DBI threshold of <0.6 during a retrospective review and prospectively studied whether this could be used *intraoperatively* to identify patients who would develop hand ischemia. Unfortunately, they concluded that it was not predictive but stated that it was a helpful target for patients requiring remedial treatment. Collectively, reduced finger pressures or DBIs can be used as additional predictors in concert with the clinical ones outlined above, but the absolute threshold value is unclear (i.e., DBI <0.45, <0.6, <1.0).[18-20]

CLINICAL PRESENTATION AND DIAGNOSIS

Patients with ARHI present with the traditional symptoms of either acute (6 P's: pain, paresthesia, paralysis, pulselessness, poikilothermia, pallor) or chronic (rest pain, tissue loss) ischemia similar to those of patients with lower extremity occlusive disease. As noted above, approximately half of our patients who required revascularization presented >30 days after the index procedure.[12] Notably, the majority of the patients who presented acutely underwent remedial revascularization within 7 days (<1 day: 19%; 1 to 7 days: 29%). It is not uncommon for these more "acute" patients to emerge from anesthesia complaining of hand pain with some type of motor or sensory compromise. The spectrum of ischemic symptoms can range from mild paresthesia to profound motor compromise. The diagnosis is fairly straightforward in the latter situation but may be more difficult in the earlier stages.

The diagnosis can usually be made based upon the history and physical examination, with additional imaging (noninvasive or invasive) reserved for equivocal cases. The differential diagnosis of postoperative hand pain/problems after an arteriovenous access is fairly limited and includes hand ischemia, peripheral neuropathy, and carpal tunnel syndrome.[21] However, foremost on this list is ARHI, and I have joked with our vascular residents that the differential diagnosis is "hand ischemia, hand ischemia, and hand ischemia." It is important to ask patients about their dialysis runs, because it is not uncommon for patients with borderline perfusion to develop symptoms on dialysis due to the associated hypotension and hypovolemia. The physical examination can occasionally confound the diagnosis, particularly for less-experienced clinicians, because it is possible to have an ischemic hand despite a palpable radial or ulnar pulse. Although a palpable pulse and an ischemic hand seem contradictory, all postoperative hand symptoms must be ascribed to ischemia until proved otherwise. Additional imaging can be helpful in this setting to support or refute the diagnosis. Although completely normal upper extremity noninvasive studies (symmetric wrist/digital pressures, triphasic radial/ulnar waveforms, normal finger photo plethysmographies (PPGs) may exclude the diagnosis, the more common scenario is to find diminished wrist pressures and a mono- or biphasic Doppler waveform (Figure 21–2). The diagnosis can be further confirmed using catheter-based or CT arteriography with the reduction or absence of contrast flow distal to the access anastomosis (Figure 21–3).

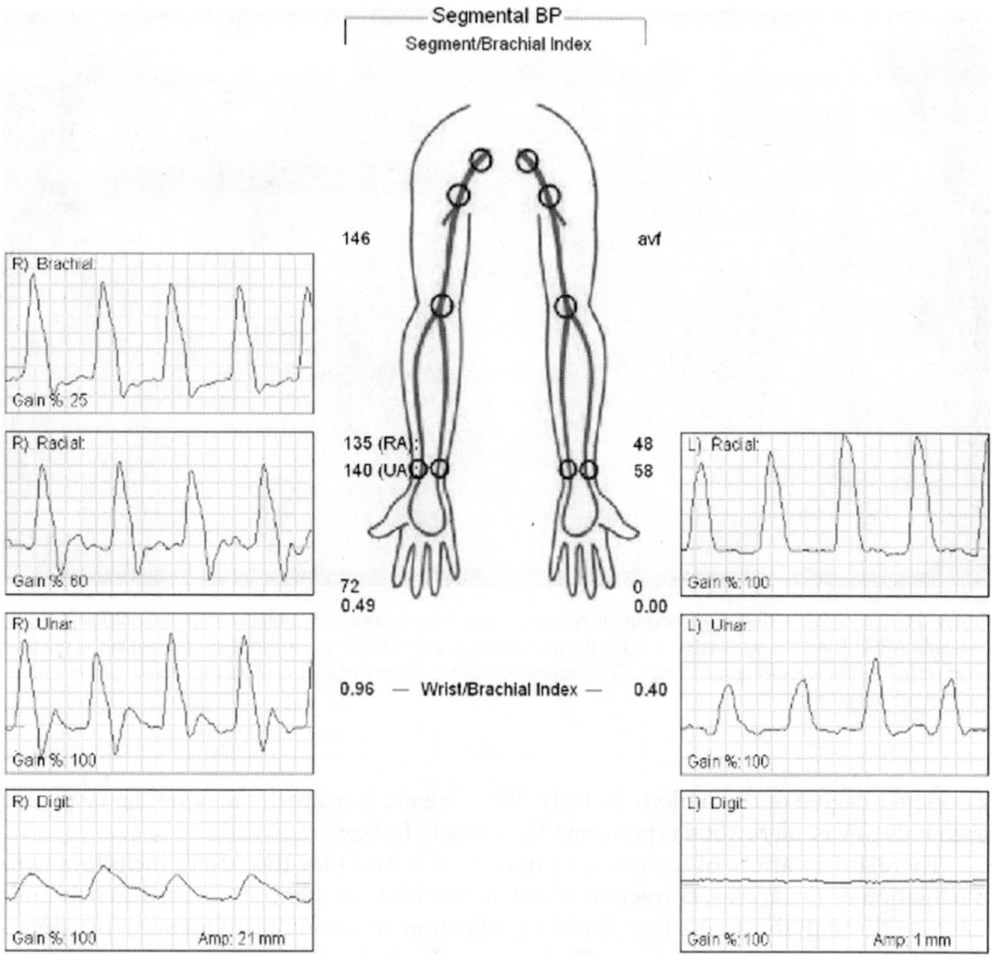

Figure 21-2. The upper extremity arterial pressures and the corresponding waveforms are shown for a patient with access-related hand ischemia (ARHI). Note the diminished pressures and waveforms on the affected side with the corresponding wrist/brachial index. The digital pressures are 0 and the digital waveforms are flat. A DBI was not calculated given the fact that the digital pressures are 0.

However, catheter-based arteriography has largely been relegated to a therapeutic study rather than a diagnostic one.

INDICATIONS AND TREATMENT STRATEGIES

The treatment goals for patients with ARHI are to reverse the underlying process and to salvage the access. However, it should be emphasized that treating the hand ischemia is foremost and that simply ligating the access will reverse the symptoms, presuming that it is performed in a timely fashion. As noted above, the natural history of ARHI is not well described, but all patients with grade 3 or severe ischemic symptoms merit definitive treatment and the majority of those with grade 2 or moderate symptoms likely merit treatment. The treatment decision is often based upon the severity of the patient's symptoms and their

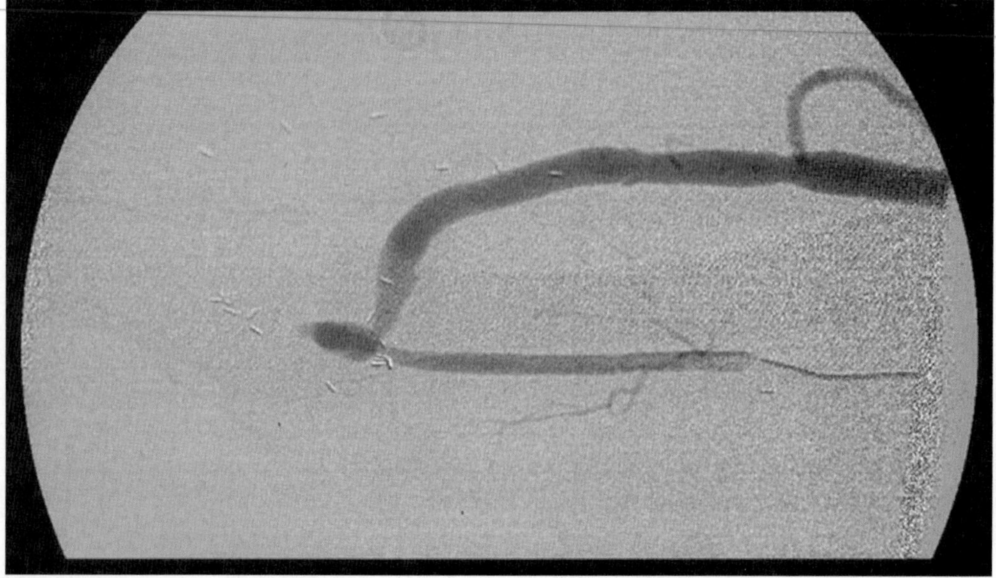

Figure 21-3. A catheter-based arteriogram is demonstrated for a patient with a brachiocephalic autogenous access and ARHI. The catheter is positioned in the mid-brachial artery. Note the absence of contrast in the brachial artery distal to the access anastomosis. The patient subsequently underwent a DRIL procedure with improvement of his symptoms.

associated degree of discomfort. Notably, the ischemic neuropathy may not be reversible even if the revascularization is performed in a timely fashion.

There are a variety of treatment options (Table 21–1) for the ARHI, including simple ligation of the access, correction of any arterial inflow stenoses, procedures to limit the flow through the access (e.g., banding, plication, anastomotic reduction), proximalization of the arterial anastomosis (PAI, Figure 21–4), ligation of the axial artery distal to the anastomosis, distal revascularization and interval ligation (DRIL, Figure 21–5), distal revascularization without ligation, and revascularization with distal inflow. Similar to other situations in which there are multiple treatment options, no single one has emerged as the definitive treatment. Indeed, they all have some advantages or disadvantages and should be viewed as complementary with different specific indications based upon the scenario.

TABLE 21-1. POTENTIAL TREATMENT OPTIONS FOR ACCESS-RELATED HAND ISCHEMIA

Access ligation
Correction of arterial inflow stenosis/occlusion
Flow-limiting procedures (banding, outflow reduction, anastomosis reduction)
Proximalization of arterial anastomosis (PAI)
Revascularization with distal inflow
Ligation of artery distal to anastomosis
Distal revascularization and interval ligation (DRIL)
Distal revascularization without interval ligation

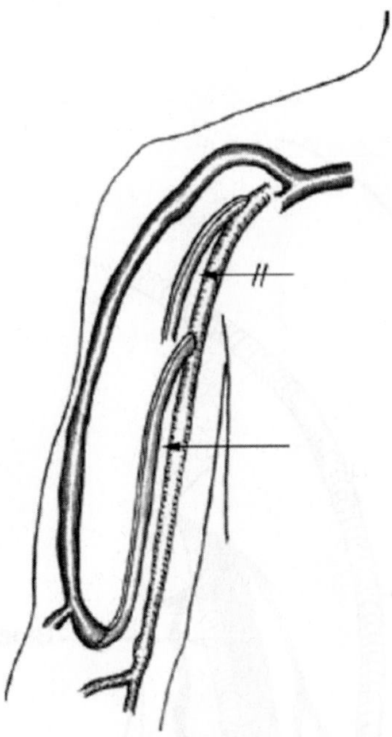

Figure 21-4. The technique described by Zanow et al.[36] for the proximalization of the arterial inflow (PAI) is shown for a brachiocephalic autogenous access. Note that the autogenous access has been dissembled and an interposition graft (4 or 5 mm PTFE) has been inserted between the more proximal brachial artery and the proximal segment of the original autogenous access. (Reproduced with permission from Zanow J, et al. Proximalization of the arterial inflow: a new technique to treat access-related ischemia. J Vasc Surg 2006; 43:1216–21.)

An appreciation of the various treatment options can be obtained by reviewing their associated hemodynamic changes. Indeed, Zanow and associates[22] have constructed a pulsatile flow circuit of an upper extremity arteriovenous access complete with collateral channels to examine these changes. Not surprisingly, they found that a decrease in the flow through the fistula (i.e., "flow-limiting" strategy) improved the distal perfusion. Placing the arteriovenous anastomosis more proximally on the arterial tree also improved the distal perfusion, whereas ligating the axial artery immediately distal to the anastomosis in an attempt to limit the retrograde perfusion had little effect. Both the DRIL and PAI resulted in a dramatic improvement in the distal perfusion, with the PAI having the greatest benefit. Interestingly, the ligation component of the DRIL only increased distal flow 10% and the overall benefit of the DRIL was reduced at higher access flow rates. Similarly, Gradman and Pozrikidis[23] constructed a flow model based upon an electrical analogue to simulate a brachioaxillary prosthetic arteriovenous access and reported that the DRIL, distal revascularization without ligation, and conversion to an axilloaxillary configuration (PAI equivalent) had the greatest impact (listed in descending order). Admittedly, these observations are based upon ex vivo models, although the theoretical calculations were supported in two patients treated for ARHI in the report by Gradman and Pozrikidis.[23] Notably, Illig et al.[24] measured arterial pressures and flow rates in nine patients undergoing the DRIL procedure. They reported that there was a "pressure sink" in the brachial artery with a mean pressure of 102±17 mm Hg in the proximal brachial artery that decreased to 47±38 mm Hg at the arteriovenous anastomosis and that the flow in the brachial

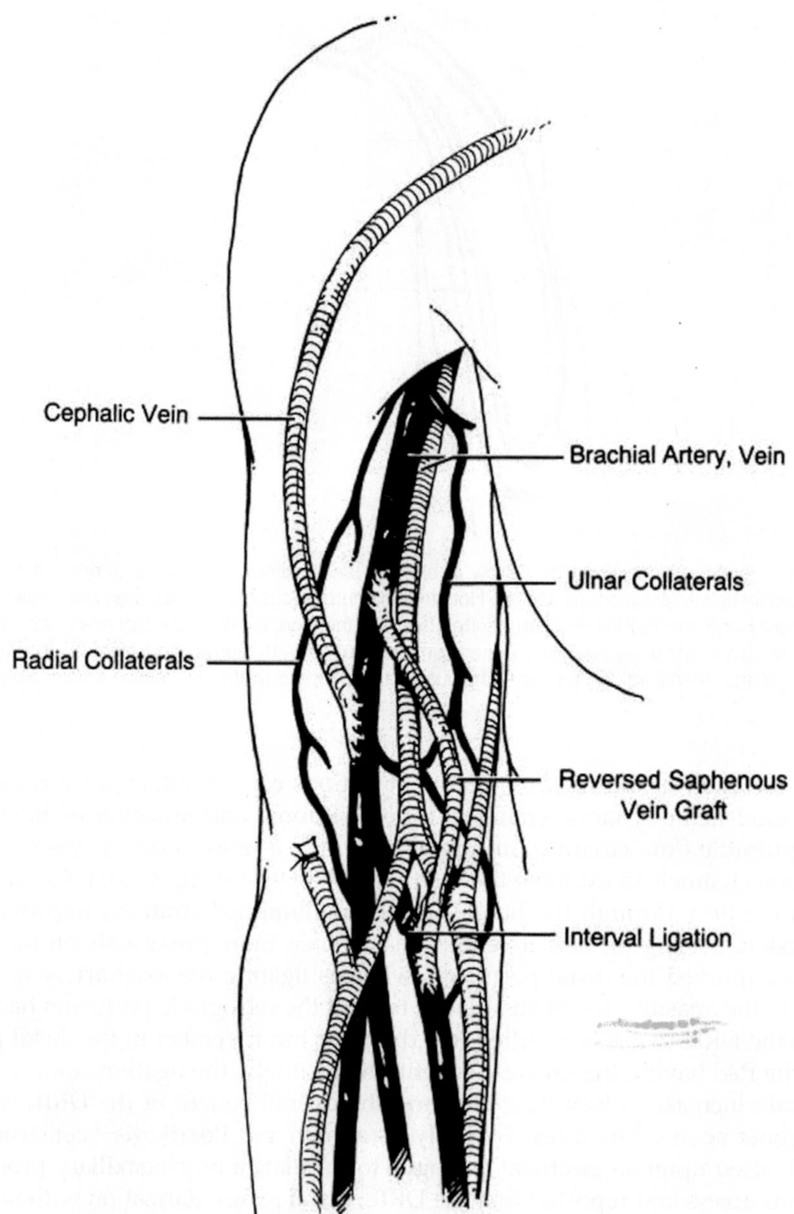

Figure 21-5. A diagram of a distal revascularization and interval ligation (DRIL) procedure is shown for a patient with an autogenous brachiocephalic hemodialysis access. Note the brachial-radial saphenous vein graft and the ligature on the proximal radial artery. (Reproduced with permission from Berman SS, et al. Distal revascularization-interval ligation for limb salvage and maintenance of dialysis access in ischemic steal syndrome. J Vasc Surg 1997;26:393–404.)

artery distal to the anastomosis was retrograde when the fistula was open. Following the DRIL procedure, the pressure gradient in the brachial artery was essentially unchanged. However, the pressure in the brachial artery bypass and the brachial artery distal to the ligation were now 104±27 mm Hg; these values did not change with compression of the arteriovenous fistula.

The ultimate clinical decision about the remedial treatment is contingent upon a variety of factors independent of the advantages/disadvantages outlined above. These include the underlying cause of the ischemia, the utility/potential utility of the access, future access options, patient comorbidities, and available conduit. Clearly, any contributory arterial inflow lesion should be corrected, and this is often a relatively easy solution for patients with proximal subclavian artery stenoses. In our own series,[12] hemodynamically significant inflow lesions were a relatively minor contributor, but this is likely secondary to our preoperative noninvasive algorithm that included arterial pressures and waveforms. Several other publications have emphasized the importance of inflow lesions as an underlying mechanism.[25-27] Regardless, an arteriogram (catheter-based or CT) should likely be part of the diagnostic/therapeutic algorithm.

Several investigators have attempted to classify ARHI into "high flow" or "low flow," although the absolute threshold for differentiating these states and their clinical significance remain unresolved.[28-30] Clearly, the flow rates in the fistula contribute to the hemodynamic changes, although it is unclear whether they are independent of the other factors involved in the adaptive/maladaptive responses.[28] Regardless, some type of "flow-limiting" procedure should be considered in this "high-flow" setting, particularly given the ex vivo observations highlighted above that the DRIL procedure may not be as effective in this scenario.[22]

The utility or potential utility of the access procedure itself is central to the treatment algorithm for the ARHI. Admittedly, this concern is somewhat irrelevant for patients with a functional autogenous access and chronic hand ischemia. However, it is very pertinent for patients with acute symptoms and either a prosthetic or an autogenous access and those with chronic symptoms and a prosthetic access. The treatment choice represents a balance between the likelihood (and potential duration) of the access being functional and the added morbidity associated with the remedial procedure. In our systemic review, the annual primary patency rates for autogenous and prosthetic access were only 60% and 40% respectively, whereas the secondary rates were 80% and 60%.[31] Furthermore, Dember and associates[32] reported from the Dialysis Access Consortium that their autogenous access maturation rate was only 40%. Although there are no absolutes, I favor revascularization (usually DRIL) for patients with acute symptoms and a reasonable autogenous access and access ligation for those with a prosthetic access. Notably, patients who develop acute symptoms after an autogenous access usually have a relatively large vein that is a major contributing factor, but it is these large veins that are more likely to mature. I have performed remedial revascularizations on patents with chronic ischemia and a function prosthetic access when it appeared that the access was going to function for a reasonable length of time.

Among the various remedial treatment options, the strategies to limit the flow through the access have been the most controversial. Although largely abandoned, they have made a comeback more recently. The fundamental problem with all of the various "flow-limiting" approaches (i.e., inflow reduction, anastomotic narrowing, outflow reduction) is striking the tenuous balance between reducing the flow sufficient to maintain distal perfusion and ensuring longer-term access patency. Furthermore, the biologic behavior and/or the associated hemodynamics may change over time (e.g., inflow artery dilation, outflow vein dilation) and, therefore, the assumptions and modifications made intraoperatively may not be sustained. Notably, the flow through a large arteriovenous fistula is independent of the communication between the vessels once the anastomosis exceeds 75% of the arterial diameter, thereby demonstrating the futility of attempting to narrow the anastomosis; reducing the anastomosis length of a brachiocephalic access to <75% for a 3-mm vessel will likely result in early thrombosis.

Part of the resurgence of these "flow-limiting" approaches has been predicated upon the use of objective measurements to quantify distal perfusion[33] and access flow.[29-30,34] Notably, Zanow et al.[30] reported a series of 95 patients with "high-flow" accesses (autogenous >800 mL/min, prosthetic >1200 mL/min) that underwent flow-directed narrowing of their access using a combination of a plicating suture line and a prosthetic cuff (Figure 21–6). Long-term relief of symptoms was achieved in 86% of the patients. Their target flow rates were 400 mL/min for the autogenous accesses and 600 mL/min for the prosthetic ones, although they stated in the discussion of their manuscript that a target of 750 mL/min may be more appropriate for the prosthetic accesses. Scheltinga and associates[29] performed a systematic review of "banding" as a "flow-reduction" procedure and reported that the success rate was <50% if performed without the guidance of flow measurements or digital pressures. However, they concluded that it was very effective when flow rate was monitored and that it was the procedure of choice for "high-flow" accesses (i.e., >1.2 mL/min). Last, Thermann et

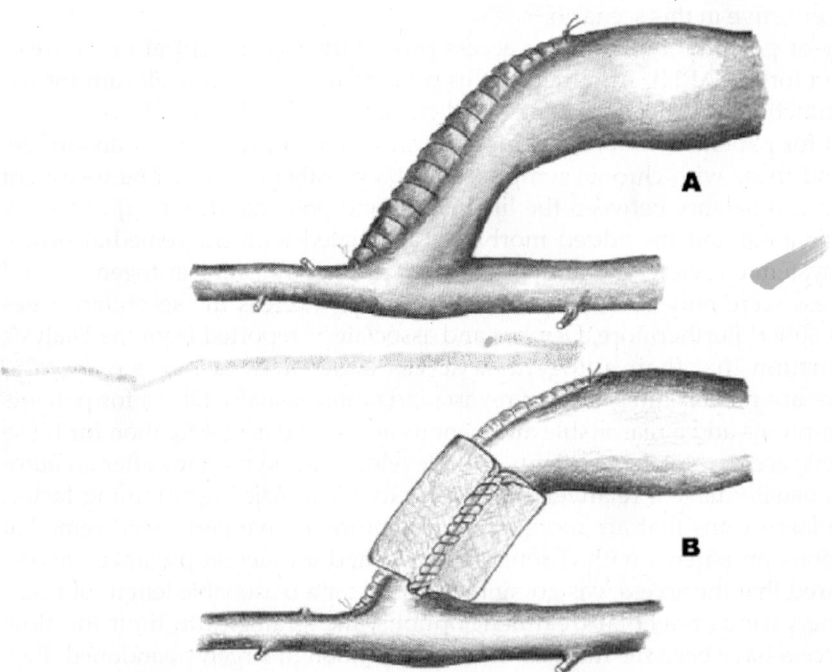

Figure 21-6. The technique described by Zanow et al.[30] to narrow the proximal autogenous access is illustrated. A. A continuous suture is used to narrow the proximal portion of the access. B. An ePTFE "cuff" is placed around the access at the proximal portion of the suture line to prevent further access dilation. (Reproduced with permission from Zanow J, et al. Flow reduction in high-flow arteriovenous access using intraoperative flow monitoring. J Vasc Surg 2006;44:1273–8.)

al.[35] reported that flow-directed banding was effective in the setting of mild, short duration skin lesions but ineffective for longer-term lesions and those with more extensive tissue loss. They concluded that more complex surgical solutions may be required in the setting of these more chronic, extensive lesions.

Proximalization of the arterial inflow or the PAI procedure (see Figure 21–3) likely represents a variant of the "flow-limiting" procedures. Although the technique does involve resiting the access anastomosis more proximal on the arterial tree, Zanow and associates[36] contended that the predominant benefit is from the flow reduction through the small-diameter prosthetic conduit. The technique has some appeal because it does not require ligating an axial artery, and it may be suitable in patients who do not have an adequate autogenous conduit for a DRIL procedure. However, the published experience is limited despite the overall magnitude of ARHI as a clinical problem. Furthermore, it requires converting an autogenous access to a composite prosthetic/autogenous access and, therefore, increases the infectious and thrombotic complications with the latter, which is particularly worrisome given the caliber of the graft (i.e., 4 or 5 mm expanded polytetrafluoroethylene (ePTFE). Notably, Zanow et al.[36] reported that the procedure was associated with the resolution of symptoms in 84% of their cases (n=30) and that the patency rates were excellent. They concluded that it was a good alternative to the DRIL procedure and recommended its use for ARHI resulting from lower flow states (i.e., autogenous access <800 mL/min, prosthetic access <1000 mL/min). Thermann and Wollert[37] reported complete resolution of symptoms in 65% of their cases encompassing both wrist (N=5) and brachial artery–based access procedures (N=18). They reported that the procedure was associated with increased radial artery flow and decreased access flow but concluded that it was not effective for patients with severe tissue loss.

A variant of the PAI procedure has been described that involves using a distal inflow site originating from the radial artery (i.e., RUDI: revision using distal inflow).[38-39] Similar to the PAI, it maintains flow through the axial arteries. However, the radial artery is not an ideal inflow source in most patients, particularly in diabetic patients with the typical forearm arterial occlusive disease.

The DRIL (see Figure 21–4) procedure likely represents the best option for most patients with ARHI and has withstood the proverbial "test of time" in terms of relief of symptoms and access salvage. However, it is worth emphasizing that Schanzer et al.[40] only first described the procedure in 1988 and the overall published experience is somewhat limited. The theoretical limitations of the procedure include the need to ligate the axial artery and the fact that the hand perfusion is dependent upon the brachial artery bypass. The hemodynamic modeling has suggested that the contribution of the "ligation" to the distal perfusion is relatively modest.[22,41] However, the clinical experience with distal revascularization alone without the interval ligation has been limited.[42]

It is worthwhile emphasizing that the management or treatment of ARHI really begins during the preoperative evaluation. The likelihood of hand ischemia should be determined with each access procedure based upon the clinical predictors outlined above and any preventive strategies to reduce the incidence should be implemented. All potential inflow arterial stenoses should be identified and corrected. The operative procedure should be selected or designed to minimize the risk of ischemia in patients deemed "at risk." This potentially includes using a small-diameter conduit (e.g., 3 mm cephalic vein vs. 6 mm basilic vein) where applicable and/or placing the arterial anastomosis as proximal as possible (e.g., proximal brachial artery vs. distal brachial artery). A remedial plan should be generated in the operating room at the time of the index procedure to address the potential hand ischemia. I frequently challenge our vascular residents during the access procedure to outline their plan to deal with the anticipated phone call from the recovery room nurse stating that the patient cannot move his or her hand and is complaining of significant pain. Occasionally, I obtain a saphenous vein survey during the preoperative work-up to identify all potential conduits for a DRIL. In the most extreme circumstances, we have performed a preemptive DRIL procedure at the time of the index access, although these have been reserved for patients with significant ipsilateral tissue loss or prior ARHI that necessitated treatment.

UNIVERSITY OF FLORIDA DRIL EXPERIENCE

We have recently documented our experience with the DRIL procedure, and indeed, it represents the largest single institutional series.[12] All patients undergoing any permanent hemodialysis access procedure between February 1998 and December 2007 were identified by review of a prospectively maintained procedural database. The patients requiring definitive treatment (i.e., ligation or DRIL) for severe (grades 2 or 3) ARHI were then identified within this larger set of access procedures. The complete hospital and outpatient medical records of those patients requiring a DRIL were then retrospectively reviewed and the perioperative and midterm outcomes determined.

All patients presenting for their initial, permanent hemodialysis access procedure were evaluated using our prospectively validated algorithm designed to optimize the use of autogenous accesses.[43] Briefly, patients underwent both arterial and venous upper extremity imaging in the noninvasive vascular laboratory. Selective invasive imaging with catheter-based arteriography and/or venography was used to confirm the initial plan. Criteria for a suitable outflow vein included a diameter $\geq$3 mm, a length spanning the forearm/arm, and the absence of ipsilateral central vein stenoses/occlusions. Criteria for a suitable inflow artery included no hemodynamically significant proximal stenoses and adequate diameter (i.e., brachial $\geq$3 mm, radial $\geq$2 mm). The hierarchy of access procedures included autogenous radiocephalic > autogenous radiobasilic > autogenous brachiocephalic > autogenous brachiobasilic > prosthetic forearm/arm > translocated femoral/popliteal vein.[16]

The diagnosis of ARHI was based primarily upon the clinical presentation and physical examination. Noninvasive imaging including upper extremity pressures and the corresponding velocity waveforms were obtained in equivocal cases. Upper extremity catheter-based arteriography with evaluation of the complete arterial tree from the aortic arch to the digits was used selectively to identify and correct any inflow lesions. Definitive treatment of persistent hand ischemia included access ligation or DRIL, with the choice contingent upon patient comorbidities, type of access, onset of ischemia, likelihood of autogenous access maturing sufficient for cannulation, and future access options.

The DRIL procedure was performed as previously described.[44-45] Briefly, the proximal anastomosis of the brachiobrachial artery bypass was placed $\geq$7 cm from the access anastomosis. The distal bypass anastomosis was placed immediately distal to that for the access and was configured end-side or end-end with ligation or transaction/oversewing of the brachial artery immediately proximal to the distal bypass anastomosis. Potential upper and lower extremity venous conduits for the DRIL were identified using ultrasound.[46] The saphenous vein (≥3 mm) was used preferentially with the alternative choices dictated by availability or surgeon preference (arm vein > femoral vein > cadaveric vein > prosthetic). Every attempt was made to preserve any available, suitable arm vein for future autogenous accesses.

Postoperative surveillance of the DRIL bypass included upper extremity arterial pressures/waveforms and duplex ultrasound scanning of the DRIL bypass.[47] Surveillance was performed at 1 month, 3 months, 6 months, 9 months, 12 months, and then every 6 months thereafter. Remedial imaging and/or treatment was performed for recurrent hand symptoms, significant decreases in the arterial pressures (i.e., 15 mm Hg), and/or abnormal grafts scans (i.e., mean graft velocity <50 cm/s, maximum velocity ratio ≥3.5).[48]

A total of 77 patients with severe ARHI were treated with a DRIL procedure (61 pts) or access ligation (16 pts) during the time course of the study. During this interval, 1519 access-related surgical procedures (exclusive of dialysis catheters) were performed, including both new constructions and revisions. The incidence of severe ARHI requiring ligation or DRIL was 6% among the new access procedures. A total of 64 DRIL procedures were performed in the 61 patients. The mean patient age was 59±13 years and the majority of patients were female, hypertensive, diabetic, and actively dialyzing (Table 21–2). Notably, 10% had had a prior episode of ARHI. The brachial artery was the inflow source for all of the index access procedures, with the brachiocephalic autogenous access configuration being the most common (Table 21–2). A significant proportion of the patients had an autogenous brachioaxillary access using the translocated femoral/popliteal vein, whereas only 2 patients had a prosthetic access. The primary ischemic symptoms that precipitated the DRIL procedures

TABLE 21-2. DEMOGRAPHICS, COMORBIDITIES, AND ACCESS CONFIGURATION

Demographics	
Age	59 ± 13
Gender (% male)	38
Comorbidities	
End-stage renal disease	92%
Hypertension	74%
Diabetes mellitus	72%
Coronary artery disease	36%
Cerebrovascular occlusive disease	23%
Congestive heart failure	20%
Peripheral vascular occlusive disease	13%
Prior access-related hand ischemia	10%
Access Configuration	
Brachiocephalic autogenous	46%
Brachiobasilic autogenous	31%
Brachioaxillary superficial femoral vein	20%
Brachioaxillary prosthetic	3%

Reproduced with permission from Huber TS, et al. Midterm outcome after the distal revascularization and interval ligation (DRIL) procedure. J Vasc Surg 2008;48:926–33.

were pain (25%), paresthesia (34%), motor dysfunction (24%), and tissue loss (17%). A preemptive DRIL was performed in 5 patients because of a prior history of ARHI and/or severe forearm arterial occlusive disease in conjunction with digital gangrene. Noninvasive vascular laboratory studies were obtained to confirm the clinical diagnosis in approximately half of the patients. The mean preoperative (i.e., pre-DRIL) wrist/brachial index (WBI) was 0.46±0.19 and the mean DBI was 0.25±0.23, with the latter used primarily for patients with noncompressible arteries at the wrist (Figure 21–7). The majority (83%) of the patients had an upper extremity arteriogram prior to their index access procedure or immediately prior to the DRIL. A hemodynamically significant arterial lesion was found proximal to the brachial artery in 6 patients; this was corrected prior to the access procedure in 3 patients and at the time of the DRIL in the others.

The DRIL procedure was performed within 7 days of the index access procedure in almost half of the cases as dictated by the acuity/severity of the symptoms: <24 hours: 19%; 1 day < DRIL ≤7 days: 29%; 7 days < DRIL ≤30 days: 8%; >30 days: 44%. The greater saphenous vein was used as the conduit in the majority of cases (greater saphenous vein – 75%, basilic/cephalic vein – 19%, cadaveric vein – 5%, femoral vein – 2%, lesser saphenous vein – 2%). The in-hospital mortality rate after the DRIL was 3%, with a single death resulting from withdrawal of hemodialysis and a second from a presumed arrhythmia. The nonfatal complication rate was 22% with the itemized breakdown including wound (14%), respiratory (3%: pneumonia, reintubation), vascular (3%: lower extremity ischemia requiring amputation from femoral/saphenous vein harvest wounds, compartment syndrome), and cardiac (2%: arrhythmia) causes. The DRIL procedure relieved the precipitating ischemic symptoms in 78% of the cases (residual symptoms: paresthesia – 13%; pain – 5%; tissue loss – 4%; motor – 2%). Notably, the residual paresthesia and motor compromise were relatively minor, with the latter associated only with very fine movements. Access ligation was required in a single patient with ongoing, severe pain despite a patent DRIL bypass. All but 2 of the patients who presented with tissue loss were able to heal their wounds; the exceptions

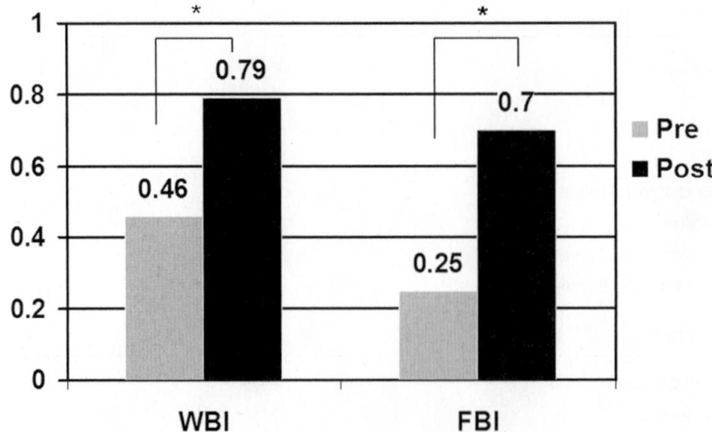

Figure 21-7. The mean preoperative (Pre) and postoperative (Post) wrist/brachial (WBI) and finger/brachial (FBI) indices are shown (alternative name for DBI). Significant increases (P<.05) were noted for both indices after the DRIL procedure. (Reproduced with permission from Huber TS, et al. Midterm outcome after the distal revascularization and interval ligation [DRIL] procedure. J Vasc Surg 2008;48:926–33.)

had severe forearm arterial occlusive disease as documented by arteriography. Both the WBIs and the DBIs increased significantly (P<.05) with postoperative values of 0.79±0.17 and 0.70 ± 0.25, respectively (see Figure 21–7). This corresponded to a mean increase (preoperative vs. postoperative) of 0.34±0.26 for the WBIs and 0.41±0.21 for the DBIs. The access maturation rate was 68% for the patients in whom the DRIL procedures were performed early after the index access procedure (i.e., prior to the index access being cannulated for dialysis). All of the accesses in use at the time of the DRIL procedure were used throughout the perioperative period without interruption.

The mean follow-up after the DRIL procedure was 12±16 mos (range 0–66). The primary DRIL patency rates (± SEM) were 77±8%, 74±9%, and 71±9% at 1 year, 3 years, and 5 years (Figure 21–8) respectively, whereas the corresponding secondary patency rates were 81±7%, 76±9%, and 76±9% (Figure 21–9). The primary assisted and secondary patency rates were identical, because all DRIL bypasses that thrombosed were abandoned. A total of 7 DRIL bypasses failed during follow-up. Three of the patients presented with recurrent symptoms (pain – 2, tissue loss) and underwent a redo DRIL bypass, 1 of which failed a second time requiring access ligation. Three other patients were asymptomatic after their DRIL bypass failed and did not require additional treatment. Notably, all 3 of the DRIL procedures performed with cadaveric vein thrombosed during follow-up. The patient survival after the DRIL procedure was 71±6%, 59±7%, and 33±9% at 1 year, 3 years, and 5 years, respectively, with a median survival time of 43 months.

The results of our study further establish the benefits of the DRIL procedure as a safe, definitive treatment for ARHI. Notably, it relieved the precipitating symptoms in the majority of patients with a success rate approaching 90% if the patients with residual paresthesias, presumably resulting from the initial ischemic injury to the nerve, were excluded. The clinical improvement was supported by the hemodynamic

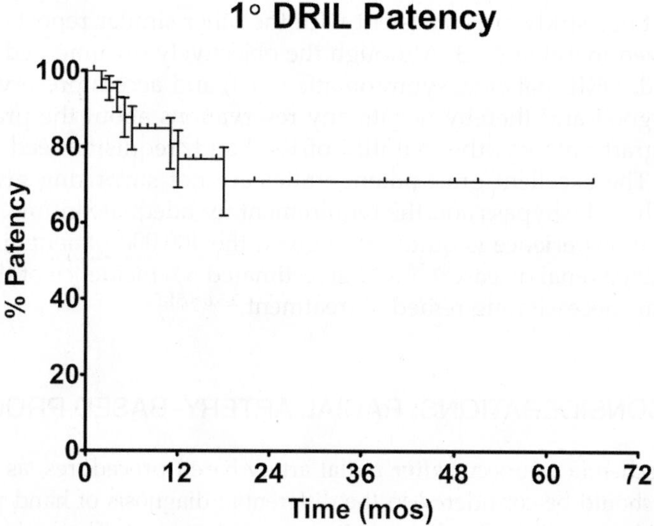

Figure 21-8. The Kaplan-Meier curve for the primary patency of the DRIL bypass is shown with the standard error bars. The standard errors were <10% throughout the time interval analyzed. (Reproduced with permission from Huber TS. et al. Midterm outcome after the distal revascularization and interval ligation (DRIL) procedure. J Vasc Surg 2008;48:926–33.)

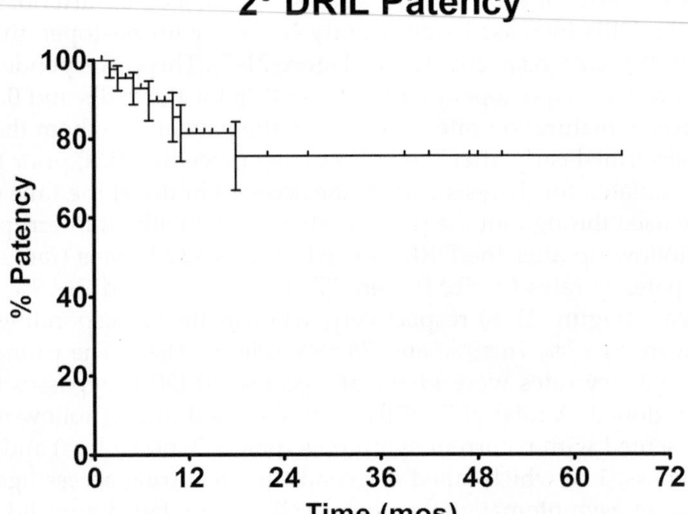

Figure 21-9. The Kaplan-Meier curve for the secondary patency of the DRIL bypass is shown with the standard error bars. The standard errors were <10% throughout the time interval analyzed. (Reproduced with permission from Huber TS, et al. Midterm outcome after the distal revascularization and interval ligation (DRIL) procedure. J Vasc Surg 2008;48:926–33.).

changes as measured by the WBIs and DBIs. Furthermore, the objectively documented, mid-term patency rates for the DRIL bypass were also very good and neither the patients' hands nor accesses appeared to be adversely affected or compromised by the procedure. Perhaps not surprisingly, the overall survival for patients requiring a DRIL was poor, thereby suggesting that the long-term durability of the DRIL may be a secondary concern.

The results of our study are consistent with the other similar reports in the literature as summarized in Table 21–3. Although the objectively documented follow-up is somewhat limited, DRIL patency, symptomatic relief, and access preservation all appear to be quite good and thereby negate any reservations about the procedure (i.e., concerns about graft patency, the viability of the hand, requisite need to ligate the brachial artery). The excellent graft patency rates are not surprising given the relatively short length of the bypass and the requirement for adequate inflow. Admittedly, the collective DRIL experience is quite small given the 400,000 patients in the United States with end-stage renal disease[49-50] and an estimated 5% incidence of those with severe hand ischemia necessitating remedial treatment.[2,5,6,8,51-52]

ADDITIONAL CONSIDERATIONS: RADIAL ARTERY–BASED PROCEDURES

Hand or digital ischemia can occur after radial artery-based procedures, as noted above. Although rare, it should be considered in the differential diagnosis of hand pain or tissue loss in patients with an ipsilateral radiocephalic autogenous access. The underlying mechanism is related to the retrograde flow from the ulnar artery and palmar arch through the access. Notably, Chemla and associates[10] documented hemodynamic improvement in terms of hand perfusion after balloon occlusion of the distal radial artery. Definitive treatment

TABLE 21-3. THE LARGER PUBLISHED DRIL SERIES

Study	Sample	DRIL Patency	Symptom Relief	Access Preservation	Patient Survival
Haimov, *Blood Purif* 1996.[55]	23	96% @ 2 yr	100% - improved 83% - resolved	46% @ 2 yr	NA
Katz, *J Am Coll Surg* 1996.[56]	5	100% (mean 7 mo)	83% - improved/resolved	100% (mean 7 mo)	NA
Stierli, *J Cardiovasc Surg* 1998.[57]	6	100% (6- 24 mo)	100% - improved/resolved	100% (6-24 mo)	NA
Knox, *J Vasc Surg* 2002.[58]	55	1° - 80% @ 4 yr (life table)	90% - improved/resolved	71% @ 3 yr (life table)	56% @ 4 yr (life table)
Lazarides, *Nephrol Dial Transplant* 2003.[4]	23	69% @ 1 yr	100% - resolved	NA	NA
Diehl, *Am J Surg* 2003.[59]	13	83% @ 2 yr	100% - improved 57% - resolved	71% @ 2 yr	NA
Korzets, *Israeli Med Assoc J* 2003.[60]	9	100% (mean 12 mos)	100% - resolved	78% (mean 12 mo)	NA
Sessa, *Ann Vasc Surg* 2004.[61]	18	94% (mean 16 mo)	100% - improved 73% - resolved	94% (mean 16 mo)	61% (mean 16 mo)
Mwipatayi, Current Surgery 2006.[62]	12	100% (median 4 mo)	83% -improved/resolved	NA	NA
Walz, *Ann Vasc Surg* 2007.[63]	38	NA	67%	NA	NA
Current Study 2008.	64	1° - 71 ± 9 @ 5 yr 2° - 76 ± 9 @ 5 yr (Kaplan-Meier)	78% - resolved	New - 68% maturation Functional – 100% continued	33 ± 9 @ 5 yr (Kaplan-Meier)

Reproduced with permission from Huber TS et al. Midterm outcome after the distal revascularization and interval ligation (DRIL) procedure. J Vasc Surg 2008;48:926–33.

includes simply occluding the distal radial artery, and this has been described using both ligatures and coils.[11,53-54]

REFERENCES

1. Sidawy AN, Gray R, Besarab A, et al. Recommended standards for reports dealing with arteriovenous hemodialysis accesses. J Vasc Surg 2002;35:603–10.
2. Papasavas PK, Reifsnyder T, Birdas TJ, et al. Prediction of arteriovenous access steal syndrome utilizing digital pressure measurements. Vasc Endovasc Surg 2003;37:179–84.
3. Keuter XH, Kessels AG, de Haan MH, et al. Prospective evaluation of ischemia in brachial-basilic and forearm prosthetic arteriovenous fistulas for hemodialysis. Eur J Vasc Endovasc Surg 2008;35:619–24.
4. Lazarides MK, Staramos DN, Kopadis G, et al. Onset of arterial "steal" following proximal angioaccess: immediate and delayed types. Nephrol Dial Transplant 2003;18:2387–90.
5. Meyer F, Muller JS, Grote R, et al. [Fistula Banding - Success-promoting Approach in Peripheral Steal Syndrome]. Zentralbl Chir 2002;127:685–8.
6. Morsy AH, Kulbaski M, Chen C, et al. Incidence and characteristics of patients with hand ischemia after a hemodialysis access procedure. J Surg Res 1998;74:8–10.
7. Schanzer H, Eisenberg D. Management of steal syndrome resulting from dialysis access. Semin Vasc Surg 2004;17:45–9.
8. Suding PN, Wilson SE. Strategies for management of ischemic steal syndrome. Semin Vasc Surg 2007;20:184–8.
9. Tordoir JH, Dammers R, Van Der Sande FM. Upper extremity ischemia and hemodialysis vascular access. Eur J Vasc Endovasc Surg 2004;27:1–5.
10. Chemla E, Raynaud A, Carreres T, et al. Preoperative assessment of the efficacy of distal radial artery ligation in treatment of steal syndrome complicating access for hemodialysis. Ann Vasc Surg 1999;13:618–21.
11. Miller GA, Khariton K, Kardos SV, et al. Flow interruption of the distal radial artery: treatment for finger ischemia in a matured radiocephalic AVF. J Vasc Access 2008;9:58–63.
12. Huber TS, Brown MP, Seeger JM, Lee WA. Midterm outcome after the distal revascularization and interval ligation (DRIL) procedure. J Vasc Surg 2008;48:926–32.
13. Scheltinga MR, van HF, Bruijninckx CM. Time of onset in haemodialysis access-induced distal ischaemia (HAIDI) is related to the access type. Nephrol Dial Transplant 2009;24: 3198–204.
14. van HF, Scheltinga MR, Krasznai AG, Cornelissen EA. Retarded hand growth due to a hemodialysis fistula in a young girl. Pediatr Nephrol 2009;24:2055–8.
15. Davidson D, Louridas G, Guzman R, et al. Steal syndrome complicating upper extremity hemoaccess procedures: incidence and risk factors. Can J Surg 2003 ;46:408–12.
16. Huber TS, Hirneise CM, Lee WA, et al. Outcome after autogenous brachial-axillary translocated superficial femoropopliteal vein hemodialysis access. J Vasc Surg 2004;40: 311–8.
17. Kusztal M, Weyde W, Letachowicz W, et al. Influence of autologous arteriovenous fistula on the blood supply to the hand in very elderly hemodialyzed patients. J Vasc Access 2005;6:83–7.
18. Valentine RJ, Bouch CW, Scott DJ, et al. Do preoperative finger pressures predict early arterial steal in hemodialysis access patients? A prospective analysis. J Vasc Surg 2002;36: 351–6.
19. Goff CD, Sato DT, Bloch PH, et al. Steal syndrome complicating hemodialysis access procedures: can it be predicted? Ann Vasc Surg 2000;14:138–44.
20. Tynan-Cuisinier GS, Berman SS. Strategies for predicting and treating access induced ischemic steal syndrome. Eur J Vasc Endovasc Surg 2006;32:309–15.
21. Namazi H, Majd Z. Carpal tunnel syndrome in patients who are receiving long-term renal hemodialysis. Arch Orthop Trauma Surg 2007;127:725–8.

22. Zanow J, Krueger U, Reddemann P, Scholz H. Experimental study of hemodynamics in procedures to treat access-related ischemia. J Vasc Surg 2008;48:1559–65.
23. Gradman WS, Pozrikidis C. Analysis of options for mitigating hemodialysis access-related ischemic steal phenomena. Ann Vasc Surg 2004;18:59–65.
24. Illig KA, Surowiec S, Shortell CK, et al. Hemodynamics of distal revascularization-interval ligation. Ann Vasc Surg 2005;19:199–207.
25. Asif A, Gadalean FN, Merrill D, et al. Inflow stenosis in arteriovenous fistulas and grafts: a multicenter, prospective study. Kidney Int 2005;67:1986–92.
26. DeCaprio JD, Valentine RJ, Kakish HB, et al. Steal syndrome complicating hemodialysis access. Cardiovasc Surg 1997;5:648–53.
27. Malik J, Slavikova M, Maskova J. Dialysis access-associated steal syndrome: the role of ultrasonography. J Nephrol 2003;16:903–7.
28. Malik J, Tuka V, Kasalova Z, et al. Understanding the dialysis access steal syndrome. A review of the etiologies, diagnosis, prevention and treatment strategies. J Vasc Access 2008;9: 155–66.
29. Scheltinga MR, van HF, Bruyninckx CM. Surgical banding for refractory hemodialysis access-induced distal ischemia (HAIDI). J Vasc Access 2009;10:43–9.
30. Zanow J, Petzold K, Petzold M, et al. Flow reduction in high-flow arteriovenous access using intraoperative flow monitoring. J Vasc Surg 2006;44:1273–8.
31. Huber TS, Carter JW, Carter RL, Seeger JM. Patency of autogenous and polytetrafluoroethylene upper extremity arteriovenous hemodialysis accesses: a systematic review. J Vasc Surg 2003;38:1005–11.
32. Dember LM, Beck GJ, Allon M, et al. Effect of clopidogrel on early failure of arteriovenous fistulas for hemodialysis: a randomized controlled trial. JAMA 2008;299:2164–71.
33. van HF, Scheltinga MR, Luirink M, et al. Access flow, venous saturation, and digital pressures in hemodialysis. J Vasc Surg 2007;45:968–73.
34. van HF, Scheltinga M, Luirink M, et al. Banding of hemodialysis access to treat hand ischemia or cardiac overload. Semin Dial 2009;22:204–8.
35. Thermann F, Ukkat J, Wollert U, et al. Dialysis shunt-associated steal syndrome (DASS) following brachial accesses: the value of fistula banding under blood flow control. Langenbecks Arch Surg 2007;392:731–7.
36. Zanow J, Kruger U, Scholz H. Proximalization of the arterial inflow: a new technique to treat access-related ischemia. J Vasc Surg 2006;43:1216–21.
37. Thermann F, Wollert U. Proximalization of the arterial inflow: new treatment of choice in patients with advanced dialysis shunt-associated steal syndrome? Ann Vasc Surg 2008;23: 485–90.
38. Chemla ES, Morsy M, Anderson L, Whitemore A. Inflow reduction by distalization of anastomosis treats efficiently high-inflow high-cardiac output vascular access for hemodialysis. Semin Dial 2007;20:68–72.
39. Minion DJ, Moore E, Endean E. Revision using distal inflow: a novel approach to dialysis-associated steal syndrome. Ann Vasc Surg 2005;19:625–8.
40. Schanzer H, Schwartz M, Harrington E, Haimov M. Treatment of ischemia due to "steal" by arteriovenous fistula with distal artery ligation and revascularization. J Vasc Surg 1988; 7:770–3.
41. Gradman WS, Pozrikidis C. Analysis of options for mitigating hemodialysis access-related ischemic steal phenomena. Ann Vasc Surg 2004;18:59–65.
42. van der MS, Zeebregts C, Tielliu I, et al. Modified distal revascularization with interval ligation procedure for steal syndrome after arteriovenous fistula creation for hemodialysis access. Vascular 2007;15:226–30.
43. Huber TS, Ozaki CK, Flynn TC, et al. Prospective validation of an algorithm to maximize native arteriovenous fistulae for chronic hemodialysis access. J Vasc Surg 2002;36: 452–9.
44. Berman SS, Gentile AT, Glickman MH, et al. Distal revascularization-interval ligation for limb salvage and maintenance of dialysis access in ischemic steal syndrome. J Vasc Surg 1997;26:393–402.

45. Schanzer H, Skladany M, Haimov M. Treatment of angioaccess-induced ischemia by revascularization. J Vasc Surg 1992;16:861–4.
46. Seeger JM, Schmidt JH, Flynn TC. Preoperative saphenous and cephalic vein mapping as an adjunct to reconstructive arterial surgery. Ann Surg 1987;205:733–9.
47. Seeger JM, Pretus HA, Carlton LC, et al. Potential predictors of outcome in patients with tissue loss who undergo infrainguinal vein bypass grafting. J Vasc Surg 1999;30:427–35.
48. Gibson KD, Caps MT, Gillen D, et al. Identification of factors predictive of lower extremity vein graft thrombosis. J Vasc Surg 2001;33:24–31.
49. Szczech LA, Lazar IL. Projecting the United States ESRD population: issues regarding treatment of patients with ESRD. Kidney Int Suppl 2004;90:S3–7.
50. Xue JL, Ma JZ, Louis TA, Collins AJ. Forecast of the number of patients with end-stage renal disease in the United States to the year 2010. J Am Soc Nephrol 2001;12:2753–8.
51. Lazarides MK, Staramos DN, Panagopoulos GN, et al. Indications for surgical treatment of angioaccess-induced arterial "steal." J Am Coll Surg 1998;187:422–6.
52. Tordoir JH, Leunissen KM. [Arterial perfusion disorders of the hand in 9 patients with arteriovenous fistula for hemodialysis]. Ned Tijdschr Geneeskd 1999;143:1093–8.
53. Plumb TJ, Lynch TG, Adelson AB. Treatment of steal syndrome in a distal radiocephalic arteriovenous fistula using intravascular coil embolization. J Vasc Surg 2007;47:457–9.
54. Porcellini M, Selvetella L, De RP, et al. [Hand ischemia due to "steal syndrome" in vascular access for hemodialysis]. G Chir 1997;18:27–30.
55. Haimov M, Schanzer H, Skladani M. Pathogenesis and management of upper-extremity ischemia following angioaccess surgery. Blood Purif 1996;14:350–4.
56. Katz S, Kohl RD. The treatment of hand ischemia by arterial ligation and upper extremity bypass after angioaccess surgery. J Am Coll Surg 1996;183:239–42.
57. Stierli P, Blumberg A, Pfister J, Zehnder C. Surgical treatment of "steal syndrome" induced by arteriovenous grafts for hemodialysis. J Cardiovasc Surg (Torino) 1998;39:441–3.
58. Knox RC, Berman SS, Hughes JD, et al. Distal revascularization-interval ligation: a durable and effective treatment for ischemic steal syndrome after hemodialysis access. J Vasc Surg 2002;36:250–6.
59. Diehl L, Johansen K, Watson J. Operative management of distal ischemia complicating upper extremity dialysis access. Am J Surg 2003;186:17–9.
60. Korzets A, Kantarovsky A, Lehmann J, et al. The "DRIL" procedure—a neglected way to treat the "steal" syndrome of the hemodialysed patient. Isr Med Assoc J 2003;5:782–5.
61. Sessa C, Riehl G, Porcu P, et al. Treatment of hand ischemia following angioaccess surgery using the distal revascularization interval-ligation technique with preservation of vascular access: description of an 18-case series. Ann Vasc Surg 2004;18:685–94.
62. Mwipatayi BP, Bowles T, Balakrishnan S, et al. Ischemic steal syndrome: a case series and review of current management. Curr Surg 2006;63:130–5.
63. Walz P, Ladowski JS, Hines A. Distal revascularization and interval ligation (DRIL) procedure for the treatment of ischemic steal syndrome after arm arteriovenous fistula. Ann Vasc Surg 2007;21:468–73.

22

Complications Associated with Hemodialysis Access

Frank T. Padberg, Jr., M.D., F.A.C.S.

INTRODUCTION

A well-functioning arteriovenous (AV) hemoaccess is a critical lifeline for the patient with chronic end-stage renal disease. Although cumulative function is frequently less than 2 to 3 years, recent efforts have concentrated upon improving this parameter; in particular, efforts have been directed toward reducing the frequency of complications. Catheters and prosthetic grafts, common in North American practice, are responsible for a disproportionate share of these problems. Considerable recent efforts have been directed toward increasing construction of functioning autogenous AV access that is less likely to produce venous thrombosis, pseudoaneurysm, or infection.

Flow-related complications may occur with any AV access constructed for hemodialysis. Life- or limb-threatening complications such as arterial steal syndrome and high-output cardiac failure represent incompletely compensated alterations in flow.

Other hemoaccess complications are related to renal insufficiency and may be seen regardless of the access. These include bleeding tendencies and neuropathy.

Recently published guidelines recommend construction of autogenous AV access prior to the need for renal replacement therapy.[1-2] Although a recent systematic review[3] was unable to make an evidence-based recommendation regarding timing of access placement, it has been a personal observation that more autogenous options remain available when the access is constructed prior to initiation of dialysis. This potentially avoids initial catheter placement, reducing the morbidity and mortality associated with prolonged catheter-based dialysis while the autogenous AV access matures. An expanded discussion and reference list on AV access complications may be found in a recent supplement of the Journal of Vascular Surgery.[4]

VENOUS HYPERTENSION—THROMBOSIS AND RELATIVE OBSTRUCTION

Venous hypertension (V-HTN) may develop in several settings. The most common of these is central venous thrombosis ipsilateral to the AV access as a result of prior brachial, axillary, and subclavian vein catheterizations. Superior vena cava or bilateral innominate vein occlusion is particularly devastating in the dialysis population. Peripheral outflow stenoses can also produce localized symptoms that are usually amenable to mechanical solutions. Venous outflow stenosis is predominantly a problem for prosthetic AV access and can result in thrombosis of the access.

Central Vein Stenosis/Thrombosis/Occlusion

Thrombosis of the central veins draining the upper extremity was once a rare clinical problem. Currently, the most common etiology is prolonged central vein instrumentation. Pacemaker wires, defibrillator leads, chemotherapy, long-term antibiotics, parenteral nutrition, and hemodialysis are common indications for prolonged central vein catheterization. Clinical evaluation for hemoaccess should include assessment for these devices. Collateralized upper extremity thrombosis is well tolerated and may not be recognized. Clinical findings include appropriate anterior chest scars and dilated collateral venous patterns, but extremity edema is uncommon when the occlusion is well compensated. Preoperative venous scans mapping veins for access should also include assessment of the outflow veins, recognizing that visualization of central thoracic components are only indirectly accessible by duplex ultrasound investigations. Placement of a new peripheral AV fistula may precipitate symptomatic venous hypertension when the collateral veins are unable to manage the increased volume flow around an otherwise well-compensated thrombotic occlusion. Although a degree of arm swelling may be tolerated, accurate puncture of the access becomes more difficult in the chronically edematous arm.

Central vein obstruction may be unilateral, but most of these devices traverse the vena cava (Figure 22–1). From an access perspective, caval obstruction/thrombosis is particularly devastating, because it usually implies loss of both upper extremities for subsequent hemoaccess sites. In severe cases, edema of the head may adversely affect cerebral and sensory functions.[5]

Recognition and management of central vein stenosis requires more than duplex imaging, that is, CT venography or fistulography. Contrast fistulography offers the option of concomitant balloon angioplasty and stenting. Although durability is less than optimal, the functional life of an access may be extended. Stents are avoided if the stenosis is in the thoracic outlet, because the scissoring action of the first rib and clavicle may lead to permanent deformation of the stent. Surgical venous bypass can be undertaken with reasonable risk if the outflow option is relatively superficial, such as the jugular, the contralateral axillary, and even the femoral vein. Intracavitary surgical interventions have been reported but, owing to the marked increase in risk, are generally reserved for true end-stage access options. If caval reconstruction is required, functional patency is better with surgical reconstruction, but the risk, is considerably greater.[6-7] Angioplasty alone is generally preferred for initial interventions unless complicated by severe recoil; it may be repeated as often as necessary to maintain functional outflow.

Implantation of lower extremity AV access is becoming increasingly common as upper extremity options are exhausted by failed previous hemoaccess or central venous obstruction. Fistulas composed of transposed femoral vein provide larger volumes of flow but several caveats are important to those considering this AV access option. Symptomatic edema is more likely if the harvested vein includes the below-knee popliteal vein. Owing to the large diameter of the femoral vein, a large anastomosis is avoided to reduce the likelihood of arterial steal syndrome. An arterial orifice limited to 4 to 6 mm is sufficient to provide excellent flow with a decreased risk of

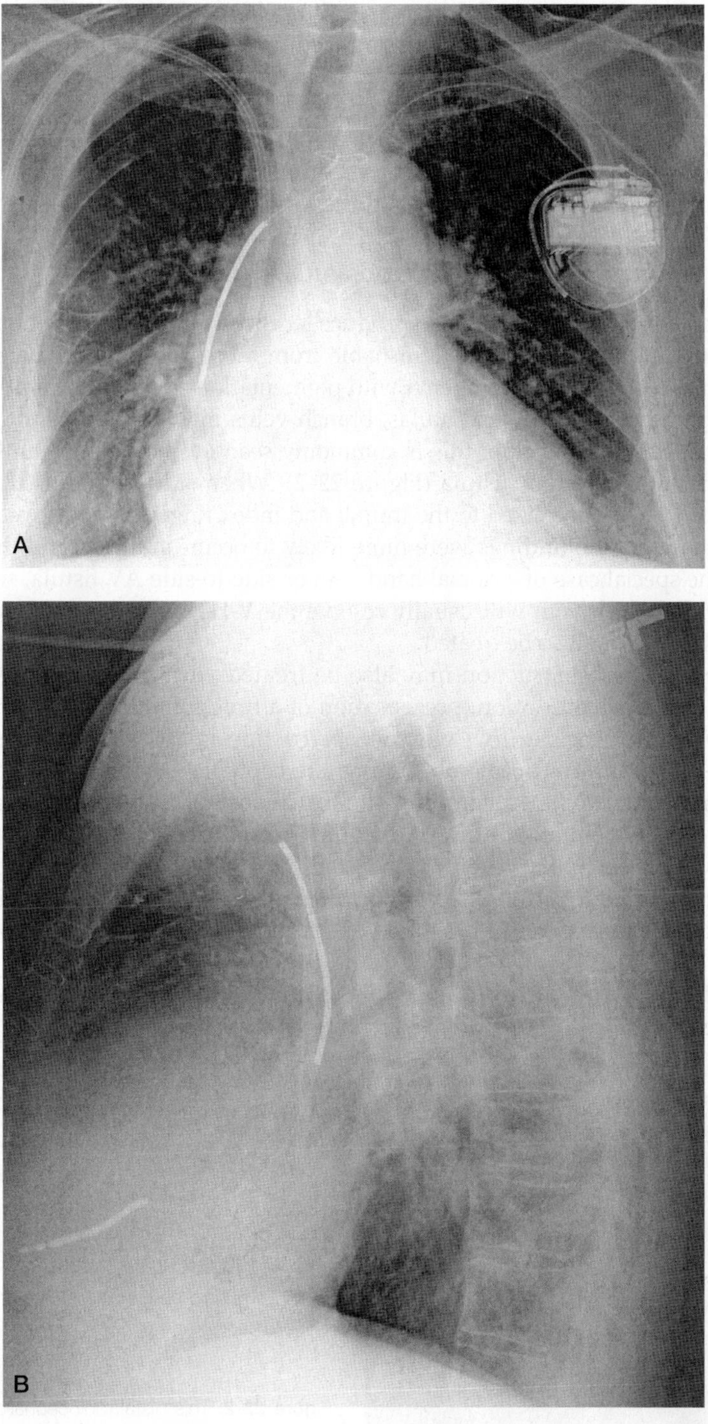

Figure 22-1. Both the defibrillator leads and the Permacath traverse the superior vena cava on this chest x-ray. For two reasons, access placement would be preferred on the right because the risk of thrombosis is decreased with the internal jugular approach and because the dialysis catheter will be removed once the access has matured.

steal.[1,8] Use of prosthetic material increases the risk of infection. When constructing a composite graft, the risk of infection is reduced by burying the prosthetic graft in the deep tissues and anastomosing it to a superficially transposed femoral vein. Whether the prosthetic graft is configured as a composite graft or as a complete prosthetic loop, originating the arterial anastomosis on the distal femoral artery is preferred unless there is extensive arterial occlusive disease; should infection occur, arterial ligation of the distal femoral artery is better tolerated than the common femoral artery.

Peripheral Venous Stenosis/Thrombosis/Obstruction

Peripheral venous obstruction may also produce localized symptoms of venous congestion. The clinical findings may be indistinguishable from those of venous hypertension in the lower extremity—brawny brown edema with pigmentation and even ulceration. With surgically constructed arteriovenous fistulas, branch veins may remain patent and dilate as more proximal stenoses develop; this is commonly seen on the dorsum of the hand with the distal wrist arteriovenous fistula (Figure 22–2). When side-to-side fistulas were common, the findings were localized to the thumb and index finger; as end-to-side fistulas became more common, the findings were more likely to occur on the second through fourth digits.[4,9] In the special case of a dorsal hand vein or side-to-side AV fistula, simple ligation of the diverting branch vein will usually resolve the V-HTN. However, concomitant outflow obstruction should also be treated.

Localized venous obstruction may also be treated with angioplasty. Although fistula ligation is always an option, preservation of a functional fistula is a preferable solution. Rerouting of the outflow past an obstruction is a particularly useful option. Consider specific outflow problems such as the cephalic arch vein. The cephalic vein empties into the subclavian, a common site for stenosis. This is best managed by ligation of the cephalic vein anatomically distal to the stenosis, with transposition and re-anastomosis onto the axillary vein; stents deployed across the cephalic arch perform poorly and may impede outflow from the entire upper extremity.[10] A similar consideration is applicable to stenosis of brachial vein outflow from basilic transpositions.

Outflow Stenosis and Thrombosis. Fibrointimal venous stenosis at the outflow of a prosthetic access will result in thrombosis rather than venous engorgement. Experienced

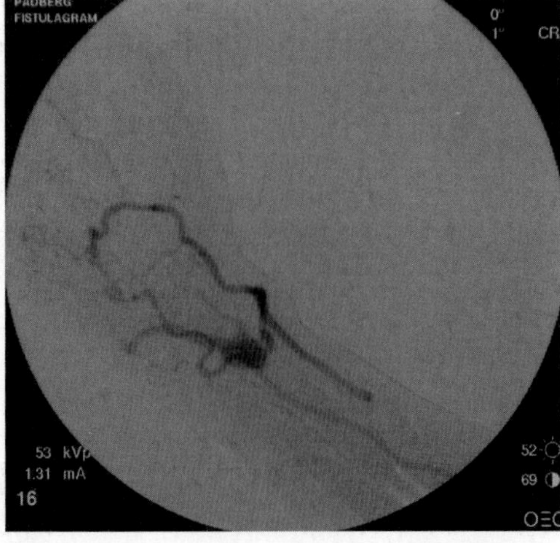

Figure 22-2. This distal radiocephalic AV fistula supported hemodialysis for over 7 years, but hand edema was produced by localized venous hypertension in this dorsal wrist vein. This was relieved by ligation and the access revised by transposition of a dilated, forearm basilic vein.

clinicians, various ultrasound-based flow measures, and duplex ultrasound will effectively detect functional stenosis in the hemoaccess. However, intervention to correct stenosis in prosthetic AV access has not resulted in prolongation of its functional life; Although this has been evaluated in a number of trials, there are no clear data to support routine surveillance and pre-emptive angioplasty for >50% stenosis, but it remains a topic of considerable interest.[1,4]

PSEUDOANEURYSM

Arteriovenous access pseudoaneurysm may be a mechanical or infectious complication. Those caused by infection are in the next section. Mechanical causes include failure of hemostasis at needle holes, breakdown of the conduit from repetitive puncture, and anastomotic disruption. Pseudoaneurysm is more commonly seen with a prosthetic graft but can still occur in autogenous access. Multiple, small pseudoaneurysms are commonly seen on prosthetic grafts that have been in use for several months, but not all will produce symptoms. A small, single pseudoaneurysm may resolve with observation. Pseudoaneurysms are often associated with concomitant venous outflow obstruction; this may explain the propensity for them to occur in the arterial end of the conduit. Enlargement and threatened compromise of the overlying skin are indications for intervention (Figure 22–3 A).

Localized pseudoaneurysm is amenable to resection and segmental replacement of a prosthetic conduit. When the proximal and distal anastomoses are uninvolved, the inflammatory fibrosis in the body of the graft may be avoided by rerouting a new prosthetic conduit around the existing aneurysmal segments and anastomosing it to both functional ends. Alternatively, covered stents may be deployed to control isolated aneurysmal segments in the conduit while retaining patency of the AV access[4,11] (Figure 22–3 B, C).

Anastomotic pseudoaneurysm will usually require revision and surgical intervention. Simple disruption of the suture line is infrequent but may be repairable; if there is no infection, the artery and conduit may be amenable to reanastomosis. When this is not possible but the conduit is still of good quality, revision of the anastomosis is the best solution.

Diffuse Autogenous Arteriovenous Access Dilation

Diffuse enlargement of a durable autogenous arteriovenous fistula should not be considered serious if there are no complications. The gradual increase in volume flow is advantageous for dialysis exchanges. Indications for intervention arise when the vein becomes acutely kinked from tortuous expansion or there is threatened skin erosion. In these situations, the conduit may be dissected free, shortened by excision of the offending section, and flow restored by end-to-end anastomosis; the overlying skin is frequently redundant from aneurysm expansion and resection of uninfected necrotic areas can often be safely excised from a well-placed skin incision; an alternative solution is placement of a remote relaxing incision to permit primary closure over the AV access.

INFECTION

AV access infection is usually localized, more likely to involve prosthetic conduit, and primarily a clinical diagnosis. Duplex imaging may be helpful by identifying extraneous

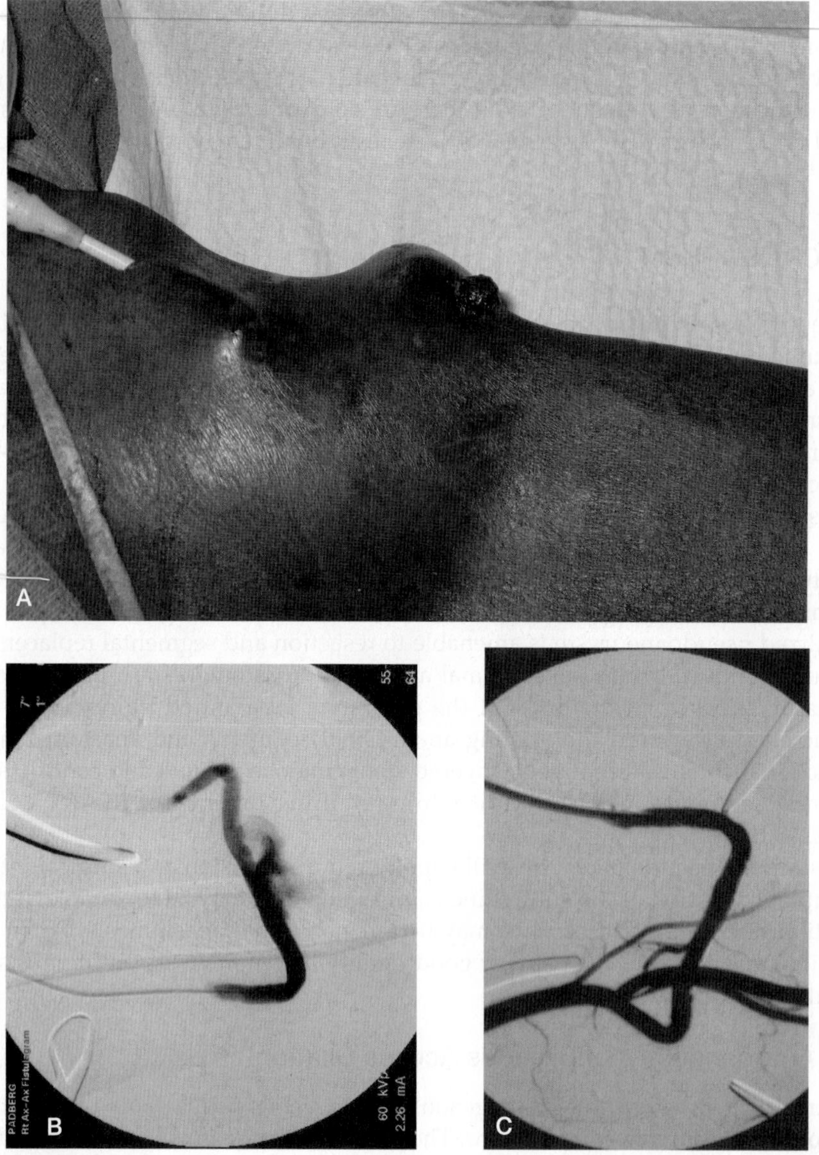

Figure 22-3. Pseudoaneurysm. A. This axillo-axillary prosthetic loop developed a pseudoaneurysm with unstable thrombus at the puncture site. Both the hemorrhagic risk and the pseudoaneurysm were controlled by percutaneous deployment of a covered stent graft. B. Fistulogram demonstrates pseudoaneurysm cavity and the site of disruption. C. Fistulogram after deployment of a covered stent demonstrates an intact graft without extravasation.

fluid collections in suspicious sites, evaluating the extent of the process, and determining integrity of the conduit or anastomosis. Purulent drainage, sinus formation, cellulitis, and localized erythema are the most common findings. Fever, bacteremia, and systemic sepsis more commonly result from indwelling hemodialysis catheters and continue to represent a major focus of morbidity for the dialysis-dependent population. In the absence of localized clinical findings, an abandoned prosthetic AV access may be responsible for systemic infection; although this is uncommon, diagnosis may require nuclear scanning with[111] In-tagged leukocytes.[12]

The organism most commonly recovered from AV access infection is *Staphylococcus* spp in 32 to 53% of cases. Enterococci and coagulase-negative *Staphylococcus* spp are the second most commonly encountered pathologic agents in 20 to 30% of cases. Gram-negative bacteria and polymicrobial infections are recovered in another 10 to 18%. The most destructive are *Staphylococcus* and *Pseudomonas* spp; in these infections, anastomotic disruption is more likely to occur. Although the clinical findings of infection may seem obvious, up to 25% of graft cultures may be reported as negative. Explanations include antibiotic suppression and bacterial biofilm adherence to prosthetic material.[4,13-15]

Management options for AV access infection require knowledge of the type of conduit, infecting organism, anastomotic involvement, the extent of the process, and whether the conduit is functional. Although uncommon, infection may involve autogenous AV access; these are usually associated with pseudoaneurysm, secondary colonization of a hematoma, or incisional complications.[4] If the mechanical problems can be controlled, the chances of salvaging a functioning access are increased. However, sacrifice of the access may be necessary if these cannot be controlled. Occasionally, with minimal mechanical issues, prolonged antibiotic therapy may successfully suppress an autogenous AV access infection.

Functional prosthetic grafts account for most of the infections in peripheral AV access sites with a reported incidence of 3.5 to 19%. If localized, the segment may be excised and a new graft implanted through a fresh tunnel utilizing uninvolved proximal and distal segments of the graft; the infected segment is resected and the original tunnels are closed. In addition to preservation of a functional access site, segmental graft resection may permit early puncture if an accessible portion of the original well-incorporated conduit remains available for percutaneous puncture. With more extensive involvement not affecting the anastomoses, partial excision is effective and avoids extensive, potentially morbid dissection of the inflow artery by oversewing the stump of the graft. Complete disincorporation of a graft or infection involving the anastomosis requires complete excision and débridement of the affected arterial wall. Primary closure, patch angioplasty, and brachial ligation are all well tolerated, and selection is based upon the extent of operative findings and destruction of the arterial wall. Several authors have reported success with these approaches to the infected AV access.[4,14,16-18]

Special Situations

Infection in the chronically occluded prosthetic graft is difficult to diagnose in the absence of obvious findings such as a chronic sinus or graft extrusion. Although subject to oversensitive detection, an[111] In-labeled leukocyte scan used to detect these may suggest occult graft infection when localized findings are sparse.[12] However, the overwhelming majority of systemic infections arise from chronic indwelling catheters for hemodialysis.[4,13]

Perigraft fluid collections are infrequent but may be mistaken for graft infection. Perigraft seromas have been observed with both Dacron and PTFE prostheses and make repetitive puncture difficult because there is little surrounding tissue to facilitate and maintain hemostasis following puncture. Lymphatic drainage or lymphoceles are less common with upper extremity graft procedures but may also require exploration for control of persistent drainage. Exploration and negative-pressure vacuum therapy has been used with some success for managing this complication.[19] Although recognized as a noninfectious problem initially, each of these collections can be secondarily complicated by infection.

ARTERIAL STEAL SYNDROME

Although a relatively infrequent complication, arterial steal syndrome probably has the greatest potential for limb dysfunction as a result of the access procedure; in addition to neuromotor disability, gangrene may lead to limb loss. Symptoms include irreversible neurologic damage leading to pain and contracture or gangrene with limb loss. Asymptomatic "steal," manifested by pulse deficits, Doppler signal attenuation, and distal flow reversal, is usually observed with AV access but becomes symptomatic only when blood flow is shunted (stolen) from tissue beds distal to the arterial anastomosis.

Unfortunately, symptomatic arterial steal can be difficult to recognize because the clinical spectrum is wide. Although it is usually associated with higher flow rates through the AV access, a low-flow version can also occur. Documented flow diversion is recognized in over 90% of hemoaccess procedures, but disabling symptoms are much less frequent.[4,20-22]

Diagnosis is predominantly clinical. Complaints of severe pain and/or sensorimotor dysfunction involving multiple peripheral forearm nerve trunks are the primary diagnostic features. Weakness of the forearm musculature and diminished sensation may be accompanied by clinical findings of distal ischemia—pallor, cyanosis, and gangrene—of the forearm musculature.[4] Symptoms will appear within a month in the majority of cases, and often immediately after the procedure. Less severe arterial steal may manifest these problems only during dialysis and may only require observation. Unilateral complaints ipsilateral to the AV access may be accompanied by reversal of flow in the distal artery.[22]

A devastating but slightly different clinical scenario occurs when symptoms are isolated to the forearm nerve trunks; labeled ischemic monomelic neuropathy (IMN), the hallmark is severe pain with sensory dysfunction and a palpable distal pulse.[23-24] Motor abnormalities in all three forearm nerve trunks occur ipsilateral to the AV access. The symptoms are commonly attributed to regional anesthetic or positioning, delaying recognition of IMN. Although infrequent, immediate deconstruction or rerouting of flow in the hemoaccess is recommended.[2]

Suspicion of arterial steal is heightened in several clinical situations. Clinical risk factors are not well defined but several studies report common associated conditions. It seems clear that the most consistent risk factor is an arterial anastomosis originating in the brachial artery. When the arterial inflow is in the forearm (most likely the radial artery), the incidence of arterial steal ranges from 0.25 to 1.8%; in contrast, the estimated risk for upper arm AV access (most likely the brachial artery) is 4 to 9%.[4,9,22-23] Unfortunately, the distinction between anatomic arterial and geographic localization is not uniformly recorded in these reports. More than half of the reported cases of arterial steal are women and/or patients with diabetes mellitus.[4,9,22-23,25] In addition, other associated factors include advancing age, prior ipsilateral AV access, and peripheral atherosclerosis. Although age, gender, and diabetes cannot be changed, there are options for anastomotic placement; a preference for forearm arterial inflow may reduce the likelihood of arterial steal.[1,4,26]

Low Flow and Arterial Steal Syndrome

Although uncommon, arterial steal may also occur in the setting of low flow. Decreased fistula flow usually results from intrinsic stenosis or thrombosis, but occasionally it will result from inadequate arterial inflow.[4,20-21] Because occlusive arterial disease in the proximal upper extremity arterial tree is unusual, it is not often considered in the initial differential diagnostic algorithm. The increased arterial flow required to support a low-resistance arteriovenous access demands greater flow than a nonexercising upper extremity. A diminished pulse is suggestive, and arteriography will identify proximal flow-reducing arterial stenosis. If recognized, correction requires an entirely different approach to arterial steal that is often endovascular (i.e., angioplasty for proximal stenosis).

Surgical management of clinically significant symptomatic arterial steal syndrome may take several different approaches. Deconstruction of the AV access by ligation is the most direct and definitive option but requires sacrifice of the AV access. In the specific instance of IMN or severe clinical symptoms of steal, immediate ligation should be considered, because permanent neuromotor damage is more likely in this setting. The only treatment associated with neurologic improvement is correction of the ischemia at the earliest opportunity after recognition.[4,23-25] However, rerouting the arterial anastomosis has successfully resolved the complaint in a number of reports. Three methods have been described and all involve moving the arterial anastomosis—either more proximally or more distally.[4,22,27-30] Restrictive banding to reduce arterial inflow has a high incidence of failure due to thrombosis and as a result is not widely employed for this indication.

HIGH-OUTPUT CARDIAC FAILURE

Cardiac failure is a common comorbidity in patients with end-stage renal disease. It is present in over 30% of those initiating dialysis and develops in another 30% during the course of their dialysis career.[31] The rarity of high-output cardiac failure is partly due to the difficulty of diagnosis and to the counterintuitive concept that failure results from increasing flow through a low-resistance fistula circuit by generating abnormally increased cardiac output. High-output failure is defined as "symptoms of cardiac failure in the presence of an above-normal cardiac index (2.3 $L/min/m^2$)."[32] The symptoms are indistinguishable from those of heart failure attributed to an inadequate cardiac pump. In theory, the low resistance of the fistula permits increased flow through the circuit until the capacity of the heart to compensate is exceeded. Thus, some investigators have attempted to define this problem by measurement of fistula flow. Greater risk of high-output failure is assigned to those with fistula flow in excess of 3.0 L/min or when AV access flow constitutes >30% of cardiac output.[32-33] A substantial decrease in cardiac output with transient fistula occlusion suggests the diagnosis. However, because cardiac function in the dialysis-dependent patient is often already compromised, a numeric classification is not always accurate. To date, this complication has been reported only with autogenous AV fistula.

Diagnosis is ultimately established by clinical improvement. Response to treatment remains the sine qua non of this diagnosis. Literature on high-output failure is sparse, essentially consisting of clinical case series. Although ligation is a definitive solution, it requires sacrifice of the fistula. Banding for this indication has a better outcome than for other AV access flow–related complications and may provide durable relief with preservation of the fistula.[34]

DYSFUNCTIONAL HEMOSTASIS

Abnormal bleeding is a common problem for patients with end-stage renal disease and is attributed to impaired platelet function. The template bleeding time is the only test that has correlated with dysfunctional hemostasis in this population and is recommended for identification of patients at risk for bleeding. In uremic individuals, these times may be prolonged for as long as 15 to 20 minutes.[35] Although dysfunctional bleeding may affect the gastrointestinal tract, intra-articular capsules, or other confined anatomic spaces, our primary focus here is on access-related bleeding.

The surgeon will encounter this when dissection planes continue to ooze during operating room procedures or when puncture sites fail to stop bleeding following dialysis. Frequently, a simple skin suture will control persistent needle hole bleeding. When the skin or the anterior wall of an AV access has degenerated, more invasive methods may be required to preserve access function. Options include interposition grafting or deployment of internal stent grafts (Figure 22–3). General preventive measures include maintaining a hematocrit >30 mL/dL and ensuring adequate interval dialysis exchanges.

Adjunctive pharmacologic therapy for excessive acute or intraoperative bleeding begins with administration of 1-deamino-8-D-arginine vasopressin (DDAVP). The dose is 0.3 μg/Kg given over 30 minutes with a 50-cc bolus of saline. The effects are thought to result from a release of von Willebrand's factor with an expected duration of 4 to 6 hours. Supplemental doses may also be given but are generally less efficacious. DDAVP may be given as subcutaneous or intranasal doses with equivalent efficacy.[36] Cryoprecipitate has also been advocated for use in this setting, although subsequent reports have been less convincing than the initial claims. Its effect is immediate and of short duration, but it has the additive risk of exposure to blood-borne disease. Infusion of conjugated estrogen (0.6 μg/kg for 4-5 days) is advocated for more chronic bleeding, because the duration of its action extends for as long as 5 to 14 days.[4,37]

NEUROPATHY

Symptoms and findings of peripheral neuropathy are present in over 70% of patients with end-stage renal disease.[38] Differentiating diabetic or uremic neuropathy from causes amenable to surgical management may be extremely difficult. Ischemic neuropathy and arterial steal were discussed previously; symptoms produced by radial or ulnar entrapment are focal mononeuropathies amenable to decompression.

Median Nerve Entrapment

Observations that may implicate the AV access include unilaterality, involvement of the nondominant hand, male gender, and duration of dialysis therapy. In the general population, nerve entrapment is more commonly seen in the female gender and in the dominant hand. Entrapment syndromes generally do not occur immediately, but the incidence increases with time and approaches 35% after 5 years on dialysis.[39] Accurate diagnosis often requires specialist assistance. A localized pressure increase in constrained fascial tunnels is thought to produce the symptoms, and this may be due to deposition and accumulation of β-amyloid.

Median nerve involvement begins with sensory complaints. The sensory distribution usually involves the thumb, index, and radial aspect of the middle finger with symptoms of numbness, tingling, and pain. Motor weakness occurs later and indicates a more advanced process. The most obvious deficiency is pinch or apposition of the thumb to the other digits and atrophy of the thenar eminence. Once the diagnosis is established, entrapment is managed by carpal tunnel release. Equivalent results are achieved with open or endoscopic procedures, although one requires a larger incision. Symptom relief is not as good in patients with renal failure; in part, this may be due to the difficulty of establishing an early diagnosis before advanced changes occur.

An unusual variant is presented by a highly calcified median artery, the bulk of which can fill the space in the carpal tunnel; in addition to the standard division of the transverse carpal ligament, treatment includes ligation and resection of the median artery. Cautious attention to the residual digital circulation is critical if the artery is patent.[40]

Ulnar Nerve Entrapment

Ulnar nerve entrapment is less common and may arise from entrapment in either the cubital or the ulnar tunnels. The sensory distribution usually involves the ulnar aspect of the ring finger and the fifth finger with symptoms of numbness, tingling, and pain. Motor weakness occurs later and indicates a more advanced process. The most obvious deficiency is weakness of ab-ad-duction of the extended fingers and of forceful grasp with atrophy of the hypothenar eminence. Once the diagnosis is established, entrapment is managed by fascial tunnel release.

The vascular surgeon may be asked about the use of a tourniquet during these short extremity procedures. Although some have used this technique successfully, thrombosis is a real risk, especially with prosthetic AV access.[41] Duplex ultrasound of the AV access is recommended prior to the procedure to determine if there are intrinsic stenoses that may increase this risk.[4]

Neuropathy Associated with Diabetes or Uremia

Uremic and/or diabetic neuropathic symptoms are frequent in this population. Electrodiagnostic studies may assist in differentiating surgically amenable problems from intrinsic diabetic or uremic neuropathy; they are not considered to offer prognostic value. When electrodiagnostic studies are performed on a routine basis, subclinical or asymptomatic abnormalities are commonly identified. Bilaterality strongly suggests a diabetic or uremic etiology. Prospective studies incorporating routine electrodiagnostic evaluations have demonstrated an equal incidence of neuropathic abnormalities bilaterally.[42] Thus, some have suggested that entrapment is really a local manifestation of a systemic problem rather than a localized problem associated with the AV access. Therefore, the presence and severity of neuropathic abnormalities before construction of AV access are important considerations, as is the method of making the diagnosis.

REFERENCES

1. Sidawy AN, Spergel LM, Besarab A, et al. The Society for Vascular Surgery: Clinical Practice Guidelines for the Surgical Placement and Maintence of Arteriovenous Access for Hemodialysis. J Vasc Surg 2008;48:2S–25S.
2. NKF-K/DOQI Clinical Practice Guidelines for Vascular Access: update 2006. Am J Kidney Dis 2006;48(suppl):S176–247.
3. Murad MH, Sidawy AN, Elamin MB, et al. Timing of referral for chronic hemodialysis vascular access placement: a systematic review. J Vasc Surg 2008;48:S31–3.
4. Padberg FT Jr, Calligaro KD, Sidawy AN. Complications of arteriovenous hemodialysis access: recognition and management. J Vasc Surg 2008;48:55S–80S.
5. Cuadra S, Padberg FT, Turbin RE, et al. Cerebral venous hypertension and blindness: a reversible complication. J Vasc Surg 2005;42:792–5.
6. Haser PB, Padberg FT Jr. Strategies for difficult hemoaccess issues, or end stage access for the end stage renal disease patient. In: Matsumura J, Pearce W, Yao JST, eds. Trends in Vascular Surgery. Chicago: Precept Press; 2003; pp. 363–74.
7. Rizvi AZ, Kalra M, Bjarnason H, et al. Benign superior vena cava syndrome: stenting is now the first line of treatment. J Vasc Surg 2008;47:372–80.
8. Gradman WS, Laub J, Cohen W. Femoral vein transposition for arteriovenous hemodialysis access: improved patient selection and intraoperative measures reduce postoperative ischemia. J Vasc Surg 2005;41:279–84.
9. Haimov M, Baez A, Neff M, Slifkin R. Complication of arteriovenous fistulae for hemodialysis. Arch Surg 1975;110:708–12.
10. Kian K, Asif A. Cephalic arch stenosis. Semin Dial 2008;21:78–82.
11. Najibi S, Bush RL, Terramani TT, Chaikof EL, et al. Covered stent exclusion of dialysis access pseudoaneurysms. J Surg Res 2002;106:15–9.
12. Brunner MC, Mitchell RS, Baldwin JC, et al. Prosthetic graft infection: limitation of indium white blood cell scanning. J Vasc Surg 1986;3:42–8.
13. Tokars JI, Miller ER, Stein G. New national surveillance system for hemodialysis associated infections: initial results. Am J Kidney Dis 2002;30:288–95.
14. Ryan SV, Calligaro KD, Scharff J, Dougherty MJ. Management of infected prosthetic dialysis arteriovenous grafts. J Vasc Surg 2004;39:73–8.
15. Padberg FT Jr, Smith SM, Eng RHK. Accuracy of disincorporation for identification of vascular graft infection. Arch Surg 1995;130:183–7.
16. Schwab DP, Taylor SM, Cull DL, et al. Isolated arteriovenous dialysis access graft segment infection: the results of segmental bypass and partial graft excision. Ann Vasc Surg 2000; 14:63–6.
17. Gifford RRM. Management of tunnel infections of dialysis polytetrafluoroethylene grafts. J Vasc Surg 1985;2:854–8.
18. Padberg FT, Lee BC, Curl RG. Management of hemoaccess site infection. Surg Gynecol Obstet 1992;174:103–8.
19. Abai B, Zickler RW, Pappas PJ, et al. Lymphorrhea responds to negative pressure wound therapy. J Vasc Surg 2007;45:610–3.
20. Khan FA, Vesely TM. Arterial problems associated with dysfunctional hemodialysis access grafts: evaluation of patients at high risk for arterial disease. J Vasc Interv Radiol 2002;13: 1109–14.
21. Duijm LEM, Liem YS, van der Rijt RHH, et al. Inflow stenoses in dysfunctional hemodialysis access fistulae and grafts. Am J Kidney Dis 2006;48:98–105.
22. Lazarides MK, Staramos DN, Panagopoulos GN, et al. Indications for surgical treatment of angioaccess induced arterial "steal." J Am Coll Surg 1998;187:422–6.
23. Hye RJ, Wolf YG. Ischemic monomelic neuropathy: an underrecognized complication of hemodialysis access. Ann Vasc Surg 1994;8:578–82.
24. Wilbourn AI, Furlan AJ, Hulley W, Ruschhaupt W. Ischemic monomelic neuropathy. Neurology 1983;33:447–51.

25. Redfern AB, Zimmerman ND. Neurologic and ischemic complications of upper extremity vascular access for dialysis. J Hand Surg [Am] 1995;20:199–204.
26. Jennings WC. Creating arteriovenous fistulas in 132 consecutive patients. Exploiting the proximal radial artery arteriovenous fistula: reliable, safe, simple forearm and upper arm access. Arch Surg 2006;141:27–32.
27. Schanzer H, Schwartz M, Harrington E, Haimov M. Treatment of ischemia due to "steal" by arteriovenous fistula with distal artery ligation and revascularization. J Vasc Surg 1988; 7:770–3.
28. Zanow J, Kruger U, Scholz H. Proximalization of the arterial inflow: a new technique to treat access-related ischemia. J Vasc Surg 2006;43:1216–21.
29. Minion DJ, Moore E, Endean E. Revision using distal inflow: a novel approach to dialysis-associated steal syndrome. Ann Vasc Surg 2005;19:625–8.
30. Berman SS, Gentile AT, Glickman MH, et al. Distal revascularization-interval ligation for limb salvage and maintenance of dialysis access in ischemic steal syndrome. J Vasc Surg 1997;26:393–404.
31. Harnett JD, Foley RN, Kent GM, et al. Congestive heart failure in dialysis patients: prevalence, incidence, prognosis, and risk factors. Kidney Int 1998;47:884–90.
32. MacRae JM, Pandeya S, Humen DP, et al. Arteriovenous fistula associated high-output cardiac failure: a review of mechanisms. Am J Kidney Dis 2004;43:E21–2.
33. Pandeya S, Lindsey RM. The relationship between cardiac output and access flow during hemodialysis. ASAIO J 1999;45:135–8.
34. Dikow R, Schwenger V, Zeler M, Ritz E. Do AV fistulas contribute to cardiac mortality in hemodialysis patients? Semin Dial 2002;15:14–7.
35. Steiner RW, Coggins C, Carvalho ACA. Bleeding time in uremia: a useful test to assess clinical bleeding. Am J Hematol 1979;7:107–17.
36. Vigano GL, Mannucci PM, Lattuada A, et al. Subcutaneous desmopressin (DDAVP) shortens the bleeding time in uremia. Am J Hematol 1989;31:32–5.
37. Livio M, Mannucci PM, Vigano GL, et al. Conjugated estrogens for the management of bleeding associated with renal failure. N Engl J Med 1986;315:731–5.
38. Bolton CF. Peripheral neuropathies associated with chronic renal failure. Can J Neurol Sci 1980;7:89–96.
39. Halter SK, DeLisa JA, Stolov WC, et al. Carpal tunnel syndrome in chronic renal dialysis patients. Arch Phys Med Rehabil 1992;62:197–201.
40. Barfred T, Hojlund AP, Bertheussen K. Median artery in carpal tunnel syndrome. J Hand Surg [Am] 1985;10:864–7.
41. Semer NB, Goldberg NJ, Cuono CB. Upper extremity entrapment neuropathy and tourniquet use in patients undergoing hemodialysis. J Hand Surg [Am] 1989;14:897–900.
42. Dyck PJ, Kratz KM, Karnes JL, et al. The prevalence of staged severity of various types of diabetic neuropathy, retinopathy, and nephropathy in a population-based cohort: the Rochester Diabetic Neuropathy Study. Neurology 1993;43:817–24.

23

Axilloaxillary Arteriovenous Access for Hemodialysis

Spence M. Taylor, M.D. and David L. Cull, M.D.

Implementation of the National Kidney Foundation Kidney/Dialysis Outcome Quality Initiative (K/DOQI) has resulted in improvements in the medical management of patients on hemodialysis and a decrease in their mortality rate.[1] Consequently, it is not uncommon for the surgeon to be confronted with patients who have "outlived" the arteriovenous (AV) access options in the upper extremity. It has been estimated that nearly 7% of access placements are located at a site other than the preferred location of the upper extremity owing to prolonged dialysis life and subsequent access failure.[2] For many of these patients, quality of life and long-term survival become primarily dependent on the surgeon's ability to provide a functional and durable AV access. To meet this challenge, the access surgeon must have a number of complex vascular access procedures in his/her surgical armamentarium and must be aware of the advantages and disadvantages of each. The most common location for AV access placement beyond the upper extremity is the femoral artery and vein. Prosthetic femoral accesses, however, are not ideal and are associated with a significant risk of infection, access-related leg ischemia, and graft failure.[3-4] The second most commonly cited alternative for AV access placement beyond the upper extremity is the chest wall axilloaxillary AV graft. Although it is apparent from the available literature that complex access procedures of the thigh and chest wall are associated with a higher complication rate, one must avoid the temptation of simply placing a cuffed dialysis catheter as an alternative. Indeed, the significant complications associated with chronic dialysis via a catheter are also well established.[5-6] The K/DOQI guidelines for vascular access recommend use of a dialysis catheter only as a bridge for AV access placement or in patients with extremely limited life expectancy.[7] In one series reporting the outcome of prosthetic femorofemoral AV accesses, the median survival for patients undergoing the procedure was 24 months.[4] Therefore, despite the challenges of complex AV access placement and treatment of their complications, their placement is usually justified in preference to a cuffed dialysis catheter.

Although the prosthetic chest wall access was first described in 1978, the literature reporting the outcome with this technique is primarily limited to case reports and small case series.[8-11] When considering axilloaxillary AV access, there are usually three options cited: axillary artery to ipsilateral axillary vein loop access, axillary artery to contralateral axillary or jugular vein straight access (necklace access), and brachial artery to jugular vein straight access (Figure 23–1). The surgeons in our group have used chest wall grafts on occasion and have reported our experience in the literature.[8] Our preference is to utilize the ipsilateral looped axilloaxillary AV access graft over the straight axilloaxillary necklace graft, although both have clinical utility. In particular, we believe that chest wall grafts may be the alternative access of choice for morbidly obese patients in whom access options in the upper extremity have been expended.

TECHNIQUE

Looped Chest Wall Graft

Most patients considered for chest wall or cervical access procedures have had previous central venous dialysis catheters and multiple upper extremity access operations and interventions; therefore, it is important that these patients undergo an imaging study to confirm central venous patency prior to surgery. If the proximal axillary, subclavian, or brachiocephalic vein has been recently angioplastied or stented, an alternative site for AV access

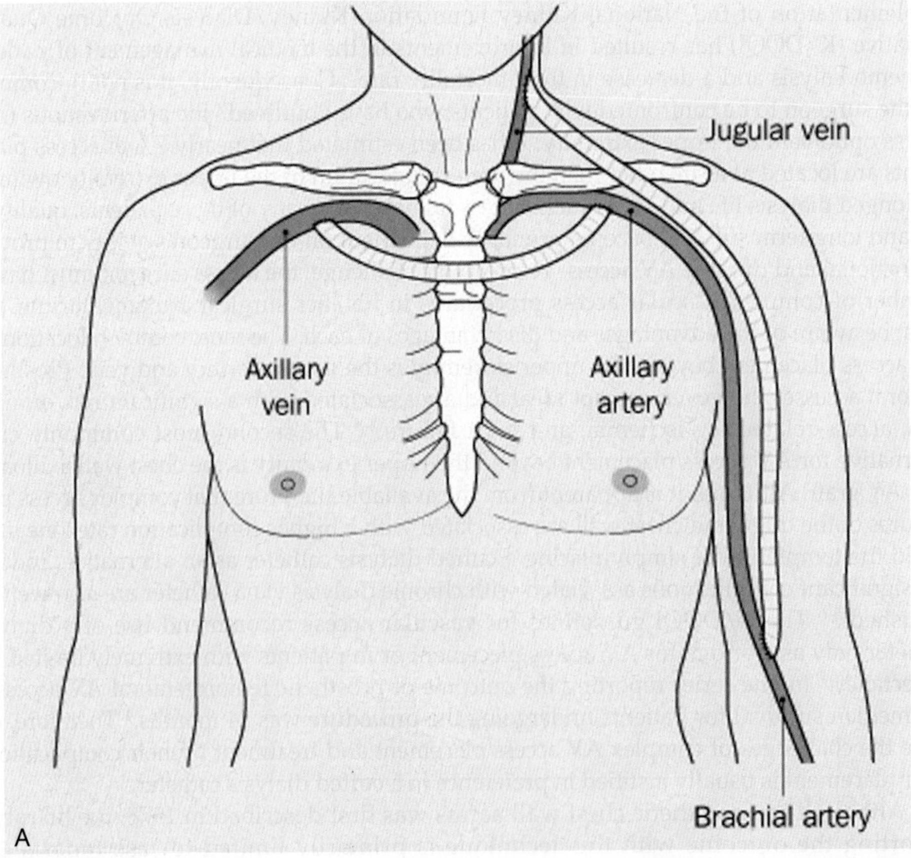

Figure 23-1. **A.** Anatomic configuration of axillary artery to contralateral axillary vein (necklace access) or jugular vein straight access (left), and **B.** the ipsilateral looped chest wall axilloaxillary AV access graft (right) *(Continued)*

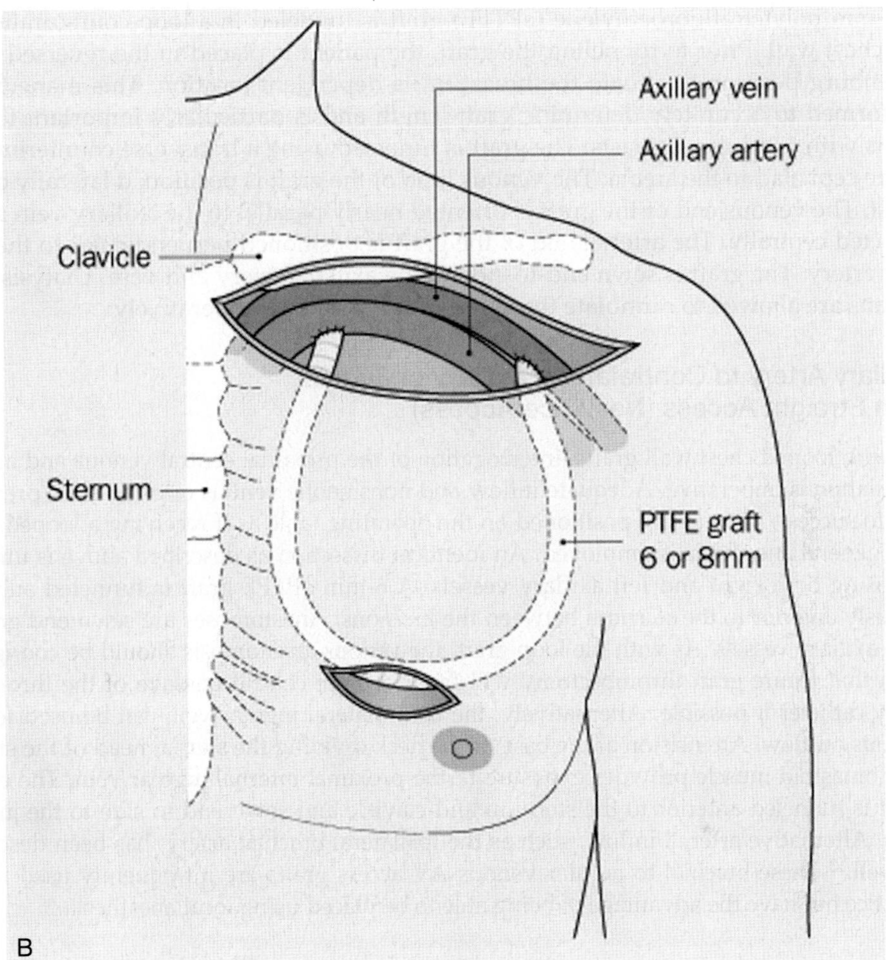

Figure 23-1. *(Continued)*

should be sought because recurrent stenosis following central venous intervention is common and may influence access patency. If a significant difference in blood pressure between the extremities exists, the axillary artery on the side with the highest pressure is the preferred donor vessel, and a contrast arteriogram or CT angiogram should be considered. In addition to anatomic considerations, the handedness of the patient also influences the choice of a right-sided or left-sided access placement.

The procedures are performed under general anesthesia. The patient is placed in the supine position with the arm extended 90 degrees on an arm board. An incision is made one fingerbreadth below the clavicle from the sternoclavicular joint to the coracoid process. The pectoralis major muscle fibers are split. The clavipectoral fascia is divided and the axillary vein is exposed and mobilized. Beneath the axillary vein, the axillary artery is exposed just distal to its exit from the thoracic outlet and medial to the insertion of the pectoralis minor muscle. The pectoralis minor muscle is not divided. Branches of the axillary artery, such as the supreme thoracic artery, are ligated and divided as necessary to achieve adequate mobilization of the axillary artery.

A 6-mm polytetrafluoroethylene (ePTFE) graft is tunneled in a loop configuration on the chest wall. Prior to tunneling the graft, the patient is placed in the reversed Trendelenburg position to situate the breast in its dependent location. This maneuver is performed to accurately determine graft length and is particularly important for patients with pendulous breasts. The graft is tunneled using a transverse counterincision made cephalad to the areola. The venous limb of the graft is positioned laterally on the chest. The venous end of the graft is oriented nearly parallel to the axillary vein and is directed centrally. The arterial end of the graft is positioned perpendicular to the axillary artery. The graft is sewn end-to-side to the axillary artery and vein. Dialysis technicians are allowed to cannulate the access 2 to 3 weeks postoperatively.

Axillary Artery to Contralateral Axillary or Jugular Vein Straight Access (Necklace Access)

As with looped chest wall grafts, interrogation of the proximal central venous and arterial circulation is imperative. Adequate inflow and nonstenotic venous outflow are a prerequisite to success. Patients are positioned on the operating table as if receiving a looped graft, and general anesthesia is employed. An identical dissection as described above is utilized, exposing both right and left axillary vessels. A 6-mm ePTFE graft is tunneled subcutaneously anterior to the sternum between the incisions. Anastomoses are sewn end graft to side axillary vessels. As with the loop graft, the venous anastomosis should be configured such that future graft thrombectomy will favor a more central passage of the thrombectomy catheter if possible. Alternatively, the contralateral jugular vein can be used for the venous outflow. An incision at the base of the neck dividing the sternal head of the sternocleidomastoid muscle provides exposure to the proximal internal jugular vein. The ePTFE graft is tunneled anterior to the sternum and clavicle and sewn end to side to the jugular vein. Alternative arterial inflow, such as the ipsilateral brachial artery, has been described as well.[12] These brachial to jugular venous AV access grafts are infrequently used in our practice but have the advantage of being able to be placed using local anesthesia.

OUTCOMES

In 1996, McCann reported outcomes for a series of 26 patients with prosthetic chest wall accesses.[10] He utilized a straight graft configuration from the axillary artery to the contralateral axillary or internal jugular vein. The secondary patency for AV accesses in his series was 60% at 2 years. There are several theoretical disadvantages to this technique. First, it is difficult to orient the venous anastomosis such that in the event of graft thrombosis, thrombectomy results in central passage of a thromboembolectomy catheter. Clearly, outflow stenosis is most likely to occur central to the venous anastomosis, making endovascular corrective intervention difficult or even impossible. Second, operative exposure of the anterior axillary vasculature can be associated with technical neurovascular complications, especially in the reoperative setting. Exposing both right and left axillary vessels obviously doubles the chances of these types of complications. Last, in the event that the patient develops operative coronary artery disease, these "necklace AV access grafts" must usually undergo division and reanastomosis at the time of median sternotomy. Although this scenario is rare, it does expose the access graft to potential bleeding and thrombotic and infectious complications. Considering all of these disadvantages, our group performs looped axilloaxillary AV grafts in preference to straight axilloaxillary neck grafts when feasible.

Two recent series, comprising 34 and 27 accesses, have reported the outcome of prosthetic axilloaxillary looped accesses utilizing the ipsilateral axillary artery and vein.[8,11] These series reported secondary patency rates of 37% and 80% at 2 years. The looped graft configuration, which utilizes the ipsilateral axillary artery and vein, preserves the contralateral axillary vessels as a site for future access placement. The authors of both of these series emphasize the importance of orienting the venous limb laterally on the chest wall, which allows the venous limb of the graft to be directed toward rather than away from the central veins. Should a subsequent stenosis develop at the venous anastomosis, this orientation toward the central veins facilitates percutaneous intervention of the access.

No case of access-related steal has been noted in any of the three largest chest wall access series.[8-9,11] In each of these series, a number of axilloaxillary vein accesses were placed in patients in whom previous accesses in the ipsilateral extremity had caused hand ischemia. Based on this experience, it appears that a history of access-related hand ischemia does not preclude access placement based off the ipsilateral axillary artery.

The chest wall access appears to be associated with a lower infection rate than prosthetic accesses in the lower extremity. The infection rates range from 4 to 15%, which compares favorably with series reporting the outcome of prosthetic accesses based off vessels in the groin. In the largest of these chest wall access series, Kendall, from our institution, noted that the infection and patency rates were not significantly different in obese compared with nonobese patients.[8] Given the technical challenge and increased complication rate associated with prosthetic access placement in the thigh position for patients who are morbidly obese, the chest wall access may be an attractive alternative to thigh access in this situation. One potential disadvantage of the chest wall access, however, is that proximal control of the axillary vessels can be extremely challenging if the chest wall graft becomes infected and needs to be excised.

Vega et al. reported a series of 51 prosthetic brachial artery–jugular vein accesses.[12] The secondary patency rate was 70% at 18 months, which is similar to the patency rate of the axilloaxillary access.

DECISION-MAKING AND ALTERNATIVE ARTERIOVENOUS ACCESS PLACEMENT

The staggering morbidity and financial burden associated with vascular access has prompted efforts, such as the K/DOQI guidelines, to use principles of evidence-based medicine to determine the outcome of access procedures and ultimately standardize AV access management.[7] These efforts have resulted in the development of clinical practice guidelines for vascular access that include an "order of preference" for AV access procedures and emphasize autogenous AV access creation. However, there is a paucity of evidence-based literature related to the outcome of "complex" access procedures that become necessary when access options in the upper extremity are expended. The literature reporting the outcome of complex AV access procedures in the lower extremity and chest wall consists only of the previously cited small series or case reports. Consequently, the K/DOQI clinical practice guidelines are silent when it comes to recommendations regarding an approach to providing access for the patient in whom AV access placement in the upper extremity is not possible. Alternative complex access procedures can involve a bridge fistula tunneled subcutaneously between any normal artery and any normal vein.

Arteries can include the aorta and any of its branches, from the great vessels to the most peripheral artery. Alternative outflow venous options are even more diverse and can include not only peripheral and central veins but also the right atrium. Truly, surgical creativity is the only limitation.

The most frequently used alternative/complex AV access site involves the femoral vessels of the lower extremity. In most patients, exposure of the femoral vessels for graft placement is relatively straightforward. The procedure can be performed under local or regional anesthesia, and compared with other complex AV access options, complications are more easily managed. However, alternative procedures must be used for patients with significant aortoiliac occlusive disease, bilateral iliofemoral venous thrombosis, or in those in whom femoral access sites have been expended. Most experts consider the chest wall AV access graft as the next alternative procedure of choice. As well, there are patients in whom a chest wall AV access graft may be preferential to a femoral thigh graft. Prosthetic femorofemoral access has significant disadvantages for patients who are obese. A previous report of prosthetic femorofemoral access from our institution found significantly higher rates of access reintervention in obese compared with nonobese patients.[4] The abdominal pannus in the obese patient that overlies the groin and the depth of the femoral vessels in the proximal thigh make femoral access placement technically difficult, with a significant risk of infection. Anecdotally, we have noticed that obese patients often have less subcutaneous fat over the axillary than the femoral vessels. The vascular exposure and tunneling for prosthetic axilloaxillary access is easier than for femoral-based access in these cases. We hypothesized that chest wall grafts might have lower infectious complications than thigh grafts in obese patients. Indeed, when we examined outcomes of our looped chest wall grafts in the obese and nonobese patients, outcomes were similar (or better in obese patients), unlike our thigh grafts (Figures 23–2 and 23–3). Given this experience,

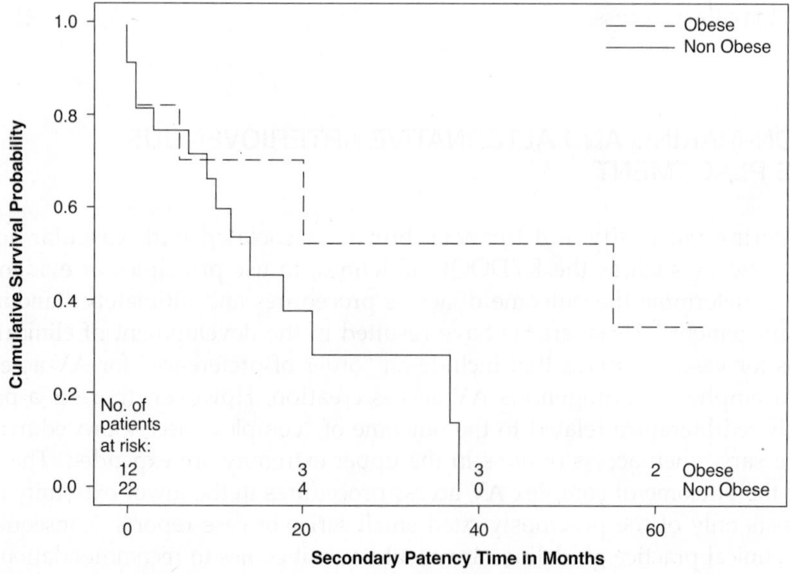

Figure 23-2. Secondary patency for a series of 34 looped axilloaxillary chest wall grafts, 12 in patients with morbid obesity (dashed line) and 22 in patients without morbid obesity (solid line). There was no statistically significant difference between curves (P=.14; log rank test).[8]

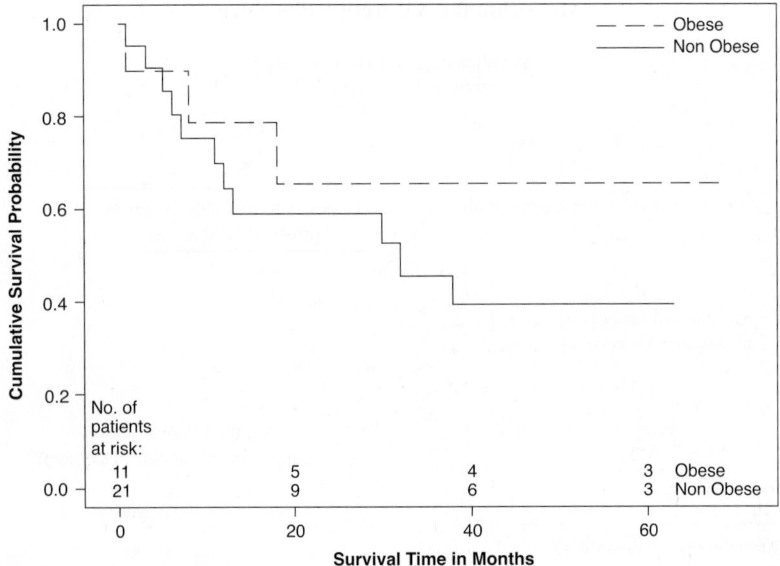

Figure 23-3. Survival for a series of 32 patients with looped axilloaxillary chest wall grafts, 11 in patients with morbid obesity (dashed line) and 21 in patients without morbid obesity (solid line). There was no statistically significant difference between curves (P=.34; log rank test).[8]

we recommend the looped chest wall graft in preference to thigh grafts in patients who are morbidly obese (Figure 23–4).

SUMMARY

Although the femoral vessels are the most common site for vascular access placement once access options in the upper extremity have been exhausted, the prosthetic axilloaxillary access can be an effective access in cases in which femoral access placement is not possible (significant aortoiliac occlusive disease, iliofemoral vein thrombosis). The prosthetic axilloaxillary access should be considered in preference to the femoral-based accesses in patients who are morbidly obese.

The femoral and axillary based prosthetic access procedures are associated with an increased incidence of complications compared with upper extremity access procedures. However, these complex access options are nearly always preferable to chronic dialysis via a permanent cuffed dialysis catheter. Indeed, current K/DOQI guidelines recommend any type of permanent AV access in preference to a cuffed venous catheter except in extreme circumstances or in scenarios in which bridging between permanent AV accesses is required.

Surgeons performing access today need to possess a working knowledge of the techniques and complications associated with axilloaxillary chest wall AV access. These grafts can be quite useful and should be employed when clinically needed.

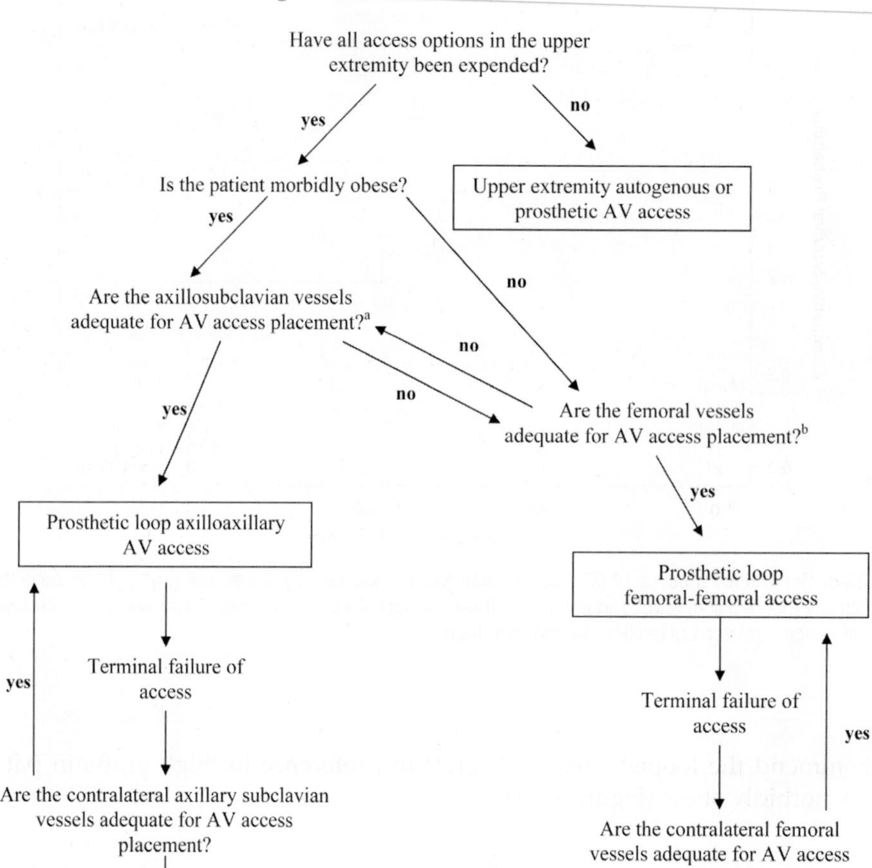

[a]Upper extremity venogram is recommended to confirm central vein patency prior to prosthetic axilloaxillary access placement.

[b]Lower extremity duplex ultrasonography is recommended to confirm adequacy of femoral vessels.

Figure 23-4. A suggested algorithm for the placement of AV access in patients where all upper extremity options have been exhausted.[8]

REFERENCES

1. U.S. Renal Data System, USRDS 2006. Annual Data Report: Atlas of End-Stage Renal Disease in the United States. Bethesda, MD: National Institutes of Health, National Institute of Diabetes and Digestive and Kidney Diseases; 2006.
2. National Kidney Foundation. K/DOQI Clinical Practice Guidelines For Vascular Access, 2000. Am J Kidney Dis 2001;37(Suppl 1):S137–81.

3. Tashjian DB, Lipkowitz GS, Madden RL, et al. Safety and efficacy of femoral-based hemodialysis access grafts. J Vasc Surg 2002;35:691–3.
4. Cull JD, Cull DL, Taylor SM, et al. Prosthetic thigh arteriovenous access: outcome using the SVS/AAVS reporting standards. J Vasc Surg 2004;39:381–6.
5. De Meester JD, Vanholder R, De Roose J, et al. Factors and complications affecting catheter and technique survival with permanent single-lumen dialysis catheters. Nephrol Dial Transplant 1994;9:678–83.
6. Saad TF. Bacteremia associated with tunneled, cuffed hemodialysis catheters. Am J Kidney Dis 1999;34:1114–24.
7. Vascular Access Work Group. Clinical practice guidelines for vascular access. Am J Kidney Dis. 2006;48:S248–78.
8. Kendall TW, Cull DL, Carsten CG, et al. The prosthetic axillo-axillary loop access: indications, technique, and outcomes. J Vasc Surg 2008;48:389–93.
9. Chuang FR, Hsieh MJ, Lee CH, et al. Axillary artery to contralateral axillary vein graft fistula in chronic hemodialysis patients. Ren Fail 2003;25:871–8.
10. McCann RL. Axillary grafts for difficult hemodialysis access. J Vasc Surg 1996;24:457–62.
11. Jean-Baptiste E, Hassen-Khodja R, Haudebourg P, et al. Axillary loop grafts for hemodialysis access: midterm results from a single-center study. J Vasc Surg 2008;47:138–43.
12. Vega D, Polo JR, Polo J, et al. Brachial-jugular expanded PTFE grafts for dialysis. Ann Vasc Surg 2001;15:553–6.

24

Access Surveillance

Audra A. Duncan, M.D.

INTRODUCTION

Routine dialysis access surveillance and subsequent intervention in an effort to prolong access patency are among the most controversial subjects in current dialysis access management. Although the literature supports the ideal type of access (autologous) and is fairly consistent in support of the timing (prior to absolute dialysis need), the data regarding surveillance are divergent. This topic is particularly of concern now, when health care costs such as surveillance imaging must be justified by proving that it reduces future adverse outcomes or decreases long-term cost.[1] The following chapter reviews the types of surveillance, indications, and results of recent studies, including a recent systematic review of the literature.[2]

Dialysis access thrombosis is the most common complication of upper extremity access procedures, occurring in 0.5 to 0.8 episodes per year in prosthetics.[3] The primary cause is venous anastomotic stenosis, although arterial inflow can contribute to thrombosis and may occur more often than previously believed. An inflow stenosis may occur at the artery-graft anastomosis (graft cases), artery-vein anastomosis (fistula cases), or juxta-anastomotic region (within 2 cm from the arterial anastomosis) with a >50% reduction in luminal diameter compared with the adjacent vessel or graft. Based on this definition, Asif et al. reported that nearly a third of 223 cases had an inflow stenosis.[4] More than 50% of cases with inflow stenosis had concomitant venous stenoses, and inflow stenosis occurred less frequently in grafts (29%) than in fistulas (40%). Therefore, access inflow stenosis is more frequent than traditionally reported and should be considered in evaluating failing access.

Because of wide ranges in luminal diameters of access vessels with varying blood flows, there is not a direct relationship between stenosis, progressing to decreased blood flow, and stenosis, leading to access failure. Rather, the blood flow likely will remain unchanged in the setting of a stenosis and then rapidly decrease when a critical point is met.[5-6] In addition, other studies have demonstrated that fistula or graft flow varies widely before and during dialysis, making interventions based purely on flow difficult.[7]

However, because of the high risk of graft or fistula thromboses in the setting of stenoses, the National Kidney Foundation (NKF) Kidney/Dialysis Outcome Quality

Initiative (K/DOQI) guidelines recommend repair of stenoses electively if there is hemodynamic dysfunction and poor delivery of dialysis or imminent thrombosis.[8] Once a stenosis is identified, treatment with surgical thrombectomy and anastomotic revision has similar outcomes to thrombolysis or mechanical thrombectomy with percutaneous transluminal angioplasty (PTA).[3] Therefore, intervention decisions can be made based on the patient's health status and anatomy.

The real question that one must ask is whether identifying an access stenosis early through scheduled surveillance will prolong the life of the fistula or graft, even in the setting of an adequately functioning fistula or graft. Several recent trials have questioned such surveillance.[2-3,9,11] In addition, controversy lies in the type of surveillance one should obtain: clinical assessment with physical examination, noninvasive flow monitoring, duplex ultrasound, dialysis venous pressures, or proceed with fistulogram based on the preceding test results.[7-8,12-14] Unfortunately, owing to the small sample size and varying indications and types of intervention, many of these studies have been criticized as inconclusive.

SURVEILLANCE TECHNIQUES

Physical Examination

The most cost-effective assessment of graft stenosis is the physical examination. Arm swelling may indicate venous anastomotic stenosis even before dialysis is instituted. In addition, NKF K/DOQI guidelines list the physical findings of the presence of collateral veins, prolonged bleeding after needle withdrawal, or altered characteristics of pulse or thrill in a graft as acceptable forms of evaluation but not the preferred technique for graft assessment.[8] However, because of the increased sensitivity of the clinical examination for assessing fistulas, physical examination criteria are considered a preferred technique for their evaluation.[8] A clinical examination should occur at least monthly by a qualified individual such as a nephrologist or dialysis nurse. At our center, access is assessed clinically at each dialysis visit or at least monthly if the patient is not yet receiving scheduled dialysis.

Flow Methods

NKF K/DOQI guidelines list multiple options for flow measurement, including the use of variable flow Doppler ultrasound, CritLine III direct transcutaneous (HemaMetrics), ultrasound dilution, or measurement with magnetic resonance angiography (MRA) or duplex Doppler ultrasound with quantitative color velocity imaging.[8] Intra-access flow measurements, directly measured static venous dialysis pressure, or duplex ultrasound flows are preferred methods of assessing grafts but unstandardized dynamic venous pressures are not recommended.[8] Direct flow measurements, physical examination, or duplex ultrasound are recommended for fistula surveillance.[1,12]

Based on K/DOQI guidelines,[8] the following findings would be an indication for further investigation with an ultrasound or fistulogram:

1. An access flow rate <600 mL/min in grafts and <400 to 500 mL/min in fistulas or a decrease of 25% in access flow from a previous stable baseline >1000 mL/min. Although some fistulas can function for years at flows <400 mL/min, treatment time may need to be extended, which is a strain on both the patient and the dialysis center.

2. A venous segment static pressure (mean pressures) ratio >0.5 in grafts or fistulas.
3. An arterial segment static pressure ratio >0.75 in grafts.

As with any screening, a patient with an isolated abnormal flow measurement in the setting of a normal physical examination or successful dialysis treatment should likely be monitored rather than referred for intervention. More important, trends in abnormal flow or difficulty in maintaining dialysis flow should be carefully considered.

Ultrasound

Although many centers may recommend proceeding directly to angiographic study after an abnormal flow measurement, duplex ultrasound may be an important study both for surveillance and/or prior to intervention or fistulogram (Figure 24–1). In centers in which duplex imaging is readily available, surveillance imaging can be done serially at regular intervals (typically once a month) in an attempt to identify failing grafts or fistulas.

Dossabhoy et al. studied 101 patients undergoing surveillance of hemodialysis grafts with duplex ultrasound. The costs of stenosis ($142/patient per year) and flow measurements ($279/patient per year) were minimal compared with the total cost of access-related care. They concluded that stenosis surveillance by duplex ultrasound combined with preemptive correction reduced hospitalization costs and the total cost of access-related care. They also found that flow surveillance did not yield a significant benefit in terms of cost reduction.[1] However, this may not be cost-effective or effective in prolonging graft survival.

At our institution, we are presently studying the effectiveness of scheduled ultrasound imaging after fistulas done at our hospital and continue to collect data on this subject. Many of our patients do not regularly receive dialysis at our hospital and return only for assessment of failing access. In these cases, ultrasound will be obtained if the physical examination is normal in order to avoid angiography if not necessary. In addition, ultrasound is recommended for patients not yet receiving dialysis in whom contrast for fistulogram is contraindicated, and ultrasound is done for preoperative anatomic mapping.

Angiography

Fistulogram is rarely done as a primary assessment. The advantages of this invasive study include the ability to both diagnose and treat concomitantly. However, in those patients who are not yet receiving dialysis, contrast angiography may be contraindicated or the onset of hemodialysis will be hastened. In patients referred for a fistulogram due to an abnormal duplex ultrasound, angioplasty is frequently (60 to 80% of patients) performed at our institution, consistent with other studies (Figure 24–2).[10] In most cases, the likelihood of needing angioplasty if an abnormality was identified only on clinical monitoring was slightly lower. As stated above, one must not disregard the potential for arterial inflow stenoses and be prepared to treat them concomitantly (i.e., prepare for femoral artery access if needed).

RECENT STUDIES

A systematic review from our institution demonstrated only a trend toward benefit in the thrombosis rate and access survival in patients who had access surveillance compared with

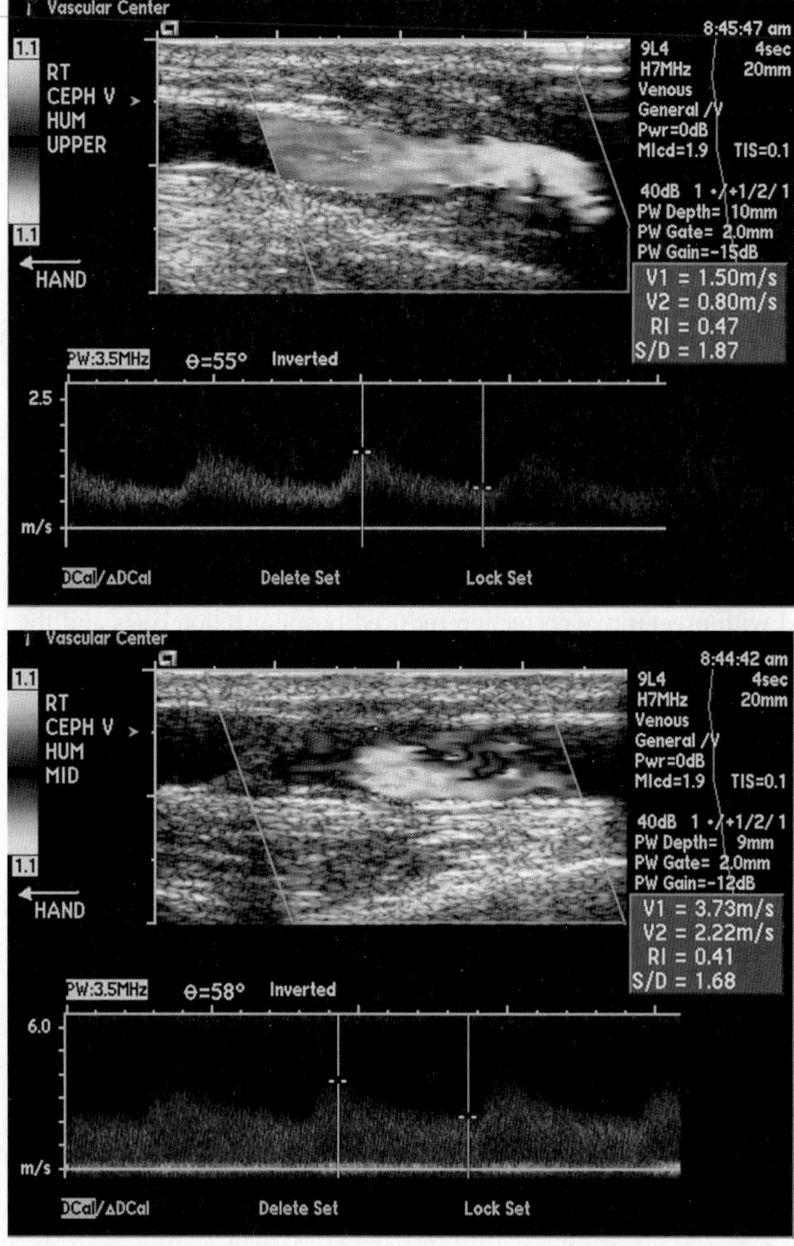

Figure 24-1. A 72-year-old man who had a brachiocephalic fistula placed 4 weeks ago but not yet accessed underwent routine duplex ultrasound surveillance. **A.** Normal appearing cephalic vein. **B.** The cephalic vein at the level of the mid-humerus has two stenoses, including the one in this image with a velocity of 373 cm/sec. He subsequently had a fistulogram and venoplasty and has had a functioning fistula for the past 6 months.

patients who had the usual clinical monitoring.[2] This review included nine studies with 1363 patients, which compared surveillance with clinical monitoring. Three studies with 207 patients compared the effect of vascular interventions with observation in patients with an abnormal surveillance result. The meta-analysis found only very low quality evidence to support the use of arteriovenous access surveillance followed by interventions and

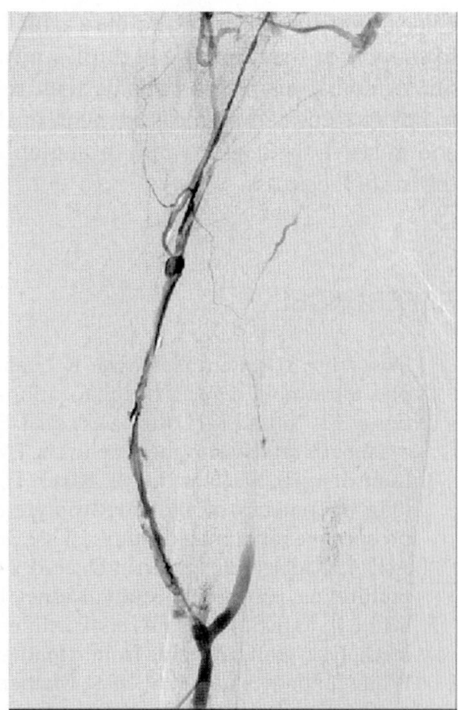

Figure 24-2. A 48-year-old man with a right brachiocephalic arteriovenous fistula underwent a fistulogram following a surveillance ultrasound 4 weeks postprocedure. The fistula thrombosed in the 3 days between ultrasound and the fistulogram, and he required thrombolysis and angioplasty, resulting in salvage of the fistula. The fistula with thrombus is shown.

recommended randomized trials of surveillance versus clinical monitoring. Of the nine reports, two studies that demonstrated significant reduction of access thrombosis in the surveillance groups had either methodologic concerns or were an early report of a 5-year cohort and therefore were not yet completed.[13-14] The review also demonstrated that patients undergoing intervention (endovascular or surgical) for a known stenosis, followed by access surveillance or usual clinical monitoring, had a decreased incidence of thrombosis but no improvement in overall graft life.[2]

Other authors have arrived at a similar conclusion that the addition of regular ultrasound surveillance to clinical monitoring increases the frequency of intervention, specifically angioplasty, but does not reduce the incidence of graft failure.[9-10] In fact, some have theorized that in select patients, angioplasty may accelerate the likelihood of flow-limiting stenosis with subsequent access thrombosis.[10]

There are several reports in support of routine surveillance.[7,13-14] It is possible that a subset of patients may benefit from surveillance, such as those 191 patients from Verona, Italy, reported by Tessitore et al.[7] In a 5-year randomized trial, they used multiple means of surveillance and concluded that active blood flow surveillance and preemptive repair of subclinical stenoses both reduce thrombosis rate and prolong the patency of forearm fistulas. Perhaps the forearm arteriovenous fistula group benefits from survelliance compared with those with an upper arm prosthetic graft, but we have not yet been able to identify the subgroups to screen on a regular basis.

CONCLUSION

Despite the conflicting reports regarding whether routine surveillance of dialysis access fistulas or grafts should be performed, most authors agree that at the very least, careful clinical assessment is safe and may actually be quite effective. In the absence of level 1 data to support or reject the use of duplex ultrasound surveillance, we are currently evaluating our hemodialysis fistula patients with serial examination. However, it is best to observe trends in clinical, flow measurement, or duplex flow data before proceeding with a costly and invasive fistulogram and/or angioplasty, because such a procedure may not prolong the life of the access.

REFERENCES

1. Dossabhoy NR, Ram SJ, Nassar R, et al. Stenosis surveillance of hemodialysis grafts by duplex ultrasound reduces hospitalizations and cost of care. Semin Dial 2005;18:550–7.
2. Casey ET, Murad MH, Rizvi AZ, et al. Surveillance of arteriovenous hemodialysis access: a systematic review and meta-analysis. J Vasc Surg 2008;48(5 Suppl):48S–54S.
3. Lumsden AB, MacDonald MJ, Kikeri D, et al. Prophylactic balloon angioplasty fails to prolong the patency of expanded polytetrafluoroethylene arteriovenous grafts: results of a prospective randomized study. J Vasc Surg 1997;26:382–92.
4. Asif A, Gadalean FN, Merrill D, et al. Inflow stenosis in arteriovenous fistulas and grafts: a multicenter, prospective study. Kidney Int 2005;67:1986–92.
5. White JJ, Ram SJ, Jones SA, et al. Influence of luminal diameters on flow surveillance of hemodialysis grafts: insights from a mathematical model. Clin J Am Soc Neph 2006;1:972–8.
6. White JJ, Jones SA, Ram SJ, et al. Mathematical model demonstrates influence of luminal diameters on venous pressure surveillance. Clin J Am Soc Neph 2007;2:681–7.
7. Tessitore N, Lipari G, Poli A, et al. Can blood fiow surveillance and pre-emptive repair of subclinical stenosis prolong the useful life of arteriovenous fistulae? A randomized controlled study. Nephrol Dial Transplant 2004;9:2325–33.
8. NKF-KDOQI Clinical Practice Guidelines and Clinical Practice Recommendations for Vascular Access, update 2006. Am J Kidney Dis 2006;48 (Suppl 1):S177–247.
9. Dember LM, Holmberg EF, Kaufman JS. Randomized controlled trial of prophylactic repair of hemodialysis arteriovenous graft stenosis. Kidney Int 2004;66:390–8.
10. Robbin ML, Oser RF, Lee JY, et al. Randomized comparison of ultrasound surveillance and clinical monitoring on arteriovenous graft outcomes. Kidney Int 2006;69:730–5.
11. Moist LM, Churchill DN, House AA, et al. Regular monitoring of access flow compared with monitoring of venous pressure fails to improve graft survival. J Am Soc Nephrol 2003; 14:2645–53.
12. Ram SJ, Work J, Caldito GC, et al. A randomized controlled trial of blood and stenosis surveillance of hemodialysis grafts. Kidney Int 2003;64:272–80.
13. Malik J, Slavikova M, Svobodova J, Tuka V. Regular ultrasonographic screening significantly prolongs patency of PTFE grafts. Kidney Int 2005;67:1554–8.
14. Roca-Tey R, Samon Guasch R, Ibrik O, et al. [Vascular access surveillance with blood flow monitoring: a prospective study with 65 patients]. Nefrologia 2004;24:246–52.

SECTION VI

Lower Extremity

25

Catheter-Based Plaque Excision: Is There a Role? Examining the SilverHawk System

Walter J. McCarthy, M.D., Chad Jacobs, M.D., and Ferenc Nagy, M.D.

As clinicians continue to expand the use of catheter-based treatment for lower extremity ischemia, numerous techniques have evolved. The comparison of competing methods is sometimes difficult, because new technology rapidly advances and is typically endorsed by groups of devotees who develop expertise then enthusiasm and publish early work. Numerous approaches have been advanced, including simple tapered dilation Dottering, laser plaque ablation,[1-2] mechanical plaque ablation, balloon angioplasty, cold balloon angioplasty, stents and drug-eluting stents, and subintimal dissection, among other ideas. For many patients with lower extremity ischemia, open surgical procedures provide excellent long-term solutions, but for some patients, percutaneous endovascular treatment is preferable.

The following discussion does not attempt to address the argument that all patients should have endovascular treatment "first" for lower extremity ischemia but does assume that some patients should and that judgment is involved. Rather, the atherectomy SilverHawk (EV3, Minneapolis, MN) method is examined, arguing that it does provide revascularization and limb salvage reliably and is a means to an end. The increase of perfusion provided by the SilverHawk technique may in some cases even be effective for patients who do not have the anatomy to support a tibial bypass. Thus, the procedure may in some cases be preferable, even in patients who do have excellent venous conduit and are good surgical candidates from a medical viewpoint. Long-term limb salvage rates will be discussed in comparison with what is likely the main competing technique, which is that of balloon angioplasty alone, with and without stents. Besides arguments to support atherectomy in selected patients, the chapter also presents useful techniques for atherectomy and representative cases.

BACKGROUND AND PUBLISHED INFORMATION

The published data related to the SilverHawk rotary atherectomy device are not extensive, but the journal articles all together are useful to review. Challenges in organizing the material from various articles involve different anatomic regions treated, different techniques, and varying endpoints of success. Thus, some authors report only femoral popliteal artery treatment and not tibial artery intervention. In all series, balloon angioplasty is used as an adjunct in areas in which the atherectomy is incomplete or is not possible, and in all articles, some stents are used. Some authors do not include calcified lesions at all and some predilate calcified tibial arteries before atherectomy. Follow-up is generally clinical, with different endpoints but with limb salvage nearly always recorded. The definitions of initial technical success and long-term treated area patency are always less rigorously established than, for example, in journal articles recording bypass graft patency. Excepting these limitations, the available articles do contain tremendously useful clinical information.

REVIEW OF THE SELECTED AVAILABLE LITERATURE

Thomas Zeller, from the Department of Angiology in Bad Krozingen, Germany, was an early practitioner with the SilverHawk device and published two papers in 2004(3). A long-term follow-up of cases came in 2007 and is very informative.[4] One hundred legs were treated but only lesions of the femoral and/or the popliteal artery were included. One third were primary cases, one third were cases with restenosis of a previously treated lesion, and one third were restenoses of previously placed stents. Low-pressure balloon angioplasty (<3 atm) was used in 59% and stents were utilized in 8% of cases. Any patient with a calcified lesion was excluded, and overall, the mean lesion length was 90 mm. All 100 procedures were reported as being initially successful. The lesions that were treated for the first time, that is, the primary lesions, had the best patency, and the restenosis cases had the worst long-term patency. For the primary treated lesions, the primary patency was 84% and 73% at 12 and 18 months. The secondary patency was better at 100% and 91% at 12 and 18 months. The restenotic lesions had lower patency. Follow-up was with duplex scanning, using a systolic peak velocity ratio of ≥2.4 as a definition of "restenosis." Rutherford categories and ankle-brachial indexes (ABIs) were both reported as improving significantly after treatment. Overall, of the 100 limbs, 3 ended up being amputated over the follow-up period. The authors' conclusions commented on the lowered durability in treating restenotic lesions in either native arteries or within stents, but overall, the authors applauded the 18-month results. They promoted the idea that atherectomy reduces vessel injury due to stretching "barotrauma," which is an inevitable result of any balloon angioplasty. They felt that barotrauma may promote intimal hyperplasia and restenosis. Clearly, this article is a review of the least difficult group of patients. It represents those with noncalcified lesions of the superficial femoral artery and/or popliteal artery only. Nevertheless, the patency for primary lesions is encouraging and the follow-up is rigorous, using a Kaplan-Meier presentation of all of the information.

In 2006, David Kandzari was instrumental in publishing two papers in the same issue of the Journal of Endovascular Therapy on the SilverHawk.[5-6] One reviews an experience with 69 patients from seven institutions, all with critical limb ischemia. The second paper outlines the findings of the TALON study (Treating Peripherals With SilverHawk: Outcomes Collection).[6] The second paper combines 601 consecutive patients treated from 19 institutions. Both papers contain valuable information. Dr. Kandzari, who was at that time at Duke University, is the corresponding author for both papers. He is currently a cardiologist at the Scripps Research Institute in La Jolla, California.

The TALON registry enrolled all patients of any type starting in August of 2003 and followed them over 18 months. This study allowed any sort of lesion, including calcified lesions, and 26.8% of the lesions treated were occlusions. Most of the lesions were in the superficial femoral or the popliteal artery, which accounted for 70% of the treated areas. Of this region, 74.8% were above the knee and 25.2% were below the knee. The study, however, did include smaller vessels, and of the 601 patients, 24.4% involved vessels below the popliteal in the tibial-peroneal or tibial arteries. The study has the advantage of large numbers, with 601 patients and 748 limbs, and addresses 1258 specific lesions. It also includes patients from 19 institutions; thus a multitude of techniques and levels of expertise are represented.

The initial success was about 95% and of those, 10.5% required predilation with balloon angioplasty before the SilverHawk device could be passed. After treatment, 26.7% required balloon angioplasty for an unsatisfactory result and 6.3% required that a stent be placed. Follow-up duplex scanning was not common but was used, and the authors commented that the ABI increased from a mean of 0.7 to a mean of 0.86 after treatment. The percentage, without need for revascularization or amputation, was used as the endpoint. At 6 months, this group was 90%, and at 12 months, it was 80%. The TALON is the largest experience with the SilverHawk and the authors correctly conclude that an 80% primary success at 12 months is fairly comparable with bypass surgery without the morbidity of bypass surgery. However, some would argue that the 80% is somewhat lower than can be achieved with venous conduit to the popliteal or tibial vessels, which does approach 90% in many series. Also, patency beyond 12 months is not demonstrated.

Kandzari's other paper in 2006 focused on patients with critical limb ischemia of Rutherford category ≥5.[5] Patients were enrolled "irrespective of the complexity of their anatomy as an alternative to balloon angioplasty, bypass surgery, and/or amputation."

All had pain at rest with ankle pressure less than 50 mm Hg and/or ulcer gangrene or nonhealing wounds. Seven institutions contributed 69 patients, totaling 76 limbs over 12 months starting in August 2003. A total of 160 lesions were addressed. Femoral and/or popliteal lesions made up 61% and tibial perioneal trunk and tibial lesions 39%. Over all, 34% were totally occluded. The authors noted that 80% of the lesions were moderate to severely calcified. Initial success defined as <50% stenosis in the target lesion was 99%. Angioplasty without a stent was used in 11% and with a stent in 6%. There were no problems with embolization, and there were no vessel perforations reported. Follow-up was only through 6 months and patency was not addressed at all. The authors used freedom from amputation as an endpoint. Of the 76 limbs involved, they initially felt 48 were in need of major amputation but actually only 16 limbs were amputated over 6 months. Thus, three quarters were saved at the 6-month point. This endpoint of "not amputated yet" at 6 months is a soft, uncertain one, as any vascular surgeon will realize. The paper, however, does support aggressive treatment of advanced lesions.

Several single-center studies and reviews[7-10] have been published by experienced vascular programs recently after presentation at major vascular meetings. Yancey et al. from the University of Kentucky Medical Center, presented 16 patients at the 2006

Southern Association for Vascular Surgery.[11] They treated TASC (Trans-Atlantic Symptomatic Stenosis Classification) type C lesions with critical limb ischemia. They reported initially good results but their stenosis-free patency of the femoral popliteal area was only 22% at 12 months. Keeling and his group from Tampa, Florida, presented 60 patients at the Peripheral Vascular Surgery Society in 2006 with 1-year primary and secondary part patency of 62% at 76%, respectively.[12]

Keeling's report contrasts with that of Chungs et al.[13] from the University of Iowa at the 2007 winter meeting of the Peripheral Vascular Surgical Society treating 20 limbs. Their 12-month primary and assistant primary patency was only 10%, and they offered a serious word of caution about the device and procedure. The Cleveland Clinic reported 73 patients at the Southern Association for Vascular Surgery in 2007 with 1-year follow-up showing 43% primary patency and 57% secondary patency along with a 75% limb salvage.[14] These authors expressed some concern about the durability of the procedure. A recent report from the University of Arizona in Tucson by Biskup et al. reported 35 patients with primary and secondary patency of 66% and 70% at 1 year.[15] The authors presented the work at the 2008 winter meeting of the Peripheral Vascular Surgery Society. They noticed the worst patency in areas in which a previous intervention had been performed in the same location of the treated artery.

James McKinsey et al. at New York Presbyterian Hospital have been early, aggressive users of the SilverHawk device. They published their intermediate results in October 2008, including work from their institution from 2004 through 2007.[16] In all, 579 lesions in 275 patients were reported and 63% were for critical limb ischemia; 218 lesions were in the tibial vessels. The 18-month data were reported with primary and secondary patencies of 58% and 82% for claudication patients and 49% and 70.8% for the limb salvage group. There was no limb loss in the follow-up period for the claudication group, and overall, the limb salvage was 93%; 4.4% went on to have bypass surgery. The authors commented that in all the patients who required bypass, follow-up angiography showed the distal vessels to be unchanged. Thus, the initial atherectomy procedure did not seem to have worsened the situation.

McKinsey has questioned if the SilverHawk has an advantage over pure balloon angioplasty alone in the lower extremity. This is a yet unaddressed and very intriguing question. Restated the question is: do we do just as well with low-profile balloons in the lower extremity, particularly in the tibial vessels, or does the SilverHawk add something? To answer this, he has compared patients over the last 2 years to SilverHawk first or balloon angioplasty alone first. He has concluded from that work that there is a unmistakable statistical advantage in patency for the SilverHawk cohort. These data, however, are still unpublished but are presented here after personal review by the senior author of this chapter. Once this information is publicly available, it will be very helpful in directing the treatment prescribed by clinicians carrying for patients with lower extremity ischemia.

SILVERHAWK ATHERECTOMY TECHNICAL ADVICE

There are several technical suggestions regarding performing SilverHawk atherectomy that can help make the difference between an efficient case with hemodynamic success versus a difficult case with a less than optimal outcome. Outlined below are several technical hints that have come from our institution's combined experience thus far with SilverHawk atherectomy. Advance planning is critical to the success of these procedures, including choice of access site, wire and sheath selection, atherectomy technique, and use of embolic protection.

Selecting femoral access is often one of the more critical decision points when performing SilverHawk atherectomy. Options include a retrograde femoral approach with percutaneous puncture of the contralateral femoral artery, antegrade ipsilateral femoral puncture, and ipsilateral surgical cutdown for an antegrade approach. The contralateral retrograde femoral approach, although initially appealing, does have limitations. Some have written that a controlateral approach is "safer" with fewer complications, but this may be because of its use in simple cases involving only the superficial femoral artery. This approach may often be more technically challenging, because it requires up-and-over access. Additionally, the length of the SilverHawk device may limit device accessibility to the infrageniculate vasculature, depending on a patient's body habitus. Thus, tibial access may mandate an antegrade puncture of the ipsilatenal common femoral artery. The additional curvature of the aortic bifurcation may provide difficulty with sheath kinking and also may cause additional difficulty with torque and manipulation of the SilverHawk device.

Using the Antegrade Approach

The antegrade ipsilateral percutaneous femoral approach has become our preferred approach, particularly for tibial lesions. Precise anatomic identification of the correct location for puncture (common femoral artery) is important to avoid complications. Fluoroscopy can be used to identify the femoral head, the inferomedial aspect of which corresponds to the location of the common femoral artery. Duplex ultrasonography can be used to visualize the common femoral artery and its bifurcation. Patients with a large, overhanging pannus may require retraction of the pannus, either by an assistant or with tincture of benzoin and tape placed to buttress the pannus preoperatively. We prefer to localize the common femoral artery with duplex ultrasound and access it in an antegrade fashion with a micropuncture kit. Once access has been obtained with a 7-French sheath, an initial hand injection is performed. If the sheath is within the profunda femoris artery, a guidewire is advanced into the distal branches of the profunda femoris. The sheath is then slowly withdrawn over the wire, and continued hand injection puffs are performed until the sheath is withdrawn into the lumen of the common femoral artery. Keeping a wire in the profunda femoris ensures that arterial access will not be lost as the sheath is withdrawn. A second guidewire can then be passed alongside the original guidewire to be directed into the superficial femoral artery. We have used an antegrade approach with increasing frequency to allow safe and easy access to the superficial femoral and infrageniculate arteries.

If body habitus or other technical factors prohibit either the ipsilateral antegrade or the contralateral retrograde percutaneous approach, a small cutdown can be performed with local anesthesia and sedation. Often, if the superficial femoral artery is patent proximally, this vessel itself can be exposed and then accessed using the Seldinger technique as in a percutaneous approach.

A third approach that has been described by various practitioners when antegrade access is technically not possible is to access the lesion from a retrograde direction, that is, from a tibial puncture. The dorsalis pedis artery can be accessed percutaneously under ultrasound guidance with a micropuncture kit, and the smallest of the SilverHawk devices can be passed retrograde without a sheath (bareback) to the target lesion.

Other Techniques

A variety of different lengths of sheaths should be on standby when performing SilverHawk atherectomy. All of the SilverHawk devices can be passed through a 7-French sheath despite markings on some of the packaging that indicate that an 8-French sheath is required. Several lengths of sheaths are useful. A short (13 cm) sheath is useful for initial access and for treatment of lesions in the proximal to mid-superficial femoral artery, particularly with antegrade access. A longer 7-French (35 cm) sheath is also useful for antegrade access when performing interventions primarily below the knee. Our approach has been to use a short sheath for initial access and, once wire access has been obtained across the lesions in the infrageniculate circulation, to advance a longer 7-French sheath positioning its tip in the popliteal artery. This has been found to provide more stability for delivery of the device and balloons, if necessary, and also protects the superficial fermoral artery during catheter exchanges.

Of additional consideration is the type of sheath to use when performing contralateral retrograde access for the up-and-over approach. Several of the standard 35- to 45-cm sheaths can to be advanced up and over the aortic bifurcation. However, nonreinforced sheaths will often kink in a patient with an acute aortic bifurcation. Certain sheaths such as the Pinnacle Destination (Terumo) sheath have adequate length to reach the contralateral common femoral artery or even the superficial femoral artery and are resistant to kinking, which otherwise can be quite troublesome when trying to pass the SilverHawk device over the aortic bifurcation.

Crossing lesions for treatment with SilverHawk atherectomy employs the same principles as crossing lesions for other types of intervention such as angioplasty and stent placement. The method most commonly used is to attempt to cross the lesion with a standard 0.035 glidewire. Use of a 5-French glide catheter is useful to add support for the glidewire. On occasion, crossed lesions require predilation with 2-, 3-, or 4-mm angioplasty balloons if the SilverHawk itself will not pass over the 0.014 wire. At times, difficult lesions can be crossed using a Dottering technique with the use of a catheter such as the Quick Cross (Spectranetics) catheter, which is a 5-French catheter with a straight but tapered tip. This catheter can help cross tight lesions or occlusions with a minimal amount of wire exposed distally, using the catheter to help Dotter across such lesions. Of course, once the catheter has been advanced across the occlusion, angiography must confirm that the catheter is intraluminal (Figures 25–1 through 25–8).

Once any target lesion has been successfully crossed with a 0.014 wire, the SilverHawk device is advanced, and it is recommended to treat the lesion in four quadrants: anterior, posterior, medial, and lateral. Depending on the size of the device and plaque burden, the cap may need to be emptied after four passes. Additional passes of the device may be then performed, focusing on specific areas of heaviest plaque burden. It is suggested that the inner wall of a bifurcation be avoided to minimize the risk of vessel perforation. Proximal lesions are treated prior to distal lesions so that the remaining devices, sheaths, and balloons, if necessary, can be passed across the previously treated lesions without risk of additional emboli (Figures 25–5 through 25–8).

It is worthwhile to be prepared to use distal embolic protection when performing SilverHawk atherectomy, particularly for calcified lesions. Filters are recommended to be used at all times when performing SilverHawk atherectomy using the RockHawk device. The RockHawk has an extra bur on its rotating blade that is useful for treating heavily calcified lesions; however, it is also much more likely to cause distal embolization. At our institution, we have, with increasing frequency, used a filter when performing any SilverHawk intervention in the superficial femoral artery. The filter is

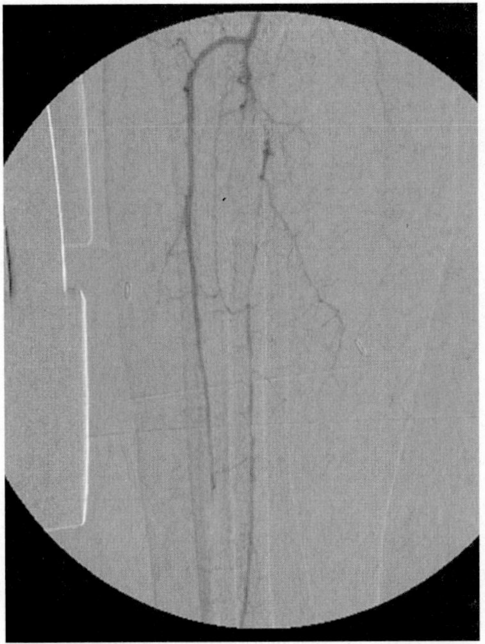
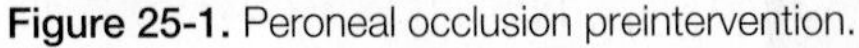

Figure 25-1. Peroneal occlusion preintervention.

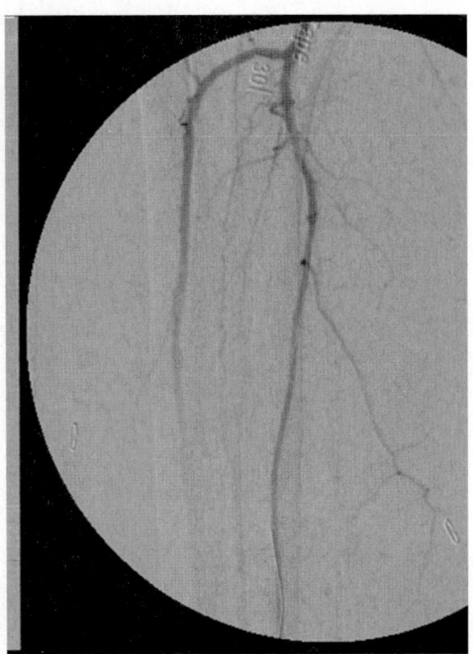

Figure 25-2. Peroneal artery post-SilverHawk atherectomy.

placed at the below-knee popliteal artery or tibioperoneal trunk and, more often than not, will return with a significant amount of atheromatous debris after completion of a superficial femoral artery SilverHawk intervention (Figures 25–9 through 25–12). Others have shown evidence of embolization in as many as 90% of lesions treated with the SilverHawk.[17-19] But fortunately most of these are of subclinical importance. Filters are less likely to be of benefit when performing tibial level intervention because the

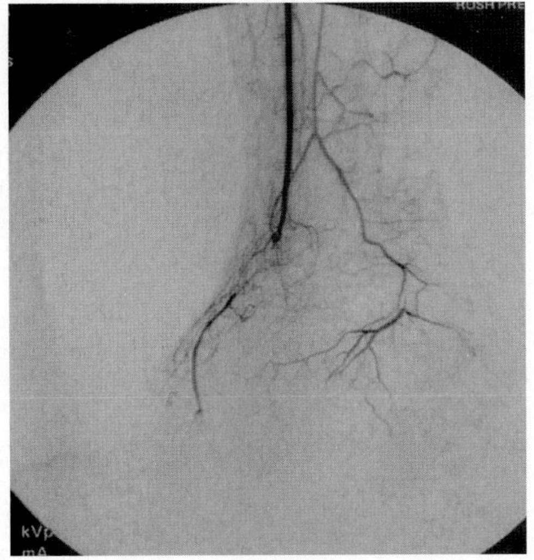

Figure 25-3. Dorsalis pedis occlusion preintervention.

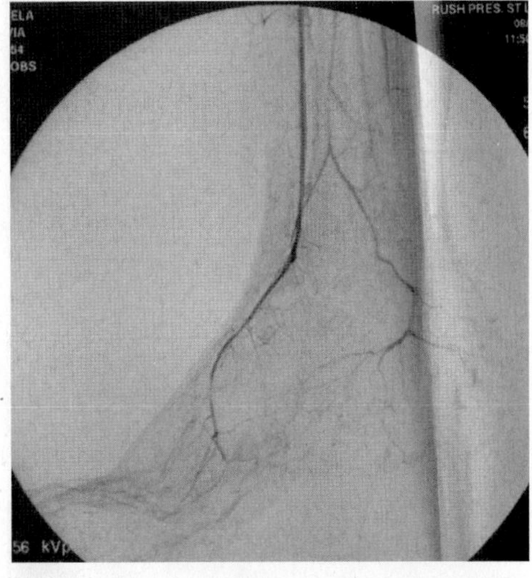

Figure 25-4. Dorsalis pedis artery post-SilverHawk atherectomy.

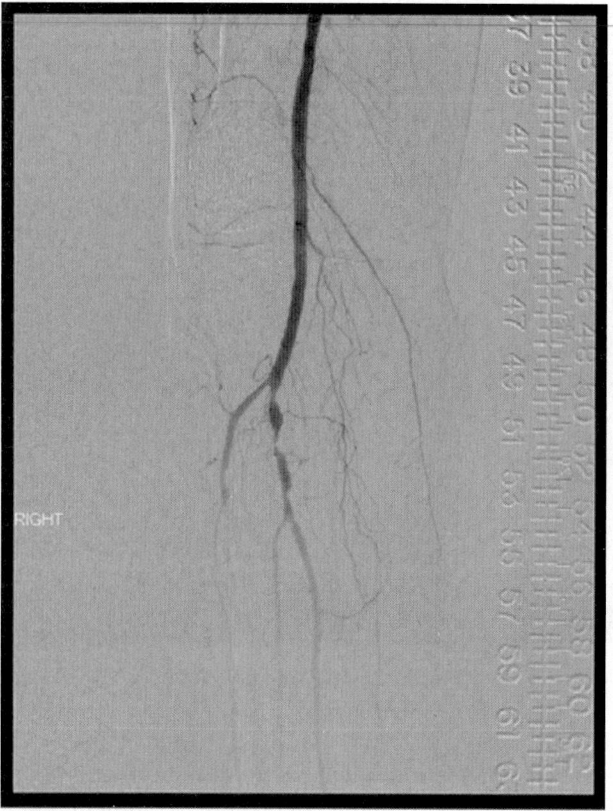

Figure 25-5. Tibioperoneal trunk stenosis preintervention.

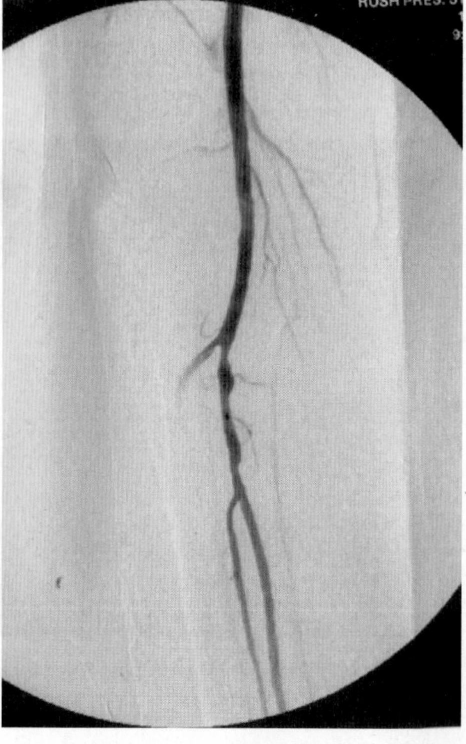

Figure 25-6. Tibioperoneal trunk stenosis post-SilverHawk atherectomy.

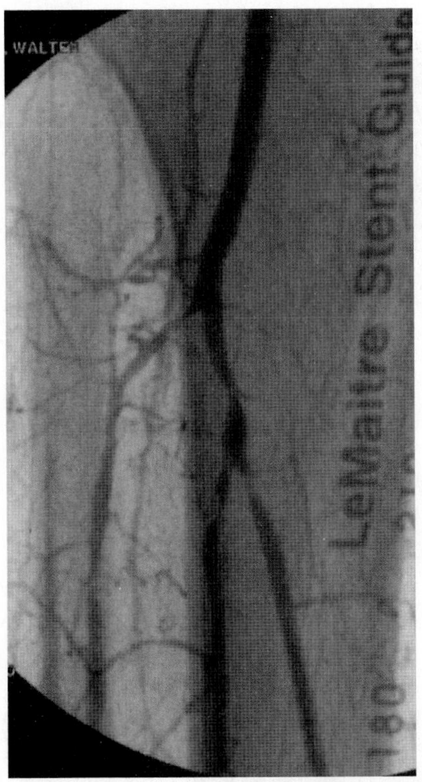

Figure 25-7. Peroneal and posterior tibial stenosis preintervention.

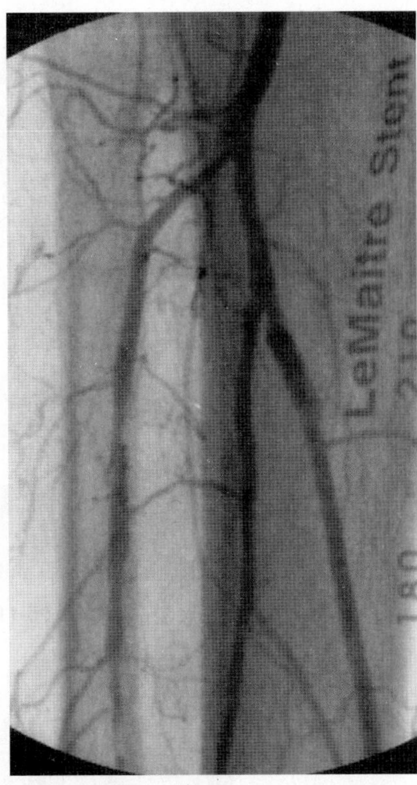

Figure 25-8. Peroneal and posterior tibial stenosis post-SilverHawk atherectomy.

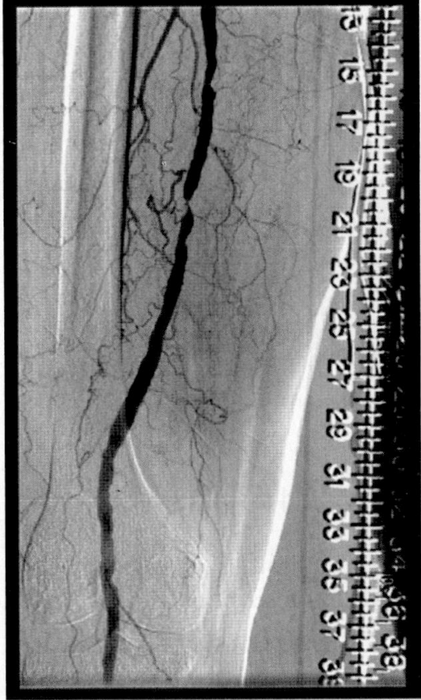

Figure 25-9. SFA stenosis preintervention.

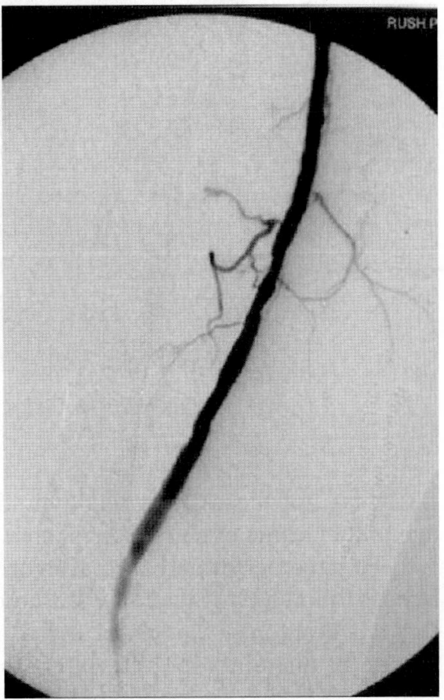

Figure 25-10. SFA post-SilverHawk atherectomy.

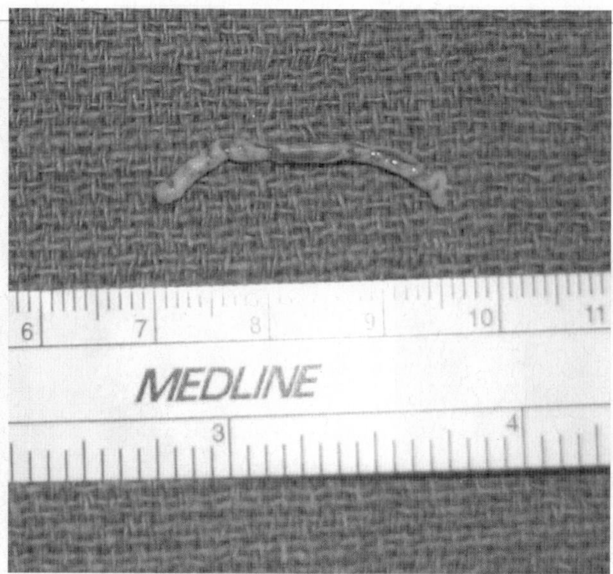

Figure 25-11. SFA atherectomy specimen.

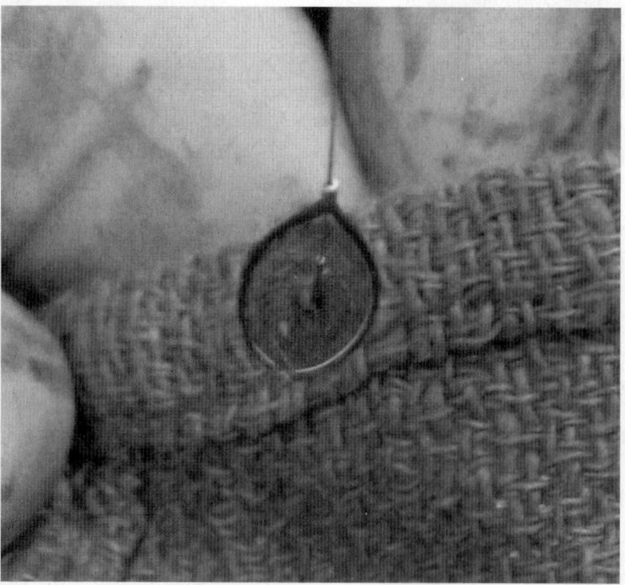

Figure 25-12. Debris in filter basket post-SFA intervention.

filter may not successfully deploy in the distal tibial vessels and may cause either damage to the intima or significant spasm in the tibial vessels.

We have performed several hybrid procedures, using a prosthetic femoropopliteal bypass followed by SilverHawk atherectomy of the tibial runoff. Experience has shown that it is best to use the SilverHawk device with pressure in the tibial arteries after completion of the femoropopliteal bypass. Passing the SilverHawk device with the inflow occluded can lead to confusing angiographic results, because the treated vessels do not distend after atherectomy as expected. We therefore perform the prosthetic bypass first and then advance the SilverHawk device through the functioning graft.

A final note is that just as with many other interventional procedures, "the enemy of good is better." A residual stenosis of 20 to 30% may be an acceptable final result for many target lesions. The risk of each additional pass of the SilverHawk device may include excessive thinning of the vessel wall with delayed pseudoaneurysm formation, severe arterial spasm, vessel perforation, occlusion, and distal embolization.

CONCLUSION

The SilverHawk directional atherectomy catheter has been studied only through a series of clinical registries and single-center database reports. Randomized trials against other means of treating lower extremity ischemia have not been conducted. The device offers the advantage of debulking atherosclerotic material and usually can be used without placing a stent or without an associated balloon angioplasty. It is useful in the femoral popliteal area and is also effective in treating tibial artery lesions. It appears that it can be reused if the patient develops restenosis and does not appear to damage the distal circulation if the patient does require a operative bypass in the future. Initial results are good, but the patency after 12-month follow-up does not compare with that of surgical bypass. The question of atherectomy versus initial balloon angioplasty remains unsolved, although initial preliminary information seems to support atherectomy in this regard.

REFERENCES

1. Wissgott C, Scheinert D, Rademaker, J, et al. Treatment of long superficial femoral artery occlusions with excimer laser angioplasty: long term results after 48 months. Acta Radiol 45:23–29, 2004.
2. McCarthy WJ, Vogelzang RL, Nemcek AA Jr, et al. Excimer laser-assisted femoral angioplasty: early results. J Vasc Surg 1991;13:5;607–14.
3. Zeller T, Rastan A, Schwarzwalder U, et al. Midterm results after atherectomy-assisted angioplasty of below-knee arteries with use of the silverHawk device. J Vasc Interv Radiol 2004;15:1391–7.
4. Zeller T, Sixt S, Schwarzwalder U, et al. Two-year results after directional atherectomy of infrapopliteal arteries with the silverHawk device. J Endovasc Ther 2007;14:232–40.
5. Kandzari DE, Kiesz RS, Allie D, et al. Procedural and clinical outcomes with catheter-based plaque excision in critical limb ischemia. J Endovasc Ther 2006;13:12–22.
6. Ramaiah V, Gammon R, Kiesz S, et al. Midterm outcomes from the talon registry: treating peripherals with SilverHawk: outcomes collection. J Endovasc Ther 2006;13:118–128.
7. Bunting TA, Garcia LA. Peripheral atherectomy: a critical review. J Interv Cardiol 2007; 20:417–24.
8. Garcia LA, Lyden SP. Atherectomy for infrainguinal peripheral artery disease. J Endovasc Ther 2009;16(Suppl II):II105–15.
9. Shrikhande GV, McKinsey JF. Use and abuse of atherectomy: where should it be used? Seminars in Vascular Surgery. J Sem vasc Surg 2008;21:204–9.
10. Ramaiah V. Endovascular Infrainguinal revascularization: technical tips for atherectomy device selection and procedural success. J Sem vasc Surg 2008;21:41–9.

11. Yancey AE, Minion DJ, Rodriguez C, et al. Peripheral atherectomy in transatlantic intersociety consensus type C femoropopliteal lesions for limb salvage. Association for Vascular Surgery. J Vasc Surg 2006;44:503–9.
12. Keeling WB, Murray LS, Stone PA, et al. Plaque excision with the SilverHawk catheter: early results in patients with claudication or critical limb ischemia. J Vasc Surg 2007;45;1; 25–31.
13. Chung SW, Sharafuddin MJ, Chigurupati R, et al. Midterm patency following atherectomy for infrainguinal occlusive disease: a word of caution. Ann Vasc Surg 2008;22:358–65.
14. Sarac TP, Altinel O, Bannazadeh M, et al. Midterm outcome predictors for lower extremity atherectomy procedures. J. Vasc Surg 2008;48;4:885–90.
15. Biskup NI, Ihnat DM, Leon LR, et al. Infrainguinal atherectomy: a retrospective review of single-center experience. Ann Vasc Surg 2008;22:776–82.
16. McKinsey JF, Goldstein L, Khan HU, et al. Novel treatment of patients with lower extremity ischemia: use of percutaneous atherectomy in 579 lesions. Ann Surg 2008;248:519–28.
17. Lam RC, Shah S, Faries PL, et al. Incidence and clinical significance of distal embolization during percutaneous interventions involving the superficial femoral artery. J Vasc Surg 2007;46;6:1155–9.
18. Shavelle DM. Plaque excision with distal protection: a logical step for superficial femoral artery SilverHawk atherectomy. J Invasive Cardiol 2009;21:11–2.
19. Shammas NW, Dippel EJ, Coiner D, et al. Preventing lower extremity distal embolization using embolic filter protection: results of the PROTECT registry. J Endovasc Ther 2008;15: 270–6.

26

Popliteal Pathology

Lindsay Kuo, B.S. and Heron Rodriguez, M.D.

INTRODUCTION

The popliteal artery is affected by a variety of diseases, ranging from atherosclerosis and its complications to lesions unique to this vessel. In this chapter, after reviewing the different surgical approaches used to expose the popliteal artery, we discuss two diseases that specifically affect this vessel: popliteal entrapment and adventitial cystic disease. Although atherosclerosis is the most common disorder affecting the popliteal artery, it is not discussed here, nor is popliteal aneurysms or traumatic injuries to the popliteal artery.

SURGICAL APPROACHES TO EXPOSE THE POPLITEAL ARTERY

The popliteal artery, positioned posterior to the knee within the popliteal fossa, is the continuation of the femoral artery after it passes through the adductor canal. It travels through the popliteal space in between the medial and the lateral heads of the gastrocnemius muscle. Within the popliteal fossa, the artery gives off numerous genicular and sural branches to supply the muscles of the calf and lower femur as well as the knee. The popliteal artery ends when it divides into the tibial-fibular trunk and the anterior tibial artery, just distal to the popliteus muscle. Three surgical approaches are used when treating popliteal artery diseases: medial, lateral, and posterior. In addition, the medial and lateral approaches can be achieved above or below the knee.

Medial Approaches

For the supragenicular medial approach, the patient is placed in a supine position. It is helpful to place a soft roll under the lower leg, creating 30 to 45 degrees of flexion and slightly externally rotating the leg. The incision is made in the distal third of the thigh parallel to the anterior border of the sartorius muscle. After incising the fascia, the popliteal vessels are found by retracting the sartorius posteriorly and the vastus medialis anteriorly. Care is taken to avoid injuring the paired popliteal veins and the saphenous branch of the femoral vein.

The infragenicular medial approach is also facilitated by the use of a soft roll, this time placed under the upper leg. A longitudinal incision is created 2 cm behind the posterior border of the tibia. After retracting the great saphenous vein and incising along the crural fascia, the popliteal veins become evident. Additional distal exposure to visualize the origin of the anterior tibialis and the tibioperoneal trunk is obtained by severing the tibial attachments to the soleus muscle.

Lateral Approaches

The lateral approach to the above-knee popliteal artery begins with a lateral incision in the distal thigh just above the knee (Figure 26–1). The iliotibial tract is opened, and the popliteal fossa is entered just behind the biceps femoris muscle. When entering the popliteal fossa, it is important to avoid injury to either the common peroneal nerve or the sciatic nerve. The sciatic nerve enters the popliteal fossa at the apex of the fossa and then gives off the common peroneal nerve.

The lateral approach to the below-knee popliteal artery (Figure 26–2) is via an incision that begins just above the head of the fibula and extends for 6 to 10 cm. The head of the fibula is an important landmark, as is the tendon of the biceps femoris. Because the common peroneal nerve is superficial and prone to injury, the patient should be warned of this prior to the procedure. Identification of the nerve is the first step of the procedure once the skin is opened. The bicep femoris muscle tendon is resected, with the peroneal nerve being protected. With the peroneal nerve being retracted, the head of the fibula is resected. The popliteal vessels and the tibial nerve are easily identified.

Posterior Approach

With the patient in the prone position, a curvilinear incision is made from the medial aspect of the leg transversely across the knee joint and then vertically in the mid-portion of the calf (Figure 26–3). With the subcutaneous tissue divided, the deep fascia of the leg is identified. The lesser saphenous vein is often found in the superficial compartment, but in most instances, it is beneath the fascia. The sural nerve is identified below the fascia, often accompanying the lesser saphenous vein. Opening the deep fascia carefully is important in order to avoid injury to these structures. Once the deep fascia is open from the apex of the popliteal fossa to the most inferior portion, the wound is retracted gently with care taken not to injure the common peroneal nerve. The common peroneal nerve takes its origin from the tibial nerve in variable locations but passes laterally through the popliteal fossa to wrap around the fibula in the lowermost aspect of the wound. Once the sural nerve and the common peroneal nerve are identified, the tissue is divided using blunt dissection down to the tibial peroneal nerve. The tibial peroneal nerve is the most superficial portion of the deepest portion of the wound (Figure 26–4). The tibial nerve is retracted, exposing the popliteal vein and artery. Working around both the vein and the nerve, it is possible to expose the popliteal artery from the adductor canal to the tibial peroneal trunk, where it passes behind the sartorius muscle. In the inferior aspect of the wound, it is sometimes difficult to control all of the blood vessels because of the remarkable arborization of the tibial peroneal nerve. Numerous nerve branches pass to the gastrocnemius and soleus muscles. In patients who are well developed, the gastrocnemius muscles also impede the view of the more distal aspects of the popliteal artery and tibial vessels.

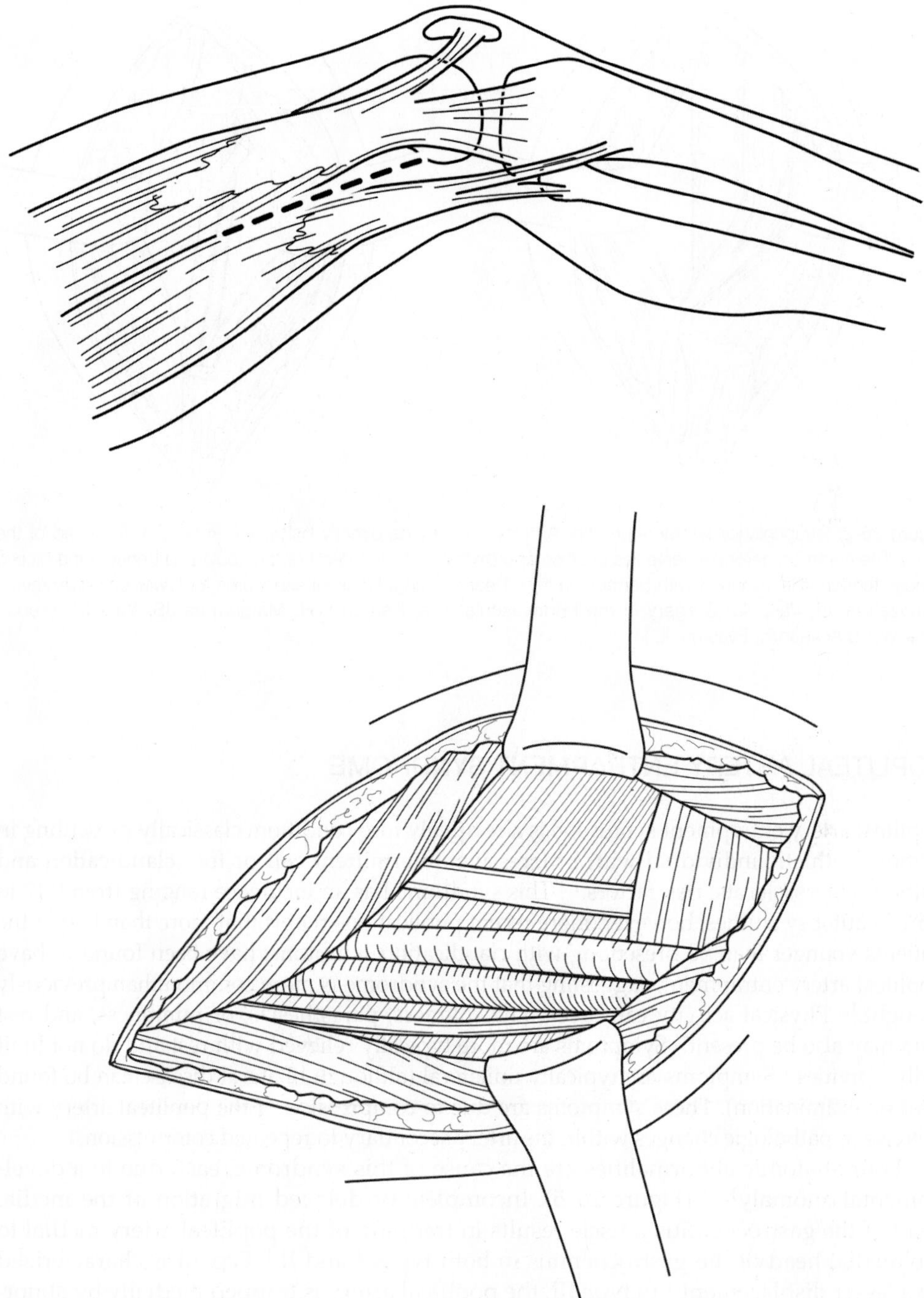

Figure 26-1. Supragenicular lateral approach. A vertical incision is made through the iliotibial tract between the vastus lateralis and the biceps femoris. The common peroneal nerve lies superficial in this wound, and care must be taken to avoid injuring it. (Reproduced with permission from Pearce, Tang. Unusual exposures for lower extremity revascularization. In: Vascular Surgery in the Endovascular Era, Pearce WH, Matsumura JS, Yao JSTY eds., Greenwood Academic, Evaston, IL.)

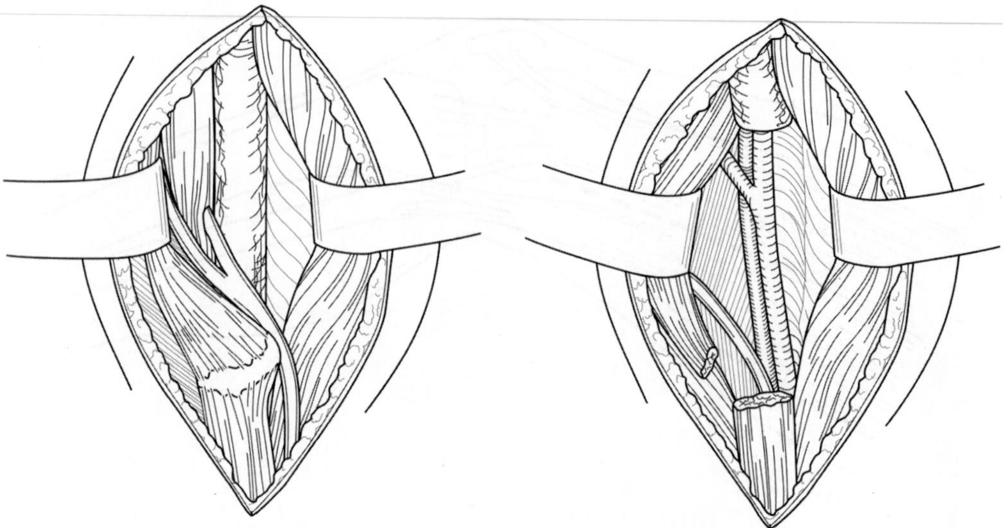

Figure 26-2. Infragenicular lateral approach. An incision is made directly below the knee over the head of the fibula. The common peroneal nerve lies in close approximation to the head of the fibula and beneath the biceps femoris tendon. (Reproduced with permission from Pearce, Tang. Unusual exposures for lower extremity revascularization. In: Vascular Surgery in the Endovascular Era, Pearce WH, Matsumura JS, Yao JSTY eds., Greenwood Academic, Evaston, IL.)

POPLITEAL ARTERY ENTRAPMENT SYNDROME

Popliteal artery entrapment syndrome is a relatively rare condition, classically presenting in a young, athletic individual with progressive, intermittent calf or foot claudication and without atherosclerotic risk factors.[1-2] This syndrome has an incidence ranging from 0.17 to 3.5% in autopsy studies; however, more recent publications report that more than half of the patients younger than 50 presenting with claudication symptoms have been found to have popliteal artery entrapment, suggesting that the syndrome is more common than previously thought.[1,3] Physical activity can precipitate coldness, paresthesias, or numbness, and rest pain may also be present.[2] Symptoms are more typically relieved with rest and do not limit daily activities.[4] Symptoms are typically unilateral (although bilateral disease can be found later on examination). These symptoms are due to compression of the popliteal artery with exercise or pathologic changes within the artery secondary to repeated compression.

Four anatomic abnormalities are the cause of this syndrome, each due to a developmental anomaly[1,5-7] (Figure 26–5). Incomplete or delayed migration of the medial head of the gastrocnemius muscle results in trapping of the popliteal artery medial to the medial head of the gastrocnemius in both types I and II.[1] Type II is characterized by a lesser displacement.[1] In type III, the popliteal artery is trapped medially by abnormal tissue bands, likely derived from the gastrocnemius, and in type IV, abnormal development of the popliteal artery (not the gastrocnemius) is responsible for the symptoms.[1-2] A type V has been proposed to describe cases in which both the popliteal artery and vein are entrapped.[8] In each of these variants, the abnormal location of the popliteal artery with respect to the musculature of the popliteal fossa results in compression of the artery with movement.

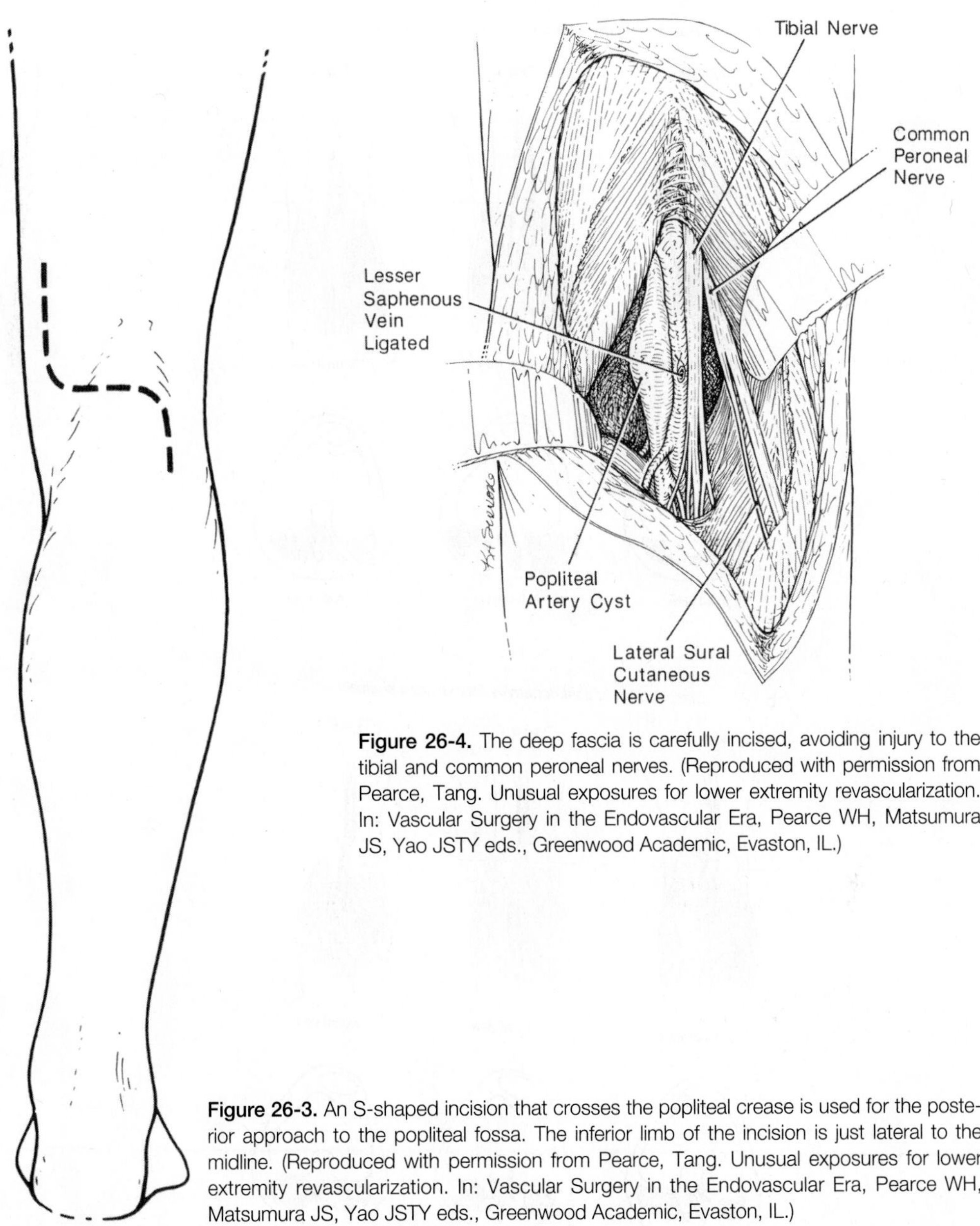

Figure 26-4. The deep fascia is carefully incised, avoiding injury to the tibial and common peroneal nerves. (Reproduced with permission from Pearce, Tang. Unusual exposures for lower extremity revascularization. In: Vascular Surgery in the Endovascular Era, Pearce WH, Matsumura JS, Yao JSTY eds., Greenwood Academic, Evaston, IL.)

Figure 26-3. An S-shaped incision that crosses the popliteal crease is used for the posterior approach to the popliteal fossa. The inferior limb of the incision is just lateral to the midline. (Reproduced with permission from Pearce, Tang. Unusual exposures for lower extremity revascularization. In: Vascular Surgery in the Endovascular Era, Pearce WH, Matsumura JS, Yao JSTY eds., Greenwood Academic, Evaston, IL.)

A sixth classification has also been described, entitled "functional entrapment" because no anatomic abnormality exists, although the popliteal artery still compresses with movement. There is no known etiology of this compression.[2] Several hypotheses have been raised, including muscle hypertrophy or compression of the popliteal artery as it passes through the distal soleus, but none has been proven.[1]

When unilateral claudication is found in a young adult without risk factors for atherosclerosis, noninvasive arterial studies can suggest the diagnosis. Ankle-brachial indexes, Doppler waveforms, duplex ultrasounds, or pulse volume recordings are

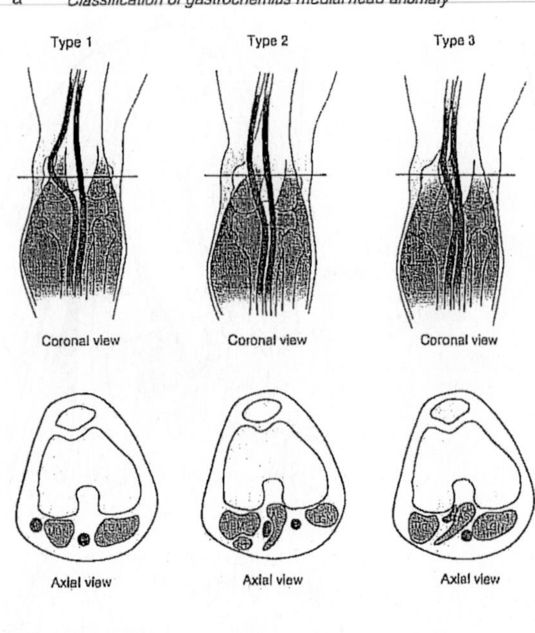

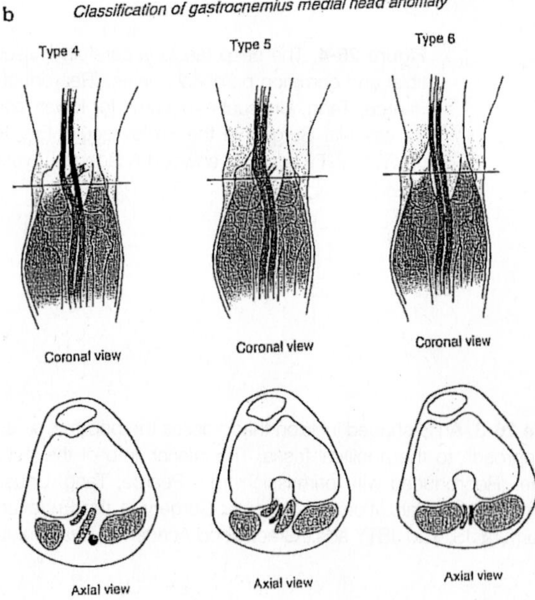

Figure 26-5. Six subtypes of gastrocnemius medial head anatomical variations causing PAES. *Type I:* an aberrant medial arterial course around normal medial head of gastrocnemius muscle. *Type 2:* abnormal head of the gastrocnemius muscle which is laterally inserted on the distal femur with medial displacement of popliteal artery. *Type 3:* an aberrant accessory slip from the medial head of the gastrocnemius muscle wraps around the normally positioned popliteal artery and entraps it. *Type 4:* the popliteal artery located deep in the popliteus muscle or beneath fibrous bands in the popliteal fossa. *Type 5:* any form of entrapment that involves the popliteal artery and vein. *Type 6:* functional type normally positioned popliteal artery which is entrapped by normally positioned gastrocnemius with hypertrophy. Reproduced with permission. Popliteal artery entrapment syndrome: morphological classification utilizing MR imaging. Kim HK, Shin MJ, Kim SM, Lee SH, Hong HJ. Skeletal Radiol (2006) 35:648–258.

used to determine artery patency while the patient is at rest as well as during active plantar flexion and passive dorsiflexion.[2,4-6,8] When these provocative measures result in decreased dorsalis pedis and posterior tibial pulses or popliteal artery narrowing or even occlusion, popliteal artery entrapment is suggested. Entrapment is also suggested when a popliteal artery is found to be occluded in a young adult. MRA has become the gold standard of diagnosis, demonstrating the anatomic abnormality responsible for entrapment.[1] Typically, a more medial course of the popliteal artery is observed (Figure 26–6). MRA, CT, and conventional angiography are also helpful in demonstrating the degree of arterial damage resulting from repeated compression. As entrapment develops over time, arterial wall scarring occurs. Severe compression, if untreated, can lead to popliteal artery occlusion or aneurysm.[6] Numerous studies have demonstrated the utility of performing bilateral screening despite unilateral symptoms and recommend bilateral imaging for all symptomatic patients.[4]

There is no role for endovascular modalities, and surgical treatment is recommended for all types of entrapment. Decompression is recommended for functional entrapment if symptoms are present.[1] Uncomplicated cases in which little arterial pathology is present or cases of functional entrapment can be treated with a myotomy, which relieves the entrapment and prevents any further disease progression. More commonly, patients present with complications caused by arterial wall degeneration, and simple releases have not been shown to be successful. Attempting a thromboendarterectomy is contraindicated. Instead, saphenous vein grafts are needed.[2]

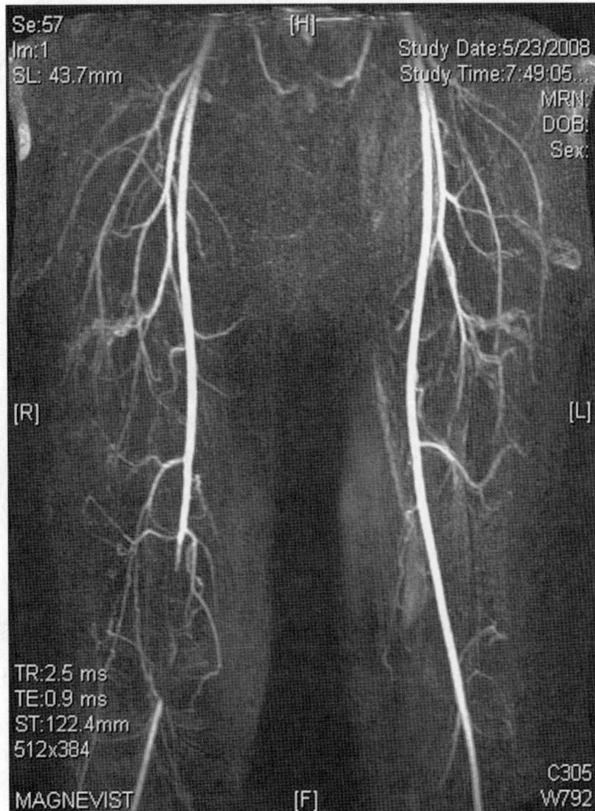

Figure 26-6. MRA showing a complete occlusion of the popliteal artery in a young male with right leg claudication. Popliteal entrapment was confirmed anatomically.

The preferred approach is generally the posterior S-shaped incision, which allows for both local arterial repair and myotomy as well as full visualization of the anatomy for classification. After exposing the popliteal vessels via the posterior approach (see above), the medial head of the gastrocnemius muscle is traced cephalad to its insertion on the femoral condyle. As one follows the tendinous insertion, it is often possible to see the entrapment caused by the lateral displacement of the medial head (Figure 26–7). The tendinous insertion is resected along with a substantial portion of the proximal muscle (Figure 26–8). In patients with damaged arteries or aneurysms, the arterial segment is replaced. A venous conduit is often harvested either from the lesser saphenous vein or by undermining the skin medially and harvesting the greater saphenous vein at the knee. With the free leg prepared, it is possible to flex and extend the leg to ensure that popliteal entrapment has been treated. The closure of the wound is often problematic. Aligning the S-shaped curve is difficult, particularly after extensive surgery when the skin may be swollen and difficult to reapproximate. Stay stitches are placed at the apex of the curvilinear incision to ensure proper alignment. The medial approach may is necessary if involvement of the superficial femoral artery (SFA) proximal to Hunter's canal or of the distal tibioperoneal trunk is present, because these segments are not accessible through the posterior approach.[4,9]

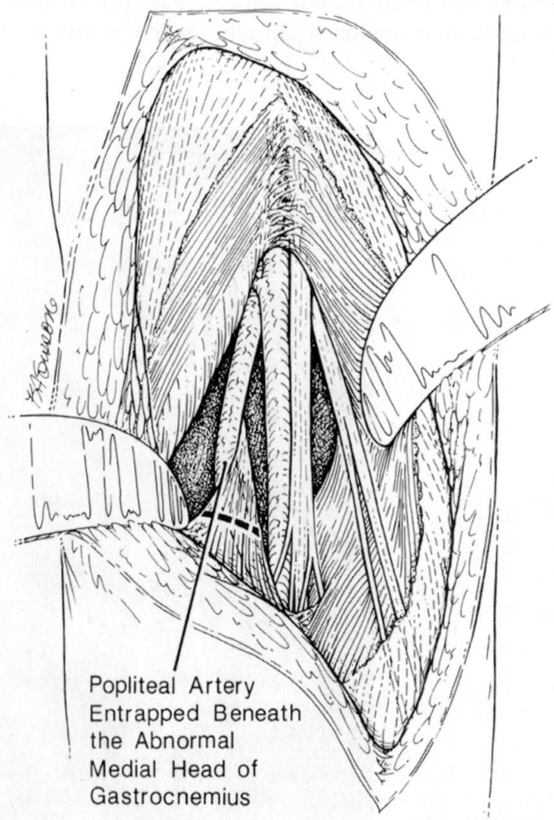

Figure 26-7. Resection of an anomalous insertion of the medial gastrocnemius muscle is made to release the entrapped popliteal artery. Note the distal branching of the tibial nerve. From: Pearce WH. Posterior approach to the popliteal artery. In: Bergan JJ, Yao JST, eds. *Techniques in Arterial Surgery*. Philadelphia: W.B. Saunders Company; 1990:180–183.

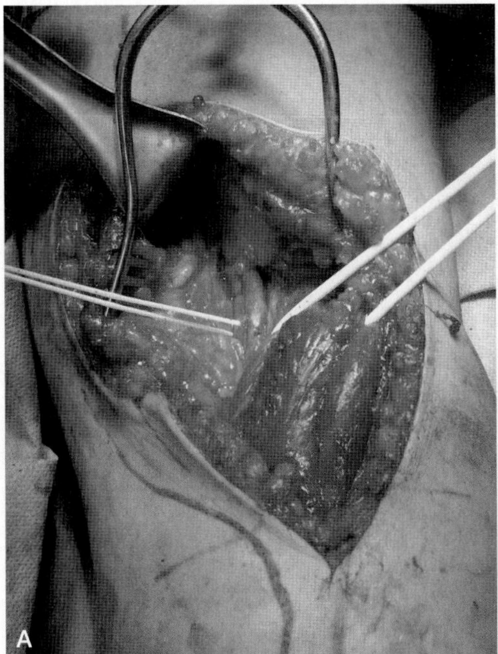

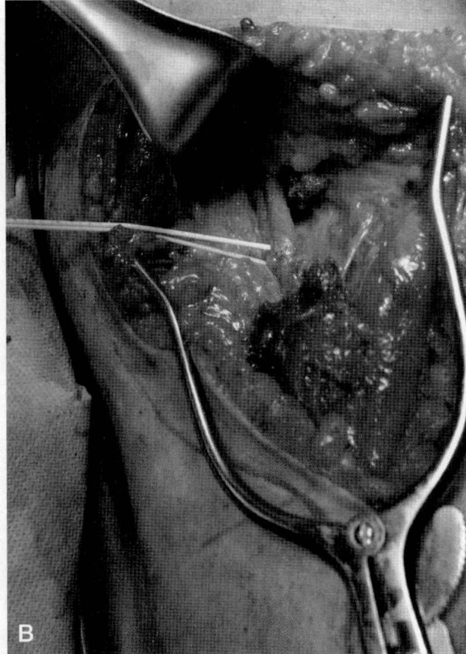

Figure 26-8. A. Surgical exposure via a posterior approach in a case of popliteal entrapment. Note the medial head of the gastrocnemius muscle with an anomalous lateral attachment causing medial displacement of the popliteal artery and vein. **B.** The same patient as in A after resection of the tendon and a portion of the muscular portion of the medial gastrocnemius head.

The relative rarity of this condition has precluded randomized studies on the effectiveness of these surgical treatments. One recent review of the literature reports that 90% of patients treated surgically return to normal sports activities within 3 months of the procedure and that most saphenous vein bypass grafts remain patent after 5 years.[2]

POPLITEAL CYSTIC ADVENTITIAL DISEASE

Popliteal cystic adventitial disease is an extremely rare condition, estimated to represent 0.1% of all vascular diseases.[10-11] In cystic adventitial disease, a cyst is present in the adventitia of the popliteal artery, causing stenosis or occlusion; however, the cyst itself is independent of the arterial lumen (Figure 26–9). The etiology of these cysts is unknown, although a few studies have indicated that cyst formation is likely joint-related and is not due to vascular, embryologic, systemic, or traumatic causes.[11]

Like popliteal artery entrapment syndrome, cystic adventitial disease is found in healthy patients, usually males, without atherosclerotic risk factors; unlike popliteal artery entrapment syndrome (PAES), cystic adventitial disease is found in a slightly older cohort, averaging 35 to 40 years old at diagnosis.[10,12-13] The typical presenting symptom is calf claudication, often abrupt in onset and beginning with vigorous activity.[14-15] The pain generally takes longer to subside than for typical claudication, and the symptoms may wax and wane over time.[15]

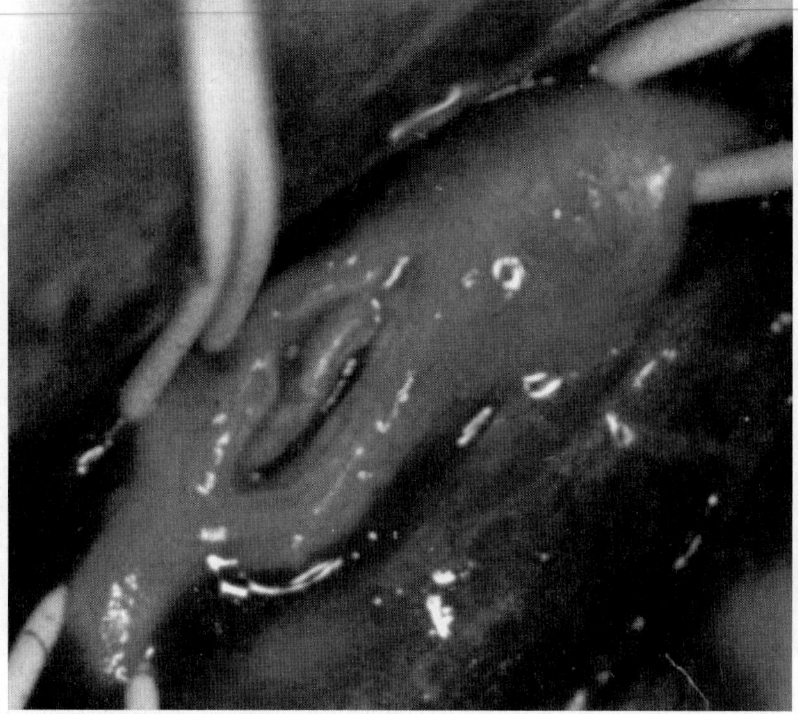

Figure 26-9. Popliteal adventitial cyst. The popliteal artery has been exposed and an arteriotomy has been created demonstrating the lumen of the vessel and the cystic cavity of the adventitial lesion.

This vague, nonspecific presentation is one factor leading to possible underdiagnosis. Another is the difficulty encountered by clinicians in confirming this disease. The patient may have normal popliteal and pedal pulses as well as normal ankle-brachial indexes; alternatively, all may be reduced.[10,16] Knee flexion can lead to a decrease in pedal pulses, known as Ishikawa sign. Duplex ultrasonography is a common technique used for screening of this condition. Duplex imaging can demonstrate a sharp line between the cyst and the lumen of the artery, representing the intima and inner media. Pulse wave velocity recordings can also demonstrate increased velocity in the narrowed lumen.[12] Doppler can also be used to diagnose this condition.[14] However, the advent of modern imaging techniques has allowed for the utilization of angiography, intravascular ultrasound, CT, and MRI to better elucidate the cause of a patient's symptoms. Typical signs on imaging are the hourglass sign, created by the presence of a concentric cyst, or the scimitar sign, due to an eccentric cyst[10] (Figure 26–10). Yet even these modalities may fail: if the cyst is so advanced that imaging demonstrates total occlusion, or if the image is uniformly cystic, the lesion may be difficult to differentiate from an aneurysm.[14,16] A recent case report by Fox and associates recommended the use of gadolinium-enhanced MRA to visualize the anatomy of the cysts in relation to the popliteal artery.[17]

The rarity of cases — reviews have suggested that a mere 300 to 400 cases are discussed in the literature — has prevented an adequate comparison of diagnostic or therapeutic modalities.[11-12,15-16] A few techniques are performed most frequently, including cyst excision and removal with artery sparing as well as saphenous vein

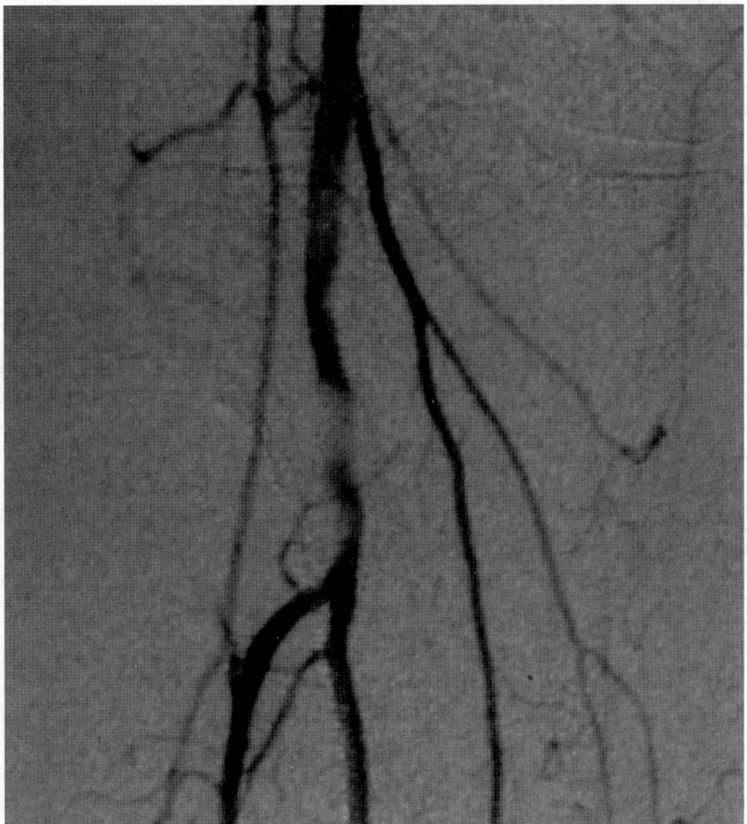

Figure 26-10. Conventional angiogram demonstrating the typical radiographic appearance of popliteal adventitial cysts. Note the eccentric, hourglass-like filling defects in the popliteal artery.

bypass grafting. Literature reviews have suggested that both of these procedures have an initial success rate of 94%.[13] One study hypothesized that total surgical replacement of the diseased portion of the vessel is superior to cyst excision, because incision into the adventitia will weaken the artery.[18] Cyst aspiration, which can now be performed with ultrasound guidance, can relieve symptoms but often fails because the cyst epithelium continues to secrete material and symptoms recur.[15] Endovascular stenting has been performed unsuccessfully, because numerous case reports note failure probably due to continued adventitial wall pressure secondary to the cyst presence.[14] Bypass grafting and cyst excision therefore seem to be the most successful means of treating cystic adventitial disease. Unfortunately, there are no long-term patency rates available.

COMMENTS

Managing popliteal pathology requires thorough anatomic knowledge of the popliteal fossa and the different approaches used to expose the popliteal artery. The clinical presentation, radiographic features, and surgical management of popliteal entrapment and adventitial cystic disease differ significantly from the features characteristic of the most commonly encountered atherosclerotic lesions affecting the popliteal artery.

REFERENCES

1. Levien LJ, Veller MG. Popliteal artery entrapment syndrome: more common than previously recognized. J Vasc Surg 1999;30:587–98.
2. Pillai JA. Current interpretation of popliteal vascular entrapment. J Vasc Surg 2008; 48:61–5.
3. Ruppert V, Verrel F, Geppert SN, et al. Results of perioperative measurements of ankle-brachial index in popliteal artery entrapment syndrome. J Vasc Surg 2004;39:758–62.
4. Turnipseed W. Popliteal entrapment syndrome, J Vasc Surg 2002;35:910–5.
5. Delaney TA, Gonzalez LL. Occlusion of the popliteal artery due to muscular entrapment. Surgery 1971;69:97–101.
6. Darling RC, Buckley CJ, Abbott WM, Raines JK. Intermittent claudication in young athletes: popliteal artery entrapment syndrome. J Trauma 1974;14:543–52.
7. Insua JA, Young JR, Humphries AW. Popliteal artery entrapment syndrome. Arch Surg 1970;101:771–5.
8. Rich NM, Collins GJ, McDonald PT, et al. Popliteal vascular entrapment: its increasing interest. Arch Surg 1979;114:1377–84.
9. Gourgiotis S, Aggelakas J, Salemis N, et al. Diagnosis and surgical approach of popliteal artery entrapment syndrome: a retrospective study. Vasc Health Risk Mgmt 2008;4:83–8.
10. Wright LB, Matchett WJ, Cruz CP, et al. Popliteal artery disease: diagnosis and treatment. Radiographics 2004;24:467–9.
11. Levien LJ, Benn CA. Adventitial cystic disease: a unifying hypothesis. J Vasc Surg 1998;28: 193–205.
12. Tsolakis IA, Walvatne CS, Caldwell MD. Cystic adventitial disease of the popliteal artery: diagnosis and treatment. Eur J Endovasc Surg 1998;15:188–94.
13. Pursell R, Torrie EPH, Gibson M, Galland RB. Spontaneous and permanent resolution of cystic adventitial disease of the popliteal artery. J Roy S Med 2004;97:77–8.
14. Rai S, Davies RSM, Vohra RK. Failure of endovascular stenting for popliteal cystic disease. Ann Vasc Surg 2009;23:410.e1–410e.5.
15. Cassar K, Engeset J. Cystic adventitial disease: a trap for the unwary. Eur J Endovasc Surg 2005;29:93–6.
16. Mino MJ, Garrigues DG, Pierce DS, Arko FR. Cystic adventitial disease of the popliteal artery. J Vasc Surg 2009;49:1324.
17. Fox CJ, Rasmussen TE, O'Donnell SD. Cystic adventitial disease of the popliteal artery. J Vasc Surg 2004;39:1351.
18. Madhavan P, Boyle T, Coyle J, et al. Cystic adventitial disease. Eur J Endovasc Surg 1998;15:456–8.

27

Long-Term Results of Combined Common Femoral Endarterectomy and Iliac Stent/Stent Grafting for Occlusive Disease

Philip P. Goodney, M.D. and Richard J. Powell, M.D.

INTRODUCTION

Endarterectomy with patch angioplasty has become the standard for treatment of isolated common femoral artery (CFA) occlusive disease.[1-2] The management of disease that extends proximally into the external iliac arteries is a more challenging problem. According to the recently modified guidelines from the Trans Atlantic Society Consensus (TASC II) document, external iliac disease involving the CFA is now classified as either TASC C or D, depending on the extent of iliac involvement. For TASC D lesions, open surgical bypass remains the recommended treatment, with consideration of endovascular options only for TASC C lesions in poor-risk patients.[3] Standard open surgical therapies include iliofemoral endarterectomy or aortofemoral bypass. Although durable, these options are associated with increased perioperative morbidity.[4-6] Less invasive but also less durable open surgical options include axillobifemoral bypass or femoro-femoral bypass for unilateral disease. In the endovascular era, endoluminal treatment has been shown in certain situations to be a comparable option for iliac occlusive disease.[7-21] However, it is not a suitable stand-alone therapy in the presence of significant common femoral artery disease.[22]

Here we describe our experience with combined common femoral endarterectomy and external iliac artery (EIA) stenting as a means to treat TASC C and D iliac lesions using both bare metal stents and stent grafts for iliac artery intervention.

Preoperative Evaluation

All patients undergo preoperative peripheral vascular evaluation with physical examination, ankle-brachial indexes (ABIs), and duplex ultrasound, computed tomographic angiography (CTA), or digital subtraction angiography (DSA) to assess iliac and CFA disease burden. Patients with significant CFA occlusive disease with proximal extension into the EIA are considered for the combined procedure. The presence of significant CFA disease is defined by greater than 2.5 times step-up increase in peak systolic velocity (PSV) across the CFA with duplex ultrasound scan, more than 50% diameter reduction with DSA or CTA, or more than 10 mm Hg systolic pressure gradient at the time of angiography. Selected patients with contralateral or distal disease requiring revascularization undergo various adjunctive procedures such as angioplasty/stenting, femoral-distal bypass, or femorofemoral crossover bypass as needed.

PROCEDURAL TECHNIQUE

Standard femoral arterial exposure is gained under general anesthesia. Needle-guided retrograde guidewire access is then obtained under fluoroscopic guidance. Standard endarterectomy and patch angioplasty are then performed with the guidewire in place. Efforts are undertaken to ensure that adequate profunda femoris artery outflow is preserved or restored. The wire is then back-fed through the center of the patch, and a retrograde working sheath is placed once inflow has been restored (Figure 27–1). Standard interventional techniques are then used to treat the proximal arterial lesion. If guidewire access cannot be obtained initially, it is then attempted after arteriotomy or endarterectomy. Rarely, contralateral iliac artery or brachial artery access is required for antegrade wire access. In recent years, re-entry devices are occasionally used for crossing chronic total

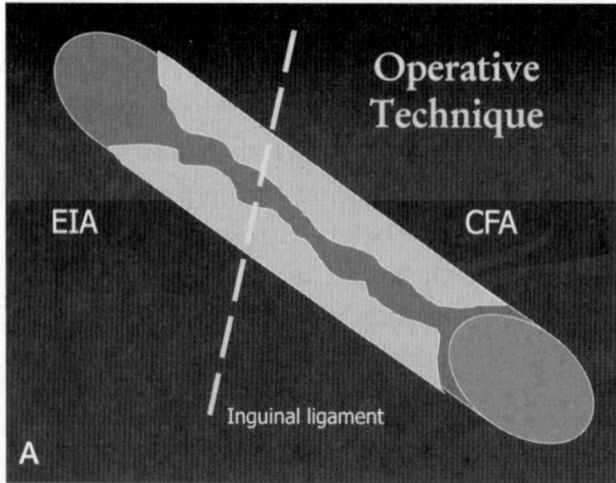

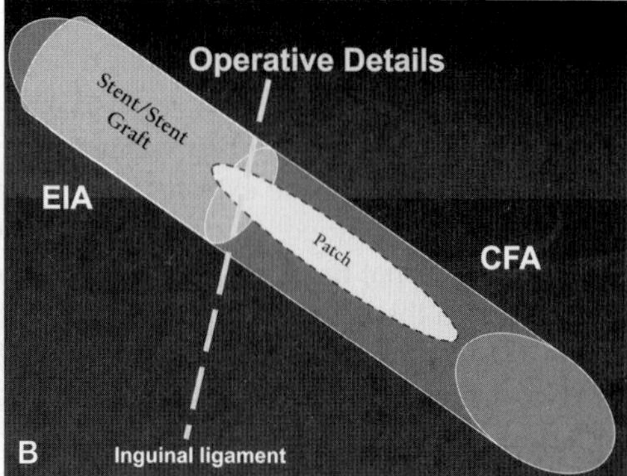

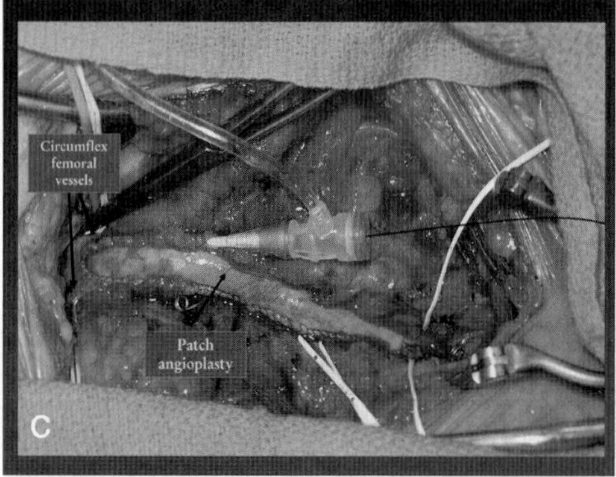

Figure 27-1. Schematic of stent graft placement with combined femoral endarterectomy and patch angioplasty. **A.** Preprocedure **B.** Postprocedure **C.** Intraoperative photograph. Note that the sheath is usually placed through the center of the patch.

occlusions of the iliac system (Pioneer Reentry Catheter, Medtronic, Santa Rosa, CA; Outback Reentry Catheter, Cordis, Miami Lakes, FL).

Arterial diameter and lesion measurements are made using preoperative CT scan measurements or calibrated using a marker catheter and fluoroscopy imaging software. The choice of device and postdeployment balloon diameter depends upon the severity of iliac artery calcification and lesion location. We generally use self-expanding stents (Wallstent, Boston Scientific, Boston, MA; Symphony, Boston Scientific, Boston, MA; SMART, Cordis, Miami Lakes, FL; Absolute, Abbott Vascular, Abbott Park, IL; Luminexx, Bard, Tempe, AZ), self-expanding stent grafts (Viabahn, W.L. Gore, Flagstaff, AZ; Fluency, Bard, Lowell, MA; Wallgraft, Boston Scientific, Boston, MA) and less frequently balloon-expandable stents (Express, Boston Scientific, Boston, MA; Palmaz, Cordis, Miami Lakes, FL) and balloon-expandable stent grafts (Icast, Atrium Medical, Hudson, NH) are used. Self-expanding devices are generally oversized by 1 to 2 mm relative to the native treated vessel. The diameter of the angioplasty balloon usually corresponds to the normal vessel size as seen on adjacent angiography or CTA. As previously described, we place the distal end of the device into the proximal portion of the patch angioplasty but above the inguinal ligament (Figure 27–2). The proximal portion of our endarterectomy and endpoint for the patch angioplasty are usually at the level of the circumflex vessels. This generally requires at most minimal division of the inguinal ligament.

RESULTS

We have now performed this procedure in over 200 patients. Patient demographics are shown in Table 27–1.

In all patients, CFA endarterectomy was performed with patch angioplasty. In 39% of cases, the EIA is the only iliac segment treated (TASC C). In 61% of cases, both the EIA and the CIA (TASC D) were treated. Forty-one percent of treated iliac vessels were occluded at the time of intervention. In 67% of cases, the SFA and profunda were patent at the completion of the procedure; in 30% of cases, only the profunda was patent; and in 3% of cases, only the SFA was patent at endarterectomy completion. There were 21 (11%) concomitant distal bypasses, 6 (3%) SFA stents, and 25 (13%) femorofemoral bypass grafts performed.

TABLE 27-1. PATIENT DEMOGRAPHICS

193 Limbs	171 Patients
Age (years)	67 (44-88)
Gender	62% male
HTN	85%
CAD	63%
Hyperlipidemia	63%
Current smokers	49%
Statin use	49%
DM	35%
COPD	31%
Renal disease (Cr > 1.6)	11%

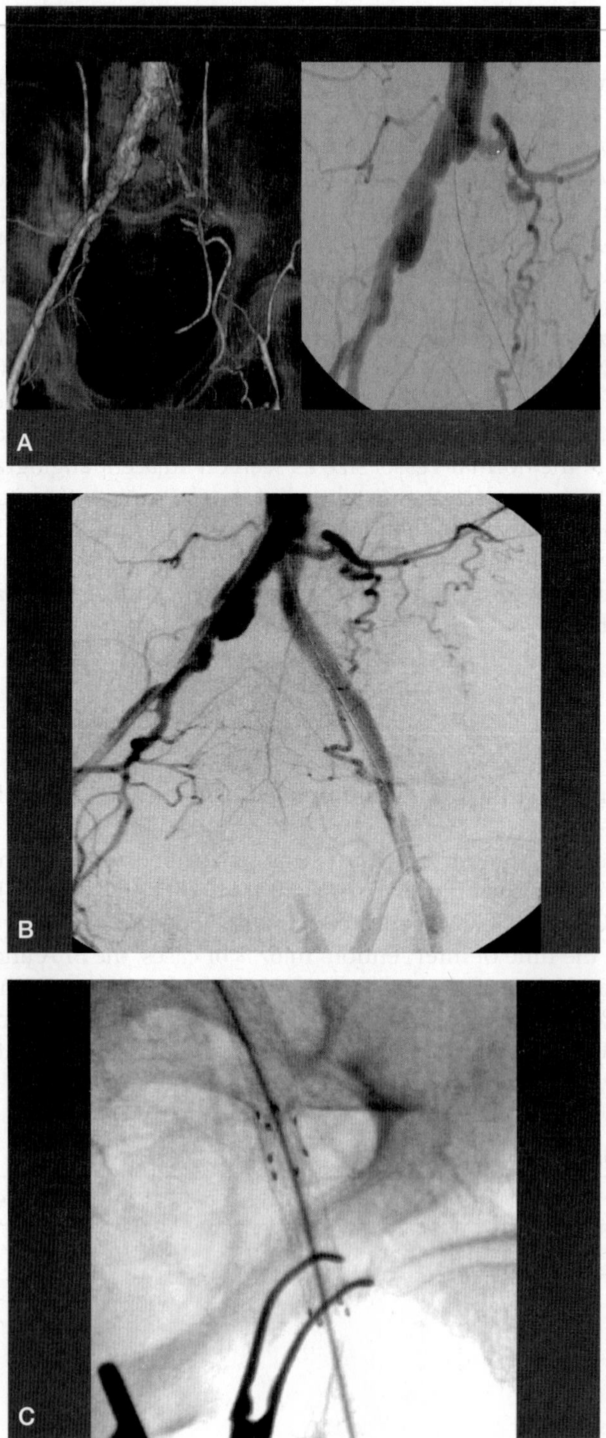

Figure 27-2. A. Total left iliac occlusion. Guidewire access obtained with retrograde sheath and re-entry device (Pioneer catheter). **B.** Stent graft treatment of iliac segment. **C.** Note extension of stent grafts into common femoral patch that is marked by vascular clamp.

Ninety percent of the iliac interventions were performed via retrograde access from the ipsilateral CFA. In 31% of cases, treatment of the CIA and EIA involved placing a bare metal stent across a patent hypogastric artery. In 3 cases, a stent graft was intentionally placed across a patent hypogastric artery. The technical success rate was 98%. There were 11 different stent or stent grafts used during the study period. During the latter part of the study period, more stent grafts were used for this application. Overall, stent grafts were used in 41% of cases.

On average, two devices (range 1 to 5) were placed in a treated EIA or EIA/CIA segment. The mean stent diameter was 8.3 mm±1.1 mm, with a mean postdilation balloon diameter of 7.4 mm±1.0 mm. The average preintervention pressure gradient in lesions that were not total occlusions was 31 mm Hg±18 mm Hg, which was reduced to 1 mm Hg±3 mm Hg after intervention. The mean preoperative ABI was 0.38±0.32, and the mean postoperative ABI was 0.72±0.24 ($P<.05$). Ninety-two percent of patients were clinically improved following the procedure. The median length of stay was 2 days (range 1 to 51 days). Median follow-up on all patients was 24 months (range 0 to 9 years).

Overall, there were 64 (33%) patients with hemodynamically significant recurrent disease. Of these, 45 patients experienced recurrent symptoms, and 19 patients remained asymptomatic but had a decrease in ABI or a diminished femoral pulse and were subsequently found to have recurrent stenoses. Twenty-eight patients (14%) eventually required a percutaneous intervention on the treated segment, and 19 patients (10%) underwent a subsequent open procedure on the treated segment. The mean time to reintervention was 21 months. Of the percutaneous reinterventions to maintain patency, 7 cases involved angioplasty of in-stent restenosis, 14 cases required restenting of the previously treated area, and 7 patients underwent more extensive stenting beyond the target lesion. Of the 19 open procedures performed, there were 6 redo endarterectomies, 4 redo endarterectomies with restenting, 1 open angioplasty, 3 redo endarterectomies with concomitant distal bypass, and 5 CFA thrombectomies with iliac recanalization or femorofemoral bypass.

Five-year survival by life-table analysis was 60±6% (Figure 27–3). Overall, there were 9 major amputations in the study group during the follow-up period.

Overall primary patency rate of the treated segment, as determined by Kaplan-Meier life-table analysis, was 60±6% at 5 years. Primary-assisted patency was 97±1% at 5 years. Secondary patency was noted to be 98±2% at 5 years.

Primary patency was significantly higher in patients receiving stent grafts versus bare metal stents (OR 0.19, 95% CI 0.08-0.45, $P<.001$). There were no additional patient or technical factors associated with failure of primary patency, including SFA, profunda, and tibial vessel patencies.

Subgroup analysis of the stent graft group versus the stent group showed significantly higher primary patency at 5 years in the stent graft group (87±5%, CI 72–94% vs. 53±7%, CI 39.5–65.2%, $P<.01$) (Figure 27–4). There were no significant differences found with primary-assisted and secondary patency rates between the groups.

There were 4 (2.3%) perioperative deaths. One patient suffered perioperative cardiogenic shock and died on the seventh postoperative day; 2 patients died from multisystem organ failure at postoperative days 18 and 22, respectively; and 1 patient died of unknown cause at home 3 days after surgery. There were 42 (22%) perioperative complications, consisting of 8 (4%) myocardial ischemic events, 5 (3%) pulmonary events, 25 (13%) wound infections, and 4 (2%) perioperative (within 30 days) thrombotic events requiring re-exploration. Three of these acute patient

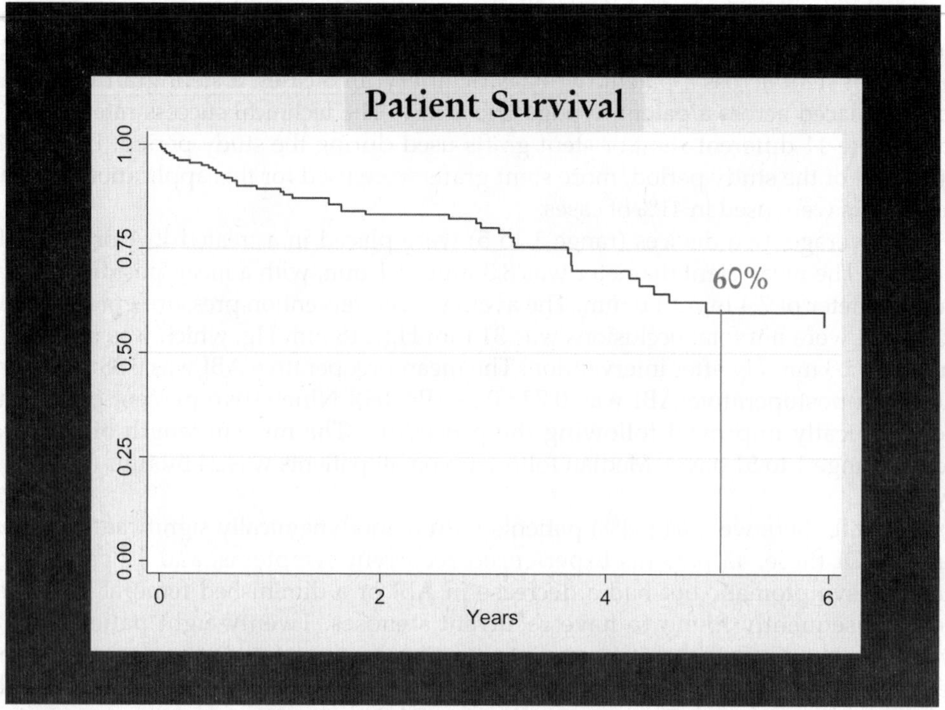

Figure 27-3. Five-year survival rates for all patients.

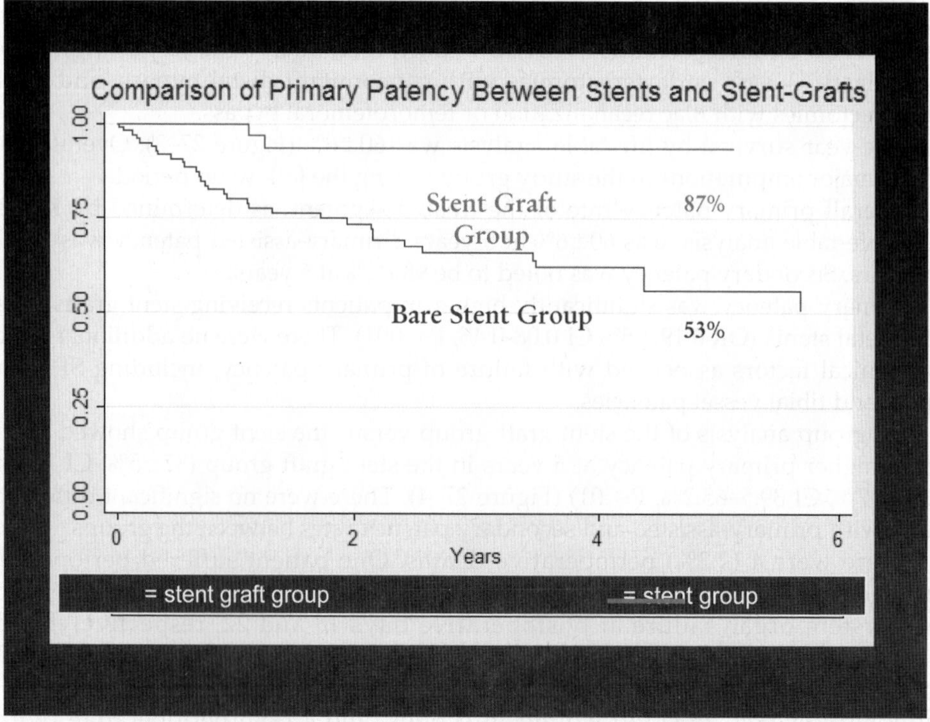

Figure 27-4. Patency for stent graft group compared with bare metal stent graft (P<.01).

occlusions occurred in the early perioperative setting, 2 of which were thrombectomized. The third perioperative occlusion patient underwent femorofemoral bypass. The fourth occlusion occurred within 30 days of the original procedure and was successfully thrombectomized with an open procedure.

DISCUSSION

In addition to our previous work,[12] several authors have published their techniques and early results with a hybrid approach to iliofemoral occlusive disease.[13,16-18] To the best of our knowledge, this report constitutes the largest series to date describing outcome and long-term patency of this procedure.

Endovascular treatment of iliac disease has radically changed management paradigms in vascular surgery over the last 2 decades. With improving technology and results, the preferred initial treatment of iliac occlusive disease is now endovascular. However, several factors such as the presence of external iliac occlusive disease, vessel calcification, and totally occluded iliac arteries have been associated with high complication rates and poor long-term durability when treatment is with bare metal stents.[19-20] Use of stent grafts in iliac occlusive disease has increased in popularity in recent years.[18,21] We have previously reported 12-month primary patency of 70% in patients treated with stent grafts for iliac occlusive disease (with and without femoral endarterectomy), which appeared to have superior patency compared with historical controls treated with bare metal stents.[22]

Despite the lack of objective evidence, these promising early results have led us to favor stent grafts over stents for the treatment of diffuse iliac occlusive disease, especially when performed in the setting of concomitant femoral endarterectomy when the larger sheath size required to place a stent graft is not a concern. The theoretical barrier to intimal hyperplasia and the ability to aggressively dilate calcified vessels are potential benefits for covered stents. Although the device sizes and postdeployment balloon diameters are not significantly different between the bare stents and the stent grafts and inflation pressures are not recorded, we believe that the lessened risk of iliac rupture leads to improved dilation with use of higher inflation pressures. These hypotheses are supported by the improved patency of stent grafts versus stents in the current study. Our preferred device is now a covered stent for this combined procedure; bare stents are usually only placed across a patent hypogastric artery. Iliac rupture, especially in small, calcified lesions, is a potentially morbid complication that can be minimized and treated by a stent graft. In our series, there were 5 iliac artery ruptures during device deployment. All were treated with a stent graft over the wire, and none required open repair.

There are several potential limitations with this technique. We do not routinely cover the hypogastric artery in treating common or external iliac lesions. The fate of a crossed hypogastric artery for treatment of adjacent disease is unknown and may eventually exacerbate or contribute to pelvic ischemia. In addition, the inability to cross long total occlusions is a potential obstacle for successful utilization of this technique. This has largely been overcome by increased use of re-entry devices.

The excellent primary-assisted patency rate reemphasizes the value of common femoral endarterectomy. This is supported by earlier work in which CFA endarterectomy with iliac stent grafting is associated with better patency rates when compared with cases undergoing iliac stent grafting alone. Nearly 50% of the failed patients in the latter group went on to have subsequent femoral endarterectomy, which might argue for a more rigorous preoperative evaluation for common femoral disease.[22] Of the patients in this series requiring subsequent intervention, more than half were managed with an outpatient percutaneous procedure to maintain patency.

It is interesting to note that treatment of EIA lesions versus more extensive treatment of EIA and CIA lesions led to a higher risk of reintervention to maintain patency. This is an unexpected finding but may relate to undertreatment of more proximal disease. Other groups have shown no significant difference in primary patency stratified by previous TASC classification, which may imply the difficult and varying nature of iliac lesions in these patients.[23]

Aortobifemoral bypass grafting remains the standard of care for diffuse aortoiliac disease.[3] Our results with this hybrid procedure cannot be directly compared with results with bypass grafting or isolated iliac stenting because of patient selection, associated comorbidities, and the varying anatomic distribution of disease. However, this procedure has comparable outcomes and is well tolerated. In addition, many of these patients would not be candidates for abdominal revascularization procedures and would benefit from the shortened hospital stay and overall decreased trauma of a limited groin exposure. Although our primary patency rates are lower than expected, many of these patients enjoy continued patency with only percutaneous reintervention. In this regard, this technique compares favorably with patency rates of extra-anatomic bypasses.[24-25] In addition, male patients are not exposed to the risks of erectile dysfunction with open iliac or aortic surgery. Although the patients in this series underwent general anesthesia, this procedure can also be performed using spinal or epidural techniques, which might improve tailored patient care.

In conclusion, we have found that CFA endarterectomy associated with iliac stenting or stent grafting is a viable alternative to more invasive open procedures in terms of both perioperative complications and long-term patency. In addition, our data suggest that stent grafts placed in the iliac position have improved primary patency compared with bare metal stents and may be the preferred device for this patient population.

REFERENCES

1. Radoux JM, Maiza D, Coffin O. Long-term outcome of 121 iliofemoral endarterectomy procedures. Ann Vasc Surg 2001;15:163–70.
2. Melliere D, Blancas AE, Desgranges P, Becquemin JP. The underestimated advantages of iliofemoral endarterectomy. Ann Vasc Surg 2000;14:343–9.
3. Norgren L, Hiatt WR, Dormandy JA, et al. Inter-society consensus for the management of peripheral arterial disease. Int Angiol 2007;26:81–157.
4. Nevelsteen a, Wouters L, Suy R. Aortofemoral Dacron reconstruction for aorto-iliac occlusive disease: a 25 year study. Eur J Vasc Surg 1991;5:179–86.
5. Malone JM, Moore WS, Goldstone J. The natural history of bilateral aortofemoral bypass grafts for ischemia of the lower extremities. Arch Surg 1975;110:1300, 1301–6.
6. de Vries SO, Hunink MG. Results of aortic bifurcation grafts for aortoiliac occlusive disease: a meta-analysis. J Vasc Surg 1997;26:558–69.
7. Marin ML, Veith FJ, Sanchez LA, et al. Endovascular repair of aortoiliac occlusive disease. World J Surg 1996;20:679–86.
8. Martin EC, Katzen BT, Benenati JF, et al. Multicenter trial of the Wallstent in the iliac and femoral arteries. J Vasc Interv Radiol 1995;6:843–9.
9. Bosch JL, Hunink MG. Meta-analysis of the results of percutaneous transluminal angioplasty and stent placement for aortoiliac occlusive disease. Radiology 1997;204:87–96.

10. Cynamon J, Marin ML, Veith FJ, et al. Stent-graft repair of aorto-iliac occlusive disease coexisting with common femoral artery disease. J Vasc Interv Radiol 1997;8:19–26.
11. De Roeck A, Hendriks JM, Delrue F, et al. Long-term results of primary stenting for long and complex iliac artery occlusions. Acta Chir Belg 2006;106:187–92.
12. Nelson PR, Powell RJ, Schermerhorn ML, et al. Early results of external iliac artery stenting combined with common femoral artery endarterectomy. J Vasc Surg 2002;35:1107–13.
13. Dosluoglu HH, Cherr GS. Pre-arteriotomy guidewire access (PAGA): a crucial maneuver for securing inflow and/or outflow in patients with bulky iliofemoral occlusive disease undergoing combined (open/endovascular) procedures. Eur J Vasc Endovasc Surg 2006;32: 97–100.
14. Rutherford RB, Baker JD, Ernst C, et al. Recommended standards for reports dealing with lower extremity ischemia: revised version. J Vasc Surg 1997;26:517–38.
15. Pentecost MJ, Criqui MH, Dorros G, et al. Guidelines for peripheral percutaneous transluminal angioplasty of the abdominal aorta and lower extremity vessels. A statement for health professionals from a special writing group of the Councils on Cardiovascular Radiology, Arteriosclerosis, Cardio-thoracic and Vascular Surgery, Clinical Cardiology, and Epidemiology and Prevention, the American Heart Association. J Vasc Interv Radiol 2003; 14:S495–515.
16. Queral LA, Criado FJ, Patten P. Retrograde iliofemoral endarterectomy facilitated by balloon angioplasty. J Vasc Surg 1995;22:742–8; discussion 748–50.
17. Ali AT, Modrall JG, Lopez J, et al. Emerging role of endovascular grafts in complex aortoiliac occlusive disease. J Vasc Surg. 2003;38:486–91.
18. Nevelsteen A, Lacroix H, Stockx L, Wilms G. Stent grafts for iliofemoral occlusive disease. Cardiovasc Surg 1997;5:393–7.
19. Powell RJ, Fillinger M, Bettmann M, et al. The durability of endovascular treatment of multisegment iliac occlusive disease. J Vasc Surg 2000;31:1178–84.
20. Powell RJ, Fillinger M, Walsh DB, et al. Predicting outcome of angioplasty and selective stenting of multisegment iliac artery occlusive disease. J Vasc Surg 2000;32:564–9.
21. Murphy TP, Webb MS, Lambiase RE, et al. Percutaneous revascularization of complex iliac artery stenoses and occlusions with use of wallstents: three-year experience. J Vasc Interv Radiol 1996;7:21–7.
22. Rzucidlo EM, Powell RJ, Zwolak RM, et al. Early results of stent-grafting to treat diffuse aortoiliac occlusive disease. J Vasc Surg. 2003;37:1175–80.
23. Park KB, Do YS, Kim DI, et al. The TransAtlantic InterSociety consensus (TASC) classification system in iliac arterial stent placement: long-term patency and clinical limitations. J Vasc Interv Radiol 2007;18:193–201.
24. Hertzer NR, Bena JF, Karafa MT. A personal experience with direct reconstruction and extra-anatomic bypass for aortoiliofemoral occlusive disease. J Vasc Surg 2007;45:527–35.
25. Passman MA, Taylor LM, Moneta GL, et al. Comparison of axillofemoral and aortofemoral bypass for aortoiliac occlusive disease. J Vasc Surg 1996;23:263–9; discussion 269–71.

28

The Cost of Patency

Dorian J. deFreitas, M.D. and
Michael C. Stoner, M.D., F.A.C.S.

INTRODUCTION

The looming crisis in health care funding stands as one of the biggest challenges facing our economy. Currently, 500 billion U.S. dollars are earmarked for Medicare and Medicaid payments this year, and the federal government predicts a 31% increase in health care spending over the next 5 years. If costs continue to grow as projected, the U.S. federal government will spend approximately 20% of its gross domestic product on health care by 2050.[1] It is thought that Medicare will no longer be solvent by 2017, and the current recession threatens to worsen our predicament. If these predictions are brought to fruition, we will be forced to ration health care or face drastic cuts in government programs and incur higher taxes.

The diagnosis, treatment, and long-term care of patients with PAD (PAD) imposes a significant burden on our health care system. PAD affects 8 to 12 million Americans and costs 151 billion dollars in direct and indirect costs per year to treat. These costs are likely to increase as the baby boomers age and hospitals and doctors realize a population of patients as a new source of revenue.

The specialty of vascular surgery has expanded with the advent of endovascular surgery, introducing an ever-increasing array of new and potentially expensive modalities to treat our patients. There has been a dramatic shift toward the use of endovascular therapy in peripheral vascular disease. There has been a 40% increase in the total number of endovascular cases in the past 7 years, with a fall in the number of open bypasses by 30%.[2] Unfortunately, many of these new treatment modalities have not been fully evaluated for either clinical efficacy or cost-effectiveness. Contemporary discussions of cost-to-benefit ratios have been hindered by a poor appraisal of the true cost involved in treatment of PAD. Often, discussions have taken into account only initial cost, involving the costs of the device and hospital stay. This is flawed and myopic, because it does not account for procedural durability, cost of reintervention, and patient longevity. Our ability as vascular surgeons to control costs while providing quality care is tantamount to our success in the future. The current administration is looking to major medical providers such as hospitals, doctors, insurance agencies, and pharmaceutical companies to cut 2 trillion dollars from health care spending over the next 10 years. We as a society of vascular surgeons must prove a significant cost-to-benefit ratio for our interventions. If not, our reimbursement and image as medical providers will be affected.

THE COMPLEXITIES OF ACCURATE COST ANALYSIS

How well do we spend our health care dollars? What is the best way to allocate health care resources? These two questions are at the root of all conversations about health care analysis and reform. Whereas these are two relatively straightforward questions, producing accurate answers is extremely difficult. At the root of the problem is defining what an acceptable cost is for a defined outcome. Determining whether a cost is justifiable is dependent on the resources available and society's perception of the value of the outcome. Owing to the complexity and philosophical nature of these questions, many cost models exist, but few of them are universally accepted or used to guide decision-making.

The most rudimentary method of cost analysis is the study of the procedural costs associated with the index procedure. Although this view may be adequate in some specialties, vascular surgery is somewhat unique in that repeated interventions are often required to maintain the desired effect. This means that the initial cost may be only a fraction of the cost over the lifetime of a procedure's being evaluated. In addition, the cost of any complication adds to the initial expense of each procedure. There are a number of other resources that must be added to taking care of vascular patients, including nursing home care, home health care, and costs of following up. It is easy to see why a direct comparison of initial cost is a poor marker of overall cost to society. Even if all the aforementioned costs were measured and then directly compared, the model would still be inadequate because it has no measure of outcomes associated with it.

Comparison of cost using quality adjusted life year (QALY) as an outcome is another commonly used method of cost analysis. QALY takes into account both quality and quantity of life generated by health care interventions. A QALY places weight on time in different health states. A year in perfect health is worth 1. A year in less than perfect health is worth less than 1, and death is considered 0. QALYs are combined with an intervention's cost to determine a cost-utility ratio. The cost-utility ratio allows for costs of interventions to be directly compared. The meaning and usefulness of QALYs are debatable. Perfect health is hard to define. It is arguable that there are states of health that are worse than death and therefore they should have a negative value. There is also a problem of accurately placing a numerical value on a subjective measure such as quality of life. Arguably, many models place too much weight on physical pain and disability over mental health. Discrimination against the elderly, chronically ill, or disabled patients is also a commonly cited flaw of QALY. QUALY-based cost analysis is an obvious improvement over a comparison of index procedure costs. Unfortunately, the many assumptions and complexity of calculating QALY affect its accuracy and reproducibility.

The Markov Decision Analysis is another method used to scrutinize expenditure. This model compares the costs of different interventions using hypothetical groups of patients. The analysis uses patency rates gleaned from previously published data and then combined with cost data to develop a marker of cost-effectiveness. The analysis often uses an arbitrary number that represents an acceptable societal cost for the desired outcome. Unfortunately, data in the literature are heterogeneous, involving different patient subsets with different comorbidities and disease severity. These same problems are seen with meta-analysis and negatively impact the validity of conclusions derived from this data. The calculations of decision analytical models are complex, require multiple assumptions, and are not easy to reproduce without expertise in the area. All of these factors make decision analysis prone to error. There are significant variations in outcomes from individual practitioners when compared with the published literature. This makes it difficult for practitioners to base their decision-making on these models. Decision analytical models offer an improvement on more rudimentary methods of cost analysis but still have many flaws.

Cost-Per-Day of Patency

In an attempt to overcome some of the failings of the aforementioned cost models, an amortized cost model was developed to examine the cost efficacy characteristics of a given revascularization procedure. Our goal was to create a model that was easy to use and understand with data that were readily available to all practicing vascular surgeons. We used patency as the outcome measure in our model for the following reasons:

- Patency is the gold standard by which outcomes are reported in peripheral vascular disease.
- Patency can be universally applied to all patient subsets.
- Patency data can be easily obtained by all practicing vascular surgeons.
- There are clear reporting standards.
- Patency is not a subjective measure.

To determine cost at any time, we calculated the summation of all costs accrued over time to maintain patency. This takes into account the initial cost and the cost of all subsequent interventions. This is then divided by time in days to give the cost per day of patency. When an intervention failed patency, the cost per day of patency remained static throughout the remaining time period of the study.

Cost per day of patency is expressed at any given time interval (*t*) as follows:

$$Cost(t) = \lim_{t \to pa} \frac{\sum_{i=o}^{t} Cost(i)}{t}$$

Where *pa* = maximum number of days of assisted patency, *Cost(i)* = total hospital costs (direct and indirect) at time interval *i* days from index procedure (*t*=*0*). With this cost model, the cost per day of patency was assessed at any given time interval from the index procedure. Hypothetical situations are illustrated in the cost-efficacy curves of Figure 28–1. The figure depicts a series of patients undergoing revascularization. Patient A undergoes a successful revascularization, without the need for subsequent reintervention throughout the follow-up time period. Patient B requires a secondary procedure to maintain patency (primary, assisted, or secondary), and subsequently maintains patency. Finally, Patient C fails patency and an assistive procedure is not undertaken. Of note, total hospital costs were accounted for at each time point. If a patient suffered a complication or adverse event from a given procedure, the financial burden of that event was included in the model (costs and indirect costs associated with treatment of that complication). Cross-over to the other mode of therapy was considered a failure to maintain patency.

THE EAST CAROLINA HEART INSTITUTE EXPERIENCE

From July 2003 to July 2006, all patients who had undergone open or endovascular treatments of femoropopliteal arterial circulation were identified in a retrospective computerized

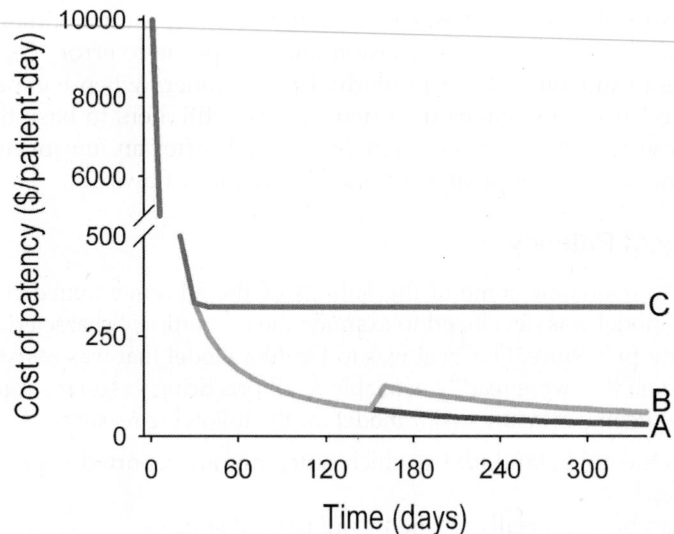

Figure 28-1. Hypothetical cost efficacy curves for the following revascularization scenarios: A – Successful initial revascularization without failure of patency or reintervention, B – Reintervention to maintain patency, C – Failure of patency without reintervention.

database. The decision to use open bypass or endovascular revascularization was based on clinical evaluation, anatomic factors, and the attending surgeon's preference.

For the purpose of this study, total costs (direct and indirect cost) for the particular encounter were used to calculate the amortized cost. Costs associated with adverse outcomes after a particular revascularization were also included for the total encounter cost calculation. Cost data were available for all patient encounters in this study. If the patient underwent a major amputation ipsilateral to the index revascularization, this was included in the cost analysis. Costs of postoperative rehabilitation, nursing home care, or lost days of work were not included in this analysis.

The primary efficacy endpoint of this study was cost per patient/day of patency 12 months following the index procedure. Primary and primary-assisted patency were the secondary endpoints in this study. Patency was determined by guidelines of the Society for Vascular Surgery.

Results

Over a 3-year period, a total of 381 femoropopliteal segments were treated in 359 patients. There were a total of 183 femoropopliteal segments treated with open revascularization and 198 treated with endovascular therapy. Both treatment groups were well matched, with no significant difference in clinical variables, including Rutherford category, age, gender, diabetes, hypertension, end-stage renal disease (ESRD) requiring dialysis, tobacco, run-off, and postoperative pharmacotherapy.

In the open group, 165 of 183 bypasses (90%) were above the knee grafts using a prosthetic conduit. Of the 198 endovascular cases, 75 (38%) were TransAtlantic Inter-Society Consensus (TASC) II classification C or D cases. Subintimal angioplasty was routinely utilized in the treatment of T ASC D cases. A luminal re-entry device was used in only 5 cases (7% of TASC C or D cases). Stents were used in 42 (21%) cases owing to a suboptimal result with standard angioplasty (>30% residual stenosis or flow-limiting dissection); and atherectomy (mechanical or laser) was used in a total of 26 (13%) cases.

Durability data demonstrated that primary-assisted patency (all indications) at 12 months was 77±0.03% for the open group and 65±0.04% for the endovascular group (P<.01). Primary assisted patency for patients with claudication at 12 months was 93±0.03% in the open group versus 80±0.04% in the endovascular group (P<.01). Primary assisted patency for patients with critical limb ischemia at 12 months was 66±0.05% in the open group and 54±0.05% in the endovascular group (P<.01).

Initial cost of open therapy was significantly higher in all subgroups. Using the model of amortized cost described above, the cost per day of patency was calculated at 1 year. A graphical representation of the cost model is shown in Figures 28–2 and 28–3. Despite the difference in initial cost, our model showed no statistically significant difference in amortized cost at 1 year between open and endovascular groups regardless of indication. For all indications, the amortized cost per day of patency at 12 months was $229±106 for claudicants and $185±124 for endovascular cases (P=.71). Claudicants treated by simple angioplasty showed the lowest cost per day of patency ($26±14), although this did not reach statistical significance when compared with open therapy.

The driving forces of this cost model are the initial procedural cost, the costs of all assistive procedures, and the durability of these procedures (Table 28–1). Failures, especially those that were not subjected to reintervention, are a very significant part of this construct. A high rate of failures and lack of reintervention is especially evident in both the open and the endovascular groups with critical limb ischemia. Failure without re-intervention resulted in a significantly higher amortized cost in the endovascular group ($551±184 (vs.) $34±4, P<.01) and a trend toward a higher cost in the open group ($418±154 (vs.) $157±122, P =.23).

Utilizing the model, subgroup analysis was undertaken to identify risk factors in which one therapy was more cost-effective. Patients with critical limb ischemia, end-stage renal disease requiring dialysis, renal insufficiency (creatinine >1.5 mg/dL), and

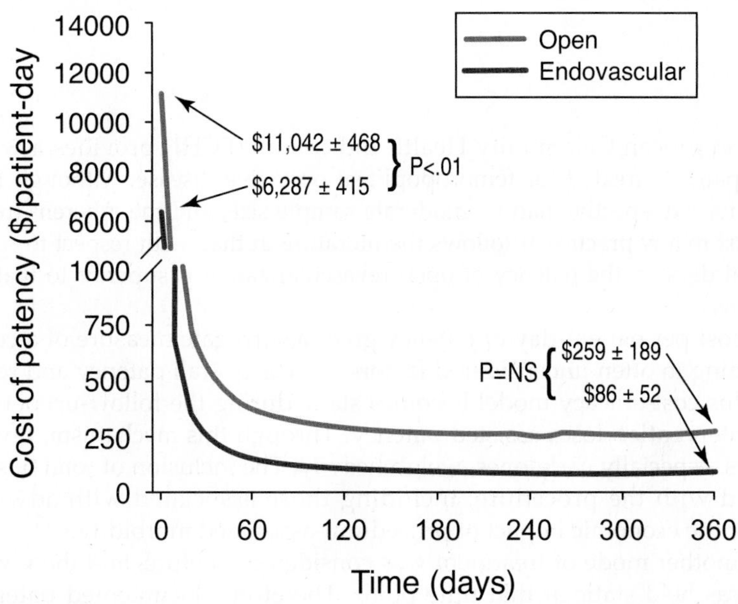

Figure 28-2. Cost efficacy curves in patients undergoing revascularization via both open and endovascular techniques for patients with claudication.

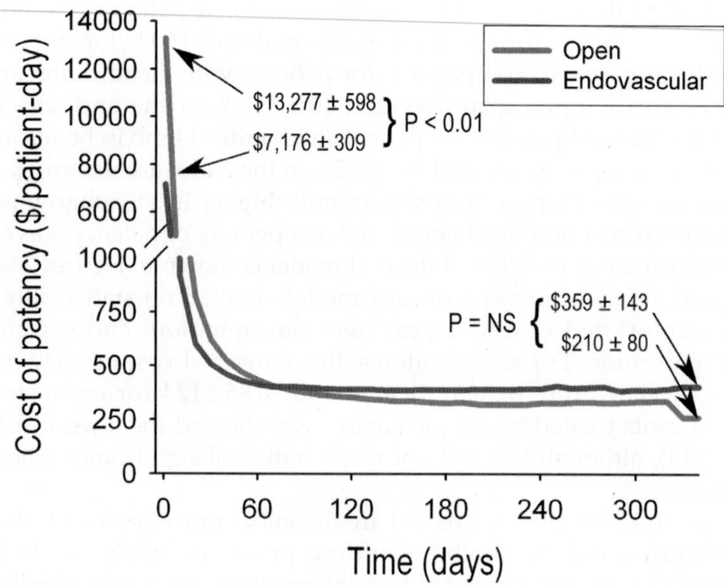

Figure 28-3. Cost efficacy curves in patients undergoing revascularization via both open and endovascular techniques for patients with critical limb ischemia.

congestive heart failure showed a trend toward open revascularization being more cost-effective; however, this did not reach statistical significance. Because early failures have a significant impact on this model, a multivariate analysis was undertaken to identify covariates associated with failure (Table 28–2). ESRD requiring dialysis was an independent risk factor for early failure in patients with critical limb ischemia for both open and endovascular therapy (OR= 3.48, P = .048). No other variable was a significant correlate of early failure.

DISCUSSION

Our experience at European Community Health Indicatiors (ECHI) provides a well-matched group of patients treated for femoropopliteal occlusive disease. Although this study is limited by its retrospective nature, moderate sample size, and the inherent treatment biases that exist in any practice, it follows the literature in that, with respect to complex femoropopliteal disease, the patency of open revascularization is superior to that of endovascular therapy.

Our model of cost per patient-day of patency gives a surrogate measure of a cost-benefit ratio by adding in often unconsidered factors such as overall patency and reintervention rates. This cost-efficacy model becomes static during the follow-up period once a particular intervention loses assisted patency. Through this mechanism, revascularization failures, especially early ones, weigh heavily. The inclusion of total hospital costs associated with the procedure, including those associated with adverse events, accounts for the economic impact of procedural-associated morbidity.

Cross-over to another mode of treatment was considered a failure, and the revascularization cost was held static at that time point. Therefore, documented patency and procedural durability become the main driving forces for economic success. The

TABLE 28-1. NUMBER OF ASSISTIVE PROCEDURES (PROC.), TOTAL COST OF ASSISTIVE PROCEDURES, AND NUMBER OF FAILED REVASCULARIZATIONS NOT UNDERGOING REINTERVENTION LISTED BY NUMBER OF MONTHS FROM INDEX PROCEDURE, STRATIFIED BY INDICATION (CLAUDICANT OR CLI) AND MODALITY (OPEN OR ENDOVASCULAR)

	Claudicants – Open (n=81)			Claudicants – Endovascular (n=112)			CLI – Open (n=102)			CLI – Endovascular (n=86)		
Time (months)	Proc. (n)	Cost (k$)	Failed (n)	Proc. (n)	Cost (k$)	Failed (n)	Proc. (n)	Cost (k$)	Failed (n)	Proc. (n)	Cost (k$)	Failed (n)
1	1	16.6	1	1	27.9	4	3	35.8	10	0	0	18
2	0	0	0	0	0	3	0	0	4	0	0	9
3	0	0	1	1	6.8	3	0	0	2	0	0	3
4	0	0	2	0	0	1	2	24.3	4	1	13.1	2
5	1	16.4	0	1	4.9	0	0	0	5	1	13.6	1
6	0	0	0	1	7.4	1	2	20.5	1	1	8.9	1
7	0	0	0	1	19.5	1	1	6.7	0	1	7.2	1
8	1	5.1	0	1	4.7	0	1	7.6	2	0	0	1
9	2	26.1	2	1	7.2	1	1	14.2	1	1	7.7	0
10	0	0	1	0	0	2	0	0	0	0	0	1
11	0	0	0	0	0	0	0	0	0	0	0	0
12	0	0	0	0	0	0	0	0	1	0	0	0

TABLE 28-2. MULTIVARIATE ANALYSIS FOR VARIABLES ASSOCIATED WITH EARLY FAILURE (<30 DAYS).

	Odds Ratio	95% Confidence Limits	P
Patient factors			
Age >80 years	1.738	0.411 – 7.359	.667
Diabetes	1.390	0.402 – 4.809	.453
Hypertension	0.455	0.058 – 3.553	.452
Hyperlipidemia	0.375	0.051 – 2.732	.332
ESRD	3.848	1.012 – 14.633	.040
CHF	2.842	0.861 – 9.380	.086
Pharmacology			
Statin	1.575	0.181 – 13.733	.681
Coumadin	1.261	0.275 – 5.771	.765
Anatomic			
Runoff <2 vessels	0.560	0.411 – 7.359	.355

ESRD = end stage renal disease, CHF = congestive heart failure.

societal definition of primary-assisted patency was utilized as our efficacy endpoint so that these data would be comparable with those of other contemporary series in the vascular surgery literature.

Interestingly, despite a nearly twofold difference in initial cost, the cost savings of endovascular therapy is not carried out over time. The loss of the cost benefit of endovascular therapy lies in its lower patency rates and need for subsequent reintervention. This is evident particularly in the critical limb ischemia cohort in whom, at 1 year, endovascular therapy is trending to become the more expensive modality. The 11% difference in patency at 1 year and the early failures of patency (<30 days) are the major influences on this high cost. This economic benefit to open revascularization in patients with critical limb ischemia has been described before for patients with complex arterial occlusive disease.[3]

Claudicants treated by endovascular therapy have a noticeable trend toward cost savings compared with open therapy, despite a 14% differential in patency at 1 year. In particular, those treated by simple angioplasty with no other adjunctive interventions showed the greatest savings. This difference is driven by the fact that there were fewer early failures in the endovascular group and the often high expense of reintervention in the open group. The improved cost-benefit ratio of angioplasty compared with bypass in the treatment of claudicants has been noted in a recent Markov decision model-based study.[4] Of course, exercise therapy is an integral component in the treatment of intermittent claudication and may possess a positive cost-efficacy profile.[5] Our current database is restricted to open and endovascular revascularizations, and therefore, we are unable to comment on the application of this cost model to exercise therapy.

Our model offers a unique method by which to assess cost in vascular disease. It is straightforward to use with the data readily available to every practitioner. It is easy to see that this amortized cost model can be tailored to investigate cost-effectiveness for interventions on other vascular beds (e.g., carotid artery, aneurysmal disease). Unfortunately, this model is not without limitations. Arguably, patency may not be the best outcome measure. The correlation between patency and freedom from symptoms and improved functional capacity is not always 100%. Brewster et al. clearly demonstrated this discrepancy.[6] In a study looking at patients with failed bypass grafts, 10% of claudicants and 21% of critical limb ischemia patients had improved symptoms despite having lost patency. Using patency as an outcome measure in this model may unnecessarily penalize interventions in certain circumstances.

While understanding the limitations of our model, we performed a subgroup analysis using limb salvage as the outcome measure. The 1-year limb salvage rates were 82% in the open group and 61% in the endovascular group (P=0.02). The amortized cost of limb salvage ($/day of limb salvage) was 127±36 in the open group versus 191±63 in the endovascular group (P=NS). The absence of statistical significance between the two groups is not surprising based on the patency data and the small sample size. Interestingly, the overall cost/day of limb salvage was lower than the cost/day of patency, reflecting that patients who lose patency but maintain limb salvage still had a successful outcome.

Other Analyses

Ultimately, it is likely that functional capacity is the most relevant outcome measure both preoperatively and postoperatively. Taylor et al. developed a novel definition of success for patients with critical limb ischemia that was defined as:[7]

- Patency up to the point of wound healing.
- Limb salvage for 1 year.
- Ambulation for 1 year.
- Survival for 6 months.

This definition nicely defines success as it relates to functional capacity of the patient. This in turn clearly demonstrates an overall benefit to the patient and society. It is easy to see how this measure of outcome could be substituted for patency in our model.

For many of the same reasons, reporting standards in claudicants should be based on improved functional capacity. There are mounting data that exercise programs have equivalent outcomes and lower costs than endovascular interventions at 1 year.[5] It is likely that interventions on claudicants will come under increasing scrutiny in the coming years. Reporting standards need to reflect the absence of lifestyle-limiting claudication, a minimum duration of patency, and the absence of lifestyle-limiting comorbidities.

It is important to note, whether using cost-per-day of patency or cost-per-day of limb salvage, that the costs are astronomical. It is likely that these costs are far beyond what would be deemed by society to be acceptable or sustainable. It is clear from this model that there must be a drive to improve patency. Efforts must be undertaken to improve technology, increase our knowledge of PAD and intimal hyperplasia, and refine patient selection criteria. Every effort should be made to reduce device costs. This can be aided by aggressive negotiations by hospitals, the government, and national vascular societies with device companies for lower costs. Some advocate that new devices should be limited to research centers until they have undergone the rigors of comparative effectiveness and are deemed acceptable. O'Brien-Irr forwarded a number of additional measures to reduce cost, including organizing vascular services within a hub, designating the radiology suite as the primary venue for endovascular interventions, and instituting selective stenting policies.[8]

FUTURE DIRECTIONS

With the looming health care crisis upon us, urgent action is needed. There is a strong need to adopt a standard cost model that looks at amortized costs and is universally understood and utilized. Information gleaned from databases can then be used to formulate strong guidelines that promote cost-effectiveness. As a society of vascular surgeons, we need to reassess reporting standards for interventions incorporating functional status and durability as outcome measures. As comparative effectiveness research gains momentum in this country, it is likely that reimbursement will be tied to procedural cost efficacy in some way. In this paradigm of health care, the most efficient and efficacious treatments will be sought. Our challenge will be to shape the system of vascular cost efficacy so that our patients and society both benefit. Ultimately, we must act to define our future lest it be defined for us.

REFERENCES

1. Contos B. Vascular Centers of Excellence - A Tactical Approach. Washington, D.C.: The Advisory Board Company; 2007.
2. Nowygrod R, Egorova N, Greco G, et al. Trends, complications, and mortality in peripheral vascular surgery. J Vasc Surg 2006;43:205–16.
3. Hunink MG, Wong JB, Donaldson MC, et al. Revascularization for femoropopliteal disease. A decision and cost-effectiveness analysis. JAMA 1995;274:165–71.
4. de Vries SO, Visser K, de Vries JA, et al. Intermittent claudication: cost-effectiveness of revascularization versus exercise therapy. Radiology 2002;222:25–36.
5. Spronk S, Bosch J, den Hoed P, et al. Cost-effectiveness of endovascular revascularization compared to supervised hospital-based exercise training in patients with intermittent claudication: a randomized controlled trial. J Vasc Surg 2008;48:1472–80.
6. Brewster DC, LaSalle AJ, Robinson JG, et al. Femoropopliteal graft failures. Clinical consequences and success of secondary reconstructions. Arch Surg 1983;118:1043–7.
7. Taylor SM, Cull DL, Kalbaugh CA, et al. Critical analysis of clinical success after surgical bypass for lower-extremity ischemic tissue loss using a standardized definition combining multiple parameters: a new paradigm of outcomes assessment. J Am Coll Surg 2007;204: 831–8.
8. O'Brien-Irr MS, Harris LM, Dosluoglu HH, et al. Lower extremity endovascular interventions: can we improve cost efficiency? J Vasc Surg 2008;47:982–7.

SECTION VII

Visceral Vessels

29

Role of Endarterectomy for Chronic Mesenteric Ischemia in the Endovascular Era

Matthew W. Mell, M.D. and William D. Turnipseed, M.D.

CMI (CMI), although uncommon, is an important diagnosis to consider in the patient with unexplained abdominal pain. CMI is the clinical manifestation of atherosclerotic occlusive disease in the mesenteric arterial circulation and frequently escapes detection because of vague complaints of intestinal dysfunction. The most severe symptoms, such as postprandial pain, weight loss, and food fear, favor the diagnosis of CMI, are almost universally associated with multivessel occlusive disease, and may herald an impending risk of acute intestinal ischemia. Diagnostic delays are common because most patients have had symptoms for more than 6 months before the diagnosis is established. Once the diagnosis of CMI is made, the goal of treatment is safe and effective revascularization that provides durable relief of symptoms, with minimal procedural risk of morbidity and mortality. Optimal treatment for patients with CMI remains controversial. Open surgical and endovascular treatment options have been well described in the published literature, but there are no level-one data or clear consensus to suggest superiority of any given treatment.

PRESENTING SYMPTOMS

Mesenteric ischemia associated with atherosclerotic occlusive disease may present with primarily chronic symptoms (CMI) or with acute-on-chronic symptoms (A-CMI). Early CMI symptoms can be confused with cholecystitis, inflammatory bowel disease, irritable bowel syndrome, or other gastrointestinal conditions. Hallmark symptoms include abdominal pain and weight loss. Characteristic pain is described as postprandial generalized abdominal aching or cramping lasting 1 to 3 hours before subsiding. Similar to ischemia in other vascular beds, the pain is reproducible with the repeated stimulation of subsequent meals.

Weight loss is present in nearly all patients, can be substantial, and is thought to be due to both decreased caloric intake and reduced nutrient absorption. Persistent postprandial pain may lead to fear of eating in 30 to 50% of patients who ameliorate symptoms by avoiding meals. Nausea and vomiting are occasionally present and may confound the diagnosis with other abdominal syndromes. Diarrhea may be present in up to 30% of patients and occurs because of intestinal malabsorption and subsequent increased osmotic load.

Patients with A-CMI are those with a history of CMI who present with signs and symptoms of AMI (abdominal pain out of proportion to examination, fever, leukocytosis, academia, and vascular collapse). Untreated A-CMI leads to intestinal infarction and death. It is important to differentiate A-CMI from AMI (AMI) because of different etiologies that may lead to the acute event. The sudden deterioration of A-CMI is associated with thrombotic occlusion of previously diseased mesenteric vessels as opposed to embolic occlusion of normal vessels in the patient with AMI. The operative strategy for revascularization should be based on intestinal viability and the etiology of the ischemic event.

DIAGNOSTIC MODALITIES

Confirmation of suspected CMI is established by vascular imaging, including duplex ultrasound, computed tomographic angiography (CTA), or magnetic resonance angiography (MRA). All have all been described for the diagnosis of CMI. Each modality has its benefits and disadvantages, and often the best diagnostic imaging is based on local availability and resources. Duplex ultrasound is noninvasive and does not expose the patient to the risks associated with invasive procedures or contrast agents; it can also identify elevated flow velocities or thrombosis associated with stenoses or occlusions of the mesenteric vessels. Image quality is dependent upon operator technique and skill and can be adversely affected by body habitus, intestinal gas, and peritonitis.

CTA provides high-resolution imaging of the aorta and mesenteric vessels, and new multislice scanners can obtain images with short breath-holds and rapid image acquisition times. Data can be reconstructed three-dimensionally, with good resolution of the more peripheral mesenteric vessels. CTA requires contrast volumes similar to those of standard angiography but avoids the need for direct arterial cannulation. CTA may be contraindicated for patients with poor renal function or contrast allergy. Additionally, CTA may overestimate disease severity in patients with heavily calcified aorta or mesenteric arteries, because intraluminal contrast and calcium have similar imaging characteristics.

MRA, like CTA, avoids the need for arterial catheterization and enjoys the same advantages of image quality as CTA. Unlike CTA, however, MRA with gadolinium-enhanced imaging can differentiate between vessel calcification and vessel occlusion. We have found this to be an important advantage of MRA for diagnosis and operative planning. As with CTA, contrast agents may be contraindicated in patients with chronic renal disease because of an increased risk of nodular sclerosing fibrosis.

We have found digital subtraction angiography (DSA), traditionally the gold standard for CMI, to be unnecessary for establishing the diagnosis in most patients. DSA is appropriate for patients with contraindications to noninvasive imaging and for those for whom the diagnosis of CMI cannot be confirmed because of poor-quality CTA or MRA visceral imaging. Angiography has assumed a greater role as a therapeutic modality with the emergence and development of percutaneous transluminal angioplasty and stent placement.

Certain information is essential to obtain when considering a treatment option such as visceral endarterectomy. The number of diseased arteries as well as disease extent within each artery must be clarified. When the pattern of disease involves the aorta as well as the origin and proximal few centimeters of the mesenteric vessels, transaortic endarterectomy may be considered. Short-segment stenosis or occlusion of the midvisceral arteries may favor angioplasty or stent placement, especially if the patient's comorbidity precludes open repair. The quality of the aorta and iliac arteries can be determined with MRA using nonreconstructed source images or with noncontrast CT. The supraceliac aorta should be free of calcification when considering aortic cross-clamp for antegrade bypass or endarterectomy. Additionally, any potential bypass inflow sites should be free of significant occlusive disease.

PATIENT SELECTION

Mesenteric endarterectomy for patients with CMI is appropriate in the absence of prohibitive comorbidity and when the anatomic disease pattern is amenable to endarterectomy. Cardiac evaluation is necessary to rule out active ischemic heart disease and confirm preserved cardiac function, thus allowing safe clamping of the supraceliac aorta. Pulmonary function tests should also be considered for active smokers and when considering a thoracoretroperitoneal approach for transaortic endarterectomy. Patients with expected intestinal infarction and those with significant reversible cardiac ischemia, severe cardiomyopathy, or severe obstructive airways disease should probably not be offered endarterectomy. Patients with CMI should have renal function studies, because impaired renal function from renal artery stenosis may benefit from renal endarterectomy in conjunction with mesenteric endarterectomy when considering the transaortic approach.

Anatomic contraindications to endarterectomy include excessive aortic disease and long-segment proximal occlusion of the mesenteric arteries. Severe calcification of the supraceliac aorta makes vascular control of the supraceliac aorta risky. CA (CA) disease that extends into the branch vessels is generally not amenable to endarterectomy. Occlusive disease in the SMA (SMA) is usually suitable for endarterectomy. Even if the disease extends 5 cm or more into the SMA, adequate exposure and endpoints can be obtained. The IMA (IMA) may be too diminutive for endarterectomy unless disease is isolated to its origin, in which case endarterectomy and Carrel patch reimplantation are feasible. Transaortic endarterectomy is our preferred treatment for CMI with concomitant occlusive disease in the visceral aortic segment if the more proximal aorta is disease-free.

OPERATIVE APPROACH

Transaortic Endarterectomy

Transaortic endarterectomy through a lateral exposure is performed using a thoracoretroperitoneal incision (Figure 29–1). The patient is placed in the right lateral decubitus position using a beanbag and axillary roll for support. The incision is made overlying the

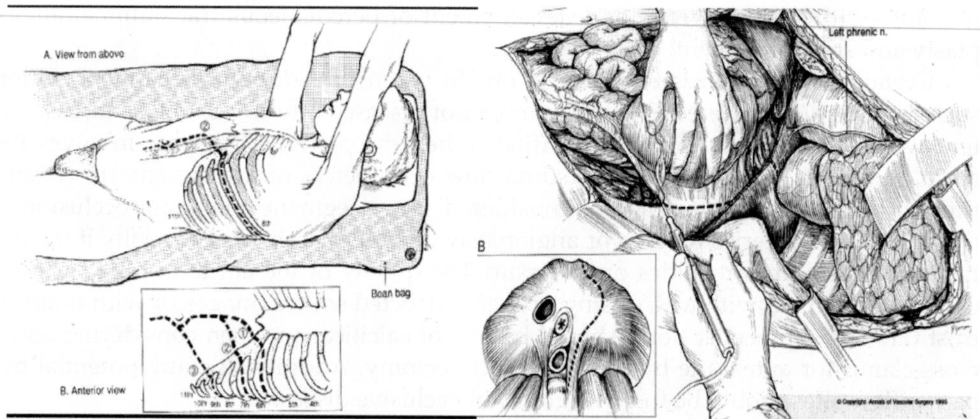

Figure 29-1. Thoracoretroperitoneal exposure of the visceral aorta. (Copyright Annals of Vascular Surgery 1995) (From Ann Vasc Surg 1995 Nov; 9:585-95.)

eighth or ninth intercostal space and carried through the muscular layers. The thoracic cavity is entered through the intercostal muscles, and the incision is carried through the costal margin. The diaphragm is divided in a circumferential manner to avoid injury to the phrenic nerve, and the median arcuate ligament is identified and divided. Proximal aortic control can easily be obtained, taking care to identify and avoid injury to the esophagus.

The retroperitoneal space can then be developed using blunt and sharp techniques. Early identification of the psoas fascia helps identify the proper tissue plane posterior to Gerota's fascia. Continued dissection allows for exposure of the left renal artery, which is an important landmark in further dissection of the visceral aorta. Exposure of the left renal artery can be helpful if renal endarterectomy is necessary. Once the origin of the left renal artery is identified and the median arcuate ligament has been divided, the visceral aorta and origins of the celiac axis and SMA can be isolated with sharp dissection. With the left kidney rotated anteriorly, the SMA can be exposed over a distance of approximately 5 cm. Additional exposure can be obtained by rotating the kidney posteriorly to expose the SMA as it courses behind the pancreas (Figure 29–2).

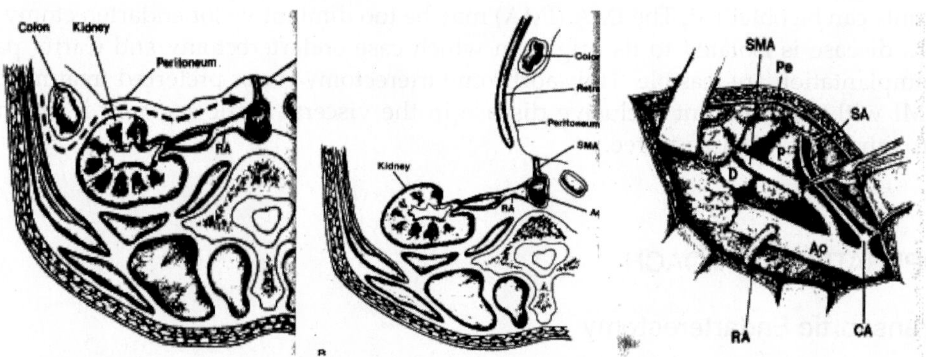

Figure 29-2. Posterior rotation of the left kidney aids exposure of the superior mesenteric artery. RA: left renal artery; Ao: aorta; CA: celiac axis; SMA: superior mesenteric artery; P: pancreas; D: duodenum; SA: splenic artery. (From J Saifi, J Cardiovasc Surg 1990 Sept; 31(5):629-33.)

The infrarenal aorta is dissected to achieve distal aortic control. If necessary, the IMA can also be identified and exposed if revascularization is indicated. With this operative method, the aorta can be exposed from the lower thorax to the common iliac arteries, allowing for potential treatment of all visceral arteries as well as the aorta.

Endarterectomy Technique

Once dissection is complete, intravenous heparin is administered, and if the renal circulation will be interrupted, the patient's core temperature is cooled to 34 degrees Centigrade. The aorta is cross-clamped and a lateral aortic incision is made corresponding to the extent of aorta to be treated. If the endarterectomy is to be confined to the SMA or celiac axis alone or in combination, the aortotomy is made in a curvilinear fashion, allowing for "trap-door" access to the aorta and origin of these vessels. The renal arteries if exposed are flushed with crystalloid cooled to 4 degrees Centigrade, and back-bleeding from visceral arteries is controlled from within using Fogarty balloons fitted with stopcocks.

Removal of atherosclerotic plaque is then begun by creating an endarterectomy plane on the aorta and performing an aortic endarterectomy. Postage stamp–sized cut-outs are made at the origins of each visceral vessel to be treated in order to achieve optimal control of the dissection. The aortic endarterectomy is completed, making sure of adequate proximal and distal transition zones and using tacking sutures when needed. Using each visceral cut-out as a handle, the endarterectomy plane is then advanced into the visceral artery. The plaque is removed taking care to create a tapered endpoint, because a distal intimal flap would most likely cause subsequent thrombosis of the artery. A tonsil clamp can be used to evaluate the patency of the artery after the endarterectomy, identifying and peeling away any loose material that remains.

Once the endarterectomy is complete, the operative site is flushed with saline to confirm adequate endpoints, and all loose debris is removed. The aortic incision is then closed primarily with 3-0 Prolene suture and flow is reestablished first to the celiac axis, then to the SMA, renal arteries, and finally the infrarenal circulation. The Fogarty balloons can be kept in place during the aortic closure. After the suture line is complete and the proximal aortic clamp has been removed, flow is established to the viscera by simply deflating the balloons and sliding them through the suture line. Any bleeding can be controlled with interrupted 4-0 Prolene sutures. Arterial flow to the lower extremities finally is returned. Intraoperative duplex ultrasound may be performed to confirm vessel patency.

Focal Visceral Endarterectomy

Some patterns of occlusive disease favor local endarterectomy with reimplantation of either the SMA or the IMA. This approach is feasible when the disease is localized to the origin of these visceral branches. Midline celiotomy is preferred for exposure. After placing appropriate self-retaining retractors, complete division of the ligament of Treitz will expose the SMA as it courses from underneath the pancreas. Dissection is carried distally to the normal artery, taking care to avoid dividing large branches to the small intestine. Dissection is continued proximally and the inferior pancreaticoduodenal arteries are isolated and ligated. This step will free the SMA from the surrounding tissue and allow it to be swung over and reimplanted without tension. The SMA is divided proximally and its stump oversewn. An inversion endarterectomy is then performed, establishing a typical feathered endpoint. The vessel can then be reimplanted into the infrarenal aorta, maintaining orientation of the SMA to avoid twisting or kinking.

The IMA can also be treated with local endarterectomy and reimplantation. Many times, this artery is diminutive and revascularization is unnecessary. Occasionally, the IMA is well developed with a robust collateral circulation to the intestinal bed via the marginal artery of Drummond and the arc of Riolan. Under these circumstances, revascularization of the IMA would be advisable. The IMA can be anatomically exposed with a standard anterior approach and dissected to the aorta. Important branches to the collateral mesenteric circulation are located near the origin of the IMA and therefore carefully identified and protected as the IMA is mobilized. The artery is divided, an endarterectomy is performed, and the IMA is reimplanted into the aorta. If the aorta is severely diseased, an aortic graft can be placed and the IMA reimplanted into the bypass as a Carrell patch.

POTENTIAL PITFALLS

Unfamiliarity with Visceral Aortic Exposure

As with all surgical procedures, a thorough knowledge of the thoracoabdominal operative approach to the visceral aorta will minimize unexpected events and allow for a safe and complete revascularization. Although some may have reservations about the rationale of this approach when other open surgical options exist, our experience has shown that with appropriate patient selection, surgical endarterectomy provides a durable repair with equivalent operative morbidity and mortality. Our comfort with the operative exposure, endarterectomy technique, and perioperative management of these patients is partly an extension of our extensive experience with open thoracoabdominal aortic aneurysm repair. Exposure and control of the visceral aorta and its branches are required for Crawford type-2, type-3, and type-4 aneurysms, and occlusive disease requiring operative treatment is found in up to 20% of these patients. Obtaining advice and assistance from a surgeon experienced with this operative approach will provide valuable support for those unfamiliar or uncomfortable with this exposure.

Injury During Endarterectomy

Identifying the appropriate endarterectomy plane is usually straightforward in the aorta and SMA but can be challenging in the CA. This artery tends to be more thin-walled, and extraction of the plaque in a too-deep plane may create an injury to the arterial wall. Limited injuries can be repaired with interrupted Prolene sutures supported with felt pledgets, but larger injuries or those with severely attenuated vessel walls may not be successfully repaired with this technique. When there are such concerns over the integrity of the CA, it should be transected and dissected to more healthy tissue, oversewing the celiac stump with pledgeted 3-0 Prolene suture placed into healthy aorta. A bypass using 8-mm or 10-mm synthetic graft can then be performed from the aorta to the transected CA, sewn in an end-to-end fashion.

Inadequate Distal Endarterectomy Endpoint

At times, plaque extends more than 5 cm into the SMA, and obtaining an adequate distal endpoint with a thoracoabdominal approach can be challenging. If there is any question of the adequacy of endarterectomy of the SMA, the artery should be exposed in its intraperitoneal portion by incising the peritoneum and dividing the ligament of Treitz. This maneuver will expose the SMA as it emerges from underneath the pancreas, usually at a place distal to the diseased segment. Inspection by palpation or with duplex ultrasound can evaluate the repair. If an incomplete endarterectomy or intimal flap is identified, an arteriotomy should be performed at this location to gain exposure of the endpoint. A sizable SMA can be transected to complete the endarterectomy; reapproximation with interrupted sutures will tack down the intima distal to the endarterectomy. Problematic endpoints in smaller vessels should be exposed with a lateral arteriotomy and subsequent patch angioplasty closure to prevent narrowing.

OUTCOMES AFTER REVASCULARIZATION

Open surgical repair has remained the standard of therapy for CMI. Because of its uncommon and varied presentation, no consensus exists with regard to the optimal surgical approach. Discussion has centered on the type of repair (endarterectomy vs. bypass), the number of arteries revascularized, the directionality of bypass (antegrade vs. retrograde), and the type of conduit (synthetic vs. autologous). All approaches have shown good overall perioperative outcomes, with mortality of 2 to 11%, symptom improvement in 90 to 100%, and complication rates of 33 to 66%.[1-5] In these studies, long-term graft patency was 63 to 90% and symptomatic recurrence occurred in 9 to 41% of patients, depending on the length of follow-up. The type of bypass did not impact survival, symptom-free survival, or graft patency.

We recently reported[6] our institutional experience with open surgical repair for CMI. Of a cohort of 80 patients, multivessel disease was present in 72. Revascularization was achieved by endarterectomy in 37 patients (34 transaortic endarterectomy, 3 local endarterectomy), visceral artery bypass in 29 patients, and combined procedures in 14 (Table 29–1). Peri-operative inpatient mortality was 3.8%. Mean follow-up was 46 months (range 1 to 206 months), and clinical follow-up was available for all patients. Estimated overall survival was 92.2%, 72.0%, and 64.5% at 1, 3, and 5 years. A total of 11 (13.8%) patients developed recurrent symptoms, 8 (28%) after surgical bypass, 3(8%) after endarterectomy, and 1 (7%) after a combined procedure. Endarectomy was independently associated with increased symptom-free survival compared with open bypass.

TABLE 29-1. TYPES OF VASCULAR REPAIR

	Repair Type		
Vessel Treated	**Endarterectomy**	**Bypass**	**Combined**
CA, SMA, IMA	4	0	3
CA, SMA	22	13	7
CA, IMA	0	0	1
SMA, IMA	0	0	3
CA only	0	5	0
SMA only	11	11	0
IMA only	0	0	0

CA: CA, SMA: superior mesenteric artery, IMA inferior mesenteric artery.

TABLE 29-2. OUTCOMES AFTER OPEN SURGICAL REVASCULARIZATION FOR CMI

	Pts (n)	# of Vessels Treated	Endarterectomy	Complications	Operative Mortality	Follow-up (months)	Symptom Recurrence
Mell 2009*[6]	80	134	46%	29%	4%	46	14%
Atkins, 2007[1]	49	88	37%	35%	2%	42	35%
English, 2004*[2]	58	80	9%	62%	29%	42	6%
Cho, 2002[3]	25	41	41%	60%	11%	60	41%
Mateo, 1999[4]	85	130	22%	33%	8%	36	24%
McAfee, 1992[5]	58	119	8%	36%	10%	40	12%
Rapp, 1986[9]	67	111	70%	21%	8%	50	8%

* Includes patients with acute-on-chronic symptoms.

The first reported repair for CMI by Shaw and Maynard in 1958[7] utilized local endarterectomy of the SMA. The feasibility of transaortic endarterectomy with a thoracoabdominal approach was demonstrated by Stoney et al. in 1977,[8] but the use of endarterectomy has declined in the past 2 decades (Table 29–2), with most studies focusing on outcomes after surgical bypass. A study by Rapp and associates[9] reported a 7% recurrence of symptoms in a cohort of 67 CMI patients who received endarterectomy (n=47) or antegrade bypass (n=20) with a mean follow-up of 4.4 years. No comparison was made between the two groups. Cho et al.[3] noted a gradual decline in the use of endarterectomy in favor of bypass. Contrary to our findings, this study did not demonstrate that type of revascularization predicted late survival, graft patency, or freedom from symptom recurrence. Failure to show any difference related to these factors is likely because this and other small series with good outcomes were underpowered to detect differences in treatment approaches.

Some studies have shown higher morbidity and mortality when mesenteric revascularization was combined with aortic reconstruction.[4,10] A recent report by Atkins et al. demonstrated no increased morbidity or mortality for combined procedures.[1] In our series, reconstruction for aortic occlusive disease was associated with increased morbidity but did not translate into increased perioperative mortality or inferior long-term outcomes. We therefore continue to offer combined procedures when clinically warranted.

Patients presenting with acute symptoms superimposed on CMI were associated with a higher morbidity, a higher incidence of reintervention, and a trend toward decreased long-term survival. Progression of mesenteric stenosis to occlusion has been estimated to account for 20 to 50% of AMI.[11-12] English et al.[2] demonstrated significantly higher peri-operative mortality for patients who presented with acute-on-chronic symptoms. Multivariate analysis identified intestinal gangrene and age as independent predictors of early death.

Increased morbidity in some subsets of patients with CMI paired with recent advances in endovascular technology has focused much of the recent attention on the potential role of percutaneous approaches to treatment. No prospective randomized trials have been reported. Many studies have demonstrated high technical success with low procedural morbidity.[3,13] Kasirajan and associates[14] compared 28 patients undergoing percutaneous angioplasty and stent (percutaneous transluminal angioplasty [PTA]/stent) to 85 historical controls. Morbidity and recurrent stenosis were not different, but patients undergoing percutaneous treatment had a higher incidence of symptom recurrence, prompting recommendation of operative revascularization for those medically fit. Atkins[1] reported no improved morbidity and mortality when comparing percutaneous with open repair. PTA/stent was associated with lower primary and clinical patency compared with open repair. Symptoms recurred in 20% of patients in both groups but sooner after PTA/stent repair. Although operative repair offers superior results for open surgical candidates, it was acknowledged that patient preference and more rapid recovery have driven practices to offering PTA/stent as initial treatment to patients with suitable anatomy provided it does not preclude later operative repair.

Brown et al.[15] noted over a mean follow-up of 13 months that their stent cohort was 7 times more likely to develop restenosis, 4 times more likely to develop recurrent symptoms, and 15 times more likely to require reintervention. They concluded that percutaneous revascularization may be best reserved for patients with severe nutritional depletion or other morbidity resulting in preclusive surgical risk and may serve as a temporizing bridge to definitive operative repair. Nearly two thirds of our patient cohort was alive at 5 years, suggesting that prolonged survival can be expected in a significant percentage of patients with CMI and therefore indicating that durable revascularization is a relevant and desirable goal.

SUMMARY

Open mesenteric revascularization can be performed with effective and durable symptom relief, low mortality, acceptable morbidity, and results in excellent long-term survival. Although endovascular treatment options have gained popularity, equivalent long-term durability has not been equivalent without close follow-up and more frequent reintervention. We therefore continue to believe that open repair should remain the standard for treatment of CMI for those patients without significant comorbid conditions or limited life expectancy. Of the surgical options, we continue to advocate the use of endarterectomy when indicated. Endarterectomy may provide the most durable repair with respect to graft patency and long-term symptom relief, and it can be performed without the use of prosthetic material. With proper experience, it can be performed without increased morbidity while achieving excellent long-term outcomes.

REFERENCES

1. Atkins MD, Kwolek CJ, LaMuraglia GM, et al. Surgical revascularization versus endovascular therapy for CMI: a comparative experience. J Vasc Surg 2007;45:1162–71.
2. English WP, Pearce JD, Craven TE, et al. Chronic visceral ischemia: symptom-free survival after open surgical repair. Vasc Endovsc Surg 2004;38:493–503.
3. Cho JS, Carr JA, Jacobsen G, et al. Long-term outcome after mesenteric artery reconstruction: a 37-year experience. J Vasc Surg 2002;35:453–60.
4. Mateo RB, O'Hara PJ, Hertzer NR, et al. Elective surgical treatment of symptomatic chronic mesenteric occlusive disease: early results and late outcomes. J Vasc Surg 1999;29:821–32.
5. McAfee MK, Cherry KJ, Naessens JM, et al. Influence of complete revascularization on CMI. Am J Surg 1992;164:220–4.

6. Mell MW, Acher CW, Hoch JR, et al. Outcomes after endarterectomy for CMI. J Vasc Surg 2008;48:1132–8.
7. Shaw RS, Maynard EP. Acute and chronic thrombosis of the mesenteric arteries associated with malabsorption: a report of two cases successfully treated by thromboendarterectomy. N Engl J Med 1958;258:974.
8. Stoney RJ, Ehrenfeld WK, Wylie EJ. Revascularization methods in chronic visceral ischemia caused by atherosclerosis. Ann Surg 1977;186:468–76.
9. Rapp JH, Reilly LM, Qvarfordt PG, et al. Durability of endarterectomy and antegrade grafts in the treatment of chronic visceral ischemia. J Vasc Surg 1986;3:799–806.
10. Foley MI, Moneta GL, Abou-Zamzam AM, et al. Revascularization of the SMA alone for treatment of intestinal ischemia. J Vasc Surg 2000;32:37–47.
11. Kwaan JHM, Connolly JE, Coutosoftides T. Concomitant revascularization of intestines during aortic-iliac reconstruction: deterrent to catastrophic bowel infarction. Can J Surg 1980;23:534–6.
12. Stoney RJ, Cunningham CG. AMI. Surgery 1993;114:489–90.
13. Matsumoto AH, Angle JF, Spinasa DJ, et al. Percutaneous transluminal angioplasty and stenting in the treatment of CMI: results and longterm followup. J Am Coll Surg 2002;194: S22–31.
14. Kasirajan K, O'Hara PJ, Gray BH, et al. CMI: open surgery versus percutaneous angioplasty and stenting. J Vasc Surg 201;33:63–71.
15. Brown DJ, Schermerhorn ML, Powell RJ, et al. Mesenteric stenting for CMI. J Vasc Surg 2005;42:268–74.

30

Spontaneous Isolated Superior Mesenteric Artery Dissection

William F. Oppat, M.D., Tamer N. Boules, M.D., and Gokulakkrishna Subhas, M.D.

BACKGROUND

Although isolated spontaneous SMA dissections are the most common type of mesenteric arterial dissection, true isolated SMA dissections are rare causes of abdominal pathology. More commonly, dissections involving the SMA result from an extension of an aortic dissection. Only 106 cases of isolated spontaneous SMA dissection without associated aortic dissection have been identified and reported in the literature.[1]

INTRODUCTION

The management of patients with abdominal pain remains a major clinical responsibility for the general surgeon. Its varied presentation and multitude of etiologies make abdominal pain one of the more difficult clinical problems that both general and vascular surgeons are asked to evaluate. Most causes of acute pain are realized after a thorough history and careful physical examination and are confirmed by laboratory testing and simple x-rays. Common clinical problems such as bowel obstructions and perforations do not require complex diagnostic imaging modalities. Elderly patients often harbor a myriad of complex medical issues that may cloud classic presentations. Furthermore, securing the etiology of abdominal pain in the elderly can be crucial for intervention and successful overall outcomes. The trend to utilize more complex imaging modalities in an attempt to rapidly diagnose the etiology of abdominal pain and precisely intervene in the care of complicated patients can be an effective strategy[2]; however, the imaging studies may also complicate a patient's care.

Many emergency rooms now have CT scanners that are dedicated for their use in the management of traumatically injured patients. In our facility, the relationship of the CT scanner to the emergency room has left the scanner even more readily available to nontrauma patients. When used appropriately, the high-resolution scanners represent an important tool of the surgeon. At times, it seems that a presumptive diagnosis based on careful history and physical examination has been supplanted by the use of such complex imaging modalities, underscoring the need for continued emphasis on the subtleties of clinical examination in resident education.

When evaluating acute mesenteric vascular pathologies, simple imaging modalities generally fail to solidify the diagnosis. Conversely, complex imaging studies, such as high-resolution CT, may reveal patterns of vascular disease that may be irrelevant to the acute clinical problem. For example, incidentally discovered abdominal aortic aneurysms identified during evaluation for diverticulitis may result in a life-preserving benefit; however, chronic occlusive disease identified at the origin of the mesenteric vessels may have no relationship to the onset of acute abdominal pain.

CLINICAL PRESENTATION

Traditionally, acute mesenteric ischemia is the result of either acute embolization or thrombosis of the celiac axis, SMA, or inferior mesenteric artery (IMA). SMA embolization is the most common presentation. Patients typically have cardiac rhythm disturbances, with midabdominal pain out of proportion to the physical examination and evidence of embolization in other vascular beds. Acute thrombosis of the SMA also manifests with midabdominal pain out of proportion to physical examination findings, but these patients tend to have typical stigmata of peripheral vascular occlusive disease in other vascular territories. SMA embolization typically occurs at the origin of the middle colic artery where a noticeable luminal caliber change occurs, sparing perfusion to the proximal small bowel through the more proximal jejunal arterial branches. Conversely, in situ thrombosis of the SMA generally occurs proximally, at its origin, and compromises blood flow to the entire small bowel and proximal colon.

In contrast, acute occlusion of the SMA secondary to dissection is most commonly the result of extension of an aortic dissection. Our group and others have identified a subset of patients with acute mesenteric ischemia who present with focal dissection of the SMA, unrelated to an adjacent aortic process. These dissections were identified with CT angiography (CTA), an immediately available modality at our institution instrumental in expediting treatment. In many cases, treatment involves anticoagulation and observation, with exploration, bowel resection, and arterial reconstruction reserved for patients with evidence of bowel infarction or peritonitis.

CASE PRESENTATION

Our clinical experience began with a middle-aged female who presented with advanced symptoms of abdominal pain. The diagnosis of isolated SMA dissection was obtained by CTA. The general surgical service had assessed the perfusion of the small bowel and colon with laparoscopic exploration and felt that no frank small bowel or colonic ischemia or infarction existed. Given the conflicting reports of management strategies in isolated mesenteric dissection, a nonoperative approach was chosen because the patient's clinical condition had stabilized.

Utilizing systemic anticoagulation as a therapy analogous to the treatment of an acute carotid artery dissection, her clinical condition dramatically improved over the next few days. Ultimately, the patient was discharged home on warfarin after reaching a target INR of 2 to 3.

Six weeks following her discharge, the patient returned with recurrent abdominal pain. Initially suspecting failure of anticoagulation, the patient was taken urgently to the angiography suite where selective mesenteric angiography was performed. To our surprise, the previously identified SMA dissection was no longer apparent, and the patient's symptoms were deemed the result of acute diverticulitis. Our service has subsequently treated others with our proposed algorithm.

DISCUSSION

The postmortem incidence of SMA dissection in a series of 6666 autopsies was 0.06%.[3] A review of the literature has revealed an increasing number of case reports[4] and small series. The first case of SMA dissection was reported by Bauersfeld[5] in 1947 at autopsy of a patient who had multiple aneurysms. From this first report until 1972, 11 more case reports identified an SMA dissection at autopsy. There were 23 cases reported between 1975 and 1999, and 71 cases have been reported since 2000. Only one death from an SMA dissection has been reported since 1972.[6]

The true incidence of isolated SMA dissection is likely underestimated because of its nonspecific presentation and laboratory findings. It is also possible that patients with SMA dissection experience a self-limited course. Physicians who assess a patient with abdominal pain should be aware of mesenteric ischemia as a potentially unusual etiology and must recognize an SMA dissection to effectively manage this rare condition. More cases are being identified as a result of increasing use of contrast-enhanced CT scans for investigating abdominal pain.

The natural course of SMA dissection would predictably include the following:[7]

1. Limited progress with cessation.
2. Progressive involvement of the vessel.
3. Reestablishment of flow into the true lumen.
4. Rupture through the true lumen.

CAUSES

The causes of spontaneous isolated SMA dissection remain elusive. The majority of patients have a history of hypertension and are smokers. Patients who were not known to have hypertension presented with a markedly elevated blood pressure higher than 160/100 mm Hg.[8] Cystic medial necrosis, segmental arterial mediolysis, vasculitis, congenital connective tissue disorders, fibromuscular dysplasia, arteriosclerosis, and trauma have been described as potential causes of an SMA dissection.[9] Histologic findings of pathologic specimens included fragmentation of elastic fibers, loss of smooth muscle tissue, fibromyxoid infiltration, areas of cystic degeneration, and atheromatous changes in the arterial wall.[10] The presumed cause of arterial dissection is a direct tear in the intima with penetration of the luminal contents into the layers of the vessel wall. Alternatively, a primary hemorrhage in the media, due to rupture of the vasa vasorum, could lead to blood between the medial and the adventitial layers of the vessel wall or in the medial laminae, which extend over a variable distance.[11-12] Iatrogenic causes of SMA dissection have been described following translumbar aortography,[13] following the use of a balloon occlusion catheter,[14] and following mesenteric angioplasty in the treatment of chronic mesenteric ischemia.[15]

SYMPTOMS

Patients with focal SMA dissection most commonly present with sudden onset of severe epigastric pain (observed in 77/84 patients). These patients presented acutely with duration of symptoms of generally less than 4 weeks. Variations in the pain syndromes included periumbilical pain, isolated back pain, diffuse abdominal pain, and epigastric pain radiating to the back. Certainly, the acute pain is related to the dissection of the SMA, acute bowel ischemia, or both.[16] Other presenting symptoms have included nausea, vomiting, melena, and abdominal distention. At least two described patients have presented with systemic hypoperfusion; the shock was ultimately attributed to a ruptured SMA dissecting aneurysm that led to the patient's demise.[17] The American Gastroenterological Association's (AGA) technical review on intestinal ischemia[18] suggests that a diagnostic work-up for acute mesenteric ischemia should be considered in every patient with a history of more than 2 to 3 hours of otherwise unexplained abdominal pain.

SIGNS

Abdominal examination in the acute setting reveals epigastric tenderness in a minority of patients. Most have complaints that outweigh their clinical examination. Patients who present with diffuse tenderness may suggest a more compromised blood supply to the gastrointestinal tract or a greater proportion of ischemic bowel. As distinct from acute mesenteric ischemia secondary to acute embolic or thrombotic causes, signs of peritonitis are much less common. Abdominal bruits are auscultated in a minority of patients.

Patients who present with frank bowel ischemia have an overall poor prognosis. Causes of bowel ischemia and necrosis are believed secondary to the narrowing of the true lumen by a rapidly expanding false lumen, causing a pressure effect, thrombotic occlusion, or distal embolization.[19-20]

INVESTIGATIONS

Ultrasound

Ultrasound, as an inexpensive and noninvasive technique, is an excellent choice for the investigation of abdominal pain, especially in the upper abdomen. The protocol used by the radiologists at our institution includes the assessment of the portal vein (for thrombosis) and the SMA (for flow). The diagnosis of an SMA dissection based on ultrasound requires the identification of an intimal flap and can be technically challenging. Thrombus within the false lumen may hinder the demonstration of an intimal flap. Also, dilation of the

SMA with an echolucent shadow in the wall may suggest the accumulation of mural thrombus. Ultrasound has limitations in obesity and patients who have air-filled and dilated bowel loops.

Contrast-Enhanced CT Scan

In developed countries, an increasing trend to use CT scanning for patients with undiagnosed abdominal pain is clearly documented. However, a noncontrast CT of the abdomen will likely miss an SMA dissection.[21] The diagnosis of an SMA dissection made by CT generally requires intravenous administration of contrast material. Contrast-enhanced CT has a better chance of assessing the origin of the mesenteric vessels, estimating dissection length, and assessing bowel perfusion. Enhanced CT scanning also helps eliminate competing etiologies of abdominal pain. Significant contrast-enhanced CT scan findings consistent with an SMA dissection include the presence of mural thrombosis, intramural hematoma, intimal flaps, enlarged SMA diameter, and an increased attenuation of fat surrounding the SMA.[22] The CT scan of a ruptured SMA dissecting aneurysm may demonstrate a hematoma in the mesentery and hemorrhagic ascites.[23] Signs of acute bowel ischemia or bowel infarction visualized by contrast enhanced CT include lack of bowel wall enhancement, mesenteric edema, and mesenteric or portal venous air.

Sakamoto et al. [24] classified SMA dissection based on contrast-enhanced CT scanning into four classes:

1. Type I: Patent false lumen with both entry and reentry.
2. Type II: Patent false lumen with entry but no reentry (cul-de-sac).
3. Type III: Thrombosed false lumen with ulcer-like projections from the true lumen.
4. Type IV: Thrombosed false lumen without ulcer-like projections.

Based upon this classification, it was felt that the Type II dissections were most likely to progress to complete SMA thrombosis and acute bowel ischemia.

CT Angiography

The CT angiogram is thought to be as accurate as conventional arteriography in the evaluation of the extent and location of a mesenteric dissection. When compared with standard angiography, many believe that the patient can avoid prolonged radiation exposure and use of high volumes of iodinated contrast medium. Unlike conventional angiography, CTA is not limited to the imaging of the intraluminal borders; it can also assess the vessels in cross-section. In our institution, it can be performed more expeditiously and without lengthy preparation or the presence of specialized and dedicated staff. Because digital subtraction angiography (DSA) is an invasive procedure, it should be utilized in patients with worsening symptoms who will likely require surgical or endovascular treatment.

Digital Subtraction Angiography

Interventionalists who favor the use of DSA argue that it has the advantage of offering therapeutic intervention in addition to solidifying a diagnosis. As experience with the deployment mesenteric stents and the infusion of thrombolytics has increased, these procedures can be accomplished with little additional contrast. Additionally, the resolution obtained with DSA allows clearer assessment of the distal anatomy of the SMA in the event that an arterial reconstruction is necessary

Other Diagnostic Modalities

Intraoperative diagnosis at the time of laparotomy was made in two patients reported in the literature.[25] Acute mesenteric ischemia resulting from embolic occlusion of the SMA at the origin of the middle colic artery results in sparing of the proximal 15 to 20 cm of jejunum due to retained perfusion of more proximal jejunal branches. Typically, SMA origin dissection that is causing significant mesenteric ischemia will involve the initial part of the jejunum. Use of intravascular ultrasound has also been described for diagnosis of SMA dissection.[26] It may be useful in demonstrating the exact condition of the vessel in the dissection region and in selecting the therapeutic strategy.

SITE AND EXTENT OF DISSECTION

Dissections of the SMA are believed to begin within 2.5 cm of its origin at the abdominal aorta in the majority of afflicted patients. Typically, the dissection extends approximately 6 cm in many of the patients. Within 2.5 cm of the origin, the SMA exits from within the pancreas at the base of the mesentery. Some authors believe that this portion of the vessel may be susceptible to acute or chronic sheer stresses, analogous to the thoracic aorta at the ligamentum arteriosum.[27-28]

MANAGEMENT STRATEGIES

Nonoperative (Conservative) Management

Our limited experience[1] and the experience of other institutions[24,29] suggest that most patients with an isolated SMA dissection and no clinical or imaging signs indicating rupture of the SMA or evidence of bowel ischemia should initially be managed conservatively. A trial of systemic anticoagulation therapy is warranted in all patients with uncomplicated, asymptomatic SMA dissection.[30-31] Conservative treatment is continued in cases in which the SMA has a good residual blood supply, if the symptoms are stable, and the true lumen compression by the false lumen does not progress. If the conservative approach fails, clinically acceptable results are still obtained when operative therapy is required.[32]

Conservative management is also effective in cases of SMA dissection even if the false lumen is completely occluded by thrombus, such as described by Sakamoto (type IV dissection).[24] Conservative treatment includes initial bowel rest, heparin infusion, antihypertensives, and vitamin K antagonists when the diet is resumed. It appears that the rationale for the initiation of systemic anticoagulation correlates with spontaneous dissections of the internal carotid artery: to prevent vessel thrombosis and limit distal embolization. However, in some reported cases, systemic anticoagulation utilized for SMA dissection does not necessarily halt the progression of the dissection or prevent aneurysmal degeneration.[32] Conservative treatment with anticoagulation has been successful even with high-grade stenosis of the main trunk of the SMA. Although some controversy exists, recommended treatment would include the administration of an intravenous heparin infusion while fasting or until the abdominal pain resolves. The patient should be transitioned to an oral anticoagulant and antiplatelet agents until imaging studies demonstrate vessel recanalization or satisfactory flow within the vessel lumen.[33]

Revascularization

Revascularization of the SMA, utilizing either an open surgical or an endovascular approach, should be considered in patients who manifest the following:

1. Signs and symptoms of intestinal ischemia or infarction.
2. Progression of dissection and expansion of aneurysm diameter.
3. Narrowing or thrombosis of the true lumen of the SMA.
4. Saccular aneurysm formation of the SMA that is likely to rupture or embolize.[34]

Surgical Treatment

The absolute indications for emergency surgical intervention are bowel infarction and arterial rupture. The first reported surgical exploration and successful reconstruction with autologus greater saphenous vein was described by Sisteron and Vieville[34] in 1975. Creative procedures for surgical revascularization of the dissected SMA have been described. Direct transposition of the SMA to the infrarenal aorta, when possible, may eliminate long-term graft-related complications. When an SMA dissection extends distally into the artery, the procedure of choice must preserve patent collateral vessel branches. Resection of the intimal flap with patch angioplasty to reconstruct the SMA has been described. Whenever possible, the undiseased proximal portion of the SMA serves as a good source of arterial inflow and has, as its advantage, the ability to avoid graft redundancy and graft kinking. Conduits of all types have been utilized; however, autologous conduits such as the greater saphenous vein, the radial artery, and the superficial femoral artery are commonly chosen. Clever reconstructions using right gastroepiploic artery have permitted the resection of a diseased SMA and ligation of SMA aneurysms proximally. The use of arterial conduits over saphenous vein or polytetrafluoroethylene (PTFE) and other prosthetic grafts was advocated because of a higher tolerance to physiologic bending and longer periods of patency as demonstrated in cardiac surgery. Additionally, prosthetic grafts have a higher propensity for infection, especially in a compromised operative field that may contain ischemic bowel.

Endovascular Treatment

Endovascular treatment can be tailored to the pathology encountered within the SMA. Various techniques have been reported, including balloon angioplasty, stent placement, intralesion thrombolytic therapy, and embolization. In selected cases, the placement of an endovascular stent can provide immediate relief of bowel ischemia and prevent further progression of the dissection. The avoidance of open surgical repair would be expected to translate into quicker recovery and shorter hospital stays, with decreased morbidity and mortality.

In most cases, self-expandable and balloon-expandable stents with diameters extending to 10 mm and overall lengths of up to 10 cm have been utilized. Currently, the choice of stent appears dependent upon operator preference and stent availability. Theoretically, in cases of advanced bowel ischemia, combining successful arterial stenting with open bowel resection would reduce the magnitude of surgery. Unstable patients may avoid lengthy arterial revascularization in a potentially hostile and possibly contaminated peritoneal cavity.

CONCLUSION

Owing to increasing use of CT scans in investigating abdominal pathology and the improvement in its resolution capabilities, the diagnosis of acute SMA dissection is occurring more frequently. The algorithm that includes systemic anticoagulation in the absence of advanced bowel ischemia and considers endovascular techniques before open surgical reconstruction may provide patients with acceptable outcomes and limit morbidity. Lack of long-term follow-up and limited numbers of patients with SMA dissection leave some uncertainty as to the ultimate benefit of various treatment algorithms for this condition.

REFERENCES

1. Subhas G, Gupta A, Nawalany M, Oppat WF. Spontaneous isolated superior mesenteric artery dissection: a case report and literature review with management algorithm. Ann Vasc Surg 2009;23:788–98.
2. Okada M, Ishiguchi T, Itoh H. Management of spontaneous dissection of the superior mesenteric artery. Intern Med 2004;43:451–2.
3. Foord AG, Lewis RD. Primary dissecting aneurysms of peripheral and pulmonary arteries. Arch Pathol 1959;68:553–77.
4. Casella I, Bosch M, Sousa W Jr. Isolated spontaneous dissection of the superior mesenteric artery by percutaneous stent placement: case report. J Vasc Surg 2008;47:197–200.
5. Baursfield RS. Dissecting aneurysm of the aorta: a presentation of fifteen cases and a review of the recent literature. Ann Intern Med 1947;26:873–89.
6. Sartelet H, Fedaoui-Delalou D, Capovilla M, et al. Fatal hemorrhage due to an isolated dissection of the superior mesenteric artery. Intensive Care Med 2003;29:505–6.
7. Yasuhara H, Shigematsu H, Muto T. Self-limited spontaneous dissection of the main trunk of the superior mesenteric artery. J Vasc Surg 1998;27:776–9.
8. Chang SH, Lien WC, Liu YP, et al. Isolated superior mesenteric artery dissection in a patient without risk factors or aortic dissection. Am J Emerg Med 2006;24:385–7.
9. Sheldon PJ, Esther JB, Sheldon EL, et al. Spontaneous dissection of the superior mesenteric artery. Cardiovasc Interv Radiol 2001;24:329–31.
10. Corbetti F, Vigo M, Bulzacchi A, et al. CT diagnosis of spontaneous dissection of the superior mesenteric artery. J Comput Assist Tomogr 1989;13:965–7.
11. Lee BM, Neiman BH. Dissecting aneurysm of superior mesenteric artery. Ill Med J 1971; 139:589–92.
12. Barmeir E, Halachmi S, Croitoru S, Torem S. CT angiography diagnosis of spontaneous dissection of the superior mesenteric artery. AJR Am J Roentgenol 1998;171:1429–30.
13. Grainger K, Aber C. Dissection of the superior mesenteric artery during aortography with recovery. Report of a case. Br J Radiol 1961;34:265–8.
14. Desgranges P, Bourriez PA, d'Audiffret A, et al. Percutaneous stenting of an iatrogenic superior mesenteric artery dissection complicating suprarenal aortic aneurysm repair. J Endovasc Ther 2000;7:501–5.
15. Allen RC, Martin GH, Rees CR, et al. Mesenteric angioplasty in the treatment of chronic intestinal ischemia. J Vasc Surg 1996;24:415–23.
16. Picquet J, Abilez O, Penard J, et al. Superficial femoral artery transposition repair for isolated superior mesenteric artery dissection. J Vasc Surg 2005;42:788–91.
17. Lee BM, Neiman BH. Dissecting aneurysm of superior mesenteric artery. Ill Med J 1971; 139:589–92.
18. Brandt LJ, Boley SJ. AGA technical review on intestinal ischemia. American Gastrointestinal Association. Gastroenterology 2000;118:954–68.

19. Ando M, Ito M, Mishima Y. Spontaneous dissecting aneurysm of the main trunk of the superior mesenteric artery: report of a case. Surg Today 1995;25:468–70.
20. Iha K, Nakasone Y, Nakachi H, et al. Surgical treatment of spontaneous dissection of the superior mesenteric artery: a case report. Ann Thorac Cardiovasc Surg 2000;6:65–9.
21. Watring NJ, Smith CM, Stokes GK, Counselman FL. Spontaneous superior mesenteric artery dissection: an unusual cause of abdominal pain. J Emerg Med 2008.
22. Kim JH, Roh BS, Lee YH, et al. Isolated spontaneous dissection of the superior mesenteric artery: percutaneous stent placement in two patients. Korean J Radiol 2004;5:134–8.
23. Suzuki S, Furui S, Kohtake H, et al. Isolated dissection of the superior mesenteric artery: CT findings in six cases. Abdom Imaging 2004;29:153–7.
24. Sakamoto I, Ogawa Y, Sueyoshi E, et al. Imaging appearances and management of isolated spontaneous dissection of the superior mesenteric artery. Eur J Radiol 2007;64:103–10.
25. Vignati PV, Welch JP, Ellison L, Cohen JL. Acute mesenteric ischemia caused by isolated superior mesenteric artery dissection. J Vasc Surg 1992;16:109–12.
26. Iwase K, Sando K, Ito T, et al. Isolated dissecting aneurysm of the superior mesenteric artery: intravascular ultrasound (IVUS) images. Hepatogastroenterology 2007;54:1161–3.
27. Solis MM, Ranval TJ, McFarland DR, Eidt JF. Surgical treatment of superior mesenteric artery dissecting aneurysm and simultaneous celiac artery compression. Ann Vasc Surg 1993;7:457–62.
28. Matsushima K. Spontaneous isolated dissection of the superior mesenteric artery. J Am Coll Surg 2006;203:970–1.
29. Yasuhara H, Shigematsu H, Muto T. Self-limited spontaneous dissection of the main trunk of the superior mesenteric artery. J Vasc Surg 1998;27:776–9.
30. Wain RA, Kwei S, Lyon RT, et al. superior mesenteric artery dissection: rationale for a conservative approach in selected patients: a case report. Vasc Surg 1999;33:641–8.
31. Sparks SR, Vasquez JC, Bergan JJ, Owens EL. Failure of nonoperative management of isolated superior mesenteric artery dissection. Ann Vasc Surg 2000;14:105–9.
32. Nagai T, Torishima R, Uchida A, et al. Spontaneous dissection of the superior mesenteric artery in four cases treated with anticoagulation therapy. Intern Med 2004;43:473–8.
33. Tsuji Y, Hino Y, Sugimoto K, et al. Surgical intervention for isolated dissecting aneurysm of the superior mesenteric artery: a case report. Vasc Endovasc Surg 2004;38:469–72.
34. Sisteron A, Vieville C. Aneurysmes des arteres a destine digestive: observations personnelles. In: Courbier R, ed. Chirurgie des arteriopathies digestives. Paris: Expansion Scientifique Francaise; 1975, pp. 197–202.

31

Visceral Artery Aneurysms Revisited

Margaret C. Tracci, M.D., J.D. and
Kenneth J. Cherry, Jr., M.D.

Visceral artery aneurysms (VAAs) are uncommon aneurysms, and yet are probably not as rare as once thought. The advent and routine use of high-resolution, noninvasive imaging modalities of computed tomography (CT) and CT angiography (CTA) and of magnetic resonance imaging (MRI) and magnetic resonance angiography (MRA) have increased the frequency of diagnosis, often as an incidental finding.[1]

Contemporary with these enhanced methods of diagnosis have been the introduction and continuing improvement of endovascular therapies to treat visceral artery aneurysms (VAAs). Embolization, covered stents, and occluding devices may all be used alone or in combination in the appropriate clinical settings to treat many of these lesions. Although long-term data are not yet available, the reduced early morbidity and mortality of these treatments, when applicable, are appealing. Endovascular intervention for visceral artery aneurysms, (VAAs) both elective and emergent, is therefore being used with increasing frequency.

Not all such aneurysms may be treated with catheter-based techniques. Anatomic considerations may mandate open repair where, for instance, major mesenteric branches arising from an aneurysm supply significant lengths of small or large bowel or major branch points arise near the site of an aneurysm. Some ruptures, depending on containment or free bleeding, location and relation to the solid or hollow organs, the presence or absence of shock, body habitus, and physiologic status, may be treated endovascularly; others still require emergent open repair.

Historically, approximately one quarter of visceral artery aneurysms (VAAs) have presented emergently, with mortalities approaching 10%.[2] Associated nonvisceral aneurysms are seen in 25 to 30% of these patients. Multiple splanchnic artery aneurysms are seen in patients with connective tissue disorders. Recently, segmental arterial mediolysis has emerged as a diagnosis — a diagnosis of exclusion — for multiple visceral artery aneurysms (VAAs). It was first proposed as a distinct entity in 1976.[3]

Whether it is distinct or part of a continuum with fibromuscular dysplasia is a matter of debate. This chapter attempts to address the current management and expected outcomes for the different visceral artery aneurysms (VAAs).

SPLENIC ARTERY ANEURYSMS

SAA remains the most common visceral aneurysm, with an incidence reported to range between 0.02 and 10.4% in the general population[4] (Figure 31–1). Although the etiology of many of these lesions remains unclear and SAAs have been associated with a wide range of conditions, these lesions have been noted to occur with greater frequency in women and in

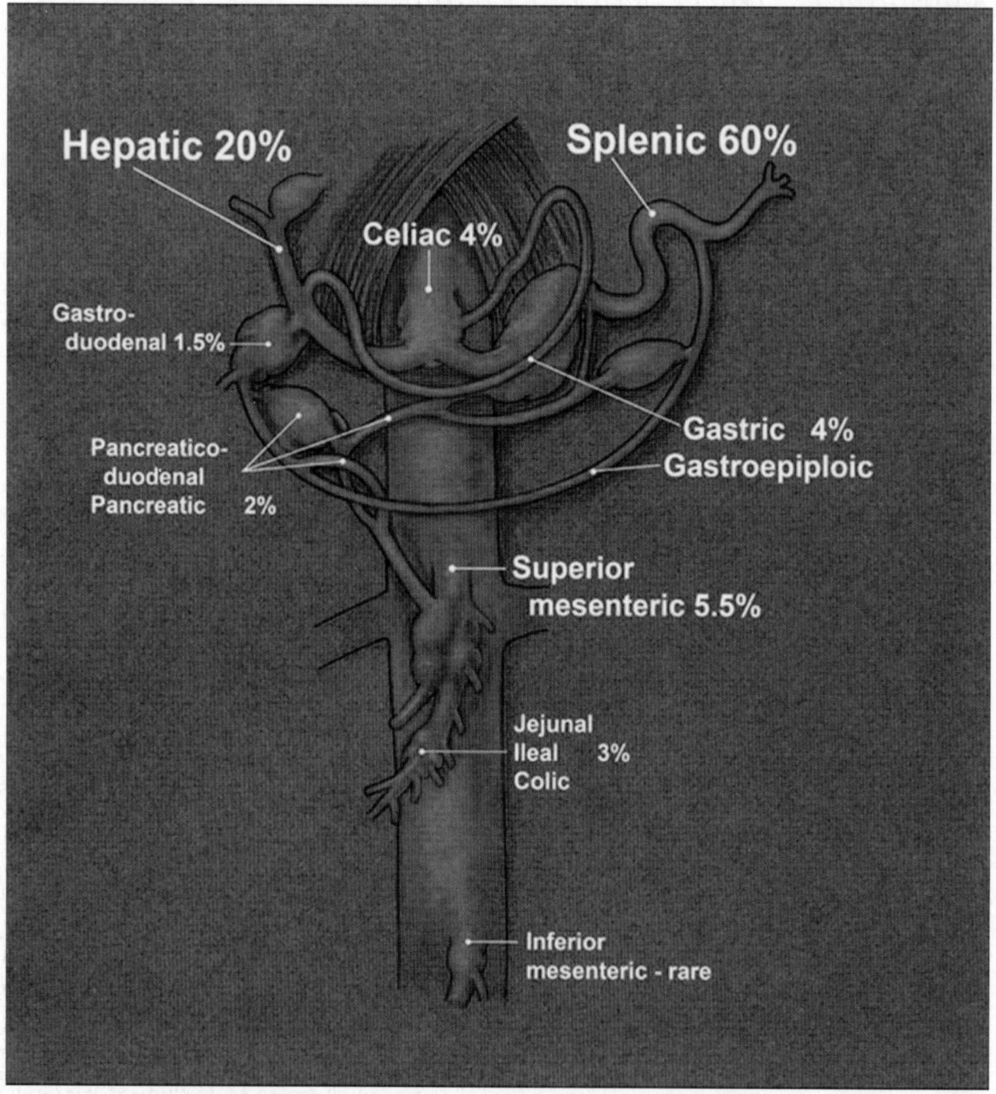

Figure 31-1. Distribution of visceral artery aneurysms. (Courtesy of Klaus D. Hagspiel, M.D.)

patients with liver disease manifesting with cirrhosis or portal hypertension. In women, aneurysms of the splenic artery become more common with increasing parity. Theories regarding the precise nature of this association implicate mechanical and hemodynamic factors accompanying the increased intravascular volume and hyperdynamic state of pregnancy as well as hormonal factors related to the effects on the arterial wall of estrogen, progesterone, and relaxin.[5] Other conditions associated with SAA include atherosclerosis, arterial fibrodysplasia, arteritis, collagen vascular disease, α-1-antitrypsin deficiency, pancreatitis and other local inflammatory states,[4] arterial fibrodysplasia with medial degeneration, trauma,[6] intravenous drug use, splenomegaly,[7] idiopathic dissection, essential hypertension, polyarteritis nodosa, Ehlers-Danlos syndrome, neurofibromatosis, and orthotopic liver transplantation.[8] Of note, many believe that the calcific atherosclerotic changes found in SAAs are secondary rather than causative events.[9]

Most SAAs are asymptomatic and are detected during radiographic examinations performed for other indications. Whereas abdominal CT remains the mainstay of diagnosis, plain radiographs may demonstrate curvilinear calcifications in the left upper quadrant of the abdomen. The differential diagnosis for this finding also includes a tortuous, calcified splenic artery, renal artery aneurysm, or calcified pancreatic masses (Figures 31–2 and 31–3). Symptomatic aneurysms frequently manifest with left upper quadrant or epigastric pain that may radiate to the left shoulder. Rupture, although relatively infrequent, may manifest with hypovolemia and rapid hemodynamic collapse. The "double-rupture phenomenon" may also be observed, in which an initial rupture into the lesser sac is relatively contained and the patient is stable until blood overflowing through the foramen of Winslow results in peritonitis and hypovolemic shock.[8] Rarely, rupture may present as gastrointestinal bleeding due to communication with the GI tract or pancreatic duct[10] or as arteriovenous fistula that may result in portal hypertension[11] or small bowel ischemia through the "mesenteric steal syndrome."[12]

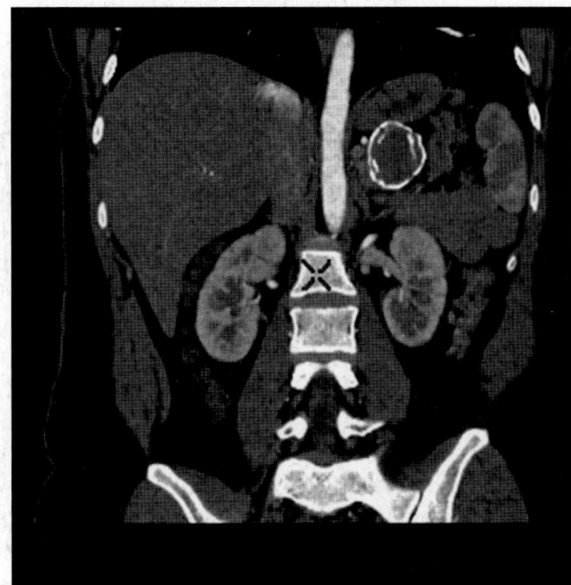

Figure 31-2. Calcified pancreatic mass, 3D reconstruction.

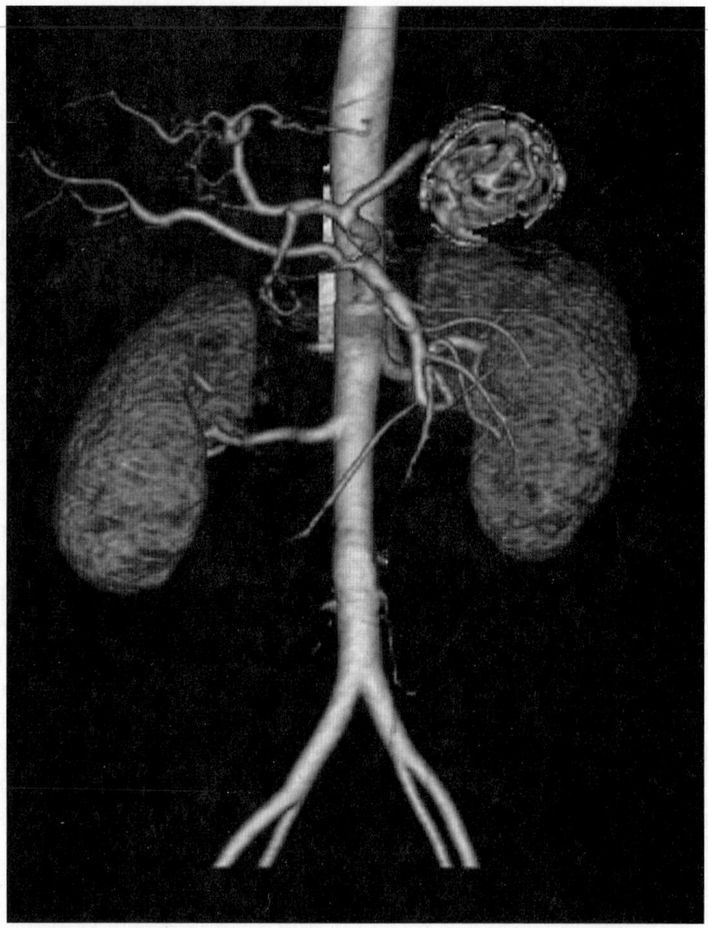

Figure 31-3. Calcified pancreatic mass on CT angiogram.

The smallest ruptured SAA noted in the largest series reported to date was 2.3 cm; the smallest observed in that institution's previously published 2 decades of experience was 2 cm.[4] Those facts suggest that the risk of rupture in small (<2 cm) aneurysms is quite low. The overall reported rate of rupture ranges from 3 to 10%.[13-14] Based on these findings, the authors advocate consideration of repair for symptomatic SAAs and those greater than 2 cm in size. When rupture does occur, it carries a mortality rate ranging from 10 to 76% in the literature, with most contemporary investigators accepting a rate of 20 to 35%.[4] In pregnant women, survival of both mother and fetus after rupture is extremely rare.[15] Overall, maternal mortality is approximately 70% and fetal mortality is reported to range from 75%[9] to higher than 90%.[4] A broad consensus exists that SAAs discovered during pregnancy or in patients of childbearing age should be considered for repair. Increased risk of rupture has also been observed in patients undergoing liver transplantation, certainly supporting the contention that SAAs detected during evaluation and preparation of the liver transplant recipient must be addressed at the time of transplantation.[4]

Several other factors have been investigated in relation to the risk of rupture. Although calcification is not protective against rupture,[4,13] beta blockers may be.[4] In addition, enhanced proteolytic activity in the setting of α-1-antitrypsin deficiency may contribute to the increased risk of rupture around the time of liver transplant in these patients.[16-17]

Traditionally, the favored modality of treatment has been surgical ligation or resection, with pancreatic or splenic resection as necessary. Aneurysms of the proximal splenic artery may be treated by resection or simple ligation, both of which have also been approached using a laparoscopic technique.[18-19] Distal lesions may be treated by splenectomy and those embedded in the body or tail of the pancreas may be treated by distal pancreatic resection with or without splenectomy, an approach particularly suited to aneurysms or pseudoaneurysms associated with pancreatitis and associated pseudocysts.[9;17]

More recently, endovascular therapy using covered stents[20] (Figures 31–4 through 31–6) or embolization with coils (Figures 31–7 through 31–10),[21] gelatin sponge (Gelfoam Pharmacia & Upjohn Co.),[22] or cyanoacrylate glue[23] has shown promise, although it remains limited by the operator's ability to selectively cannulate the target vessels and by a 20% failure rate in patients presenting with pancreatic pseudocyst and a 10 to 15% overall failure rate. In addition, several reports suggest that percutaneous thrombin injection performed under CT or ultrasound guidance may prove to be an effective and minimally morbid method of therapy for splenic artery pseudoaneurysm, although publication of longer-term follow-up of these patients is necessary for valid comparison of techniques. The major known complications of thrombin injection include immune reaction to bovine thrombin (factor V antibody) or distal thromboembolic complications.[24]

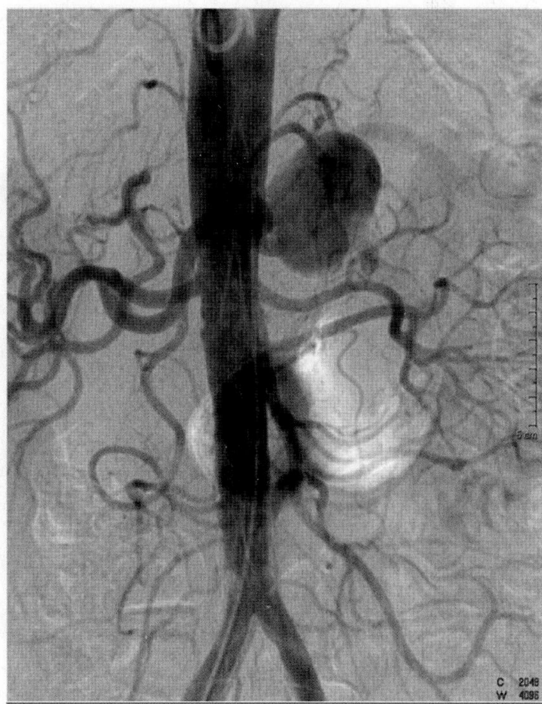

Figure 31-4. Splenic artery aneurysm (SAA). (Courtesy of Klaus D. Hagspiel, M.D.)

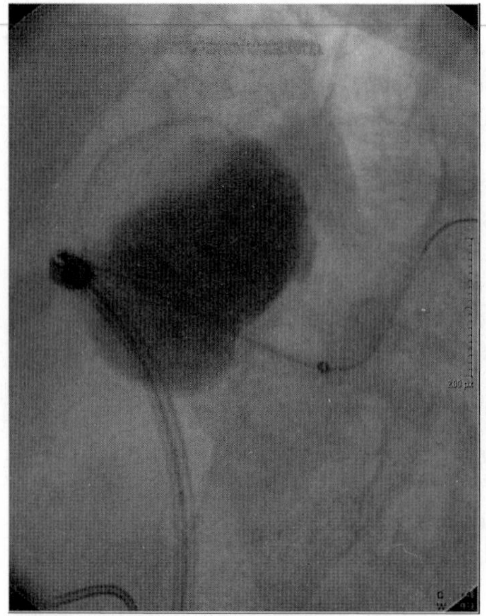

Figure 31-5. Deployment of covered stent. (Courtesy of Klaus D. Hagspiel, M.D.)

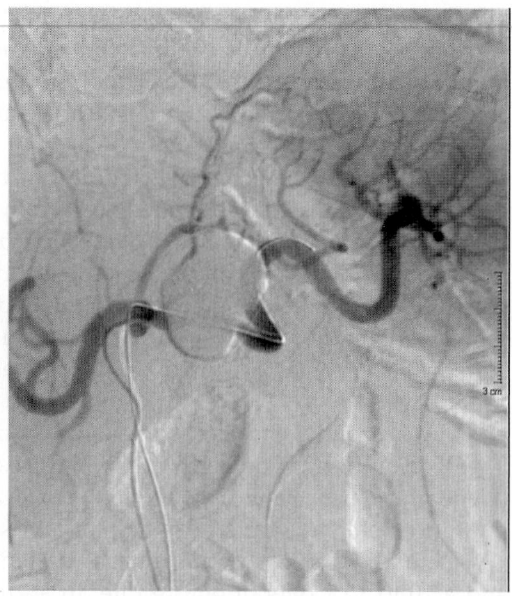

Figure 31-6. Exclusion of splenic artery aneurysm using covered stent. (Courtesy of Klaus D. Hagspiel, M.D.)

HEPATIC ARTERY ANEURYSMS

Historically, aneurysms of the hepatic artery represent the second most common visceral artery aneurysm VAAs and 20% of all VAAs.[6] Recent reports that include false aneurysms of the hepatic arterial system suggest that these lesions may represent an even greater pro-

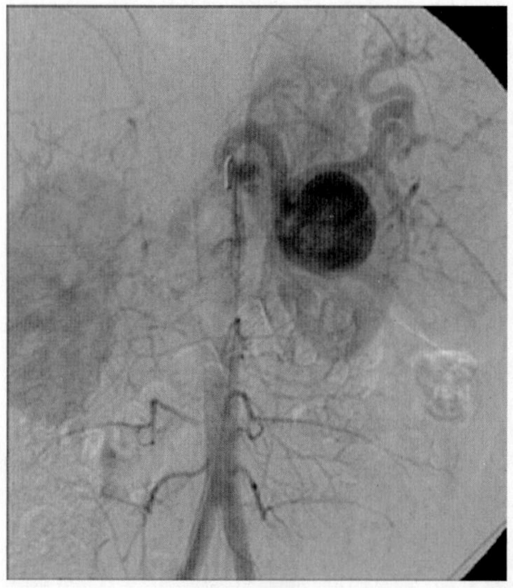

Figure 31-7. Splenic artery aneurysm. (Courtesy of Alan H. Matsumoto, M.D.)

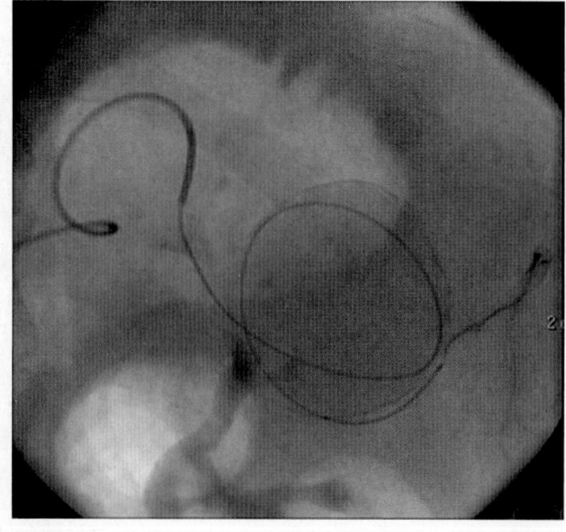

Figure 31-8. Embolization of distal branch vessels. (Courtesy of Alan H. Matsumoto, M.D.)

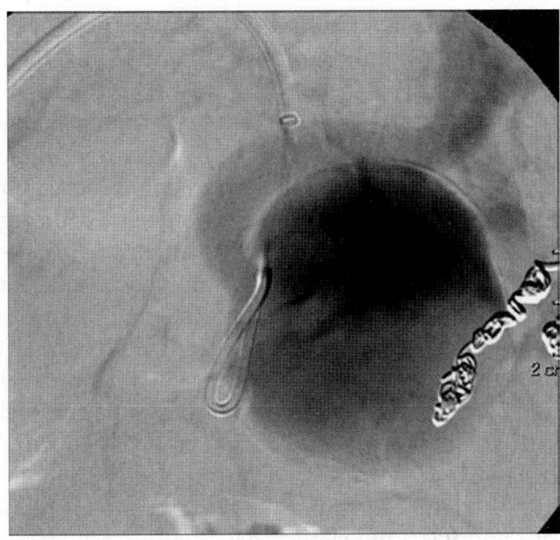

Figure 31-9. Embolization of main afferent artery. (Courtesy of Alan H. Matsumoto, M.D.)

portion of visceral aneurysms. This increase is commonly attributed to the increased use of percutaneous techniques for biliary procedures and to improved detection of iatrogenic and traumatic injuries with CT imaging.[25]

True and false aneurysms of the hepatic artery have been attributed to etiologies including trauma or iatrogenic injury, intravenous drug use, vasculitis, local inflammatory processes,[7] medial degeneration, liver transplant,[8] atherosclerosis, infective endocarditis, arterial fibrodysplasia, polyarteritis nodosa, systemic lupus erythematosus; congenital causes such as Marfan syndrome, Ehlers-Danlos syndrome, Osler-Weber-Rendu syndrome, and hereditary hemorrhagic telangiectasia; or, rarely, Takayasu arteritis, Kawasaki disease, von Recklinghausen neurofibromatosis, or Wegener

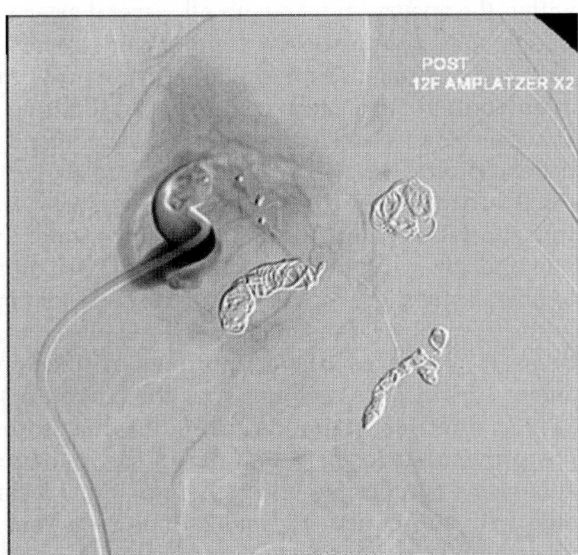

Figure 31-10. Splenic artery aneurysm postembolization. (Courtesy of Alan H. Matsumoto, M.D.)

granulomatosis.[4] Of note, the shift in etiology over time also reflects a decrease, in the modern era of antibiotics, in the incidence of mycotic aneurysms related to bacterial endocarditis.[26-27]

Hepatic artery aneurysms are frequently asymptomatic. However, symptomatic aneurysms may manifest with right upper quadrant or epigastric pain or obstructive jaundice from bile duct compression. Biliary colic, hemobilia, and obstructive jaundice are considered to represent a classic, although relatively uncommon, presenting triad.[28] Rupture may occur into either the peritoneum or the biliary tract. The former is generally associated with extrahepatic aneurysms and typically presents with hypovolemic shock, and the latter is associated with intrahepatic aneurysms and may manifest as hemobilia and gastrointestinal bleeding.[6,8]

Indications for the repair of hepatic artery aneurysms include rupture, symptoms, and size. Unsurprisingly, given the relative rarity of this lesion and the limited data available on the natural history and risk of rupture of asymptomatic aneurysms, institutions vary with regard to size criteria for repair. The authors consider aneurysms over 2 cm in diameter to be appropriate for repair in a patient who is a good operative risk and has a life expectancy of at least 2 years. Although the risk of rupture certainly increases for aneurysms over 2 cm in size, it must be noted that rupture has been reported of aneurysms smaller than 2 cm.[29] Among asymptomatic patients, other risk factors have been identified as predictive of complications, including the presence of multiple hepatic artery aneurysms and etiology other than ASO, such as fibromuscular dysplasia, polyarteritis nodosa, or mycotic aneurysm.[4]

Traditional operative management for extrahepatic aneurysms includes excision with or without saphenous vein or synthetic conduit reconstruction, whereas intrahepatic aneurysms have been treated with ligation or, where necessary, partial hepatic resection. Whereas collateral circulation generally permits excision or ligation without reconstruction of aneurysms of the common hepatic artery, those of the proper hepatic artery generally require arterial reconstruction to preserve flow.[6] The repair of more distal hepatic artery aneurysms may be rendered more technically difficult by the proximity of the bile duct. In the case of large aneurysms or those attended by significant inflammation, proximal and distal control may be more easily achieved from within the aneurysm.[4] As with all visceral artery aneurysms (VAAs), open repair has traditionally been associated with significant morbidity and mortality rates, particularly in the setting of rupture. In the event of rupture, the emergent nature of the operation and patient factors contribute to reported mortality rates of 20% or higher.[9] However, even elective operations must contend with significant patient comorbidities and difficulties of exposure and control.[30]

A broad range of endovascular therapies has been applied to the treatment of true and false aneurysms of the hepatic artery. The relatively high technical success rate and low morbidity and mortality rates of these procedures have contributed to liberalization of many clinicians' criteria for repair, leading some to conclude that in the absence of unusual risk factors, all hepatic artery aneurysms should be addressed.[9]. Endovascular techniques utilized in the treatment of hepatic artery aneurysms include coil embolization, covered stent exclusion (Figures 31–11 and 31–12), and percutaneous thrombin injection. Transcatheter coil embolization has proven particularly popular in the management of intrahepatic true or false aneurysms but, despite relatively high initial technical success rates, has been associated with subsequent recanalization, aneurysm rupture, hepatic necrosis, hepatic abscess, and cholecystitis.[4]

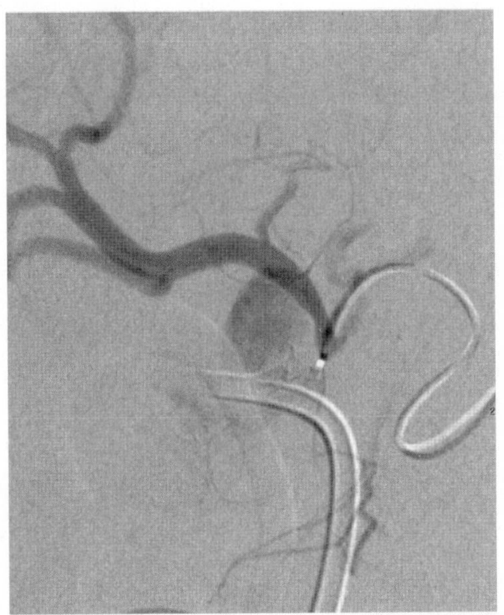

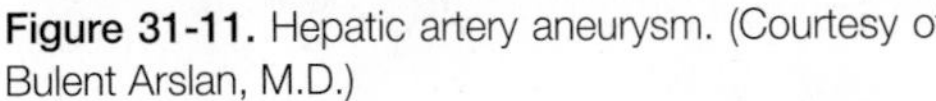

Figure 31-11. Hepatic artery aneurysm. (Courtesy of Bulent Arslan, M.D.)

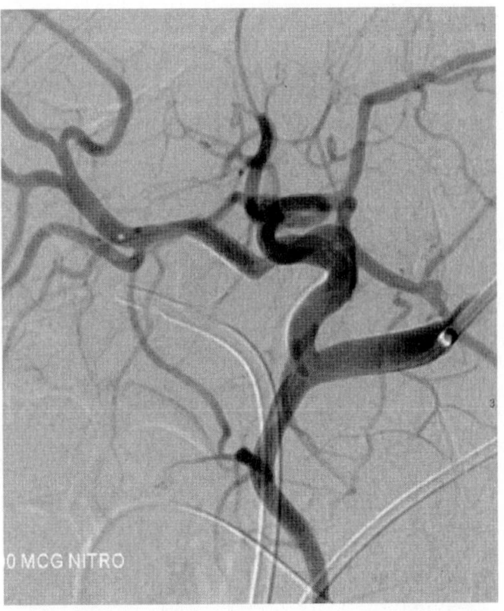

Figure 31-12. Exclusion of hepatic artery aneurysm using covered stent. (Courtesy of Bulent Arslan, M.D.)

SUPERIOR MESENTERIC ARTERY ANEURYSMS

Aneurysms of the superior mesenteric artery account for approximately 5.5% of visceral artery aneurysms (VAAs). Historically, infectious etiologies of these lesions, often related to bacterial endocarditis, have frequently been reported. However, in modern series, noninfectious factors such as atherosclerosis, medial dysplasia, collagen vascular disease, polyarteritis nodosa, Behçet's syndrome,[31] dissection, trauma, local inflammatory processes,[32] or neurofibromatosis[8] predominate. Unlike many other visceral artery aneurysms, (VAAs) those of the superior mesenteric artery are typically symptomatic at presentation and may manifest as epigastric pain or mesenteric ischemia.[8] Ischemic symptoms may be attributable to dissection, intraluminal thrombus, or thromboembolism.[9] Although the incidence of rupture varies widely among reports in the literature, a relatively large recent series suggests a rate as high as 38%. Rupture was, in this series, accompanied by a 37.5% operative mortality rate.[31]

In the Mayo series, the authors embraced the widely shared conclusion that repair should be considered in all cases in which the patient presents a reasonable operative risk. Four of the five aneurysms observed through the study period without surgical treatment were <1.5 cm in size.[31] Emergent repair carries significant risk of complications, most commonly related to bowel ischemia. Despite that, others have reported that in the emergent setting, ligation without revascularization is the procedure of choice in the absence of preoperative symptoms or intraoperative signs of mesenteric ischemia. Opening of the aneurysm with ligation of inflow and outflow branches may be the most practical approach in this setting. Where evidence of ischemia exists and the patient's condition permits, revascularization using an interposition or aortomesenteric graft may be attempted. In the emergent setting, this reconstruction should preferentially utilize the saphenous vein, because a large proportion of patients presenting

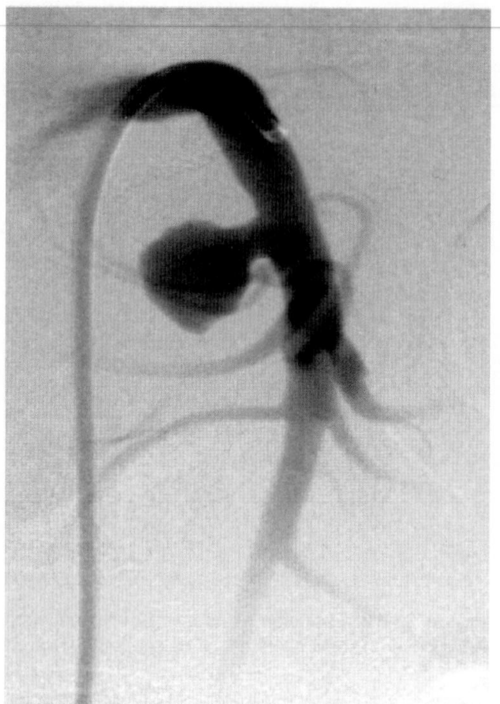

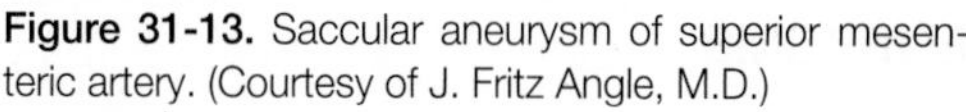

Figure 31-13. Saccular aneurysm of superior mesenteric artery. (Courtesy of J. Fritz Angle, M.D.)

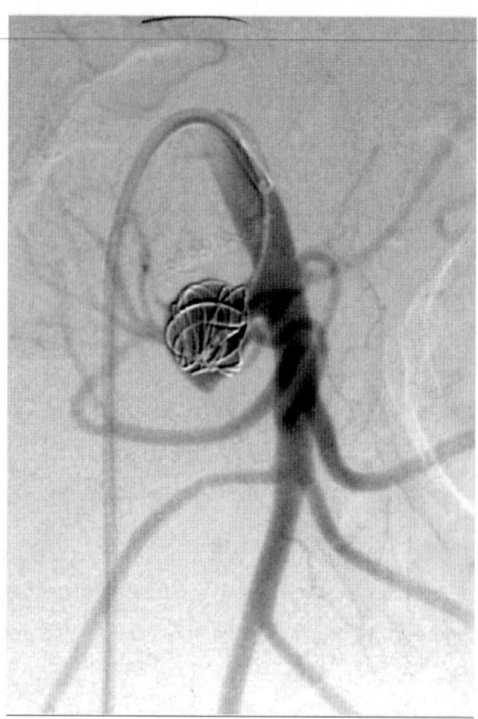

Figure 31-14. Placement of detachable coils in superior mesenteric artery aneurysm. (Courtesy of J. Fritz Angle, M.D.)

with rupture ultimately require bowel resection.[31] Elective repair permits more careful evaluation, based on preoperative anatomic evaluation, of the need for revascularization. Where collateral visceral perfusion does not appear adequate, reconstruction using prosthetic graft or saphenous vein may be selected. Most vascular surgeons, ourselves included, recommend formal reconstruction.

Transcatheter embolization of superior mesenteric artery aneurysms has been reported and seems well suited to the treatment of saccular aneurysms, particularly in the setting of a hostile abdomen (Figures 31–13 to 31–15).[33] Concern regarding the risk of distal embolization that attends this technique is particularly pertinent in the treatment of superior mesenteric artery lesions. Covered stent treatment has also been described, although it may increase the risk of segmental ischemia requiring resection and is certainly contraindicated in the setting of infection (Figures 31–16 and 31–17). Several reports exist as well of percutaneous thrombin treatment of visceral aneurysms, including those of the superior mesenteric artery.[34]

CELIAC ARTERY ANEURYSMS

Although relatively rare, celiac artery aneurysms pose a substantial risk of rupture, ranging from 10 to 20%.[31] The literature also suggests that rupture continues to be attended by a 50 to 100% mortality rate.[25] Associated conditions include atherosclerotic disease, medial dysplasia, collagen vascular disease,[31] Takayasu arteritis,[8] trauma, aortic dissection, post-

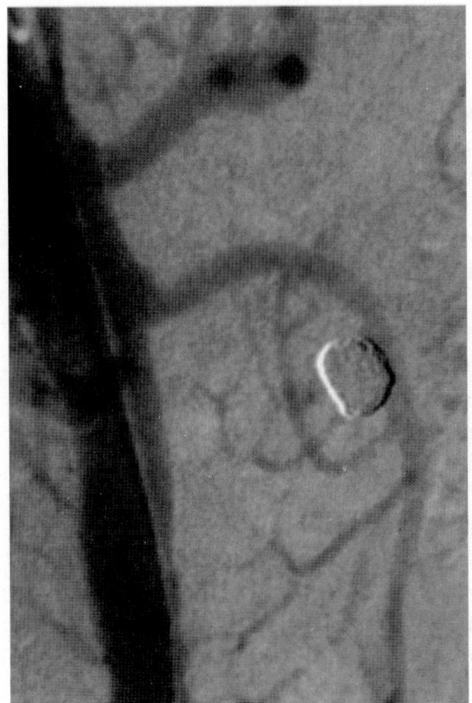

Figure 31-15. Successful embolization of saccular superior mesenteric artery aneurysm. (Courtesy of J. Fritz Angle, M.D.)

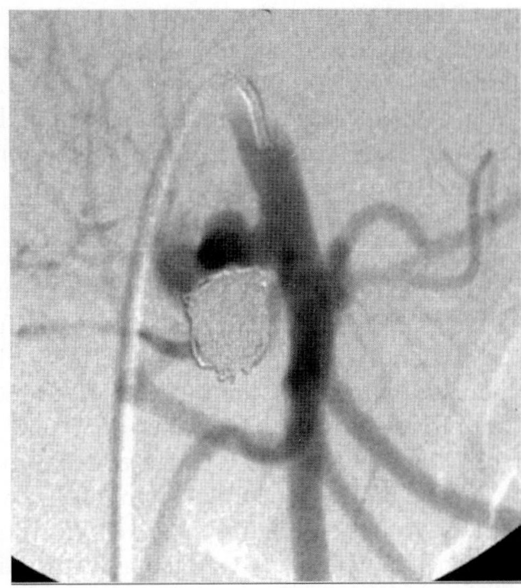

Figure 31-16. Superior mesenteric artery aneurysm with gastrointestinal bleeding 2 years following coil embolization. (Courtesy of Alan H. Matsumoto, M.D.)

stenotic dilation[9] and infections, including *Salmonella, Streptococcus, Staphylococcus,* syphilis, and tuberculosis.[35-36] In the modern era, atherosclerosis and medial dysplasia have emerged as the primary etiologies of these lesions, with a concomitant reduction in the incidence of celiac aneurysms of infectious etiology, particularly those associated with syphilis and tuberculosis.[36] In the Mayo Clinic series, two thirds of patients presenting with

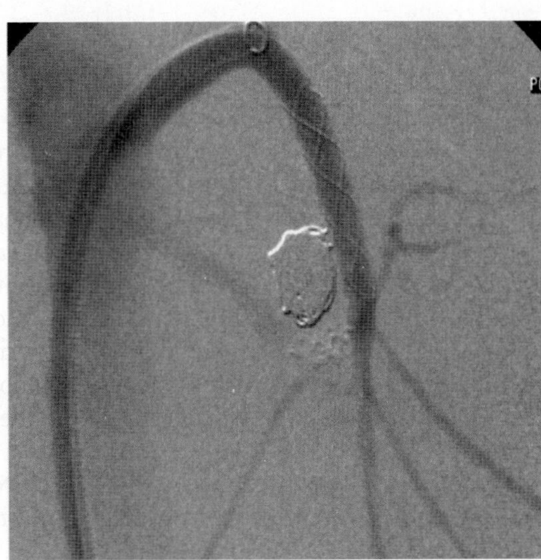

Figure 31-17. Exclusion of superior mesenteric artery aneurysm using covered stent (Courtesy of Alan H. Matsumoto, M.D.)

celiac artery aneurysms were male,[35] although others have found a ratio closer to 1:1 in recent series.[36] Interestingly, celiac artery aneurysms may have coexistent visceral artery aneurysms (VAAs) in 22 to 38% and nonvisceral aneurysms in 18 to 67% of cases.[35-36]

Celiac artery aneurysms may manifest with abdominal pain alone, abdominal pain radiating to the back, back pain, or nausea and vomiting. Recent series suggest that 24 to 44% of patients will present with symptoms, with the remainder discovered incidentally during other radiographic examinations or at laparotomy. An upper abdominal bruit or palpable pulsatile mass may also be noted on physical examination. Whereas rupture frequently presents as hemoperitoneum with rapid hemodynamic collapse, the "double-rupture" phenomenon previously described in SAA may also occur. These aneurysms may rupture into the transverse colon or other hollow viscera, with resultant gastrointestinal bleeding.

The authors support treatment of celiac artery aneurysms that are either symptomatic or greater than 2 cm in size. Rupture has been described in relatively small lesions, leading to some investigators' preference to repair all celiac aneurysms unless the patient has a prohibitive operative risk.[9] Historical efforts to treat celiac artery aneurysms include attempts in the late 1800s to induce thrombosis through the application of electric current and, in 1910 and 1911, to accomplish the same end by the introduction of lengths of intra-aneurysmal wire.[36] Modern operative management typically consists of aneurysmectomy with concomitant revascularization using either synthetic or saphenous vein conduit or simple ligation.[35] Other operative approaches have included direct reconstruction through aortic implantation of the celiac artery or its branches or aneurysmectomy with end-to-end arterial anastomosis.[36] Revascularization is generally favored over ligation alone, because the latter approach relies on adequate collateral circulation and may be complicated by hepatic, gastric, splenic, or small bowel necrosis. Mycotic aneurysm and Ehlers-Danlos syndrome present two rare circumstances in which ligation may be preferable to revascularization. Rare reports exist of endovascular treatment of celiac artery aneurysms using covered stents[37] and/or embolization.[38-39] Endovascular therapy of celiac artery lesions is, however, significantly limited by local anatomy. In addition, subsequent treatment failures, including not only reperfusion but also actual rupture, have been reported for endovascular embolization.[40]

RARE VISCERAL ANEURYSMS

Beyond those entities described above, there are also a range of exceedingly rare aneurysms of the smaller visceral branch arteries, including the inferior mesenteric, colic, jejunal, ileal, gastric, gastroepiploic, pancreaticoduodenal, and gastroduodenal. Because the literature regarding aneurysms consists of isolated case reports and very small series, management is guided largely by extrapolation and anecdote. The first six of these may present with gastrointestinal bleeding from erosion into adjacent viscera or with frank intraperitoneal bleeding. Jejunal, ileal, inferior mesenteric, and colic arteries may also rupture into the mesentery. Whereas these aneurysms historically presented with rupture, the wider use of various imaging modalities has led to the more frequent diagnosis of asymptomatic lesions.[17]

Multiple lesions are unusual and may result from a connective tissue disorder (Figure 31–18), vasculitis, segmental arterial mediolysis, or an infectious etiology.[41-42]

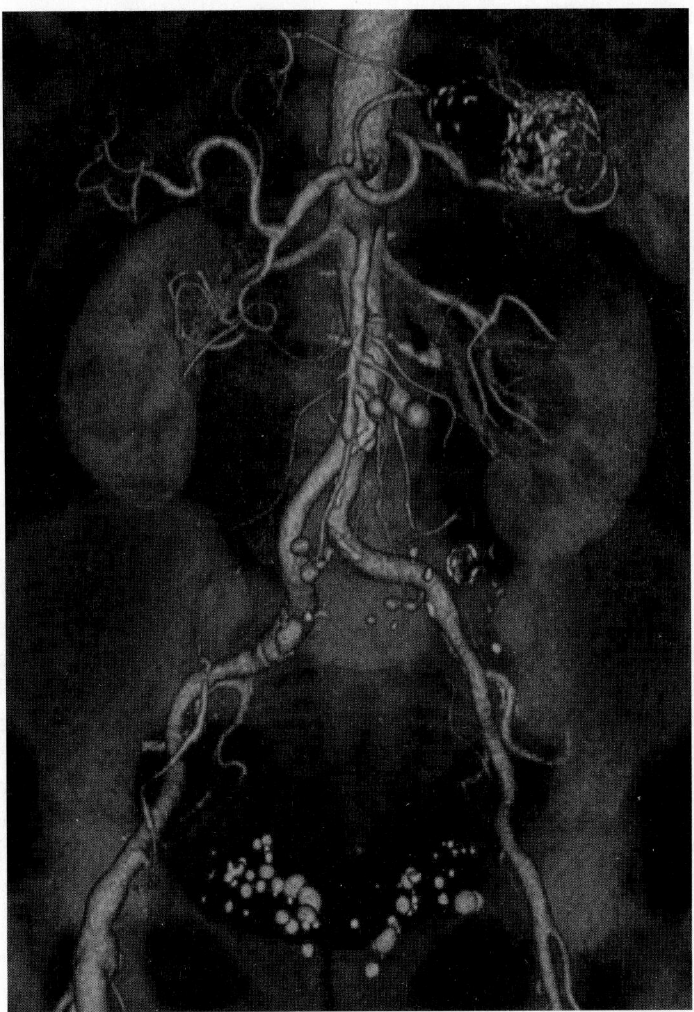

Figure 31-18. Multiple aneurysms in patient with type 4 Ehlers-Danlos syndrome. (Courtesy of Alan H. Matsumoto, M.D.)

Evidence of medial dysplasia and atherosclerosis has been found in these aneurysms, although many remain of unclear etiology.[17] Pancreaticoduodenal and gastroduodenal aneurysms may be associated with peripancreatic inflammation or pseudocyst or may arise as a complication of pancreaticoduodenectomy or transplantation.[9] These aneurysms may present with gastrointestinal hemorrhage, "abdominal apoplexy" related to rupture into the stomach or duodenum or, less frequently, into the pancreatic or biliary systems. As with all visceral artery aneurysms, (VAAs) rupture carries a significant risk of mortality, which appears to be somewhat higher in pancreatitis-related lesions.[9,17,25] Rarely, aneurysmal change of vessels constituting collateral circulation between the celiac and the superior mesenteric arteries, including the arc of Buehler, has been observed in the setting of mesenteric occlusive disease, representing a local flow phenomenon similar to the poststenotic dilation observed in the setting of atherosclerotic disease.[43]

Traditionally, surgical therapy has consisted of ligation with resection of any resultant nonviable bowel. Particularly in the setting of pancreatitis-associated lesions, ligation from within the aneurysm or even pancreatic resection may be necessary. Endovascular intervention in the smaller branch vessels, particularly coil embolization, provides an appealing alternative. Therapy must focus on completely addressing all branches supplying the aneurysm to minimize the risk of recanalization. Percutaneous thrombin injection has also been described. (REFS) When asymptomatic aneurysms are detected, elective ligation or embolization is recommended where feasible.[17,34]

In approximately 0.25 to 0.5% of the population, the celiac and superior mesenteric arteries arise from the aorta as a common celiomesenteric trunk. There are now several reports in the literature of aneurysms of this common trunk.[44-45] Both atherosclerosis and medial degeneration have been observed in these lesions.[44] Repairs have included interposition graft, aneurysmectomy with primary or patch repair,[44] and prosthetic bypass from the thoracic aorta following interposition graft of a very tortuous supraceliac aorta.[45]

In summary, visceral artery aneurysms (VAAs) represent a relatively rare but clinically important variant of aneurysmal vascular disease. Whereas the traditional mainstay of therapy has been surgical, a trend toward increasing use of endovascular therapy has been widely noted. Potential advantages in terms of operative morbidity and mortality are evident in the early literature and are bound to be clarified as experience is accrued in this area. However, it must be remembered that endovascular therapy is not without complications or limitations on its application imposed by anatomy and technical considerations. Furthermore, clinical presentations that are confounding to traditional open surgical therapy are often equally unappealing to endovascular operators. Catheter-based therapy for type 4 Ehlers-Danlos syndrome, for instance, carries daunting morbidity and mortality rates ranging from 17 to 67% and 6 to 19%, respectively, primarily related to frequent and severe access site complications, dissection, perforation, or pseudoaneurysm formation.[46]

REFERENCES

1. Horton KM, Smith C, Fishman EK. MDCT and 3D CT angiography of splanchnic artery aneurysms. Am J Roentgenol 2007;189:641–7.
2. Stanley JC. Abdominal visceral aneurysms. In: Haimovici H, ed: Vascular Emergencies. New York, Appleton-Century-Crofts; 1981;387–96.
3. Slavin RE, Gonzales-Vitale JC. Segmental mediolytic arteritis: a clinical pathologic study. Lab Invest 1976;35:23–9.
4. Abbas MA, Stone WM, Fowl RJ, et al. Splenic artery aneurysms: two decades experience at Mayo Clinic. Ann Vasc Surg 2002;16:442–9.
5. Hallett JW. Splenic artery aneurysms. Semin Vasc Surg 1995;8:321–6.
6. Stanley JC. Mesenteric arterial occlusive and aneurysmal disease. Cardiol Clin 2002;16:442–9.
7. Hiramoto JS, Messina LM. Visceral artery aneurysms. Curr Treat Options Cardiovasc Med 2005;7:109–17.
8. Pasha SF, Gloviczki P, Stanson AW, Kamath PS. Splanchnic artery aneurysms. Mayo Clin Proc 2007;82:472–9.
9. Upchurch GR, Zelenock GB, Stanley JC. Splanchnic artery aneurysms. In: Rutherford RB, ed. Vascular Surgery. 6th ed. Philadelphia: Elsevier Saunders; 2005;1565–81.
10. Harper PC, Gamelli RL, Kaye MD. Recurrent hemorrhage into the pancreatic duct from a splenic artey aneurysm. Gastroenterology 1984;87:417–20.

11. Brothers TE, Stanley JC, Zelenock GB. Splenic arteriovenous fistula. Int Surg 1995;80:189–94.
12. Sendra F, Safran DB, McGee G. A rare complication of splenic artery aneurysm. Mesenteric steal syndrome. Arch Surg 1995;130:669–72.
13. Trastek VA, Pairolero PC, Joyce JW, et al. Splenic artery aneurysms. Surgery 1982;91:694–9.
14. Angelakis EJ, Baer WE, Barone JE, Lincer RM. Splenic artery aneurysm rupture during pregnancy. Obstet Gynecol Surg 1993;48:145–8.
15. Caillouette JC, Merchant EB: Ruptured splenic artery aneurysm in pregnancy: twelfth reported case with maternal and fetal survival. Am J Obstet Gynecol 1993;168:1810–1.
16. Gaglio PJ, Regenstein F, Slakey D, et al. Alpha-1-antitrypsin deficiency and splenic artery aneurysm rupture: an association? Am J Gastroenterol 2000;95:1531–4.
17. Tessier DJ, Stone WM, Fowl RJ, et al. Clinical features and management of splenic artery pseudoaneurysm: case series and cumulative review of literature. J Vasc Surg 2003; 38: 969–74.
18. Leung KL, Kwong KH, Tam YH, et al. Laparoscopic resection of splenic artery aneurysm. Surg Endosc 1998;12:53.
19. Trias M, Targarona EM, Espert JJ et al. Laparoscopic surgery for splenic disorders. Lessons learned from a series of 64 cases. Surg Endosc 1998;12:66–72.
20. Brountzos EN, Vegenas K, Apostolopoulou SC, et al. Pancreatitis-associated splenic artery pseudoaneurysm: endovascular treatment with self-expandable stent-grafts. Cardiovasc Intervent Radiol 2003;26:88–91
21. Hung RK, Loh C, Goldstein L. Selective use of electrolytic detachable and fibered coils to embolize a wide-neck giant splenic artery pseudoaneurysm. J Vasc Surg 2005;41:889–92.
22. Guan Y-S, Sun L, Zhou X-P, et al. Polyvinyl alcohol and gelatin sponge particle embolization of splenic artery pseudoaneurysm complicating chronic alcoholic pancreatitis. World J Gastroenterol 2005;11:2684–6.
23. Kim BS, Do HM, Razavi M. N-butyl cyanoacrylate glue embolization of splenic artery aneurysms. J Vasc Interv Radiol 2004;15:91–4.
24. Krueger K, Zaehringer M, Lackner K. Percutaneous treatment of a splenic pseudoaneurysm by thrombin injection. J Vasc Intervent Radiol 2005;15:91–4.
25. Shanley CJ, Shah NL, Messina LM. Common splanchnic artery aneurysms: splenic, hepatic, and celiac. Ann Vasc Surg 1996;10:315–22.
26. Senocak F, Cekirge S, Senocak ME, Karademir S. Hepatic artery aneurysm in a 10-year-old boy as a complication of infective endocarditis. J Pediatr Surg 1996;31:1570–2.
27. Lal RB, Strohl JA, Piazza S, et al. Hepatic artery aneurysm. J Cardiovasc Surg 1989;30: 509–13.
28. Zachary K, Geier S, Pellecchia C, Irwin G. Jaundice secondary to hepatic artery aneurysm: radiological appearance and clinical features. Am J Gastroenterol 1986;81:295–8.
29. Erskine JM. Hepatic artery aneurysm. Vasc Surg 1973;7:106–25.
30. Kasirajan K, Greenberg RK, Clair D, Ouriel K. Endovascular management of visceral artery aneurysm. J Endovasc Ther 2001;8:150–5.
31. Stone WM, Abbas M, Cherry KJ, et al. Superior mesenteric artery aneurysm: is presence an indication for intervention? J Vasc Surg 2002;36:234–7.
32. Messina LM, Shanley CJ. Visceral artery aneurysms. Surg Clin North Am 1997;77:425–42.
33. Stambo GW, Hallisey MJ, Gallagher JJ. Arteriographic embolization of visceral artery pseudoaneurysms. Ann Vasc Surg 1996;10:476–80.
34. Kemmeter P, Bonnell B, VanderKolk MD, et al. Percutaneous thrombin injection of splanchnic artery aneurysms: two case reports. J Vasc Intervent Radiol 2000;11:469–72.
35. Stone WM, Abbas MA, Gloviczki P, et al. Celiac artery aneurysms: a critical reappraisal of a rare entity. Arch Surg 2002;137:670–4.
36. Graham LM, Stanley JC, Whitehouse WM, et al. Celiac artery aneurysms: historic (1745–1949) versus contemporary (1950–1984) differences in etiology and clinical importance. J Vasc Surg 1985;2:757–64.
37. Atkins BZ, Ryan JM, Gray JL. Treatment of a celiac artery aneurysm with endovascular stent-grafting: a case report. Vasc Endovasc Surg 2003;37:367–73.

38. Carroccio A, Jacobs TS, Faries P, et al. Endovascular treatment of visceral artery aneurysms. Vasc Endovasc Surg 2007;41:373–82.
39. Schoder M, Cejna M, Langle F, et al. Glue embolization of a ruptured celiac trunk pseudoaneurysm via the gastroduodenal artery. Eur Radiol 2000;10:1335–7
40. Onohara T, Okadome K, Yasumori K, et al. Rupture of embolized celiac artery pseudoaneurysm into the stomach: is coil embolization an effective treatment of celiac anastomotic pseudoaneurysm? Eur J Vasc Surg 1992;6:330–2.
41. Trevisani MF, Ricci MA, Michaels RM, Meyer KK. Multiple mesenteric aneurysms complicating subacute bacterial endocarditis. Arch Surg 1987;122:823–4
42. Sellke FM, Williams GB, Donovan DL, Clarke RE. Management of intra-abdominal aneurysms associated with periarteritis nodosa. J Vasc Surg 1986;4:294.
43. Suzuki K, Tachi Y, Ito S, Maruyama K, et al. Endovascular management of ruptured pancreaticoduodenal artery aneurysms associated with celiac axis stenosis. Cardiovasc Intervent Radiol 2008;31:1082–7.
44. Kalra M, Panneton JM, Hofer JM, Andrews JC. Aneurysm and stenosis of the celiomesenteric trunk: a rare anomaly. J Vasc Surg 2003;7:679–82.
45. Ailawadi G, Cowles RA, Stanley JC, et al. Common celiacomesenteric trunk: aneurysmal and occlusive disease. J Vasc Surg 2004;40:1040–3.
46. Bade MA, Queral LA, Mukherjee D, Kong LS. Endovascular abdominal aortic aneurysm repair in a patient with Ehlers-Danlos syndrome. J Vasc Surg 2007;46:360–2.

32

Infectious Aortitis

Paul J. Speicher, B.A. and Heron E. Rodriguez, M.D.

INTRODUCTION

Aortitis is described as inflammation involving at least one layer of the aortic wall and is caused by a number of mechanisms. Confusion remains in the literature regarding how to best categorize the various etiologies of aortic wall inflammation, which can be broadly grouped as infectious and inflammatory. Noninfectious aortitis can be a component of many systemic connective tissue diseases and vasculitides, primarily Takayasu disease and giant cell arteritis, among others.[1] Further, ever since Osler coined the term mycotic aneurysm to describe an aortic wall infection secondary to endocarditis,[2] there has been significant confusion regarding the various types of infectious aortitis. The most common form of infectious aortitis is a secondary infection from a previously placed surgical graft.[3] We refer to this as prosthetic-associated aortic infection. Abdominal aortic aneurysms (AAAs) can also manifest with evidence of severe periaortic inflammation and local and systemic signs of infection. Very often, these aneurysms are saccular instead of fusiform, and we refer to those as mycotic aneurysms, even in the absence of endocarditis (Figure 32–1). Theoretically, seeding of a pre-existing AAA and formation of a saccular aneurysm after infection are possible mechanisms. Less frequently, infection of the aorta can present without an aneurysm and in the absence of any pre-existing known vascular surgery or graft placement. This is thought to result from several mechanisms, all of which lead to the common result of invasion of a pathogen into the aortic wall. During the last 10 years, we have treated 10 patients with systemic signs of infection, periaortic inflammation. and disruption of the aortic wall without aneurysms. As such, primary infectious aortitis has no universally accepted definition. Because the point of entry of infectious agents is presumably always a tissue or organ different than the aorta, true primary infectious aortitis may not exist. In this paper, we use the term secondary infectious aortitis for all types of aortic infection for which a primary infectious source is clinically identified (Table 32–1). We limit the use of the term primary infectious aortitis for the rare cases when after extensive diagnostic work-up, no source of infection is found other than the infected tissue in the aorta and no pre-existing aneurysm was known. Speculatively, an episode of undetected transient bacteremia is responsible for aortic seeding. In two otherwise healthy patients re-

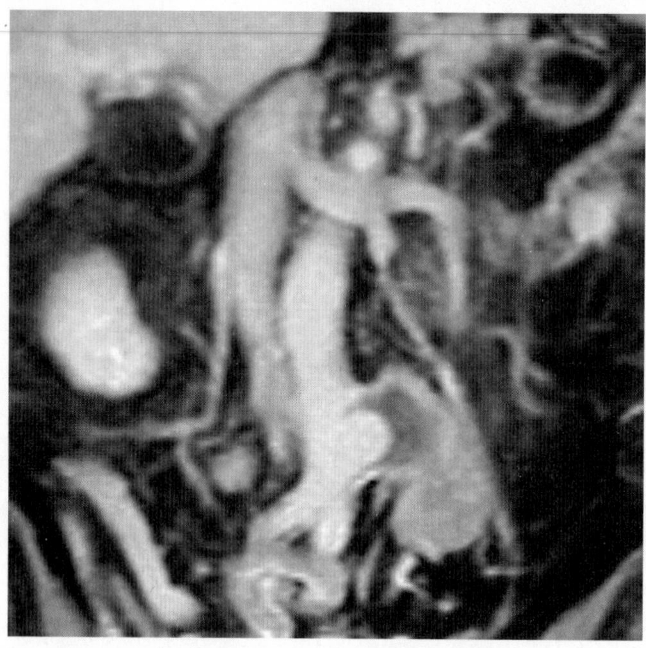

Figure 32-1. MRA showing an infected, saccular aneurysm of the infrarenal aorta.

cently treated in our institution in which no evident source of infection was found after exhaustive testing, the antecedent of prophylactic dental cleaning within 10 days of presentation was observed. This would support such speculation.

PRESENTATION

Prosthetic-associated aortic infection is an increasingly common condition. Many reports have been published describing the management of infected prosthesis after open and endovascular aneurysm repair. Conversely, infectious aortitis not associated with a prosthetic device is a relatively rare entity. Its true incidence is unknown. Given the rarity and notoriously nonspecific clinical manifestations of early aortitis, diagnosis requires a high index of suspicion.[4-5]

TABLE 32-1. ETIOLOGIES OF PRIMARY AND SECONDARY AORTIC INFECTION

Primary aortic infections	Primary aortitis
	Infectious, saccular aneurysm (mycotic)
	Seeding of pre-existing AAAs
Sources for secondary aortic infection	Postoperative aortic stent/graft infection
	Aortic trauma
	Infectious endocarditis
	Oral abscess
	IV drug use
	Infected dialysis graft
	Local spread of contiguous infection

Patients can present with a wide range of symptoms that are notably nonspecific, including fever of unknown origin, back or abdominal pain, leukocytosis, anemia, and elevated erythrocyte sedimentation rate or C-reactive protein levels. Diagnosis of infectious aortitis is difficult and often occurs only after an imaging study reveals periaortic inflammation and disruption of the aortic wall (Figure 32–2). Interestingly, we have noted a predisposition for the visceral segment of the abdominal aorta to be involved in cases of infectious aortitis (Figure 32–3). Similarly, MRI is often able to depict periaortic fluid and localized inflammation, which is suggestive of purulence but not diagnostic of infection. MRI is limited, however, to patients who are hemodynamically stable without signs of impending sepsis. Unfortunately, aortic imaging is often nonspecific in cases of aortitis and is unable to definitively differentiate among infectious, inflammatory, and idiopathic etiologies. The diagnosis of infectious aortitis is complicated by the fact that blood cultures are often negative. Unfortunately, blood cultures are specific but their sensitivity has been poor with reported ranges in the literature of 50 to 69%.[6-8] Once a radiographic study raises the suspicion for an aortic infection, attempts should be made to identify a possible source. History of any prior prosthetic vascular device in the aorta or in a remote location should be noted. A thorough physical examination is performed, looking for signs of infectious endocarditis, oral infections, evidence of intravenous drug use, or any chronic skin lesions. In addition to blood cultures, a transesophageal echocardiogram and dental consultation are performed. A patient labeled as having primary infectious aortitis was found to have a source of infection in his mouth only after x-ray of the mouth

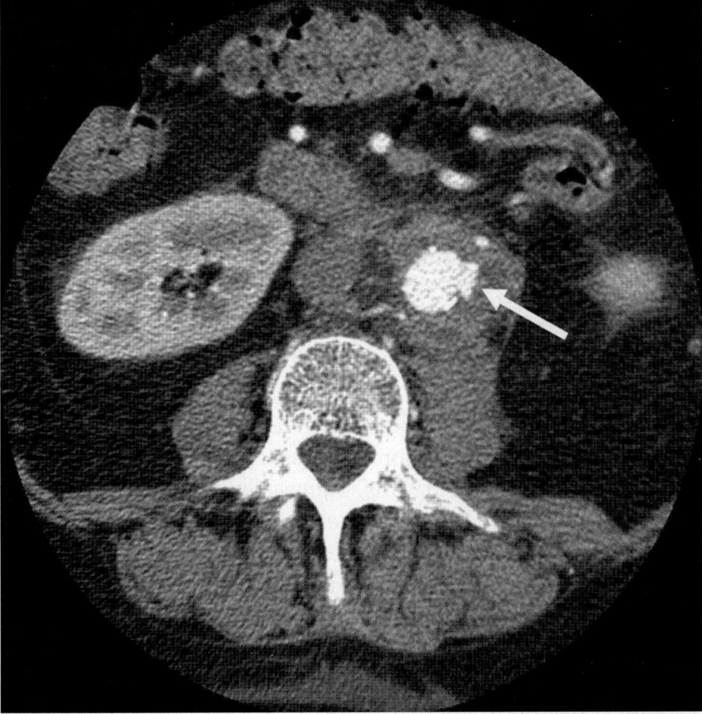

Figure 32-2. CTA showing severe periaortic inflammation with disruption of the aortic wall (arrow).

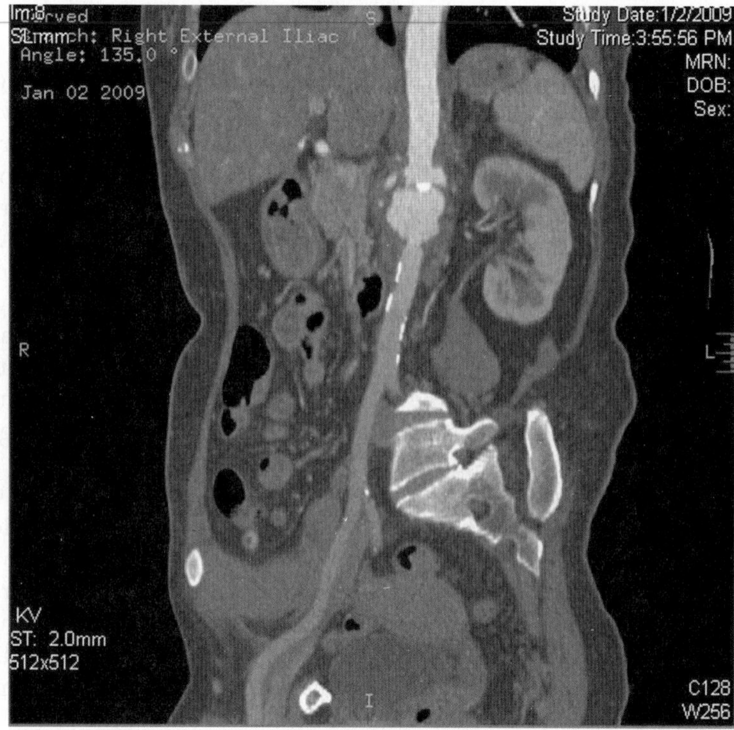

Figure 32-3. CTA showing disruption of the visceral segment of the aorta with severe inflammatory changes.

showed an abscess without any external manifestations on oral mucosal examination. The differential diagnosis for infectious aortitis is broad, including systemic connective tissue disease, atherosclerotic ulceration, and primary aortic tumors. Systemic connective tissue diseases, such as Takayasu disease and giant cell arteritis, should be ruled out in cases of aortitis without clear etiology. Despite their extremely rare nature, primary aortic tumors must also be considered, because intraoperative tumor appearance has been reported to be indistinguishable from that of aortitis.[9]

MICROBIOLOGY

The decline of rheumatic fever and endocarditis over the past century with the advent of antibiotics has led to a shift in the microbiology associated with aortic infections. In more recent studies of infected aortic aneurysms, *Salmonella*, *Staphylococcus*, and *Streptococcus* species are involved most often, and outcomes have been shown to be very pathogen-dependent.[4-5,10-12] Anaerobic infections are also thought to play a role, and their incidence is believed to be underestimated because to difficulties with isolation and culture.[10]

At Northwestern Memorial, since 1998 we have treated 10 patients diagnosed with infectious aortitis not associated with a prosthetic device and without an aneurysm. Five patients were diagnosed with true primary infectious aortitis, because no cause of infection was found after a thorough clinical work-up. One of these patients was found to have intraoperative cultures positive for methicillin-resistant *Staphyloccus aureus* (MRSA)

TABLE 32-2. ETIOLOGIES AND MICROBIOLOGY OF NORTHWESTERN MEMORIAL HOSPITAL (NMH) EXPERIENCE

Patient	Location	Etiology	Culture Results
1	Pararenal	Primary	Negative
2	Paravisceral	Primary	Negative
3	Paravisceral	Primary	Negative
4	Paravisceral	Primary	*S. pneumoniae*
5	Paravisceral	Primary	Methicillin-resistent *S. aureus*
6	Infrarenal	Endocarditis	Methicillin-resistent *S. aureus*
7	Pararenal	Endocarditis	Methicillin-resistent *S. aureus*
8	Paravisceral	Prostatitis	*Escherichia coli* + *S. aureus*
9	Paravisceral	Dialysis catheter	Pan-sensitive *S. aureus*
10	Infrarenal	Dental abscess	Negative

but with negative blood cultures subsequently and no identifiable source of infection. Another patient was transferred from an outside hospital with *Streptococcus pneumoniae* bacteremia and CT scan demonstrating a periaortic stranding suspicious for infection but with no other source of infection and subsequent negative cultures. The 3 remaining patients with primary aortitis had clinical and radiographic evidence suggestive of infection, but no pathogen was isolated. Of the other 6 patients, a pathogen was isolated and a potential source of infection was found (Table 32–2).

MANAGEMENT

Early and aggressive treatment is essential to minimize morbidity and mortality in patients with infectious aortitis. When no definitive source of infection can be determined, laparoscopic or open surgical exploration or CT-guided periaortic aspiration should be performed to establish a diagnosis. Similar to issues with blood cultures, aortic tissue cultures are also not particularly sensitive, and reports indicate that in patients with infectious aortitis, 8 to 25% had negative aortic wall cultures.[7,10,13] When infectious aortitis is suspected, broad-spectrum antibiotics should be initiated immediately, with later treatment tailored to specific blood and tissue cultures and sensitivities.

The surgical management of infectious aortitis is similar for prosthetic-associated aortic infection, mycotic aneurysms, or infectious aortitis. It involves removal of the inflamed or diseased aortic segment with arterial reconstruction to retain distal perfusion. Two broadly defined techniques have been described and implemented for aortic repair and reconstruction: extra-anatomic bypass grafting and in situ reconstruction.

Extra-anatomic Techniques

Extra-anatomic grafting followed by excision of the diseased aortic segment has been widely accepted and remains the classic conservative management for aortic infections. In this approach, arterial reconstruction is carried out via axillobifemoral bypass through tissue planes unaffected by infection. Then, the aorta is exposed and the diseased portion resected using thorough débridement. The obvious advantage of the extra-anatomic bypass approach is that it avoids placing a graft in the infected retroperitoneal space, which is a significant risk factor for postoperative graft infection. The downside to this strategy is that the axillobifemoral bypass is less durable than in situ interposition grafts and runs the risk of subsequent limb thrombosis from the axillofemoral conduit in approximately 25% of patients.[7,14-15] Of even graver consequence is the rare complication of aortic stump blow-out, wherein the proximal aortic stump closure is oversewn or contaminated and eventually fails, leading to rapid internal hemorrhage.[16] Although some clinicians consider extra-anatomic bypass to be the continued gold standard in the surgical management of aortitis, other methods of reconstruction are steadily gaining popularity.

In Situ Techniques

In situ reconstruction in the surgical treatment of aortitis has gained favor among vascular surgeons in recent decades. This approach eliminates concerns regarding aortic stump blow-out while at the same time providing improved vessel patency. Considering that the graft is being placed in an infected tissue field, this approach was originally hampered by unfavorable infection rates with early synthetic prostheses. More recently, however, many concerns have been alleviated by more favorable results with newer graft compositions and techniques.[17] In situ reconstruction has also become more feasible as a result of increased access to advanced pre- and postoperative imaging assessment as well as continued advances in antibiotic therapy. Although the general concept of in situ reconstruction is conserved, there are a number of options available regarding graft compositions: drug-bonded synthetic grafts, autogenous tissue grafts, and either fresh or cryopreserved cadaveric allografts.

Drug-bonded synthetic grafts were created in an attempt to address the classically high infection rates associated with in situ prosthetic graft placement. Prosthetic grafts have the advantage of being technically the most simple, with uniform fabrication and improved patency. Despite direct binding of antibiotics to the synthetic material, increased propensity to postoperative infection remains, and prosthetic grafts are mainly used as a temporizing measure. In studies of antibiotic-soaked grafts by Young and Bandyk, reinfection rates were found to be 7 to 11%, with perioperative mortality rates of 8%.[18-19]

Autogenous tissue grafts are the most favorable from a microbiologic perspective.[20] For autogenous in situ grafting, the patient's femoropopliteal veins are used to reconstruct a portion of the aorta. This allows for significantly increased resistance to infection as well as improved vessel patency compared with extra-anatomic bypass. Studies by Clagett and Nevelsteen have reported graft reinfection rates of 0%, with operative mortality rates of 7% and long-term patency of 83 to 94%.[21-22] This approach is complicated, however, by the increased operating time required to harvest deep veins in the leg, most commonly the superficial femoropopliteal vein. Autogenous grafting also carries its own set of unique morbidities as a result of major manipulation of the venous system in the legs, including permanent leg edema, paresis, fasciotomy, and postoperative deep veini thrombosis (DVT).[23] As a result, autogenous in situ grafting has failed to gain widespread acceptance as a primary repair technique.

Cadaveric allografts were first reported in the late 1940s[24] but have more recently gained significant popularity for in situ repair and have been studied considerably. Historically, cryopreserved and fresh allografts have been plagued by postoperative infections and a lack of adequate tissue typing and pathogen screening in fresh samples. More recently, short-term outcome studies have shown acceptable morbidity and mortality results, and some authors have shown significant benefits when compared with other techniques.[25] The majority of published series include mainly patients with prosthetic-associated aortic infections. A study by Chiesa looking at 44 patients with cryopreserved conduits demonstrated a 0% reinfection rate at 40 months' follow-up.[26] In our own series, we compared 52 patients receiving cryopreserved allografts in various arterial beds to 53 patients receiving either extra-anatomic prosthetic bypass or autogenous in situ reconstruction. In our experience, we demonstrated a 30-day mortality for cryopreserved allografts of 5.2% compared with 7.5% for the combined extra-anatomic and autogenous group. Similarly, 1-year procedure-related mortality was found to be 7.0% and 13.2% in the cryopreserved allograft and nonallograft groups, respectively.[27] Further, Vogt et al. were able to show benefits in survival, duration of hospitalization, ICU care, cost-effectiveness, and postoperative infection when comparing cryopreserved allograft placement with traditional extra-anatomic bypass.[28] As a result, the use of cryopreserved grafts has become a popular alternative as a temporizing measure, allowing for complete resolution of infection before placement of a permanent prosthetic graft. Based on better than expected long-term results, some investigators now consider the use of cryopreserved allografts as a primary alternative in the treatment of aortic infections.[25]

CURRENT SURGICAL APPROACH AT NORTHWESTERN MEMORIAL

Our current preference is the use of cadaveric allografts for in situ replacement of all cases of aortic infections (prosthetic-associated infections, mycotic aneurysms, and primary aortitis). In a few cases, we have used rifampin-soaked Dacron grafts and rarely femoropopliteal venous reconstructions. We reserve the use of extra-anatomic bypasses for patients with severe comorbidities or very elderly patients. All cases of primary aortitis have been treated with homografts. Because most of our patients have had involvement of the visceral segment of the abdominal aorta, a retroperitoneal approach with proximal control of the supraceliac aorta along with dissection and control of the proximal segment of the visceral arteries has been used most frequently. In one patient with concomitant infectious aortitis limited to the infrarenal segment and a ruptured infected femoral aneurysm, a transperitoneal approach was used. After proximal and distal control is achieved, extensive débridement of the involved segment of the aorta and perioartic tissues is carried out (Figure 32–4). Once healthy arterial tissue is obtained at both proximal and distal ends, the homograft is implanted (Figures 32–5 and 32–6). Regarding the use of homografts, several technical points are worth mentioning. When selecting the homograft to be used, the most important determinant is the length and not the diameter of the segment to be replaced. We have found no difficulties in matching the diameter of the native vessels to the diameter of the homograft. In general, homografts expand in diameter about 30 to 40% once pulsatile flow enters their lumina, and we do not hesitate to use homografts with smaller diameters compared with those of the measured native vessels. Conversely, the available length of the homograft usually becomes a limiting factor, and a graft of appropriate length should be chosen. Intraoperatively, it is important to appropriately time the preprocessing of the homograft, because thawing and preparation take no less than 45 minutes. All efforts are made to avoid the placement of clamps in the homograft and to minimize the creation of needle holes. Aortoiliac homografts are placed with the suture-tied visceral branches facing the prevertebral tissues, because more often than not, open holes are present in the posterior aspect of the homograft where untied lumbar vessels are present. This allows for

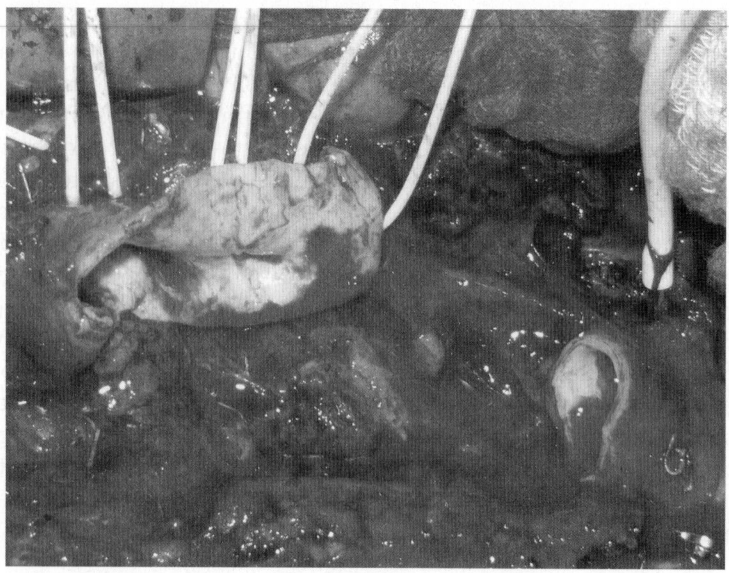

Figure 32-4. Intraoperative view after débridement of the paravisceral aorta in a case of primary aortitis. The origin of the visceral vessels was preserved in an anterior "tongue" of aorta, whereas the supraceliac aorta was removed circumferentially along with the posterior aspect of the visceral aorta.

suture ligation of these defects once flow is allowed to enter the homograft. Finally, we avoid suturing homografts to anything other than healthy arterial tissue (i.e., vein grafts, prosthetic grafts, homograft to homograft anastomosis), because anecdotally, we have had poor results when deviating from this principle.

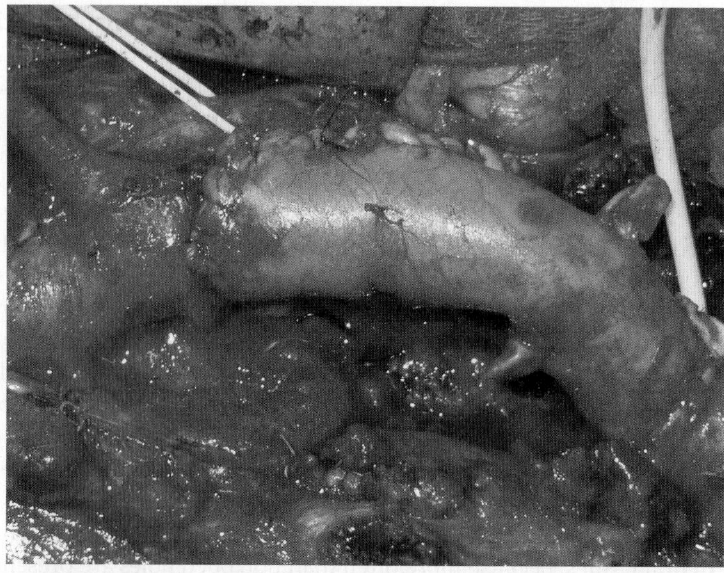

Figure 32-5. Interposition aortic homograft placed in the patient shown in Figure 32-4.

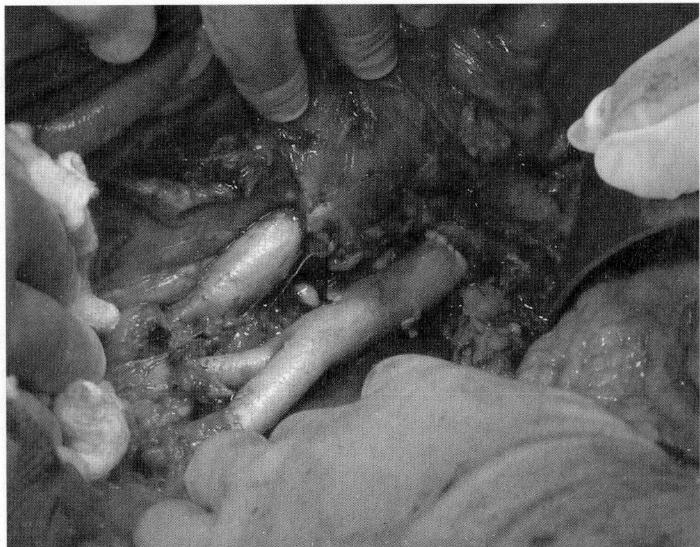

Figure 32-6. Aortic homograft in situ after extensive débridement of an infected aorta and periaortic tissues.

OUTCOMES

Historically, regardless of its cause, infectious aortitis has been associated with poor outcomes. There are no series reporting outcomes after treatment of infectious aortitis that are not associated with pre-existing aneurysms. Less than 50 years ago, infected aortic aneurysms were considered uniformly fatal.[8] Since then, survival rates have been steadily improving. In a series published in 2001 of 43 patients with infected aortic aneurysms, Oderich et al. reported survival rates of 82% and 50% at 1 and 5 years, respectively.[29] Similarly, a 2005 review of six series by Reddy and Weaver of 149 total patients with infected aortoiliac aneurysms revealed an early postoperative survival rate of 77%.[30]

Some recent studies have indicated that certain factors appear to be associated with worse outcomes, including aneurysm rupture, extensive periaortic inflammation, female gender, and both *Salmonella* and *S. aureus* infection.[4,29] Similarly, Fillmore and Valentine[31] have recently stressed the important role of the patient's own immune response in terms of clinical outcome. In terms of surgical approach, compared with in situ repair, extra-anatomic bypass has traditionally been associated with superior outcomes. Recent evidence is mounting, however, to indicate that if done properly, in situ repair may actually have similar or even better results.

CONCLUSIONS

Aortic infections are challenging problems that require complex surgical management. The most common presentation is a prosthetic-associated aortic infection, but infected aneurysms and aortitis without aneurysm formation are also seen. A high level of suspicion is required, and diagnosis depends on imaging studies. Aggressive antibiotic therapy and surgical débridement are the cornerstones of therapy. Several methods for aortic reconstruction are available, each associated with advantages and complications.

REFERENCES

1. Hoffman GS. Determinants of vessel targeting in vasculitis. Clin Dev Immunol. 2004; 11:275–9.
2. Osler W. The Gulstonian lectures on malignant endocarditis. BMJ 1885;1:467.
3. Rojo-Leyva F, Ratliff NB, Cosgrove DM, et al. Study of 52 patients with idiopathic aortitis from a cohort of 1204 surgical cases. Arthritis Rheum. 2000;43:901–7.
4. Sessa C, Farah I, Voirin L, et al. Infected aneurysms of the infrarenal abdominal aorta: diagnostic criteria and therapeutic strategy. Ann Vasc Surg 1997;11:453–63.
5. Teng W, Sarfati MR, Mueller MT, Kraiss LW. Pneumococcal aortitis: a difficult preoperative diagnosis. J Vasc Surg 2006;43:177–9.
6. Anderson CB, Butcher HR, Ballinger WF. Mycotic aneurysms. Arch Surg 1974;109:712.
7. Reddy DJ, Shepard AD, Evans JR, Wright DJ. Management of infected aortoiliac aneurysms. Arch Surg 1991;126:873.
8. Bennett DE, Cherry JK. Bacterial infection of aortic aneurysms: a clinicopathologic study. Am J Surg 1967;113:321.
9. Bohner H, Luther B, Braunstein S, et al. Primary malignant tumors of the aorta: clinical presentation, treatment, and course of different entities. J Vasc Surg 2003;38:1430–3.
10. Brown SL, Busuttil RW, Baker JD, et al. Bacteriologic and surgical determinants of survival in patients with mycotic aneurysms. J Vasc Surg 1984;1:541–7.
11. Maclennan AC, Doyle DL, Sacks SL. Infectious aortitis due to penicillin-resistant *Streptococcus pneumoniae*. Ann Vasc Surg 1997;11:533–5.
12. Bronze MS, Shirwany A, Corbett C, Schaberg DR. Infectious aortitis: an uncommon manifestation of infection with *Streptococcus pneumoniae*. Am J Med 1999;107:627–30.
13. Bitseff EL, Edwards WH, Mulherin JL Jr, et al. Infected abdominal aortic aneurysms. South Med J 1987;80:309–12.
14. Reddy DJ, Lee RE, Oh HK. Suprarenal mycotic aortic aneurysm: surgical management and follow-up. J Vasc Surg 1986;3:917.
15. Trairatvorakul P, Sriphojanart S, Sathapatayavongs B. Abdominal aortic aneurysms infected with *Salmonella*: problems of treatment. J Vasc Surg 1990;12:16.
16. Perera GB, Fujitani RM, Kubaska SM. Aortic graft infection: update on management and treatment options. Vasc Endovasc Surg 2006;40:1–10.
17. Vogt PR, von Segesser LK, Goffin Y, et al. Eradication of aortic infections with the use of cryopreserved arterial homografts. Ann Thorac Surg 1996;62:640–5.
18. Young, RM, Cherry KJ Jr, Davis PM, et al. The results of in situ prosthetic replacement for infected aortic grafts. Am J Surg 1999;178:136–40.
19. Bandyk DF, Novotney ML, Johnson BL, et al. Use of rifampin-soaked gelatin-sealed polyester grafts for in situ treatment of primary aortic and vascular prosthetic infections. J Surg Res 2001;95:44–9.
20. Knosalla C, Goëau-Brissonnière O, Leflon V, et al. Treatment of vascular graft infection by in situ replacement with cryopreserved aortic allografts: an experimental study. J Vasc Surg 1998;27:689–98.
21. Clagett GP, Bowers BL, Lopez-Viego MA, et al. Creation of a neo-aortoiliac system from lower extremity deep and superficial veins. Ann Surg 1993;218:239–48.
22. Nevelsteen A, Lacroix H, Suy R. Autogenous reconstruction with the lower extremity deep veins: an alternative treatment of prosthetic infection after reconstructive surgery for aortoiliac disease. J Vasc Surg 1995;22:129–34.
23. Clagett GP, Valentine RJ, Hagino RT. Autogenous aortoiliac/femoral reconstruction from superficial femoral-popliteal veins: feasibility and durability. J Vasc Surg 1997;25:255–70.
24. Gross RE, Hurwitt ES. Preliminary observation on the use of human arterial grafts in the treatment of certain cardiovascular defects. N Engl J Med 1948;239:578–9.
25. Kieffer E, Gomes D, Chiche L, et al. Allograft replacement for infrarenal aortic graft infection: early and late results in 179 patients. J Vasc Surg 2004;39:1009–17.

26. Chiesa R, Astore D, Piccolo G, et al. Fresh and cryopreserved arterial homografts in the treatment of prosthetic graft infections: experience of the Italian Collaborative Vascular Homograft Group. Ann Vasc Surg 1998;12:457–62.
27. Brown KE, Heyer K, Rodriguez HE, et al. Arterial reconstruction with cryopreserved human allografts in the setting of infection: a single-center experience with midterm follow-up. J Vasc Surg 2009;49:660–6.
28. Vogt PR, Brunner-La Rocca HP, Carrel T, et al. Cryopreserved arterial allografts in the treatment of major vascular infection: a comparison with conventional surgical techniques. J Thorac Cardiovasc Surg 1998;116:965–72.
29. Oderich GS, Panneton JM, Bower TC, et al. Infected aortic aneurysms: aggressive presentation, complicated early outcome but durable results. J Vasc Surg 2001;34:900.
30. Reddy DJ, Weaver MR. Infected aneurysms. In: Rutherford RB, ed., 6th edition. Vascular Surgery. Philadelphia: Elsevier; 2005:1581–96.
31. Fillmore AJ, Valentine RJ. Surgical mortality in patients with infected aortic aneurysms. J Am Coll Surg 2003;196:435–41.

33

Vascular Laboratory Evaluation Following Superior Mesenteric Artery Stenting

Dae Y. Lee, M.D., Erica L. Mitchell, M.D., and Gregory L. Moneta, M.D.

INTRODUCTION

Chronic mesenteric ischemia (CMI) is a rare but potentially lethal disorder. The incidence of the disease is quite low and accounts for less than 5% of all intestinal ischemic diseases. Consequently, the optimal treatment remains poorly defined, and many of the issues regarding the optimal number of vessels to be revascularized and the means of revascularization remain debatable.

ETIOLOGY AND PATHOPHYSIOLOGY

More than 95% of cases of CMI are caused by aortic atherosclerosis encroaching on the ostia of the visceral arteries. A variety of other causes have been implicated in this disease, including collagen vascular disease, inflammatory vasculopathy, and vasoconstrictive drugs, all of which merit investigation in the appropriate clinical setting. In most but not all cases, symptomatic CMI results from high-grade stenosis or occlusion of both the celiac and the SMAs, reflecting the rich collateral network of the three primary mesenteric arteries.

The pathophysiology of CMI is explained by increased demand for oxygenated blood by the intestines and insufficient supply of oxygenated blood to the intestines in response to food. At rest, the splanchnic circulation receives about 20% of the cardiac output and uses about 20% of the body's oxygen consumption. Both blood flow and oxygen demand nearly double after a large meal.[1] In patients with significant occlusive disease of the splanchnic circulation, there is a relative imbalance between tissue supply and demand for oxygen following ingestion of a meal. The result is postprandial pain, so-called intestinal angina. Untreated, the natural history of the disease can be progression to severe cachexia and/or intestinal infarction.

PRESENTATION AND DIAGNOSIS

Two thirds of all patients diagnosed with CMI are women, and the majority have risk factors for systemic atherosclerotic disease. Indeed, most have manifestations of systemic atherosclerotic disease, as evidenced by carotid, femoral, or abdominal bruits, intermittent claudication, diminished peripheral pulses, decreased ankle-brachial systolic pressure ratios, coronary artery disease, and stroke. There is no specific association between CMI and smoking, but the vast majority of the patients with CMI have a history of smoking.[2] The classic presentation of chronic intestinal ischemia is postprandial epigastric pain. The abdominal cramping discomfort usually occurs 30 minutes after eating, gradually increases in severity, and then slowly resolves over 1 to 3 hours.[3-4] Although the pain may be minimal at first, the abdominal pain typically progressively increases in severity over weeks to months. Patients may develop a fear of eating (sitophobia) with resultant weight loss and malnutrition. Diarrhea, nausea, and vomiting are other common nonspecific manifestations of the disease.

Diagnosis of CMI can be difficult owing to the vague nature of the complaints initially. Abdominal plain films and CT scans are usually normal, although vascular calcification may be present. Many patients are misdiagnosed as having biliary colic, gastritis, peptic ulcer disease, or even diverticulitis. Patients therefore often experience months of symptoms prior to diagnosis or bowel infarction. A high index of suspicion is therefore needed for a timely diagnosis and lifesaving intervention.

Virtually all patients with CMI have high-grade stenosis or occlusion of the superior mesenteric artery (SMA), and therefore, detection of SMA lesions is the cornerstone of the diagnosis of CMI. Angiography remains the gold standard for identifying the visceral artery lesions associated with CMI. However, owing to the invasive nature of the procedure and the nephrotoxicity of the contrast material, other modalities of detecting mesenteric artery disease are frequently utilized when initially evaluating a patient for CMI. In particular, the initial diagnosis of significant native artery visceral artery stenoses associated with CMI can be made using duplex ultrasound.[5-6] There are well-established duplex ultrasound criteria for identification of high-grade stenosis in the SMA and celiac arteries, with duplex evaluation of the SMA having very high levels of sensitivity and specificity. Studies performed at our institution comparing mesenteric duplex scans and arteriograms, demonstrated that a SMA peak systolic velocity (PSV) of ≥ 275 cm/sec or no flow signal are reliable indicators of a 70% or greater angiographic stenosis of the SMA.[3,7-8] Similar studies performed at Dartmouth have validated the accuracy of duplex ultrasound criteria for a ≥50% SMA stenosis, using a PSV of ≥300 cm/sec.[9-10] Because the negative predictive value of duplex ultrasonography approaches 99%, it is justifiable to pursue other etiologies of abdominal pain after a negative duplex study.[11]

TREATMENT STRATEGIES

Once the diagnosis of CMI is made based on symptoms and high-grade stenosis of the SMA and/or celiac arteries as indicated by duplex ultrasound criteria, arteriography should be performed in planning mesenteric revascularization for CMI (Figure 33–1). Medical management alone is not effective. The goals of revascularization in symptomatic patients are to improve symptoms and nutritional status and prevent intestinal infarction.

Rarely is such intervention emergent, allowing the appropriate medical work-up to be undertaken to minimize the morbidity of surgery.

Open surgical repair employing either antegrade or retrograde bypasses or transaortic endarterectomy has been the gold standard of treatment for CMI since the first successful repair reported by Shaw from the Massachusetts General Hospital in 1958.[12] Open surgical repair has been successful in most patients with excellent long-term relief of symptoms. Park and associates[13] showed that the rate of symptomatic recurrences was not different for single-vessel versus multiple-vessel reconstructions or for antegrade versus retrograde grafts. Operative repair, although effective, is associated with significant morbidity. Such morbidity is not surprising in this patient population, because many patients with CMI have advanced generalized atherosclerosis, significant weight loss, malnutrition, and low albumin levels, all predictors of increased morbidity after major surgical procedures.[14]

In recent years, endovascular revascularization has emerged as an alternative treatment for CMI in the elderly or particularly in higher-risk patient. In a recent study, Schermerhorn et al.[15] found endovascular revascularization for CMI has been increasing in frequency for all patients with CMI. In appropriate patients with two- or three-vessel mesenteric artery disease, including that of the SMA, the preferential endovascular intervention is usually treatment of the SMA with angioplasty and stenting

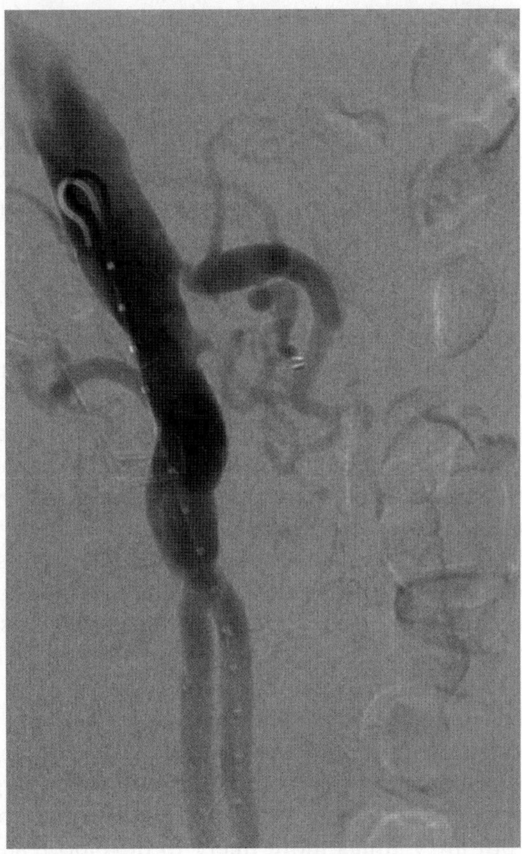

Figure 33-1. Preoperative arteriogram showing celiac and superior mesenteric artery stenosis (SMA).

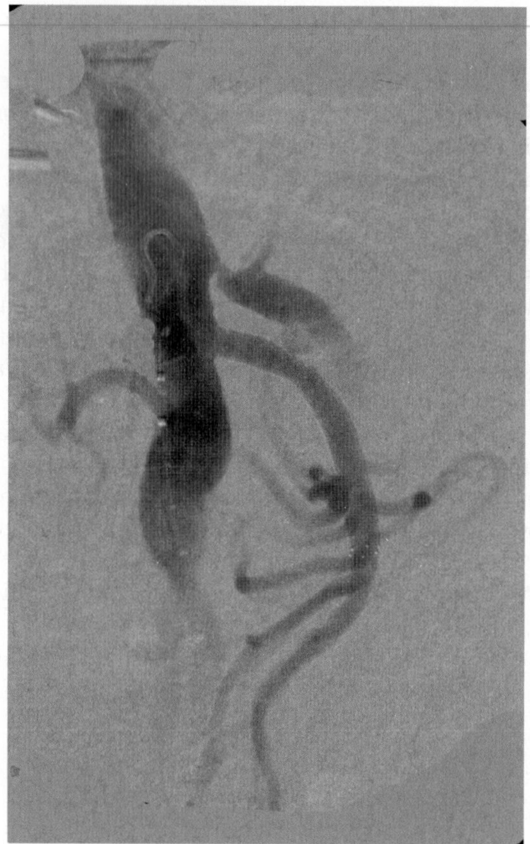

Figure 33-2. Postprocedure arteriogram showing an SMA stent with resolution of stenosis.

(Figure 33–2). If the SMA cannot be treated endoluminally, the celiac artery can also be treated with endovascular techniques. Because of the risk of stent crushing due to repeated extrinsic compression from the median arcuate ligament, balloon-expanded stents are avoided in the celiac artery, unless one is confident that there is only an atherosclerotic etiology of the celiac artery stenosis. Self-expanding nitinol stents are probably the most appropriate choice in this location, given the metal's shape memory and its ability to withstand repetitive compression stresses.[16]

There are no randomized controlled trials comparing open versus endovascular treatment for CMI. The general consensus is that angioplasty or stenting for CMI is a less morbid but also less durable alternative to open surgical intervention. Reports of percutaneous transluminal angioplasty (PTA) of visceral atherosclerotic lesions indicate initial technical success is achieved in up to 90 to 100%.[16-21] The overall periprocedural mortality rate of the endovascular approach is between 0 and 13%, and the complication rate is between 0 and 25%. Durability is in question, with reported recurrence rates of symptoms ranging from 0 to 60%.[22-23]

Brown and associates[18] found that compared with open surgery, SMA stent patients have lower perioperative major morbidity and shorter hospital and intensive care lengths of stay but are 7 times more likely to develop restenosis, 4 times more likely to develop recurrent symptoms, and 15 times more likely to require reintervention. Landis et al. [24] also found that percutaneous intervention had durable early and midterm clinical success but frequently required repeated interventions to maintain assisted primary patency. However, in one of the largest series of CMI patients treated with endovascular therapy to date, Silva et al.[25] found results supportive of endovascular therapy. Long-term benefits and symptom recurrence were comparable with those reported with surgical revascularization. The authors in this study evaluated 59 patients with CMI who underwent stent placement in 79 stenotic mesenteric arteries. Fifty of the 59 patients had relief of symptoms, and only 17% of the patients had recurrence of symptoms, with a mean follow-up time of 38±15 months.

POSTPROCEDURE SURVEILLANCE

Owing to the high costs associated with CTA and MRA, the invasive nature of arteriography, and the nephrotoxicity of contrast medium associated with arteriograms and CTAs, duplex ultrasound has been used for postoperative surveillance of mesenteric artery bypass grafts. A recent study performed at our institution characterized duplex-derived flow velocities in mesenteric artery bypass grafts to serve as standards for postoperative surveillance of mesenteric bypass grafts.[26]

Similarly, investigational efforts have recently shifted to using duplex scanning as a follow-up tool for patients with splanchnic artery stents.[27] Ultrasound criteria for stenosis within mesenteric artery stents are currently not available. Duplex-derived PSVs and end-diastolic velocities may depend on the caliber of the artery beyond the stent, the diameter of the stent, and the length of native artery that is stented. Despite the lack of validation data, it is routine in many centers to use post–stent duplex scanning to assess patency of mesenteric artery stents.

There are a few studies that used duplex scanning to evaluate for restenosis in stented mesenteric arteries. AbuRahma et al.[17] evaluated 22 patients who underwent angioplasty and stenting of the celiac or SMAs for symptomatic chronic visceral ischemia. These authors obtained high initial technical (96%) and clinical (95%) success rates; however, PTA and stenting were associated with a high incidence of late restenosis based on strict Doppler criteria. Freedom from recurrent stenosis (≥70%) at 1, 2, 3, and 4 years was 65%, 47%, 39%, and 13%; freedom from recurrent symptoms was 67% at all 4 intervals. Fenwick and associates[28] also found high restenosis rates based on Doppler criteria for their patients treated with SMA stents. In their study, restenosis also did not correlate with recrudescence of symptoms.

Although follow-up of endovascularly treated mesenteric vessels is said to be important because of the high incidence of restenosis in stented vessels, there is no evidence that intervention on the basis of duplex-defined restenosis improves long-term patency or prevents recurrence of symptoms.[29] This may in part be because the criteria used to define stenosis in native nonstented arteries are not applicable to stented SMAs. It does appear that higher velocity levels are required for identification of stenosis in stented internal carotid arteries and renal arteries than would be expected from criteria developed for identifying stenosis in these native arteries.[30-33] A similar situation may exist for the mesenteric vessels. Therefore, we felt additional work evaluating flow velocities in mesenteric arteries treated with angioplasty and stenting was required. Investigation is also necessary to determine whether these changes in mesenteric flow velocities can be associated with change in symptoms and the need for further intervention in patients with CMI treated with percutaneous angioplasty/stents.

In a recent study, we evaluated whether traditional duplex criteria for high-grade native artery mesenteric artery stenosis can be extrapolated to stented SMAs.[34] We reviewed combined interventional radiology and vascular surgery registries for all visceral arterial angiography procedures performed from January 1997 to December 2007 at Oregon Health & Science University (OHSU). Patients who underwent SMA stenting for atherosclerotic lesions were identified and selected for review. Specific angiographic data extracted included percent angiographic SMA, celiac and inferior mesenteric artery stenosis prior to stent placement, pressure gradients measured across the SMA lesion prior to stent placement, and pressure gradients measured across the SMA lesion after stent placement. Pressure gradients were obtained with a coaxial system with the aortic pressure obtained from the sheath in the aorta and the SMA pressure obtained from the catheter tip placed beyond the stenosis. Vascular laboratory data included fasting duplex determination of the maximal native artery SMA PSV prestenting, and the maximal PSV in the region of the SMA stent (proximal and distal ends of the stent as well as intrastent) poststenting of the SMA.

Early clinical failures were evaluated with repeat angiography. We did not perform follow-up angiography in the absence of clinical indications. Duplex scans, angiographic images, and catheter-derived pressure gradients in the SMA prior to and after stenting of SMA stenoses were compared. Technical success of SMA stent placement was defined as <30% angiographic SMA stenosis after stent placement. Pressure gradients were not used to judge technical success of the SMA stent procedure.

During the study period, 35 patients considered high risk for open surgical intervention underwent SMA stent placement for either acute or chronic symptoms of visceral ischemia. Symptoms included acute onset of abdominal pain, postprandial abdominal pain, diarrhea, vomiting, weight loss, and sitophobia (fear of food). Excluding procedures performed for debranching of the aorta for stent graft repair of thoracoabdominal aneurysm, there were also 86 open mesenteric revascularizations performed during this same time frame.

Angiographic degree of SMA stenosis was determined in 10% increments using calibers from lateral aortograms in all patients both pre- and poststenting. All patients except 3 had ≥70% diameter stenosis of the SMA prior to stenting. Two of these patients had occlusion of the SMA prior to stent placement. Twenty-four patients (69%) had concomitant ≥70% celiac artery stenosis or occlusion, 2 patients had aberrant hepatic arteries arising off the stenotic SMA, and all but 2 patients had high-grade IMA stenosis (≥70%) or occlusion. Overall, 31 patients (89%) had high-grade stenosis of two of the three principal mesenteric arteries. The 3 patients with <70% SMA stenosis had approximately 60% diameter reduction of the SMA and prestent pressure gradients measuring more than 47 mm Hg. Two had concomitant celiac artery occlusion or 90% stenosis.

No celiac artery or inferior mesenteric artery stenoses or occlusions were treated. The technical success of SMA stent placement was defined by angiographic criteria in all cases, with all 36 patients treated having <30% angiographic residual SMA stenosis following stenting. A single SMA stent was placed in 28 patients, and two stents were placed in 6 patients; 1 patient had four stents placed.

Preintervention pressure gradients across the SMA stenosis were obtained in 20 stenotic but patent SMAs (two occluded SMAs were stented) and averaged

57±38 mm Hg (range 15 to 187 mm Hg). Poststent pressure gradients were obtained in 22 patients and averaged 11±13 mm Hg (range 0 to 45 mm Hg). In 15 cases, poststent pressure gradients were <15 mm Hg, with 8 patients having poststent measured pressure gradients >15 mm Hg (17, 18, 20, 20, 25, 40, and 45 mm Hg). When pre- and poststenting pressure gradients were compared using a paired t-test in the 18 patients with stenotic SMAs that were stented, the pressure gradients fell significantly from a mean of 57 mm Hg to 10 mm Hg (P<.001) (Figures 33–3 and 33–4).

There were 6 patients with <50% celiac artery stenosis who had pressure gradients measured in the SMA following stent placement. In all but 1 of these patients, the post-SMA stent pressure gradient was 0, and in the remaining patient, it was only 7 mm Hg. Sixteen patients with ≥60 to 99% celiac artery stenosis or occlusion had SMA pressure gradients measured postplacement of the SMA stent. The mean post-SMA stent pressure gradient in these patients was 14 mm Hg (range 0 to 45 mm Hg). Comparing pre- and poststent pressure gradients in patients with <60% celiac stenosis with those with >60% celiac stenosis showed that the presence of a celiac stenosis of ≥60% was associated with an increased SMA pressure gradient post-SMA stenting (P=.006).

Fasting prestent screening duplex scans were performed in 18 patients. PSVs in the native SMA were <275 cm/sec in 16. Mean PSV was 450±152 cm/sec in patients with patent arteries (range 256 to 770 cm/sec). Two patients had occluded SMAs with no demonstrated flow in the vessels by ultrasonography prior to stent placement. Thirteen patients underwent poststent surveillance ultrasonography between 1 and 45 days (mean 11.5 days) following placement of the SMA stent. Peak systolic

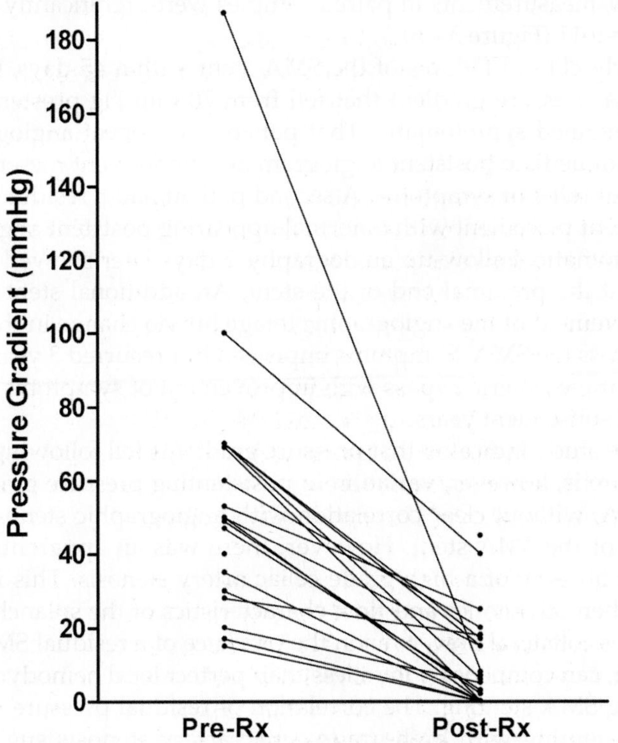

Figure 33-3. Dot plot of pressure gradients pre- and poststenting of the SMA.

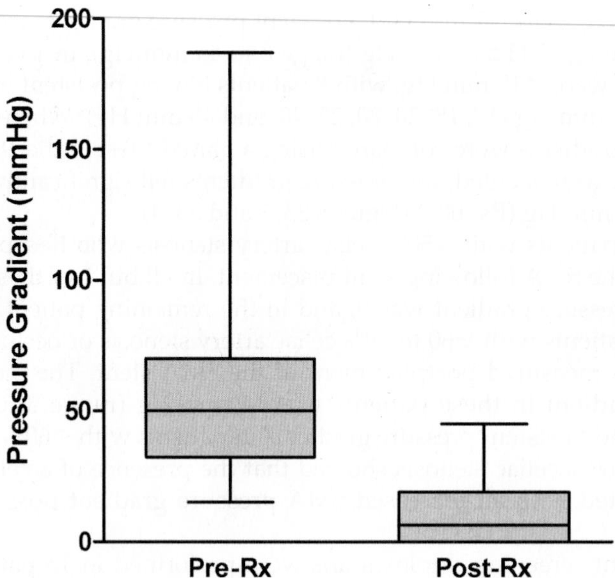

Figure 33-4. Box plot showing pressure gradient in the SMA pre- and poststenting. Thick horizontal lines, boxes, and error bars denote median, interquartile range, and range respectively; P<0.001.

velocities exceeded criteria for ≥70% native SMA stenosis (≥275 cm/sec) in every post-stent velocity measurement (mean 336±45 cm/sec, range 279 to 416 cm/sec [Figure 33–5]). However, PSV measurements in paired samples were significantly lower post-stent than present; P=.011 (Figure 33–6).

There were 2 early clinical failures of the SMA stent within 45 days. One patient had a measured SMA pressure gradient that fell from 70 mm Hg prestent to 17 mm Hg poststent and remained symptomatic. That patient had repeat angiography with no change from the immediate poststent angiogram and underwent mesenteric artery bypass with long-term relief of symptoms. A second patient had a residual 20 mm Hg gradient following stent placement with a normal-appearing poststent angiogram and also remained symptomatic. Follow-up angiography 2 days later showed a questionable weblike defect at the proximal end of the stent. An additional stent was placed with apparent improvement of the angiographic image but no change in the measured pressure gradient across the SMA. Symptoms improved but recurred 3 years later, and the patient underwent mesenteric bypass with improvement of symptoms and no further procedures for 4 subsequent years.

The data from the study indicated that pressure gradients fell following placement of an SMA stent. There is, however, variation in poststenting pressure gradients measured across the SMA, without clear correlation with angiographic stenosis or short-term clinical failure of the SMA stent. However, there was an apparent correlation with the presence or absence of a high-grade celiac artery stenosis. This result likely reflects the complex hemodynamics and flow characteristics of the splanchnic circulation, in which perhaps collateral flow, even in the presence of a residual SMA pressure gradient poststenting, can compensate for a less than perfect local hemodynamic result in the SMA following SMA stenting. The correlation of residual pressure gradients in the SMA following stenting with high-grade celiac artery stenosis suggests that a stented SMA by itself is insufficient to normalize the splanchnic circulation. However,

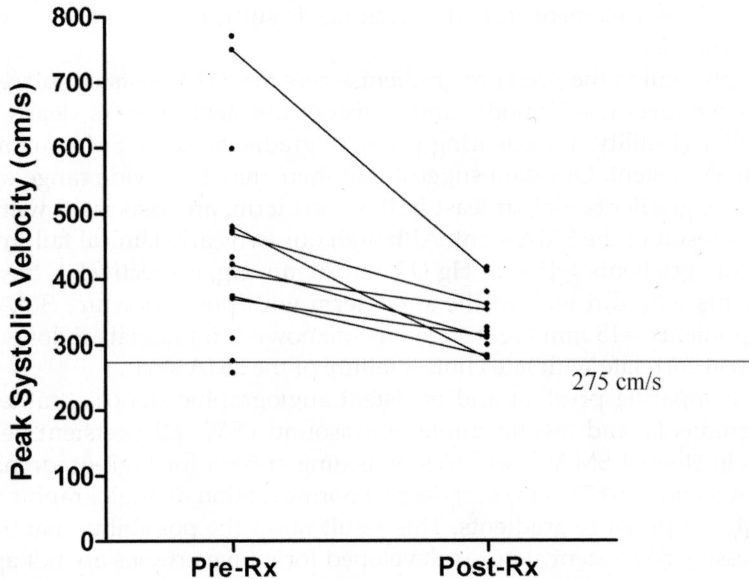

Figure 33-5. Dot plot of SMA PSVs prior to and after SMA stent placement.

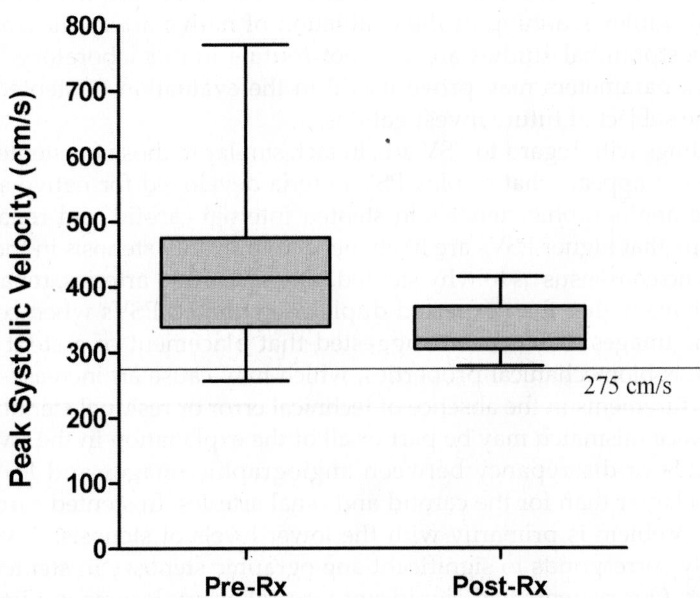

Figure 33-6. Box plot showing SMA PSVs pre- and poststenting. Thick horizontal lines, boxes, and error bars denote median, interquartile range, and range, respectively; P=.011. Dashed line represents >70% SMA stenosis for PSV>275 cm/sec.

in most cases, improvement in hemodynamics is sufficient to improve symptoms of intestinal ischemia.

Although a fall in the pressure gradient across the SMA poststent placement likely indicates some favorable hemodynamic effect of the stent, there is clearly no consensus as to clinical utility of measuring pressure gradients in the SMA following placement of an SMA stent. Our data suggest that there may be a wide range of post-SMA stent pressure gradients that, at least in the short term, are associated with an acceptable clinical result of the SMA stent. Although our two early clinical failures had post-stent pressure gradients >15 mm Hg (17 and 20 mm Hg, respectively), there were five other patients who did well in the short term with postprocedure SMA measured pressure gradients >15 mm Hg. It remains unknown if immediate follow-up pressure gradients will correlate with late clinical failure of the SMA stent.

When comparing prestent and poststent angiographic stenosis, catheter-derived pressure gradients, and fasting duplex ultrasound PSVs, all poststent velocity measurements in stented SMAs had PSVs exceeding criteria for high-grade native artery ≥70% SMA stenosis (≥275 cm/sec) despite normalization of angiographic images and greatly reduced pressure gradients. This result raises the possibility that duplex criteria for assessing SMA stent stenosis developed for native arteries are not applicable to stented arteries.

Other duplex parameters may be more useful than PSVs in the evaluation of the stented SMA. Because of our long-standing use of PSVs in the evaluation of mesenteric artery stenosis, other duplex parameters, such as poststenotic turbulence or measurements of residual stenosis from B-mode images are not routinely recorded in our laboratory. Also, previous studies from our institution have shown limited utility of postprandial duplex scanning in the evaluation of native artery mesenteric stenosis. Therefore, postprandial studies are also not routine in our laboratory.[35] These additional duplex parameters may prove useful in the evaluation of stented arteries and should be the subject of future investigations.

Our findings with regard to PSV are, in fact, similar to those for stented carotid and renal arteries. It appears that duplex PSV criteria developed for native artery stenosis overestimate angiographic stenosis in stented internal carotid and renal arteries.[22-23] It also appears that higher PSVs are likely needed to stratify stenosis in these vessels.

There is no consensus as to why stented internal carotid arteries, renal arteries, and now SMAs have higher than expected duplex determined PSVs when compared with angiographic images. It has been suggested that placement of a stent into a native artery alters its biomechanical properties, which may cause an increase in ultrasound velocity measurements in the absence of technical error or residual stenotic disease.[31-32]

Compliance mismatch may be part or all of the explanation in the SMA. However, the magnitude of discrepancy between angiographic images and PSVs in stented SMAs seems larger than for the carotid and renal arteries. In stented carotid and renal arteries, the problem is primarily with the lower levels of stenosis. A very high PSV still generally corresponds to significant angiographic stenoses in stented carotid and renal arteries. Our patients had significant visceral artery lesions in virtually all their primary mesenteric arteries but only the SMA was treated. It may be that high flow levels through the stented SMA under such circumstances account, in part, for the large discrepancy between ultrasound and angiographic findings in stented SMAs.

There are no standardized ultrasound criteria for the detection of high-grade stenosis in stented SMAs. Our recent study showed that angiographic pressure gradients in stented SMAs are affected by the presence or absence of high-grade celiac artery stenoses. In addition, although fasting duplex-measured SMA PSVs are reduced after stenting, they remain above criteria levels that predict high-grade native artery SMA stenosis. It appears that duplex ultrasound PSV criteria for nonstented SMAs cannot be applied to stented SMAs and new duplex ultrasound criteria are required to predict high-grade stenosis in stented SMAs. Prospective studies and poststent surveillance protocols are needed to more systematically address this question and to develop new ultrasound criteria for the evaluation of stented SMAs. In the interim, studies utilizing only ultrasound follow-up of stented SMAs may be overestimating rates of recurrent stenosis in the stented SMA.

CONCLUSION

It appears that the use of duplex scanning in the evaluation of mesenteric arteries after stenting is feasible. However, there are no precise ultrasound criteria for stenosis within stented mesenteric arteries. Despite the lack of validation data, we routinely use poststent duplex scanning, at baseline and to serve as comparisons for follow-up evaluation of stent patency. We believe increasing markedly elevated, focal peak systolic velocities on serial examinations within the stented regions should lead to a contrast angiogram to confirm in-stent or distal native arterial stenosis. A stable isolated PSV elevation in a stented SMA without recurrence of symptoms perhaps can be safely followed.

REFERENCES

1. Bell DR. Special circulations. In: Rhoades RA, Bell DR, 3rd ed. Medical Physiology: Principles for Clinical Medicine. Philadelphia: Lippincott Williams & Wilkins; 2008, p. 296.
2. Moawad J, Gewertz BL. Chronic mesenteric ischemia: clinical presentation and diagnosis. Surg Clin North Am 1997;77:357–69.
3. Moneta GL, Taylor DC, Helton WS, et al. Duplex ultrasound measurement of postprandial intestinal blood flow: effect of meal composition. Gastroenterology 1988;95:1294–301.
4. Poole JW, Sammartano RJ, Boley SJ. Hemodynamic basis of the pain of chronic mesenteric ischemia. Am J Surg 1987;153:171–6.
5. Jäger KA, Fortner GS, Thiele BL, et al. Noninvasive diagnosis of intestinal angina. J Clin Ultrasound 1984;12:588–91.
6. Nicholls SC, Kohler TR, Martin RL, et al. Use of hemodynamic parameters in the diagnosis of mesenteric insufficiency. J Vasc Surg 1986;3:507–10.
7. Moneta GL, Lee RW, Yeager RA, et al. Mesenteric duplex scanning: a blinded prospective study. J Vasc Surg 1993;17:79–84; discussion 85–6.
8. Moneta GL, Yeager RA, Dalman R, et al. Duplex ultrasound criteria for diagnosis of splanchnic artery stenosis or occlusion. J Vasc Surg 1991;14:511–8; discussion 518–20.
9. Bowersox JC, Zwolak RM, Walsh DB, et al. Duplex ultrasonography in the diagnosis of celiac and mesenteric artery occlusive disease. J Vasc Surg 1991;14:780–6; discussion 786–8.
10. Zwolak RM, Fillinger MF, Walsh DB, et al. Mesenteric and celiac duplex scanning: a validation study. J Vasc Surg 1998;27:1078–87; discussion 1088.
11. Nicoloff AD, Williamson WK, Moneta GL, et al. Duplex ultrasonography in evaluation of splanchnic artery stenosis. Surg Clin North Am 1997;77:339–55.
12. Shaw RS, Maynard EP. Acute and chronic thrombosis of the mesenteric arteries associated with malabsorption; a report of two cases successfully treated by thromboendarterectomy. N Engl J Med 1958;258:874–8.

13. Park WM, Cherry KJ, Chua HK, et al. Current results of open revascularization for chronic mesenteric ischemia: a standard for comparison. J Vasc Surg 2002;35:853–9.
14. Gibbs J, Cull W, Henderson W, et al. Preoperative serum albumin level as a predictor of operative mortality and morbidity: results from the National VA Surgical Risk Study. Arch Surg 1999;134:36–42.
15. Schermerhorn ML, Giles KA, Hamdan AD, et al. Mesenteric revascularization: management and outcomes in the United States, 1988–2006. J Vasc Surg 2009;50:341–8.e341.
16. Sharafuddin MJ, Olson CH, Sun S, et al. Endovascular treatment of celiac and mesenteric arteries stenoses: applications and results. J Vasc Surg 2003;38:692–8.
17. AbuRahma AF, Stone PA, Bates MC, et al. Angioplasty/stenting of the superior mesenteric artery and celiac trunk: early and late outcomes. J Endovasc Ther 2003;10:1046–53.
18. Brown DJ, Schermerhorn ML, Powell RJ, et al. Mesenteric stenting for chronic mesenteric ischemia. J Vasc Surg 2005;42:268–74.
19. Razavi M, Chung HH. Endovascular management of chronic mesenteric ischemia. Tech Vasc Interv Rad 2004;7:155–9.
20. Schaefer PJ, Schaefer FK, Mueller-Huelsbeck S, et al. Chronic mesenteric ischemia: stenting of mesenteric arteries. Abdom Imaging 2007;32:304–9.
21. Yazdi HR, Youness F, Laroia S, et al. Mesenteric artery stenting for chronic mesenteric ischemia. J Vasc Dis Manag.
22. Matsumoto AH, Tegtmeyer CJ, Fitzcharles EK, et al. Percutaneous transluminal angioplasty of visceral arterial stenoses: results and long-term clinical follow-up. J Vasc Interv Radiol 1995;6:165–74.
23. Sheeran SR, Murphy TP, Khwaja A, et al. Stent placement for treatment of mesenteric artery stenoses or occlusions. JVIR 1999;10:861–7.
24. Landis MS, Rajan DK, Simons ME, et al. Percutaneous management of chronic mesenteric ischemia: outcomes after intervention. JVIR 2005;16:1319–25.
25. Silva JA, White CJ, Collins TJ, et al. Endovascular therapy for chronic mesenteric ischemia. J Am Coll Cardiol 2006;47:944–50.
26. Liem TK, Segall JA, Wei W, et al. Duplex scan characteristics of bypass grafts to mesenteric arteries. J Vasc Surg 2007;45:922–7; discussion 927–8.
27. Armstrong PA. Visceral duplex scanning: evaluation before and after artery intervention for chronic mesenteric ischemia. Pers Vasc Surg Endov Ther 2007;19:386–92; discussion 393–94.
28. Fenwick JL, Wright IA, Buckenham TM. Endovascular repair of chronic mesenteric occlusive disease: the role of duplex surveillance. Aust N Z J Surg 2007;77:60–3.
29. Morvay Z, Nagy E, Bagi R, et al. Sonographic follow-up after visceral artery stenting. J Ultrasound Med 2004;23:1057–64.
30. AbuRahma AF, Abu-Halimah S, Bensenhaver J, et al. Optimal carotid duplex velocity criteria for defining the severity of carotid in-stent restenosis. J Vasc Surg 2008;48:589–94.
31. Armstrong PA, Bandyk DF, Johnson BL, et al. Duplex scan surveillance after carotid angioplasty and stenting: a rational definition of stent stenosis. J Vasc Surg 2007;46:460–5; discussion 465–6.
32. Lal BK, Hobson RW, Goldstein J, et al. Carotid artery stenting: is there a need to revise ultrasound velocity criteria? J Vasc Surg 2004;39:58–66.
33. Setacci C, Chisci E, Setacci F, et al. Grading carotid intrastent restenosis: a 6-year follow-up study. Stroke 2008;39:1189–96.
34. Mitchell EL, Chang EY, Landry GJ, et al. Duplex criteria for native superior mesenteric artery stenosis overestimate stenosis in stented superior mesenteric arteries. J Vasc Surg 2009;50:335–40.
35. Gentile AT, Moneta GL, Lee RW, et al. Usefulness of fasting and postprandial duplex ultrasound examinations for predicting high-grade superior mesenteric artery stenosis. Am J Surg 1995;169:476–9.

34

Complex Abdominal Aortic Diseases and Reconstruction in Children

Ying Zhuge, M.D. and
Omaida C. Velazquez, M.D., F.A.C.S.

Diseases of the aorta and its branches in the pediatric population manifest in the form of two major groups: aneurysms and stenoses. These two processes can occur in either the thoracic or the abdominal aorta. Patients with aneurysms can present with a pulsatile abdominal mass and abdominal pain and be diagnosed incidentally or after rupture has occurred. Stenosis, conversely, usually manifests with hypertension and its sequelae, which can range from headaches to seizures, to cardiomyopathy, to renal failure. Causes of these diseases include congenital, inflammatory, traumatic, and idiopathic processes.[1] In the following chapter, we review the epidemiology, pathophysiology, diagnosis, and treatment of the more common vascular pathologies that afflict the pediatric abdominal aorta: abdominal aortic aneurysm, renovascular hypertension, middle aortic syndrome (MAS), and traumatic vascular processes.

ANEURYSMS

Arterial aneurysms in childhood are extremely rare and usually acquired.[2-3] Common causes of acquired aneurysmal disease include infection (mycotic aneurysms), trauma (umbilical artery catheterization), connective tissue disease (e.g., Marfan syndrome, Ehlers-Danlos syndrome, and tuberous sclerosis), and vasculitis (e.g., Takayasu arteritis).[3-5] In 1991, Sarkar et al. developed a classification system for these aneurysms (Table 34–1).[6]

Mycotic aneurysms develop from septic emboli from the heart, and in neonates, umbilical artery catheterization is becoming an increasingly important factor.[3] The usual culprits are *Streptococcus*, methicillin-resistant *Staphylococcus aureus*, *Pseudomonas*,

TABLE 34-1. CLASSIFICATION OF CHILDHOOD ARTERIAL ANEURYSMS

Class	Peripheral Artery Affected	Clinical Characteristics
I. Arterial infection	Aorta (especially thoracic), iliac	Cardiovascular anomalies and umbilical catheterization; predisposing factors; dyspnea, cough, chest pain with progression to rupture, and death if untreated
II. Giant cell aortoarteritis	Aorta (peripheral arteries, rare)	Signs and symptoms vary from being absent to shock; untreated aortic lesions progress to rupture
III. Autoimmune vasculitis	Renal, hepatic, and splenic arterial branches	Usually asymptomatic but may cause hematuria, perirenal hematomas, or death with rupture
IV. Kawasaki disease	Coronary (20–30%), axillo-brachial, iliofemoral, hepatic	Often asymptomatic; myocardial infarction or tamponade (coronary), limb ischemia (extremity), and obstructive jaundice (hepatic) may occur
V. Medial degeneration, Marfan, and Ehlers-Danlos syndromes	Aorta	Aortic rupture or dissection common; arteriography and vascular reconstruction hazardous in type IV Ehlers-Danlos syndrome
VI. Medial degeneration—other forms	Aorta (peripheral arteries, rare)	Associated with cardiac and aortic anomalies; often present with aortic dissection or rupture
VII. Arterial dysplasia	Renal	Usually asymptomatic, detected during arteriography for renovascular hypertension
VIII. Idiopathic, congenital	Iliofemoral, brachial, aorta	Often asymptomatic but may cause limb ischemia; rupture unreported
IX. Extravascular causes	Aorta, visceral, and extremity arteries	Aortic aneurysms often rupture; peripheral lesions asymptomatic; visceral lesions may cause gastrointestinal bleeding

Reprinted with permission from Kaye AJ, Slemp AE, Chang B, et al. Complex vascular reconstruction of abdominal aorta and its branches in the pediatric population. J Pediatr Surg 2008:43:1082–8.

(Excerpt from Sarkar R, Coran A, Cilley R, et al. Arterial aneurysms in children: clinicopathologic classfication. J Vasc Surg 1991; 13:47–56.)

and *Salmonella*.[3,7] Affected vessels usually have underlying disease such as atheroma, cystic medial necrosis, congenital abnormalities, or trauma, and bifurcations and coarctations are sites of predilection.[3] These aneurysms must be surgically repaired to prevent rupture, which may be imminent in some presentations. Conventional aneurysmorrhaphy (as in adult open aneurysm repair) may be an option, but many presentations, particularly in mycotic conditions, require aneurysm excision and formal bypass reconstruction.[3] In a few selected patients, endovascular repair has been successfully performed, but the size limitations, durability concerns, and associated connective tissue disorders all tend to severely limit the use of current endovascular technology to treat aortic aneurysms in the pediatric population.

Mutations in the collagen, elastin, and glycoproteins that make up the framework of the vascular system can lead to weakened walls that are more prone to aneurysmal dilation. In Marfan syndrome, the defect is in the gene for fibrillin-1, and typical vascular symptoms include ascending aortic aneurysm and dissection and aortic regurgitation from retrograde dissection. In Ehlers-Danlos syndrome, the defect is in the triple helix arrangement of collagen.[3] Repair of the aorta in these patients with connective tissue disorders carries high risk and can be extremely problematic because of their vessel wall friability; hence, great care must be taken when handling these diseased vessels with clamps and sutures.

Tuberous sclerosis is an autosomal dominant disorder characterized by seizures, mental retardation, and facial adenoma sebaceum.[8] It is also associated with renal hamartomas, cardiac malformations, and periventricular sclerotic and calcification in the brain.[8] It has been hypothesized that vascular lesions occur secondary to nodular fibrosis, hamartomatous formation in the vasculature, and ischemia or an underlying collagen disorder or a combination of systemic hypertension and vascular dysplasia.[1] In aortic aneurysms associated with tuberous sclerosis, fragmentation of the media, loss and clumping of elastic fibers, and accumulation of mucopolysaccharides have been found.[8]

Takayasu arteritis is characterized by aortic irregularity (stenosis, occlusion, or aneurysmal dilation) with involvement of the major branches combined with an elevated erythrocyte sedimentation rate and a positive tuberculin skin test.[3] The etiology of this disease is not clear, although there is a strong correlation with tuberculosis and it primarily affects females. The treatment of choice in an arteritis is immunosuppressive therapy. The prognosis depends on the presence of its major complications, which consist of retinopathy, hypertension, aneurysm, and aortic regurgitation.[3]

Congenital aneurysms, which are distinct entities from acquired aneurysms, also occur, although far less commonly.[4,9] On pathologic examination, the diseased aorta typically shows medial degeneration (cystic medial necrosis) with fragmentation of elastic fibers, intimal fibrosis, and deposition of myxoid material (hyaluronic acid) in the intima.[3-4]

Patients with aortic aneurysms typically present in the preteen years, with a large pulsatile abdominal mass and an audible epigastric bruit.[3-4] Other complaints include local pain, hematemesis, and painless obstructive jaundice.[6] They can also be asymptomatic, with the diagnosis made incidentally, or in some unfortunate cases after rupture.[1,3] True aneurysms most commonly occur in the aorta, with the major branches of the aorta such as the renal and iliac arteries the next most common,[9] and most false aneurysms occur in the extremities.[9] Concurrent aneurysms can also occur in multiple places, including intracranial vessels.[1,4] Therefore, a complete preoperative work-up is important, and it includes total body imaging with computerized tomographic angiography (CTA) and/or magnetic resonance angiography (MRA) (Figure 34–1).[1] In addition, laboratory studies may guide preoperative diagnosis. For example, elevated erythrocyte sedimentation rate or C-reactive protein may suggest vasculitis or inflammatory processes; serum creatinine levels reflect adequate or compromised renal function; and an echocardiogram is used to evaluate cardiac function and look for possible aortic arch disease.[1]

Owing to the risk of rupture,[2,9-10] embolism, or thrombosis, standard practice at most institutions is immediate surgical repair and reconstruction with preservation of blood flow to vital organs (Figure 34–2). The exception is if the aneurysm is caused by an arteritis, which is managed (at least initially) with steroids and antihypertensives and frequent follow-up imaging. In children younger than 6 years old, adequate autologous options for graft construction are usually not available and cryopreserved arterial autografts can be used in this population.[1,8] The graft is sutured to the native artery with both running and interrupted sutures to allow for future transverse growth, and a gentle C-shape configuration is given to the reconstruction conduit to allow for longitudinal growth.[1] In addition, management of hypertension is an essential part in the treatment of these patients, because hypertension plays a role in the formation of the aneurysms as well as their progression. For patients who are managed with

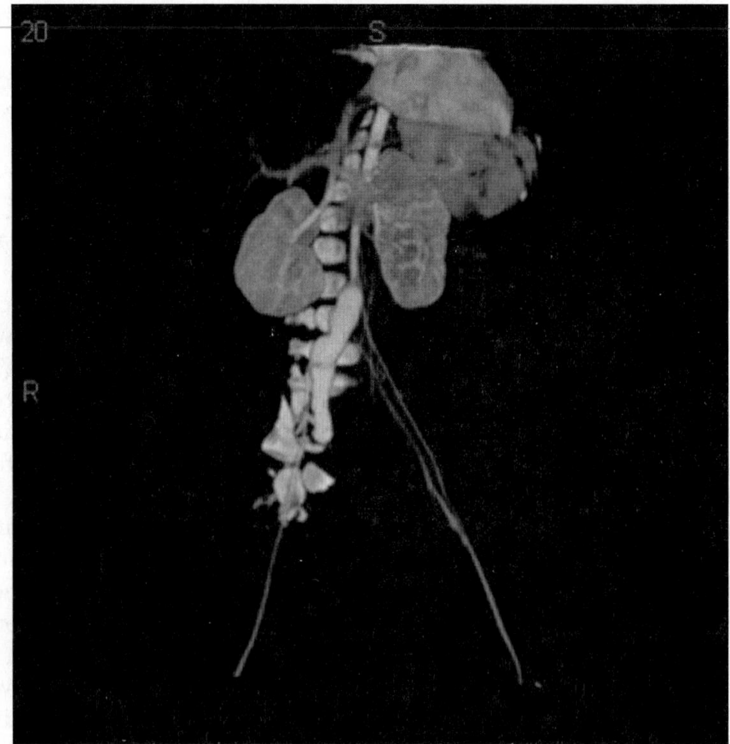

Figure 34-1. A 4-month-old girl with a history of prenatal hydronephrosis also has a large aneurysm extending from the right common iliac artery to the right internal iliac artery.

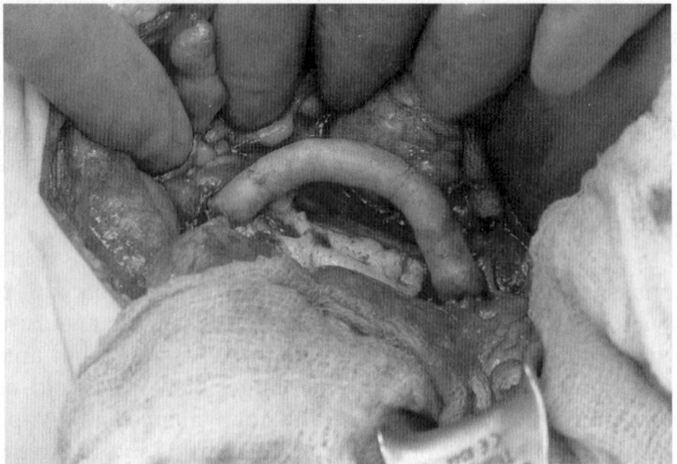

Figure 34-2. The aneurysm is seen splayed open and a 4-mm cryopreserved superficial saphenous artery graft is used as the conduit.

medications, close follow-up with serial imaging is important. Children with the highest survival rates are those with focal aneurysmal disease of the aorta or extremities when compared with those with diffuse and/or intracranial disease.[1] In the case of mycotic aneurysms, the source of infection must be controlled aggressively.

STENOSIS

Stenotic lesions of the aorta, also known as coarctations, occur in the thoracic and abdominal aorta, although far less frequently in the latter.[11] These children are treated medically for hypertension and followed closely while awaiting optimal size and availability of an autogenous conduit for reconstruction.[1] Prosthetic conduits may also be an acceptable option, depending on the size of the child and the size of the aorta proximal and distal to the coarctation. Occasionally, only medical therapy is necessary if adequate control of hypertension can be achieved with minimal side effects. As the child grows, the abdominal aortic caliber may also grow and operative reconstruction for stenosis of the abdominal aorta is not uniformly needed, particularly when the diagnosis is made in the neonate or infant age groups. Prompt operative intervention may be required for poorly controlled symptoms, that is, hypertension, progressive ventricular hypertrophy, severe claudication or vertical growth delay, and/or renal/mesenteric ischemia.[1] Diseases found to be associated with stenosis include idiopathic MAS, Takayasu disease, neurofibromatosis, and fibromuscular dysplasia. Any of these diseases may present with associated renovascular hypertension. We discuss the most commonly encountered stenotic problems in the abdominal aorta: MAS and renovascular hypertension.

Middle Aortic Syndrome

MAS is an uncommon condition characterized by narrowing of the abdominal aorta, often with involvement of its visceral branches, including renal and splanchnic arteries.[1,12-13] It accounts for 0.5 to 2.0% of all coarctations,[11,14-16] and usually presents in the second to third decade of life.[13,17-18] Most lesions are found at the renal artery, although they can be suprarenal, infrarenal, or diffuse. Critical renal artery stenosis occurs in 80 to 90% of cases, and visceral arteries are affected 35% of the time.[1,18] Histopathologic examination of the artery specimen often reveals intimal fibromuscular dysplasia consisting of focal and irregular intimal thickening with fibrosis of the muscular media and no inflammation.[11,13] The etiology of MAS is unknown, although developmental, immunologic, and inflammatory causes have been proposed.[11-12] Some have proposed that idiopathic MAS arises from failure of two dorsal aortas to fuse during embryonic development[19], rubella infection,[20] or abnormal migration of the kidney.[21] Table 34–2 lists secondary causes of MAS.[13,22] Associations with neurofibromatosis, Williams, and Alagille syndromes have also been described.[13,23-24]

Neurofibromatosis is an autosomal dominant disorder characterized by café au lait spots, freckling, dermal neurofibromas, optic nerve gliomas, Lisch nodules, learning disabilities, and skeletal abnormalities, including scoliosis.[25] The mutation occurs in the NF1 gene, whose gene product neurofibromin is expressed in endothelial and smooth muscle cells of blood vessels. The vascular lesions of neurofibromatosis can be classified into five different types: pure intimal lesions, advanced intimal lesions with medial changes, nodular aneurysmal lesions with loss of medial elements, periarterial

TABLE 34-2. ETIOLOGY OF MIDDLE AORTIC SYNDROME

Etiology
Idiopathic
Aortitis
Atherosclerosis
Neurocutaneous syndrome
Williams syndrome
Other

Reprinted with permission from Sethna CB, Kaplan BS, Cahill AM, et al. Idiopathic mid-aortic syndrome in children. Pediatr Nephrol 2008:23:1135–42.

nodule lesions, and epithelioid lesions with cellular proliferation.[1] Williams syndrome is an autosomal dominant disease characterized by supravalvular aortic stenosis, dysmorphic facies known as "elf face," mental retardation, transient infantile hypercalcemia, and growth retardation.[26] Studies show that the mutation is in the elastin gene on chromosome 7. Alagille syndrome is a genetic disorder characterized by a paucity of interlobular bile ducts, butterfly vertebrae, characteristic facies, and ocular posterior embryotoxin.[18] Cardiovascular malformations can also occur, such as tetralogy of Fallot and ventricular septal defects, and peripheral pulmonary stenosis has also been associated with this disorder.[18]

Hypertension is the most common clinical symptom in MAS and it occurs in 94% of patients.[13] It is often asymptomatic, but patients can present with malignant hypertension and such symptoms as hypertensive retinopathy and hypertensive encephalopathy (mental status changes, headache, nosebleeds).[11,13,24] Other clinical presentations include lower extremity claudication, renal failure, mesenteric ischemia (abdominal angina), growth discrepancy, left ventricular hypertrophy, and congestive heart failure.[1,11,13,18] Physical examination findings include abdominal bruits, heart murmurs (characteristic of left ventricular hypertrophy or heart failure), decreased femoral and/or pedal pulses, leg length discrepancy, elevated blood pressure in the upper extremities and lower blood pressure in the lower extremities, and in severe cases growth deceleration.

Accurate imaging, such as arteriography, CTA, or MRA, is essential to allow planning of vascular reconstruction as well as follow-up postoperatively. The gold standard for diagnosis of MAS is angiography examining the aorta and bilateral renal arteries, which is nearly 100% accurate.[1,11,27-28] However, in complete coarctations and in small children, CTA or MRA carries much less risk and can be an equally effective diagnostic tool. In addition, renal function needs to be assessed with serum creatinine levels, renin levels, and renal ultrasound. The heart must also be assessed by echocardiography. Secondary causes should be ruled out. For example, the erythrocyte sedimentation rate reflects an inflammatory cause, and the level should be normalized before surgery because it is best not to operate during the active phase of arteritis.[28]

In MAS, primary treatment goals are preservation of functional renal tissue and improvement of hypertension.[12] Prior to the development of effective antihypertensives, 45% of patients died from hypertensive emergencies.[22] Therefore, initial management involves antihypertensives, with close follow-up, including ultrasound of the heart and kidneys to evaluate for end-organ damage until definitive treatment can be

TABLE 34-3. INDICATIONS FOR SURGERY FOR MIDDLE AORTIC SYNDROME

Uncontrolled hypertension
Compromised renal function
Claudication
Failure to thrive
Mesenteric ischemia

carried out.[13] Medical therapy is also used in patients whose surgical risk is unacceptably high. Onset of end-organ damage such as congestive heart failure or renal failure indicates failure of medical therapy and need for operative intervention.[1] Other indications for surgery include intractable claudication and mesenteric ischemia and failure to thrive (Table 34–3). In the absence of a definitive indication for surgery, however, invasive intervention should be postponed until after puberty to allow for full growth to be achieved and to reduce the risk of secondary revision procedures in the long-term follow-up.

Operative treatment is dictated by native vessel size, age at operation, potential for further growth, and degree of renovascular involvement.[1,12] Thus, the timing of surgery should also be individualized and based on severity of symptoms, response to medical treatment, the surgical risk, and the size and age of the patient.[13] Surgical options include aorto-aortic bypass, patch aortoplasty, aortorenal bypass, renal autotransplantation, and in the extreme case of an unsalvageable kidney, partial or total nephrectomy. Although percutaneous transluminal angioplasty (PTA) may occasionally be an option, this form of treatment is seldom possible and/or durable to treat aortic stenosis in the pediatric population. With isolated renal artery stenosis, however, renal artery PTA can be effective in the pediatric age group and is often used as an initial treatment. PTA may need to be repeated for recurrence of symptoms, but renal artery stenting is not recommended in this age group. PTA is usually reserved for isolated, nonocclusive, nonostial lesions. The disadvantages of angioplasty, however, include (1) fragmentation of the vessel and subsequent thrombus formation, leading to persistent hypertension and eventual need for further intervention; and (2) rapid restenosis due to the excess elastin fibers in these lesions after balloon dilation.[29] Some have proposed the use of a metallic stent after angioplasty.[30] However, this technique has largely fallen out of favor with the advent of techniques with better outcomes.[11]

Single-staged aorto-aortic bypass with or without renal and splanchnic revascularization is the procedure of choice in patients with diffuse disease throughout the aorta.[13,23] The hypogastric artery (internal iliac artery) has been used as interposition grafts with minimal subsequent dilation and appropriate prospective growth,[1,12] but it can be difficult to acquire adequate length for this autogenous conduit. Also, the hypogastric artery is sometimes involved in the disease process, causing stenosis later in life.[11] Therefore, prosthetic material such as Dacron is usually used in this setting as the conduit. Patch aortoplasty can be used for short-segment stenosis and for young patients who may need bypass later in life. In younger patients who do not have adequate autologous graft material, a Dacron patch can be used.[1,12] Cryo-preserved allograft conduits are also an option, but their long-term patency is unclear.

Aside from the aortic stenosis, renal artery stenosis must also be addressed to prevent further renal damage. Renal autotransplantation can be performed into nondiseased iliac vessel without introduction of exogenous tissue.[12] However, finding a segment of nondiseased iliac vessel may not be possible in some cases, because the disease is often diffuse. Some have proposed reimplantation of the renal artery into the arch of Riolan when it is highly developed as an alternative.[31] Renal artery bypass can also be performed using autologous grafts or reverse saphenous vein graft, although placement within a Dacron mesh tube is recommended in the latter to avoid aneurysmal dilation of the vein grafts.[1,11,32] Much debate has ensued regarding the optimal bypass material. Some studies advocate the use of autologous material for repair of renal artery bypass to ensure adequate size during development. They have shown high reintervention rates 20 or 30 years after treatment when prosthetic material or venous grafts were used.[12] The hypogastric artery, external iliac artery, superficial femoral artery, and splenic arteries have all been proposed as possible graft candidates.[33-34] Stanley et al. , for example, prefer to use the hypogastric artery as the conduit.[29,34] If the hypogastric artery is used, a bifurcation branch at the distal end should be included to allow for a wide branch-patch orifice by incising the crotch between the branch and the trunk of the artery.[34] It is important to note that late stenosis of hypogastric artery aortorenal grafts, although rare, can occur, and the process is usually similar to the original disease process, because disease, especially in MAS, tends to be diffuse. Conversely, O'Neill prefers the use of reverse saphenous vein grafts reinforced with Dacron mesh, citing possible future impotence in male patients as another reason for not using the hypogastric artery as the conduit.[28] In the extreme case in which irreversible renal damage has already occurred, nephrectomy or embolization has been performed in an effort to alleviate renal vascular hypertension, although this is done only in extreme cases because as much renal tissue as possible should be preserved due to the possibility of recurrence of disease.[11]

Finally, although some have advocated prophylactic revascularization in asymptomatic patients of the celiac artery or SMA,[35-36] mesenteric reconstructions are rarely necessary because of the high level of collaterals that have usually formed in these patients.[11-12]

Like all pediatric vascular surgery, a dilemma occurs in children who have not yet undergone puberty because subsequent radial and longitudinal growth of vessels poses a problem. Similar to the aneurysm repair techniques described above, interrupted sutures allow for radial growth while curving the graft in a C-shape that will straighten out over time, permitting longitudinal growth (Figure 34–3). In addition, reinforcing the anastomosis externally with a band of Dacron has also been successfully used by some groups.[31]

Several case series have shown that the bypass graft techniques described above in this patient population have good long-term results and few complications.[1,11] Occasional graft thrombosis can occur, but immediate reoperation by replacement or declotting of the graft has been successful.[11] After treatment, hypertension is usually relieved or improved, although occasionally the use of an antihypertensive is still necessary.[1,11] It is important to continue follow-up of these patients to examine for possible future complications, such as aneurysm formation, chronic graft stenosis, thrombosis, and suture line disruption.[13]

Renovascular Hypertension

The overall incidence of hypertension in children ranges between 1 and 5%.[28] Pediatric renal artery occlusive disease is the third most common cause of hypertension in infants and children after thoracic isthmic coarctation of the aorta and parenchymal renal disease.[29,34] Renovascular lesions account for nearly one third of children with hypertension,

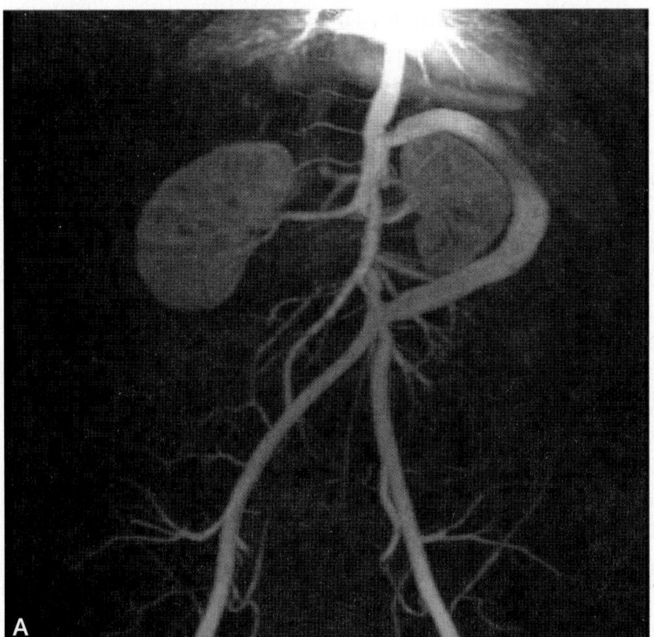

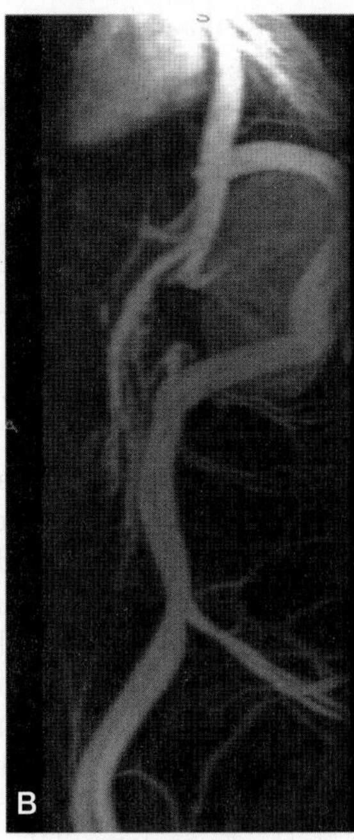

Figure 34-3. A 4-year-old boy presented with abdominal pain and was diagnosed with middle aortic syndrome of unknown etiology. He was treated with an aorto-aortic Dacron bypass. Because of the need to account for future growth, interrupted sutures were used to allow for radial growth while curving the graft in a C-shape that will straighten out over time, permitting longitudinal growth.

and 75% of toddlers with hypertension can be corrected surgically.[28,30] Although most occur unilaterally, bilateral involvement is common. Up to one third of cases also present with aortic narrowing (see above).[12,24,27-28,34,37] Similar to the lesions in the MAS, renal artery disease displays concentric stenosis, whose histologic appearance is one of disruption of normal medial architecture and fragmentation of internal elastic lamina as well as excess elastic tissue in the adventitia.[34] Also similar to MAS, causes of renovascular hypertension include fibromuscular hyperplasia, Williams syndrome, neurofibromatosis, vasculitis, and trauma.[28]

Renovascular hypertension presents similarly to MAS, with hypertension, often silent, as the main symptom. However, when left untreated, uncontrolled hypertension can cause strokes, seizures, impaired mental development from encephalopathy, failure to thrive, left ventricular hypertrophy, flash pulmonary edema, congestive heart failure, and oliguric renal failure.[28-29] Because essential hypertension is rare in this patient population, the presence of hypertension warrants a work-up to find its cause, with an angiogram being the most important diagnostic study.[28-29,34] Similar to MAS, surgical options for treatment include PTA, renal autotransplantation, renal artery resection and reimplantation or reanastomosis, aortorenal bypass (with autogenous vein grafts or internal iliac artery grafts), iliorenal bypass with vein grafts, thoracoabdominal aorto-aortic bypass, patch aortoplasty, and nephrectomy.[30,34]

Renal autotransplantation, preferably bilateral, has been shown to abolish the renin-angiotensin vicious cycle and alleviate hypertension in these patients, although its routine use is controversial.[34,38] Renal artery reimplantation is a more commonly used surgical approach. It is accomplished by resection of the diseased portion of the renal artery and reimplanting the renal artery to another section of the normal renal artery or the aorta.[29,34] This is useful for patients with disease limited to the main renal artery or a segmental artery.[34] The transected normal renal artery can be spatulated anteriorly and posteriorly, and the aortotomy made twice the length of the renal artery diameter to ensure a sufficiently large anastomosis.[34] Aortorenal bypass is technically difficult due to the need for a disease-free aorta, consideration for the patient's future growth, and graft durability. When the aorta was involved in past decades, thoracoabdominal aorto-aortic bypass to serve as inflow to bilateral renal bypass grafts was a common procedure for renovascular hypertension, and it has fallen out of favor with the advent of less invasive procedures. However, it is sometimes used, employing a Dacron tube graft tailored to patient size and potential for future growth. Patch aortoplasty with polytetrafluoroethylene (PTFE) is often used in patients who are young, but this may need further intervention in the future. Finally, nephrectomy is reserved for patients with persistent hypertension for whom all other means of revascularization have been exhausted.

As is the case with aneurysmal disease as well as MAS, in patients who are growing, interrupted absorbable sutures or running sutures that are not tied to each other are used to allow future radial growth of the anastomosis.[30] It is also important to note that owing to the smaller scale of the pediatric patient, small mural thrombi that may be insignificant in the adult may have devastating consequences in the neonate. Therefore, it is important to prevent intimal damage in these patients with delicate vessel manipulation, clamping with minimal force, and avoiding stretching and desiccation of the graft and native vessel.[39] Systemic anticoagulation based on patient weight should be used during the revascularization. Properly performed, it has been shown that operative intervention benefits over 95% of the patient population, with hypertension either cured or improved.[28-29,34]

TRAUMA

Causes of pediatric vascular injuries include motor vehicle accidents, falls, stabs, and gunshot wounds.[30,40-41] These injuries can occur in the arterial system as well as the venous system, the central nervous system as well as the peripheral system. For example, vascular injuries can occur in the neck from penetrating trauma, in the thoracic aorta, the vena cava, and the common femoral artery (CFA).

Traumatic aortic injury due to blunt trauma includes transections, intimal flaps, and pseudoaneurysms, which can occur in both the thoracic aorta and the abdominal aorta.[40] Patients who are restrained tend to present with abdominal aortic injury, whereas those who are unrestrained present more with thoracic aortic injury.[40] Diagnostic studies include computed tomography, angiography, and in some cases transesophageal echocardiography. Patients who are hemodynamically stable can be managed nonoperatively, with good outcome, although close long-term follow-up is necessary.[40] Open surgical repair by vascular occlusion and rapid repair (the "clamp and sew technique") using interposition grafts with or without bypass or shunting is the standard of therapy when surgical intervention is necessary.[30]

Complications of surgery include paraplegia, pneumonia, sepsis, renal failure, recurrent laryngeal nerve injury, and pulmonary embolus.[40] Outcome also depends on the presence of associated injuries, such as hollow viscous injuries, extremity injuries, solid organ injuries, spine injuries, and head injuries, which are present in up to 80% of patients due to the immense force necessary to bring about aortic injuries.[42]

Recent advances in endograft repair are promising, and successful deployment of an endograft has been documented in a high-risk child with traumatic pseudoaneurysm of the aorta.[10,43] Szeto and associates describe a case of a 16-year-old boy with a history of radiotherapy for mediastinal T-cell lymphoma, subsequent tracheal stenosis, multiple tracheal reconstructive surgeries, tracheal-innominate fistula requiring ligation, pseudoaneurysm formation at the site of ligation, multiple coilings, and emergency presentation with an expanding pulsatile mass at the tracheostomy site. Owing to adhesions and poor anatomy in the neck region from previous radiation and multiple surgeries, an endovascular approach was taken with an excellent outcome (Figure 34–4).[44]

CONCLUSION

With advancement of technology, pediatric patients who undergo vascular surgery in their youth have prolonged survival. Issues that need to be examined in these patients include their quality of life, physical and emotional development, future sexual function, as well as

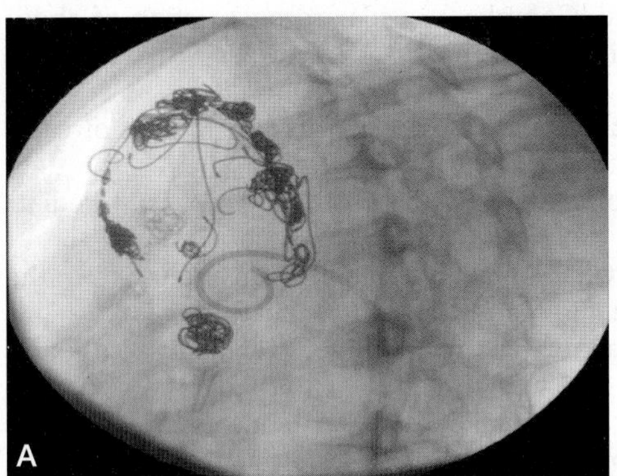

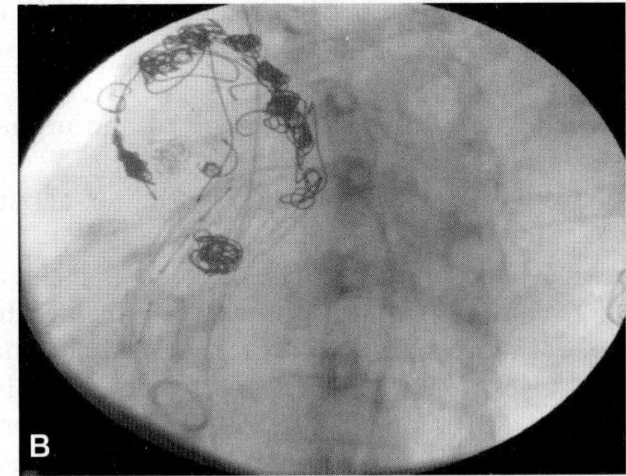

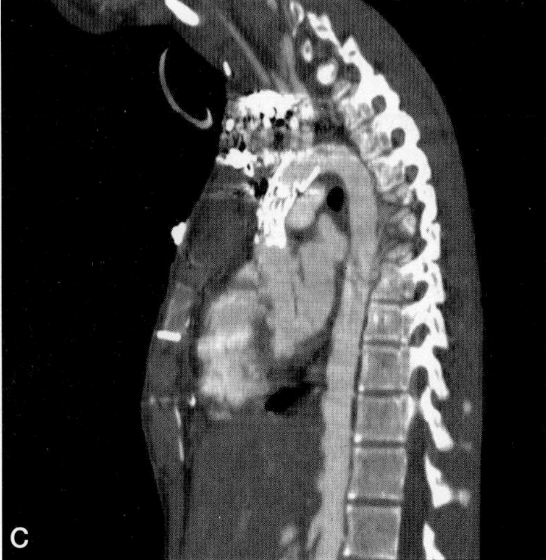

Figure 34-4. A 16-year-old boy status postchemotherapy and radiation for mediastinal T-cell lymphoma presented with tracheal stenosis and needed multiple tracheal reconstructive surgeries. He then developed tracheoinnominate fistula requiring ligation, pseudoaneurysm formation at the site of ligation, and multiple coilings. He presented emergently with an expanding pulsatile mass at the tracheostomy site after the pseudoaneurysm blew out, displacing the coils (A). An endovascular approach was used because of adhesions and poor anatomy in the neck region from previous radiation and multiple surgeries (B). The patient had an excellent outcome (C). (Reprinted with permission from Szeto WY, Fairman RM, Acker MA, et al. Emergency endovascular deployment of stent graft in the ascending aorta for contained rupture of innominate artery pseudoaneurysm in a pediatric patient. Ann Thorac Surg 2006;81:1872–5.)

graft integrity with time and growth. Barral et al. conducted a 17-year follow-up of eight patients who underwent vascular surgery for such causes as MAS, aortic aneurysm, and Takayasu disease. They found that certain patients needed further surgical intervention for such complications as fibrosis of an implanted renal artery, deterioration of graft, and formation of aneurysm. All patients had normal physical development, normal sexual function, and excellent quality of life with scores ranging from 78 to 83% on the Short Form 36 questionnaire.[31,45]

Optimal management of aortic disease in the pediatric population requires a multidisciplinary approach, including pediatric, general, and transplant surgeons as well as nephrologists, geneticists, rheumatologists, and cardiologists. In addition, the surgeon needs to take into consideration the child's growth potential. Taking into account the numerous resources, personnel, and expertise that are necessary to manage these complex disease processes, children with complex vascular diseases are best managed at tertiary institutions with a significant volume of pediatric vascular experience to ensure optimal outcome.[46]

REFERENCES

1. Kaye AJ, Slemp AE, Chang B, Mattei P, et al. Complex vascular reconstruction of abdominal aorta and its branches in the pediatric population. J Pediatr Surg 2008;43: 1082–8.
2. Howorth MB Jr. Aneurysm of abdominal aorta in the newborn infant. Report of case. N Engl J Med 1967;276:1133–4.
3. Millar AJ, Gilbert RD, Brown RA, et al. Abdominal aortic aneurysms in children. J Pediatr Surg 1996;31:1624–8.
4. Mehall JR, Saltzman DA, Chandler JC, et al. Congenital abdominal aortic aneurysm in the infant: case report and review of the literature. J Pediatr Surg 2001;36:657–8.
5. Sarkar R, Cilley RE, Coran AG. Abdominal aneurysms in childhood: report of a case and review of the literature. Surgery 1991;109:143–8.
6. Sarkar R, Coran AG, Cilley RE, et al. Arterial aneurysms in children: clinicopathologic classification. J Vasc Surg 1991;13:46–56; discussion 56–7.
7. Lobe TE, Richardson CJ, Boulden TF, et al. Mycotic thromboaneurysmal disease of the abdominal aorta in preterm infants: its natural history and its management. J Pediatr Surg 199; 27:1054–9; discussion 1059–60.
8. van Reedt Dortland RW, Bax NM, Huber J. Aortic aneurysm in a 5-year-old boy with tuberous sclerosis. J Pediatr Surg 1991;26:1420–2.
9. Guzzetta PC, Congenital and acquired aneurysmal disease. Semin Pediatr Surg 1994,3: 97–102.
10. Saad SA, May A. Abdominal aortic aneurysm in a neonate. J Pediatr Surg 1991;26: 1423–4.
11. O'Neill JA Jr, Berkowitz H, Fellows KJ, Harmon CM. Midaortic syndrome and hypertension in childhood. J Pediatr Surg 1995;30:164–71; discussion 162–171.
12. Lillehei CW, Shamberger RC. Staged reconstruction for middle aortic syndrome. J Pediatr Surg 2001;36:1252–4.
13. Sethna CB, Kaplan BS, Cahill AM, et al. Idiopathic mid-aortic syndrome in children. Pediatr Nephrol 2008;23:1135–42.
14. Connolly JE, Wilson SE, Lawrence PL, Fujitani RM. Middle aortic syndrome: distal thoracic and abdominal coarctation, a disorder with multiple etiologies. J Am Coll Surg 2002;194: 774–81.

15. Lewis VD 3rd, Meranze SG, McLean GK, et al. The midaortic syndrome: diagnosis and treatment. Radiology 1988;167:111–3.
16. Sen PK, Kinare SG, Engineer SD, Parulkar GB. The Middle Aortic Syndrome. Br Heart J 1963;25:610–8.
17. De Bakey M, Garrett HE, Howell JF, Morris GC Jr. Coarctation of the abdominal aorta with renal arterial stenosis: surgical considerations. Ann Surg 1967;165:830–43.
18. Shefler AG, Chan MK, Ostman-Smith I. Middle aortic syndrome in a boy with arteriohepatic dysplasia (Alagille syndrome). Pediatr Cardiol 1997;18:232–4.
19. Maycock W. Congenital stenosis of the abdominal aorta. Am Heart J 1937;13:633–46.
20. Siassi B, Klyman G, Emmanouilides GC. Hypoplasia of the abdominal aorta associated with the rubella syndrome. Am J Dis Child 1970;120:476–9.
21. Graham LM, Zelenock GB, Erlandson EE, et al. Abdominal aortic coarctation and segmental hypoplasia. Surgery 1979;86:519–29.
22. Onat T, Zeren E. Coarctation of the abdominal aorta. Review of 91 cases. Cardiologia 1969; 54:140–57.
23. Panayiotopoulos YP, Tyrrell MR, Koffman G, et al. Mid-aortic syndrome presenting in childhood. Br J Surg 1996;83:235–40.
24. Robinson L, Gedroyc W, Reidy J, Saxton HM. Renal artery stenosis in children. Clin Radiol 1991;44:376–82.
25. Rosser TL, Vezina G, Packer RJ. Cerebrovascular abnormalities in a population of children with neurofibromatosis type 1. Neurology 2005;64:553–5.
26. Onis Vilches MC, Rubio Cuadrado MV, Martinez de la Iglesia J, Lopez Granados A. [William's syndrome. Report of a case with family involvement]. Rev Clin Esp 1998;198: 91–4.
27. Guzzetta PC, Potter BM, Ruley EJ, et al. Renovascular hypertension in children: current concepts in evaluation and treatment. J Pediatr Surg 1989;24:1236–40.
28. O'Neill JA Jr. Long-term outcome with surgical treatment of renovascular hypertension. J Pediatr Surg 1998;33:106–11.
29. Stanley JC, Criado E, Upchurch GR Jr, et al. Pediatric renovascular hypertension: 132 primary and 30 secondary operations in 97 children. J Vasc Surg 2006;44:1219–28; discussion 1219–28.
30. St Peter SD, Ostlie DJ. A review of vascular surgery in the pediatric population. Pediatr Surg Int 2007;23:1–10.
31. Barral X, de Latour B, Vola M, et al. Surgery of the abdominal aorta and its branches in children: late follow-up. J Vasc Surg 2006;43:1138–44.
32. Berkowitz HD, O'Neill JA Jr. Renovascular hypertension in children. Surgical repair with special reference to the use of reinforced vein grafts. J Vasc Surg 1989;9:46–55.
33. Lacombe M. [Role of surgery in the treatment of renovascular hypertension in the child]. Bull Acad Natl Med 2003;187:1081–93; discussion 1093–4.
34. Stanley JC, Zelenock GB, Messina LM, Wakefield TW. Pediatric renovascular hypertension: a thirty-year experience of operative treatment. J Vasc Surg 1995;21:212–26; discussion 226–7.
35. Messina LM, Reilly LM, Goldstone J, et al. Middle aortic syndrome. Effectiveness and durability of complex arterial revascularization techniques. Ann Surg 1986;204:331–9.
36. van Dongen RJ. Renal and intestinal artery occlusive disease. World J Surg 1988; 12:777–87.
37. Stanley JC, Fry WJ. Pediatric renal artery occlusive disease and renovascular hypertension. Etiology, diagnosis, and operative treatment. Arch Surg 1981;116:669–76.
38. Ellis D, Shapiro R, Scantlebury VP, et al. Evaluation and management of bilateral renal artery stenosis in children: a case series and review. Pediatr Nephrol 1995;9:259–67.
39. Mansfield PB, Hall DG, Di Benedetto G, et al. The care of vascular endothelium in pediatric surgery. Ann Surg 1978;188:216–28.
40. Anderson SA, Day M, Chen MK, et al. Traumatic aortic injuries in the pediatric population. J Pediatr Surg 2008;43:1077–81.

41. Aspalter M, Domenig CM, Haumer M, et al. Management of iatrogenic common femoral artery injuries in pediatric patients using primary vein patch angioplasty. J Pediatr Surg 2007;42:1898–902.
42. Harris LM, Hordines J. Major vascular injuries in the pediatric population. Ann Vasc Surg 2003;17:266–9.
43. Aidinian G, Karnaze M, Russo EP, Mukherjee D, Endograft repair of traumatic aortic transection in a 10-year-old—a case report. Vasc Endovascular Surg 2006;40:239–42.
44. Szeto WY, Fairman RM, Acker MA, et al. Emergency endovascular deployment of stent graft in the ascending aorta for contained rupture of innominate artery pseudoaneurysm in a pediatric patient. Ann Thorac Surg 2006;81:1872–5.
45. Beattie DK, Golledge J, Greenhalgh RM, Davies AH: Quality of life assessment in vascular disease: towards a consensus. Eur J Vasc Endovasc Surg 1997;13:9–13.
46. Cox CS Jr., Black CT, Duke JH, et al. Operative treatment of truncal vascular injuries in children and adolescents. J Pediatr Surg 1998;33:462–7.

SECTION VIII

Venous

35

Combined Superficial and Deep Venous Reflux: What Do We Do?

Brian S. Knipp, M.D. and
Thomas W. Wakefield, M.D., F.A.C.S.

BACKGROUND

Chronic venous insufficiency (CVI) encompasses a spectrum of disease states. Although technically speaking, telangiectasias and venous varicosities are early manifestations, most investigators limit CVI to severe edema, trophic skin changes, and venous ulceration. The pathophysiology of this disease is complex, involving the interaction between the superficial and the deep venous systems as well as the communicating or perforating veins. Both active (muscle pump mechanisms) and passive (valvular) mechanisms contribute toward centripetal flow in the normal physiologic state. Any disturbance to this normal flow pattern can lead to progressive overload and failure of other aspects of the system, which manifests as venous stasis.

Venous reflux, which leads to venous insufficiency, is a common problem. The risk of development of venous stasis ulceration has been estimated to be 1% in developed nations.[1] In a population-based cross-sectional study of over 3000 subjects, Maurins documented pathologic reflux (valve closure times >500 msec) in 35.3% of the population; deep reflux was present in 20.0%; in 7.2% of subjects, deep reflux >1000 msec duration was detected.[2] Males were more likely to have deep vein insufficiency in this study, whereas women were more likely to have superficial vein insufficiency. Risk factors for CVI include advanced age and severity of reflux.[3-4] Age may correlate with symptoms owing to the fact that prolonged exposure to ambulatory venous hypertension leads to chronic degeneration of the venous system and eventually CVI. In a more detailed analysis, age correlated with superficial but not deep system reflux. Both superficial and deep reflux correlated with severity of symptoms (or clinical, etiologic, anatomic, and pathophysiologic [CEAP] stage). This study also documented a higher association between severe CVI (C4-C6 disease) and reflux in males.[2]

The etiology of venous insufficiency can be divided into primary reflux due to gradual degeneration of the vein wall and valves starting in the superficial system, progressing to perforators, and finally the deep system or secondary reflux due to combined outflow obstruction and valvular damage following deep venous thrombosis (DVT). In the first major report using this classification, approximately 80% of patients with CVI were noted to have primary reflux and 20% had secondary reflux.[5]

The lower extremity venous system can be conceptualized as a parallel pump arrangement consisting of the superficial and deep veins. The deep system, being larger, has a greater capacitance and therefore under normal circumstances can handle moderate increases in volume of venous return by dilation and increased flow rates. The superficial system similarly can tolerate increased volume, although to a lesser degree. Smaller vessel size and greater restriction due to overlying dermis lead to valvular incompetence when the superficial system is chronically volume overloaded. Varicosities subsequently develop, followed by trophic skin changes as proinflammatory leukocytes and mediators become extravasated into the interstitium.

The deep and superficial systems communicate through a series of perforating veins with unidirectional valves. Incompetence of these valves tends to lead to increased volume in the superficial system, especially in situations in which the deep system is plagued with outflow obstruction or volume overload secondary to valvular reflux.

The primary focus of this discussion is the complex problem of combined venous reflux. This is not an uncommon problem. Twenty to 30% of patients with symptomatic CVI are found to have combined superficial and deep venous reflux on duplex testing. In a study of 138 limbs with class C5 or C6 CVI, 27.5% were found to have combined superficial and deep reflux.[6] Another study documented a 22% rate of combined superficial and deep vein reflux; 27 of 31 cases were segmental.[7] In a recent study by Marsten et al., of 336 patients undergoing EVA for superficial reflux, 75 (22%) had concomitant deep system reflux; 19 of 75 (25%) of the deep reflux condition were axial, the remainder segmental central visual field [CVP] or popliteal vein [PV] alone).[8]

Although combined insufficiency could result from post-thrombotic DVI combined with primary superficial insufficiency, the more common presentation is progressive primary venous insufficiency. In the overload theory of Bergan, superficial insufficiency develops due to a milieu of inflammation and damage of valves and venous dilation, thought to be secondary to chronic ambulatory venous hypertension in the superficial system. Reflux and varicosities in the superficial system lead to increased blood return to the deep system.[9] Eventually, the capacitance of these vessels is exhausted, and deep valvular reflux develops due to the inability of the valve leaflets to coapt properly. It therefore makes intuitive sense that eradication of the incompetent superficial vessels would allow the deep system to return to a normophysiologic state and deep reflux would improve or even cease.

There are three basic approaches to the management of patients with CVI with combined superficial and deep venous reflux. Graded compression therapy is the mainstay of management and has been shown in many trials to provide nearly equivalent wound healing to surgical intervention. However, the drawback of compression therapy, aside from patient noncompliance (which can be substantial), is the fact that compression does not directly correct the physiologic abnormality but only manages it. Surgical options, therefore, may be necessary in recalcitrant cases and even favored in most circumstances. Surgical procedures can be divided into three categories: superficial surgery (flush ligation, saphenous stripping, endovenous ablative techniques), perforator interruption (surgical ligation or SEPS), and deep venous reconstruction (valve transplant, valvuloplasty, or external banding).[10]

Deep venous reconstruction has shown moderate clinical utility and should be reserved for a select group of patients who have exhausted other options, and we do not discuss this topic in detail in this review.[11] Superfical and/or perforator surgery, conversely, addresses the source of overflow in the Bergan model and would seem to be an appropriate intervention in addition to compression therapy.

Although there is growing evidence that superficial surgery for combined reflux improves hemodynamics, symptoms, and wound healing, randomized clinical trials (RCTs) failed to conclusively demonstrate the merits of this approach. One of the major problems with these trials is that none were designed to answer the problem of combined reflux and are underpowered to do so. The other substantial problem is that not all deep insufficiency is the same. There is likely a regional variation in the effect of superficial ablation on deep insufficiency. In the study by Padberg and associates, patients with proximal segmental deep venous incompetence had the best result from saphenous ablation and perforator ligation.[3] There is also evidence that reflux velocity may have a role in the response of the deep venous system to superficial ablation.[8]

The fact that DVI may be either primary or secondary to a post-thrombotic state further complicates the issue. Poor ulcer healing and high recurrence rates were found in patients treated with superficial and perforator surgery in the presence of DVI.[12-13] Sottiurai demonstrated improvement in outcomes by adding deep venous reconstruction to superficial and perforator surgery in patients with combined reflux.[14] However, these studies fail to differentiate the etiology of the deep insufficiency. Glovickzki demonstrated that in the absence of post-thrombotic syndrome and venous outflow obstruction, DVI did not have a detrimental effect on wound healing.[15] Rhodes documented that patients with post-thrombotic states failed to demonstrate hemodynamic improvements postsurgery.[16]

NONRANDOMIZED TRIALS

Prior to 2003, no RCTs of superficial surgery for combined insufficiency had been performed; all trials were observational or retrospective cohort studies. In many cases, evaluation of the role of superficial surgery on deep reflux was included as a subset analysis in the context of a larger study.

One of the clinical endpoints evaluated by early trials was resolution of venous reflux by duplex imaging. In a study of 29 limbs with saphenous and deep system reflux, saphenous vein stripping led to abolishment of femoral reflux in 27 patients. Three patients were noted to have both femoral and popliteal reflux; this reflux was abolished in all 3.[17] In another study of 17 patients with femoral reflux, removal of the proximal saphenous vein and stab avulsions of venous varicosities led to resolution of deep reflux.[18] In a study of 42 limbs with combined deep and superficial reflux, Dix et al. found that patients with segmental reflux had resolution of deep reflux approximately 50% of the time (11 out of 21 limbs), whereas in patients with multisegment disease, only approximately 30% (6 out of 21 limbs) demonstrated resolution.[19] Puggioni et al. also documented a 30% rate of deep reflux resolution with superficial venous surgery in their subgroup of 17 patients with combined superficial and axial

TABLE 35-1. NONRANDOMIZED TRIALS

Study	n	Severity	Reflux	Intervention	Resolution of Reflux [%]
Sales 1994	17	Class I-III	SR + DS	LSV stripping and phlebectomy	94.1
Walsh 1994	29	N/A	SR + DS/A	LSV stripping and phlebectomy	93.1
Puggioni 2003	22	CEAP 1-6	SR + DS	LSV stripping or RFA	36.4
	17	CEAP 1-6	SR + A	LSV stripping or RFA	11.8
Dix 2005	21	CEAP 4-6	SR + DS	LSV or SSV stripping	52.4
	21	CEAP 4-6	SR + A	LSV or SSV stripping	28.6

Rates of resolution of reflux by duplex ultrasonography documented by different investigators. SR: superficial reflux. DS: deep segmental reflux. A: deep axial reflux. LSV: long saphenous vein. RFA: radiofrequency ablation.

reflux; however, in the subgroup with combined superficial and segmental deep reflux (n=21), 36% exhibited resolution of deep reflux with superficial venous surgery (Table 35–1).[20]

One of the factors complicating evaluation of surgical intervention for combined reflux disease, however, has been the fact that various clinical endpoints have been evaluated. Padberg et al. demonstrated in 11 limbs with combined superficial and deep system reflux that surgical ablation of the saphenous system and perforators led to substantial improvements in the hemodynamics of the deep venous system, including improvements in the venous filling index (VFI) from 12±5 mL/sec to 2.7±1 mL/sec, the venous clinical severity score (VCSS) from 10 to 1.4, and the calf muscle pump ejection fraction from 43%±11% to 59%±13%. These relationships were true regardless of the distribution of reflux (proximal segmental, distal segmental, or axial). It is interesting to note that only 3 of 11 limbs in this study demonstrated abolition of deep system reflux, but substantial improvements in venous hemodynamics were noted. The authors concluded that "surgical correction of [superficial and perforator incompetence] significantly improves clinical symptoms and venous hemodynamics [and therefore] superficial and perforator ablation is an appropriate initial step in the management of combined deep and superficial venous incompetence."[3] Ahmed et al. studied 64 patients undergoing aggressive superficial surgical therapy compared with 36 patients undergoing less aggressive treatment. Follow-up duplex scanning after aggressive treatment of superficial venous disease showed improvement or complete reversal of deep vein insufficiency in over 80% of patients versus 28% of patients receiving less aggressive treatment.[21] Other authors have noted that the presence of multisegment or axial reflux predicts recalcitrance of deep reflux after superficial ablation. In a series of patients undergoing saphenofemoral or popliteal disconnect procedures, all patients with superficial reflux alone demonstrated healing of their ulcers without compression therapy, whereas none of the patients with combined reflux were able to heal ulcers without compression. Importantly, all nine patients in this study had axial reflux.[22]

RANDOMIZED CLINICAL TRIALS

Owing to clinical equipoise in the management of CVI, five RCTs were attempted to address the utility of superficial surgery in addition to compression therapy. One study failed to accrue sufficient numbers to yield a meaningful result.[23] One RCT specifically excluded patients with deep system obstruction or reflux.[1] In a third RCT, superficial surgery did not show any benefit in time for healing of ulcers, healing rate, or quality of life.[24]

In 2004, Barwell et al. published the results of the Effect of Surgery and Compression on Healing and Recurrence (ESCHAR) trial, a RCT enrolling 500 patients of an eligible 765 in a well-designed intention-to-treat analysis.[25] Gohel subsequently reported on the long-term outcomes of this trial at 3 years[26]: 242 patients were randomized to surgery plus compression, and 252 patients underwent compression alone. In subgroup analysis, 76 patients were found to have both superficial and deep segmental reflux. In patients in the surgery plus compression arm (n=37), the ulcer recurrence rate was 24% at 3 years versus patients in the compression only arm (n=39), who had a significantly higher recurrence rate, 52% at 3 years (P=.044). A similar trend was seen in the 49 patients with superficial plus axial reflux. In patients treated with surgery plus compression (n=20), there was a 24% recurrence rate; those treated with compression alone (n=29) had a higher recurrence rate of 46%, although significance was not reached (P=.23). In no subgroup (superficial reflux alone, superficial plus deep segmental reflux, or superficial plus deep axial reflux) was there a difference in ulcer healing rate. Therefore, the authors concluded that compression therapy is necessary and sufficient for healing; however, correction of the underlying venous abnormality is required to decrease the risk of recurrence. Whereas the effect on patients with DVI was less than that seen in superficial reflux only, the sample size was substantially smaller and therefore the authors concluded that "deep venous reflux should not be considered an absolute contraindication to superficial venous surgery as patients may experience significant hemodynamic and clinical benefits."[26]

Another study of 200 limbs randomized patients to subfacial endoscopic peforator surgery (SEPS) and surgical ablation of the incompetent saphenous system with compression versus compression only. The trial was a well-designed intention-to-treat analysis with only 4 patients lost to follow-up (3 surgical, 1 compression only) and 3 patients crossing over (all surgical patients electing for compression only). DVI was present in 49 of 94 patients (52%) in the surgical arm and 57 of 102 patients (56%, difference not significant) in the compression only arm. Notably, these investigators elected not to differentiate segmental from axial deep venous reflux. In patients with DVI, ulcer-free rates were 64% in the surgical group versus 43% in the compression group (P=NS) over the 3-year study period. Ulcer healing was 82% in the surgical arm and 74% in the compression arm (P=NS). Recurrence rates were not reported but were stated to be no different regardless of treatment arm (Table 35–2).[27]

The major shortfalls of these RCTs were small patient populations, evaluation of combined insufficiency as a subgroup analysis, and inconsistent definition of study populations.

RECENT INVESTIGATIONS

Despite the performance of the previously mentioned RCTs, there is still insufficient evidence to conclusively recommend a therapeutic approach for combined superficial and deep venous reflux.[28] The strongest evidence continues to come from the previously and subsequently published uncontrolled series. However, it is becoming clear that superficial surgery has a salutary effect on DVI. It remains unclear whether there is a subset of patients who will benefit most from superficial surgery for treatment of deep venous reflux.

TABLE 35-2. RANDOMIZED CONTROLLED TRIALS

Study	n	Severity	Reflux	Intervention	Healing Rate	Recur Rate	Ulcer-Free Rate
ESCHAR	37	CEAP 5-6	SR + DS	Superficial surgery and compression		24.0%	
	39	CEAP 5-6	SR + DS	Compression alone		52.0%*	
	20	CEAP 5-6	SR + A	Superficial surgery and compression		24.0%	
	29	CEAP 5-6	SR + A	Compression alone		46.0%	
van Gent 2006	49	CEAP 6	SR + DS/A	Superficial surgery and compression	82.0%		64.0%
	57	CEAP 6	SR + DS/A	Compression alone	74.0%		43.0%

Rates of healing, recurrence, and ulcer-free time in two RCTs.
*P<.05. SR: superficial reflux. DS: deep segmental reflux. A: deep axial reflux. ESCHAR, CEAP

Marsten et al. attempted to address this issue by defining a maximal reflux velocity (MRV) that was shown to be predictive of the resolution of symptoms. Several enlightening observations may be gleaned from this study. First, in all cases of isolated common femoral reflux (combined with superficial reflux), superficial surgery led to substantial improvement in VCSS and VFI (P<.001 for both observations). The MRV had no effect on this finding. In the other subset of patients in this study with either popliteal or multisegment reflux combined with superficial reflux, superficial surgery produced significant improvement in both VCSS and VFI as well. The magnitude of improvement, however, was dependent on MRV. In patients with MRV <10 cm/sec, the VCSS improved from 7.1±2.1 to 1.6±0.9 (P<.001) and the VFI improved from 5.4±2.3 mL/sec to 2.2±2.3 mL/sec (P<.001). In patients with MRVs >10 cm/sec, the VCSS improved from 8.2±2.7 to 3.5±3.5 (P<.001), significantly less improvement than for low MRV (P=.03). Similarly, the VFI for these patients improved from 6.9±4.7 mL/sec to 4.4±3.2 (P=.007), less improvement than for low MRV (P=.01). The authors concluded that superficial surgery should still be offered to all patients with combined reflux in addition to appropriate compression therapy, but patients with popliteal or multisegment deep reflux and high MRVs should be counseled that their likelihood of benefit is less than for other subsets of patients.[8]

In 2008, our group published a series of endovenous laser ablations for saphenous reflux in 460 limbs. We specifically analyzed our results comparing patients with DVI with those without DVI.

The first significant finding of our research was that the presence of DVI (regardless of whether it was segmental or axial) had no effect on the duration of superficial venous occlusion. Occlusion rates were over 90% at 30 months regardless of the presence of DVI. Second, there was no effect of DVI (segmental or axial) on complications such as DVT, saphenofemoral thrombus extension, superficial thrombophlebitis, paresthesias, or bruising.

Importantly, significant improvements were noted in symptoms for both superficial and combined disease in VCSS scores (decrease from 6 [IQR 5 – 8] to 3 [IQR 2 – 5] over 1 year). The presence of deep insufficiency was not a barrier to improvement in clinical severity scores. Of note, we evaluated both segmental and axial reflux and found similar results for both. Incidentally, DVI had no effect on the rate of venous recannalization in the superficial system (P=.117).[29] In patients with superficial reflux only, VCSS decreased from 6.8±3.1 to 3.8±2.0 (P<.001), whereas in patients with superficial and deep insufficiency, VCSS decreased from 6.7±3.2 to 3.6±2.0 (P<.001). In subgroup analysis of segmental deep reflux, VCSS decreased from 6.6±3.0 to 3.4±1.7 (P<.001), whereas in patients with axial reflux, VCSS decreased from 6.9± 4.0 to 4.1±2.6 (P=.003) (Table 35–3).

The primary conclusion that should be gleaned from these studies is that in the properly selected patients, superficial venous surgery adds substantially to the management of combined deep and superficial reflux.

CONCLUSIONS

Whereas the randomized data are currently sparse for a true Level 1 recommendation for superficial venous surgery in the setting of combined venous reflux, the weight of evidence seems to suggest that ablation of the superficial venous system has a salutary effect on deep venous reflux in the non-PTS setting. Bergen's overload hypothesis is supported by hemodynamic studies based on air plethysmographic data demonstrating decreased VFI, increased EF, and decreased RVF following superficial ablation. Although not all subclasses of deep venous reflux seem to respond as well as others to this type of therapy, it is clearly efficacious in proximal segmental reflux and at the very least nonharmful in the

TABLE 35-3. RECENT INVESTIGATIONS

Study	n	Severity	Reflux	Intervention	VCSS pre	VCSS post	VFI pre	VFI post
Marsten 2008	75	CEAP 5-6	SR + DS/A	EVA and Trivex	7	1.9 ± 2.2†	6.37 ± 3.9	2.67 ± 2.3*
	35	CEAP 5-6	SR + CFV	EVA and Trivex	N/A	N/A†	N/A	N/A†
	40	CEAP 5-6	SR + FV and/or PV	EVA and Trivex	7.7 ± 2.5	2.6 ± 2.7†	6.2 ± 3.8	3.3 ± 3.0†
	N/A	CEAP 5-6	SR + FV and/or PV and MRV <10 cm/sec	EVA and Trivex	7.1 ± 2.1	1.6 ± 0.9†	5.4 ± 2.3	2.2 ± 2.3†
	N/A	CEAP 5-6	SR + FV and/or PV and MRV >10 cm/sec	EVA and Trivex	8.2 ± 2.7	3.5 ± 3.5†	6.9 ± 4.7	4.4 ± 3.2*
Knipp 2008	132	CEAP 1-6	SR	EVLT ± phlebectomy	6.8 ± 3.1	3.8 ± 2.0†		
	311	CEAP 1-6	SR + DS/A	EVLT ± phlebectomy	6.7 ± 3.2	3.6 ± 2.0†		
	250	CEAP 1-6	SR + DS	EVLT ± phlebectomy	6.6 ± 3.0	3.4 ± 1.7†		
	61	CEAP 1-6	SR + A	EVLT ± phlebectomy	6.9 ± 4.0	4.1 ± 2.6*		

Hemodynamic and clinical parameters in patients undergoing superficial venous surgery with combined reflux.
SR: superficial reflux. DS: deep segmental reflux. A: deep axial reflux. EVA: endovenous ablation. EVLT: endovenous laser therapy. VCSS: venous clinical severity score. VFI: venous filling index. CEAP: clinical, etiologic, anatomic, and pathophysiologic. CFV: central visual field. PV: popliteal vein. MRV: maximal reflux velocity.
*Signifies P<.05;
†signifies P<.001.

more advanced cases. Further work is necessary in defining exactly which populations will most benefit from superficial venous surgery in addition to compression therapy. A randomized clinical trial specifically addressing this question would be appropriate; a priori subset analysis could be used to define particular patients likely to benefit. However, at this time, we feel it is appropriate to offer superficial venous ablation to all patients with combined superficial and DVI, except for those patients in whom the superficial system is compensating for persistent deep venous obstruction or severe post-thrombotic changes. Patients with multisegment or distal deep reflux should, however, be counseled that superficial surgery is less likely to achieve complete benefit in their case.

There are a variety of new approaches to the management of severe manifestations of CVI on the horizon. Christensen recently presented a series combining eradication of superficial reflux with ulcer débridement, subcutaneous fasciotomy, and skin grafting. They achieved excellent results in the group of patients receiving both fasciotomy and skin grafting; in patients with ulceration secondary to severe superficial venous insufficiency, skin grafting was unnecessary, indicating the utility of local fasciotomy in this patient population.[30] Another approach recently published by Italiano et al. describes creation of venous neovalves.[31] Eagerly awaited is the endovenous delivery of implantable artificial valves. Until these techniques become more mature, however, standard superficial venous surgical strategies should continue to be employed in the majority of patients with combined superficial and deep venous reflux.

REFERENCES

1. Zamboni P, Cisno C, Marchetti F, et al. Minimally invasive surgical management of primary venous ulcers vs. compression treatment: a randomized clinical trial. Eur J Vasc Endovasc Surg 2003;25:313–8.
2. Maurins U, Hoffmann BH, Losch C, et al. Distribution and prevalence of reflux in the superficial and deep venous system in the general population—results from the Bonn Vein Study, Germany. J Vasc Surg 2008;48:680–7.
3. Padberg FT Jr, Pappas PJ, Araki CT, et al. Hemodynamic and clinical improvement after superficial vein ablation in primary combined venous insufficiency with ulceration. J Vasc Surg 1996;24:711–8.
4. Christopoulos D, Nicolaides AN, Szendro G. Venous reflux: quantification and correlation with the clinical severity of chronic venous disease. Br J Surg 1988;75:352–6.
5. Eklof B, Rutherford RB, Bergan JJ, et al. Revision of the CEAP classification for chronic venous disorders: consensus statement. J Vasc Surg 2004;40:1248–52.
6. Marston WA, Carlin RE, Passman MA, et al. Healing rates and cost efficacy of outpatient compression treatment for leg ulcers associated with venous insufficiency. J Vasc Surg 1999; 30:491–8.
7. Labropoulos N, Tassiopoulos AK, Kang SS, et al. Prevalence of deep venous reflux in patients with primary superficial vein incompetence. J Vasc Surg 2000;32:663–8.
8. Marston WA, Brabham VW, Mendes R, et al. The importance of deep venous reflux velocity as a determinant of outcome in patients with combined superficial and deep venous reflux treated with endovenous saphenous ablation. J Vasc Surg 2008;48:400–5; discussion 405–6.
9. Bergan JJ. Venous insufficiency and perforating veins. Br J Surg 1998;85:721–2.
10. Raju S, Neglen P. Chronic venous insufficiency and varicose veins. N Engl J Med 2009;360:2319–27.
11. Hardy SC, Riding G, Abidia A. Surgery for deep venous incompetence. Cochrane Database Syst Rev 2004;3:CD001097.

12. Browse NL, Burnand KG. The cause of venous ulceration. Lancet 1982;2:243–5.
13. Bradbury AW, Stonebridge PA, Callam MJ, et al. Foot volumetry and duplex ultrasonography after saphenous and subfascial perforating vein ligation for recurrent venous ulceration. Br J Surg 1993;80:845–8.
14. Sottiurai VS. Surgical correction of recurrent venous ulcer. J Cardiovasc Surg (Torino) 1991; 32:104–9.
15. Gloviczki P, Bergan JJ, Rhodes JM, et al. Mid-term results of endoscopic perforator vein interruption for chronic venous insufficiency: lessons learned from the North American Subfascial Endoscopic Perforator Surgery Registry. The North American Study Group. J Vasc Surg 1999;29:489–502.
16. Rhodes JM, Gloviczki P, Canton LG, et al. Factors affecting clinical outcome following endoscopic perforator vein ablation. Am J Surg 1998;176:162–7.
17. Walsh JC, Bergan JJ, Beeman S, Comer TP. Femoral venous reflux abolished by greater saphenous vein stripping. Ann Vasc Surg 1994;8:566–70.
18. Sales CM, Bilof ML, Petrillo KA, Luka NL. Correction of lower extremity deep venous incompetence by ablation of superficial venous reflux. Ann Vasc Surg 1996;10:186–9.
19. Dix FP, Picton A, McCollum CN. Effect of superficial venous surgery on venous function in chronic venous insufficiency. Ann Vasc Surg 2005;19:678–85.
20. Puggioni A, Lurie F, Kistner RL, Eklof B. How often is deep venous reflux eliminated after saphenous vein ablation? J Vasc Surg 2003;38:517–21.
21. Ahmad I, Ahmad W, Dingui M. Prevention or reversal of deep venous insufficiency by aggressive treatment of superficial venous disease. Am J Surg 2006;191:33–8.
22. Scriven JM, Hartshorne T, Thrush AJ, et al. Role of saphenous vein surgery in the treatment of venous ulceration. Br J Surg 1998;85:781–4.
23. Davies AH, Hawdon A J, Greenhalgh RM, Thompson, S., on behalf of the USABLE trial participants. Failure of a trial evaluating the effects of venous surgery on healing and recurrence rates in venous ulcers? The USABLE trial: rationale, design, and methodology, and reasons for failure. Phlebology 2004;19:137–42.
24. Guest MG, Smith J J, Tripuraneni G, et al. Randomised clinical trial of varicose vein surgery with compression versus compression alone for the treatment of venous ulceration. 2003;18:130–6.
25. Barwell JR, Davies CE, Deacon J, et al. Comparison of surgery and compression with compression alone in chronic venous ulceration (ESCHAR study): randomised controlled trial. Lancet 2004;363:1854–9.
26. Gohel MS, Barwell JR, Taylor M, et al. Long term results of compression therapy alone versus compression plus surgery in chronic venous ulceration (ESCHAR): randomised controlled trial. BMJ 2007;335:83.
27. van Gent WB, Hop WC, van Praag MC, et al. Conservative versus surgical treatment of venous leg ulcers: a prospective, randomized, multicenter trial. J Vasc Surg 2006;44:563–71.
28. Howard DP, Howard A, Kothari A, et al. The role of superficial venous surgery in the management of venous ulcers: a systematic review. Eur J Vasc Endovasc Surg 2008;36:458–65.
29. Knipp BS, Blackburn SA, Bloom JR, et al. Endovenous laser ablation: venous outcomes and thrombotic complications are independent of the presence of deep venous insufficiency. J Vasc Surg 2008;48:1538–45.
30. Christenson JT. Postthrombotic or non-postthrombotic severe venous insufficiency: impact of removal of superficial venous reflux with or without subcutaneous fasciotomy. J Vasc Surg. 2007;46:316–21.
31. Lugli M, Guerzoni S, Garofalo M, et al. Neovalve construction in deep venous incompetence. J Vasc Surg 2009;49:156–62, 162 e151–2; discussion 162.

36

Isolated Gastrocnemius and Soleal Vein Thrombosis

Timothy Lautz, M.D. and Melina R. Kibbe, M.D.

INTRODUCTION

In 1960, Barritt and Jordan first showed the benefit of anticoagulation in patients with symptomatic deep vein thrombosis (DVT) or pulmonary embolism (PE) to reduce the incidence of recurrent PE and mortality.[1] Multiple subsequent clinical trials have confirmed the risk for PE and post-thrombotic syndrome in patients with proximal DVT and further defined the optimal management strategy for these patients.[2-7] Over the past 50 years, the favorable risk versus benefit profile for therapeutic anticoagulation in patients with progressively more distal DVT has been recognized.[3,8-9] Furthermore, recent studies have demonstrated the clinical significance of calf vein thrombosis in the spectrum of venous thromboembolism (VTE) disorders.[10-12] However, studies on calf vein thrombosis have largely focused on the axial veins: the anterior tibial (AT), posterior tibial (PT), and peroneal veins. Isolated gastrocnemius and soleal vein thrombosis (IGSVT) is a newly recognized problem whose clinical significance remains debated. IGSVT is being diagnosed with increasing frequency owing to improved venous duplex technology with higher-resolution scans that allow for accurate assessment of these small vessels as well as heightened awareness of the morbidity and mortality associated with calf DVT. This chapter reviews the epidemiology, natural history, clinical presentation, treatment options, and our institution's experience with IGSVT.

EPIDEMIOLOGY

DVT and PE remain major causes of morbidity and mortality. According to the 2009 statistics from the American Heart Association, a new diagnosis of VTE occurs in approximately 1 in 1000 persons each year.[13] The 30-day mortality has been reported to be 6 to 9% for DVT and 12 to 15% for PE.[13-15] The 1-year mortality rate for all VTEs has been reported to be 20 to 31%.[16-18] Furthermore, nearly 30% of patients with DVT will develop chronic venous insufficiency with resultant complications, including swelling, discomfort, and ulceration.[19] Calf thrombi account for nearly half of all newly diagnosed DVTs in some studies, although epidemiologic data distinguishing outcomes for proximal versus calf DVT are quite limited. A 20 to 30% rate of proximal propagation is widely cited for calf DVT managed without anticoagulation.[20-21] There is controversy in the literature, however, with some prospective studies citing a much lower rate of proximal DVT extension from calf DVT.[22] In a study of 1913 patients with VTE followed for an average of 1.5 years, 47% of all patients had DVT limited to the calf veins.[16] Although lower than for proximal or bilateral calf thrombi, unilateral calf DVT was associated with a 29% rate of PE, a 20% 2-year mortality, and a 7.7% recurrence rate at 2 years.[16] A prospective randomized controlled trial showed that the risk of VTE recurrence for patients with calf DVT was 2% with 6 weeks and 3.4% with 12 weeks of oral anticoagulation therapy, and there was no significant difference in outcomes between the treatment groups.[9]

The incidence of IGSVT is less well defined. In an analysis of the patterns and distribution of calf thrombi, Labropoulos et al. noted that isolated calf DVTs were found in 4.8% of lower extremity venous duplex studies and accounted for 34% of positive examinations.[10] The soleal and gastrocnemius veins were involved in 39% and 29% of positive studies, respectively. Thrombus was limited to a single vein in 64% of affected limbs, including the soleal vein in 20% and the gastrocnemius vein in 17% of limbs. Kerr et al. identified the soleal vein as the site for 20% of single-vessel thrombi.[23] Krunes and associates noted that the gastrocnemius and soleal veins were involved in 79% of all patients found to have a DVT by sonography and phlebography, and thrombus was limited to these veins in 25% of cases.[24]

CLINICAL PRESENTATION

IGSVT may be slightly more common in women.[10,25] The mean age at presentation is between 57 and 71 years, but IGSVT occurs in people of all ages, including adolescents as young as 16 years of age.[10,25-26] Symptoms, including pain and/or swelling, are reported in 70 to 86% of patients diagnosed with IGSVT.[10,25] Asymptomatic patients are typically diagnosed during routine duplex screening for high-risk situations. The percentage of patients who are symptomatic versus asymptomatic in any clinical series is dependent upon the indications for obtaining duplex examinations at different institutions and is therefore difficult to determine. The mean duration of symptoms prior to the diagnosis of IGSVT has been reported to be approximately 10 days.[25] IGSVT is frequently diagnosed in both the inpatient and the outpatient settings, with between 42 and 68% of cases occurring in patients receiving acute inpatient care.[10,25]

IGSVT can occur in any combination of the gastrocnemius and/or soleal veins and in one or both legs. Soleal vein thrombosis was much more common than gastrocnemius vein thrombosis in two studies, occurring in 78 to 82% of IGSVT cases.[25-26] One study examined the number of thrombotic veins involved in each muscle and found that 83% of patients with gastrocnemius thrombus and 44% with soleal thrombus had two or more involved veins.[27] In the same study, the diameter of the thrombosis was

≥8 mm in 59% and 56% of patients with isolated gastrocnemius and soleal vein thrombi, respectively.

The same acquired and inherited criteria known to be risk factors for DVT are also believed to predispose patients to IGSVT. These risk factors include cancer, thrombophilia, prior history of VTE, smoking, hormone replacement therapy or oral contraceptive therapy, recent surgery or trauma, and prolonged immobilization. The presence of cancer is the only individual risk factor that has been identified as an independent predictor of IGSVT propagation to proximal DVT or PE.[25] No model exists using risk factors to predict the development of IGSVT or the progression from IGSVT to VTE. The incidence of specific risk factors in patients diagnosed with IGSVT are reported in Table 36–1.

NATURAL HISTORY

Studies on the natural history of patients with IGSVT are limited by relatively small sample size. MacDonald et al. prospectively followed 135 limbs with IGSVT managed without anticoagulation and monitored with serial duplex examination for 3 months.[25] Complete thrombus resolution occurred in 10% of patients at 2 weeks and 46% of patients at 3 months. IGSVT remained stable or resolved in 84% of limbs at 3 months. Thrombus extension to the deep system was quite rare, occurring in only 16% of patients. The vast majority of thrombus extension that occurred did so during the first 2 weeks of follow-up. No patients developed femoral veins or more proximal DVT, and only 3% extended to the popliteal vein. The authors concluded that IGSVT appeared to be more benign than other calf vein thrombi.

The relationship between IGSVT and PE is also poorly defined. The incidence of progression from IGSVT to PE has been quoted at 0 to 7%.[11] Additionally, several authors have reported a 5 to 11% rate of symptomatic PE concurrent with the diagnosis of IGSVT.[11,27-29] Although a cause-and-effect mechanism cannot be assumed, the frequent association of IGSVT with a new diagnosis of PE may be clinically relevant. It is possible that PE in these patients is caused by complete embolization of a more proximal DVT, leaving no remaining trace on subsequent duplex study. However, IGSVT cannot be ruled out as a direct source of these PEs.

TABLE 36-1. VENOUS THROMBOEMBOLISM RISK FACTORS IN PATIENTS WITH ISOLATED GASTROCNEMIUS AND SOLEAL VEIN THROMBOSIS

Risk Factor	Incidence
Recent surgery or trauma	30–65%
Prior VTE	10–47%
Smoking	37%
Cancer	5–29%
Prolonged immobilization	29%
HRT/OCP	3–25%
Thrombophilia	3–15%

HRT = hormone replacement therapy; OCP = oral contraceptive pill VTE.

TREATMENT

There are currently no data from large randomized controlled prospective clinical trials available to guide management decision for patients with IGSVT, and as a result, treatment is inhomogeneous. The most recent guidelines from the American College of Chest Physicians Evidence-Based Clinical Practice Guidelines (8th edition) do not specifically address patients with IGSVT.[3] Potential treatment options include observation with or without serial duplex examinations, prophylaxis with compression stockings and/or anticoagulation, therapeutic doses of anticoagulation, or inferior vena cava filters. For each patient, the risks of major bleeding with anticoagulation (2 to 4% yearly with an international normalized ratio (INR) of 2 to 3 and higher in certain patient populations) must be weighed against the morbidity and mortality of potential DVT and PE.[7,30]

Observation

Advocates of conservative management for patients with IGSVT contend that the disease has a benign natural history and the risks of anticoagulation outweigh the benefits. Some go so far as to argue against even searching for thrombosis in the distal leg.[31] Citing the aforementioned natural history data, these authors argue that propagation to the deep system occurs in only 10 to 15% of patients with IGSVT. Therefore, if all patients with IGSVT are anticoagulated, 85% will be unnecessarily overtreated.[10]

Follow-up duplex examinations are clearly indicated for patients with IGSVT who are managed conservatively. However, the optimal timing and duration of follow-up remain unresolved. Current recommendations include initial repeat duplex within 4 to 14 days of IGSVT diagnosis. MacDonald et al. followed patients at 5, 9, 14, 30, and 90 days and found that 91% of thrombus extension occurred within 2 weeks of initial diagnosis.[25] Other studies, however, have identified higher rates of VTE recurrence well beyond 2 weeks, including a 9% rate between 3 to 9 months and a 14% rate between 9 and 36 months.[27] For this reason, we believe that patients should be followed serially until the thrombus resolves, propagates, or shows sonographic features of chronicity.

Anticoagulation

Mounting evidence suggests that therapeutic anticoagulation reduces the risk of VTE in patients with IGSVT. Schwarz et al., in a nonrandomized prospective study, reported a 0% rate of DVT in 52 patients with IGSVT treated with therapeutic doses of heparin and compression for 10 days versus a 25% rate of DVT in 32 patients who received compression with or without prophylactic doses of heparin ($P<.0002$).[26] Recruitment of patients into the group managed without therapeutic anticoagulation was stopped early because a significant difference in outcome was observed with planned interim analysis. No patients in either group developed symptomatic PE or major bleeding. Gillet et al. likewise demonstrated the importance of therapeutic anticoagulation in their prospective study of 128 patients with IGSVT.[27] They observed a 19% rate of VTE recurrence despite 1 to 3 months of therapeutic anticoagulation.

At present, there are no data to suggest an advantage of any one anticoagulant over another (i.e., unfractionated heparin, low-molecular-weight heparin [LMWH], or vitamin K antagonist), and there is conflicting evidence about the optimal duration of therapy. In the study by Schwarz et al., a 10-day course of LMWH was successful in preventing VTE recurrence during 3 months of follow-up.[26] However, Gillet and associates showed that VTE recurrence is not uncommon despite 1 to 3 months of therapeutic anticoagulation.[27] A randomized controlled trial comparing 6 versus 12 weeks of anticoagulation demonstrated that 6 weeks was sufficient for patients with calf vein thrombosis.[9] Although this study included patients with calf DVT (tibial and peroneal veins), the results should be translatable to patients with IGSVT, which affects nonaxial muscular veins. As in all patients with venous thrombosis, an individualized assessment of the risks and benefits of anticoagulation is required before deciding on the optimal management.

Inferior Vena Cava Filters

Those patients with IGSVT who are considered to have a contraindication to anticoagulation and felt to be at high risk of VTE or those in whom a PE would be potentially catastrophic should be considered for an inferior vena cava filter. In one study of all distal DVTs, inferior vena cava filter was the initial treatment in 6.9% of patients.[11] There are currently no data to support or refute this practice in patients with IGSVT.

NORTHWESTERN UNIVERSITY EXPERIENCE

We recently reviewed 38,426 lower extremity venous duplex studies performed during a 5-year period from 2002 to 2007 and identified 7522 studies that were positive for thrombosis.[32] From this cohort, 784 patients with IGSVT in one or more limbs were identified. After excluding patients with contralateral DVT, concurrent PE, or lack of follow-up, 406 patients with IGSVT in 452 limbs were included in our analysis.

We found that IGSVT occurred in 2.0% (784/38,426) of all lower extremity duplex examinations and accounted for 10.4% (784/7522) of positive studies.[32] The mean age of patients with IGSVT was 60.7±16.4 years and 53% of subjects were male. The majority of patients were symptomatic (65%) and inpatients (55%) at the time of diagnosis. In contrast to the previously cited studies, the gastrocnemius vein was involved more frequently (60%) than the soleal vein (37%), and both veins were involved in 3% of patients. The left limb alone was involved in 47% of patients, the right alone in 41% of patients, and both limbs were affected in 11% of patients. DVT risk factors included cancer (29%), thrombophilia (4%), recent surgery (55%), limb trauma (10%), prior VTE (10%), and smoking (37%).

Among our cohort, 30% of patients with IGSVT who received no anticoagulation and 27% who received prophylactic anticoagulation developed VTE events. This included significant rates of proximal DVT extension as well as PE. Interestingly, we observed 14.6% and 11.8% rates of common femoral vein DVT as well as 4.2% and 5.9% rates of PE in patients managed with prophylactic or no anticoagulation, respectively. VTE occurrences frequently happened many months after IGSVT diagnosis. In multivariate analysis, a prior history of VTE was the only clinical factor that predicted VTE occurrence. Over the duration of follow-up, approximately 40% of patients who received prophylactic or no anticoagulation experienced complete thrombus resolution. As in other studies, PE at the time of IGSVT diagnosis was not rare, occurring in 5.6%

of patients. For these cases, lower extremity duplex was performed to locate a source of embolism in patients with radiographically confirmed PE.

As described above, the incidence of VTE was unacceptably high for patients with IGSVT who were observed or given prophylactic doses of heparin. However, treatment with therapeutic anticoagulation reduced the rate of VTE significantly from 30 to 12% ($P<.05$). This included a significant decrease in proximal DVT extension, including to the common femoral vein. A nonsignificant trend toward reduction in PE was also observed in patients who received therapeutic anticoagulation (3.7%) compared with those who received no anticoagulation (5.9%). In multivariate analysis, when controlled for all other factors, treatment with therapeutic anticoagulation independently predicted a reduction in VTE events. Finally, therapeutic anticoagulation significantly increased the likelihood of complete thrombus resolution. Over the entire duration of the study, IGSVT resolved in 61% of the group that received therapeutic anticoagulation but only 40% of those who received no anticoagulation.

FUTURE DIRECTION

Although mounting data suggest that therapeutic anticoagulation reduces the risk of VTE in patients with IGSVT, further studies are needed to confirm the positive risk versus benefit profile. The data supporting this management strategy are based on retrospective and small prospective studies, and the conclusions are not universal (Table 36–2). A randomized controlled trial is required to prove that the reduced morbidity and mortality resulting from therapeutic anticoagulation, including death, symptomatic PE, and/or post-thrombotic syndrome, outweigh the low but real risk of clinically significant bleeding that occurs with anticoagulation. Ideally, a randomized trial would also clarify the optimal duration of therapy. Ultimately, however, the goal is to delineate factors that predict which patients with IGSVT will develop VTE and reserve anticoagulation for the 30% of patients who fall into this subset.

CONCLUSION AND RECOMMENDATIONS

IGSVT is associated with a clinically significant rate of progression to proximal DVT and PE and cannot be considered a totally benign process. In the absence of major bleeding risk factors, we recommend therapeutic anticoagulation for 6 weeks in patients diagnosed with IGSVT. Patients who cannot be anticoagulated should be followed with serial duplex examinations. The high incidence of VTE events, frequently occurring many weeks to months after initial diagnosis, highlights the need for vigilance in monitoring and caring for this patient population.

TABLE 36-2. SUMMARY OF KEY FINDINGS FROM STUDIES ON ISOLATED GASTROCNEMIUS AND SOLEAL VEIN THROMBOSIS

Study	# Limbs Studied	Study Design	Study Criteria	Treatment Group(s)	Follow-Up	Finding	Recommendation
Schwarz 2001[26]	84	Prospective, nonrandomized	Symptomatic only	Therapeutic vs no anticoagulation	3, 5, 10 days, 1, 3 months	0% vs 25% DVT	Short course anticoagulation
MacDonald 2003[25]	135	Prospective, observational	All	No anticoagulation	5, 9, 14 days 1, 3 months	16.3% distal DVT 0% proximal DVT	Serial duplex for 2 weeks
Gillet 2007[27]	131	Prospective, observational	Symptomatic only	1–3 months therapeutic anticoagulation	1, 3, 9 & up to 36 months	18.8% symptomatic VTE recurrence	Anticoagulation
Lautz 2009[32]	452	Retrospective, cohort	All	Therapeutic vs prophylactic vs no anticoagulation	Variable, mean 7.5 months	12% vs 27% vs 30% VTE	Anticoagulation

DVT = deep vein thrombosis; VTE = venous thromboembolism,

REFERENCES

1. Barritt DW, Jordan SC. Anticoagulant drugs in the treatment of pulmonary embolism. A controlled trial. Lancet 1960;1:1309–12.
2. Hull RD, Raskob GE, Hirsh J, et al. Continuous intravenous heparin compared with intermittent subcutaneous heparin in the initial treatment of proximal-vein thrombosis. N Engl J Med 1986;315:1109–14.
3. Kearon C, Kahn SR, Agnelli G, et al. Antithrombotic therapy for venous thromboembolic disease: American College of Chest Physicians Evidence-Based Clinical Practice Guidelines (8th Edition). Chest 2008;133:454S-545S.
4. Prandoni P, Lensing AW, Cogo A, et al. The long-term clinical course of acute deep venous thrombosis. Ann Intern Med 1996;125:1–7.
5. Strandness DE Jr, Langlois Y, Cramer M, et al. Long-term sequelae of acute venous thrombosis. JAMA 1983;250:1289–92.
6. Palareti G, Cosmi B, Legnani C, et al. D-dimer testing to determine the duration of anticoagulation therapy. N Engl J Med 2006;355:1780–9.
7. Kearon C, Gent M, Hirsh J, et al. A comparison of three months of anticoagulation with extended anticoagulation for a first episode of idiopathic venous thromboembolism. N Engl J Med 1999;340:901–7.
8. Lagerstedt CI, Olsson CG, Fagher BO, et al. Need for long-term anticoagulant treatment in symptomatic calf-vein thrombosis. Lancet 1985;2:515–8.
9. Pinede L, Ninet J, Duhaut P, et al. Comparison of 3 and 6 months of oral anticoagulant therapy after a first episode of proximal deep vein thrombosis or pulmonary embolism and comparison of 6 and 12 weeks of therapy after isolated calf deep vein thrombosis. Circulation 2001;103:2453–60.
10. Labropoulos N, Webb KM, Kang SS, et al. Patterns and distribution of isolated calf deep vein thrombosis. J Vasc Surg 1999;30:787–91.
11. Meissner MH, Caps MT, Bergelin RO, et al. Early outcome after isolated calf vein thrombosis. J Vasc Surg 1997;26:749–56.
12. Lohr JM, James KV, Deshmukh RM, Hasselfeld KA, et al. Calf vein thrombi are not a benign finding. Am J Surg 1995;170:86–90.
13. Lloyd-Jones D, Adams R, Carnethon M, et al. Heart disease and stroke statistics—2009 update: a report from the American Heart Association Statistics Committee and Stroke Statistics Subcommittee. Circulation 2009;119:e21–181.
14. White RH. The epidemiology of venous thromboembolism. Circulation 2003;107:I4–8.
15. Cushman M, Tsai AW, White RH, et al. Deep vein thrombosis and pulmonary embolism in two cohorts: the longitudinal investigation of thromboembolism etiology. Am J Med 2004; 117:19–25.
16. Seinturier C, Bosson JL, Colonna M, et al. Site and clinical outcome of deep vein thrombosis of the lower limbs: an epidemiological study. J Thromb Haemost 2005; 3:1362–7.
17. Anderson FA Jr, Wheeler HB, Goldberg RJ, et al. A population-based perspective of the hospital incidence and case-fatality rates of deep vein thrombosis and pulmonary embolism. The Worcester DVT Study. Arch Intern Med 1991;151:933–8.
18. Heit JA, Silverstein MD, Mohr DN, et al. Predictors of survival after deep vein thrombosis and pulmonary embolism: a population-based, cohort study. Arch Intern Med 1999;159: 445–53.
19. Eklof B, Rutherford RB, Bergan JJ, et al. Revision of the CEAP classification for chronic venous disorders: consensus statement. J Vasc Surg 2004;40:1248–52.
20. Philbrick JT, Becker DM. Calf deep venous thrombosis. A wolf in sheep's clothing? Arch Intern Med 1988;148:2131–8.
21. Kearon C. Natural history of venous thromboembolism. Circulation 2003;107:I22–30.
22. Masuda EM, Kessler DM, Kistner RL, et al. The natural history of calf vein thrombosis: lysis of thrombi and development of reflux. J Vasc Surg 1998;28:67–73; discussion 73–4.

23. Kerr TM, Cranley JJ, Johnson JR, et al. Analysis of 1084 consecutive lower extremities involved with acute venous thrombosis diagnosed by duplex scanning. Surgery 1990;108: 520–7.
24. Krunes U, Teubner K, Knipp H, Holzapfel R. Thrombosis of the muscular calf veins—reference to a syndrome which receives little attention. Vasa 1998;27:172–5.
25. MacDonald PS, Kahn SR, Miller N, Obrand D. Short-term natural history of isolated gastrocnemius and soleal vein thrombosis. J Vasc Surg 2003;37:523–7.
26. Schwarz T, Schmidt B, Beyer J, Schellong SM. Therapy of isolated calf muscle vein thrombosis with low-molecular-weight heparin. Blood Coagul Fibrinolysis 2001;12:597–9.
27. Gillet JL, Perrin MR, Allaert FA. Short-term and mid-term outcome of isolated symptomatic muscular calf vein thrombosis. J Vasc Surg 2007;46:513–9; discussion 519.
28. Lohr JM, Kerr TM, Lutter KS, et al. Lower extremity calf thrombosis: to treat or not to treat? J Vasc Surg 1991;14:618–23.
29. Ohgi S, Tachibana M, Ikebuchi M, et al. Pulmonary embolism in patients with isolated soleal vein thrombosis. Angiology 1998;49:759–64.
30. Schulman S, Granqvist S, Holmstrom M, et al. The duration of oral anticoagulant therapy after a second episode of venous thromboembolism. The Duration of Anticoagulation Trial Study Group. N Engl J Med 1997;336:393–8.
31. Righini M, Bounameaux H. Clinical relevance of distal deep vein thrombosis. Curr Opin Pulm Med 2008;14:408–13.
32. Lautz T, Abbas F, Novis S, et al. Isolated gastrocnemius and soleal vein thrombosis (IGSVT): Should these patients receive therapeutic anticoagulation. Ann Surg 2009; in press.

37

Lymphedema: Current Udate and Management

Gail L. Gamble, M.D.

Few practitioners are interested in the condition of lymphedema, its pathophysiology, diagnosis, or available treatment options. It is often considered a benign "nuisance" condition, not a medical problem, with few treatments offered for the bewildered and frustrated patient. Primarily thought of as nonoperative in management, the surgeon may also consider this condition as an area of nonexpertise. A consultation is often sought with the vascular surgeon, who remains a primary resource for generalists facing the problem of new-onset limb edema. Detailed knowledge of the lymphatic system is important to the surgeon for this diagnosis as well as for the interrelationship of lymphatic integrity to the venous system. When proper diagnosis and appropriate treatment result in volume reduction, the results can be life-changing for the chronically afflicted patient.

LYMPHATIC ANATOMY, PATHOPHYSIOLOGY, AND MOLECULAR GENETICS

Anatomy

The primary function of the lymphatic system is absorption and homeostatic transport of protein-rich fluid not transported within the veins. Other important functions include the mediation of local immune response and interconnection of the lymphoid tissues.[1] Lymph flow is initiated in loosely arranged capillaries within the interstitium. The endothelial lining of the lymphatic capillary lacks a tight junction, which allows for distention during increased interstitial pressures to create valve-like openings allowing uptake of extra fluid and large macromolecules, including interstitial proteins. The lymph fluid then drains into precollecting and collecting vessels that have a basement membrane layer, with the collecting vessels also having a smooth muscle layer and valve-like structures that aid in propulsion of the lymph forward. Similar to the venous system, there are both superficial and deep networks of lymphatics serving the skin and subcutaneous tissues as well as the fascial and subfascial compartments. These two systems interconnect via the perforating vessels. Ultimately, the lymph drains into the thoracic duct or the right lymphatic duct of the proximal venous system.[2-3]

Pathophysiology

When a homeostatic balance exists, lymph flow is dictated by the balance between the hydrostatic pressures manifested by increased blood flow, the oncotic pressures of the interstitium, and the lymphatic system's ability to regulate its own outflow to avoid significant variation in the local tissue environment. When a mal-development, disruption, or blockage of lymph flow occurs, it should be noted that the physiologic characteristics of the arterial and venous capillaries initially remain normal. This increases intralymphatic pressures distal to the lymphatic abnormality, with lymph vessel dilation, valvular structural loss, and poor lymphatic transport.[4]

Lymphedema, which by practical definition is reduced lymph transport or low output failure of the lymphatic system, may be classified as primary or secondary.[3] Primary lymphedema denotes decreased or nondevelopment of some component of the lymphatic vascular tree. Secondary lymphedema occurs when the architecture of normal functioning lymphatics is altered in some way by tumor obstruction, trauma, surgical disruption, radiation-induced fibrosis, or infection-related lymphatic vessel destruction.

The development of lymphedema may not be clinically noticeable for several years, as chronic change with slowing of lymphatic transport impacts the local tissue environment over time. Recent studies have measured increased lymphatic fluid volume in limbs contralateral to a previously thought normal limb that had developed acute erysipelas.[5-6] Thus, it is now felt that a subclinical or latency stage exists, which requires recognition as a lymphedema precursor or Grade 0 lymphedema (Table 37–1).[7] With persistent lymphatic (protein-rich) interstitial stasis, there occurs thickening of the dermal/epidermal junctions, regional tissue inflammation, and fibrosis with dilation of the distal collecting lymphatics. Chronic lymphatic stasis over time often results in the development of significant adipose tissue, for reasons that remain unclear.[8-9] Cytokines as well as cellular elements of lymph or chyle that chronically persist within the lymphedematous tissues may stimulate resident cells, including adipocytes and fibroblasts to proliferate and undergo fibrosis and altered function as a result of chronic lymph stasis.

Molecular Genetics

Considerable progress into the molecular basis of lymphatic development, function, and disease has been forthcoming over the past decade. There have been major advances in our understanding of the pathogenesis of several primary forms of lymphedema as well as lymphedema-associated syndromes, largely owing to cutting-edge genetic and genomic

TABLE 37-1. CLINICAL GRADES OF LYMPHEDEMA

Grade 0	Latent, preclinical, lymphedema not visible or palpable
Grade I	Reversible, pitting edema present, reduces with elevation
Grade II	Not reversible, no reduction with elevation, fibrosis present
Grade III	Not reversible, severe skin changes with fibrosis, sclerosis, papillomatosis

technologies that have allowed much more refined localization of the loci and genes involved in lymphatic vasculogenesis as well as regeneration. In addition, there are a variety of more common to rare, complex-combined vascular malformations of the extremities that involve perturbation of the lymphatics. These include more purely lymphatic as well as mixed lymphatic in combination with arterial and/or venous malformations that are considered mixed anomalies.

The capillary heme-angio as well as lymph-angio vascular syndromes can be classified by anatomic and pathologic features as well as functional vascular syndromic disorders encompassing both fast-flow and slow-flow anomalies.[10] Fast-flow developmental disorders include the capillary arteriovenous malformation (CAVM) as well as the related but less common malformation in which lymphedema and lymphatic vesicles are also present, which is classified as capillary lymphatic AVM (CLAVM). This includes the Parkes Weber and Stewart-Bluefarb syndromes. The majority of complex-combined vascular malformations are of slow-flow type, with either overgrowth or undergrowth of involved limbs. These would include the CLM and CLVM types with overgrowth, such as Klippel-Trenaunay syndrome, as well as the CLVM with limb undergrowth, known as Servelle-Martorell syndrome. Each of these involves as yet not fully defined genetic mutations that in combination with growth factors and other trophic regulators of cell development and growth, contribute to the complex and varied phenotypic alterations typically seen in each of these distinct forms of disease. In the case of Klippel-Trenaunay syndrome, there is genetic evidence that dysregulation of the angiogenic factor, AGGF-1 (VG5Q), plays a significant role in the development of this type of complex-combined vascular syndrome.[11]

The classic inherited lymphedema disorders, including Milroy (autosomal dominant, inherited, congenital lymphedema) and Meige disease (pubertal onset tending toward autosomal dominant inheritance) as well as lymphedema-distichiasis syndrome, have revealed important new findings in recent years concerning the molecular pathology underlying the development of the disrupted lymphatics (reviewed in Connell et al.).[12] These seminal observations have paralleled the remarkable new discoveries into the vascular endothelial growth factor (VEGF) family of mitogenic and developmentally important ligands and VEGF receptor (VEGFR) family as well as developmental factors regulating lymphatic vasculogenesis and lymphatic remodeling, maturation, regeneration, and overall lymphatic function. Milroy disease has been identified to be caused by mutations within the VEGFR3 gene product, which prevents development of the initial superficial lymphatics of skin in the animal model of the disease.[13] However, in the human disease, Connell et al.[12] report that involved skin of patients with Milroy disease demonstrates an abundance of cutaneous lymphatics in contrast to the animal model of the disease. In nonedematous skin, expression of VEGFR3 appears to be preserved. By contrast, there has been controversy as to the molecular cause of Meige disorder. Early reports had suggested that the transcription factor, Fox C2, was mutated. However, more recent studies have not been able to confirm the implication that this gene is responsible for Meige disease.[14] By contrast, the lymphedema-distichiasis syndrome is due to mutations within the Fox C2 gene. Elegant animal and in vitro studies have complemented these family studies to more fully understand the complex molecular biology and biology of lymphangiogenesis. At least 18 genes, ranging from VEGF and VEGFR to transcription factors prox I and sox 18, have been implicated in lymphatic vascular development and maturation. Many of these have been further characterized in specific screening assays to be critical in normal lymphatic function as well.[2]

INCIDENCE

The primary lymphedemas are extremely rare, prevalence being reported from the British literature at approximately 1 in 6000.[15] Incidence data are reported very rarely other than a 1985 report from the Mayo Clinic that cites the incidence of primary lymphedema as 1.15 per 100,000 up to age 20.[16] For the condition of secondary lymphedema, most studies are from the breast cancer literature, which cites from 6 to 50% incidence with some study variation.[17] A recent population-based study of 631 breast cancer patients, following patients for 5 years using a validated self-report questionnaire, revealed a lymphedema incidence of 42 per 100 women or 42%.[18] A review of available literature for multiple tumor types further reveals variable but significant incidence rates (several studies as high as 40%) in patients with groin dissection for melanoma as well as in the gynecologic tumor population postgroin dissection and radiation.[19] It was widely anticipated that increasingly conservative surgical intervention, including sentinel lymphadenectomy and more focused radiation, would virtually eradicate the development of lymphedema, but that has not been realized.[20] This strongly implicates a multifactorial etiology for lymphedema development, even in the secondary setting. In the non-Western world, the most common secondary lymphedema is lymphatic filariasis, which occurs subsequent to infection from *Wuchereria bancrofti*. Although its true incidence is not clearly documented, it is reported that approximately 120 million people in at least 83 endemic countries suffer from this condition.[21]

RISK FACTORS AND PREVENTIVE MEASURES

Risk Factors

The risk factors for clinical expression of primary lymphedema, other than known genetic risk, are similar to those now documented for secondary lymphedema. Multiple conditions are associated with the clinical onset of secondary lymphedema as documented in various studies (Table 37–2). Although traditionally the presence of extensive surgery (lymphadenectomy) and sites of radiation come to mind as being risk factors,[22] the incidence of weight gain since treatment and prior infection in the regional area are strong links noted in recent literature.[17,24] The multiplicity of risk factors identified, coupled with the variable and frequent long latency between lymphatic insult at surgery and development of clinical lymphedema, challenge the clinician. One should consider early the patient's comorbidities and the unique risks presented by individual disease and treatment processes when counseling any patient regarding the likelihood of lymphedema development in the immediate or distant future.[9]

TABLE 37-2. LYMPHEDEMA-ASSOCIATED RISK FACTORS

Infection (remote or recent, severe or mild)[17,23]
Weight gain (since cancer treatments)[17,24]
Limb trauma (e.g., surgery, fracture, burn)[25]
Chronic venous Insufficiency (stasis ulceration, chronic inflammation)[26]
Surgical extent/location (lymphadenectomy, tumor location)[27]
Radiation location (over lymphatic beds)[23]

Preventive Measures

Preventive measures are largely empirical and poorly studied. There have been lists of restrictions and limb protections promulgated through the patient literature without substantial evidence base.[28] There are several precautions that are widely accepted and seem reasonable to follow:

1. Rigorous skin care: Avoidance of dried fissured skin remains critical, risking barrier breakdown with increased potential for bacterial access. Daily moisturizing with nonalcohol-based cream rubbed into dampened skin will trap the water for better hydration and lubrication. Regular skin assessment of feet and hands to avoid fungal infection can be helpful to minimize associated episodes of cellulitis.[29]
2. Reduction of body mass index (BMI): Weight management with attention to good nutrition is also key to minimize the effects and risks of obesity in the limb at risk. The documentation for increased lymphedema occurrence with increased BMI is clear. Statistically significant lymphedema (arm volume) reduction has also been associated with weight loss at 12-week follow-up in a small but prospective study that followed patients who were subjected to an individualized reduced calorie diet compared with controls who did not formally attempt weight loss.[30] In educating patients who desire to proactively minimize risk for lymphedema, weight management may be a valuable self-management tool within the patient's control.
3. Exercise: Perhaps the greatest change in philosophy for treatment of limbs at risk or those with early lymphedema is in the realm of limb exercise. For years, exercise or significant weight-bearing through the upper or lower extremities was frowned upon and thought to increase lymphedema risk. The literature of the past decade has pointed increasingly against this.[31-34] Although sample sizes were small, these studies reported that upper extremity exercise results in no increased incidence of lymphedema development or exacerbation of swelling. Most recently, a prospective randomized trial of 141 women with breast cancer–related lymphedema reported no greater limb volume change than controls, less self-reported severity, fewer lymphedema exacerbations, and increased strength.[35] It appears that a slowly progressive exercise regimen is well tolerated without lymphedema exacerbation and has many documented positive benefits, including increased quality of life.[36-37]

CLINICAL PRESENTATION AND ASSESSMENT

The assessment for and diagnosis of lymphedema are largely clinical in nature. The presentation is often nondramatic and insidious, with an episode of mild edema that resolves and then reappears sometime later. Early attention to prevention of edema recurrence is important, so single incidents should be valued and treated as early lymphedema with prophylactic measures of light compression. Evaluation should investigate a history of limb trauma, perioperative or other infections in affected areas, and history of previous malignancy requiring radiation. The examiner must rule out other etiologies of limb edema, including other organ pathology such as renal or hepatic insufficiency, protein-losing syndromes, thyroid disease, cardiovascular or pulmonary disease, obesity-related edema, the condition of lipedema, or other rarer systemic disease such as amyloidosis. Imaging to assist in focusing the diagnosis should include duplex ultrasound to exclude occult deep venous thrombosis and ensure venous integrity and CT of the abdomen and pelvis in order to rule out undiscovered proximal obstruction if lower limbs are affected. Bone x-rays could exclude bony overgrowth in lymphovascular syndromes. The physical examination should include a thorough evaluation of all limbs and trunk, not just the suspected area of edema. Close scrutiny of all palpable lymph nodes should be undertaken, including cervical, axillary, and groin areas, also checking for lymphatic "cording" along these areas. The subtle clinical Stemmer's sign (mild edema on dorsum of the foot between the first two toes) is a clinical indication of early lymph stasis. It should be noted that lymphedema is not found only in the extremity but occurs in the trunk, genitals, neck, and facial areas as well. The character of the edema should be recorded, including pitting, firmness/fibrosis of tissue, skin integrity (including dryness or cracking), skin temperature, color, and hyperkeratosis/papillomatosis if present.

In the United States, the most common reason for lymphatic failure is tumor and related treatments, and in these instances, clinical history and examination may be sufficient for diagnosis (other than ultrasound). In cases of new-onset nontrauma-related unilateral limb edema, lymphoscintigraphy is noted to be a very useful tool to clarify the integrity of the lymphatic system in question. This technique involves the intradermal injection of radiolabeled colloid between two digits of feet or hands with subsequent timed measurement of lymphatic uptake and transport.[38] When considering the etiology of new-onset unilateral lymphedema, the lymphoscintigraphic test is important not only for visualizing the affected limb but also for investigating the lymphatic integrity of the presumed opposite normal limb as well.

Measurement of extent of lymphedema is not standardized to date. Serial circumferential measurements and volumetric recordings have traditionally been utilized. Recent other measurement options include bioelectric impedance tissue analysis[39-40] and perometry (opto-electric infrared measurement with calculated volume).[41] Unfortunately, to date, no one measurement tool has been accepted as the overall standard that would enable both individual clinical progress and methodologic research comparisons with greater ease.

MANAGEMENT OPTIONS

Pharmacologic Intervention

Traditionally, there have been few pharmacologic agents routinely used in the care of chronic lymphedema. Historically, diuretics have been used without much success when lymphedema alone is the primary cause for swelling. Because the etiology of the edema is related to increased interstitial oncotic pressure secondary to macromolecule concentration rather than to increased hydrostatic pressure, the diuretic has little effect on fluid reduction. When a component of venous failure exists concurrently, it is appropriate to initiate a low-dose trial to see if the local environment may be decompressed. Additionally, in the clinical setting, in the rare instance of hospitalization for aggressive reduction management, a short course of intense diuretic therapy may be used in conjunction with elevation and compression techniques. In the early 1990s, a benzopyrone agent, coumarin, was reported to have a significant effect in lymphedema reduction, an effect thought to occur by stimulating local tissue macrophage activity with resultant proteolysis.[42] A meta-analysis has supported the success of these agents in reducing edema volumes.[43] However, increased liver enzyme levels noted in another study have precluded widespread use, and these drugs are not available in the United States to date.[44]

Lymphedema as a chronic disease poses increased risk of acute and chronic recurrent infectious cellulitis. The elevated risk is due to several factors, including potential disruption of the skin barrier by fungal infection and trauma as well as by the protein-rich accumulation of fluid within the limb that predisposes to an environment conducive to bacterial growth. The condition must, therefore, be treated promptly and effectively with antimicrobial therapy. The usually invasive organisms are members of the streptococcal bacterial family. Antibiotics found to be most effective, therefore, are penicillins, cephalosporins, and clindamycin orally or parenterally if progression of disease or systemic symptoms and signs warrant this route of administration. If the frequency or severity of recurrent episodes dictates, prophylactic longer-term or regular intermittent antibiotic use is routinely administered, although there are no controlled studies to show preferred efficacy of one regimen or another or, in fact, definite clinical benefit in overall outcomes of morbidity or mortality associated with lymphedema.

Manual Therapy

The accepted gold standard of treatment for lymphedema currently is decongestive lymphatic therapy.[7] This group of treatments includes both an aggressive reduction phase and a more long-standing maintenance phase (Table 37–3) and has been documented to be effective in multiple descriptive and controlled studies.[45-48] Specially trained therapists are required for the techniques utilized in this program.

Manual drainage (Figures 37–1 and 37–2) is performed with the patient supine and relaxed and is a very light first truncal massage to presumably open and clear proximal lymph channels, then proceeding to a more distal massage to propel lymph across superficial plexes from drainage beds not functioning to those more proximal that are. After clearing the lymph with massage, the second component involves a skilled multilayer bandaging process (Figures 37–3 and 37–4) to provide a rigid resistance to subcutaneous fluid deposition. The concept of the low-stretch bandage is one of low pressure at rest but high "working" pressure with muscle pump action. This is in contrast to the typical elastic bandage that has a higher pressure at rest but yields with muscle contraction and movement. Exercises within the bandage system work to assist in moving fluid into the lymphatic vessels, transporting the fluid proximally while the resistance of the bandage is applied. Other forms of exercise are also important, including range of motion, stretching, and aerobic conditioning.[49] Meticulous skin hygiene is critical in minimizing the risks of skin breakdown, with the inherent risk of infection (cellulitis). The maintenance phase consists of a pressure garment worn to maintain fluid reduction during the day with continued bandaging at night.

TABLE 37-3. COMPLEX DECONGESTIVE THERAPY COMPONENTS

Phase I: Reduction	Phase II: Maintenance
Manual lymphatic massage/drainage	Daily use of pressure garments
Complex multilayered low-stretch wrapping	Nightly use of pressure system (wrap or rigid sleeve)
Specific lymphatic exercises	Continued exercise regimen
Skin care education and techniques	Continued skin monitoring

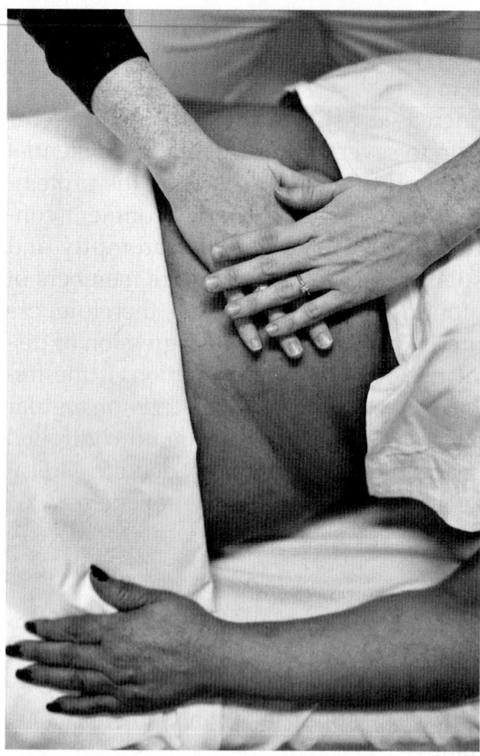

Figure 37-1. Light compression manual massage of trunk stimulates and opens proximal trunk lymph channels preceding lymphatic drainage of the limb.

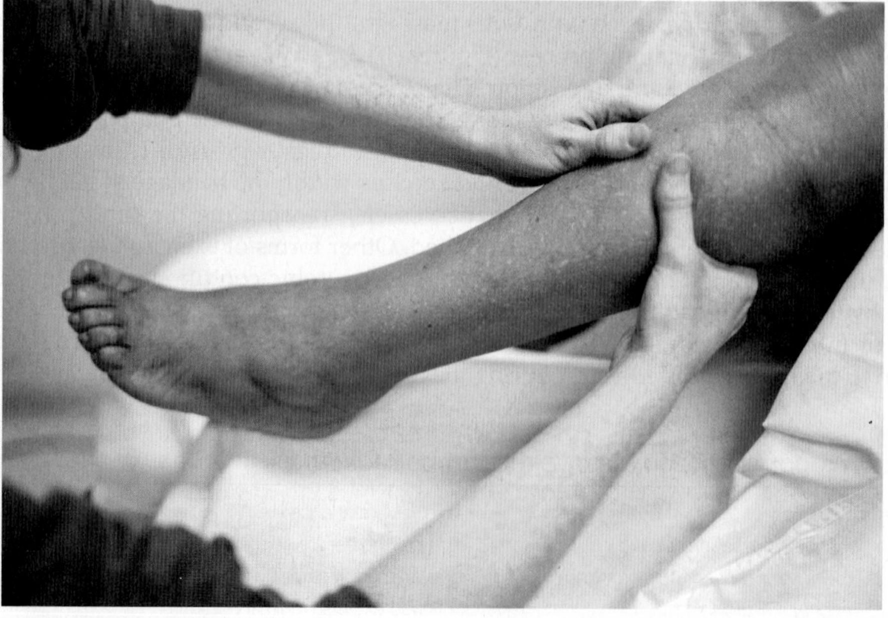

Figure 37-2. Manual drainage of limb is performed proximal to distal, small area distal to proximal, massage moving fluid toward the cleared proximal trunk channels.

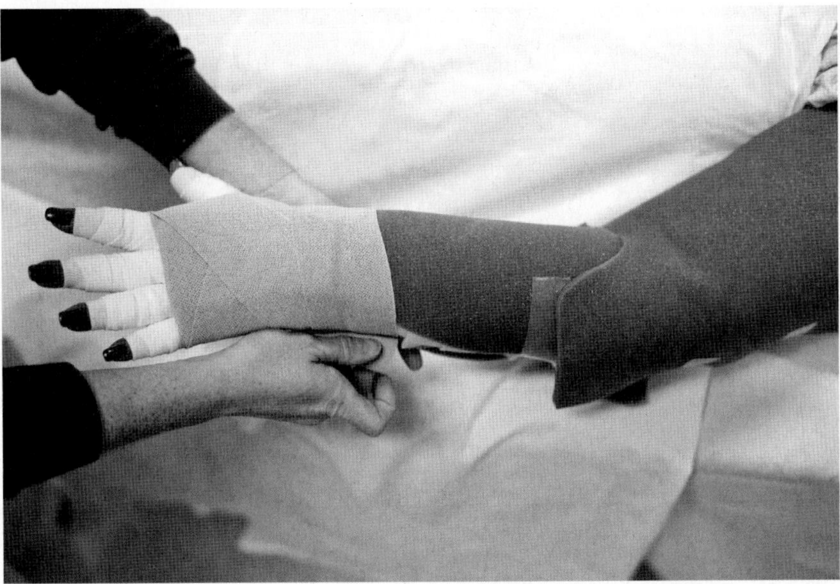

Figure 37-3. Multilayered compression system through foam placement allows maximal pressures over areas of recalcitrant edema without creating discomfort.

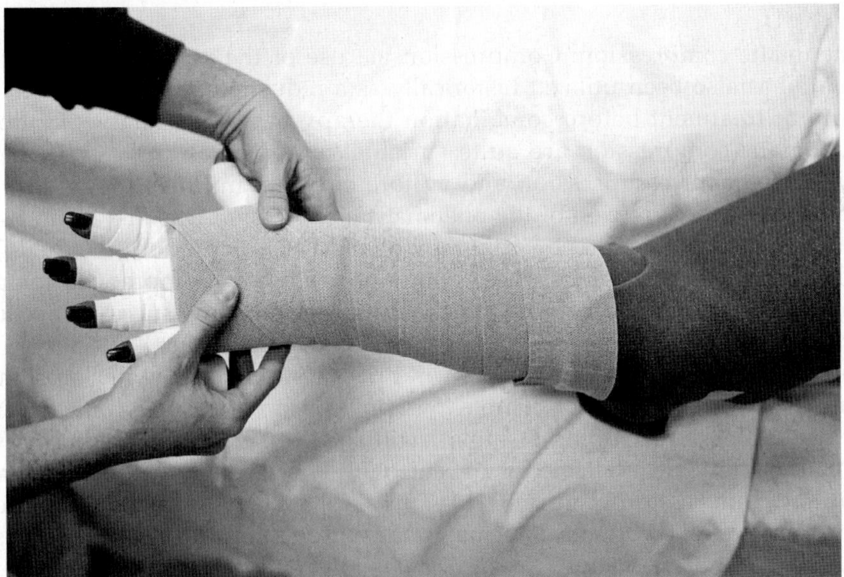

Figure 37-4. Completing the multilayered compression with low-stretch bandaging allows comfort at rest but provides increased resistance with muscle pumping to enhance lymph transport proximally.

Compression

Compression of some type is critical to maintain the success of reduction regardless of the intervention used. Many patients have multifactorial edema, with dependency and minimal muscle pumping function of inactivity working against gains made during the reduction phase.

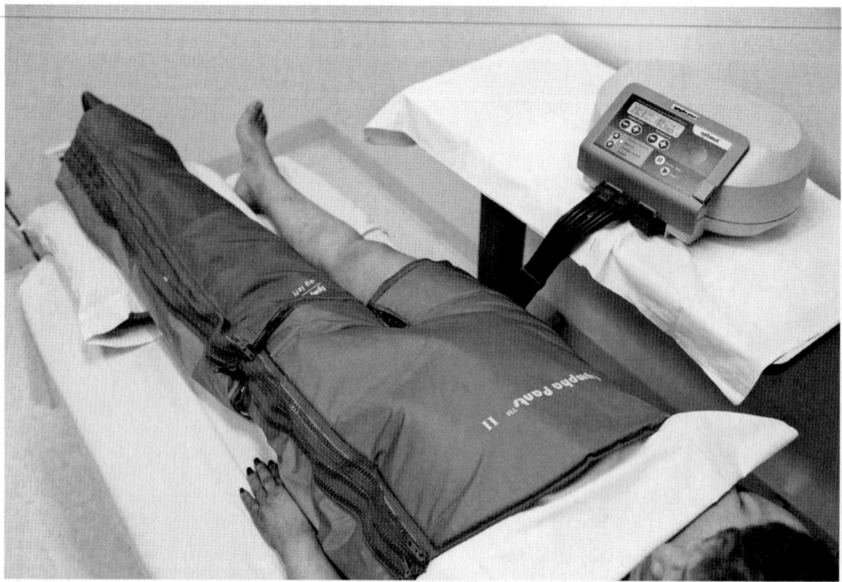

Figure 37-5. Newer-concept sequential pneumatic devices approximate pattern of manual drainage lymph transport by stimulating first truncal areas, then limb. Several different commercial options are available for upper and lower limbs.

1. Pneumatic compression: Compression via use of the pneumatic compression pump has also been utilized historically as a reduction tool and was the major form of treatment before combination therapy became available. Options for pneumatic compression are quite variable, with pumps being available with single-chamber compression and a more complex multichambered option.[49] Historically, the direction of the pneumatic compression was in a distal to proximal direction, but recent newer pump options aim to reproduce the fluid flow of the manual lymph massage. These pumps have a truncal compression component that precedes the limb compression component and some success in reduction, and certainly patient comfort is being reported (Figure 37– 5).[50]
2. Rigid compression devices: After over 2 decades of success with the somewhat cumbersome techniques of complex wrapping procedures, a significant number of new products providing a similar rigid compressive resistance but easy donning capability are available for patients with lymphedema who have a need for chronic compression (Figure 37–6). There are multiple options for upper and lower limb, trunk, and facial edema. In the author's clinical experience, these easily worn compression systems seem to be tolerated better by the patient, especially during the long-standing patient-managed maintenance phase. It should be noted that contrary to strict philosophies of several decades ago, there is now more often a blend of massage and bandaging utilized for Phase I reduction, combined with options for different compression types developed within an individual's lymphedema chronic Phase II maintenance management program.
3. Compression garments. Elastic compression stockings, often initially considered in edema treatment planning, should normally be reserved for ongoing maintenance of limb volume after reduction in the lymphedema patient. This is in distinction to the patient with minor venous insufficiency whom the vascular

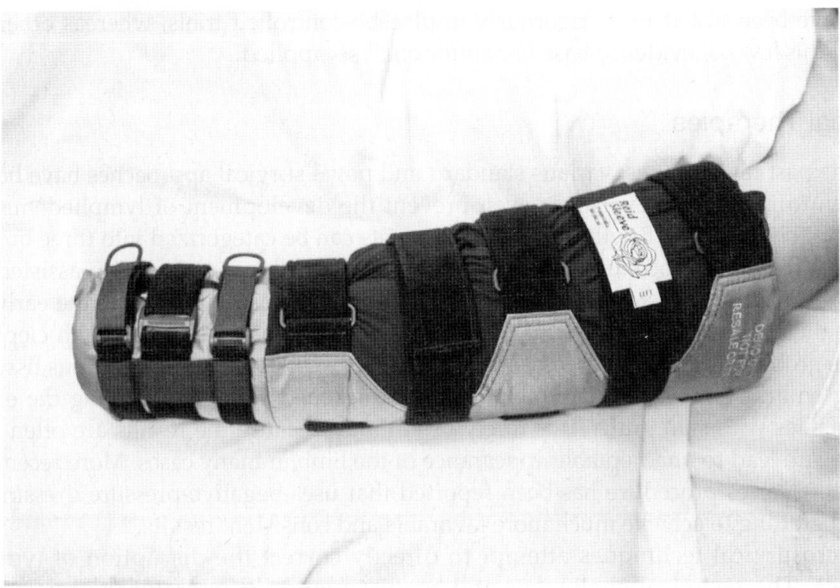

Figure 37-6. Static compression device requires minimal effort for application. Multiple commercial options of padded or quilted compression devices are available for upper and lower limb and trunk.

surgeon evaluates more frequently. Rather than a simple prescription handed to the patient for procurement at any local pharmacy, the lymphedema maintenance compression garment, its fit, durability, and efficacy are among the most important components of any lymphedema management program. Currently, there are multiple commercial firms fabricating garments for upper and lower extremity, trunk, and face. Garments may be prefabricated or custom fit. The multiplicity of prefabricated sizes available minimizes the necessity for custom fitting. The increasing occurrence of multifactorial edema, including phlebolymphatic edema, associated with chronic obesity has required innovation and creativity in development of well-fitting garment options attempting to preserve edema reduction that has been achieved. Although many donning assists are now commercially available, patients with severe obesity may still have difficulty with an independent donning program, and patient's donning challenges must be an important consideration when ordering any garment. Although patients with peripheral venous disease usually may require only a 20- to 30-mmHg pressure garment, patients with lymphatic failure usually require a 30- to 40-mmHg pressure garment system. This also adds difficulty to donning capability. In our experience, innovation with "layered" compression, overlapping distal and separate proximal garment systems, may be necessary to allow for independent donning. Development of relationships with an excellent lymphedema therapy team along with creative vendors is a necessity for the vascular specialist.

Novel Nonsurgical Therapies

In addition to the more commonly used regimens described above, other types of treatments have appeared in the literature, including aqua therapy,[51] deep breathing,[52] hyperbaric oxygen,[53] low-level laser,[54] kinesio tape,[55] microwave heating,[56] and others. Some of these have been tested more rigorously in placebo-controlled trials, whereas others have not had this level of evidence-based scientific analysis applied.

Surgical Therapies

Over the past few decades, various standard and novel surgical approaches have been undertaken to minimize, reverse, or even prevent the development of lymphedema of the upper or lower limbs.[57] Briefly, surgical treatments can be categorized into three broad approaches: resection procedures, microsurgical reconstructions, and suction-assisted lipectomy or liposuction. Historically, the Charles procedure was developed in the early 1900s to treat the most severe forms of lymphedema, namely Grade III disease with elephantiasis. This procedure consists of radical excision of the excessive lymphedematous tissues, including en bloc removal of papillomatous and thickened skin and covering the exposed surgical sites with skin grafts. It is rarely used today because the results are often unpredictable and lead to unacceptable appearance of the limb in many cases. More recently, the modified Charles procedure has been reported that uses negative-pressure dressings and delayed grafting to achieve much more favorable and consistent results.[58]

Microsurgical techniques attempt to directly correct the disruption of lymphatic channels. The technical challenges and requirements for operator experience have limited more widespread adoption of this approach worldwide. It is a surgical treatment performed mainly in Europe and Asia, with few centers in the United States offering patients this procedure. Campisi et al. from Italy have developed and successfully reduced lower limb lymphedema of primary and secondary cause using the lymphatic-venous-lymphatic plasty (LVLA).[59] Others have suggested that the results are dependent on the operator and patient population, and the extent of reduction may be limited in many cases.[60] More recently, Boccardo and associates have examined the efficacy of lymphatic venous microsurgery in the prevention of lymphedema following axillary dissection for breast cancer.[61] Although preliminary, extension of these surgical approaches to prophylactic prevention of lymphedema may offer earlier treatment options to counteract the inherent risks associated with axillary dissection and other oncologic surgical interventions. Another related prevention measure at the time of surgery that warrants further investigation has been the technique of axillary reverse mapping performed at the time of sentinel lymph node biopsy.[62]

Various surgical approaches to transfer tissues that may restore or improve lymphatic function or fluid resorption have been proposed. These include free muscle flap, lymph-fascia grafting or omentoplasty as well as vascularized lymph node transfers to limbs in which lymphadenectomy had been performed as part of surgical intervention for treatment of malignancy.[63-69]

Most recent in the armamentarium of techniques for the surgeon to relieve limb overgrowth as a result of lymphedema is removal of subcutaneous fibrofatty tissue by means of circumferential liposuction. Suction-assisted lipectomy has been developed and investigated over the past decade as a more innovative approach for the more advanced and irreversible grades of lymphedema. Long-term results have been reported and show considerable promise, particularly for chronic, upper limb lymphedema. It should be noted that the success of this surgical approach includes the use of a long-term compression garment postoperatively.[70-72]

This brief review has touched upon only a few of the many issues facing the patient with lymphedema and the practitioner who must command knowledge of the appropriate anatomy, potential pathologies, diagnostic tools, and myriad management options, conservative and surgical. Multiple excellent reviews are available for further study.[1,3,49,73-77] Through a multidisciplinary approach, including the vascular researcher, clinician, surgeon, and rehabilitation professional, the patient currently has options for a brighter future of lymphatic disease management.

REFERENCES

1. Rockson SG. Lymphedema. Am J Med 2001;110:288–95.
2. Karpanen T, Alitalo K., Molecular biology and pathology of lymphangiogenesis. Annu Rev Pathol 2008;3:367–97.
3. Rockson S. Diagnosis and management of lymphatic vascular disease. J Am Coll Cardiol 2008;52:799–806.
4. Strick DM, Gamble GL. Lymphedema in the cancer patient. In: Stubblefield MD, O'Dell MW, eds. Cancer Rehabilitation Principles and Practice. New York: Demos Publishing; 2009, pp. 1011–22.
5. Damstra RJ, van Steensel MAM, Boomsma JHB, et al. Erysipelas as a sign of subclinical primary lymphoedema: a prospective quantitative scintigraphic study of 40 patients with unilateral erysipelas of the leg. Br J Dermatol 2008;158:1210–5.
6. Soo JK, Bicanic TA, Heenan S, et al. Lymphatic abnormalities demonstrated by lymphoscintigraphy after lower limb cellulitis. Br J Dermatol 2008;158:1350–3.
7. The diagnosis and treatment of peripheral lymphedema. 2009 Consensus Document of the International Society of Lymphology. Lymphology 2009:42:51–60.
8. Brorson H, Ohlin K, Olsson G, et al. Adipose tissue dominates chronic arm lymphedema following breast cancer: an analysis using volume rendered CT images. Lymphat Res Biol 2006;4:199–210.
9. Rockson SG. Addressing the unmet needs in lymphedema risk management. Lymphat Res Biol 2006;4:42–6.
10. Enjolras O, Chapot R, Merland JJ. Vascular anomalies and the growth of limbs: a review. J Pediatr Orthop 2004;13:349–57.
11. Tian XL, Kadaba R, You SA, et al. Identification of an angiogenic factor that when mutated causes susceptibility to Klippel-Trenaunay syndrome. Nature 2004;427:640–5.
12. Connell F, Brice G, Mortimer P. Phenotypic characterization of primary lymphedema. Ann N Y Acad Sci 2008;1131:140–6.
13. Connell FC, Ostergaard P, Carver C, et al. Analysis of the coding regions of VEGFR3 and VEGFC in Milroy disease and other primary lymphoedemas. Hum Genet 2009;124:625–31.
14. Rezaie T, Ghoroghchian R, Bell R, et al. Primary non-syndromic lymphoedema (Meige disease) not caused by mutations in FOXC2. Eur J Hum Genet 2008;16:300–4.
15. Dale RF. The inheritance of primary lymphoedema. J Med Genet 1985;22:274–8.
16. Smeltzer DM, Stickler GB, Schriger A. Primary lymphedema in children and adolescents: a follow-up study and review. Pediatrics 1985;76:206–18.
17. Petrek JA, Senie RT, Peters M, et al. Lymphedema in a cohort of breast carcinoma survivors 20 years after diagnosis. Cancer 2001;92:1368–77.
18. Norman SA, Localio AR, Potashnik SL, et al. Lymphedema in breast cancer survivors: incidence, degree, time course, treatment, and symptoms. J Clin Oncol 2009;27:390–7.
19. Williams AF, Franks PJ, Moffatt CJ. Lymphoedema: estimating the size of the problem. Palliat Med 2005;19:300–13.
20. Sener SF, Winchester DJ, Martz CH, et al. Lymphedema after sentinel lymphadenectomy for breast carcinoma. Cancer 2001;92:748–52.
21. Ottesen EA. Lymphatic filariasis: treatment, control and elimination. Adv Parasitol 2006; 61:395–441.

22. Tsai RJ, Dennis LK, Lynch CF. The risk of developing arm lymphedema among breast cancer survivors: a meta-analysis of treatment factors. Am Surg Oncol 2009;16:1959–72.
23. Segerstrom K, Bjerle P, Graffman S, et al. Factors that influence the incidence of brachial oedema after treatment of breast cancer. Scand J Plast Reconstr Surg Hand Surg 1992;26: 223–7.
24. Werner RS, McCormick B, Petrek J, et al. Arm edema in conservatively managed breast cancer: obesity is a major predictive factor. Radiology 1991;180:177–84.
25. Pavoltsky F, Amrani S, Trau H. Recurrent erysipelas: risk factors. J Dtsch Dermatol Ges 2004:2:89–95.
26. Mortimer PS. Implications of the lymphatic system in CVI-associated edema. Angiology 2000;51:3–7.
27. Herd-Smith A, Russo A, Muraca MG, et al. Prognostic factors for lymphedema after primary treatment for breast carcinoma. Cancer 2001;92:1783–7.
28. Nielson I, Gordon S, Selby A. Breast cancer related lymphoedema risk reduction advice: a challenge for health professionals. Cancer Treat Rev 2008;34:621–8.
29. Semel JD, Goldin H. Association of athlete's foot with cellulitis of the lower extremities: diagnostic value of bacterial cultures of ipsilateral interdigital space samples. Clin Infect Dis 1996;23:1162–4.
30. Shaw C, Mortimer P, Judd PA. A randomized controlled trial of weight reduction as a treatment for breast cancer-related lymphedema. Cancer 2007;10:1868–74.
31. Harris SR, Niesen-Vertommen SL. Challenging the myth of exercise-induced lymphedema following breast cancer: a series of case reports. J Surg Oncol 2000;74:95–9.
32. McKenzie DC, Kalda AL. Effect of upper extremity exercise on secondary lymphedema in breast cancer patients: a pilot study. J Clin Oncol 2003;21:463–6.
33. Ahmed RL, Thomas W, Yee D, et al. Randomized controlled trial of weight training and lymphedema in breast cancer survivors. J Clin Oncol 2006;24:2765–72.
34. Courneya KS, Segal RJ, Mackey JR, et al. Effects of aerobic and resistance exercise in breast cancer patients receiving adjuvant chemotherapy: a multicenter randomized controlled trial. J Clin Oncol 2007;25:4396–404.
35. Schmitz KH, Ahmed RL, Troxel A, et al. Weight lifting in women with breast-cancer–related lymphedema N Engl J Med 2009;361:664–73.
36. Ohira T, Schmitz KH, Ahmed RL, et al. Effects of weight training on quality of life in recent breast cancer survivors: the Weight Training for Breast Cancer Survivors (WTBS) Study. Cancer 2006;106:2076–83.
37. Bicego D, Brown K, Ruddick M, et al. Effects of exercise on quality of life in women living with breast cancer: a systemic review. Breast J 2009;15:45–51.
38. Witte CL, Witte MH. Diagnostic and interventional imaging of lymphatic disorders. Int Angiol 1999;18:25–30.
39. Ward LC. Bioelectrical impedance analysis: proven utility in lymphedema risk assessment and therapeutic monitoring. Lymphat Res Biol 2006;4:51–6.
40. Cornish B. Bioimpedance analysis: scientific background. Lymph Res Biol 2006;4:47–50.
41. Spillane AJ, Saw RP, Tucker M, et al. Defining lower limb lymphedema after inguinal or ilio-inguinal dissection in patients with melanoma using classification and regression tree analysis. Ann Surg 2008;248:286–93.
42. Casley-Smith JR, Morgan RG, Piller NB. Treatment of lymphedema of the arms and legs with 5,6-benzo-[a]–pyrone. N Engl J Med 1993;329:1158–63.
43. Casley-Smith JR. Benzo-pyrones in the treatment of lymphoedema. Int Angiol 1999;18: 31–41.
44. Loprinzi CL, Kugler JW, Sloan JA, et al. Lack of effect of coumarin in women with lymphedema after treatment for breast cancer. N Engl J Med 1999:340:346–50.
45. Foeldi E, Foeldi M, Weissleder H. Conservative treatment of lymphedema of the limbs. Angiology 1985;36:171–80.
46. Ko DS, Lerner R, Klose G, et el. Effective treatment of lymphedema of the extremities. Arch Surg 1998;133:452–8.

47. Szuba A, Achalu R, Rockson SG. Decongestive lymphatic therapy for patients with breast carcinoma–associated lymphedema. Cancer 2002;95:2260–7.
48. Mondry TE, Riffenburgh RH, Johnstone PA. Prospective trial of complete decongestive therapy for upper extremity lymphedema after breast cancer therapy. Cancer J 2004;10:42–8.
49. Cheville AL, McGarvey CL, Petrek AJ, et al. Lymphedema management. Semin Radiat Oncol 2003;13:290–301.
50. Wilburn O, Wilburn P, Rockson, SG. A pilot, prospective evaluation of a novel alternative for maintenance therapy of breast cancer-associated lymphedema. BMC Cancer 2006;6: 84–93.
51. Tidhar D, Katz-Leurer M. Aqua lymphatic therapy in women who suffer from breast cancer treatment-related lymphedema: a randomized controlled study. Support Care Cancer 2009;Jul 15, epub.
52. Moseley AL, Piller NB, Carati CJ. The effect of gentle arm exercise and deep breathing on secondary arm lymphedema. Lymphology 2005;38:136–45.
53. Gothard L, Stanton A, MacLaren J, et al. Non-randomised phase II trial of hyperbaric oxygen therapy in patients with chronic arm lymphoedema and tissue fibrosis after radiotherapy for early breast cancer. Radiol Oncol 2004;70:217–24.
54. Carati CK, Anderson SN, Gannon, BJ, et al. Treatment of postmastectomy lymphedema with low-level laser therapy. A double blind, placebo-controlled trial. Cancer 2003;98: 1114–22.
55. Tsai HJ, Hung HC, Yang JL, et al. Could kinesio tape replace the bandage in decongestive lymphatic therapy for breast-cancer-related lymphedema? A pilot study. support care cancer 2009; epub DOI 10.1007/s00520–009–0592–8.
56. Chang TS, Han LY, Gan JL, et al. Microwave: an alternative to electric heating in the treatment of peripheral lymphedema. Lymphology 1989;22:20–4.
57. Warren AG, Brorson H, Borud L, et al. Lymphedema. A comprehensive review. Ann Plast Surg 2007;59:464–72.
58. van der Walt J, Perks TJ, Zeeman B, et al. Modified Charles procedure using negative pressure dressings for primary lymphedema. Ann Plast Surg 2009;62:669–75.
59. Campisi C, Boccardo F, Zilli A, et al. The use of vein grafts in the treatment of peripheral lymphedemas: long-term results. Microsurgery 2001;21:143–7.
60. Damstra RJ, Voesten HGJ, van Schelven S, et al. Lymphatic venous anastomosis (LVA) for treatment of secondary arm lymphedema. A prospective study of 11 LVA procedures in 10 patients with breast cancer related lymphedema and a critical review of the literature. Breast Cancer ResTreat 2009;113:199–206.
61. Boccardo F, Casabona F, De Cian F, et al. Lymphedema microsurgical preventive healing approach: a new technique for primary prevention of arm lymphedema after mastectomy. Ann Surg Oncol 2009;16:703–8.
62. Boneti C, Korourian S, Bland K, et al. Axillary reverse mapping: mapping and preserving arm lymphatics may be important in preventing lymphedema during sentinel lymph node biopsy. J Am Coll Surg 2008;206:1038–42.
63. Ngan HYS, Tam KF, Ng TY. Prevention of lymphoedema using omentoplasty after pelvic lymphadenectomy: a prospective randomised controlled trial. Hong Kong Med J 2008;14 (suppl 5):S43–6.
64. Parrett BM, Sepic J, Pribax JJ. The contralateral rectus abdominis muscutaneous flap for treatment of lower extremity lymphedema. Ann Plast Surg 2009;62:75–9.
65. Lin, GH, Ali R, Chen SC, et al. Vascularized groin lymph node transfer using the wrist as a recipient site for management of postmastectomy upper extremity lymphedema. Plast Reconstr Surg 2009;123:1265–75.
66. Qi F, Gu J, Shi Y, et al. Treatment of upper limb lymphedema with combination of liposuction, myocutaneous flap transfer and lymph-fascia grafting: A Preliminary Study. Microsurgery 2009;29:29–34.
67. Medgyesi S. A successful operation for lymphoedema using a myocutaneous flap as a "wick." Br J Plast Surg 1983;36:64–6.

68. Classen DA, Irvine L. Free muscle flap transfer as a lymphatic bridge for upper extremity lymphedema. J Reconstr Microsurg 2005;21:93–9.
69. Slavin SA, Van den Abbeele AD, Losken A, et al. Return of lymphatic function after flap transfer for acute lymphedema. Ann Surg 1999;299:421–7.
70. Brorson H. Liposuction in arm lymphedema treatment. Scand J Surg 2003;92:287–95.
71. Damstra RJ, Voersten HGJM, Klinkert P, et al. Circumferential suction-assisted lipectomy for lymphoedema after surgery for breast cancer. Br J Surg 2009;96:859–64.
72. Eryilmaz T, Kaya B, Ozmen S, et al. Suction-assisted lipectomy for treatment of lower-extremity lymphedema. Aesthetic Plast Surg 2009;33:671–3.
73. Cheville AL. Current and future trends in lymphedema management: implications for women's health. Phys Med Rehabil Clin North Am 2007;18:539–53.
74. Lawenda BD, Mondry TE, Johnstone PAS. Lymphedema: a primer on the identification and management of a chronic condition in oncologic treatment. CA Cancer J Clin 2009; 59:8–24.
75. Warren AG, Brorson H, Borud LJ, et al. Lymphedema: a comprehensive review. Ann Plast Surg 2007;59:464–72.
76. Moseley AL, Carati CJ, Piller NB. A systematic review of common conservative therapies for arm lymphoedema secondary to breast cancer treatment. Ann Oncol 2007;18:639–6.
77. Tiwari A, Cheng K-S, Button M, et al. Differential diagnosis, investigation, and current treatment of lower limb lymphedema. Arch Surg 2003;138:152–61.

38

Chronic Venous Disease: Scientific Basis for Patient Management

Anthony J. Comerota, M.D., F.A.C.S., F.A.C.C.

INTRODUCTION

Chronic venous disease (CVD) refers to abnormalities of the superficial and/or deep venous system, leading to the spectrum of symptoms ranging from itching, heaviness, pain, aching, swelling, and cramps of the lower extremity to signs such as varicosities (reticular and overt varicose veins), edema, pigmentation, eczema, and ultimately ulceration.

The clinical, etiologic, anatomic, and pathophysiologic (CEAP) classification is an international reference that has been broadly accepted to allow standardized classification of the lower extremity affected with CVD.[1] CVD is the most common medical affliction worldwide. In the United States, five million people suffer with CVD.[2] Approximately 500,000 have an active venous ulcer at any given time, and approximately 1% of the population in industrialized countries will develop a venous ulcer some time during their lifetimes. Risk factors leading to advanced CVD include age, increased body mass index (BMI), a history of leg injury, lower socioeconomic class reflected by lack of health insurance, and male gender.[3] However, the single most profound risk is a history of deep venous thrombosis (DVT). Individuals with DVT have a 26-fold increased risk of developing CVD. The recent San Diego Population Study[4] documented that family history, flat feet, multiple pregnancies, and hours standing were risk factors for women. Interestingly, African-American ethnicity was protective.

Post-thrombotic (secondary) CVD is generally more virulent and more difficult to manage than primary venous disease. The incidence and severity of post-thrombotic venous disease depends upon the magnitude and distribution of the acute DVT as well as the number of episodes. Kahn et al.[5] reported an overall risk of chronic post-thrombotic syndrome in 37% of patients with acute DVT followed for a mean of 2.2 years. They reported that factor V Leiden and prothrombin gene mutation were independent predictors of a *lower* risk of post-thrombotic syndrome. This interesting observation requires confirmation by other investigators.

PATHOPHYSIOLOGY

Ambulatory Venous Hypertension

Simply put, the underlying pathophysiology of CVD is *ambulatory venous hypertension.* In individuals with a normal venous system, ambulatory venous pressures at the ankle fall to 30 to 40% of the standing venous pressures. As venous valve function deteriorates and reflux occurs, the exercising venous pressure cannot fall to its normal nadir. If venous obstruction is superimposed, the normal drop in exercising venous pressure is substantially compromised. The combination of valvular incompetence and luminal obstructions produces the highest ambulatory venous pressure and the most severe morbidity. Figure 38–1 shows a normal ambulatory venous pressure, dropping to 30% of the standing venous pressure (which was approximately 100 mm Hg). The subject with CVD shows an abnormally high ambulatory venous pressure, only dropping to 55% of the standing venous pressure.

Most physicians understand the simple physics of high venous pressure leading to increased capillary hydrostatic pressure, resulting in both a transudation and ultimately an exudation of tissue fluid, producing edema. As capillary pressure rises, larger molecules, especially proteins, enter the interstitial space. Therefore, a persistently elevated venous pressure results in the production of tissue fluid having a high protein content.[6] As long as the lymphatic system functions normally, limb elevation and compression can control and eventually eliminate the edema. However, if the high protein content of the tissue fluid and the subsequent inflammatory process obliterate lymphatic channels, secondary lymphedema occurs.

Activation of Cellular and Enzymatic Pathways

The importance of white blood cells (WBCs) and their activation and adhesion have been elucidated in the pathophysiology of CVD, especially in patients with advanced CVD. White cells take 1000 times longer than red cells to deform upon entering the capillary bed and are responsible for approximately 50% of peripheral vascular resistance, despite their comparatively small numbers in the circulation.[7] When white cells become activated and attach to capillary endothelium, they release free radical cytoplasmic granules containing

Chronic Venous Disease

Pathophysiology

Ambulatory Venous Hypertension

(A) Normal **(B)** CVD

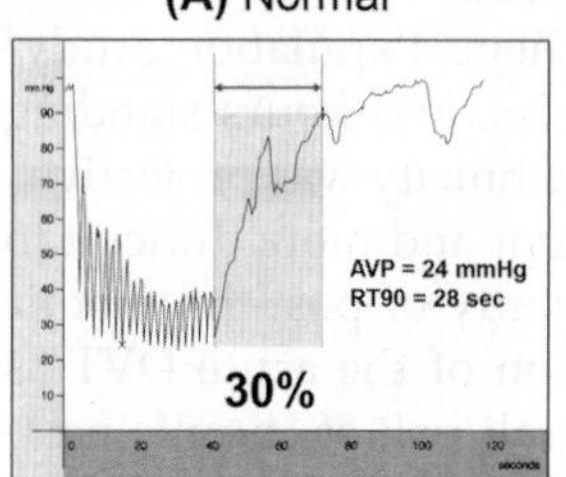

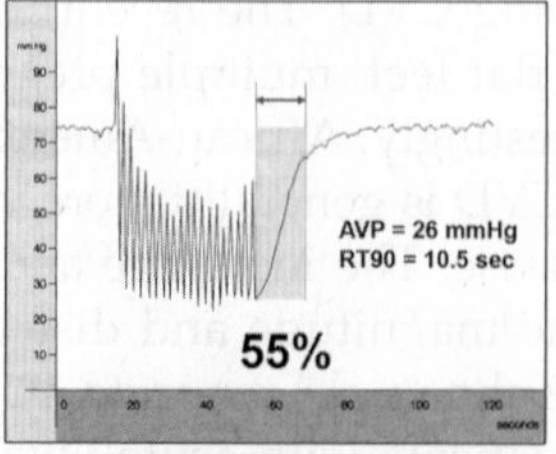

AVP of Normal
- Low Pressure
- Long Refill Time
(Normal Valve Fct.)

AVP of Patients with CVD
- High Pressure
- Short Refill Time
(Valve Incompetence)

Figure 38-1. Ambulatory venous hypertension is the underlying pathophysiology of chronic venous disease (CVD). A Normal ambulatory venous pressure (AVP) tracing showing a 70% fall in pressure with ambulation and a slow refill time due to normally functioning venous valves. B The pressure tracing of a patient with CVD showing only a 45% fall in venous pressure (ambulatory venous hypertension) and rapid venous refill due to venous valvular incompetence.

proteolytic enzymes,[8] which have a destructive effect on lipid membranes, proteins, and connective tissues.

In general, physicians have not appreciated the connection between venous hypertension and leukocyte activation, although this has been well studied in both animals and humans. When neutrophils degranulate, lactoferrin (a neutrophil granule enzyme) is released. In human models of venous hypertension, plasma lactoferrin concentrations are increased after a 30-minute period of induced venous hypertension.[9]

Lalka et al.[10] demonstrated that an animal model of venous hypertension stimulated significant increases in myeloperoxidase activity as a result of leukocyte trapping. Other biomarkers such as plasma L-selectin (a marker of leukocyte activation) and CD11b (a marker of WBC endothelial adhesion) have been studied in a human model of induced venous hypertension. Plasma L-selectin significantly increased, confirming leukocyte activation, and CD11b significantly decreased, reflecting endothelial adhesion of leukocytes after the onset of venous hypertension (Figure 38–2).

The increased white cell adhesion and emigration through capillary endothelium results in protease production and increased capillary permeability. The increased capillary permeability has been shown with micrographic images demonstrating macro-molecular leakage and microhemorrhages.[11] The enzymatic results of these cascading events include increased production of matrix metalloproteinases (MMPs), decreased tissue inhibitors of metalloproteinases (TIMPs), and increased transforming growth factor beta (TGFβ). The endothelium is perturbed, leading to increased expression of factor VIII-related antigen and adhesion molecules intercellular adhesion molecule-1 (ICAM-1), endotnelial leukocyte adhesion molecule-1 (ELAM-1), and vascular cell adhesion molecule-1 (VCAM-1).[12-13] There is upregulation of vascular endothelial growth factor (VEGF) in the epidermis of patients with venous disease, most prominently observed in patients with skin changes. VEGF likely accounts for at least

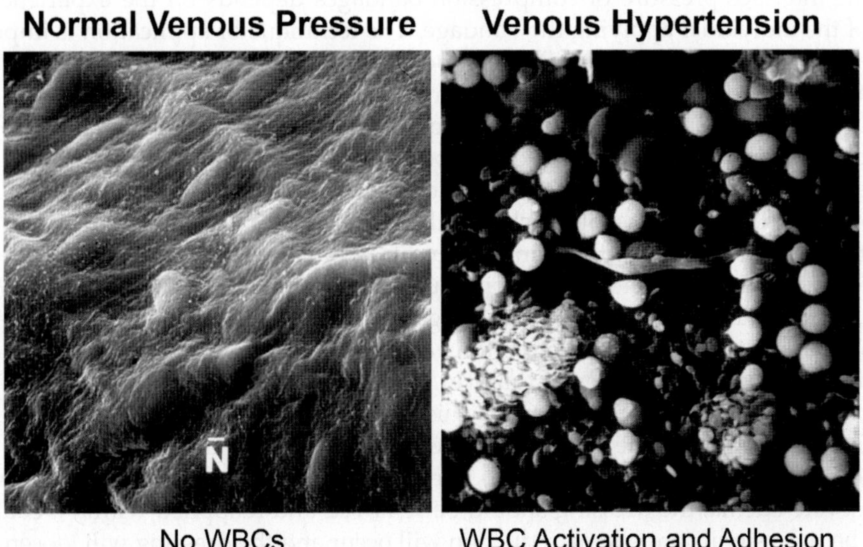

Figure 38-2. Venous hypertension increases white blood cell (WBC) activation and adhesion in an animal model. Scanning electron micrographs of venous endothelium from a vein with no increased pressure and showing WBC adhesion after induced venous hypertension.

some of the vascular proliferation observed in the skin of patients with venous disease and is responsible for increased microvascular permeability to large molecules, which is a feature of the skin microangiopathy observed in capillary microscopy studies.[14]

It seems apparent that if CVD is to be successfully treated, venous hypertension needs to be reduced or, ideally, avoided.

PATIENT MANAGEMENT

Compression

Sustained Compression. Compression is the cornerstone of treatment of patients with CVD. With the exception of patients with isolated superficial venous disease, CVD should be considered as controllable but not curable. Application of the proper amount of compression is key to the control of CVD. It is often difficult to identify the "proper" amount of applied pressure; however, a simple rule of thumb is to use whatever amount of pressure is required to control edema. As mentioned earlier, venous hypertension stimulates leukocyte activation and adhesion. External compression has an anti-inflammatory effect.[15]

Elastic stockings and elastic bandages exert pressure when they are stretched. With exercise, only small elevations in pressure occur, because the elastic material stretches with each step. Therefore, the working (ambulatory) external pressure is not much higher than the resting pressure. Because of the elasticity of the garment fibers, there is sustained pressure when the patient assumes a supine position, which may lead to discomfort.

Inelastic compression, such as the multilayered compression bandages or the rigid, nonelastic Velcro strap bandages, apply a sustained pressure and demonstrate high interface pressure peaks during ambulation, thereby reducing ambulatory venous hypertension.[16-17]

The interface pressure of compression bandages depends on the experience and skill of the individual applying the bandage. The technique of application is important for patient comfort and therefore compliance. The bandage should be applied with the foot dorsiflexed and the instep and anterior ankle padded with cotton gauze. The wrap should be applied from the base of the toes to the anterior tibial tubercle with sustained, even, multilayered pressure. My preference is to use a pure zinc oxide paste gauze on the skin, thereby avoiding the occasional allergic reaction to the paraben preservative, bismuth, and other chemicals in the Unna paste. The zinc oxide paste gauze is applied directly to the skin (and ulcer), with additional bulk over areas of ulceration and skin depression. A cotton gauze roll is then applied over the zinc oxide wrap, overlapping each turn of the bandage by approximately 50%. A Coban self-adherent dressing is applied over the cotton gauze, again overlapping each rotation of the dressing by about 50%. The result is a firm, inelastic pressure dressing from the base of the toes to the anterior tibial tubercle. This functions as a nonelastic graduated compression dressing when the patient is in the upright position, and is similar to an intermittent pneumatic compression (IPC) garment during ambulation. In patients who have severe edema, the dressing should be removed and reapplied within a couple of days, because significant edema reduction will occur and the dressing will loosen.

A 15-year review of 998 patients with venous ulceration treated with multilayer compression dressings revealed that 73% of the ulcers healed in patients who returned for more than one treatment.[18] The median time to healing was 9 weeks. When multilayer compression dressings were compared with elastic compression stockings in the management of ulcers, both were effective, demonstrating 70% healing. However, the multilayer dressings required less than half the time to achieve healing.[19]

Intermittent Pneumatic Compression. The mainstay of treatment of patients with venous ulcers is multilayered compression dressings as described previously. However, as shown in randomized trials and nonrandomized series, the application of IPC speeds ulcer healing and may heal otherwise difficult ulcers.[20-21]

Investigators have elucidated the mechanism of benefit of IPC. High-pressure, short-duration IPC significantly increases venous velocity[22] and reduces the arterial-venous pressure gradient. Physiologic effects of properly applied IPC include reduction in edema and increased $TcPO_2$,[23] arterial blood flow, and foot-skin perfusion,[24] which result in improved healing of venous ulcers.[20-21] The proper IPC is high-pressure, rapid-inflation, which cycles at 2 to 3 times per minute. Lower pressures and slower cycle times have less hemodynamic effect, resulting in less clinical benefit.[25]

Topical Wound Oxygen

An interesting report recently surfaced from Ireland indicating distinct advantages of topical wound oxygen (TWO_2) in patients with refractory venous ulcers. Tawfick and Sultan[26] recently reported a parallel observational comparative study. Eighty-three patients with refractory venous ulcers were studied. Forty-six were managed using TWO_2, whereas 37 were treated with conventional compression dressings (CCD). At the end of 12 weeks, the mean reduction in ulcer surface area was 96% in the TWO_2 group compared with 61% in the CCD group. Eighty percent of the TWO_2 ulcers were healed compared with 35% of the CCD-treated ulcers ($P<.0001$). Median time to healing was 45 days in TWO_2-treated patients and 182 days in CCD patients ($P<.0001$). Thirty-two TWO_2 ulcers showed reverse gradient healing (midwound outward), suggesting that TWO_2 may change the biology of wound healing. Nine of 19 MRSA-positive ulcers managed with TWO_2 were rendered MRSA-negative after 5 weeks compared with 0/17 MRSA-positive CCD ulcers. After 24 months of follow-up, 8 out of 13 healed CCD ulcers recurred compared with 0/37 TWO_2 healed ulcers, suggesting a difference in the biology of the healed wound. No local or systemic complications were encountered in either treatment group.

This interesting report requires confirmation with a full description of treatment details. A randomized trial appears warranted, and if this benefit can be reproduced, TWO_2 may become an important adjunct in the management of patients with venous ulcers.

Pharmacotherapy

Pentoxifylline. The pharmacotherapeutic options for the management of CVD are limited in the United States. The benefit of pentoxifylline has been recognized for patients with venous ulcers.[27] Initially, pentoxifylline was thought to act by improving red cell deformability, thereby also improving oxygen delivery to ischemic and damaged tissues. More recently, it appears that pentoxifylline has an effect on inhibition of cytokine-mediated neutrophil activation.[28] Pentoxifylline was also been shown to reduce both endothelial white cell adhesion and the release of superoxide free radicals. Therefore, it appears that pentoxifylline interrupts the white cell activation occurring in patients with chronic venous disease.

A double-blind, placebo-controlled trial with 59 patients with venous ulcers was performed by Weitgasser et al.[29] Of 30 patients on active treatment, 26 improved compared with only 13 out of 29 patients on placebo. A multicenter, placebo-controlled trial was performed by Colgan and associates[30] comparing 1200 mg per day of pentoxifylline versus placebo in patients with venous ulcers. All patients received local care and conventional compression hose. At 6 months, 23 out of 38 pentoxifylline-treated patients healed versus 12 out of 42 placebo patients ($P<.05$).

A more recent Cochrane analysis summarized eight randomized trials evaluating pentoxifylline versus placebo in patients with venous ulcers.[31] Compression therapy was used in five of the eight trials. The results indicated that pentoxifylline increased overall healing of venous ulcers ($P=.003$) and speed of ulcer healing ($P=.001$); however, there was a nonsignificant increase in gastrointestinal side effects.

Micronized Purified Flavonoid Fraction. Hydroxyrutosides are a class of flavonoid drug derived from plant glycosides. A number of animal studies document the cellular and anti-inflammatory effect of these compounds, which have translated into clinical benefit. The most extensively studied is the micronized purified flavonoid fraction (MPFF) compound. Although it is not yet available in the United States, MPFF is used and has been studied extensively in Europe.

Animal studies have shown that MPFF inhibits leukocyte activation and adhesion, reduces leukocyte emigration, and reduces capillary permeability with hypertension.[32] MPFF has also been shown to improve lymphatic flow in an animal model.[33] Juteau et al.[34] have shown that MPFF increases venous tone of diseased saphenous veins, and Behar et al.[35] showed reduced capillary filtration of albumin; Belcaro et al.[36] demonstrated that MPFF improved skin $TcPO_2$. Randomized clinical trials have demonstrated that MPFF improves the healing of venous ulcers.[37-38]

Surgical and Endovenous Intervention

Superficial Disease and Incompetent Perforators. Advances in technology have resulted in the percutaneous endovenous obliteration of superficial venous insufficiency. Using radiofrequency ablation[39-40] and endovenous laser therapy,[41-42] superficial venous disease can be safely and effectively eliminated. These same techniques have been used to obliterate incompetent perforators.

Foam sclerotherapy has several advantages compared with liquid sclerosing agents.[43] There is minimal if any dilution with blood, homogeneous distribution along the injected vein, and a sclerosant that is easily identified with ultrasound. Foam sclerotherapy is predominantly used for the management of superficial venous insufficiency in branch varicosities, although it has occasionally been used for the management of incompetent perforators.

Venous Valve Reconstruction/Transplantation

From the late 1970s through the late 1990s, a number of clinicians actively pursued surgical correction of deep vein valve incompetence. Techniques included vein segment transfer, direct valve reconstruction, and axillary vein valve transplantation.

Vein segment transfer rapidly fell into disfavor. Results of transposition series (83 limbs) revealed that only 35% of patients with venous ulcers healed, and in those, there was a 36% recurrent rate. Therefore, it is difficult to show clinical benefit. Hemodynamics were improved in only 35% of patients.[44]

O'Donnell[44] reviewed the results of 15 reports of vein valve transplantation in 420 limbs. Seventy-nine percent of the patients with venous ulcers had their ulcers healed postoperatively; however, there was a 28% recurrence rate. Only 27% of patients improved their venous hemodynamics compared with preoperative evaluation.

Because the most severe CVD and the most recalcitrant venous ulcers occur in post-thrombotic patients, venous valve transplantation into a diffusely sclerotic and recanalized venous system will do little to improve the pathophysiology. Direct vein valve reconstruction and vein valve transplantation are best used in patients with primary deep vein valvular incompetence. These patients represent a minority of patients with CVD.

Treatment of Chronic Venous Obstruction

The most impressive advance in the management of patients with incapacitating venous disease has been the correction of chronic venous obstruction. Many of these patients have post-thrombotic venous obstruction. The majority of patients have involvement of the iliocaval segments. Similar to patients with advanced arterial disease, multisegment venous occlusive disease produces the most severe morbidity.

Patients present with pain, edema, and discoloration, and many have already suffered ulceration. Often, patients are limited in their physical activity, and young patients are often on disability.

A complete noninvasive evaluation including physiologic studies as well as venous duplex is followed by ascending phlebography, including iliocavography. Restoring unobstructed venous outflow from the inguinal ligament to a patent vena cava is critical to restoring quality of life to these patients. The patient illustrated in Figure 38–3 is an example of the aforementioned. This patient was an officer in the Royal Air Force when he developed iliofemoral venous thrombosis. Treated with anticoagulation, he developed severe post-thrombotic morbidity, which resulted in his inability to perform his duties. Therefore, he was placed on disability.

Ascending phlebography reveals obstruction of the iliofemoral venous system. Percutaneous endovenous recanalization was achieved following successful venoplasty and stenting. All pressure gradients were eliminated, and normal venous return was restored. The patient resumed full activity, demonstrated normal venous outflow, and was asymptomatic after maximal activity at 1-year follow-up.

A more extensive example is illustrated by the patient summarized in Figure 38–4. This patient likewise had incapacitating post-thrombotic morbidity following iliofemoral and femoropopliteal venous thrombosis treated with anticoagulation alone. She had C5 venous disease and suffered with incapacitating venous claudication, tense swelling of her limb, and persistent discomfort. Ascending phlebography showed extensive post-thrombotic venous disease throughout her left infrainguinal and suprainguinal venous system. Her iliofemoral segment was occluded with severe disease of the infrainguinal venous segment. In patients such as this, a common femoral endovenectomy is performed from the confluence of the femoral and profunda femoris veins to the external iliac vein (see Figure 38–4). The venotomy is closed with a bovine pericardial patch. Through the caudal aspect of the patch closure, a sheath is placed for access into the iliocaval venous segment. Transluminal venous recanalization is then achieved with subsequent stenting. Stents are extended from the endovenectomized common femoral vein to the inferior vena cava, if necessary. Restoring unobstructed drainage into the vena cava significantly reduces venous

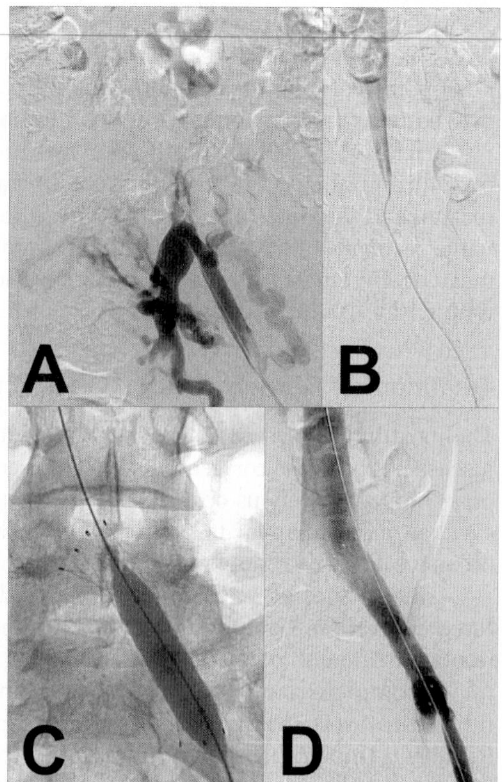

Figure 38-3. A Iliocavagram showing occlusion of the left common femoral vein following iliofemoral DVT in a 26-year-old man. B Following guidewire penetration and contrast injection demonstrating a normal vena cava, balloon angioplasty and stenting C were performed, resulting in a patent iliofemoral venous segment D with unobstructed venous outflow. The patient returned to full function with no further symptoms of venous claudication.

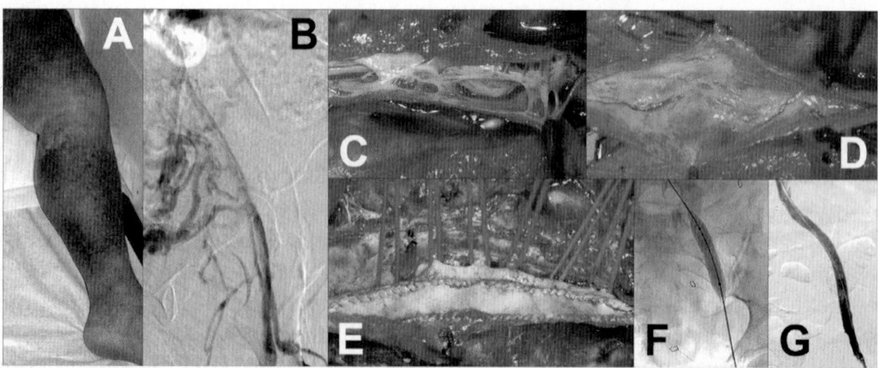

Figure 38-4. A A patient with severe, chronic, post-thrombotic syndrome had extensive iliofemoral DVT 10 years earlier. B A phlebogram showing severe occlusive disease of the left common femoral vein and chronic occlusion of the external and common iliac veins. C Following exposure and venotomy of the left common femoral vein, one can appreciate the extensive endoluminal scarring, obstructive webs, and synechia of the post-thrombotic vein. D Following endovenectomy, the lumen is restored and, E after patch venoplasty, F endovascular recanalization of the external and common iliac veins is achieved with balloon dilation and stenting, G restoring unobstructed venous drainage into the vena cava. The patient's symptoms and quality of life were markedly improved.

pressure and improves lower extremity venous drainage. The clinical result is extremely gratifying.

Neglen and Raju[45] have reported the largest series of endovenous recanalization procedures for chronic iliofemoral venous occlusion. They reported that venous stenting can be performed with low morbidity and mortality in the spectrum of patients, including post-thrombotic and morbidly obese patients. Long-term patency rates were good and clinical outcomes gratifying. They showed, however, that long-term failures occurred more frequently and repeat interventions were more common in patients with post-thrombotic obstruction. This is not surprising, considering that patients with post-thrombotic obstruction generally have long-segment disease and are more likely to be prothrombotic.

SUMMARY

Significant advances have been made in the management of patients with CVD. Whereas sustained compression remains the foundation of care, it is now recognized that all compression is not the same. Inelastic compression has distinct advantages and IPC further improves venous physiólogy.

Although pharmacotherapy is limited in the United States, pentoxifylline appears to have a role in patients with venous ulceration, and MPFF affects cellular function, reduces inflammation and edema, and also appears to speed ulcer healing.

Operative techniques have been refined and their limitations recognized. Most important, however, is the recognition that treating and eliminating venous outflow obstruction significantly reduces CVD and can substantially improve quality of life.

REFERENCES

1. Eklof B, Rutherford RB, Bergan JJ, et al. Revision of the CEAP classification for chronic venous disorders: consensus statement. J Vasc Surg 2004;40:1248–52.
2. Alguire PC, Mathes BM. Chronic venous insufficiency and venous ulceration. J Gen Intern Med 1997;12:374–83.
3. Scott TE, Mendez MV, LaMorte WW, et al. Are varicose veins a marker for susceptibility to coronary heart disease in men? Results from the Normative Aging Study. Ann Vasc Surg 2004;18:459–64.
4. Criqui MH, Jamosmos M, Fronek A, et al. Chronic venous disease in an ethnically diverse population: the San Diego Population Study. Am J Epidemiol 2003;158:448–56.
5. Kahn SR, M'Lan CE, Lamping DL, et al. The influence of venous thromboembolism on quality of life and severity of chronic venous disease. J Thromb Haemost 2004;2: 2146–51.
6. Landis EM, Jonas L, Angevine M, Erb W. The passage of fluid and protein through the human capillary wall during venous congestion. J Clin Invest 1932;11:717–34.
7. Braide M, Amundson B, Chien S, Bagge U. Quantitative studies on the influence of leukocytes on the vascular resistance in a skeletal muscle preparation. Microvasc Res 1984;27: 331–52.
8. Weissmann G, Smolen JE, Korchak HM. Release of inflammatory mediators from stimulated neutrophils. N Engl J Med 1980;303:27–34.
9. Shields DA, Andaz S, Sarin S, et al. [Neutrophil activation in experimental venous hypertension]. Phlebologie 1993;46:687–9.

10. Lalka SG, Unthank JL, Nixon JC. Elevated cutaneous leukocyte concentration in a rodent model of acute venous hypertension. J Surg Res 1998;74:59–63.
11. Schmid-Schonbein G. Molecular basis of venous insufficiency. In: Bergan JJ, ed. The Vein Book. Burlington: Elsevier; 2007, pp. 67–79.
12. Wilkinson LS, Bunker C, Edwards JC, et al. Leukocytes: their role in the etiopathogenesis of skin damage in venous disease. J Vasc Surg 1993;17:669–75.
13. Veraart JC, Verhaegh ME, Neumann HA, et al. Adhesion molecule expression in venous leg ulcers. Vasa 1993;22:213–8.
14. Bates DO, Curry FE. Vascular endothelial growth factor increases hydraulic conductivity of isolated perfused microvessels. Am J Physiol 1996;271:H2520–8.
15. Junger M, Steins A, Hahn M, Hafner HM. Microcirculatory dysfunction in chronic venous insufficiency (CVI). Microcirculation 2000;7:S3–12.
16. Partsch H. Improvement of venous pumping function in chronic venous insufficiency by compression depending on pressure and material. Vasa 1984;13:58–64.
17. Partsch B, Partsch H. Calf compression pressure required to achieve venous closure from supine to standing positions. J Vasc Surg 2005;42:734–8.
18. Lippmann HI, Fishman LM, Farrar RH, et al. Edema control in the management of disabling chronic venous insufficiency. Arch Phys Med Rehabil 1994;75:436–41.
19. Hendricks WM, Swallow RT. Management of stasis leg ulcers with Unna's boots versus elastic support stockings. J Am Acad Dermatol 1985;12:90–8.
20. Coleridge-Smith PD, Sarin S, Hasty J, Scurr JH. Sequential gradient pneumatic compression enhances venous ulcer healing: a randomized trial. Surgery 1990;108:871–5.
21. Kumar S, Samraj K, Nirujogi V, Budnik J, Walker MA. Intermittent pneumatic compression as an adjuvant therapy in venous ulcer disease. J Tissue Viability 2002;12:42–4, 46, 48.
22. Malone MD, Cisek PL, Comerota AJ, Jr., et al. High-pressure, rapid-inflation pneumatic compression improves venous hemodynamics in healthy volunteers and patients who are post-thrombotic. J Vasc Surg 1999;29:593–9.
23. Kolari PJ, Pekanmaki K, Pohjola RT. Transcutaneous oxygen tension in patients with post-thrombotic leg ulcers: treatment with intermittent pneumatic compression. Cardiovasc Res 1988;22:138–41.
24. Eze AR, Comerota AJ, Cisek PL, et al. Intermittent calf and foot compression increases lower extremity blood flow. Am J Surg 1996;172:130–4.
25. Nikolovska S, Arsovski A, Damevska K, et al. Evaluation of two different intermittent pneumatic compression cycle settings in the healing of venous ulcers: a randomized trial. Med Sci Monit 2005;11:CR337–43.
26. Tawfick W, Sultan S. Does topical wound oxygen offer an improved outcome over conventional compression dressings in the management of refractory nonhealing venous ulcers? [Abstract]. Vascular 2009;17:S82.
27. Kearon C, Kahn SR, Agnelli G, et al. Antithrombotic therapy for venous thromboembolic disease: ACCP Evidence-Based Clinical Practice Guidelines (8th ed). Chest 2008;133:454S-545S.
28. Sullivan GW, Carper HT, Novick WJ Jr, Mandell GL. Inhibition of the inflammatory action of interleukin-1 and tumor necrosis factor (alpha) on neutrophil function by pentoxifylline. Infect Immun 1988;56:1722–9.
29. Weitgasser H. The use of pentoxifylline (Trental 400) in the treatment of leg ulcers: results of a double-blind trial. Pharmatherapeutica 1983;2:143–51.
30. Colgan MP, Dormandy JA, Jones PW, et al. Oxpentifylline treatment of venous ulcers of the leg. BMJ 1990;300:972–5.
31. Jull AB, Waters J, Arroll B. Pentoxifylline for treating venous leg ulcers. Cochrane Database Syst Rev 2002;1:CD001733.
32. Korthuis RJ, Gute DC. Postischemic leukocyte/endothelial cell interactions and microvascular barrier dysfunction in skeletal muscle: cellular mechanisms and effect of Daflon 500 mg. Int J Microcirc Clin Exp 1997;17(Suppl 1):11–7.

33. Cotonat A, Cotonat J. Lymphagogue and pulsatile activities of Daflon 500 mg on canine thoracic lymph duct. Int Angiol 1989;8:15–8.
34. Juteau N, Bakri F, Pomies JP, et al. The human saphenous vein in pharmacology: effect of a new micronized flavonoidic fraction (Daflon 500 mg) on norepinephrine induced contraction. Int Angiol 1995;14:8–13.
35. Behar A, Lagrue G, Cohen-Boulakia F, Baillet J. Study of capillary filtration by double labelling I131–albumin and Tc99m red cells. Application to the pharmacodynamic activity of Daflon 500 mg. Int Angiol 1988;7:35–8.
36. Belcaro G, Cesarone MR, De Sanctis MT, et al. Laser Doppler and transcutaneous oximetry: modern investigations to assess drug efficacy in chronic venous insufficiency. Int J Microcirc Clin Exp 1995;15(Suppl 1):45–9.
37. Glinski W, Chodynicka B, Roszkiewicz J, et al. [Effectiveness of a micronized purified flavonoid fraction (MPFF) in the healing process of lower limb ulcers. An open multicentre study, controlled and randomized]. Minerva Cardioangiol 2001;49:107–14.
38. Coleridge-Smith PD. Daflon 500 mg and venous leg ulcer: new results from a meta-analysis. Angiology 2005;56(Suppl 1):S33–9.
39. Merchant RF, Pichot O, Myers KA. Four-year follow-up on endovascular radiofrequency obliteration of great saphenous reflux. Dermatol Surg 2005;31:129–34.
40. Lurie F, Creton D, Eklof B, et al. Prospective randomized study of endovenous radiofrequency obliteration (closure procedure) versus ligation and stripping in a selected patient population (EVOLVeS Study). J Vasc Surg 2003;38:207–14.
41. Min RJ, Khilnani NM. Endovenous laser treatment of saphenous vein reflux. Tech Vasc Interv Radiol 2003;6:125–31.
42. Proebstle TM, Moehler T, Gul D, Herdemann S. Endovenous treatment of the great saphenous vein using a 1,320 nm Nd:YAG laser causes fewer side effects than using a 940 nm diode laser. Dermatol Surg 2005;31:1678–83.
43. Guex J-J. Sclerofoam for treatment of varicose veins. In: Bergan JJ, ed. The Vein Book. Burlington: Elsevier; 2007, pp. 201–10.
44. O'Donnell TF. Venous valve transplantation and vein transposition for valvular incompetence of deep veins. In: Gloviczki P, Yao JS, eds. Handbook of Venous Disorders, 2nd ed. London:Arnold; 2001, pp. 336–45.
45. Neglen P, Hollis KC, Olivier J, Raju S. Stenting of the venous outflow in chronic venous disease: long-term stent-related outcome, clinical, and hemodynamic result. J Vasc Surg 2007; 46:979–90.

SECTION IX

Tevar

39

TEVAR following FDA Approval: Results of the TAG 05-02 Post marketing Study

Mark D. Morasch, M.D., F.A.C.S.

In March 2005, the Gore TAG® Thoracic Endoprosthesis (TAG®) became the first device approved in the United States for use in the primary treatment of descending thoracic aortic aneurysms (DTAA). Since approval, the technology has been dispersed with some uniformity throughout the United States. As part of the approval process, the manufacturer agreed to conduct a postmarketing study of the device used to treat patients with DTAA from multiple geographically disbursed sites and by physicians from three distinct tiers of device training. The purpose of the postapproval study is to evaluate the long-term performance of the TAG® in the primary treatment of DTAA as utilization of the technology has become diffusely disbursed. The study has also been designed to assess the effectiveness of the Gore TAG® Physician Training Program (GTPTP) as designed with regards to new physician training.

TAG 05-02 is a multicenter, nonrandomized observational study. A total of 150 subjects diagnosed with DTAA were enrolled and treated between January 2006 and April 2008. Subjects were enrolled both prospectively and retrospectively from 25 geographically distributed investigational sites. No limit was set on the number of subjects who could be enrolled per site (Figure 39–1). The experience of the implanting physicians varied considerably between and within sites. Implanting physicians were categorized into three tiers depending upon experience level.

Complete pre- and post-treatment data have been collected out to 1 year. One year data lock took place in July of this year. Data will continue to be collected annually for 5 years post-treatment. Patient follow-up, including diagnostic studies and physical examinations, are completed at predetermined time points, with windows for compliance and with the impact of loss to follow-up assessed.

To be enrolled, patients had to have a DTAA that otherwise required surgical repair and aortic anatomy that had to meet Instructions for Use (IFU). Mycotic and uncontained ruptured aneurysms were excluded. Patients were excluded if they had

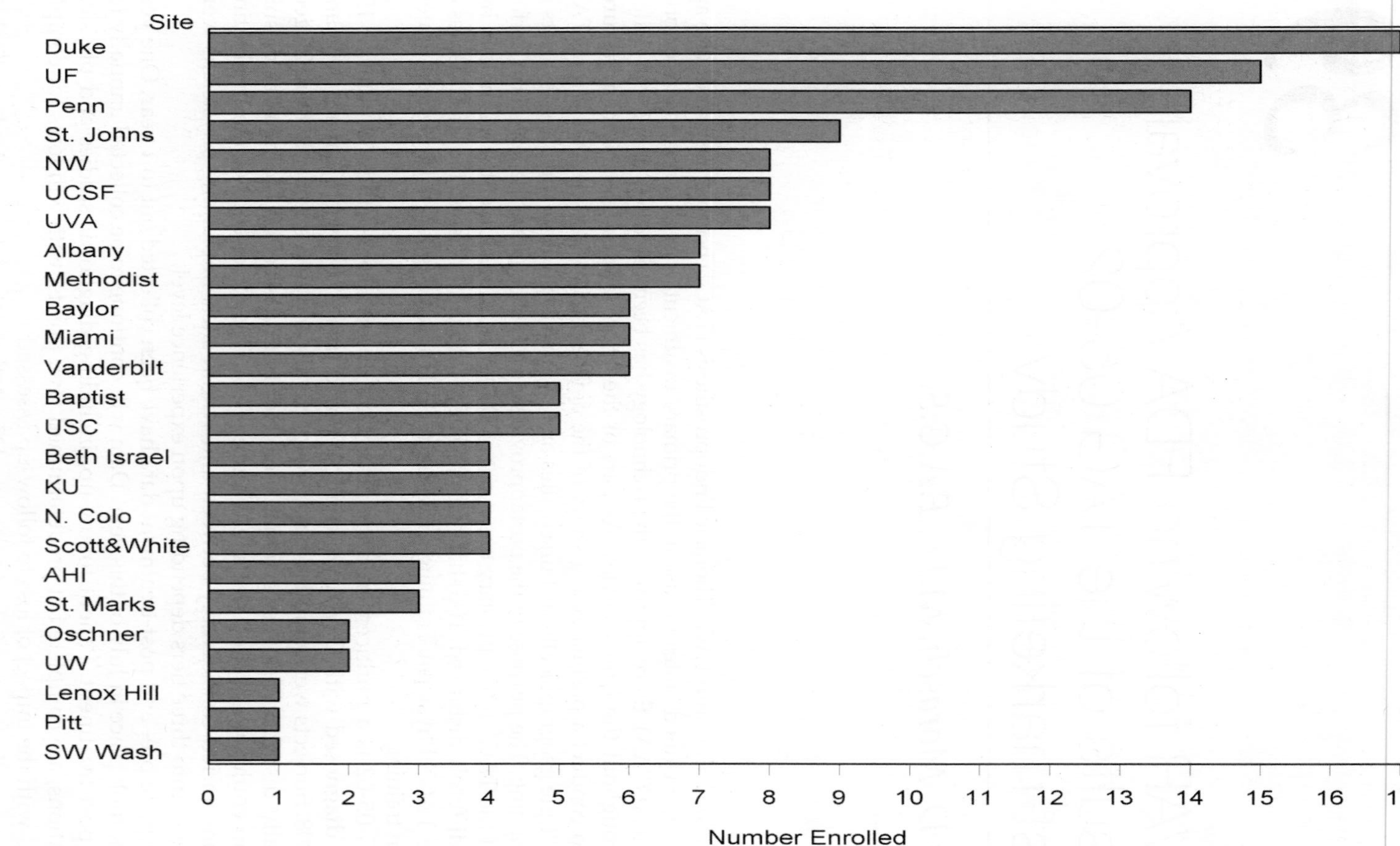

Figure 39-1. Subjects enrolled per site.

evidence of acute or chronic dissection or a degenerative connective tissue disorder. Coverage of major aortic branch vessels, exclusive of the left subclavian artery, would exclude the patient from enrollment. Management of a covered left subclavian artery was left up to the discretion of the implanting surgeon.

Sixty-eight percent of patients implanted were male. Average age at implantation was 74. Eighty percent of patients met strict inclusion/exclusion criteria. Average procedure time was just over 2 hours. Average blood loss was estimated at 200 cc. All 150 patients were successfully accessed and all had a device successfully delivered to the target pathologic area. There were no immediate surgical conversions.

Thirteen patients did not return for the 30-day evaluation. There were 4 deaths (from bowel ischemia, respiratory failure, AAA rupture, cardiac tamponade) for a 30-day all-cause mortality of 2.7%. The major adverse event rate was 21% (including 2 strokes and 6 cases of paraplegia/paresis), and the major device-related event rate was 8.0%. Twelve patients required endoluminal intervention within the window for 30-day follow-up for device-related events. Reinterventions included the placement of additional thoracic devices, coil embolization of leaks, and branch vessel stenting. No conversions were required.

At 1 year, a total of 14 patients had died, and 2 additional patients were lost to follow-up. A total of 14 patients died from the time of implantation to the end of the 1-year window. The 10 deaths occurring between 30 days and 1 year were categorized as the result of cardiac complications (n=3), pulmonary complications (n=3), vascular complications (n=1), neoplasm (n=1), or other/unknown (n=2). There was an additional 25% major adverse event rate. Nearly half that rate was due to cardiac complications unrelated to the aneurysm or to the device. Seven patients required additional thoracic aortic device implantation procedures. At 1 year, the major device-related event rate was 13%, with 10 patients experiencing clinically important endoleaks, 1 patient experiencing device migration, and 1 patient sustaining aneurysm rupture.

The Gore TAG® Thoracic Endoprosthesis can be used successfully to treat DTAA by physicians trained in the GTPTP with limited major adverse events and with few major device related events.

40

Chronic Aortic Dissections: Management and Outcomes

Charles Acher, M.D., F.A.C.S. and Girma Tefera, M.D., F.A.C.S.

There is an extensive clinical literature on the treatment of acute aortic dissection, but little is written about the clinical course of patients with chronic aortic dissections. Most of the information available is contained in a few series in which late outcomes of acute dissection are documented.[1-3] From the few papers that detail the natural history of chronic dissection, it is estimated that 25 to 50% of late deaths occur from rupture as a result of late aneurysm formation. This of course implies that patients with acute dissections should be followed indefinitely for aortic enlargement. Other factors that affect late morbidity are renal function, stroke, and cardiac disease at the time of acute dissection. In this chapter, we attempt to establish why and when chronic dissections should be treated and some of the many variations and problems encountered in their surgical treatment.

The most common indication for repair is aneurysmal dilation. The incidence of aneurysmal dilation increases with time and becomes clinically significant (>6 cm) in 30 to 40% of patients within 5 years of the acute event. In our experience, the size at which an aneurysm from dissection should be repaired is similar to other thoracic or thoracoabdominal aneurysms, that is, between 6 and 7 cm. The rate of aortic expansion in those requiring surgery is relatively rapid, occurring within 36 months of the acute dissection in most of the patients we have followed.

OPERATIVE CONSIDERATIONS

There are several points to consider when repairing chronic dissections that range from how much aorta to replace to whether hypothermic arrest is needed. With chronic dissections, the use of sequential clamping of the aorta is essential because these patients tend to have many open intercostal arteries, and back bleeding from these vessels can result in significant blood loss and in some cases can be torrential enough to cause exsanguination before intercostal ligation can be completed. In order to highlight some considerations in repair, we present several cases that demonstrate specific points.

CASE 1. THE BASIC REPAIR: ANEURYSMAL DILATATION IN CHRONIC DISSECTION

RP presented at age 41 with an acute type B dissection that was treated medically but required a mesenteric revascularization with an iliac to SMA bypass because of intestinal ischemia from malperfusion. He had severe underlying essential hypertension requiring four-drug therapy after surgery for blood pressure control. He was followed with MR angiography (MRA) of his thoracoabdominal aorta at 1, 6, and 12 months after discharge and then every 6 months. By the 36th month postdissection, his aortic diameter had increased to 6.3 cm and he was having more episodes of back and chest pain (Figure 40–1). At that point, he had a spinal artery MR angiogram, thallium stress test, echocardiogram, and pulmonary function tests as part of the preoperative evaluation for surgical repair of his aorta.

This is a typical time course for patients who continue to have aortic expansion after acute dissection. Several issues arise during this observation period, including the difficulty of blood pressure control (antihypertensive management should include a beta blocker) and the patient's or physician's anxiety about observation. It is not uncommon to have urgent admissions during the observation period because a hypertensive crisis leads to chest and back pain. Not uncommonly, these episodes are precipitated by noncompliance with medications because of undesirable side effects. If the aorta is within the observation range (<6 cm), patient education and resumption of antihypertensive medications are the goals. Our judgment is that the disease risk should exceed the surgical risk before surgical correction is undertaken. Once the dilation is more than 5 to 6 cm, surgery is indicated. Preoperative evaluation is a comprehensive cardiopulmonary assessment to determine the extent of comorbidities such as chronic obstructive pulmonary disease (COPD), reduced ejection fraction, or cardiac valve dysfunction. Preoperative cessation of smoking is encouraged.

The Surgery

Our surgical technique has been described in detail previously[4-5] and consists of graft inclusion, moderate hypothermia (31 to 33 degrees Centigrade), selective renal cooling (each renal artery is rapidly perfused with 300 to 400 mL of 4 degrees Centigrade Ringer's lactate), spinal fluid drainage, neurochemical protection (naloxone, steroids, and thiopental), optimizing blood pressure and cardiac function, and for the last 6 years, reimplanting some intercostal arteries. We do not routinely use assisted circulation, but hypothermic circulatory arrest is used in very proximal aneurysms in which there is no place to clamp the arch. A dedicated team of vascular surgeons and cardiac anesthesiologists who all use the same protocol for surgical and anesthetic management perform all emergencies as well as all elective surgeries. This team approach is invaluable for managing these complex patients and is a major factor in optimizing results.

The level of thoracoabdominal incision is modified based on the location of the aneurysm. For an aneurysm this proximal, a fifth intercostal incision is made and taken to the midline and then down the midline to below the umbilicus. In this patient, there was not room to clamp distal to the left subclavian artery, and therefore, the aorta was cleared between the left carotid and the left subclavian arteries for applying the cross-clamp. Because the initial aortic clamp was proximal to the subclavian artery, it was exposed and controlled in its proximal portion so it could be easily cross-clamped during the proximal anastomosis. When dissecting the distal arch, special care is taken to iden-

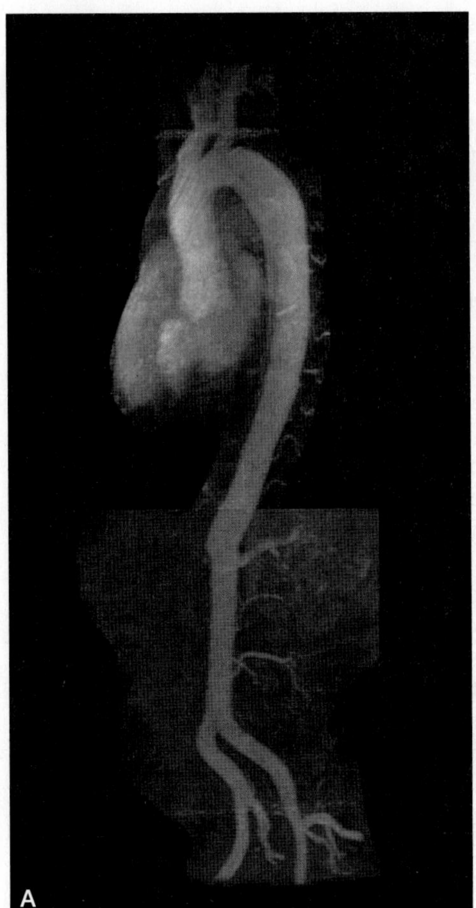

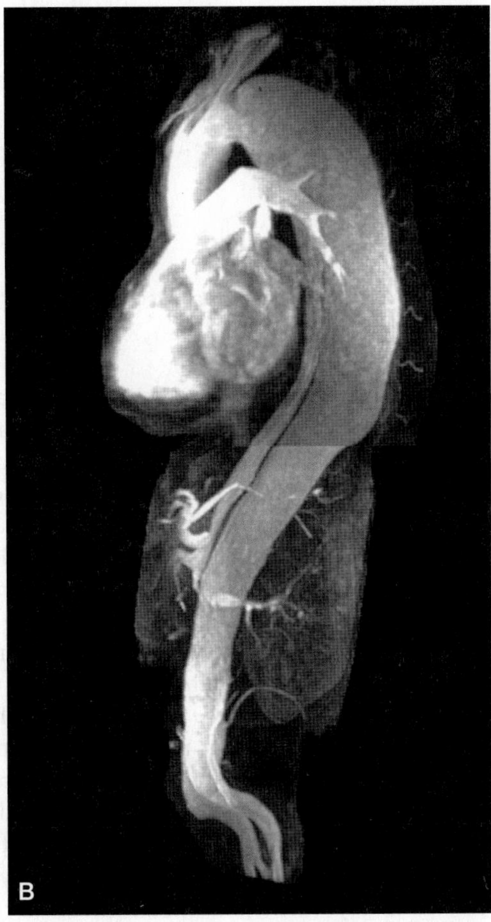

Figure 40-1. A. Type B dissection treated medically with minimal aortic dilatation initially. B. By 36 months after initial dissection, the patient's aorta had expanded from 3.8 cm to 6.5 cm.

tify and preserve the phrenic nerve and the vagus nerve with its recurrent branch, which is dissected off the underside of the aorta to minimize possible injury from inclusion in the anastomosis. Preventing vocal cord paralysis when possible reduces postoperative pulmonary complications. Care must be taken to avoid injury to the phrenic nerve insertion on the diaphragm. The diaphragm is incised by staying very close to the chest wall until past the area of possible injury. The phrenic nerve can be easily injured here and doing so greatly increases pulmonary problems postoperatively.

Exposure of the abdominal portion of the aorta in this case included the celiac artery, SMA, and left renal arteries as well as both iliac arteries. The diaphragm was incised radically through the aortic hiatus in making the initial thoracoabdominal incision and the inferior pulmonary ligament was taken down. In exposing the abdominal portion of the aorta and iliac arteries, the periaortic lymphatics and sometimes the large lumbar vein coming off the renal vein are ligated. The final part of the exposure is to identify and dissect the intercostal arteries to be reimplanted. In this patient, three intercostal arteries were reattached from T8, 9, and 10 as separate buttons (Figure 40–2).

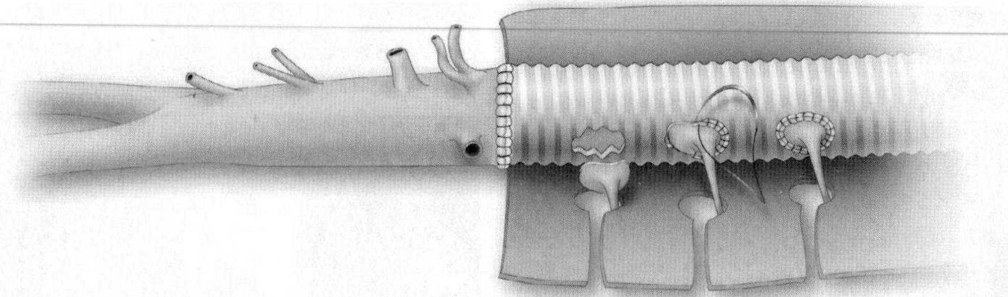

Figure 40-2. Attaching intercostal arteries with aortic "buttons" after completing aortic replacement minimizes renal and visceral ischemic times.

Once the exposure is complete, the patient's core temperature must be below 34 degrees Centigrade, the spinal fluid pressure below 6 mm Hg, and the systolic blood pressure below 100 mm Hg before cross-clamping the aorta. The anesthetic management during the cross-clamping is quite complex and requires considerable experience; it has been described in detail previously.[4]

The proximal clamp is applied over 20 to 25 seconds to allow accommodation and coordinate with the anesthesiologist to ensure that the heart tolerates the clamp and increase in blood pressure. When opening a chronic dissection, the false lumen is entered first because the true lumen is compressed medially; therefore, it is important to open the dissecting septum to gain access to the true lumen, where many of the intercostal arteries are located. After opening the septum up to the clamp or its origin, the intercostals are oversewn rapidly and then the septum is excised, giving a clear view of the anastomotic sewing ring. We use a large MH needle on a 2-0 Prolene suture with an imbricating vertical and horizontal mattress running suture line with frequent large (1.5 x 2 cm) felt pledgets where reinforcement is needed. In this case, where the dissection went up to the subclavian artery, the suture line included the lip of the subclavian artery with the mattress suture invaginating the graft into the aortic lumen for a tight seal. Once the proximal anastomosis is completed, the patient is put in the Trendelenburg position, and the graft is flushed first from the subclavian and then from the aorta to remove any air or debris. Then a clamp is placed on the graft and flow is opened to the graft and then to the subclavian artery while the patient is positioned head-down. If the anastomosis is hemostatic, the graft is reclamped below the anastomosis, the sequential clamp is removed, and the aorta is opened to below the visceral vessels. The remaining intercostals are quickly oversewn, the ones preselected for reimplantation are microbulldogged, and balloon catheters (No. 4 short Fogarty) are placed in the celiac artery and SMA. The renal arteries are then perfused with 300 to 400 mL of cold (4 degrees Centigrade) renal perfusate (Lactate Ringer's solution with 25 Gmmannitol and 1000 U heparin/L), and the Fogarty occluding catheters are inserted. Renal perfusion usually lowers the core temperature another 1.5 to 2 degrees Centigrade. Visceral and renal vessels are next attached to the graft as a Carrel patch. In this case, the right renal artery was occluded with the original dissection and was shrunken and nonfunctional; therefore the left renal artery was perfused with 600 mL of renal perfusion. Because of the distance between visceral vessels, the SMA and celiac artery were attached as one visceral patch and the left renal artery as a separate patch. We make the visceral patch a narrow as possible ellipse to avoid aneurysmal patch dilation later, and the left renal window is circular. The graft windows are created using a hand-held disposable fine-tipped cautery (ACU) to avoid fraying the woven graft material. After completing visceral and renal attachment, the patient is placed in the Trendelenburg position, and the graft is flushed of clot or debris and then reclamped below the renal anastomosis; the proximal clamp is then removed, establishing flow to the visceral patch. Following this, the Fogarty catheters are removed, establishing flow to these vessels, which are then examined for a palpable pulse and Doppler flow. Indigo carmine is used after reestablishing renal blood flow to document time of resumption of urine production. The renal ischemia time was 64 minutes and the urine reappearance time was <15 minutes in this patient.

The distal aortic anastomosis is then completed, again excising the dissecting septum and a similar flushing and irrigating with heparin saline to remove clot or debris is done before reestablishing flow to the legs. Upon completing aortic reconstruction, the anesthesiologist administers pooled fresh frozen plasma and, if indicated, platelets to reverse the coagulopathy that is always present. Once there is no major surgical bleeding, attention is turned to reattaching the selected intercostal arteries.

In this patient, we reattached three intercostal arteries from T8-9, 9-10, and 10-11 (see Figure 40–2). The preoperative spinal artery MRA identified the greater radicular artery (GRA) coming off the left T8-9 intercostal artery. A side-biting Satinsky clamp is used to reattach the intercostal buttons, which are sewn on with 4-0 Prolene (see Figure 40–2). Before closing, flow is confirmed in all vessels by Doppler auscultation. We did nothing to the previous visceral bypass, which continued to function in spite of a normal open SMA (Figure 40–3).

Commentary

The final decision about where to clamp is made after exposing the aorta, but the preoperative imaging is very important in understanding what the options might be. Three-dimensional imaging is very helpful but gives just the flow lumen image, and in some cases, especially with dissections that involve the arch, the possibilities for clamping are

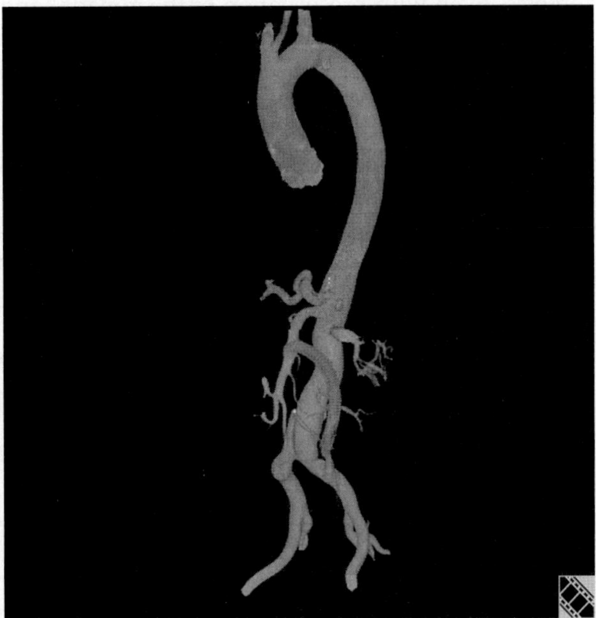

Figure 40-3. In Case 1, the aorta was replaced from the left subclavian to the distal abdominal aorta. Even with a widely patent superior mesenteric artery (SMA), after aortic reconstruction the iliac SMA bypass remained patent.

not always clear. In cases in which it is not totally clear whether or in which the aorta can be clamped, the decision to use hypothermic arrest is made after opening the chest. A dissected arch can tolerate clamping if it is not too large, but determining tolerance for clamping is a subjective decision. Sewing a graft into a chronically dissected aorta requires excising the septum to create a common channel so the true and false flow lumina are not compromised. For the proximal anastomosis, this septal excision is relatively limited because of the clamp proximity, but at a distal anastomosis, the septal excision can be more extensive, particularly in the visceral portion of the aorta so that all vessels come off the same lumen. In dissections, it is especially important to identify and prepare areas for sequentially clamping the descending thoracic aorta during the proximal anastomosis. Usually, as in this case, only one such sequential clamp is needed before exposing the visceral segment for renal cooling. However, even with sequential clamping, significant blood loss can occur from back bleeding intercostals before they can be ligated, and Cell Saver scavenging with retransfusion is essential. A little extra dissection of the intercostal arteries for external control prior to opening the aorta can be helpful if such a surgical dissection is not too difficult or traumatic, and the intercostal arteries to be reattached are dissected out for some length from the aorta so they can be controlled with microbulldogs prior to opening the aorta.

Other Issues

The location of an "elephant" trunk for cross-clamping is not always obvious because it is usually pushed to one wall of the aneurysm and is difficult to palpate. Therefore, an extra long aortic clamp as close to the subclavian artery as possible usually captures the elephant trunk, which can then be reclamped for better positioning and control after the aorta is opened.

Occasionally, the patient has a retroaortic left renal vein that is in the way of the repair. Using straight short DeBakey clamps, we divide the retroaortic renal vein after completing the proximal anastomosis and resuture it after completing the distal anastomosis. Even with preservation of the gonadal and adrenal veins, after reestablishing renal artery flow, the renal vein frequently needs decompression to avoid venous congestion of the kidney, which can adversely affect renal function. In cases in which vein reanastomosis fails for technical reasons, we create an interposition graft with bovine pericardium.

Preoperative imaging of important intercostal arteries is helpful, but this identification is inexact and operative findings are very important in deciding which intercostals, if any, to reattach. Intercostal artery reattachment can be tedious because of the quality of the aortic wall for creating the buttons. If the aorta has very heavy plaque, endarterectomy can make anastomosis easier, but patency is reduced, probably because of platelet adhesion or dissection. Therefore, we prefer to create a larger button (nickel to quarter size) and sew full thickness if there is not too much calcification. The Satinsky clamp should be placed posterior enough so that there is no tension on the intercostal artery.

This patient was hospitalized for 8 days and had no serious complications and was discharged on three antihypertensive medications and with normal renal function. This case demonstrates our standard approach to the many chronic dissections we follow and treat.

Thirty-seven patients like this were treated from 1985 to 2008, with paraplegia in 2 out of 37 (5.4%, O/E ratio of 0.14), with 1 recovering enough motor function to ambulate. The mortality rate was 8% (3/37), from acute MI with cardiogenic shock in 1, major stroke with pulmonary complications in 1, and pulmonary failure in 1. The mean length of hospital stay was 19.6 days (median 13.4 days). Eleven percent (4/37) of patients required hypothermic arrest for repair. Long-term survival was 88%, 81%, and 73% at 1, 3, and 5 years, respectively, in these elective patients.

We recently reviewed our experience with acute Type B aortic dissections. Of 79 patients who presented with acute type B dissection, 19 (23%) required emergency surgery. The remaining 60 were successfully medically treated. Our follow-up protocol includes CTA or MRA of the chest and abdomen at 3, 6, 9, 12 months and yearly thereafter. During follow-up, elective surgery for chronic aneurysmal dilation occurred in 18 patients (30%). Of these 18, 90% developed their aneurysm within 24 months.

ACUTE-ON-CHRONIC DISSECTION

Of the 63 patients (9%) we have treated with chronic dissections, 26 (41%) presented acutely, usually with back or chest pain, uncontrolled hypertension, and large ruptured aneurysms. In some of these patients, controlling blood pressure relieves their pain and there is time to do a complete preoperative cardiopulmonary work-up. However, in many patients, a more acute issue requires urgent attention.

CASE 2. RECURRENT DISSECTION

KP was a 31-year-old male when he first presented with an acute Type B dissection. He had severe essential hypertension but was erratic and unreliable in taking his medications. He presented with severe chest and back pain and a blood pressure of 240/140 mm Hg. At the time of dissection, he lost motor function in his lower extremities, which returned spontaneously after about 45 minutes. This was interpreted as transient spinal cord ischemia. CT scan at his initial dissection showed a classic Type B dissection with true and false lumina in a nondilated aorta and involved the distal arch. He was treated medically with antihypertensives in the ICU and required intubation and sedation because of alcohol and heroin withdrawal. After 18 days in the hospital, he was discharged on four antihypertensive medications with well-controlled blood pressure.

He had no more acute episodes until 10 years later, when he again presented with malignant hypertension (260/130) and transient loss of lower extremity motor function, which returned after about 30 minutes. However, this time he had weakly palpable femoral pulses, reduced urine output, and abdominal pain consistent with mesenteric ischemia. His CT scan showed a progressive dissection of his old dissection with near aortic occlusion of the true lumen cephalad to the visceral vessels. He clearly had a malperfusion of his distal aorta and branch vessels (Figure 40–4). His dissection extended proximally to a bovine arch, making a cross-clamp impossible. He was repaired under hypothermic arrest after reaching a core temperature of 15 degrees Centigrade, and the aorta was replaced down to the renal arteries with a beveled graft sewn across from the visceral arteries. At the time of surgery, there were no open intercostal arteries, and the proximal anastomosis was flush with the bovine origin of the innominate and left carotid arteries with a bypass to the left sublcavian artery (Figure 40–5). The patient awoke paraplegic and remained so in spite of attempted

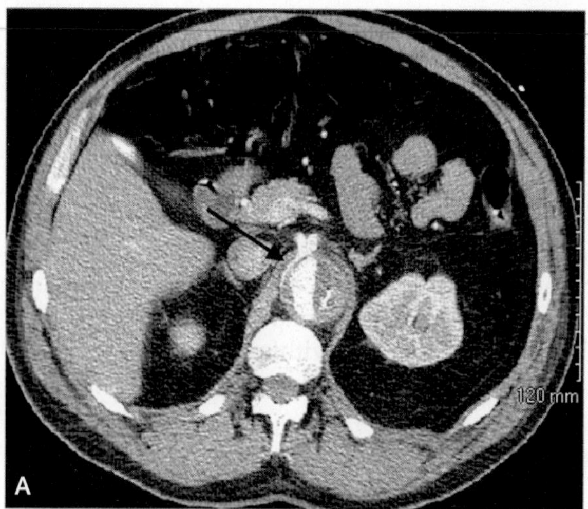

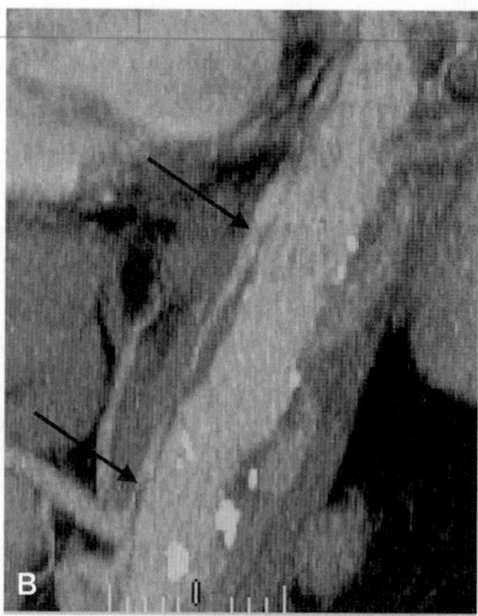

Figure 40-4. A. In the patient with redissection of a Type B dissection that occurred 10 years previously with transient paraplegia, the axial CT angiogram images show that the true lumen is severely compressed, resulting in symptoms of acute mesenteric ischemia, ischemic nephropathy, and reduced femoral pulses. B. The lateral view shows the true lumen compressed for most of its course, resulting in a functional coarctation.

rescue with spinal fluid drainage. His recovery was relatively uncomplicated because he was young and strong enough to transfer in and out of a wheelchair and he resumed his life teaching music.

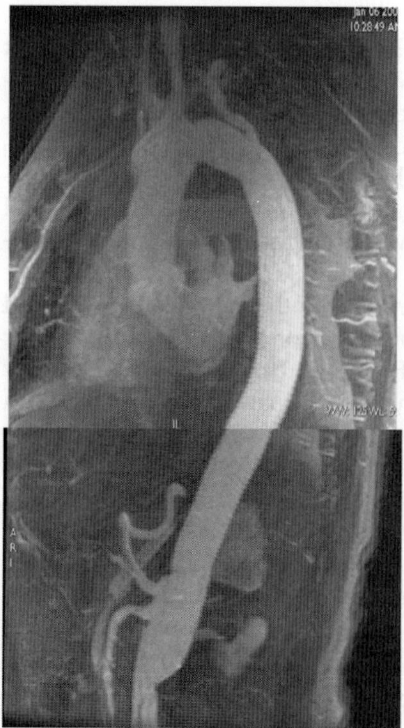

Figure 40-5. In the Case 2 patient, aortic repair necessitated hypothermic circulatory arrest because the distal portion of the "bovine" arch was involved in the dissection, requiring bypass of the left subclavian artery and a proximal anastomosis flush with the right carotid artery.

Commentary

We use hypothermic circulatory arrest for anatomic reasons, and in our experience, it is a much more complicated procedure with higher mortality and morbidity. The spinal drain is placed using fluoroscopy. Because of the thoracoabdominal incision, arterial and venous cannulation are through the femoral vessels with the bicaval venous cannula inserted over a guidewire to the level of the junction of the atrium and superior vena cava using transesophageal echo guidance. The left ventricular sump is placed through the left atrial appendage, and there is no cardioplegia with cardiac protection dependent on the profound hypothermia. Twenty-five percent of the patients repaired using circulatory arrest have postoperative bleeding from coagulopathy that requires reoperation, usually some days after surgery, for hematoma evacuation after correction of the coagulopathy. Operative mortality is also higher. What the technique allows is an unobstructed view into the arch, and the proximal anastomosis can be parachuted deep into the arch, which avoids the need for another surgery to replace the arch. This technique is used often in patients who have had a previous Type A dissection repair without arch replacement. This case also illustrates our observation that if a patient presents with transient spinal cord ischemia, paraplegia is almost a certain outcome of surgical repair no matter what surgical technique is used, and therefore, surgical correction is used only under the most extreme circumstances.

CASE 3. MYCOTIC ANEURYSM AFTER DISSECTION

RA is a 26-year-old woman who suffered a Type B dissection while taking an early morning walk. She felt sudden chest and back pain that was followed quickly by loss of strength in her lower extremities. After some delay, she was diagnosed with acute occlusion of her aorta at the renal and infrarenal levels with loss of perfusion to her left kidney. She was treated with an emergency axillobifemoral bypass to restore pelvic and lower extremity circulation but experienced severe myonecrosis requiring thigh and leg fasciotomies and temporary dialysis for myoglobin-induced renal failure. She recovered from this terrible insult with loss of much of her left quadriceps, but with intensive rehabilitation, she was eventually able to walk unassisted. Four months after her original dissection and 1 month after her last skin graft, she developed a 7-cm MRSA mycotic aneurysm of the thrombosed portion of her infrarenal aorta, presenting with fever, malaise, and positive blood cultures (Figure 40–6).

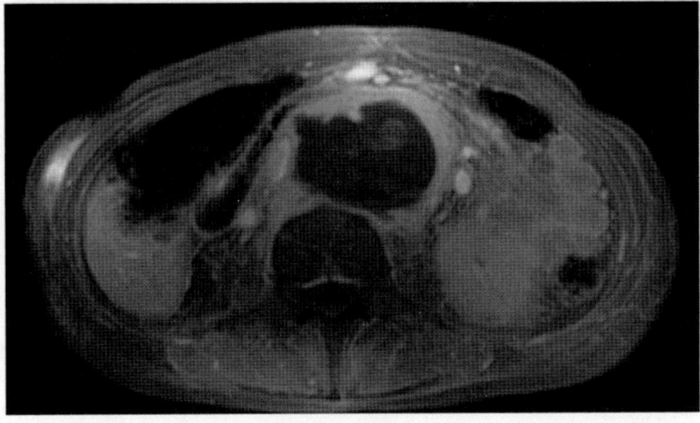

Figure 40-6. A 7.5-cm mycotic aneurysm from MRSA in the thrombosed abdominal aorta of a 26-year-old female who had an acute Type B dissection 3 months prior that required an emergency axillobifemoral bypass.

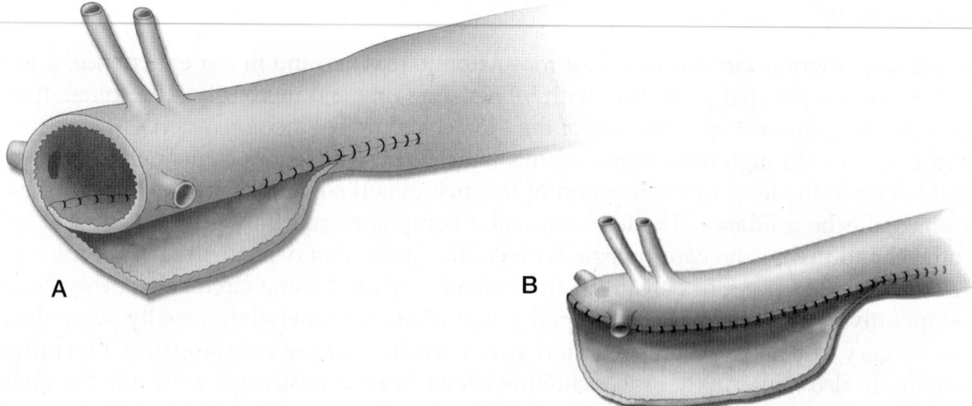

Figure 40-7. A and B. To reconstruct the aorta, the aortic wall was imbricated after débriding all of the infected clot and debris in order to avoid use of a synthetic graft in such a severely MRSA-infected aorta.

She was treated with radical débridement of her infected aorta and reconstruction of the visceral segment using her own chronically dissected aortic wall. This reconstruction required clamping above the celiac artery, removing the dissection septum, and imbricating the suture line to reduce aortic diameter (Figure 40–7). Pledgets of bovine pericardium were used to reinforce the suture line. An autogenous reconstruction was done because of the MRSA infection, which we felt precluded synthetic or homograft as a curative solution. This patient survived intact and has been followed for 4 years with minimal dilation of her aortic reconstruction and proximal type B dissection (Figure 40–8).

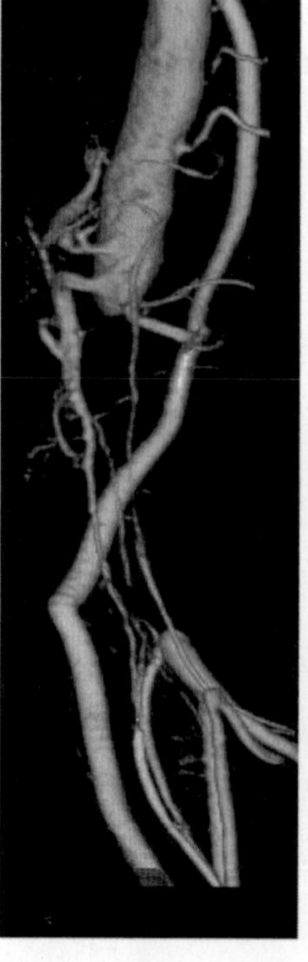

Figure 40-8. The patient's aorta reconstruction has remained stable without significant dilation for the last 4 years.

CASE 4. RUPTURED CHRONIC DISSECTION

GS is a 66-year-old male who was treated medically and followed serially for a Type B aortic dissection 2 years prior to presenting with acute back and chest pain accompanied by severe hypertension (180/95). CTA showed what appeared to be a rupture of the aorta contained in the aortic hiatus of the diaphragm, but his aortic diameter was only 3 to 4 cm and, except for the leak, was unchanged from his CT scan 6 months earlier (Figure 40–9). He was a very large man (BMI 40) with advanced COPD, pulmonary hypertension, and a history of a Type A dissection repair 4 years prior. Because of what we felt was a very high pulmonary risk for surgery, we controlled his blood pressure in the ICU and rescanned him in 36 hours, and it was clear that the hematoma had enlarged. In order to maximize his survival chances, we elected to repair the ruptured portion of his aorta, sewing it to his proximal and distal dissected aorta. This allowed an approach through the eighth intercostal space using an extraperitoneal dissection and leaving the central portion of the diaphragm intact. The aorta was replaced from the mid-descending aorta to the celiac artery with a 26-mm Dacron graft, and no intercostals were reattached (Figure 40–10). Large felt pledgets (1.5 × 2 cm) were used to secure the suture line and the dissecting septum was excised proximally and distally in order to sew to a common channel. Pulmonary issues complicated the patient's postoperative recovery, but he was eventually weaned from the ventilator and discharged 21 days after surgery on three antihypertensive medications. His remaining chronic dissection is monitored.

Commentary

For most surgeons, there is significant uncertainty about what will be encountered when trying to sew a chronically dissected aorta and when an acute dissection actually heals

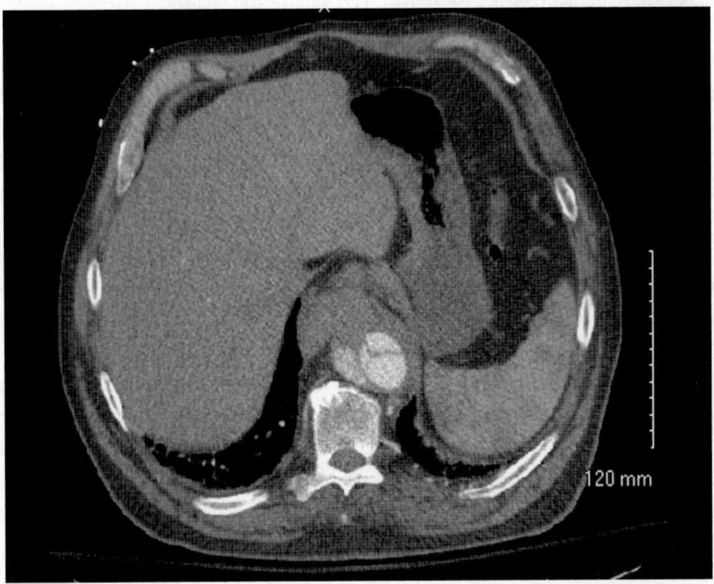

Figure 40-9. A spontaneous rupture in a chronic aortic dissection that had been followed for 3 years without significant aortic enlargement. It is unusual for an aortic dissection to rupture with so little enlargement, and it remained unexplained why this aorta failed.

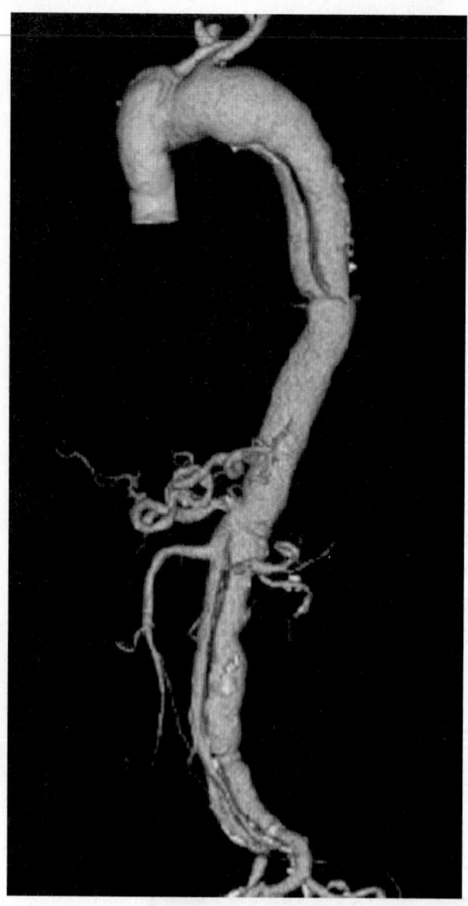

Figure 40-10. Because of severe pulmonary hypertension and COPD, just the ruptured portion of the aorta was replaced to allow a lower intercostal incision that we felt would give the patient a better chance of survival. The graft was sutured to chronically dissected aorta proximally and distally.

enough to take on the sewing characteristics of a chronic dissection. The technical definition of when an acute dissection becomes chronic is arbitrary and not defined by healing of the aortic wall. There are no firm guidelines on this, but our judgment is that within 6 weeks of the acute event, there is significant remodeling (thickening and healing) of the dissected aortic wall that might give it the "feel" of a chronic dissection. Even with that significant remodeling of the dissection, the use of large felt pledgets (2 × 1 cm) or strips externally, especially when sewing the false lumen, is often required. In Case 3, there was significant preoperative uncertainty about the integrity of the aortic wall because of both the mycotic aortitis and the recent dissection. After radical débridement of the infected clot, wall, and debris, we found aortic wall in the visceral segment that was sewable, and because of the infection, bovine pericardial pledgets were used. Felt pledgets are contraindicated in an infected field. If we had been forced to use a graft, it would have been Gore-Tex with Gore-Tex hand-made pledgets instead of felt. In both cases, the patient's blood pressure was kept lower than we normally would during aortic occlusion because the aortic clamp was applied to the dissected aorta.

It is unusual for a chronic dissection to rupture, as happened in Case 4, if it has not become a significant aneurysm. An exception to this is dissection in a patient with Ehlers-Danlos syndrome that usually ruptures acutely if medical management is attempted. This is unlike our experience with Marfan syndrome patients who can be reliably followed like any medically managed Type B or postoperative Type A dissection. It was unclear why this patient ruptured a nonaneurysmal chronic dissection, but his uncontrolled hypertension may have played a role.

Of the 26 patients with chronic dissections who presented acutely, 5 (19%) died perioperatively and 4 (15%, O/E ratio 0.24) had paraplegia. Mortality was 50% (2/4) in the paralyzed patients and 13.6% (3/22) in the patients without paralysis. The cause of death was cardiac in 2 patients (1 intraoperatively), pulmonary in 2 patients, and postoperative GI bleeding with shock and arrest in 1 patient. Four (15%) patients required hypothermic arrest for repair. The mean length of hospital stay was 29 days (median 19).

SUMMARY

We have tried to present a realistic picture of the presentations in chronic dissection and some of the major issues and problems surgeons face in treating these complex patients. This sampling of the wide variety of problems that may be encountered hopefully illuminates some of the basic principles in the management of chronic aortic dissection that can be applied generally. The fundamental anesthetic principles of hypothermia, hemodynamic management, spinal fluid drainage, and neurochemical protection, with or without assisted circulation and intercostal reimplantation, applied consistently by a dedicated and experienced anesthetic team, are essential for optimal outcomes.

Preparing for the surgery carefully, with adequate imaging and contingency planning for unexpected intra-operative findings, is important for even the very experienced surgeon but essential for the less experienced. Operating on chronic dissections requires awareness of aortic handling properties and the liberal use of pledgets for suture line support to be successful. Intercostal mapping preoperatively can be helpful in identifying potentially important intercostal arteries. However, even with the best preparation and planning, this is a high-risk patient population and should be approached cautiously and electively. This requires consistent long-term follow-up after the initial acute episode.[6]

REFERENCES

1. Miller DC. Improved follow-up for patients with chronic dissections. Semin Thorac Cardiovascular Surg 1991;3:270–6.
2. Haverich A, Miller DC, Scott WC, et al. Acute and chronic aortic dissections—determinants of long-term outcome for operative survivors. Circulation 1985;72:1122–34.
3. Masuda Y, Yamada Z, Morooka N, et al. Prognosis of patients with medically treated aortic dissections. Circulation 1991;84:III7–13.
4. Acher CW, Wynn MM. Technique of thoracoabdominal aneurysm repair. Ann Vasc Surg 1995;9:585–95.
5. Acher CW, Wynn MM, Mell MW, et al. A quantitative assessment of the impact of intercostal artery reimplantation on paralysis risk in thoracoabdominal aortic aneurysm repair. Ann Surg 2008;248:529–40.
6. Acher CW, Wynn MM. Thoracoabdominal Aneurysm Surgery: Scientific Principles and Practice, 3rd ed. Philadelphia: Lippincott: Williams & Wilkins; 2001, pp. 1790–803.

41

Current Treatment of Type B Thoracic Aortic Dissections

P. A. Naughton, M.D., M. Garcia-Toca, M.D., and Mark K. Eskandari, M.D.

INTRODUCTION

Acute thoracic aortic dissection is an uncommon but potentially fatal condition with an incidence of 3 cases per 100,000 patients. Based on the Stanford classification, 60% of aortic dissections are Type A and 40% Type B.[1] Management and outcome differ between Types A and B; therefore in this chapter we focus on Type B dissections.

The pathogenesis of Type B dissection is multifactorial. Risk factors for developing dissection include male gender, arterial hypertension, connective tissue diseases, steroid and cocaine use, bicuspid aortic valve, and iatrogenic and deceleration trauma.[2] Clinical presentation is diverse, ranging from asymptomatic, incidental diagnosis to thoracic aortic rupture. In contrast to Type A dissection, uncomplicated acute Type B dissection has a relatively favorable prognosis, with 90% survival to hospital discharge after receiving antihypertensive therapy.[3] However, when acute Type B dissections are complicated by rupture, end-organ malperfusion, or signs of impending rupture, urgent intervention is indicated.[4] Chronic Type B dissection (survival >14 days after onset of dissection) is an entirely different entity and management options are considered separately.[5]

ACUTE TYPE B DISSECTION

Medical Management

Intensive medical management controlling hypertension and pulse with beta blockers and nitrates and appropriate pain relief are the preferred therapeutic approaches to uncomplicated aortic Type B dissection.[6] Monitoring blood pressure and reducing systolic pressure to 100 to 120 mmHg in the intensive care setting while maintaining renal perfusion is a priority.[7] One possible exception to this approach are patients with underlying connective tissue disease; this cohort of patients may be considered for prompt operative repair.

Much information on acute Type B dissections regarding management, prognosis, and treatment outcome can be ascertained from the International Registry of Acute Aortic Dissection (IRAD)[8]: 242 consecutive patients presented with acute Type B dissection; 189 were treated medically, 27 were treated with endovascular intervention, and 26 underwent open surgical repair. In-hospital mortality was significantly greater in those patients who underwent open surgical repair (29%, P<.001) compared with those treated with endovascular (11%) and medical management (10%). Interestingly, in those who survived, there was no significant mortality differences at 3 years regarding open surgery (76%), endovascular treatment (82%), and medical management (76%). Predictors of follow-up mortality included age 70 yrs, female gender, hypertension, renal failure, atherosclerosis, previous aortic surgery, and patients who presented with signs of rupture or impending rupture.

Endovascular Intervention

Intervention is indicated in patients with intractable pain, signs of impending rupture, or distal malperfusion. In complicated dissections, 30 to 50% of patients have lower limb and visceral ischemia, and 50 to 80% mortality is reported in the absence of prompt intervention.[8] Malperfusion may result from direct extension of the dissection flap into the orifice of a visceral or lower extremity artery (static obstruction) or by the dissection flap's prolapsing into the vessel origin (dynamic obstruction).[9]

Over the last 10 years, endovascular techniques, including stent graft deployment, stenting obstructed aortic side branches, and percutaneous fenestration, have emerged as feasible, less invasive alternatives to open surgical repair for patients with acute, complicated Type B dissections.[10-12] Endovascular intervention obviates the need for aortic cross-clamping, reduces intraoperative blood loss, avoids a thoracotomy and single-lung ventilation, has a more rapid procedural time compared with open surgery, and may be associated with a lower risk for perioperative paraplegia.

Stent Grafts. The primary objective of endografting for acute Type B dissections is to cover the primary entry tear in the hope of obliterating flow in the false-lumen and preferentially directing flow back into the true lumen. In the acute setting, this facilitates end-organ perfusion and controls hemorrhage.[13-14] In the middle to long term, it is anticipated that stent grafts depressurize the false-lumen, thereby promoting false-lumen thrombosis and subsequently diminishing the risk of future aneurysmal dilation. The incidence of false-lumen thrombosis is variable, but when it occurs, it is associated with an improved prognosis.[15]

U.S. Food and Drug Administration Approved-Stent Grafts

GORE TAG Thoracic Endograft (Figures 41–1 and 41–2). This endograft is composed of an ePTFE graft supported by an outer self-expanding nitinol stent. It was the first commercially available thoracic stent graft approved by the U.S. Food and Drug Administration in March 2005. Flexibility makes this stent graft an attractive option in treating challenging, tortuous anatomy. The Gore TAG Pivotal trial was a multicenter, nonrandomized prospective trial comparing treatment of descending thoracic aortic aneurysms with stent grafts versus open repair.[17] Benefits conferred by TAG stent grafts compared with open surgery

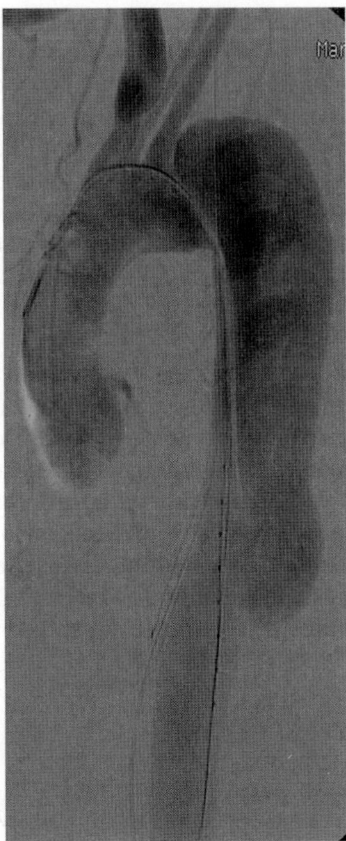

Figure 41-1. Arch aortogram demonstrating a Type B aortic dissection commencing just beyond the left subclavian artery. Note the Pigtail catheter is within the true aortic lumen. There is rapid filling of the false lumen and aneurysm formation of the descending thoracic aorta.

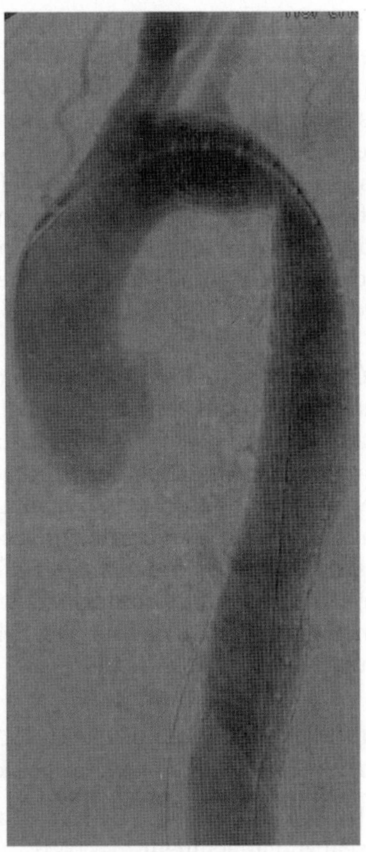

Figure 41-2. Arch aortogram following deployment of a TAG (Gore) stent graft. The proximal landing zone is just beyond the left subclavian artery, with the distal landing zone low in the descending thoracic aorta. There is no evidence of an endoleak and no filling of the false lumen. Note the kink within the proximal aspect of the stent-graft, this was not flow limiting.

included decreased paraplegia or paraparesis (14% vs. 3%), decreased early mortality (10% vs. 2%), and decreased intensive care and hospital stay. On a cautionary note, at 2-year follow-up 15% of patients experienced endoleak. In addition, fracture of the longitudinal support wire was reported in 20 patients. This longitudinal wire was subsequently removed in the redesign of the TAG stent graft. One complication of the redesigned TAG device is stent graft infolding, which may occur when the stent graft is excessively oversized. To date, this device has labeling only for the treatment of thoracic aortic aneurysms. Its use for the treatment of acute/chronic aortic dissections either is part of a clinical trial or is off-label.

Cook Zenith Stent Graft. The TX2 stent graft is a full-thickness woven polyester fabric sewn to self-expanding stainless steel Z-stents with braided polyester and hand-stitched monofilament polyprolene suture. In addition, the Z-stents contain barbs at the distal and proximal ends to augment aortic attachment and seal. FDA approval was based on the results of the TX2 trial comparing 160 patients with descending thoracic aortic aneurysms and penetrating ulcers treated with TX2 with 60 patients who had open surgical repair.[18] Patients treated endovascularly had significantly less major morbidity at 30 days compared with the open group. At 1 year follow-up in the endovascular group, there were no ruptures or open conversions and the incidence of endoleak and migration was 3.9% and 2.8%, respectively. Areas of ongoing development with Zenith stent grafts include branched devices and fenestrations. Limitations of this device include a multistep delivery system and less flexibility compared with other endografts. The STABLE trial is an ongoing trial investigating a dissection device specific to the treatment of Type B dissections; otherwise, this device currently is labeled for the treatment of thoracic aortic aneursyms or penetrating aortic ulcers.

Medtronic Stent Grafts. The Talent device is composed of a Dacron graft sewn to a self-expanding nitinol stent. The proximal and distal ends contain bare-spring design to facilitate attachment and seal. The use of the Talent device to treat thoracic aortic pathology is reported in the vascular talent thoracic stent graft system for the treatment of thoracic aortic aneurysms (VALOR) trial, a large prospective, multicenter, nonrandomized observational trial.[19] The European experience was reported in the Talent Thoracic Retrospective Registry. In Europe, the Valiant device is a refinement of the Talent device, conferring improved trackability, conformability, and deployment.[20] As is the case with TX2, the Talent thoracic device is currently labeled only for the treatment of aneurysms and penetrating ulcers.

Limitations of Thoracic Aortic Stent Grafting for Dissections

Several limitations of thoracic aortic stent grafting exist.

1. Lack of disease-specific endograft designs enabling flexible delivery with durable seal and attachment.
2. Access restrictions. All commercially available stent grafts require large-caliber delivery systems. Verhoye et al[14] report a 25% incidence of arterial injury requiring surgical repair in patients undergoing thoracic stent graft deployment.
3. Landing zone. A 2 cm proximal and distal landing zone is necessary to achieve fixation. A proximal landing zone may be augmented by additional hybrid procedures, including left carotid-subclavian bypass or transposition.[21] Some also advocate temporarily lowering arterial pressure during stent graft deployment to prevent distal migration of the endograft.[22]
4. Stent graft balloon dilation should be avoided because of the risk of retrograde extension of the dissection converting to a Type A.
5. Risk of stroke. Stroke may occur from embolic events precipitated by guidewire- or catheter-induced intimal trauma. Air embolization at the time of endograft deployment is also a recognized risk for stroke with current devices. Periprocedureal stroke was more commonly seen in first-generational stent graft devices; yet in current device trials, the stroke rate ranged from 3 to 8%.[19]
6. Despite improved results, compared with open repair in-patient mortality remains high for acute Type B dissections. Dias et al[23] report a 16% 30-day mortality, and Verhoye et al[14] report a 25% early mortality.
7. Multiple distal re-entry fenestrations may allow continued perfusion of the false-lumen with aneurysmal dilation. Distal extension of the stent graft to seal these fenestrations increases the risk of spinal ischemia. Some also advocate the PETTICOAT (provisional extension to induce complete attachment) concept of ex-

tending the stent graft scaffold distally with open-cell bare-metal stents.[24] The deployment of bare metal stents or "paving" may also be used as an adjunct to ameliorate flow into the visceral or iliac vessels.

8. Stent-specific complications: endoleaks, migration, stent graft fracture, and infolding. Parker et al,[25] in a review article, report that the incidence of endovascular reintervention for endoleaks in patients with Type B dissections treated with stent grafts is 7.6% and the incidence of open surgical reintervention is 2.8%. Dias et al[23] report a series of 31 patients treated with endografts for acute complicated Type B dissection. They report a 6.5% incidence of stent graft–related late deaths. Verhoye et al[14] report that freedom from treatment failure (aortic rupture, device fault, reintervention, aortic death) was 67% at 5 years. In view of this evidence and also from information from stent graft treatment of infrarenal aneurysms, there is a clear need to complete long-term surveillence of the stent grafts.
9. Patents with an underlying connective tissue disease, such as Marfan syndrome, pose a relative contraindication to stent graft deployment.[4] Although apparently successful stent graft deployment has been reported in this cohort of patients, concern regarding the impact of persistent radial forces of a stent graft on the weak aorta of patients with Marfan syndrome means most surgeons favor open repair if the patient is deemed fit for surgery.

Aortic Fenestration. Surgical aortic fenestration was first described in 1935 and the endovascular technique in 1990.[26] The use of endovascular stent grafts has largely superseded aortic fenestration; however, it remains an important technique in our armamentarium for the urgent treatment of acute malperfusion secondary to dissection. It is particularly useful in treating dynamic obstructing lesions and dissections near the arch that are difficult to treat with stent graft deployment.[12]

The use of intravascular ultrasound is a beneficial adjunct in percutaneous fenestration, enabling accurate differentiation of true and false lumina, positioning of aortic side branches, and re-entry tears. The principle of fenestration entails fashioning a wide orifice of communication between the false and the true lumina.[27]

Various fenestration techniques are described. The most commonly described technique involves puncturing the intimal flap from the true to false-lumen with a trans-septal needle and enlarging the communication with a large-diameter balloon.[28] (Figures 41–3 to 41–6) Multiple fenestrations can be done along the dissection to achieve equalization of pressures between the true and the false lumina. Some interventionalists also place a stent to maintain the fenestration, but this is not our preference because of concern regarding stent collapse or crush. Stents, however, can be used to optimize flow into the branch vessel ostia.

A second approach, the "scissor" technique, involves cannulating the true and false lumina with rigid guidewires.[29] One wire is placed through the proximal tear; this wire is then snared from the opposing lumen and retrieved caudally. Both ends of the wire are then pulled caudally simulataneously to create a "cheese-wire" effect on the intimal flap, thus slicing through the flap to create free communication between the two lumina. It is important that in the absence of a distal re-entry site in the false channel, a distal exit site is fashioned to prevent rupture from high pressures in the false channel.

Complications of fenestration include the risk that the torn intimal flap may occlude the iliac arteries.[30] Also the risk of future aneurysmal dilation of the thin-walled false lumina is a concern for long-term surveillance.

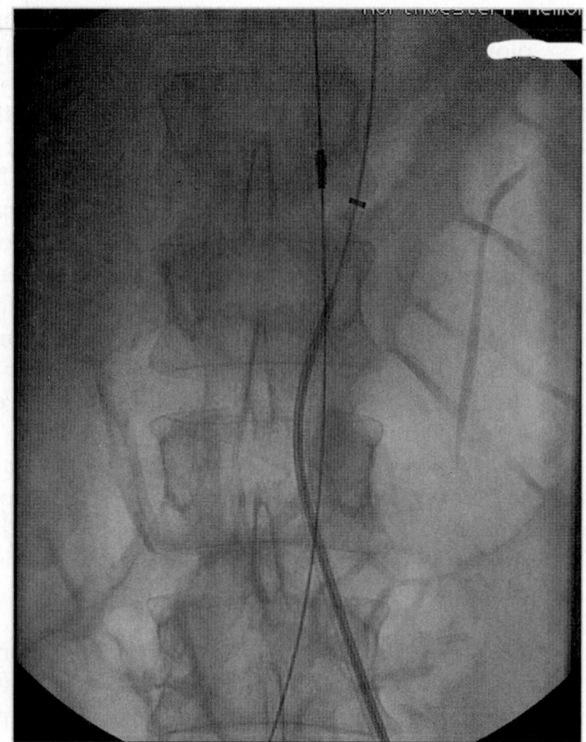

Figure 41-3. Figure a: Initial digital subtraction angiogram demonstrates contrast filling of the true aortic lumen, with contrast opacification of the right renal artery, celiac artery and superior mesenteric artery. Note only vague filling of the false lumen and no filling of the left renal artery.

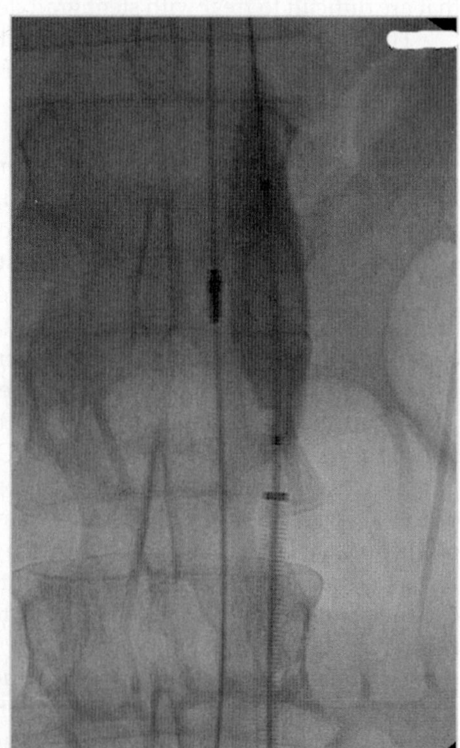

Figure 41-4. Fluoroscopic image showing a guidewire from the right common femoral artery within the true lumen. The guiding catheter, from the left common femoral artery, has crossed from the true lumen intó the false lumen, following fenestration with a Rosch-Uchida needle. The guidewire from the guiding catheter is within the false lumen.

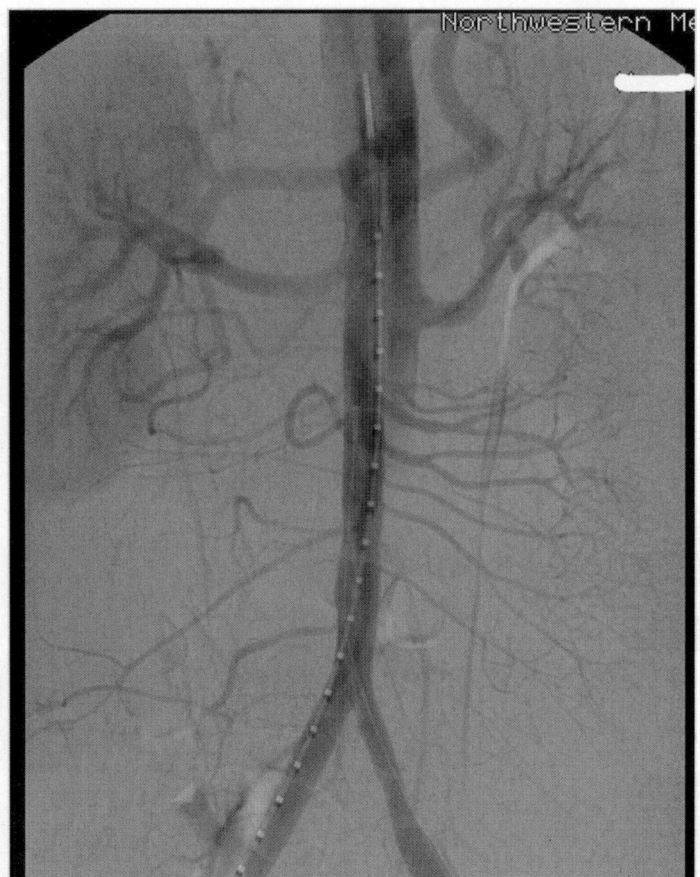

Figure 41-5. Following fenestration a 14 mm x 40 mm balloon was inflated across the site of fenestration to enable creation of a large communication between the true and false lumen in order to equalize pressures between the two lumen and to allow more flow into the false lumen to perfuse any visceral arteries arising from the false lumen.

Uncovered Stents. Uncovered stents can be successfully used to treat static or dynamic obstruction of the aortic side branches or iliac arteries. Stents may be used in isolation or in combination with stent graft deployment or aortic fenestration.

Open Surgical Repair

At present, no randomized trials have compared open and endovascular repair for complicated acute Type B dissections. Table 41–1 contains the recent results of contemporary open repair, but most studies combine the results of acute and chronic presentations and combine differing pathologies, for example, dissection, degenerative aneurysms.

One of the most devastating complications of open thoracoabdominal surgery is ischemic spinal cord injury. Much recent attention has focused on improved outcome by augmenting peri-operative spinal perfusion. Useful adjuncts include cerebrospinal fluid (CSF) drainage and maintaining distal body perfusion by bypass. Coselli et al,[31] in a randomized controlled trial, report that the incidence of postoperative paraplegia

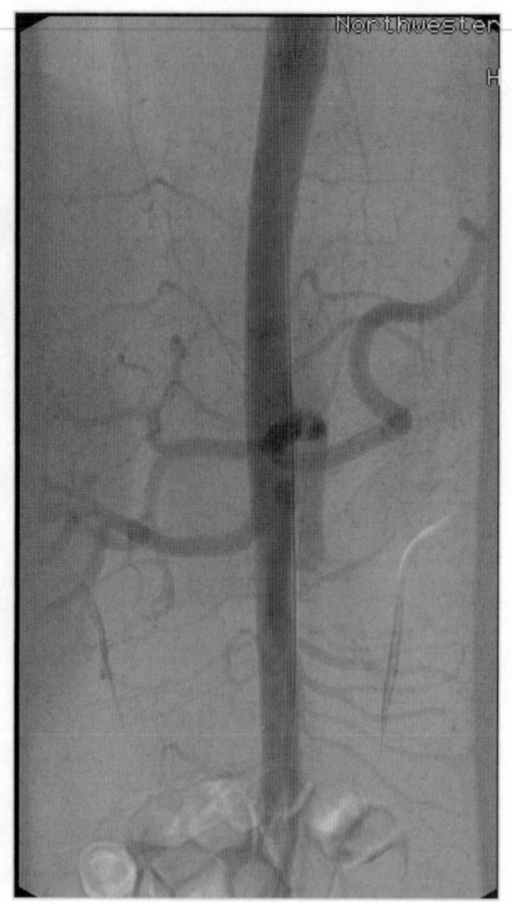

Figure 41-6. Completion angiogram with a graduated Pigtail catheter within the true lumen. Note the left renal artery now fills promptly from the false lumen.

was significantly less in the group treated prophylactically with CSF drainage (2.6% vs. 13%). However, Dardik et al[32] and Wynn et al[33] underline the need for careful monitoring of drainage volume and content with risks of subdural hematoma in cases of excessive drainage.

TABLE 41-1. OPEN SURGICAL REPAIR OF DESCENDING THORACIC AORTA

Author	No of patients	Acute dissection No. (%)	Hospital Mortality	Renal Failure	Paralysis/ paraplegia	Stroke
Estrera[43]	300	18(6)	24 (8)	12 (2.1)	7 (2.3)	6 (2.1)
Coselli[44]	387	48 (12)	11 (4.4)	29 (7.5)	10 (2.6)	
Borst[45]	132	5 (4)	4 (3)	2 (1.3)	12 (9)	
Svensson[46]	832	50 (6)	63 (8)	58 (6.9)	90 (10.4)	29 (3.5)
Verdant[47]	267	33 (12)	39 (15)	1 (0.4)	0	

Chronic Dissection

Chronic thoracic aortic dissection occurs in patients who survive >14 days after acute dissection. Risk of aneurysmal dilation and rupture of the thoracic aorta are the main concerns on long-term follow-up. Management options consist of medical, endovascular, and open surgical management and should be balanced on the basis of the patient's prognosis vs. the risks of intervention. Thoracic aortic aneurysms secondary to dissection are reported to have a more rapid growth rate and increased risk of rupture due to a thinner restraining wall compared with degenerative aneurysms.[34] Growth rates of 0.1 to 0.74 cm per year are reported among patients with chronic dissection. Juvonen et al[35] followed 50 patients with chronic dissection who were operated on when thoracic aortic diameter exceeded 5.5 cm. Despite this aggressive approach to intervention, they reported an 18% mortality rate secondary to rupture. In the absence of level 1 evidence, most surgeons advocate the need for intervention on aneurysms of a diameter of 5.5 to 6 cm.[4] In patients with underlying connective tissue disorder, most surgeons intervene at a diameter of 5 to 5.5 cm. Patients with symptomatic aneurysms presenting with pain, dyspnea, hoarseness, or dysphagia should also be considered for intervention.

Medical Management

Although the medical management of acute uncomplicated dissection has a favorable survival outcome, the long-term results are not so encouraging. The majority of patients are of an advanced age and succumb to comorbidities, but it is estimated that 20 to 50% eventually develop late aortic complications by 4 years.[36] Predictors of late aortic complications include aortic diameter, persistence of flow in the false-lumen, and arterial hypertension.[1] For this reason, strict management of blood pressure is the backbone of medical management of chronic Type B dissections.

The INSTEAD trial[37] (INvestigation of STEnt grafts in patients with Type B Aortic Dissections) is an ongoing prospective, multicenter, randomized trial comparing the outcome of uncomplicated chronic Type B dissections treated medically versus those treated with Medtronic Talent stent grafts. This trial aims to provide evidence regarding the management of uncomplicated chronic dissections. Initial results report a mortality of 10% in the endovascular group compared with 3% in the medical group.

Endovascular Intervention

Similar to acute dissections, the rationale behind endograft treatment of chronic dissections is sealing the proximal entry site, thereby promoting false-lumen thrombosis and aortic remodeling. Spontaneous thrombosis of the false-lumen will occur in <4% of patients.[38]

However, chronic dissection differs anatomically from acute dissections. First, the chronic intimal flap gets progressively thicker due to fibrosis. Second, there are more intimal tears reported in chronic dissections. Although Eggebrecht et al[39] report that operative mortality is less in patients with chronic dissection compared with those with acute dissection, these anatomic characteristics may make endovascular treatment of chronic dissections technically more challenging. Based on these anatomic differences, it is reported that the elimination of flow in the false-lumen is much lower in stent grafting chronic dissections compared with acute dissections.[40] This may increase the rate of reintervention in patients treated endovascularly for chronic dissections.[41]

Sstent grafting chronic dissection is also limited by the fact that any residual, uncovered aorta is at long-term risk for degeneration and rupture.

Open Surgery

In the absence of level 1 evidence, several observational studies compare endovascular with open surgery treating chronic dissections. Nienaber et al[42] prospectively compared 12 patients treated with stent graft deployment with 12 matched surgical controls. Proximal seal and complete lumen thrombosis were achieved in all endovascularly treated patients at 3 months. No major morbidity or mortality was reported in the endovascular group compared with a 33% incidence of death (P=.04) and major morbidity incidence of 42% (P=.04) after open surgery.

CONCLUSION

Acute complicated Type B dissection is one of the most attractive applications of stent graft management. The ongoing INSTEAD trial will provide important information to address the controversy surrounding the treatment of uncomplicated acute Type B dissections. Further improvements in stent graft design and technology may improve results and increase the number of acute and chronic dissections successfully treated by endovascular intervention.

REFERENCES

1. Hagan PG, Nienaber CA, Isselbacher EM, et al. The International Registry of Acute Aortic Dissection (IRAD): new insights into an old disease. JAMA 2000;283:897–903.
2. Larson EW, Edwards WD. Risk factors for aortic dissection: a necropsy study of 161 cases. Am J Cardiol 1984;53:849–55.
3. Estrera AL, Miller CC 3rd, Safi HJ, et al. Outcomes of medical management of acute type B aortic dissection. Circulation 2006;114:1384–9.
4. Svensson LG, Kouchoukos NT, Miller DC, et al. Expert consensus document on the treatment of descending thoracic aortic disease using endovascular stent-grafts. Ann Thorac Surg 2008;85:S1–41.
5. Crawford ES. The diagnosis and management of aortic dissection. JAMA 1990;264:2537–41.
6. Kodama K, Nishigami K, Sakamoto T, et al. Tight heart rate control reduces secondary adverse events in patients with type B acute aortic dissection. Circulation 2008;118:S167–70.
7. Akin I, Kische S, Ince H, et al. Indication, timing and results of endovascular treatment of type B dissection. Eur J Vasc Endovasc Surg 2009;37:289–96.
8. Tsai TT, Fattori R, Trimarchi S, et al. Long-term survival in patients presenting with type B acute aortic dissection: insights from the International Registry of Acute Aortic Dissection. Circulation 2006;114:2226–31.
9. Peterson BG, Eskandari MK. Endovascular repair of descending aortic dissections. Semin Thorac Cardivasc Surg 2005;17:268–73.
10. Dake MD, Miller DC, Semba CP, et al. Transluminal placement of endovascular stent-grafts for the treatment of descending thoracic aortic aneurysms. N Engl J Med 1994;331: 1729–34.
11. Barnes DM, Williams DM, Dasika NL. et al. A single-center experience treating renal malperfusion after aortic dissection with central aortic fenestration and renal artery stenting. J Vasc Surg 2008;47:903–10.

12. Beregi JP, Haulon S, Otal P, et al. Endovascular treatment of acute complications associated with aortic dissection: midterm results from a multicenter study. J Endovasc Ther 2003;10: 486–93.
13. Eggebrecht H, Nienaber CA, Neuhäuser M, et al. Endovascular stent-graft placement in aortic dissection: a meta-analysis. Eur Heart J 2006;27:489–98.
14. Verhoye JP, Miller DC, Sze D, Complicated acute type B aortic dissection: midterm results of emergency endovascular stent-grafting. J Thorac Cardiovasc Surg 2008;136:424–30.
15. Tsai TT, Evangelista A, Nienaber CA, et al. Partial thrombosis of the false lumen in patients with acute type B aortic dissection. N Engl J Med 2007;357:349–59.
16. Bernard Y, Zimmermann H, Chocron S, et al. False lumen patency as a predictor of late outcome in aortic dissection. Am J Cardiol 2001;87:1378–82.
17. Makaroun MS, Dillavou ED, Kee ST, et al. Endovascular treatment of thoracic aortic aneurysms: results of the phase II multicenter trial of the GORE TAG thoracic endoprosthesis. J Vasc Surg 2005;41:1–9.
18. Matsumura JS, Cambria RP, Dake MD, et al. International controlled clinical trial of thoracic endovascular aneurysm repair with the Zenith TX2 endovascular graft: 1-year results. J Vasc Surg 2008;47:247–57.
19. Fairman RM, Criado F, Farber M, et al. Pivotal results of the Medtronic Vascular Talent Thoracic Stent Graft System: the VALOR trial. J Vasc Surg 2008;48:546–54.
20. Fattori R, Nienaber CA, Rousseau H, et al. Results of endovascular repair of the thoracic aorta with the Talent Thoracic stent graft: the Talent Thoracic Retrospective Registry. J Thorac Cardiovasc Surg 2006;132:332–9.
21. Peterson BG, Eskandari MK, Gleason TG, Morasch MD. Utility of left subclavian artery revascularization in association with endoluminal repair of acute and chronic thoracic aortic pathology. J Vasc Surg 2006;43:433–9.
22. Lupattelli T, Garaci FG, Basile A, et al. Emergency stent grafting of type B aortic dissection: technical considerations. Emerg Radiol 2008;15:375–82.
23. Dias NV, Sonesson B, Koul B, et al. Complicated acute type B dissections—an 8-years experience of endovascular stent-graft repair in a single centre. Eur J Vasc Endovasc Surg 2006; 31:481–6.
24. Nienaber CA, Kische S, Zeller T, et al. Provisional extension to induce complete attachment after stent-graft placement in type B aortic dissection: the PETTICOAT concept. J Endovasc Ther 2006;13:738–46.
25. Parker JD, Golledge J. Outcome of endovascular treatment of acute type B aortic dissection. Ann Thorac Surg 2008;86:1707–12.
26. Williams DM, Brothers TE, Messina LM. Relief of mesenteric ischemia in type III aortic dissection with percutaneous fenestration of the aortic septum. Radiology 1990;174:450–2.
27. Williams DM, Andrews JC, Marx MV, et al. Creation of reentry tears in aortic dissection by means of percutaneous balloon fenestration: gross anatomic and histologic considerations. J Vasc Interv Radiol 1993;4:75–83.
28. Chavan A, Hausmann D, Dresler C, et al. Intravascular ultrasound-guided percutaneous fenestration of the intimal flap in the dissected aorta. Circulation 1997;96:2124–7.
29. Beregi JP, Prat A, Gaxotte V, et al. Endovascular treatment for dissection of the descending aorta. Lancet 2000;356:482–3.
30. Lookstein RA, Mitty H, Falk A, et al. Aortic intimal dehiscence: a complication of percutaneous balloon fenestration for aortic dissection. J Vasc Interv Radiol 2001;12:1347–50.
31. Coselli JS, Lemaire SA, Köksoy C, et al. Cerebrospinal fluid drainage reduces paraplegia after thoracoabdominal aortic aneurysm repair: results of a randomized clinical trial. J Vasc Surg 2002;35:631–9.
32. Dardik A, Perler BA, Roseborough GS, et al. Subdural hematoma after thoracoabdominal aortic aneurysm repair: an underreported complication of spinal fluid drainage? J Vasc Surg 2002;36:47–50.
33. Wynn MM, Mell MW, Tefera G, et al. Complications of spinal fluid drainage in thoracoabdominal aortic aneurysm repair: a report of 486 patients treated from 1987 to 2008. J Vasc Surg 2009;49:29–34.

34. Davies RR, Goldstein LJ, Coady MA, et al. Yearly rupture or dissection rates for thoracic aortic aneurysms: simple prediction based on size. Ann Thorac Surg 2002;73:17–27.
35. Juvonen T, Ergin MA, Galla JD, et al. Risk factors for rupture of chronic type B dissections. J Thorac Cardiovasc Surg 1999;117:776–86.
36. Winnerkvist A, Lockowandt U, Rasmussen E, et al. A prospective study of medically treated acute type B aortic dissection. Eur J Vasc Endovasc Surg 2006;32:349–55.
37. Nienaber CA, Zannetti S, Barbieri B, et al. INvestigation of STEnt grafts in patients with type B Aortic Dissection: design of the INSTEAD trial—a prospective, multicenter, European randomized trial. Am Heart J 2005;149:592–9.
38. Erbel R, Oelert H, Meyer J, Puth M, et al. Effect of medical and surgical therapy on aortic dissection evaluated by transesophageal echocardiography. Implications for prognosis and therapy. The European Cooperative Study Group on Echocardiography. Circulation 1993;87:1604–15.
39. Eggebrecht H, Herold U, Kuhnt O, et al. Endovascular stent-graft treatment of aortic dissection: determinants of post-interventional outcome. Eur Heart J 2005;26:489–97.
40. Kusagawa H, Shimono T, Ishida M, et al. Changes in false lumen after transluminal stent-graft placement in aortic dissections: six years' experience. Circulation 2005;111:2951–7.
41. Sayer D, Bratby M, Brooks M, et al. Aortic morphology following endovascular repair of acute and chronic type B aortic dissection: implications for management. Eur J Vasc Endovasc Surg 2008;36:522–9
42. Nienaber CA, Fattori R, Lund G, et al. Nonsurgical reconstruction of thoracic aortic dissection by stent-graft placement. N Engl J Med 1999;340:1539–45.
43. Estrera AL, Miller CC III, Chen EP, et al. Descending thoracic aortic aneurysm repair: 12-year experience using distal aortic perfusion and cerebrospinal fluid drainage. Ann Thorac Surg 2005;80:1290–6.
44. Coselli JS, LeMaire SA, Conklin LD, et al. Left heart bypass during descending thoracic aortic aneurysm repair does not reduce the incidence of paraplegia. Ann Thorac Surg 2004;77:1298–303.
45. Borst HG, Jurmann M, Buhner B, et al. Risk of replacement of descending aorta with a standardized left heart bypass technique. J Thorac Cardiovasc Surg 1994;107:126–33.
46. Svensson LG, Crawford ES, Hess KR, et al. Variables predictive of outcome in 832 patients undergoing repairs of the descending thoracic aorta. Chest 1993;104:1248–53.
47. Verdant A. Descending thoracic aortic aneurysms: surgical treatment with the Gott shunt. Can J Surg 1992;35: 493–6.

42

Combining Open and Endovascular Approaches to Complex Aneurysms

Joseph S. Coselli, M.D., Susan Y. Green, M.P.H., Ourania Preventza, M.D., and Scott A. LeMaire, M.D.

INTRODUCTION

The groundbreaking experience of endovascular repair of the infrarenal portion of the abdominal aorta[1] and the promising contemporary results in the descending thoracic aorta[2] have led to the increased application of endovascular approaches in certain aortic segments—namely, the aortic arch and thoracoabdominal aorta—that traditionally have been repaired solely with open surgical techniques because of the anatomic complexity imposed by the major branch vessels. When considering the three primary options for aortic repair, Greenberg et al.[3] suggest assessing the two major factors that affect each patient's outcome: physiologic reserve and anatomic complexity. Patients with poor physiologic reserve and complex aortic anatomy that precludes purely endovascular repair with simple tube stent grafts are ideally suited for combined or "hybrid" approaches that use open surgical procedures to reroute branch vessel circulation, enabling subsequent placement of the stent-graft to exclude the entire aortic aneurysm (Table 42–1).[4] This chapter describes several combined approaches to the repair of aneurysms of the aortic arch or thoracoabdominal aorta.

HYBRID APPROACH TO AORTIC ARCH REPAIR

Typical Complications of Traditional Open Arch Repair

Conventional surgical repair of the aortic arch is generally performed through a median sternotomy; cardiopulmonary bypass, hypothermic circulatory arrest, and cerebral perfusion are used to protect the brain while normal blood flow through the brachiocephalic

TABLE 42-1. TREATMENT APPROACHES CHOSEN ACCORDING TO PHYSIOLOGIC RESERVE AND ANATOMIC COMPLEXITY

Physiologic Risk	Anatomic Complexity	Approach
Low	Low	Well served by open or endovascular repair
Low	High	Ideal for open repair
High	Low	Ideal for endovascular repair
High	High	Ideal for a combined approach

Adapted from Greenberg RK, Clair D, Srivastava S, et al. Should patients with challenging anatomy be offered endovascular aneurysm repair? J Vasc Surg 2003;38:990–6.

vessels is temporarily halted. However, despite the use of protective adjuncts, arch replacement continues to carry substantial risk. Prolonged cardiopulmonary bypass and hypothermic circulatory arrest are associated with increased mortality, neurologic morbidity, and other complications. Contemporary series have shown excellent results, particularly in highly experienced centers; published early mortality rates range from 0 to 5%, and permanent stroke rates range from 0 to 4%.[5-7] However, patient-specific comorbidities such as advanced age, chronic renal dysfunction, previous cardiac damage, or history of stroke can greatly increase a patient's risk of these adverse outcomes,[8-9] and such patients are often considered inoperable because they are unable to withstand traditional aortic arch repair. In very high-risk patients, a combined approach has been advocated as an effective alternative that produces acceptable mortality rates and fewer neurologic, cardiac, and pulmonary complications.

Debranching to Lengthen the Proximal Landing Zone

The aortic arch has been anatomically mapped by Criado and associates[10] into five zones to facilitate procedure planning as well as to document the location of the proximal landing zone (Figure 42–1). In day-to-day practice, endovascular repair of the descending thoracic aorta frequently incorporates the more distal aspects of the aortic arch (Zone 3); however, hybrid arch repair necessitates landing in more proximal aspects of the aortic arch (Zones 0, 1, and 2). Combined arch repairs involve debranching and reimplantation of the supra-aortic vessels to increase the length of the branchless aortic "tube" and subsequently facilitate adequate sealing between the stent-graft and the aorta. Typically, fully rerouting the brachiocephalic vessels is approached through a median sternotomy, but cardiopulmonary bypass and hypothermic circulatory arrest are only rarely needed.[11] The supra-aortic vessels can be rerouted by using a variety of custom or commercially available branched grafts and are usually brought forward to the ascending aorta, which is used as an inflow source. Alternatively, for less extensive arch-debranching, one may transpose the native left subclavian artery (LSCA) and left common carotid artery (LCCA) onto the innominate artery or perform end-to-side bypass grafts between vessels; such bypasses can be constructed by using prosthetic grafts or reversed saphenous vein grafts. The endovascular portion of the repair is performed simultaneously or is briefly delayed to facilitate recovery, and deployment is approached in either a retrograde or an antegrade fashion. Performing the repair in one stage avoids between-stage rupture—an important problem in two-stage aortic repairs.[12]

The first report of hybrid arch repair described a physically compromised patient who needed reoperation for a leaking aortic arch patch graft. A custom trifurcated graft was prepared; two branches were used to bypass the LCCA and LSCA, and the third branch was used as a conduit to deliver a stent-graft in an antegrade fashion into the

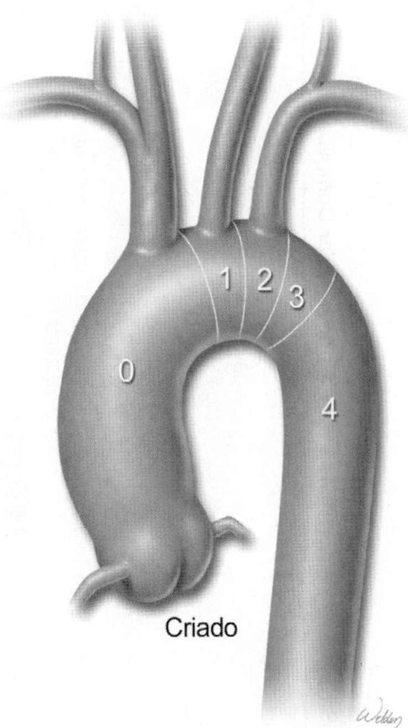

Figure 42-1. The Criado landing zones used to describe the proximal anatomy during an endovascular repair. Zone 0 includes the ascending aorta and the origin of the innominate artery. Zone 1 includes the origin of the left common carotid artery. Zone 2 includes the left subclavian artery origin. Zone 3 is within 2 cm immediately distal to the left subclavian artery, and Zone 4 is more than 2 cm distal to the origin of this vessel.

aortic arch.[13] This repair and a similar repair performed in Japan by Kato et al.[14] opened up the possibility of performing hybrid arch repair in high-risk patients.

Expanding on these distal two-vessel arch-debranching techniques, several authors have reported using total arch rerouting and proximal two-vessel debranching techniques to repair both aortic arch aneurysm and acute ascending aortic dissection (Table 42–2).[11,13,15-24] These repairs incorporate the innominate artery and LCCA into the debranching process (Zones 0 and 1) and may also include the LSCA. Exposure is typically accomplished via median sternotomy, as described above; after a partial occluding clamp is applied to the ascending aorta, a bifurcated or trifurcated graft is anastomosed. Then, the innominate artery is sewn to one of the graft's branches, usually in an end-to-end fashion; the proximal portion of this artery is ligated, oversewn, or merely left to be occluded by the stent-graft.[16-17,19] Next, the LCCA is attached to the graft and ligated proximally. When exposure is compromised by a large arch aneurysm, the branch grafts may be anastomosed to the arteries in an end-to side fashion. In cases of significant displacement of the LCCA or LSCA due to arch disease, one can make additional small neck incisions for these bypasses. When Zone 1 is used for the landing zone, the LCCA can be rerouted by performing a right common carotid artery (RCCA)-to-LCCA bypass through two small vertical neck incisions, thereby avoiding the need for a median sternotomy.[11]

The options for managing the LSCA include coverage of the origin with the stent-graft, revascularization and proximal ligation, and ligation without revascularization. Although simply occluding the LSCA with the stent-graft is generally well tolerated, risks include back-bleeding and Type II endoleak formation as well as arm ischemia, which may be more prevalent than originally thought.[17,25] Type II endoleaks related to LSCA back-bleeding can be successfully treated with coil embolization. If upper extremity ischemia develops after LSCA coverage or ligation, then an LCCA-to-LSCA bypass can be performed through a lateral neck incision (Figure 42–2). Weigang et al. employ a selective approach to LSCA revascularization and advocate revascularizing

TABLE 42-2. REVIEW OF SELECTED REPORTS OF HYBRID ARCH REPAIRS

First Author, Year	Zone 0 or 1 Arch Patients n	Most Common Deployment	1- or 2-Stage Repair	Incision	TIA n (%)	Stroke n (%)	Early Death n (%)	Endovascular Complications
Buth, 1998[13]	1	Antegrade	1	Median sternotomy	0	0	0	None
Bergeron, 2005[31]	11	Retrograde	2	Transverse sternotomy	1 (9)	0	1 (9)	Guidewire perforated left ventricle, leading to death
Saleh, 2006[20]	15	Retrograde	2	Median sternotomy	0	0	0	None
Zhou, 2006[24]	16	Antegrade (8) or retrograde (8)	Both	Not specified	0	0	1 (6)	Anastomoses disturbed by delivery sheath, leading to bleeding and death
Melissano, 2007[18]	26	Retrograde	1	Not specified	—	2 (8)	2 (8)	1 unresolved Type Ia endoleak 2 ruptures resulting in late death
Szeto, 2007[21]	8	Retrograde	1	Median sternotomy	2 (25)	0	1 (13)	None
Chan, 2008[11]	16	Retrograde	1	Median sternotomy (Zone 0) 2 neck incisions with tunneling (Zone 1)	3 (19)	0	0	Type Ib endoleak treated with an additional distal stent-graft
Chen, 2008[15]	6	Retrograde	1	Partial sternotomy with neck incision near LSCA	0	0	0	None
Gottardi, 2008[16]	49	Retrograde	2	Median sternotomy (Zone 0) or upper hemisternotomy (Zone 1)	1 (2)	0	5 (10)	1 death before endovascular stage could be completed
Hughes, 2008[17]	7	Antegrade	1	Median sternotomy	—	0	0	1 case late type II endoleak from retrograde filling by LSCA
Riesenman, 2008[19]	25	Retrograde	Both	Median sternotomy	0	5 (20)	3 (12)	30-day endoleak present in 8 patients 5 type 1a 2 type II 1 type 1a/II combo Authors stated that these were related to incomplete ligations
Wang, 2008[22]	15	Retrograde	Both	Median sternotomy	1 (7)	0	1 (7)	The 1 death resulted from ballooning after a type I endoleak in a case of dissection
Wiegang, 2009[23]	26	Antegrade	1	Upper right L-shaped hemisternotomy	1 (4)	0	4 (15)	1 type II endoleak due to filling from a left vertebral artery arising off the aortic arch

Excludes isolated left subclavian artery (LSCA) bypasses, hybrid elephant trunk repairs, and hybrid prosthetic device implantations; n = number; TIA = transient ischemic attack

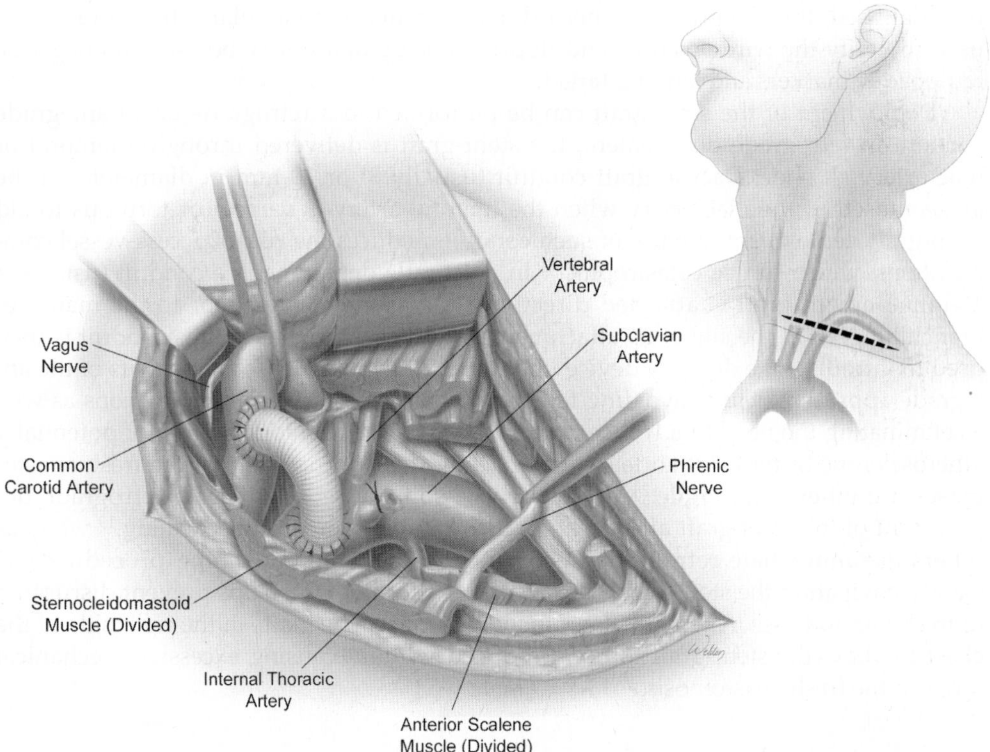

Figure 42-2. Left carotid–to–subclavian artery bypass is performed through a supraclavicular incision (inset). The subclavian artery is exposed by dividing the anterior scalene muscle while the overlying phrenic nerve is gently displaced with a vessel loop. (Used with permission of Elsevier: Bozinovski J, LeMaire SA, Weldon SA, et al. Hybrid repairs of the distal aortic arch and proximal descending thoracic aorta. Op Tech Thorac Cardiovasc Surg 2007;12:167–77.)

the LSCA in patients with the following situations: a dominant left vertebral artery, an incomplete circle of Willis, previous or pending coronary artery revascularization with the left internal thoracic artery; or left upper extremity arteriovenous fistula.[23] In contrast, Gottardi et al. routinely revascularize the LSCA as part of their standard repair protocol.[16]

A few additional technical considerations regarding arch-debranching procedures deserve mention. First, when there is an anomalous left vertebral artery arising from the arch, this artery may be divided at its origin and transposed onto another vessel to prevent the formation of an endoleak.[23,26] Second, although its use is not yet widespread, near-infrared spectroscopy can be used to monitor cerebral perfusion during debranching procedures to prevent brain ischemia.[27] Third, during full arch-debranching, some authors caution against merely ligating the relocated vessels and instead prefer to divide and oversew them to reduce endoleak risk.[19] Fourth, aortic banding can be used in hybrid arch repairs to establish an adequate "neck" and achieve a better seal with the endograft.[15,20,28-29]

The endovascular portion of the repair is performed with the patient under systemic heparinization and controlled hypotension. Adenosine-induced bradycardia and rapid cardiac pacing are two adjunctive techniques that can be used to facilitate precise deployment of the stent-graft.[29-30] In an effort to minimize the amount of contrast material used, transesophageal echocardiography and intravascular ultrasound can be used to verify the wire position, and fluoroscopic guidance may be used to image the radiopaque markers and landing target.

Deployment of the stent-graft can be performed in a retrograde or an antegrade fashion. In retrograde deployment, the stent-graft is delivered through a femoral or iliac artery. A short Dacron graft conduit (usually 8- or 10-mm in diameter) can be anastomosed to the iliac artery when the femoral artery is narrow or tortuous to aid stent-graft deployment; the use of such conduits reduces the risk of access-vessel complications, which can be catastrophic.[31] In antegrade deployment, a conduit (usually a 10-mm Dacron) graft is attached directly to the ascending aorta or to the main debranching graft at the site of its attachment to the ascending aorta; this conduit is then used to introduce the delivery device into the arch (Figure 42–3). The benefits of the antegrade approach include avoiding femoral or iliac access-vessel complications as well as eliminating the need to advance the stent-graft through a long section of potentially atherosclerotic or tortuous aorta. A drawback of this approach is that the fresh anastomoses are inherently fragile.[24] Consequently, some authors advocate retrograde deployment of the stent-graft after a short delay to allow for vascular healing,[19] whereas others use immediate retrograde deployment after the debranching procedure.[11,18] Gently navigating the stent-graft over a super-stiff guidewire helps prevent disruption of fresh anastomoses. Alternatively, a small incision can be made in the right side of the chest to allow the stent-graft to be introduced without causing excessive mechanical force on the fresh anastomosis.[23]

Hybrid Elephant Trunk Approach

Another Type of combined open and endovascular repair is the hybrid elephant trunk technique. The traditional open elephant trunk procedure is used to repair extensive aortic aneurysms and is performed in two stages. The first stage involves a full arch replacement that leaves a 10-cm "trunk" of Dacron graft hanging beyond the distal anastomosis into the proximal descending thoracic aorta. During the second-stage completion repair—which is usually performed several weeks later—the elephant trunk is used to facilitate the proximal anastomosis of a descending or thoracoabdominal aortic replacement procedure (Figure 42–4). In the hybrid approach to the elephant trunk procedure, the trunk is used as a proximal landing zone during an endovascular completion repair. Placing marker clips or a wire at the distal end of the elephant trunk during the first stage facilitates the placement of the stent-graft during the retrograde second procedure. The hybrid elephant trunk procedure may be performed immediately after the elephant trunk arch replacement, thus eliminating the risk of between-stage aneurysm rupture, which is usually fatal.

Outside the United States, some surgeons use a variation of this approach known as the frozen elephant trunk, which involves a hybrid prosthesis that is part Dacron graft and part stent-graft. The stent-graft end of the device is generally deployed through the open aortic arch into the proximal descending thoracic aorta under direct vision. The proximal Dacron end is then anastomosed to the ascending aortic graft used in the conventional open arch repair.[32-33]

Results

As shown in Table 42–2, outcomes from hybrid arch repair are generally quite good. In these small series of hybrid arch repairs (many of which were abstracted from larger series to focus on proximal arch repair), early mortality rates range from 0 to 15%, and stroke

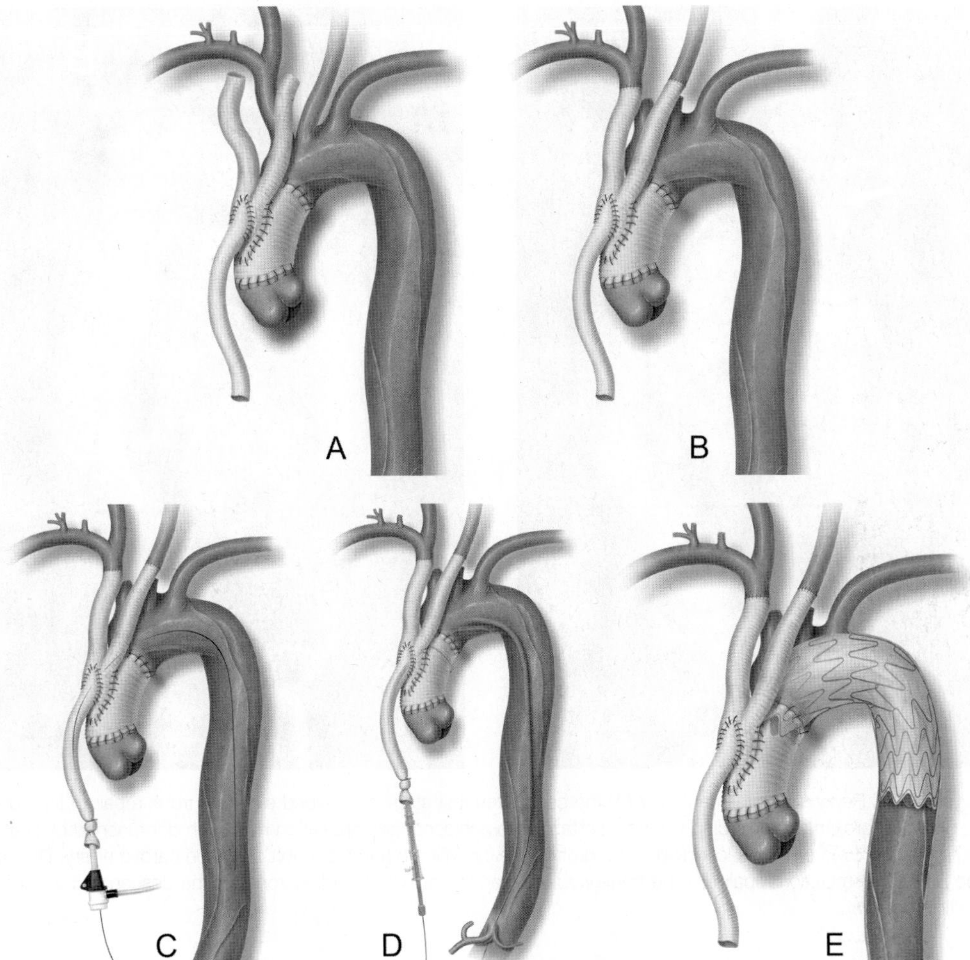

Figure 42-3. Illustration of an antegrade approach to a Zone 0 stent-graft deployment in a hybrid repair of aortic dissection. A. A 10-mm conduit has been attached to a bifurcated debranching graft, which has been anastomosed to the ascending aortic graft. B. The bifurcated graft is anastomosed to the left common carotid and innominate arteries. C. After a 9-Fr sheath is introduced into the conduit, D. the stent-graft is positioned and E. deployed in an antegrade fashion. Note that the proximal portion of the stent-graft lies within the ascending aortic graft. The delivery conduit is transected and oversewn to complete the repair. (Used with permission of Allen Press Publishing Services and Dr. Edward B. Diethrich: Diethrich EB, Ghazoul M, Wheatley GH III, et al. Great vessel transposition for antegrade delivery of the TAG endoprosthesis in the proximal aortic arch. J Endovasc Ther 2005;12:583–7; Diethrich EB, Ghazoul M, Wheatley GH III, et al. Surgical correction of ascending type A thoracic aortic dissection. J Endovasc Ther 2005;12:660–6.)

rates range from 0 to 20%[11,13,15,17,19,20,23]; several of the studies report no early death or stroke. Greenberg et al. reported a 2-year mortality rate of 16% after endovascular elephant trunk completion procedures.[34]

Complications resulting in death include between-stage rupture,[16] aneurysm rupture during balloon angioplasty treatment for endoleak,[22] acute kinking of the stent-graft,[35] stent-graft migration,[18,35] and perforation of the left ventricle by a guidewire.[31] Infrequent complications include sternal wound infection and dehiscence,[23] conversion to open surgery after stent-graft fracture and collapse,[18] bleeding from suture lines necessitating re-exploration,[11] postoperative local dissection,[16,31] spinal cord ischemia,[18-19]

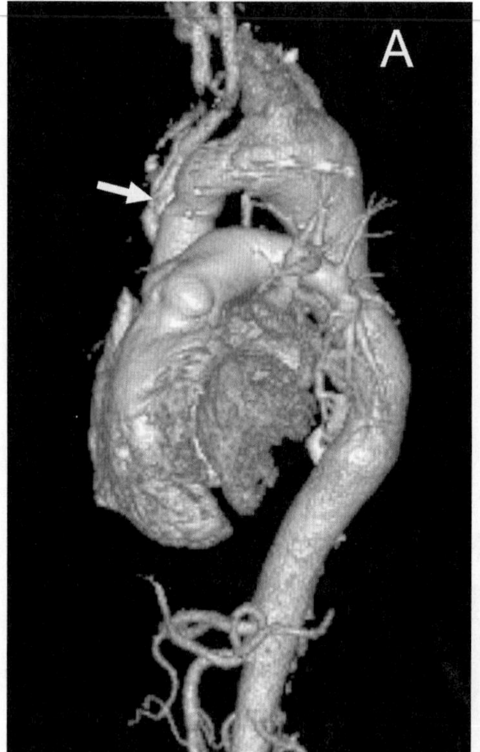

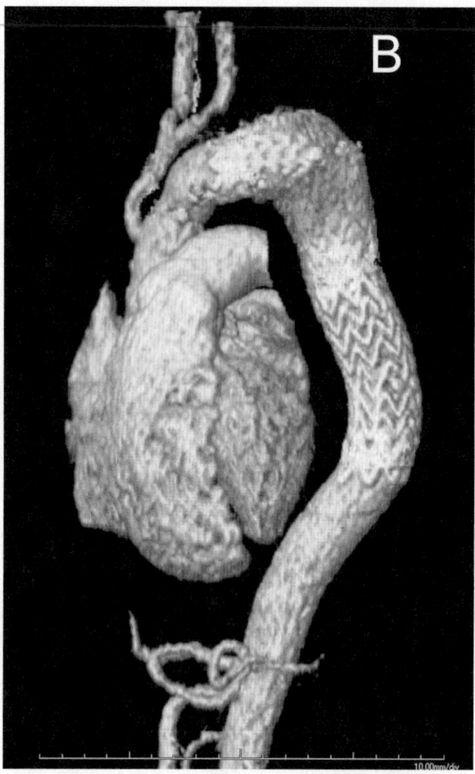

Figure 42-4. Reconstructive imaging of (A) the completed first stage of a hybrid elephant trunk repair of the aortic arch and proximal descending thoracic aorta. The brachiocephalic circulation has been debranched by placing a graft (arrow) from the ascending aortic graft to the innominate artery and left common carotid artery. During the Stage 2 completion repair (B), the trunk was used as the proximal landing zone for the descending thoracic aortic stent-graft.

and acute renal failure.[18,24,36] Erosion of the Dacron graft by the stent-graft is a rare complication after hybrid elephant trunk repairs.[37]

In our experience with nine hybrid arch repairs performed since November 2005, including one case with concomitant hybrid thoracoabdominal aortic aneurysm (TAAA) repair (Figure 42–5), many of the patients had chronic dissection and previous aortic repair. There were three early deaths (33%) and one perioperative stroke (11%). Although there were no early endoleaks in the six survivors, both Type I and Type II endoleaks developed in one survivor almost 2 years postoperatively; these endoleaks were treated with a secondary stent-graft procedure and coil embolization, respectively.

We have performed 14 hybrid elephant trunk procedures since February 2006, with 1 early death (7%). Although there were no cases of paraplegia, there was 1 case of stroke (7%) and 1 of renal failure (7%). Early endoleak occurred in 4 cases (3 Type II endoleaks and 1 Type IV endoleak). The Type II endoleaks necessitated conversion to open repair in the first case, a secondary intervention with coil embolization and deployment of a Palmaz stent in the second case, and observation only in the third case. The patient with the Type IV endoleak underwent a secondary stent-graft placement 4 months later. There were 2 late deaths, at 24 and 27 months postoperatively.

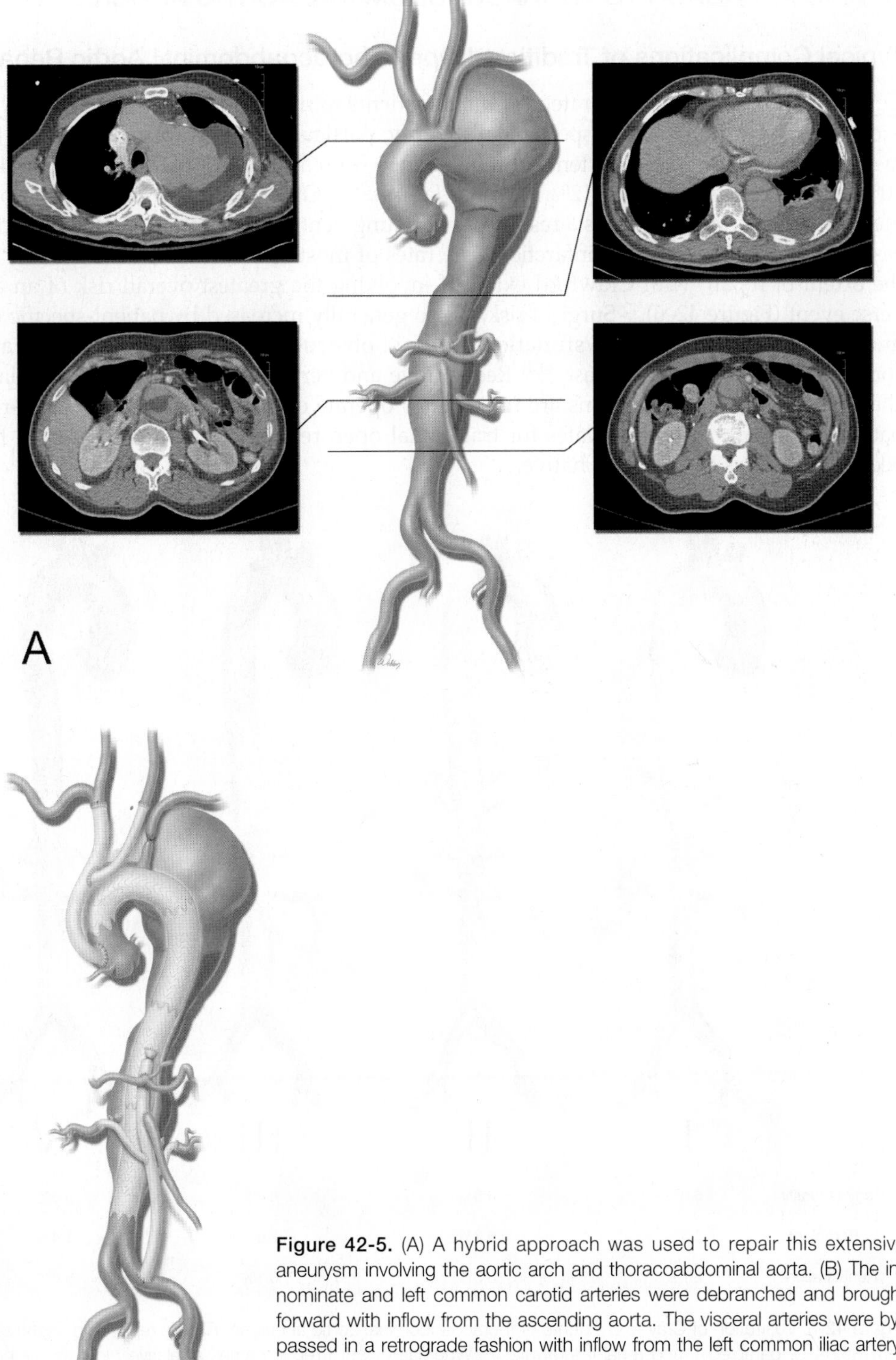

Figure 42-5. (A) A hybrid approach was used to repair this extensive aneurysm involving the aortic arch and thoracoabdominal aorta. (B) The innominate and left common carotid arteries were debranched and brought forward with inflow from the ascending aorta. The visceral arteries were bypassed in a retrograde fashion with inflow from the left common iliac artery. Four stent-grafts were deployed to exclude an extensive aneurysm and cover nearly the entire aorta.

HYBRID APPROACH TO THORACOABDOMINAL AORTIC REPAIR

Typical Complications of Traditional Open Thoracoabdominal Aortic Repair

Contemporary management strategies enable patients to undergo open TAAA repair with excellent early survival and respectable morbidity, particularly in experienced centers; the overall primary risks for all extents of repair range from 5 to 12% for early mortality, 4 to 10% for paraplegia, and 4 to 12% for renal failure.[38-40] Other complications include pulmonary dysfunction (largely as a result of single-lung ventilation and preexisting lung disease), stroke, and myocardial infarction. The rates of most complications differ greatly by the extent of repair, with Crawford extent II involving the greatest overall risk of an adverse event (Figure 42–6).[40] Surgical risk is also generally increased by patient-specific comorbidities such as renal dysfunction, chronic obstructive pulmonary disease, and coronary artery occlusive disease.[39,41] Reoperative and very elderly patients are especially challenging, and many surgeons are reluctant to operate on them. In these very high-risk patients, who are poor candidates for traditional open repair, a combined approach has been suggested as a viable alternative.

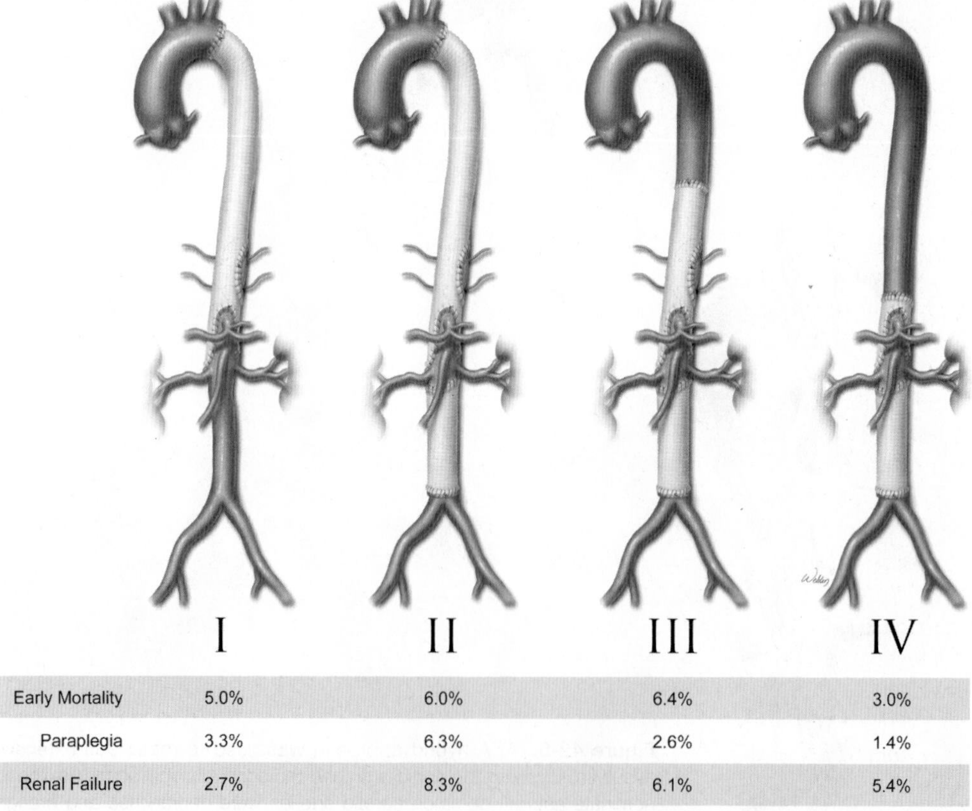

	I	II	III	IV
Early Mortality	5.0%	6.0%	6.4%	3.0%
Paraplegia	3.3%	6.3%	2.6%	1.4%
Renal Failure	2.7%	8.3%	6.1%	5.4%

Figure 42-6. Illustration of Crawford extents of thoracoabdominal aortic aneurysm (TAAA) repair and associated early mortality, paraplegia, and renal failure rates.[40] Whereas extent I repair carries a relatively low risk of both paraplegia and renal failure, extent II repair carries a much higher risk of paraplegia and renal failure. (Used with permission of Elsevier: Coselli JS, Bozinovski J, LeMaire SA. Open surgical repair of 2286 thoracoabdominal aortic aneurysms. Ann Thorac Surg 2007;83:S862–4.)

Debranching to Enable Coverage of the Visceral Artery Origins

Hybrid thoracoabdominal aortic repair involves rerouting some or all of the visceral arteries (i.e., the celiac axis, superior mesenteric, and renal arteries), such that blood flow to the viscera is not interrupted by subsequent stent-graft exclusion of the TAAA. Complexity of repair increases when longer lengths of the aorta are covered and greater numbers of vessels require debranching. In 1998, the first hybrid TAAA repair was performed by Quinones-Baldrich et al.[42] in a patient with an extent IV TAAA. They performed open extra-anatomic bypasses to the renal, superior mesenteric, and celiac arteries, followed by endovascular exclusion of the aneurysm. Since then, several small series and case reports have been published; a summary of selected studies is presented in Table 42–3.[17,24,43-52]

Advantages of the hybrid TAAA approach include the avoidance of aortic cross-clamping and single-lung ventilation as well as the reduction of visceral ischemia times, which may benefit patients with cardiopulmonary comorbidities, prevent reperfusion injury, and protect against associated complications such as renal dysfunction and cardiac strain. Many groups use cerebrospinal fluid drainage during hybrid TAAA repairs to reduce the risk of paraplegia.[36,46,53] Although renal ischemic times are shorter than those required by open TAAA repairs, renal injury may be exacerbated by the large amounts of contrast media that are generally necessary to obtain the detailed images needed to plan and conduct the repair. Some centers use cold crystalloid renal perfusion during renal artery clamping to protect against renal dysfunction.[46]

Although a less extensive incision is used (as compared with that used in standard open repair), exposure for TAAA debranching usually requires substantial retroperitoneal or transperitoneal exposure.[17] However, there are a few reports of minimally invasive laparoscopic or laparorobotic hybrid TAAA procedures,[54-55] and these approaches may gain appeal.

There are many ways in which visceral-vessel debranching procedures can vary, including the Type of inflow, the Type of debranching graft used, and the approach to selecting and bypassing target arteries. Inflow can be provided from an antegrade source (e.g., proximal aortic segments) or a retrograde one (e.g., an iliac artery) and can be established by creating one or multiple proximal anastomoses (Figure 42–7).[24,46] The approach to rerouting the visceral circulation is extensively tailored to the individual patient and may include both antegrade and retrograde bypasses within the same repair.[56] The inflow origin should be selected such that it is not compromised during or after stent-graft deployment and is relatively free of disease such as atherosclerosis or heavy calcification. The inflow anastomosis is usually end-to-side.

There are several potential configurations for visceral debranching grafts. Options include the "Lazy C" as popularized by Black,[44] inverted bifurcated grafts,[48] Y grafts as preferred by Chiesa,[46] and any number of custom grafts.[17,57-58] Most often, 8- or 10-mm Dacron or polytetrafluoroethylene (PTFE) grafts are used for the bypasses, but occasionally a saphenous or deep vein graft may be incorporated into the repair or a vessel may be transposed.[52,59-61] Uncommon strategies for visceral debranching have included using an "octopus" graft from the ascending aorta to revascularize the visceral arteries because of diseased iliac arteries,[62] using a pedicled right iliac artery with a saphenous vein graft to revascularize the superior mesenteric and common hepatic arteries,[60] and reimplanting the visceral arteries as a patch on a short section of a 20-mm Dacron tube graft.[63] Additional options include a newly developed, commercially available branched graft (designed to reroute the arch vessels) that has been modified by

TABLE 42-3. SELECT SERIES OF CONTEMPORARY HYBRID TAAA REPAIRS

First Author, Year	Hybrid TAAA Patients n	1- or 2-Stage Repair	Extent of Repair	Early Endoleak n (%)	Paraplegia n (%)	Renal Dysfunction n (%)	Early Death n (%)	Comment
Black, 2006[44]	29	1	I-IV	11 (38)	0	4 (14)	7 (24)	Procedure was abandoned in 3 patients, 1 of whom had rupture on postoperative day 10
Resch, 2006[51]	13	Both	II, III, IV	8 (62)	2 (15)	2 (15)	3 (23)	1 patient had between-stage rupture that resulted in early death
Zhou, 2006[24]	15	Both	I, III, IV	NR	0	2 (13)	0	2 patients (33) had renal artery thrombosis that necessitated hemodialysis
Chiesa, 2007[46]	13	1	I, II, IV, VAP	0	1 (8)	2 (15)	3 (23)	Early deaths were related to respiratory failure, coagulopathy, and pancreatitis
Donas, 2007[47]	8	Both	I, II, IV, V	NR	0	1 (13)	1 (13)	1 patient (13) had mesenteric bypass occlusion that later necessitated reoperation
Gawenda, 2007[48]	6	1	II, III, IV	0	0	0	0	2 patients (33) had renal artery thrombosis during follow-up period
Lee, 2007[49]	17	2	II, III, IV	1 (6)	0	1 (6)	4 (24)	A 17-year-old patient was later suspected of having a connective tissue disorder after an additional aneurysm developed All early deaths occurred after the debranching procedure
Böckler, 2008[50]	28	Both	I-IV	5 (18)	4 (14)	8 (29)	4 (14)	3 patients (11) had peripheral graft occlusion within 30 days of procedure
Hughes, 2008[17]	6	1	II, V, VAP	0	0	0	0	2 patients (33) needed renal dialysis preoperatively
Siegenthaler, 2008[52]	10	Both	I-IV	0	0	NR	1 (10)	5 cases (50) were selective revascularizations of celiac axis after coverage during the endovascular repair
Aguiar Lucas, 2009[43]	10	Both	IV, V	0	0	2 (20)	1 (10)	1 patient died 3 months postoperatively due to an infected graft
Quinones-Baldrich, 2009[50]	15	Both	I-IV	4 (27)	1 (7)	1 (7)	0	2 patients (13) had small bowel obstruction that necessitated reoperation

n = number; NR = not reported; TAAA = thoracoabdominal aortic aneurysm; VAP = visceral artery patch.

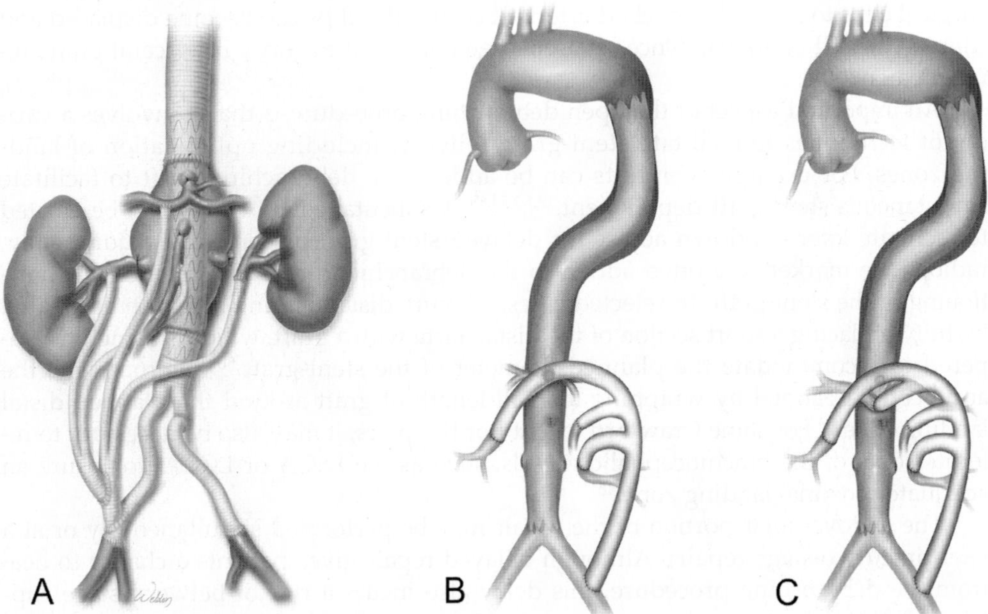

Figure 42-7. Options for visceral debranching by using retrograde inflow from the common iliac artery include (A) using a homemade graft attached end-to-end to the left renal artery and end-to-side to the remaining visceral arteries; and using commercially available custom-fabricated grafts attached end-to-side (B) or end-to-end (C) to the celiac axis and end-to-end to the remaining visceral arteries. (Used with permission of Elsevier: Zhou W, Reardon M, Peden EK, et al. Hybrid approach to complex thoracic aortic aneurysms in high-risk patients: surgical challenges and clinical outcomes. J Vasc Surg 2006;44:688–693), and Dr. Chad Hughes (Hughes GC, Nienaber JJ, Bush EL, et al. Use of custom Dacron branch grafts for "hybrid" aortic debranching during endovascular repair of thoracic and thoracoabdominal aortic aneurysms. J Thorac Cardiovasc Surg. 2008;136:21–28).

lengthening one branch so that the conduit can be used to bypass the celiac axis[57] and a commercially available custom-fabricated branched graft that has side branches for each of the visceral arteries and a conduit for subsequent endovascular deployment.[17]

The selection of target vessels for debranching is also highly variable. One highly controversial topic is how to manage the celiac axis. Several authors state that the celiac axis can be safely occluded, provided that there is sufficient collateral circulation, as can be demonstrated by a balloon occlusion test or, theoretically, by a gastric pH calculation.[64-65] However, others conclude that a balloon occlusion test does not guarantee that the celiac axis can be safely occluded, and they report numerous complications associated with not revascularizing the celiac axis, such as foregut ischemia, choledocholithiasis, and endoleak.[66] Still others suggest taking a minimal approach to repair whenever possible, and they freely occlude the celiac axis if no additional visceral rerouting is required, despite the risk of late reintervention for Type I endoleak; they then selectively revascularize as needed.[52] In some patients, it is necessary to reroute the inferior mesenteric artery.[52,61] The visceral vessels are typically debranched sequentially to minimize the duration of end-organ ischemia. Although the distal anastomoses are most often created in an end-to-end fashion, end-to-side anastomoses can be useful in some graft configurations.[17] After the target artery is bypassed, the proximal aspect of the artery is ligated. Black et al.[44] have cautioned against using surgical clips to ligate debranched arteries because the clips can become displaced and cause a Type II endoleak. Once revascularized, the vast majority of visceral grafts remain patent.[67]

An important aspect of the open debranching procedure is that it involves a variety of techniques to facilitate stent-graft delivery, including optimization of landing zones. For example, conduits can be added to a debranching graft to facilitate simultaneous stent-graft deployment.[17,50,58,68] A subcutaneous conduit can be created to facilitate later cut-down access for delayed stent-graft placement.[53] Additionally, radiopaque markers are often added to the debranching graft to facilitate later positioning of the stent-graft. In selected cases, a secure distal landing zone can be created by fully replacing a short section of the distal aorta with a graft, which is sometimes tapered to accommodate the planned diameter of the stent-graft.[50] Alternatively, the aorta can be banded by wrapping a small length of graft around the planned distal landing zone.[69] For some Crawford extent I or II repairs, it may also be necessary to relocate some of the brachiocephalic vessels, such as the LSCA or LCCA, to ensure an adequate proximal landing zone.[48]

The endovascular portion of the repair may be performed simultaneously or at a later time (two-stage repair). Although delayed repair gives patients a chance to heal from the debranching procedure, this delay also incurs a risk of between-stage rupture.[45,49-50] Rarely, the endovascular stage of repair precedes the debranching procedures, as in the case of an emergent repair.[47] Endovascular deployment, with or without a facilitating conduit, is most commonly performed retrograde (i.e., through the femoral or iliac arteries) but may be performed in an antegrade manner (e.g., through the common carotid arteries), especially if the femoral or iliac arteries are heavily calcified or tortuous.[47,63] In hybrid repairs, a simple "tube" graft is most commonly used, although a bifurcated module may be added distally.[49,59,70] The endograft is deployed as it is in thoracic endovascular aortic repair (TEVAR), with at least a 2-cm section of normal aorta for the proximal and distal landing zones. Commonly, more than one stent-graft is used because the length of aorta to be covered in a TAAA hybrid repair tends to be much greater than that covered in TEVAR; sequential stent grafts generally overlap by at least 5 cm.

Results

The technical success of endovascular deployment during hybrid TAAA repairs ranges from 70% up to 100%.[44-45,49,67] Clinical outcomes from select series of hybrid TAAA repairs are presented in Table 42–3, with early mortality rates ranging from 0 to 24%, paraplegia rates ranging from 0 to 15%, and renal dysfunction rates ranging from 0 to 29%. In a systematic review of 13 series with 58 patients, Donas et al.[67] found that elective and urgent repairs were associated with a mortality rate of 11%, no cases of paraplegia, a renal dysfunction rate of 9%, and an overall endoleak rate of 21%. Pre-existing morbidities clearly affect outcomes after hybrid TAAA repair, much as they influence traditional open TAAA repair.[49] For example, Böckler et al.[45] identified chronic obstructive pulmonary disease as an independent predictive risk factor for mortality in hybrid TAAA repairs.

Paraplegia and paraparesis remain poorly understood in hybrid TAAA repair. Reported cases are presented in Table 42–4. The extent of repair (i.e., the amount of aorta covered by the stent-graft) affects the likelihood of paraplegia, as does postoperative hypotension, which has been associated with several cases of delayed deficits.[17,45,50-53,62,68,71] Other complications include ischemic bowel,[52] myocardial infarction,[47]

TABLE 42-4. REVIEW OF SPINAL CORD ISCHEMIA IN HYBRID TAAA REPAIR

First Author, Year	Hybrid TAAA n	Paraplegia	Paraparesis	Prophylactic CSF Drain	CSF Drain Placed after Deficit	Reported Hypotension	Disease	Staged Repair	Comment
Resch, 2006[51]	13	2 (15%)	2 (15%)	Yes	No	Yes	Extent II and III	NR	Death in 2 with paraplegia and 1 with paraparesis Resolved at 12 months in the remaining patient
Chiesa, 2007[46]	13	1 (8%)	0	Only in I and II	Yes	No	VAP	No	Onset delayed 2 days Resolved after CSF drain placed
Lawlor, 2007[68]	2	1 (50%)	0	Yes	No	No	Extent I aneurysm with infrarenal aneurysm	No	Onset delayed 24 hours Persisted at 8 weeks with significant motor deficit
Torsello, 2007[62]	1	0	1 (100%)	No	Yes	No	Extent II aneurysm with dissection	Yes	Onset delayed 24 hours Resolved after 3 days of CSF drainage
Ballard, 2008[53]	4	0	2 (50%)	Yes	No	No	Type II dissection Extent II aneurysm	Yes	Persisted at 12 months in dissection patient Resolved at 3 months in aneurysm patient
Böckler, 2008[45]	28	4 (14%)	0	NR	NR	Yes	NR	NR	Persisted at publication in 3 patients Resolved in 1 patient Moved toward staged repair to reduce risk of paraplegia
Hughes, 2008[17]	6	0	1 (17%)	Yes	Yes	No	Extent II	No	Onset after CSF drain clamped Resolved after additional drainage
Siegenthaler, 2008[52]	13	0	1 (8%)	Yes	No	Yes	NR	NR	Onset delayed 3 weeks Resolved with discontinuation of antihypertensive medications Ambulation recovered Mild unilateral deficit persisted at publication Also used evoked potentials as protective measure
Tshomba, 2008[71]	7	1 (14%)	0	No	Yes	No	VAP	No	Onset delayed 2 days Resolved after CSF drainage
Quinones-Baldrich, 2009[50]	15	1 (7%)	0	Yes	No	Yes	Extent III	No	Onset delayed 24 hours Fatal MI 6 months postoperatively

CSF = cerebrospinal fluid; MI = myocardial infarction; NR = not reported; VAP = visceral artery patch; TAAA = thoracoabdominal aortic aneurysm; n = number.

stroke,[52] pancreatic fistula leading to late death,[51] interim rupture,[49,51] renal failure,[45] prolonged ileus,[24] and infection.[43,49,52] The risk of endoleak is not insignificant for hybrid TAAA procedures. Patent intercostal and lumbar arteries covered by the stent-graft may back-bleed, causing a Type II endoleak; such bleeding near a landing zone can compromise the seal, leading to a Type I endoleak. Reintervention for endoleak is not uncommon and usually involves performing a secondary endovascular procedure to insert additional devices, using balloon dilation to achieve a better seal or using coil embolization.

Our experience with TAAA hybrid repair involves four patients who underwent these procedures since February 2007. As previously mentioned, one of these patients also underwent arch-vessel debranching (see Figure 42–5). All four patients required Crawford extent II repairs but had substantial comorbidities and were therefore not considered satisfactory candidates for open repair. Despite technically successful procedures (all aneurysms were excluded upon endograft deployment and no endoleaks occurred), clinical outcomes were disappointing. There were two early deaths, one case of paraplegia, and two late deaths that occurred on postoperative days 152 and 244.

CONCLUSIONS

These innovative approaches to treating complex aortic aneurysms offer several potential advantages over standard open repairs and purely endovascular repairs. For example, compared with standard open surgical repair, a hybrid repair typically involves less blood loss, less transfused blood, fewer pulmonary complications, and shorter intensive care and hospital stays, and patients are more likely to be discharged home rather than to extended care. In theory, hybrid repairs also reduce the risk of Type 1 endoleak by increasing surgeons' ability to select appropriate landing zones that are well away from the aneurysmal aortic segment and critical branch arteries.

However, there may not be a benefit in terms of early mortality, spinal cord ischemia, or stroke. There is conflicting evidence regarding whether or not renal complications are reduced in endovascular repair, and although one could infer that the reduced amount of renal ischemia should be accompanied by a reduction in renal complications, this benefit may be offset by inflammatory processes, contrast administration, embolization, and other factors that adversely affect the kidneys.[72] Additionally, because hybrid approaches are relatively new, there are limited long-term data on their outcomes, although 10-year reports are now emerging.[50] Despite these current limitations, combined repair offers the opportunity to capitalize on the beneficial aspects of open and endovascular repair and thus maximize the benefit of repair for the individual patient. Importantly, hybrid repairs are extending the treatment options for high-risk patients who do not have adequate physiologic reserve to undergo traditional open repairs.

ACKNOWLEDGMENTS

The authors thank Scott A. Weldon, M.A., C.M.I., and Carol P. Larson, C.M.I., for creating the medical illustrations, and Stephen N. Palmer, Ph.D., E.L.S., for invaluable editorial support.

REFERENCES

1. Parodi JC, Palmaz JC, Barone HD. Transfemoral intraluminal graft implantation for abdominal aortic aneurysms. Ann Vasc Surg 1991;5:491–9.
2. Rodriguez JA, Olsen DM, Shtutman A, et al. Application of endograft to treat thoracic aortic pathologies: a single center experience. J Vasc Surg 2007;46:413–20.
3. Greenberg RK, Clair D, Srivastava S, et al. Should patients with challenging anatomy be offered endovascular aneurysm repair? J Vasc Surg 2003;38:990–6.
4. LeMaire SA. Combining open and endovascular approaches to complex aneurysms. Ann N Y Acad Sci 2006;1085:208–12.
5. Kamiya H, Hagl C, Kropivnitskaya I, et al. Quick proximal arch replacement with moderate hypothermic circulatory arrest. Ann Thorac Surg 2007;83:1055–8.
6. Kazui T, Bashar AH. Aortic arch replacement using a trifurcated graft. Ann Thorac Surg 2006;81:1552.
7. Suzuki K, Kazui T, Bashar AH, et al. Total aortic arch replacement in patients with arch vessel anomalies. Ann Thorac Surg 2006;81:2079–83.
8. Czerny M, Fleck T, Zimpfer D, et al. Risk factors of mortality and permanent neurologic injury in patients undergoing ascending aortic and arch repair. J Thorac Cardiovasc Surg 2003;126:1296–301.
9. Shah PJ, Estrera AL, Miller CC III, et al. Analysis of ascending and transverse aortic arch repair in octogenarians. Ann Thorac Surg 2008;86:774–9.
10. Criado FJ, Clark NS, Barnatan MF. Stent graft repair in the aortic arch and descending thoracic aorta: a 4-year experience. J Vasc Surg 2002;36:1121–8.
11. Chan YC, Cheng SW, Ting AC, et al. Supra-aortic hybrid endovascular procedures for complex thoracic aortic disease: single center early to midterm results. J Vasc Surg 2008;48: 571–9.
12. Diethrich EB, Ghazoul M, Wheatley GH III, et al. Great vessel transposition for antegrade delivery of the TAG endoprosthesis in the proximal aortic arch. J Endovasc Ther 2005; 12:583–7.
13. Buth J, Penn O, Tielbeek A, et al. Combined approach to stent-graft treatment of an aortic arch aneurysm. J Endovasc Surg 1998;5:329–32.
14. Kato M, Kaneko M, Kuratani T, et al. New operative method for distal aortic arch aneurysm: combined cervical branch bypass and endovascular stent-graft implantation. J Thorac Cardiovasc Surg 1999;117:832–4.
15. Chen IM, Wu FY, Shih CC. Banding technique for endovascular repair of arch aneurysm with unsuitable proximal landing zone. Circ J 2008;72:1981–5.
16. Gottardi R, Funovics M, Eggers N, et al. Supra-aortic transposition for combined vascular and endovascular repair of aortic arch pathology. Ann Thorac Surg 2008;86:1524–9.
17. Hughes GC, Nienaber JJ, Bush EL, et al. Use of custom Dacron branch grafts for "hybrid" aortic debranching during endovascular repair of thoracic and thoracoabdominal aortic aneurysms. J Thorac Cardiovasc Surg 2008;136:21–8, 28 e21–6.
18. Melissano G, Civilini E, Bertoglio L, et al. Results of endografting of the aortic arch in different landing zones. Eur J Vasc Endovasc Surg 2007;33:561–6.
19. Riesenman PJ, Tamaddon HS, Farber MA. Surgical bypass procedures to facilitate endovascular repair of aortic arch pathology. J Cardiovasc Surg (Torino) 2008;49:461–9.
20. Saleh HM, Inglese L. Combined surgical and endovascular treatment of aortic arch aneurysms. J Vasc Surg 2006;44:460–6.
21. Szeto WY, Bavaria JE, Bowen FW, et al. The hybrid total arch repair: brachiocephalic bypass and concomitant endovascular aortic arch stent graft placement. J Card Surg 2007;22: 97–102; discussion 103–4.
22. Wang S, Chang G, Li X, et al. Endovascular treatment of arch and proximal thoracic aortic lesions. J Vasc Surg 2008;48:64–8.
23. Weigang E, Parker J, Czerny M, et al. Endovascular aortic arch repair after aortic arch debranching. Ann Thorac Surg 2009;87:603–7.

24. Zhou W, Reardon M, Peden EK, et al. Hybrid approach to complex thoracic aortic aneurysms in high-risk patients: surgical challenges and clinical outcomes. J Vasc Surg 2006;44:688–93.
25. Reece TB, Gazoni LM, Cherry KJ, et al. Reevaluating the need for left subclavian artery revascularization with thoracic endovascular aortic repair. Ann Thorac Surg 2007;84: 1201–5; discussion 1205.
26. Gottardi R, Seitelberger R, Zimpfer D, et al. An alternative approach in treating an aortic arch aneurysm with an anatomic variant by supraaortic reconstruction and stent-graft placement. J Vasc Surg 2005;42:357–60.
27. Santo KC, Barrios A, Dandekar U, et al. Near-infrared spectroscopy: an important monitoring tool during hybrid aortic arch replacement. Anesth Analg 2008;107:793–6.
28. Antona C, Vanelli P, Petulla M, et al. Hybrid technique for total arch repair: aortic neck reshaping for endovascular-graft fixation. Ann Thorac Surg 2007;83:1158–61.
29. Bergeron P, Mangialardi N, Costa P, et al. Great vessel management for endovascular exclusion of aortic arch aneurysms and dissections. Eur J Vasc Endovasc Surg 2006;32:38–45.
30. Slovut DP, Sullivan TM. Combined endovascular and open revascularization. Ann Vasc Surg 2009;23:414–24.
31. Bergeron P, Coulon P, De Chaumaray T, et al. Great vessels transposition and aortic arch exclusion. J Cardiovasc Surg (Torino) 2005;46:141–7.
32. Di Bartolomeo R, Di Marco L, Armaro A, et al. Treatment of complex disease of the thoracic aorta: the frozen elephant trunk technique with the E-vita open prosthesis. Eur J Cardiothorac Surg 2009;35:671–5; discussion 675–6.
33. Karck M, Kamiya H. Progress of the treatment for extended aortic aneurysms: is the frozen elephant trunk technique the next standard in the treatment of complex aortic disease including the arch? Eur J Cardiothorac Surg 2008;33:1007–13.
34. Greenberg RK, Haddad F, Svensson L, et al. Hybrid approaches to thoracic aortic aneurysms: the role of endovascular elephant trunk completion. Circulation 2005;112:2619–26.
35. Palma JH, Guilhen JS, Gaia DF, et al. Early complication after hybrid thoracic aortic aneurysm repair. Interact CardioVasc Thorac Surg 2008;7:441–3.
36. Brueck M, Heidt MC, Szente-Varga M, et al. Hybrid treatment for complex aortic problems combining surgery and stenting in the integrated operating theater. J Interv Cardiol 2006;19:539–43.
37. Fehrenbacher JW, McCready RA. Erosion of elephant trunk Dacron graft limb by thoracic endograft causing acute aneurysm expansion. J Vasc Surg 2009;49:491–3.
38. Chiesa R, Melissano G, Civilini E, et al. Ten years experience of thoracic and thoracoabdominal aortic aneurysm surgical repair: lessons learned. Ann Vasc Surg 2004;18:514–20.
39. Conrad MF, Crawford RS, Davison JK, et al. Thoracoabdominal aneurysm repair: a 20-year perspective. Ann Thorac Surg 2007;83:S856–61; discussion S852–90.
40. Coselli JS, Bozinovski J, LeMaire SA. Open surgical repair of 2286 thoracoabdominal aortic aneurysms. Ann Thorac Surg 2007;83:S862–4.
41. LeMaire SA, Miller CC III, Conklin LD, et al. A new predictive model for adverse outcomes after elective thoracoabdominal aortic aneurysm repair. Ann Thorac Surg 2001;71:1233–8.
42. Quinones-Baldrich WJ, Panetta TF, Vescera CL, et al. Repair of type IV thoracoabdominal aneurysm with a combined endovascular and surgical approach. J Vasc Surg 1999;30: 555–60.
43. Aguiar Lucas L, Rodriguez-Lopez JA, Olsen DM, et al. Endovascular repair in the thoracic and abdominal aorta: no increased risk of spinal cord ischemia when both territories are treated. J Endovasc Ther 2009;16:189–96.
44. Black SA, Wolfe JH, Clark M, et al. Complex thoracoabdominal aortic aneurysms: endovascular exclusion with visceral revascularization. J Vasc Surg 2006;43:1081–9; discussion 1089.
45. Böckler D, Kotelis D, Geisbusch P, et al. Hybrid procedures for thoracoabdominal aortic aneurysms and chronic aortic dissections—a single center experience in 28 patients. J Vasc Surg 2008;47:724–32.

46. Chiesa R, Tshomba Y, Melissano G, et al. Hybrid approach to thoracoabdominal aortic aneurysms in patients with prior aortic surgery. J Vasc Surg 2007;45:1128–35.
47. Donas KP, Schulte S, Krause E, et al. Combined endovascular stent-graft repair and adjunctive visceral vessel reconstruction for complex thoracoabdominal aortic aneurysms. Int Angiol 2007;26:213–8.
48. Gawenda M, Aleksic M, Heckenkamp J, et al. Hybrid-procedures for the treatment of thoracoabdominal aortic aneurysms and dissections. Eur J Vasc Endovasc Surg 2007;33: 71–7.
49. Lee WA, Brown MP, Martin TD, et al. Early results after staged hybrid repair of thoracoabdominal aortic aneurysms. J Am Coll Surg 2007;205:420–31.
50. Quinones-Baldrich W, Jimenez JC, DeRubertis B, et al. Combined endovascular and surgical approach (CESA) to thoracoabdominal aortic pathology: a 10-year experience. J Vasc Surg 2009;49:1125–34.
51. Resch TA, Greenberg RK, Lyden SP, et al. Combined staged procedures for the treatment of thoracoabdominal aneurysms. J Endovasc Ther 2006;13:481–9.
52. Siegenthaler MP, Weigang E, Brehm K, et al. Endovascular treatment for thoracoabdominal aneurysms: outcomes and results. Eur J Cardiothorac Surg 2008;34:810–9.
53. Ballard JL, Razavi M, Harward TR, et al. Visceral/renal artery debranching for complex thoracoabdominal hybrid procedures via retroperitoneal abdominal aortic exposure: a preliminary report. Ann Vasc Surg 2008;22:173–8.
54. Bakoyiannis C, Cagiannos C, Wasilljew S, et al. Totally laparoscopic aortohepatic bypass for aortic debranching during endovascular thoracoabdominal aneurysm repair. Eur J Vasc Endovasc Surg 2007;34:173–5.
55. Wahlgren CM, Skelly C, Shalhav A, et al. Hybrid laparorobotic debranching and endovascular repair of thoracoabdominal aortic aneurysm. Ann Vasc Surg 2008;22:285–9.
56. Fulton JJ, Farber MA, Marston WA, et al. Endovascular stent-graft repair of pararenal and type IV thoracoabdominal aortic aneurysms with adjunctive visceral reconstruction. [erratum appears in J Vasc Surg 2005 May;41(5):906]. J Vasc Surg 2005;41:191–8.
57. Esposito G, Marullo AG, Pennetta AR, et al. Hybrid treatment of thoracoabdominal aortic aneurysms with the use of a new prosthesis. Ann Thorac Surg 2008;85:1443–5.
58. Kpodonu J, Shennib H, Wheatley GH III, et al. A novel technique of deployment of a thoracic endograft in the hybrid treatment of a patient with thoracoabdominal aneurysm. Ann Thorac Surg 2008;85:666–8.
59. Flye MW, Choi ET, Sanchez LA, et al. Retrograde visceral vessel revascularization followed by endovascular aneurysm exclusion as an alternative to open surgical repair of thoracoabdominal aortic aneurysm. J Vasc Surg 2004;39:454–8.
60. Iguro Y, Yotsumoto G, Ishizaki N, et al. Endovascular stent-graft repair for thoracoabdominal aneurysm after reconstruction of the superior mesenteric and celiac arteries. J Thorac Cardiovasc Surg 2003;125:956–8.
61. Murphy EH, Beck AW, Clagett GP, et al. Combined aortic debranching and thoracic endovascular aneurysm repair (TEVAR) effective but at a cost. Arch Surg 2009;144:222–7.
62. Torsello G, Can A, Umscheid T, et al. Hybrid thoracoabdominal aneurysm repair with simultaneous antegrade visceral revascularization and supra-aortic debranching from the ascending aorta. J Endovasc Ther 2007;14:342–6.
63. Murray D, Ghosh J, Khwaja N, et al. Staged open and endovascular repair of thoracoabdominal aneurysms using the common carotid artery. Ann Vasc Surg 2005;19:103–7.
64. Gawenda M, Brunkwall J. When is it safe to cover the left subclavian and celiac arteries. Part II: celiac artery. J Cardiovasc Surg (Torino) 2008;49:479–82.
65. Waldenberger P, Bendix N, Petersen J, et al. Clinical outcome of endovascular therapeutic occlusion of the celiac artery. J Vasc Surg 2007;46:655–61.
66. Leon LR Jr, Mills JL Sr, Jordan W, et al. The risks of celiac artery coverage during endoluminal repair of thoracic and thoracoabdominal aortic aneurysms. Vasc Endovasc Surg 2009;43:51–60.

67. Donas KP, Czerny M, Guber I, et al. Hybrid open-endovascular repair for thoracoabdominal aortic aneurysms: current status and level of evidence. Eur J Vasc Endovasc Surg 2007;34: 528–33.
68. Lawlor DK, Faizer R, Forbes TL. The hybrid aneurysm repair: extending the landing zone in the thoracoabdominal aorta. Ann Vasc Surg 2007;21:211–5.
69. Lawrence-Brown M, Sieunarine K, van Schie G, et al. Hybrid open-endoluminal technique for repair of thoracoabdominal aneurysm involving the celiac axis. J Endovasc Ther 2000;7:513–9.
70. Yoshida M, Mukohara N, Shida T, et al. Combined endovascular and surgical procedure for recurrent thoracoabdominal aortic aneurysm. Ann Thorac Surg 2006;82:1099–101.
71. Tshomba Y, Bertoglio L, Marone EM, et al. Visceral aortic patch aneurysm after thoracoabdominal aortic repair: conventional vs hybrid treatment. J Vasc Surg 2008;48:1083–91.
72. Chang CK, Chuter TA, Niemann CU, et al. Systemic inflammation, coagulopathy, and acute renal insufficiency following endovascular thoracoabdominal aortic aneurysm repair. J Vasc Surg 2009;49:1140–6.

43

Connective Tissue Disorders for the Vascular Surgeon

James H. Black III, M.D.

INTRODUCTION

Connective tissues serve as a framework or matrix to hold the cells and structures of our body together. The primary structural proteins of connective tissue are composed of collagen and elastin, which vary in type and amount within each of the body's tissues (Table 43–1). A connective tissue disorder is a disease in which the primary target is either collagen or elastin proteins. Whereas inflammation may affect these proteins and induce structural damage, such conditions often imply some element of autoimmunity and are termed collagen vascular diseases or mixed connective tissue diseases. Such conditions and arteritides related to the vascular tree quite often have weaker genetic factors that predispose to their development. Although clustering of aneurysms in multiply affected family members may indicate some element of an inheritance pattern, there are often greatly varying levels of expressivity and penetrance and no defined genetic test available to assist treatment. This chapter defines the common connective tissue disorders affecting the arterial tree that have a studied natural history, a defined basis for genetic inheritance, and sufficiently understood pathophysiologic mechanisms to guide treatment paradigms. These "heritable disorders of connective tissue"[1] have severe vascular manifestations and include most commonly Marfan syndrome (MFS), vascular type of Ehlers-Danlos syndrome (EDS IV), Loeys-Dietz syndrome (LDS), and familial thoracic aortic aneurysm and dissection (TAAD).

MARFAN SYNDROME

> "I present to the Society a little girl five and one-half years old, suffering from a congenital deformation of the four limbs, for which I have not found a precedent from the authors whom it was possible for me to consult."
>
> - A.B. Marfan, 1896[2]

TABLE 43-1. STRUCTURAL ELEMENTS OF BLOOD VESSELS

Structural proteins	Approximate Amount (% dry wt)	Function
Type I collagen	20-40	Fibrillar network
Type III collagen	20-40	Thin fibrils
Elastin, fibrillin	20-40	Elasticity
Type IV collagen, laminin	<5	Basal lamina
Types V and VI collagen	<2	Function unclear
Proteoglycans (>30 types)	<3	Resiliency

Antonin-Bernard Marfan was a Professor of Pediatrics in Paris, and the patient who so puzzled him was named Gabrielle. A follow-up of her initial report at age 11 revealed thoracolumbar kyphoscoliosis, pectus carinatum, and signs of tuberculosis.[3] Indeed, she would succumb to infection at age 16 and no autopsy was performed to document vascular involvement. The first description of aortic pathology in MFS was published a year after the death of Professor Marfan in 1943.[4] Whereas Marfan correctly identified the many mendelian features of the condition that would eventually bear his name, the pleiotropic disorder has benefited from decades of further description of clinical manifestations, molecular pathogenesis, and emerging therapeutic options.

Epidemiology and Natural History

The incidence of MFS is about 2 to 3 per 10,000 individuals, although this estimate relies on proper recognition of all affected and genetically predisposed individuals.[5] A population-based study in Scotland demonstrated the incidence at 1 in 9802 live births.[6] although this number would underestimate the true incidence, because features, particularly skeletal, of MFS become more apparent with growth. Furthermore, although the disorder is passed as a dominant mendelian trait, about 25% of cases are due to sporadic de novo mutations.[7] The disease has no gender predisposition, and the tall stature with long bone overgrowth (dolichostenomelia) leads to an increased incidence in athletes, particularly in those who play basketball and volleyball.

Life span of individuals affected with MFS was significantly shortened before the widespread and successful refinement of aortic root surgery. Before adoption of thresholds for aortic root replacement, the cause of death was cardiovascular (aortic rupture, dissection, or valvular) in 90% of cases.[8] A report in the 1970s on the life expectancy in MFS individuals described longevity as only two thirds that of unaffected individuals, with the life table mortality curves deviating in infancy.[8] However, a more recent assessment of longevity in MFS describes a near-normal life expectancy, indicating improvement and refinement in diagnosis and treatment of the many manifestations of the disorder.[9]

Pathogenesis

As early as 1955, it was suggested that the basic structural defect in MFS was localized to the elastic fiber,[10] with skin and aorta from patients showing decreased elastin content and fragmentation of elastic fibers.[11-12] Yet the elastin gene and molecule were poor targets to explain the clinical manifestations of MFS in tissues that are devoid of elastin, such as bone and the ciliary zonules in the eye. Further analysis demonstrated that the amorphous fragmented elastin tissues were surrounded by a rodlike material with a distinct staining pattern and distinguishable susceptibility to enzymatic digestion.[13] These so-called microfibrils are 10 to 14 nm in diameter and are constituents of all connective tissues. Fibrillin-1 (FBN1) was then identified as the principal component of the extracellular matrix microfibril, present in all tissues with the phenotypic manifestations of MFS.[13] Additional linkage analysis mapped the MFS locus to 15q21.1.[14] In 1991, Dietz et al. performed mutational analysis of FBN1 in patients with MFS and identified two unrelated patients with identical, denovo, missense mutations.[7] To date, all of the mutation analyses have identified the FBN1 gene as the sole locus for the classic MFS disorder, and most families have unique or private mutations. Neither the location of the mutation nor the type of amino acid altered is sufficient to predict phenotype, with the exception of mutations within exons 24-32 that are associated with a severe form of MFS diagnosed in early childhood.[15-16] The mutation is passed in an autosomal dominant manner with complete penetrance. Therefore, 50% of offspring of an affected individual can inherit a genetic predisposition to the disorder (Figure 43–1).[5]

The FBN1 gene contains 65 exons spanning 235kb of genomic DNA.[17-18] The gene encodes a 350-kDa glycoprotein that is highly conserved among different species.[18] Murine models of MFS have provided the opportunity to study the earliest pathogenetic abnormalities in elastogenesis and aortic aneurysm formation.[19-20] These models demonstrated that FBN1 molecules are not needed to assemble an elastic fiber; rather, microfibrils are required to maintain elastic fibers during postnatal life. If proper connections among elastic fibers and vascular smooth muscles cells are not maintained, then cells adopt matrix degrading enzymes such as matrix metalloproteinase 2 and 9. The cleavage point for these enzymes is in domain C (Figure 43–2). Thereafter, aortic wall homeostasis is perturbed; inflammation and elastic fiber calcification and structural weakening may ensue. This pathology has been observed in large muscular arteries from MFS patients.[21]

Recent discovery of the role of microfibrils in regulating cytokine has further advanced our understanding of the pathogenesis of MFS and raised the possibility of a

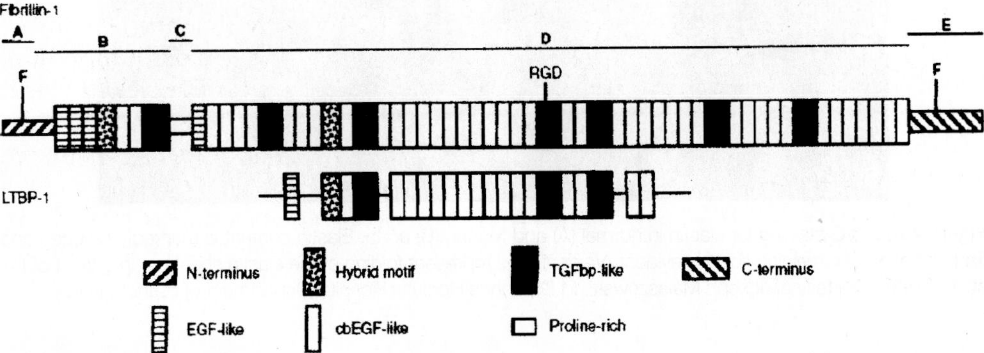

Figure 43-1. Domain organization of fibrillin-1 and LTBP-1 proteins. The bulk of the fibrillin-1 protein is contained in regions B and D. These regions have repetitive cysteine-rich domains, including those first identified with epidermal growth factor precursor (EGF-like) and latency-inducing transforming growth factor β-binding proteins (TGFbp-like). Protein structure is maintained in a "pleat" by disulfide bonds among cysteine residues and calcium binding to promote protein-protein interactions (cbEGF-like domain) in a rigid rodlike fashion.

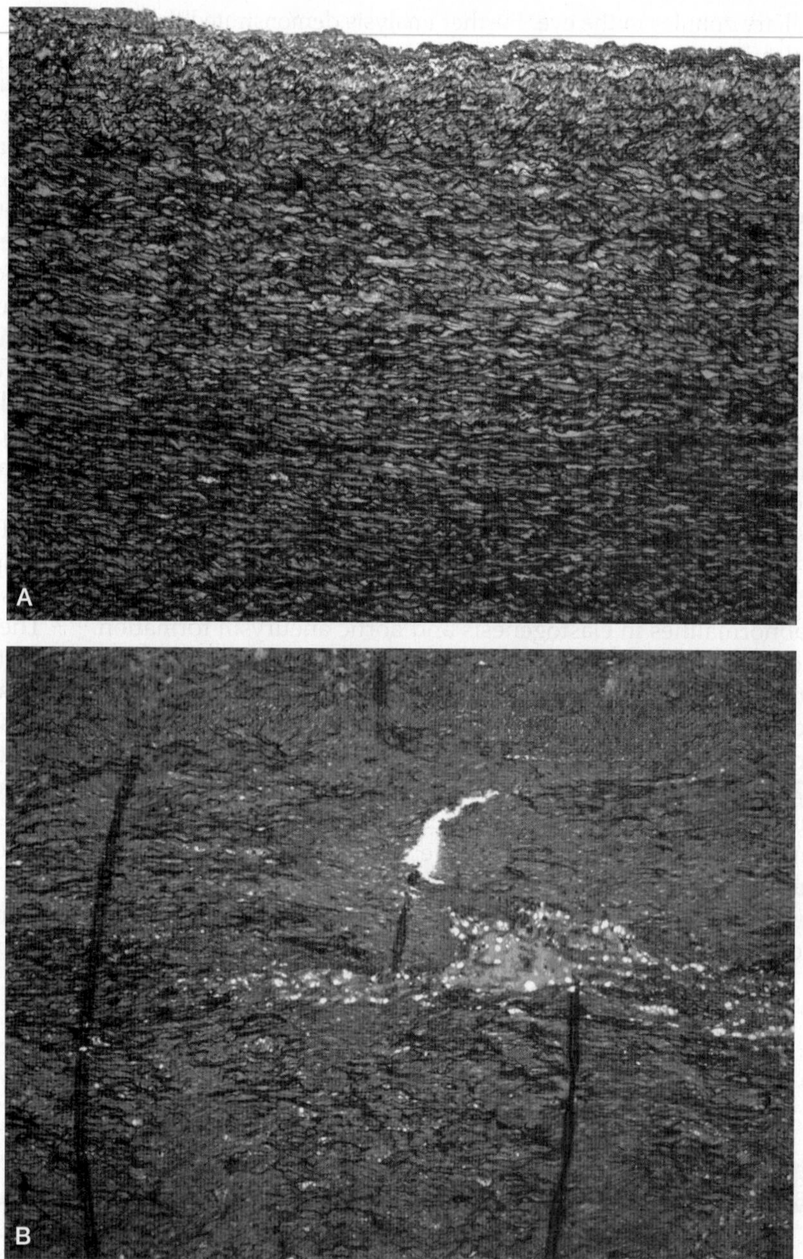

Figure 43-2. VVG staining for elastin in normal (A) and Marfan (B) aorta. Elastin content is markedly reduced and fragmentation of remaining fibrils is evident. Vertical lines represent folding of the elastin sheet as an artifact of fixation. (Plates courtesy of Joseph Maleszewski, M.D., Johns Hopkins Hospital Department of Pathology.)

new treatment paradigm. Fibrillin 1 shares a high degree of homology with the latent transforming growth factor β (TGF-β) binding proteins (see Figure 43–1). The TGF-β cytokines are secreted as large latent complexes consisting of TGF-β, a latency-associated peptide, and one of three latent TGF-β binding proteins.[22] On release, the large latent complex is sequestered within the extracellular matrix, and once the mature cytokine is released from the binding proteins, interactions with cell surface receptors and downstream signaling can occur. The homology between fibrillins and latent TGF-β binding proteins prompted the hypothesis that microfibrils may play a role in trafficking of TGF-β and its activation. Credence has been lent to this hypothesis with the demonstration of elevated TGF-β activity and free TGF-β levels in FBN1-deficient mice during developmental septation of the lung[23] and development of myxomatous cardiac valvular changes.[24] Furthermore, administration of TGF-β neutralizing antibody could rescue the phenotype.[23] This additional pathogenetic mechanism of dysregulated TGF-β activity seems more plausible to explain clinical features of MFS that are poorly reconciled with structural failure, such as long bone overgrowth, craniofacial abnormalities, and muscle hypoplasia.[24]

Clinical Manifestations and Diagnostic Evaluation

MFS is a multisystem disorder with manifestations principally within the cardiovascular, ocular, and skeletal systems. Diagnostic clinical criteria were outlined at the International Nosology of Heritable Connective Tissue Disorders of Connective Tissue Meeting in Berlin in 1986.[25] However, the recognition that many individuals diagnosed under these criteria did not have the FBN1 mutation (genetic testing became possible after 1986) carried in their more affected family members led to revision in 1996.[26] Termed the Ghent Criteria, greater emphasis was placed on diagnostic use of clinical findings and family history that are divided into major and minor criteria. A "major criterion" is one that carries high diagnostic specificity because it is so infrequent in the general population.[27] Once an individual is diagnosed with MFS, all first-degree relatives should be evaluated for the presence of the condition. In children, this may require repeated evaluations to avoid missing the disorder in evolution (Table 43–2).

The role of clinical genetic testing in establishing a diagnosis remains limited, because over 500 mutations have been found, and 90% of the mutations are private within a pedigree.[15] Even within families in which the same mutation is shared, phenotypic variation is prominent. Thus, exacting a genotype-phenotype correlation is difficult.[28] Furthermore, approximately 25% of patients with the disorder have a de novo mutation, limiting feasibility of a more focused analysis. In addition, it is estimated that 10% of the mutations in the FBN1 gene that cause MFS are missed by conventional screening methods.[29] At present, the diagnosis of MFS rests primarily on physical clinical assessment.

Differential Diagnosis

Other conditions are associated with FBN1 mutations and may be considered in the differential diagnosis of MFS. The MASS phenotype is based on the association of **m**itral valve prolapse, myopia, mild **a**ortic root dilation, **s**triae, and mild **s**keletal changes.[30] The skeletal features of MASS often include the mild manifestations of tall stature, mild dolichostenomelia (long bone growth), and scoliosis. Occasionally, a major Ghent criteria may be met from the skeletal system, but no other major criteria are noted. For patients with MASS, mutations in the FBN1 gene have generally created premature termination codons and the mutant transcript can be easily and rapidly degraded. Congenital contractural arachnodactyly shares many skeletal features with MFS, but no ocular and cardiovascular manifestations are present. The mutation in the few patients in the literature is located in the fibrillin-2 gene,[31] and physical therapy is key to maintain joint range of motion. The overlap of LDS and MFS are considered later in this chapter.

TABLE 43-2. GHENT CRITERIA FOR DIAGNOSIS OF MARFAN SYNDROME

Index Case

- If the family/genetic history is not contributory, major criteria in two or more different organ systems and involvement of a third organ system are required.
- If a genetic mutation known to cause Marfan syndrome in others is identified, one major criterion in an organ system and involvement of a second organ system are required.

Relative of an Index Case Who Has Met Criteria for Diagnosis

- With the presence of a major criterion in the family history, one major criterion in an organ system and involvement of a second organ system are required.

Genetic/Family History

Major criteria (any one of the following)

- Having a parent, child, sibling who meets these diagnostic criteria independently
- Presence of a mutation in FBN1 which is known to cause Marfan syndrome
- Presence of haplotype around FBN1, inherited by descent, known to be associated with unequivocally diagnosed Marfan syndrome in the family

Minor criterion

- None

Organ Systems

CARDIOVASCULAR

Major criteria (either)

- Dilation of the ascending aorta, with or without aortic regurgitation and involving at least the sinuses of Valsalva.
- Dissection of the ascending aorta.

Minor criteria (only one need be present)

- Mitral valve prolapse with or without mitral valve regurgitation
- Dilation of the main pulmonary artery in the absence of valvular or peripheral pulmonic stenosis, younger than 40 years old
- Calcification of the mitral annulus, younger than 40 years old
- Dilation or dissection of the descending thoracic or abdominal aorta, younger than 50 years old

For involvement of the cardiovascular system, only one of the minor criteria must be present.

SKELETAL

Major criteria (at least four of the following constitute major criteria in the skeletal system)

- Pectus carinatum
- Pectus excavatum, requiring surgery
- Reduced upper segment to lower segment ratio or arm span to height ratio >1.05
- Wrist and thumb signs (wrist: ability to overlap fifth finger and thumb around wrist, thumb: thumb extends across ulnar border of hand when folded inward)
- Scoliosis of >20 degrees or spondylolithesis
- Reduced extension at the elbows (<170 degrees)
- Medial displacement of the medial mallelolus, causing pes planus (flat feet)
- Protrusion acetabuli (medial socket wall protrudes/bows into ring of pelvis)

(Continued)

TABLE 43-2. ***(Continued)***

Minor criteria
- Pectus excavatum of moderate severity
- Joint hypermobility
- High arched palate with dental crowding
- Facial appearance (dolichocephaly: long and narrow face, malar hypoplasia, enopthalmos, retrognathia, down-slanting palpebral features)

For involvement of the skeletal system, at least two features contributing to major criteria or one feature from the list contributing to the major criterion and two minor criteria must be present.

OCULAR SYSTEM

Major criterion
- Ectopia lentis (lens dislocation)

Minor criteria
- Abnormally flat cornea
- Increased globe length
- Hypoplastic iris or ciliary muscle causing decreased miosis (leading to near sightedness)

For involvement of the ocular system, at least two minor criteria must be present.

PULMONARY SYSTEM

Major criterion
- None

Minor criteria
- Spontaneous pneumothorax
- Apical blebs

For involvement of the pulmonary system, only one minor criterion must be present.

SKIN AND INTEGUMENT

Major criterion
- None

Minor criteria
- Striae atrophicae (stretch marks) without marked weight gain, pregnancy, or repetitive stress)
- Recurrent hernia

For involvement of the skin and integument, only one minor criterion must be present.

DURA

Major criterion
- Lumbosacral dural ectasia

Minor criterion
- None

Surveillance

MFS is a pleiotropic disorder and surveillance of the many systems at risk for abnormality is prudent. The cardinal manifestations are ocular, skeletal, and cardiovascular. Regular slit-lamp examinations by an ophthalmologist, a cardiologist for imaging of the aortic root, and an orthopedist for development of scoliosis should be performed on an annual basis. In this section, the focus is placed on aortic and vascular pathology. For recommendations in regard to the other body systems, the readers may find useful information at the National Marfan Foundation Website (www.marfan.org). The clinical manifestations within the cardiovascular system that require attention are the atrioventricular valves, annuloaortic valve mechanism, and the aortic root and ascending aorta.

Thickening of the atrioventricular valves is very common and is often associated with mitral or tricuspid valve prolapse.[5] In about 25% of patients, the mitral valve prolapse may progress to severe mitral regurgitation[32]. Mitral regurgitation is the most common indication for cardiac surgery in infants and children with the disorder.[32] Children with early onset of MFS may develop congestive heart failure, pulmonary hypertension, and death due to this mitral insufficiency, and this is the leading cause of morbidity and mortality in young children with the disorder.[32] Interestingly, twice as many women have progression of their mitral valve prolapse to severe regurgitation as men.[32] Calcification of the mitral annulus in individuals younger than 40 years constitutes a minor criterion in the cardiovascular system.

Aortic valve dysfunction likely represents a late event in the continuum of annuloaortic ectasia due to root degeneration. The aortic valve, like the mitral, may also develop calcification at an early age.[32] Dilated cardiomyopathy, beyond explanation by associated valvular incompetence, is also seen in MFS. The mutant FBN1 protein in the cardiac ventricles has been implicated, but overall, the rates of cardiomyopathy are low. In a study of 234 patients with MFS without significant aortic or atrioventricular valvular disease, 17 patients (8%) had left ventricular enlargement, but none had an ejection fraction of less than 25%.[33]

Aortic aneurysm and dissection are the most life-threatening manifestations of MFS. The threat is age-dependent, and dilation at the sinuses of Valsalva can begin in utero; thus life-long transthoracic echocardiography is needed. For patients with poor visualization of the aortic root and ascending aorta due to anterior chest deformity, CTA or magnetic resonance angiography (MRA) (to avoid radiation exposure) is a viable substitute. In contrast to degenerative aneurysm, the dilation may be confined to only the aortic root and not the ascending aorta. Normal aortic dimensions can vary widely with both age and size, and proper interpretation in patients affected by MFS requires age-dependent nomograms.[34] Surgical repair of the aortic root and ascending aorta is recommended when its greatest diameter exceeds 50 mm in adults.[35] Earlier intervention may be warranted with a family history of early dissection. Thresholds for replacement of the aortic root in children are not established given the observation that dissection is very rare in the young.[5] However, if the aortic root is noted to grow >1 cm over consecutive annual assessment, or if significant aortic regurgitation is present, early surgery may be necessary.[27]

Lifestyle modifications are routinely recommended to patients once the diagnosis of MFS is established. On the basis of data from the United States, genetic cardiovascular diseases account for 40% of deaths in young athletes.[36-37] A recent consensus document cited that "burst" exertion such as sprinting, weight-lifting, basketball, and soccer should generally be avoided. Favored are recreational sports in which energy expenditure is stable and consistent over long periods of time, such as informal jogging, biking, and lap swimming.[38] Symptoms potentially referable to a cardiovascular cause, such as shortness of breath, presyncope, and chest discomfort, should prompt immediate withdrawal from activity and evaluation. Recent litigation suggests physician reliance on consensus statements to determine medically reasonable levels of activity in patients with cardiovascular abnormalities as appropriate.[39]

Medical Treatment

Medical treatment with β-adrenergic receptor blockade to delay aortic root growth or prevent aortic dissection in MFS is currently considered a standard of care.[27] General recommendations are for resting heart rate <70 bpm and submaximal exercise <100 bpm. The rationale for this treatment paradigm is focused on decreasing proximal aortic shear stress and dp/dT. The only randomized trial assessing the effect of beta blockade studied 70 patients of whom 32 received propanolol.[40] Treated patients were titrated using an open-label approach to keep HR 100 bpm during exercise or resulting in a 30% rise in systolic time interval. Serial echocardiograms were performed and accounted for by age, height, and weight over a mean follow-up of 7 years. Fewer patients in the propanolol- treated group reached the primary endpoint of aortic regurgitation, aortic dissection, surgery, heart failure, or death (five in treatment group and nine in control group). Aortic growth after normalization was lower in the propanolol treated group (0.023/year) (vs.) the control group (0.084/year, P<.001).[40] For patients with increased body weight or end-diastolic aortic diameter >40 mm, the response to beta blockade was worse, suggesting that beta blockers must be given at an adequate dose and early in the course of the disorder to optimize benefit.[27,40] Approximately 10 to 20% patients will be intolerant of beta blockade due to asthma, fatigue, or depression. For these patients, a calcium channel blocker may be justified.[41]

Recent publication of the ability of losartan, an FDA-approved antihypertensive medication and selective AT-1 receptor antagonist, to inhibit aortic aneurysm in murine models of MFS[42] has opened a potential new medical treatment paradigm. The exact mechanisms by which losartan inhibits TGF-β in the aortic wall are not completely understood, but a variety of feedback mechanisms are likely.[43] A multicenter trial comparing betablockade and losartan therapy in MFS in children and young adults has been initiated through the National Institutes of Health. Currently, there are no specific recommendation for losartan dosing or long-term therapy in individuals with MFS.

Surgical Treatment

The traditional threshold for surgical repair of the aortic root is 5 cm in patients with MFS. The association between aortic diameter and the risk of aortic catastrophe is clearly established, and aortic aneurysm size >6 cm predicts a fourfold increase in risk for aortic rupture or dissection in patients with MFS.[44] Although the aortic root is the site most often affected, once a dissection has occurred, degeneration of an aneurysm may affect other segments of the aorta or its branches. Indeed, as the life expectancy of individuals affected by MFS has increased with prophylactic root replacement, it is plausible that the remaining aorta or other large arteries may progress to require repair in the absence of antecedent dissection. For aortic arch and descending thoracic or thoracoabdominal aneurysm, standard criteria for repair generally follow that of atherosclerotic aneurysms with a threshold of 5.5 to 6.0 cm.[45]

Surgical Treatment of the Aortic Root

Composite surgical replacement of the aortic root and valve was pioneered by Bentall and De Bono in 1968.[46] Prior to this, the outlook for repair of MFS patients with dissections or aneurysm in the aortic root was dismal, with high bleeding rates and excessive mortality. The Bentall technique has proven to be safe and durable. Long-term survival was significantly improved when compared with the natural history of aortic disease in patients, with a 91% 10-year survival rate.[35] At follow-up of 6.7 years, 36% of the deaths were attributable to the "downstream" aorta. Although reoperative root replacement was rare after composite valve graft (CVG), 10% of the patients required distal aortic surgery.[35]

Owing to the risks of thromboembolism and the lifetime requirement for warfarin anticoagulation, recent efforts have been directed at maintaining the native aortic valve. This valve-sparing root replacement (VSRR) approach has the additional benefit of avoiding warfarin embryopathy in women with MFS who may desire later pregnancy. To date, there has been no randomized trial comparing CVG and VSRR techniques, but the available data are encouraging with low rates of valve dysfunction (20 to 25% with 3-4+ AR) and few reoperations.[47-48]

Surgery of the Descending Thoracic and Thoracoabdominal Aorta

The first successful replacement of the thoracoabdominal aorta in a patient with MFS was performed by Crawford in the 1980s.[49] Elective surgical repair of descending thoracic aortic aneurysms and thoracoabdominal aortic aneurysms in MFS has benefited from the general refinements and introduction of adjuncts to reduce spinal cord injury and other major complications in a manner similar to that for standard atherosclerotic aneurysms. Prophylactic aortic replacement is indicated when the aortic diameter reaches 5.5 to 6.0 cm or if symptoms appear suspicious for aortic cause. Because of the frequent involvement of the descending aorta by extensive aortic dissections, surgery in these regions in MFS is often indicated for aortic diameter and chronic underlying dissection. As such, the extent of repairs in MFS tends to be greater, with 42 to 78% of all TAAAs being DeBakey extent II.[45,50] As expected, the mean age of MFS patients undergoing repair of TAAA is 34 to 48 years of age, younger than nonconnective tissue disorder patients.[45,50-51] In comparison with patients with degenerative TAAA presenting for repairs, there was no higher rate of acute presentation with dissection or rupture in patients with MFS TAAA (6 to 8%, each).[45,51] Paraparesis and paraplegia rates after TAAA repair in MFS patients compare favorably with results from those with nonconnective tissue disorders when matched for extent of repair required.[45,50-51] Owing to the very young mean age of the MFS patients undergoing TAAA repair (vs.) the older mean age of degenerative TAAA patients, overall long-term survival was better in MFS patients (Figure 43–3).[45]

Given the preponderance of Type II TAAA repairs in the available series, the freedom from further aortic repair is very low owing to the fact that there is little aorta remaining to degenerate. As such, secondary aortic procedures in patients with MFS are often performed for pseudoaneurysm or aneurysm degeneration of the inclusion or Carrel patches (see Figure 43–3). In a series of 107 patients who had TAAA repair. including creation of visceral patches, 17 were known to have a connective tissue disorder.[52] With a mean time to diagnosis of 6.5 years, 3 of these 17 patients (17.6%) returned with aneurysmal degeneration of the visceral patch. By comparison, visceral patch aneurysms were noted in only 5.6% of atherosclerotic TAAA repairs.[52] All of these MFS patients had inclusion patches that encompassed the celiac axis, superior

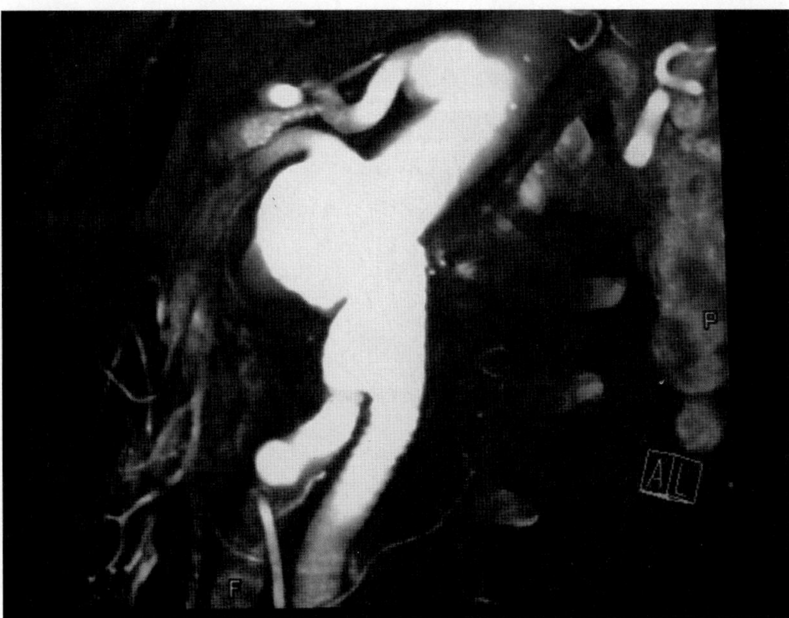

Figure 43-3. Visceral patch aneurysm in a patient with Marfan syndrome and prior thoracoabdominal aortic aneurysm repair with visceral inclusion technique.

mesenteric artery, and both renal arteries, suggesting the visceral patch should be greatly reduced in all connective tissue disorder patients to prevent late degeneration. Symptomatic presentation was noted in the series with a ruptured aneurysm appreciated in a patient (non-connective tissue disease) with a 6.1-cm patch aneurysm. Given the morbidity of the repair of the patch aneurysm (two intraoperative deaths among five patients taken to the operating room), the authors recommend maintaining an indication for repair of >6.0 cm.[52] We have changed our reconstruction to include prefabricated Dacron grafts with four branches for direct anastomosis to the origins of the renal and visceral vessels, thereby eliminating any retained aorta in the abdomen (Figure 43–4).

Endovascular Treatment

In general, aortic stent-grafts should not be used in the thoracic or abdominal aorta or for patients with other connective tissue diseases. The current approved devices have never been studied in the fragile milieu of the MFS aorta (connective tissue disorder was an exclusion criteria), and the question of persistent radial force on the aorta remains unanswered. A recent publication recommended endovascular repair *only* in instances of late localized pseudoaneurysm and stenting across native tissue aneurysm from "graft to graft."[27] A recent Society for Thoracic Surgery Consensus Statement recommended strongly against endovascular repair unless operative risk was deemed truly prohibitive by a center experienced in the management of complex aortic disease.[53] A recent report of thoracic endovascular repair in eight patients with connective tissue disorder (six with MFS, two with Ehlers-Danlos syndrome) [EDS] demonstrated initial success with few major complications, but the authors narrowly propose that the technique may be justified in emergencies as a "bridging" method.[54] No long-term follow-up is provided.

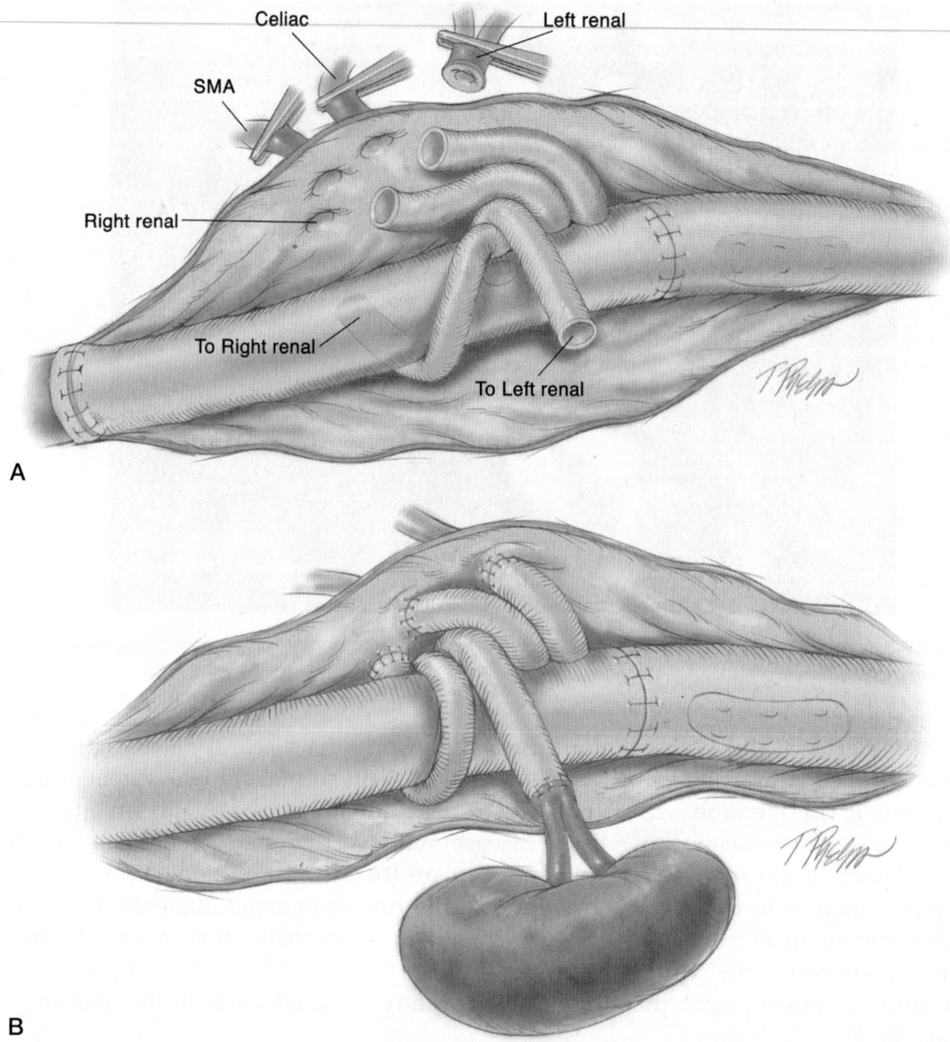

Figure 43-4. Reconstruction of thoracoabdominal aorta in a patient with connective tissue disorder totally eliminating retained aortic tissue. (A) Prefabricated polybranch graft is sewn to the thoracic graft and distally to the infrarenal aorta to provide orientation. (B) Orientation of branches allows redundancy to accommodate return of abdominal contents to the left retroperitoneum.

Conclusions

MFS has benefited from a century of progress in the study of its pathogenesis and more recent refinements in surgical techniques to handle the cardinal manifestations within the cardiovascular system that have plagued affected individuals. Proper genetic counseling, surveillance, and prudent application of modern surgical techniques have greatly modified the natural history of the disorder. As individuals with MFS begin to age, our understanding of accelerated joint disease and primary descending aortic involvement must evolve. Undoubtedly, new treatment paradigms can be expected with increasing sophistication of experimental approaches to uncover the operant pathogenetic mechanisms.

VASCULAR TYPE EHLERS-DANLOS SYNDROME

EDS is a heterogeneous group of heritable disorders of connective tissue characterized by joint hypermobility, skin hyperextensibility, and tissue fragility affecting skin, ligaments, joints, blood vessels, and internal organs. There are many subtypes of the disorder (Table 43–3), with the classic EDS (Types I and II) being the most common, inherited as an autosomal trait and having some repute as the "Elastic Man" and "India Rubber Man" of the late 19th century side-shows and Barnum circuses.[55] The importance of identifying the correct type cannot be underestimated because the natural history and modes of inheritance differ among the subtypes. Historically, the older literature did not clearly differentiate among the types, and the severe complications of the vascular type of Ehlers-Danlos syndrome were cited as representative as the whole syndrome, thereby creating unnecessary anxiety. For this review, we focus on the vascular type (EDS IV), its pathogenesis in defective type III procollagen encoded by the COL3A1 gene, and its management.

Epidemiology and Natural History

The prevalence of EDS IV is currently estimated to be 1:50,000 and is inherited in an autosomal dominant manner.[56] Approximately 50% of cases represent new mutations, and as a rule, each patient or family carries a unique mutation in the COL3A1 gene, which codes for type III procollagen.[57]

The overall life expectancy in EDS IV is dramatically shortened, largely as a result of vascular rupture, with a median life span of 48 years (range 6 to 73 years).[58] In a study of 220 patients with EDS IV, confirmed by abnormal type III procollagen molecules and 199 relatives with clinical diagnoses of EDS IV, major complications in childhood were rare, but 25% of the subjects suffered medical or surgical complications by

TABLE 43-3. SUBTYPES OF EHLERS-DANLOS SYNDROME

Nomenclature		Skin (0-4+)	Joint Laxity (0-3+)	Features	Inheritance
NEW	*TYPE*	*ELASTIC/FRAGILE*			
Classic	I, II	+++/+++	+++	Vascular complications rarely	AD
Hypermobile	III	+/+	+++	Arthritis	AR
Vascular	IV	−/++++	+	Rupture of arteries, uterus, intestine, thin skin	AD
Kyphoscoliotic	VIA, VIB	+++/++	+++	Hypotonia, osteoporosis, kyphoscoliosis, rupture of arteries, globe of eye	AR
Arthrochalasic	VIIA, VIIB	++/+	+++	Hip luxations, osteoporosis	AD
Dermatosparactic	VIIC	−/++++	+	Skin doughy and lax	AR
Other	V	++/++			X-linked
	VIII	+/++	++	Periodontal disease	AD
	IX	+/−	+	Lax skin, osteoporosis, bladder diverticula, retardation	X-linked
	X	+/+	++	Petechiae	?

age 20. By age 40, 80% had developed major complications.[58] Death occurred in 131 subjects, with vascular rupture of thoracic or abdominal vessels in 78 (59%), central nervous system hemorrhages in 9 (7%), and an unspecified bleeding source in 16 (12%). Organ rupture (heart, uterus, spleen, liver) caused death in 13 (10%) of the cases, and intestinal rupture led to demise in 10 (8%) subjects.[58]

Pathogenesis

EDS IV is due to mutations in the COL3A1 gene, located at 2q31-q32, which encodes 51 exons distributed over 44 kb. The gene encodes a procollagen molecule, proα1(III), with 1467 amino acids, of which 1029 are located within the central triple helical domain.[55] Basic collagen synthesis requires three polypeptide procollagen chains, referred to as α chains,. to be folded tightly into a triple helix. Each chain of proα1(III) has a simple repetitive sequence of approximately 1000 amino acids wherein a glycine residue occurs every third amino acid (Gly-X-Y). The glycine, the smallest of all the amino acids, fits sterically into the restricted space where the three chains of the triple helix come together. The X and Y amino acids are frequently proline and hydroxyproline, which by virtue of their ring structure provide rigidity to the triple helix final type III collagen protein. The majority of published mutations in the COL3A1 gene are simple glycine substitutions within the triple helical domain.[58-59]

Because procollagen III is a homotrimer, the synthesis of an equal number of normal and mutant α1(III) chains results in seven eighths of the collagen III molecules being abnormal and containing one or more mutant chains. The abnormal collagen III molecule cannot fold stably into a triple helix and is slowly degraded in the rough endoplasmic reticulum of the fibroblast and never secreted extracellularly.[60] The abnormal collagen III leads to a quantitative deficiency of collagen III and sometimes to disturbed fibril formation by the remaining normal collagen III. As such, tissues rich in collagen III, such as skin, blood vessels, and internal organs, are most affected.

Morphologically, proα1(III) mutations result in greatly reduced extractable collagen III, with 10 to 25% normal levels noted in lung, skin, and blood vessels.[61-62] Although collagen III is a minor component of adult skin, its deficiency has a dramatic effect, likely owing to its presence as the dominant collagen in a fetus <20 weeks old. It seems likely that collagen III is the primary scaffold in the developing fetus for subsequent matrix deposition by dermal fibroblasts.[63] Skin in EDS IV may measure only a quarter of the normal thickness, thereby appearing translucent and revealing the extensive network of subcutaneous veins, a major criterion of affected individuals.[64] Arterial vessels are also appreciated to have a thin wall with a markedly reduced collagen content.[65] The average collagen fibril cross-sectional area was decreased in the media of all arteries and the adventitia is thinned.[66]

Clinical Evaluation

EDS IV has the worst prognosis among the EDSs, and for this reason, examination of the patient is mandatory. Physical findings may mimic other EDS subtypes or other connective tissue disorders (Table 43–4). The presence of any two or more of the major criteria is highly indicative of the diagnosis, and laboratory testing is strongly recommended. Such testing is both labor- and time-intensive but should be considered strongly before any treatment course is chosen for the possibly affected individual.

The diagnosis of EDS IV is confirmed by demonstration of structurally abnormal collagen III and/or direct mutation analysis. Biochemical testing seeks to define abnor-

TABLE 43-4. DIAGNOSTIC CRITERIA OF EHLERS-DANLOS SYNDROME, VASCULAR TYPE[66]

Major Diagnostic Criteria
Thin, translucent skin
Arterial/intestinal/uterine fragility or rupture
Extensive bruising
Characteristic facial appearance (thin delicate nose, thin lips, hollow cheeks)
Minor Diagnostic Criteria
Acrogeria
Hypermobility of small joints
Tendon and muscle rupture
Talipdes equinovarus (clubfoot)
Early-onset varicose veins
Arteriovenous, carotid-cavernous sinus fistula
Pneumothorax/pneumohematothorax
Gingival recession
Positive family history, sudden death in (a) close relatives

mal collagen III produced by ascorbate-stimulated cultured skin fibroblasts. The abnormal collagen III leads to decreased overall production (from intracellular digestion), defective secretion, or to post-translational modifications as judged by slower mobility on gel or abnormal sensitivity to proteases.[67] Direct molecular genetic analysis of the COL3A1 gene is also possible from a blood/serum sample; yet this approach is not widely used owing to labor-intensive mutation analyses.

The differential diagnosis of EDS IV includes disorders of bruisability and wound healing such as von Willebrand's disease, platelet disorders, and scurvy. Bruisability is often elicited in children and may mimic nonaccidental injury ("battered child syndrome").[68] Indeed, excessive bruising and hematoma formation are common first presentations. In EDS IV, rupture or dissection of arteries occurs most often in medium-sized vessels (vs.) the predominant occurrence of the same in the aorta of the MFS patient. Vessel tortuosity and elongation may be similar to arterial tortuousity syndrome or LDS, but vascular surgery is often much more tolerated in the latter. Multiple aneurysms through the visceral vessels may also be noted in polycystic kidney disease and hereditary forms of cerebral cavernous malformations.[69]

Treatment Selection

Although no therapies exist for the condition of EDS IV, knowledge of the diagnosis can influence the management strategies, assist in reproductive counseling, and direct treatment of major complications. All patients with a confirmed diagnosis of EDS IV should carry a medical alert bracelet, papers noting information of the condition, and their blood group. General recommendations for anesthesia also exist; these include cross-match of adequate blood, avoidance of intramuscular injection, adequate peripheral access, avoidance of arterial lines and central venous catheters, and gentle intubation maneuvers.[70] If central access is required, then ultrasound-guided access (i.e., "sono-site") is mandatory.

Vascular catastrophe in EDS IV is not predictable, and vessel rupture can occur at any vessel diameter. Given the difficulty of handling the fragile tissues and vessels, management of spontaneous bleeding should be conservative as long as possible, especially in interstitial (muscular, retroperitoneal) spaces.[71-72] Bleeding within the peritoneal cavity usually requires immediate transfusion; if surgery is required, vessel ligation with umbilical tapes appears to be the safest course (vs.) direct repairs.[71] Direct reconstructions must be tensionless, often using pledgets to reduce suture trauma, and reinforced circumferentially (Figures 43–5 and 43–6). Angiography should be avoided because of severe morbidity and the risk of vessel dissection and/or perforation during selective catheterization or from the puncture site itself. In one study, the major complication rate from arteriography was 67% with a 12% mortality rate,[-72] although the benefit of a more contemporary lower-profile catheter and endovascular devices may favorably impact this historically high percentage. If endovascular and arteriographic approaches are needed, direct repair of the femoral artery should be strongly considered.

Gastrointestinal perforations account for 25% of all EDS IV complications.[58] The sigmoid colon is the location of most perforations and prompt diagnosis and immediate colostomy are favored.[58] For small bowel intestinal rupture, ostomy is also preferred, and most patients have restoration of bowel continuity in a staged fashion without complication.[58] Recurrent bowel perforation is always a risk and occurred between 2 weeks to 26 years after the first event in 17% of the patients.[58]

Medical Therapy

No effective medical therapy exists for EDS IV. Prophylactic measures to control blood pressure and reduce atherosclerotic risk factors are recommended, but there are no studies demonstrating impact on the natural history of the disease or time to first major complica-

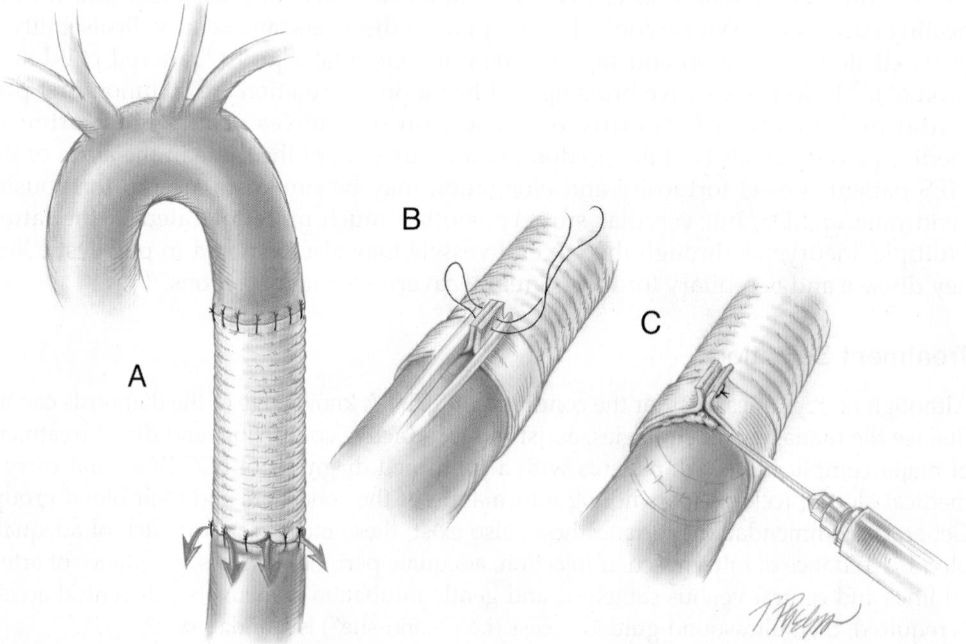

Figure 43-5. Technique for reinforcement of weak adventitial and medial tissue leading to uncontrolled needle track bleeding with cirumferential felt reinforcement.

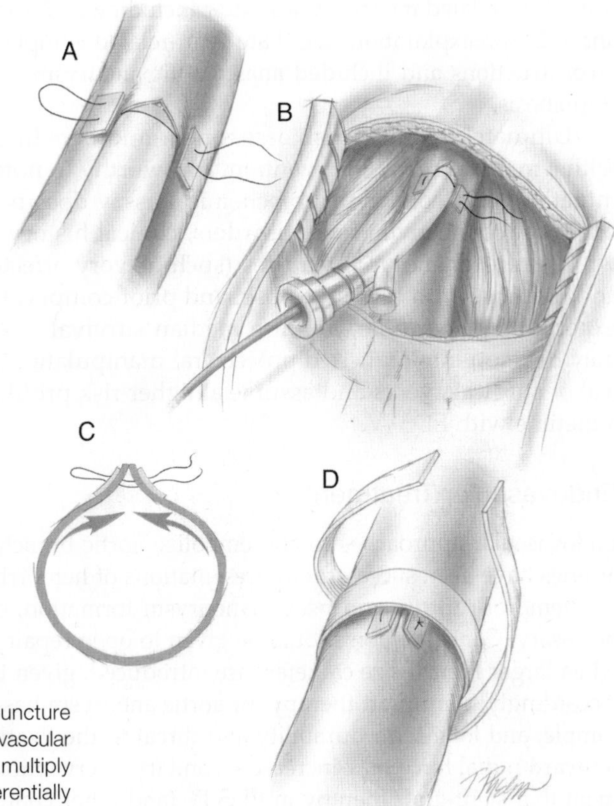

Figure 43-6. Direct repair of femoral puncture site during endovascular intervention for vascular Ehlers-Danlos syndrome. Repair site is multiply buttressed for hemostasis and circumferentially reinforced to reduce late pseudoaneurysm.

tion. Lifestyle modifications for EDS IV follow the general recommendations of other genetic diseases, as reviewed in the section within MFS earlier in this chapter.[38] Daily doses of ascorbic acid (vitamin C) have been offered on the theoretical basis of improving procollagen stability by conversion of proline residues in the Y position within the Gly–X–Y sequences to hydroxyproline via prolyl hydroxylase. This enzyme requires ascorbic acid as a cofactor, and the resulting hydroxylation event allows the mature collagen molecule to fold into the triple helix stably at body temperature.

Surgical Treatment

Surgical management of EDS IV is a formidable challenge. The traditional risk assessment paradigm cites invasive procedures so fraught with complications that intervention should be performed only when the patient is faced with imminent risk of death.[73-74] The presentation of patients with EDS IV can include arterial manifestations throughout the entire vascular tree. The outcomes of 31 patients over a 30-year period were studied retrospectively at a tertiary referral center.[75] Among 24 patients, there were 132 with vascular complications that prompted presentation for evaluation. While 85 of 132 complications were present before or during the first evaluation, 47 additional complications arose during a 6.3-year median follow-up. Fifteen of 31 patients underwent a vascular intervention with 2 operative deaths (1 from an ascending aortic repair and the other after a series of eight operations by anastomotic rupture of a carotid-subclavian graft). Overall procedure-related morbidity was 46%, including a 37% incidence of postoperative bleeding and a 20% reexploration rate. Late graft-related complications occurred in 40% of arterial reconstructions and included anastomotic aneurysm, anastomotic disruptions, and graft thrombosis.

Ultimately, patient risk assessment and benefit compel any decision to proceed with a major surgical intervention. It is worthy to note that genetic analysis of specific mutations and collagen III biochemical assay does not predict clinical course.[55,75] But like most connective tissue disorders, clinical history can be informative. For patients with severe phenotypic features (such as very affected skin and facial morphology) and for those with early age onset and prior complicated courses, complications can be expected. Furthermore, because median survival is 48 to 54 years,[58,75] older patients may develop intolerance to procedural manipulations (vs.) prior uncomplicated medical or surgical events and assume a higher risk profile as vessel fragility worsens over a lifetime with EDS IV.

Endovascular Treatment

Endovascular approaches to coil embolize aortic branch vessels and other medium-sized arteries have been successful in presentations of hemorrhage.[75] Arterial access can precipitate femoral rupture and pseudoaneurysm formation, especially when large devices are necessary. Consideration should be given to open repair of any access puncture, especially when larger French size catheters are introduced, given the rate of complications reported. Accordingly, stent-graft therapy for aortic aneurysm has not been reported in a significant sample, and long-term durability and threat to the fixation zones in the setting of chronic outward radial force may increase secondary interventions. As such, there is general agreement that stent-graft therapy in EDS IV (and other connective tissue disorders) should be avoided (see Figure 43–6).[53]

Pregnancy in EDS IV

Pregnancy in women with EDS IV should be closely monitored. Whether elective cesarean section is warranted before labor or to allow spontaneous vaginal delivery is not known.[76] In the largest study of 220 patients with EDS IV, 81 women had 183 deliveries. Twelve women (15%) died during the peripartum period or within 2 weeks postpartum.[58] The cause of death in these women was five uterine ruptures, two vessel ruptures during labor, and five deaths in the postpartum period from vessel rupture. Women with Ehlers-Danlos syndrome who become pregnant should be considered high risk and should be followed at high-risk centers. Genetic counseling is also mandatory, because the disorder is inherited as an autosomal dominant trait and 50% of offspring of an affected individual will inherit the disease.

Conclusions

There are no specific therapies for EDS IV, and life expectancy is shortened most often by vascular catastrophe. Proper identification of patients presenting with major diagnostic criteria should prompt biochemical investigation of type III procollagen production. Patient self-education in this disorder, often to inform treating physicians, may influence management of specific vascular complications as well as pregnancy and reproductive counseling. With the advent of newer scientific methodologies using genetically defined animal models to discover new pathophysiologic pathways, it is hoped that novel medical paradigms may evolve to favorably impact patients affected by EDS IV.

LOEYS-DIETZ SYNDROME

LDS is a newly described aortic syndrome characterized by aortic aneurysm and vascular tortuousity, craniofacial abnormality of the bifid uvula or cleft palate, and hypertelorism.[77] The disease is caused by heterozygous mutations in the genes encoding transforming growth factor beta receptors 1 and 2 (TGFβR1 and TGFβR2, respectively). Since the original report, two subtypes of LDS have been delineated. LDS Type I has both severe craniofacial features and aortic aneurysm. LDS Type II is typified by less severe craniofacial abnormality, usually only a bifid uvula or high palate, and the aortic aneurysm. Whereas the primary aneurysm involvement is in the aortic root, the aggressive nature of the root aneurysm to dissect and/or rupture at small diameters and in childhood separates this condition from MFS and EDS IV. Identification of affected patients and testing of all first-degree relatives are of paramount importance to motivate prophylactic surgery.

Epidemiology

In a study of 52 probands and 38 relatives, the median survival of the cohort was 37.0 years. Of these 90 patients, there were 27 deaths before or during the study interval, with a mean age of death of 26.0 years (range 0.5 to 47.0). The leading cause of death was thoracic aortic dissection in 67%, followed by abdominal aortic dissection in 22%, and cerebral hemorrhage in 7%. The mean age at the first vascular dissection was 26.7 years, and the mean age of first vascular surgery, usually for ascending aortic pathology, was 19.8 years.[77]

Comparison of survival in the two subtypes of LDS was also reported.[77] In LDS Type I, mean age of death was lower (22.6 years) (vs.) LDS Type II (31.8 years, P=.06), Mean age of first surgery was 10 years, younger in LDS Type I (vs.) Type II (16.9 years (vs.) 26.9 years, P=.03). Craniofacial abnormalities when scored into a craniofacial severity index correlated inversely with time of first surgery (more severely affected individuals indicated more aggressive aortic pathology).[77]

Pathogenesis

Ultrastructural analysis of the aortic wall demonstrates collagen deposition in excess of that appreciated in MFS in LDS patients. Elastin fibers are disarrayed and fragmented, with reduced total elastin content noted.[78] Two major genetic perturbations have been described in the TGF-β signaling pathway leading to LDS.[77-78] Approximately two thirds of LDS patients have mutations in the gene encoding TGFβR2, and the remainder have mutations in the gene encoding TGFβR1.[77] With rare exception, the mutations were germline heterozygous missense mutations affecting the amino acids in the functionally critical intracellular kinase domain of the receptor.[78] Indeed, truncation of the intracellular domain of the TGF-β receptor would be expected to preclude signal transduction, but a paradoxical increase in TGF-β activity is observed.[77] Tissues from affected individuals shows nuclear enrichment of SMAD2, suggesting increased TGF-β signaling.[78] The mechanism by which mutations in the TGF-β receptor cause the multisystem manifestations of LDS are poorly understood and remain to be fully elucidated. There are no firm genotype-phenotype correlations to predict more aggressive aortic pathology.

Clinical Evaluation

LDS is a multisystem disorder with a classic triad of craniofacial abnormality (90%), hypertelorism (wide-set eyes, 90%), and arterial tortuousity/aneurysm (98%). Within 40 LDS patients who underwent complete anthropometric evaluation, besides the classic triad, there were additional findings throughout the craniofacial, skeletal, and cutaneous systems.[77] Developmental delay was infrequent (15%) and was occasionally associated with craniosynostosis, hydrocephalus, or Arnold-Chiari malformation—suggesting that learning disability is a rare primary manifestation.[77]

Craniofacial manifestations are most commonly hypertelorism and cleft palate or bifid uvula. Craniosynostosis was present in 48%, malar hypoplasia (flat mid face) in 60%, and blue sclera in 40%. In contradistinction to MFS, lens dislocation (ectopia lentis) was not recorded in any patient with LDS.[77]

Skeletal manifestations included arachnodactyly in 70% and pectus deformity (excavatum or carinatum) in 68%. Clubfoot malformations were noted in 45% and joint laxity was common, occurring in 68% of subjects.[77] Importantly, this joint laxity was also noted in the cervical spine, and cervicoatlanto instability could render standard intubation maneuvers a threat to spinal cord compression. As such, flexion and extension views of the cervical spine are recommended, with >30% slip indicating a need for cervical fusion for safety. Dolichostenomelia, seen often in MFS, was infrequently noted in LDS (18%).[77]

Cardiovascular involvement is a hallmark of LDS, but aneurysms are not limited to the aortic root but can occur throughout the vascular tree. Arterial tortuousity, particularly of the supra-aortic vessels, should prompt consideration of the disease.[79] Vessel elongation within tortuous segments can be difficult to diagnose without three-dimensional imaging (Figure 43–7) and centerline measurement.

Patients, especially children, affected by LDS have high rates of severe allergy, with food allergy and inflammatory bowel disease noted in many. There remains no distinct mechanistic insight into this preponderance, which is not seen in any other connective tissue disorder. Increased levels of TGF-β are proposed to interfere with normal CD4+T helper-cell differentiation, thereby yielding T-helper cells which produce interleukin-17 (IL-17). The Th-17 T cells are implicated in the development of autoimmune inflammatory conditions.

The differential diagnosis of LDS includes arterial tortuousity syndrome (ATS), in which medial degeneration of elastic fibers can lead to elongation, stenosis, tortuosity, and eventual aneurysm formation. Interestingly, ATS is an autosomal recessive disorder caused by mutation of the glucose transporter GLUT10 and is the only connective tissue disorder recognized to stem from defective glucose metabolism. GLUT10 deficiency is associated with upregulation of TGF-β in the arterial wall, also observed in LDS.[80] Cardiovascular prognosis seems much more favorable in ATS than LDS.[80] Owing to the early age of presentation of dramatic pathology, EDS IV is often considered along with the LDS disease. It could not be more critical to differentiate between the two, either on clinical examination to determine the LDS triad or with biochemical testing to confirm EDS IV, because surgical management and tissue fragility are dramatically more challenging in EDS IV than LDS patients.

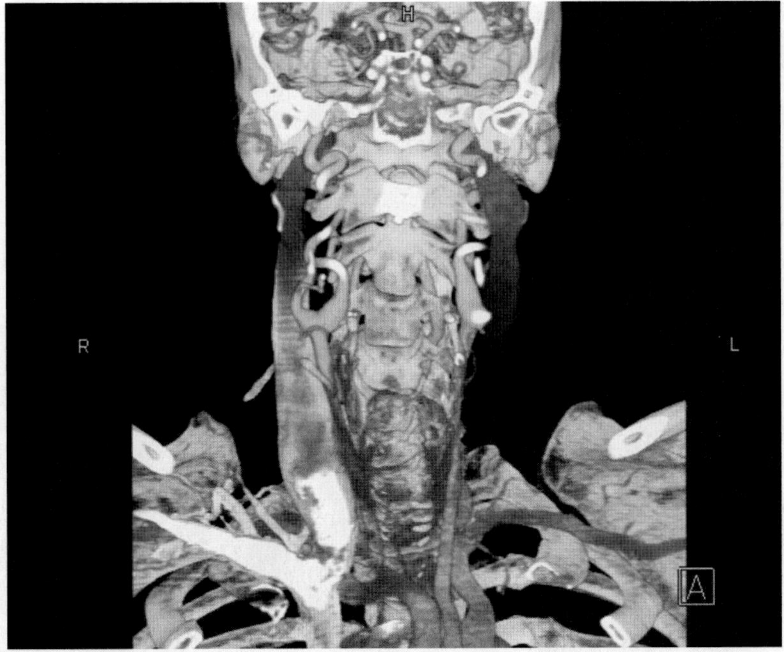

Figure 43-7. Typical vessel tortuousity in Loeys-Dietz syndrome can include carotid, vertebral, and subclavian arteries.

Treatment Selection

Patient risk assessment for prophylactic repair in LDS must account for the aggressive nature of aneurysms in the disorder. Certainly, each patient should be evaluated individually, and for those with marked craniofacial abnormality, an aggressive posture should be maintained toward repair. The new diagnosis of a patient as affected by LDS should prompt a head-to-toe CT or MR imaging study to determine the presence of arterial pathology outside the aortic root.[80] Because involvement of supra-aortic trunks and vertebral vessels is not uncommon, surgical exposure may be difficult, and embolization approaches considered. Given the widespread involvement of the arterial pathology in this disorder, multiple operations or interventions on a single patient are not uncommon.[77,81-82]

Surgical Treatment

Early results after surgical treatment of aneurysm in LDS are now emerging owing to the very recent characterization of clinical and genetic features specific to the disease. Tissue handling and aortic anastomoses are favorable, and a small series of aortic root replacement patients of adults and children demonstrated no operative mortality; however, 3 of 21 patients died in follow-up of thoracic aorta (n=2) and abdominal aorta (n=1) rupture.[79] In the author's institution, there have been five patients who returned for descending thoracic aortic replacement after prior ascending/VSRR repairs. Three of these patients returned thereafter with patch aneurysms after prior thoracoabdominal repairs and were confirmed as LDS on subsequent TGFβR testing. As in MFS, this limited experience suggests patch size should be limited or preferably avoided by direct anastomosis with a

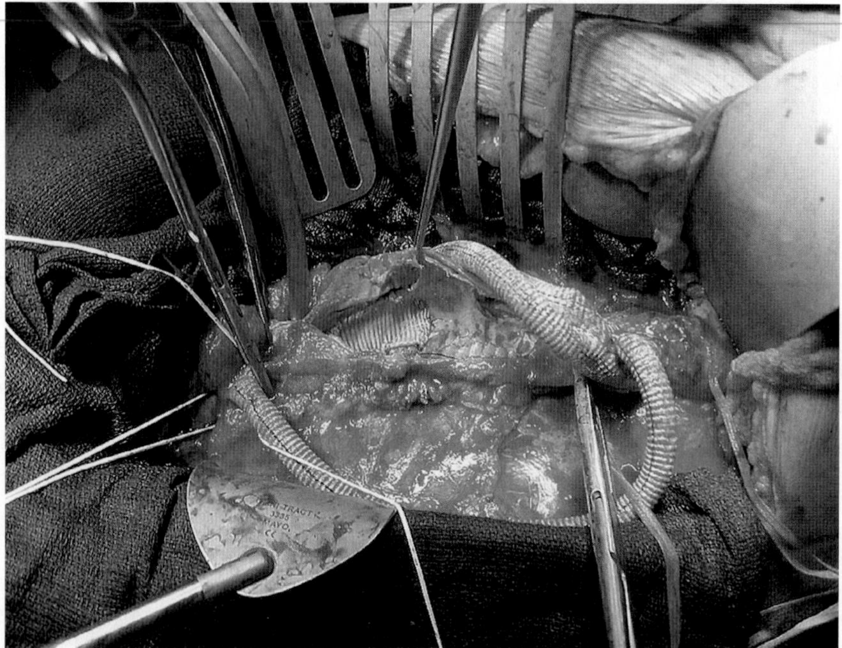

Figure 43-8. Intraoperative photo of patch aneurysm repair with individual bypass to branch vessels and patching of defect from within the abdominal graft.

multiple branched Dacron graft (see Figure 43–4). Based upon the experience in the aortic root with premature rupture at small diameters, a general recommendation for repair of any aortic segment in adults would be 4 cm or growth of aneurysm by more than 0.5 cm in 1 year.[79,81] Recommendations for repair of peripheral aneurysms in LDS have not been determined, but rate of growth and absolute size both factor into the decision, making regular surveillance with high-quality imaging critica (Figure 43–8).

Medical Therapy

Current recommendations for medical management and surveillance in LDS are predicated upon the beta blockade regimen recommended in MFS, with the threshold for repair postured more aggressively in LDS. Nonetheless, the pathophysiologic mechanism of increased TGF-β activity in the vessel wall compels some to initiate losartan therapy for the disease. However, randomized trials are lacking and preliminary data for losartan therapy are not conclusive to date. Lifestyle modifications also should restrict "burst" activity per MFS restrictions.[38]

Conclusions

LDS is unique among connective tissue disorders in the aggressive nature of aneurysms that rupture and/or must be dissected at very young patient age, the widespread involvement of the arterial tree, and characteristic craniofacial features. Age at presentation and subtle cutaneous changes may first raise EDS IV as a critical lead diagnosis in the differential, separating the diagnosis of LDS, and management paradigms move aggressively toward prophylactic repairs in LDS while EDS IV remains very conservative. Ongoing research into the role of TGF-β overactivity in LDS in newly defined genetic animal models should yield medical treatment paradigms for the disorder in the near future.

FAMILIAL THORACIC AORTIC ANEURYSM AND DISSECTION

Although it has been recognized that TAAD occur in individuals with known genetic syndromes, a genetic basis for TAAD in patients who do not have a defined connective tissue disorder has recently been investigated. Familial studies suggest that 11 to 19% of all non-syndromic TAAD patients have a first-degree relative with TAAD.[83-84] Pedigree analysis suggests familial TAAD is inherited as a predominantly autosomal dominant disorder with decreased penetrance and variable expression yielding considerable clinical heterogeneity.[85] Genetic mapping of loci in familial TAAD had provided new insights into the pathogenesis of aneurysms throughout the aorta.

Pathogenesis

Five loci have been mapped for familial TAAD to date, including three identified genes. Despite locus heterogeneity, the final common pathologic change in the aortic wall is medial degeneration.[85-86] Smooth muscle cell disarray and proteoglycan accumulation are also typically present.[86] The first loci mapped for familial TAAD was the *TAAD1* locus at 5q13-14.[87] The initial genetic screen identified the location of the defective gene by using two families with similar phenotype for mapping. Subsequent to this mapping, 15 families were found with familial TAAD patterning, segregated as an autosomal dominant disease, with reduced penetrance primarily in women to 5q13-14.[88] Involvement is primarily in the ascending aorta.[88] A second locus for familial TAAD was mapped to 11q23-24, designated *FAA1*. Linkage to this region was established using a single large family.[89] In contrast to *TAAD1, FAA1* was associated with more diffuse vascular disease with both thoracic and abdominal aortic aneurysms as well as other arteries. *FAA1* appears to be rare as a cause of familial TAAD, because no additional families have been linked to the *FAA1* locus.[88] A third locus for familial TAAD, termed *TAAD2,* was mapped to 3p24-25, and it was determined that TGFβR2 is the mutant gene at this locus.[90-91] The TGFβR2 gene was screened in 80 unrelated families with familial TAAD, and mutations were discovered in the TGFβR2 gene in 4 (5%), suggesting TGFβR2 mutations are an uncommon cause of familial TAAD. All 4 affected families carried mutations that affected arginine at amino acid 460 in the intracellular kinase domain, suggesting a "hot-spot" for familial TAAD and mutations. These families developed ascending aortic pathology but also aneurysms and dissections in the descending aorta and other vessels.[91]

A fourth locus was mapped to 16p12.2-13.13 in a family with TAAD associated with patent ductus arteriosus. [92] The defective gene was identified as smooth muscle cell myosin heavy chain 11 (MYH11). MYH11 is a major contractile protein specific to smooth muscle cells. Affected individuals heterozygous for MYH11 mutations have marked aortic stiffness with a substantial decrease in aortic compliance.[92] It is estimated that MYH11 mutations account for approximately 2% of familial TAAD.[93]

α-Actin mutations have recently been discovered to cause 14% of familial TAAD.[93] The actin proteins are highly conserved and are critical cytoskeletal elements. There are six tissue-specific actin isoforms: two in striated smooth muscle cell (ACTA 1 in skeletal muscle and ACTC in cardiac muscle), two in smooth muscle cells (ACTA 2 in vascular smooth muscle cells and ACTG2 in visceral smooth muscle), and two in non-muscle cells (ACTB, ACTG1). Aortic tissue demonstrates cystic medial degeneration with focal areas of marked vascular smooth muscle proliferation. Interestingly, familial TAAD patients with ACTA2 mutations also are noted to have significant livedo reticularis, a physical finding not encountered in the other connective tissue disorders. Overall penetrance of familial TAAD in individuals with ACTA2 mutations was low (0.48) and did not increase with age. This fact distinguishes ACTA 2 mutations from other genes in familial TAAD, where penetrance is clearly age-related.[93]

Conclusion

Familial TAAD is noted in approximately 20% of thoracic aneurysms or dissections. Although penetrance is low after autosomal dominant inheritance and variability is common, it remains challenging for the clinician to separate familial TAAD from sporadic TAAD events. The recent discovery of myosin and actin mutations within familial TAAD opens a new paradigm of nonsyndromic TAAD stemming from perturbations of the smooth muscle cell contractile unit. In time, hopefully, treatment paradigms will evolve based upon discovery, but for now, recommendations for surgical interventions in familial TAAD follow the standards of MFS.

SUMMARY

Research into the pathogenesis of connective tissue disorders over the past 2 decades has rapidly evolved to discover new treatment paradigms. Indeed, information from the Human Genome Project has facilitated genetic discovery in connective tissue disorders, and the benefits of this landmark effort are now beginning the process of translation to the clinical arena. As these patients age, portions of the vascular tree other than the ascending aorta may become affected, placing vascular surgeons in the management paradigm of these challenging patients. Whereas progress is certain, patients with connective tissue disorders currently should maintain regular surveillance, seek expert opinion when intervention is contemplated, and receive genetic counseling to maintain reproductive health. When intervention is chosen, proper operative preparation and use of adjunctive techniques may foster a more successful outcome.

REFERENCES

1. McKusick V, Heritable Disorders of Connective Tissue. St. Louis: CV Mosby; 1956.
2. Marfan A-B. Un cas de deformation congenitale des quarte members plus prononcee aux extremites caracterisee par l'allongement des os avec un certain degree d'amincissement. Bull Mem Soc Med Hop Par (Ser 3) 1896;13:220–6.
3. Mery H, Baboneix L. Un cas de deformation congenitale des quatres members: Hyperchondroplasie. Bull Mem Soc Med Hop Par (Ser 3) 1902;19:671–6.
4. Baer RW, Taussig HB, Oppenheimer EH. Congential aneurysmal dilatation of the aorta associated with arachnodactyly. Bull Johns Hopkins Hosp 1943;72:309–31.
5. Judge DP, Dietz HC. Marfan's syndrome. Lancet 2005;366:1965–76.

6. Gray JR, Bridges AB, Faed MJ, et al. Ascertainment and severity of Marfan syndrome in a Scottish population. J Med Genet 1994;31:51–4.
7. Dietz HC, Cutting GR, Pyeritz RE, et al. Marfan syndrome caused by a recurrent de-novo missense mutation in the fibrillin gene. Nature 1991;352:337–9.
8. Murdoch JL, Walker BA, Halpern BL, et al. Life expectancy and causes of death in the Marfan syndrome. N Engl J Med 1972;286:804–8.
9. Silverman DJ, Burton KL, Gray J, et al. Life expectancy in the Marfan syndrome. Am J Cardiol 1995;75:157–60.
10. McKusick VA. The cardiovascular aspects of Marfan syndrome: a heritable disorder of connective tissue. Circulation 1955;11:321–42.
11. Halme T, Savunen T, Aho H, et al. Elastin and collagen in the aortic wall: changes in the Marfan syndrome and annuloaortic ectasia. Exp Mol Pathol 1985;43:1–12.
12. Tsuji T. Marfan syndrome: demonstration of abnormal elastic fibers in skin. J Cutan Pathol 1986;13:144–53.
13. Sakai LY, Keen DR, Engvall E. Fibrillin, a new 350-kD glycoprotein, is a component of extracellular microfibrils. J Cell Biol 1986;103:2499–509.
14. Kainulainen K, Pulkkinen L, Savolainen A, et al. Location of chromosome 15 of the gene defect causing Marfan syndrome. N Engl J Med 1990;323:935–9.
15. Collod-Beroud G. Beroud C, Ades L, et al. Marfan database: new mutations and new routines for the software. Nucl Acids Res 1998;26:229–33.
16. Putnam EA, Cho M, Zinn AB, et al. Delineation of the Marfan phenotype associated with mutations in exons 23–32 of the FBN-1 gene. Am J Med Genet 1996;62:233–42.
17. Corson GM, Chalberg SC, Dietz HC, et al. Fibrillin binds calcium and is coded by cDNAs that reveal a multidomain structure and alternatively spliced exons at the 5″ end. Genomics 1993;17:476–84.
18. Biery NJ, Eldadah ZA, Moore CS. Revised genomic organization of FBN1 and significance for regulated gene expression. Genomics 1999;56:70–7.
19. Periera L, Andrikolopouluos K, Tian J, et al. Targetting of the gene encoding fibrillin-1 recapitulates the vascular aspect of Marfan syndrome. Nat Genet 1997;17:218–22.
20. Periera L, Lee Sy, Gayraud B, et al. Pathogenetic sequence for aneurysm revealed in mice underexpressing fibrillin-1. Proc Natl Acad Sci U S A 1999;96:3819–23.
21. Bunton TE, Biery NJ, Gayraud B: Phenotypic alteration of vascular smooth muscle cells precedes elastolysis in a mouse model of Marfan syndrome. Circ Res 2001;88:37–43.
22. Saharinen J, Hyytianen M, Taipale J, et al. Latent transforming growth factor β binding proteins (LTBPs)—structural extracellular matrix proteins for targeting TGF-β action. Cytokine Growth Factor Rev 1999;10:99–107.
23. Neptune ER, Frischmeyer PA, Arking, et al. Dysregulation of TGF-β activation contributes to pathogenesis in Marfan syndrome. Nat Genet 2003;33:407–11.
24. Ng CM, Cheng A, Myers LA, et al. TGF-β dependent pathogenesis of mitral valve prolapse in a mouse model of Marfan syndrome. J Clin Invest 2004;114:1586–92.
25. Beighton P, de Paepe A, Danks D, et al. International nosology of heritable disorders of connective tissue, Berlin, 1986. Am J Med Genet 1988;29: 581–94.
26. De Paepe A, Devereaux RV, Dietz HC, et al. Revised diagnostic criteria for the Marfan syndrome. Am J Med Genet 1996;62:417–26.
27. Milewicz DM, Dietz HC, Miller C. Treatment of aortic disease in patients with Marfan syndrome. Circulation 2005;111:e150-e157.
28. Loeys B, Nutyinck L, Delvaux I, et al. Genotype and phenotype analysis of 171 patients referred for the molecular study of the fibrillin-1 gene because of suspected Marfan syndrome. Arch Intern Med 2001;161:2447–554.
29. Loeys B, De backer J, Van Acker P, et al. Comprehensive molecular screening of the FBN1 gene favors locus homogeneity of classical Marfan syndrome. Hum Mutat 2004;24:140–46.
30. Glesby MJ, Pyeritz RE. Association of mitral valve prolapse and systemic abnormalities of connective tissue. A phenotypic continuum. JAMA 1989;262:523–8.

31. Wang M, Clericuzio CL, Godfrey M. Familial occurrence of typical and lethal congenital contractural arachnodactyly caused by misplacing of exon 34 in FBN2. Am J Hum Genet 1997;59:1027–34.
32. Pyeritz RE, Wappel MA. Mitral valve dysfunction in Marfan syndrome. Clinical and echocardiographic study of prevalence and natural history. Am J Med 74:797–807.
33. Meijboom LJ, Timmermans J, van Tintelen JP, et al. Evaluation of left ventricular dimensions and function in Marfan syndrome with significant valvular regurgitation. Am J Cardiol 2005;95:795–7.
34. Roman MJ, Devereuax RB, Kramer-Fox R, et al. Two-dimensional echocardiographic aortic root dimensions in normal children and adults. Am J Cardiol 2005;95: 795–7.
35. Gott VL, Greene PS, Alejo DE, et al. Replacement of the aortic root in patients with Marfan syndrome. N Engl J Med 1999;340:1307–13.
36. Maron BJ, Shirani J, Poliac LC, et al. Sudden death in young athletes: clinical, demographic, and pathologic profiles. JAMA 1996;276:199–204.
37. Yeatman AT, Bornemeier RA, McCrindle BW, et al. Long-term outcome in patients with Marfan syndrome: is aortic dissection the only cause of death? J Am Coll Cardiol 2003;41:329–32.
38. Maron BJ, Chaitman BR, Ackerman MJ, et al. Recommendations for physical activity and recreational sports participation for young patients with genetic cardiovascular diseases. Circulation 2004;109:2807–16.
39. Maron BJ, Mitten MJ, Quandt EF, et al. Competitive athletes with cardiovascular disease: the case of Nicholas Knapp. N Engl J Med 1998;339:1632–5.
40. Shores J, Berger KR, Murphy EA, et al. Progression of aortic dilatation and the benefit of long-term β-blockade in Marfan syndrome. N Engl J Med 1994;330:1335–41.
41. Rossi-Foulkes R, Roman MJ, Rosen SE, et al. Phenotypic features and impact of β-blockade or calcium anatagonist therapy on aortic lumen size in Marfan syndrome. Am J Cardiol 1999;83:1364–8.
42. Habashi JP, Judge DP, Holm TM, et al. Losartan, an AT-1 antagonist, prevents aortic aneurysm in a mouse model of Marfan syndrome. Science 2006;312:117–21.
43. Matt P, Habashi JP, Carrel T, et al. Recent advances in Marfan syndrome: should we now treat surgical patients with losartan? J Cardiovasc Thor Surg 2008;135:389–94.
44. Davies RR, Goldstein LJ, Coady MA, et al. Yearly rupture or dissection rates for thoracic aortic aneurysm: simple prediction based on size. Ann Thorac Surg 2003;73:17–27.
45. Lemaire SA, Carter SA, Volguina IV, et al. Spectrum of aortic operations in 300 patients with confirmed or suspected Marfan syndrome. Ann Thorac Surg 2006;81:2063–78.
46. Bentall H, De Bono A. A technique for complete replacement of the ascending aorta. Thorax 1968;23:338–9.
47. deOliviera NC, David TE, Ivanov J, et al. Results of surgery for aortic root aneurysm in patients with Marfan syndrome. J Thorac Cardiovasc Surg 2003;125:789–96.
48. Bethea BT, Fitton TP, Alejo DE, et al. Results of aortic valve-sparing operations: experience with remodeling and reimplantation procedures in 65 patients. Ann Thorac Surg 2004;78:767–72.
49. Crawford ES. Marfan's syndrome: broad spectral surgical treatment of cardiovascular manifestations. Ann Surg 1983;198:487–505.
50. Coselli JS, LeMaire SA, Buket S. Marfan syndrome: the variability and outcome of operative management. J Vasc Surg 1995;21:432–43.
51. Dardik A, Krosnick T, Perler BA, et al. Durability of thoracoabdominal aortic aneurysm repair in patients with connective tissue disorders, J Vasc Surg 2002;36:696–703.
52. Dardik A, Perler BA, Roseborough GS, et al. Aneurysmal expansion of the visceral patch after thoracoabdominal aortic replacement: an argument for limiting patch size? J Vasc Surg 2001;34:405–10.
53. Expert consensus document on the treatment of descending thoracic aortic disease using endovascular grafts. Ann Thorac Surg 2008;85:S1–41.

54. Geisbusch P, Kotelis D, von Tengg-Kobligk, et al. Thoracic aortic endografting in patients with connective tissue diseases. J Endovasc Ther 2008;15:144–9.
55. Steinman B, Royce PM, Superti-Furga: Ehlers-Danlos syndrome. In: Connective Tissue and Its Heritable Disorders. Wiley-Liss; Philadelphia; 2002, pp. 431–523.
56. Superti-Furga A, Steinman B, Byers PH. Type III collagen deficiency. Lancet 1989;1:903–4.
57. Pope FM, Martin GR, McKusick VA. Inheritance of Ehlers-Danlos type IV syndrome. J Med Genet 1977;14:200–4.
58. Pepin M, Schwarze U, Superti-Furga A, Byers PH. Clinical and genetic features of Ehlers-Danlos Type IV, the vascular type. N Engl J Med 2000;342:673–80.
59. Pope FM, Narcisi P, Nicholls AC, et al. COL3A1 mutations cause variable clinical phenotypes including acrogeria and vascular rupture. Br J Dermatol 1996;135:163–81.
60. Prockop DJ. Osteogenesis imperfecta: phenotypic heterogeneity, protein suicide, short and long collagen. Am J Hum Genet 1984;36:499–505.
61. Clark JG, Kuhn C, Uitto J. Lung collagen in type IV Ehlers-Danlos syndrome. Am Rev Respir Dis 1980;122:971–8.
62. Nerlich AG, Stoss H, Lehman H, et al. Pathomorphological and biochemical alterations in Ehlers-Danlos syndrome type IV. Pathol Res Pract 1994;190:697–706.
63. Epstein EH. $\alpha 1$(III) Human skin collagen, release by pepsin digestion and preponderance in fetal life. J Biol Chem 1974;249:3225–31.
64. Holbrook KA, Byers PH. Ultrastructural characteristics of the skin in a form of the Ehlers-Danlos syndrome type IV. Lab Invest 1981;44:342–50.
65. Crowther MA, Lach B, Dunmore PJ, et al. Vascular collagen fibril morphology in type IV Ehlers-Danlos syndrome. Connect Tissue Res 1980;25:209–17.
66. Beighton P, De Paepe A, Danks D, et al. Ehlers-Danlos syndromes: revised nosology, villefranche, 1997. Am J Med Genet 1997;77:31–7.
67. Nuytinck L, Narcisi P, Renard JP, et al. Detection and characterization of an overmodified type III collagen by analysis of non-connective tissues in a patient with Ehlers-Danlos syndrome IV. J Med Genet 1992;29:375–80.
68. Roberts DL, Pope FM, Nicholls AC, et al. Ehlers-Danlos syndrome type IV mimicking non-accidental injury in a child. Br J Dermatol 1984;111:341–5.
69. Leblanc R, Lorenzo A, van der Rest M. Type III collagen mutations and cerebral aneurysms. Stroke 1989;20:1432–3.
70. Dolan P, Sisko F, Riley E. Anesthetic considerations for Ehlers-Danlos syndrome. Anesthesiology 1980;52:266–9.
71. Freeman RK, Swegle J, Sise MJ. The surgical complications of Ehlers-Danlos syndrome. Am Surg 1996;62:869–73.
72. Cikrit DF, Miles JH, Silver D. Spontaneous arterial perforation: the Ehlers-Danlos specter. J Vasc Surg 1987;5:248–55.
73. Germain DP. Clinical genetic features of vascular Ehlers-Danlos syndrome. Ann Vasc Surg 2002;16:391–7.
74. Berqvist D. Ehlers-Danlos type IV syndrome: a review from a vascular surgical point of view. Eur J Surg 1996;162:163–70.
75. Oderich GS, Panneton JM, Bower TC. The spectrum, management and clinical outcome of Ehlers-Danlos syndrome type IV: a 30 year experience. J Vasc Surg 2005;42:98–106.
76. Weinbaum PJ, Cassidy SB, Campbell WA. Pregnancy management and successful outcome of Ehlers-Danlos syndrome type IV. Am J Perinatol 1987;4;134–7.
77. Loeys BL, Schwarze U, Holm T. Aneurysm syndromes caused by mutations in the TGF-β receptor. N Engl J Med 2006;355:788–98.
78. Loeys B, Chen J, Neptune E, et al. A syndrome of altered cardiovascular, craniofacial, neurocognitive, and skeletal development caused by mutations in TGFBR1 and TGFBR2. Nat Genet 2005;37:275–81.
79. Williams JA, Loeys BL, Nwakanma LU, et al. Early surgical experience with Loeys-Dietz: a new syndrome of aggressive thoracic aortic aneurysm disease. Ann Thorac Surg 2007;83: s757–63.

80. Coucke PJ, Willaert A, Wessels MW, et al. Mutations in the facilitative glucose transporter GLUT10 alter angiogenesis and cause arterial tortuousity syndrome. Nat Genet 2006;38: 452–7.
81. Black JH, Loeys BL, Oswald G, Dietz HC. Peripheral vascular manifestations of Loeys-Dietz syndrome. Presented at Society for Vascular Surgery Annual Meeting, San Diego, 2008.
82. Lemaire SA, Pannu H, Tran-Fadulu, et al. Severe aortic and arterial aneurysms associated with TGFBR2 mutation. Nat Clin Pract Cardiovasc Med 2007;4:167–71.
83. Albornoz G, Coady MA, Roberts M, et al. Familial thoracic aortic aneurysms and dissections—incidence, modes of inheritance, and phenotypic patterns. Ann Thorac Surg 2006;82: 1400–6.
84. Biddinger AM, Rcklin J, Coselli JS, et al. Familial thoracic aortic dilatations and dissections: a case control study. J Vasc Surg 1997;25:506–11.
85. Pannu H, Avidian N, Tran-Fadulu V, et al. Genetic basis of thoracic aortic aneurysms and dissections, potential relevance to abdominal aortic aneurysms. Ann N Y Acad Sci 2006;1085:242–55.
86. Pannu H, Tran-Fadulu V, Papke C, et al. MYH11 mutations result in a distinct vascular pathology driven by insulin-like growth factor 1 and angiotensin 2. Hum Mol Genet 2007;16:2453–62.
87. Guo D, Hasham SQ, Kuang, et al. Familial thoracic aortic aneurysms and dissections: genetic heterogeneity with major locus mapping to 5q13–14. Circulation 2001;103:2461–8.
88. Tran-Fadulu V, Chen JH, Lemuth D, et al. Familial thoracic aortic aneurysms and dissections: three families with early-onset ascending and descending aortic dissections in women. Am J Med Genet 2006;140A:1196–202.
89. Kakko S, Raisanen T, Tamminen M, et al. Candidate locus analysis of familial ascending aortic aneurysms and dissections confirms the linkage to chromosome 5q13–14 in Finnish families. J Thor Cardiovasc Surg 2003;126: 106–13.
90. Hasham SN, Willing MC, Guo DC, et al. Mapping a locus for familial thoracic aortic aneurysms and dissections (TAAD2) to 3p24–25. Circulation 2003;107:3184–90.
91. Pannu H, Tran-Fadulu V, Chang J, et al. Mutations in transforming growth factor β receptor type II case familial thoracic aortic aneurysms and dissections. Circulation 2005;112:513–20.
92. Zhu L, Vranckx R, Khau Van Kien P, et al. Mutations in myosin heavy chain 11 cause a syndrome associating thoracic aortic aneurysm/aortic dissection and patent ductus arteriosus. Nat Genet 2006;38:343–9.
93. Guo DC, Pannu H, Tran-Fadulu V, et al. Mutations in smooth muscle α-actin (ACTA-2) lead to thoracic aortic aneurysms and dissections. Nat Genet 2007;39:1488–93.

44

Renal Malperfusion Following Aortic Dissection

Dawn M. Barnes, M.D., David M. Williams, M.D., Nara L. Dasika, M.D., Himanshu J. Patel, M.D., John E. Rectenwald, M.D., Jonathan L. Eliason, M.D., Guillermo A. Escobar, M.D., G. Michael Deeb, M.D., and Gilbert R. Upchurch, Jr., M.D.

INTRODUCTION

Acute dissection is a common lethal aortic disease.[1-5] Current literature suggests that aortic dissection results in visceral, renal, cerebral, spinal, or limb ischemia in approximately one third of cases, and that peripheral vascular insufficiency increases overall patient morbidity and early mortality.[1-2,6-13] The anatomic and physiologic variables at the foundation of any compromised vascular bed include (1) the percentage of aortic circumference dissected, (2) the presence of a distal reentrant focus in the false lumen or true lumen outflow, and (3) the relationship of branch ostia to the true lumen versus the false lumen.[14-15] However, specific treatment guidelines have yet to be established, and the optimal initial management of these patients remains controversial in terms of the use of a surgical versus an endovascular approach as well as the timing of central aortic repair.

PATHOPHYSIOLOGY

Immediately following dissection, there is "intrinsic true lumen collapse" to a variable degree, the false lumen subsequently dilates, resulting in an increased aortic cross-sectional area. The degree of increase correlates with blood pressure, the depth of the dissection plane within the media (i.e., residual wall thickness), and the percentage of the wall circumference involved in the dissection. Because the false lumen (outer aortic wall) is thinner and elastin-poor, it expands to generate the necessary wall tension required to balance

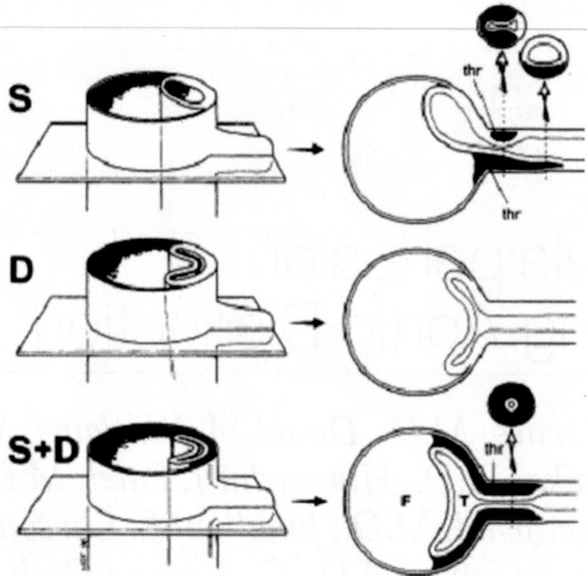

Figure 44-1. Drawing depicting two types of branch vessel obstruction at aortic dissection. In static obstruction (*S*), the dissection flap intersects or enters the branch vessel origin. In dynamic obstruction *(D),* the mural flap spares the branch vessel wall but prolapses across the branch vessel origin, covering it like a curtain. A mixed-type (static and dynamic) obstruction *(S+D)* is also shown. (Permission for reproduction granted by the Radiological Society of North America [RSNA]: From Williams DM, Lee DY, Hamilton BH, et al. The dissected aorta: Part III. Anatomy and radiologic diagnosis of branch vessel compromise. Radiology 1997;203:37–44.)

a given blood pressure, and the true lumen collapses secondary to the loss of transmural pressure across the dissection flap combined with elastic recoil and shortening of the flap.[16]

Williams et al. classified branch vessel compromise secondary to aortic dissecting hematoma as either static or dynamic[17] (Figure 44–1). Static obstruction occurs when the course of dissection coincides with the origin of a branch vessel and the aortic hematoma propagates into that vessel wall, thereby constricting the lumen. Dynamic obstruction results from prolapse of the dissection flap across the branch vessel origin. Additionally, a dynamic narrowing proximal to a branch ostia may compromise a vessel otherwise spared by the dissection flap. Finally, a mélange of any of these mechanisms may also be present. The distinction between obstruction types clinically (by IVUS and/or arteriography) determines the indicated course of interventional therapy. Although dynamic obstruction has historically been the most common type of obstruction,[15] our series analyzed 71 patients with 104 renal arteries demonstrating obstructions that were classified as 43 static, 30 dynamic, and 22 combined static and dynamic.[18]

CLINICAL PRESENTATION

Renal malperfusion presents clinically as progressive hypertension, evolving renal insufficiency, and/or evidence of impaired blood flow on CT imaging. Renal malperfusion may complicate both acute and chronic type A and type B dissections. It may also accompany alternate patterns of visceral malperfusion. Interestingly, clinically unsuspected renal malperfusion is not uncommon and can be diagnosed in patients in whom renal malperfusion is not clinically suspected with the aid of intravascular ultrasound, manometry, and angiography.[18] Patients who suffer renal artery obstruction early in the course of aortic dissection but who spontaneously reperfuse the kidney may suffer from unilateral or bilateral acute tubular necrosis (ATN) with no ongoing anatomic abnormality at the time of angiography. In putting numerous clinical papers in context, especially with non-operated type B dissections, it should be noted that "renal dysfunction" does not distinguish between simple ATN, mechanical obstruction by a static or dynamic mechanism, or a combination of the two.

APPROACH TO THERAPY

Miller et al. identified both renal dysfunction and renal/visceral ischemia as significant independent predictors of operative mortality in both acute and chronic type A and B aortic dissections.[19] What is not well established and remains controversial is the optimal treatment strategy for patients suffering aortic dissection complicated by peripheral vascular malperfusion. Some advocate immediate aortic reconstruction in the setting of an acute type A dissection. This is supported by the observation that the majority of cases of peripheral malperfusion (up to 80%) will resolve with restoration of blood through the true lumen.[1-2,8,11] Others, including our own practice, advocate delaying surgery on acute type A dissections in preference for percutaneous correction of the peripheral vascular malperfusion to allow for recovery from reperfusion to reduce overall mortality.[1,7-8,17,20-21] Most will advocate medical management for acute type B dissections, reserving surgery (aortic graft replacement or extra-anatomic bypass) for patients with intractable pain, uncontrolled hypertension, severe aortic branch malperfusion, or aneurysm expansion.[21] Studies have recognized that renal failure with anuria and bowel ischemia in the setting of acute aortic dissection have been associated with lethal multiorgan failure, making resolution of these symptoms a major priority.[9,20] Fann and associates demonstrated that impaired renal perfusion is associated with a high operative mortality rate (50% with renal ischemia compared with 23% for those without compromised renal perfusion) and that both impaired renal perfusion and renal dysfunction were significant independent predictors of operative death.[8,22] These authors maintain that compromised renal perfusion is the only peripheral vascular complication that was a significant independent predictor of operative death.[8]

Recently, Shiiya et al. recognized various mechanisms of malperfusion and found that although a central aortic operation alone successfully reversed all aortic-type malperfusion in acute type A and B dissections (100%), it was not effective for every branch-type malperfusion. Specifically, they noted that surgical fenestration did not successfully reverse branch-type renal malperfusion in all of their patients (2 of 13 patients, or 15%); however, percutaneous stenting was successful in all vessels with branch-type malperfusion.[23]

Finally, Estrera et al. have reinforced that end-organ malperfusion is the most common cause of significant morbidity during the acute presentation of type B aortic dissection, presumably resulting from thrombosis, ischemia-reperfusion injury, or a systemic inflammatory response syndrome.[2,24-25] Additionally, they showed that low glomerular filtration rate was an independent risk factor for mid-term mortality.[25]

STENT GRAFTING

Endovascular stent graft placement at the site of the aortic intimal tear has rapidly evolved as a technique increasingly employed in approaching the dissected aorta in an effort to redirect flow into the true aortic lumen.[1,26-27] In 1999, Dake et al. reported on 19 patients with aortic dissection, 37% of whom suffered symptomatic branch compromise. These authors demonstrated a 100% technical success rate in covering the aortic tear, resulting in resolution of peripheral ischemia in 76% of their cohort. The resolution of peripheral ischemia applied to 22 of 22 patients with dynamic obstruction and 6 of 15 patients with combined static and dynamic obstruction. Since this early report, there have been several additional reports supporting the utility and safety of aortic stent grafts.[26-27] Feezor et al. recently published their experience with thoracic endovascular aortic aneurysm repairs utilizing the TAG device. Fifteen percent of their 216 patient cohort had acute, complicated type B dissections. Eleven of these patients suffered branch vessel malperfusion (75% of which required branch vessel stenting), and 15 underwent endovascular repair for rupture. Of those patients who underwent endovascular repair for rupture, 27% required adjunctive branch vessel stenting. The authors cited a 76% morbidity rate and 21% early mortality rate with this approach.[28] Whereas stent grafting can be quite successful when directed at relieving a dynamic obstruction, the benefit in the setting of a branch-obstructing flap (i.e., static obstruction) remains unclear.

PERCUTANEOUS PROCEDURAL DETAILS

At the University of Michigan, all patients between June 1996 and March 2004 with suspected visceral malperfusion of any type underwent angiographic and IVUS studies. Angiographic evaluation of renal malperfusion is directed at finding and treating an ongoing anatomic renal artery obstruction. IVUS is performed from the ascending aorta to the iliac arteries to define the relationship of the dissection flap to branch arteries, and to determine which lumen each major branch arises from (Figure 44–2). Pressures in the SMA, bilateral renal arteries, and bilateral external iliac arteries are measured simultaneously with pressures in the aortic root. Bilateral renal and superior mesenteric arteriograms with hand injections of contrast are obtained to establish that the location of each measurement is peripheral to the distal extent of the false lumen. Aortic injections are almost never performed, thereby minimizing dye load. True renal malperfusion is confirmed by a systolic gradient between the aortic root and the renal hilum of >10 mm Hg (the threshold at which renal artery stenosis is typically treated by these operators), failure of the artery to fill during injection of contrast in the true and false lumen of the aorta, or evidence of a "curtain-like" occlusion of the vessel origin or the true lumen above the origin by IVUS.

The systematic approach to renal artery compromise at the University of Michigan is corroborated by Beregi and associates' "aortic dissection treatment algorithm" set forth for acute malperfusion complicating acute aortic dissection.[20] As aortorenal gradients are determined by the total obstructive lesion, treatment is directed initially at dynamic obstruction if present. In this case, aortic fenestration is attempted close to the origin of the compromised vessel. The false-lumen pressure in a classic aortic dissection is generally greater than or equal to the true-lumen pressure. Therefore, a fenestration procedure does not reduce pressure in the false lumen but at best raises the

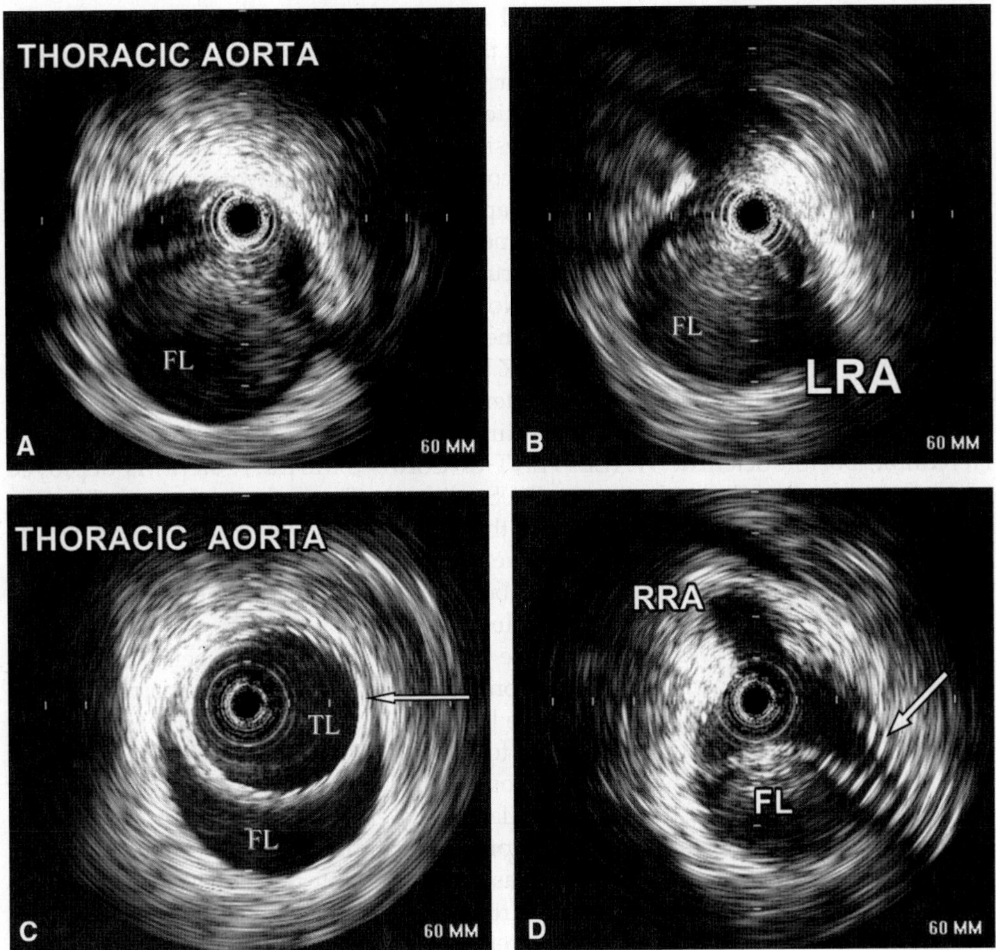

Figure 44-2. Intravascular ultrasound (IVUS) imaging of the thoracic aorta of a patient with an acute type B aortic dissection. A, The false lumen (FL) is hyperechoic and fully distended, obliterating the true lumen (TL) of the aorta except for a slit-like envelope anteriorly. B, In this image of the same patient's left renal artery (LRA), it appears to arise from the FL, but selective arteriography demonstrated that the renal artery was narrowed but remained tethered to the TL. C, IVUS imaging of the thoracic aorta after fenestration and placement of a Wallstent (Boston Scientific). The TL has been stented (arrow), with only some continued mild narrowing in the unstented region across the superior mesenteric and bilateral main renal arteries (not illustrated). After aortic fenestration and aortic stenting, a 17 mm Hg systolic gradient was measured across the renal artery origin, despite a re-entry tear at the origin. D, Final IVUS images of the bilateral renal arteries after aortic fenestration, aortic wall stent, and LRA stenting. Selective stenting of the LRA reduced the systolic gradient to 6 mm Hg. (From Barnes DM, Williams D, Dasika N, et al. A single-center experience treating renal malperfusion after aortic dissection with central aortic fenestration and renal artery stenting. J Vasc Surg 2008;45:903–10.)

true-lumen pressure to match that of the false lumen, thus providing local blood flow across the dissection flap at physiologic pressures.[17]

As an example, if a "curtain-type collapse" of the abdominal aorta is noted at the level of the renal arteries, a fenestration is performed near that level. An Amplatz wire is typically advanced through a Cobra catheter. The catheter is then withdrawn over the wire and exchanged for a Rosch-Uchida introducer set that is subsequently placed in the true lumen. The wire is removed and the trocar, in its encasing 5-French catheter, is advanced and thrust through the dissection flap using fluoroscopic and IVUS guidance. The trocar is exchanged for the Amplatz wire to allow balloon dilation of the flap and creation of the fenestration tear with a 14-mm diameter balloon. Typically, during balloon dilation, little resistance is encountered and little "waist" is noted. Following creation of the tear, the configuration of the two lumina is observed using IVUS. If the true lumen remains collapsed or, in questionable cases, if a gradient between the root and the abdominal aorta persists, a large-diameter (16 to 22 mm) self-expanding stent is deployed in the aortic true lumen, taking care not to cover the renal artery or SMA origins (see Figure 44–2). Note that compromise of the SMA should be treated before addressing compromise of the renal (or iliac) arteries.

If there is evidence of Cordis PALMAZ balloon-expandable stent or static obstruction, branch vessel stenting should be attempted (Figure 44–3). A Cordis PALMAZ balloon-expandable stent or self-expanding bare stent (i.e., Cook Zilver, Guidant Herculink, Boston Scientfic WALLSTENT or Cordis S.M.A.R.T. stent) is deployed under fluoroscopic and, in select cases, IVUS guidance. The stents are extended further into the aortic lumen (up to 5 to 10 mm) than is necessary when treating atherosclerotic stenoses. Early in our experience, we observed balloon-expanded stents being crushed even by small residual gradients between the true and the false lumina, and we presently use self-expanding stents exclusively.

Reassessment with IVUS and pressure measurements must be performed before terminating the procedure, because occasionally revascularization of a major vessel results in proximal collapse of the aortic true lumen with resultant dynamic obstruction. If dynamic obstruction results secondary to treating a branch artery narrowing, it is treated in standard fashion with fenestration and aortic stenting. Procedural success is confirmed by resolution of true-lumen collapse and elimination of, or at least significant improvement in, aortobranch artery pressure gradients as determined by IVUS, branch arteriography, and manometry. Reasons to defer intervention at the time of initial angiography include dissection or thrombosis extending into the lobar arteries such that distal cannulation of the renal artery's true lumen or other intervention is apt to cause further renal compromise, inability to access accessory branches for stenting, and an aortorenal pressure gradient considered "borderline" and unlikely to result in refractory hypertension or renal insufficiency. These same factors are also the reasons why small residual post-treatment pressure gradients are not always pursued therapeutically.

Our prospective study cohort included 165 patients with aortic dissection (both acute and chronic types A and B). Renal malperfusion was confirmed in 90 patients, 71 of whom underwent endovascular therapy including isolated unilateral or bilateral renal artery stenting (31), proximal aortic fenestration with or without aortic stenting (24), or both renal artery stenting and proximal aortic fenestration with or without aortic stenting[16]. This approach yielded a 90% success rate in resolving the aortorenal gradient (to <10 mm Hg) and was associated with five procedure-related complications and a periprocedural mortality rate of 21%.

SUMMARY

Renal malperfusion complicates one third of aortic dissections and increases associated morbidity and mortality. Branch vessel obstruction can be defined as static or dynamic —

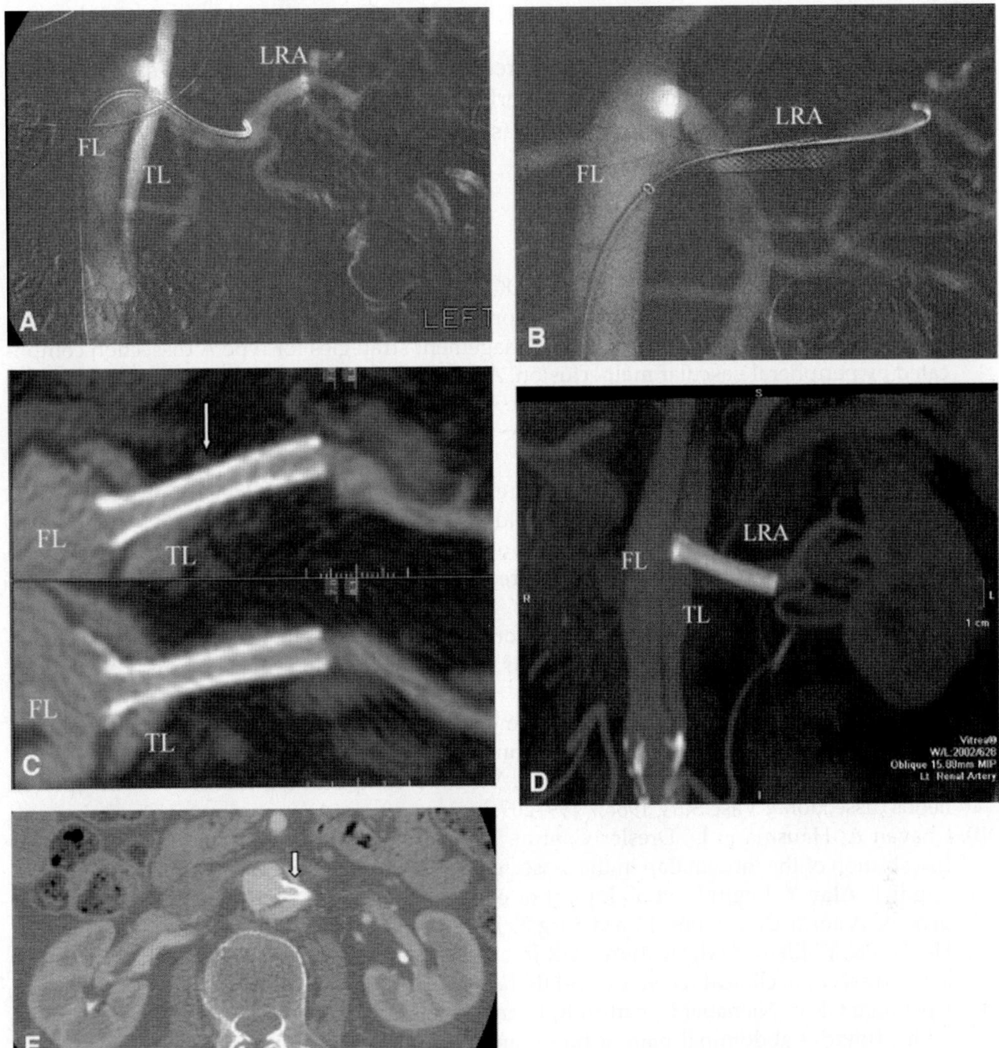

Figure 44-3. A, Carbon dioxide angiogram of a patient with aortic dissection shows static left renal artery (LRA) obstruction and the true lumen (TL), false lumen (FL), and the dissection flap prolapsing into the LRA. Note that the catheter is in the FL. B, Carbon dioxide angiogram of the LRA after fenestration and LRA stenting. C and D, Three-dimensional reformats of the LRA stent (arrow). The true and false aortic lumina are identified. Note the stent extending through the aortic TL. E, Cross-sectional computed tomography image of the same patient at the 4-month follow-up. The arrow is directed at the previously placed LRA stent; note the bright and symmetric left renal contrast enhancement supporting adequate perfusion. (From Barnes DM, Williams D, Dasika N, et al. A single-center experience treating renal malperfusion after aortic dissection with central aortic fenestration and renal artery stenting. J Vasc Surg 2008;47:903–10.)

the distinction is important because it determines the therapeutic approach. Renal artery stenting is appropriate for static obstructions, and proximal central aortic fenestration or endograft repair is appropriate for a dynamic obstruction. It is clear that percutaneous aortic fenestration and renal artery stenting in aortic dissections with renal artery obstruction are technically feasible and adaptable to numerous clinical situations.

Acknowledgment

The data from this chapter primarily appeared in manuscript form in Barnes DM, et al. A single-center experience treating renal malperfusion after aortic dissection with central aortic fenestration and renal artery stenting. J Vasc Surg 2008;47:903–10.

REFERENCES

1. Lauterbach SR, Cambria RP, Brewster DC, et al. Contemporary management of aortic branch compromise resulting from acute aortic dissection. J Vasc Surg 2001;33:1185–92.
2. Girardi LN, Krieger KH, Lee LY, et al. Management strategies for type A dissection complicated by peripheral vascular malperfusion. Ann Thorac Surg 2004;77:1309–14.
3. Pate JW, Richardson RJ, Estridge CE. Acute aortic dissections. Ann Surg 1976;42:395–404.
4. Hirst AE, Johns VJ, Klime SW. Dissecting aneurysm of the aorta: a review of 505 cases. Medicine 1958;37:217–9.
5. Hagan PG, Nienaber CA, Isselbacher EM, et al. The International Registry of Acute Aortic Dissection (IRAD)—new insights into an old disease. JAMA 2000;283:897–903.
6. DeBakey ME, McCollum CH, Crawfor ES, et al. Dissection and dissecting aneurysms of the aorta: twenty-year follow-up of five hundred twenty-seven patients treated surgically. Surgery 1982;92:1118–34.
7. Slonim SM, Nyman U, Semba CP, et al. Aortic dissection: percutaneous management of ischemic complications with endovascular stents and balloon fenestration. J Vasc Surg 1996;23:241–53.
8. Fann JI, Sarris GE, Mitchell RS, et al. Treatment of patients with aortic dissection presenting with peripheral vascular complications. Ann Surg 1990;212:705–13.
9. Cambria RP, Brewster DC, Gertler J, et al. Vascular complications associated with spontaneous dissection. J Vasc Surg 1988;7:199–209.
10. Chavan A, Hausmann D, Dresler C, et al. Intravascular ultrasound-guided percutaneous fenestration of the intimal flap in the dissected aorta. Circulation 1997;96:2124–7.
11. Yagdi T, Atay Y, Engin C, et al. Impact of organ malperfusion on mortality and morbidity in acute A aortic dissections. J Card Surg 2006;21:363–9.
12. Henke PK, Williams DM, Upchurch GR Jr, et al. Acute limb ischemia associated with type B aortic dissection: clinical relevance and therapy. Surgery 2006;140:532–9.
13. Upchurch GR Jr, Nienaber C, Fattori R, Evangelista, et al. Acute aortic dissection presenting with primarily abdominal pain: a rare manifestation of a deadly disease. Ann Vasc Surg 2005;19:367–73.
14. Cambria RP. Surgical treatment of complicated distal aortic dissection. Semin Vasc Surg 2002;15:97–107.
15. Black JH, Cambria RP. Aortic dissection: perspectives for the vascular/endovascular surgeon – pathogenesis of malperfusion syndromes. In: Rutherford RB, ed. Vascular Surgery. 6th ed. Philadelphia: Elsevier Saunders;2005, pp. 1515–17.
16. Williams DM, LePage MA, Lee DY. The dissected aorta: Part I. Early anatomic changes in an in vitro model. Radiology 1997;203:23–31.
17. Williams DM, Lee DY, Hamilton BH, et al. The dissected aorta: Part III. Anatomy and radiologic diagnosis of branch-vessel compromise. Radiology 1997;203:37–44.
18. Barnes DM, Williams D, Dasika N, et al. A single-center experience treating renal malperfusion after aortic dissection with central aortic fenestration and renal artery stenting. J Vasc Surg 2008;47:903–10.
19. Miller DC, Mitchell RS, Oyer PE, et al. Independent determinants of operative mortality for patients with aortic dissections. Circulation 1984;70:I153–64.
20. Beregi JP, Haulon S, Otal P, et al. Endovascular treatment of acute complications associated with aortic dissection: midterm results from a multi-center study. J Endovasc Ther 2003;10:486–93.

21. Hsu RB, Ho YL, Wang SS, et al. Outcome of medical and surgical treatment in patients with acute type B aortic dissection. Ann Thorac Surg 2005;79:790–4.
22. Fann JI, Smith JA, Miller DC, et al. Surgical management of aortic dissection during a 30-year period. Circulation 1995;92:II113–21.
23. Shiiya N, Matsuzaki K, Kunihara T, et al. Management of vital organ malperfusion in acute aortic dissection: proposal of a mechanism-specific approach. Gen Thorac Cardiovasc Surg 2007;55:85–90.
24. Deeb GM, Williams DM, Bolling SF, et al. Surgical delay for acute type A dissection with malperfusion. Ann Thorac Surg 1997;64:1669–75.
25. Estrera AL, Miller CC, Goodrick J, et al. Update on outcomes of acute type B aortic dissection. Ann Thorac Surg 2007;83:S842–5.
26. Dake MD, Kato N, Mitchell RS, Semba et al. Endovascular stent-graft placement for the treatment of acute aortic dissection. N Engl J Med 1999;340:1546–52.
27. Dake MD, Wang DS. Will stent-graft repair emerge as treatment of choice for acute type B dissection? Semin Vasc Surg 2006;19:40–7.
28. Feezor RJ, Martin TD, Hess PJ, et al. Early outcomes after endovascular management of acute, complicated type B aortic dissection. J Vasc Surg 2009;49:561–7.

SECTION X

Abdominal Aortic Aneurysm I

45

Pharmacological Therapy: The Treatment of Small Abdominal Aortic Aneurysms

Mathew G. Longo, M.D. and B. Timothy Baxter, M.D.

INTRODUCTION

A 50% increase in the diameter of a vessel in comparison to its expected normal diameter is defined as an aneurysm.[1] The aneurysmal degeneration of the abdominal aorta and the iliac vessels, if untreated, is a frequent, lethal, age-related process. The prevalence of an abdominal aortic aneurysm (AAA) in men over the age of 60 years is anywhere from 4 to 8%, and in women of the same age group, 0.5% to 1.5%.[2-8] Risk factors consistent with AAA development include advanced age, cigarette smoking, male gender, and family history.[9-10]

Currently, the only treatment effective in preventing AAA rupture as well as aneurysm-related death is mechanical intervention through open operative aneurysmorrhaphy or endovascular aortic aneurysm repair. Ruptured AAAs and complications following repair of aortic aneurysms account for at least 15,000 deaths per year in the United States. The estimate of the actual mortality rate is potentially as high as 30,000 deaths per year.[8]

The approach to the management of AAAs is based on a surveillance protocol with the recommendation of elective surgical repair once the aneurysm reaches a size of 5.5 cm or greater or elective repair based upon rapid expansion or development of symptoms.[11] Currently, there are a lack of diagnostic biomarkers or effective nonsurgical therapies to halt the progression of early-stage disease. There is also a substantial amount of debate regarding the etiology of AAA initiation and growth. Several investigators are actively pursuing a more proactive strategy involving both the detection of small AAAs and therapeutic intervention using various pharmacologic therapies to retard or halt AAA growth. There are three important features of AAAs that lend themselves to this approach:

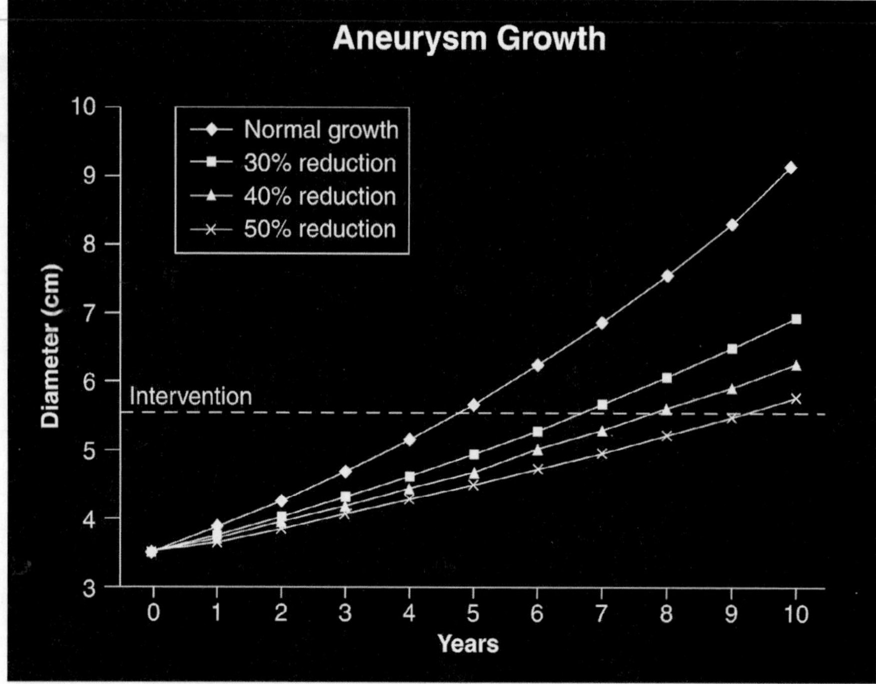

Figure 45-1. Average change in aneurysm diameter as a function of time is indicated by the diamond markers. The other growth rates show the effects of a medical therapy that inhibited growth by 30% (square markers), 40% (triangle markers), and 50% (x markers).

1. Inexpensive and accurate methods for detection.
2. Long periods of surveillance prior to intervention.
3. Life expectancy of the affected population.

With the knowledge that small AAAs grow anywhere from 0.3 to 0.5 cm per year, a 50% decrease in the aortic expansion rate of 3 cm AAA would stretch the time from initial diagnosis to surgical intervention to longer than a decade[12-13] (Figure 45–1).

PATHOGENESIS OF AORTIC ANEURYSMS

In an attempt to devise various medical treatments for AAAs, the therapies have been targeted to address one or multiple theories regarding the pathogenesis of AAAs. Most investigators believe that there is a combination of inflammation and/or an abnormal immune response, proteolytic degradation of the aortic wall, and unique biomechanical wall stresses placed on the infrarenal abdominal aorta and that these are contributory elements to aortic aneurysm development and expansion.

Inflammation

Samples of aortic aneurysm tissue taken at the time of operative repair or autopsy demonstrate an inflammatory cell infiltrate consisting of T cells, B cells, dendritic cells, plasma cells, and macrophages.[14-16] The cells are located throughout the intima, media, and adventitia. This contrasts with samples of normal aortic tissue or atherosclerotic aortic tissue, which typically shows only T cells and macrophages located within the intima and media.[16] Furthermore, as aneurysms increase in size, there is a corresponding increase in the inflammatory cell infiltrate.[17] The stimulus for the recruitment of inflammatory cells into the aorta is unknown. It continues to be an area of ongoing research. Theories behind the recruitment of inflammatory cells range from a belief that the immune response is a nonspecific versus an autoimmune process driven by immunoglobulin G and plasma cells.[18] Other theories rest with the belief that *Chlamydia pneumoniae* infection is a contributor to the formation of AAAs.[19] However, there is a high prevalence of chlamydial infection in the general population, and strong evidence for the specificity of this agent in the development of AAAs is lacking.[20] Another theory of inflammatory cell recruitment is based on animal research. It involves the action of the chemokines, interleukin-8 (IL-8), and monocyte chemoattractant protein-1.[21] These are upregulated in animal aneurysm models, and these chemokines are present in the aortic smooth muscle prior to the influx of inflammatory cells during experimental AAA development.[22] In human AAA tissue, there are also noted to be greater amounts of both IL-8 and monocyte chemoattractant protein-1.[21]

Once inflammatory cells are present in the aorta, they dictate both the coordination and the direction of the ongoing immune response. They orchestrate this response through the action of cytokines, which are produced by both invading inflammatory cells and the resident of the mesenchymal cells. Based on studies of AAA tissue culture explants, the overexpression of the proinflammatory cytokines such as tumor necrosis factor alpha (TNF-γ), IL-6, and IL-1 β have been noted.[23-24] The Th-1 cytokine, interferon gamma (IFN-γ), has also been implicated in human AAA development. Most notably, elevated circulating levels of IFN-γ appear to correlate with more rapid aneurysm expansion.[25]

The presence of inflammatory cells and the upregulation of various cytokines also result in decreased medial smooth muscle cell density. AAA specimens taken at the time of open repair reveal a paucity of medial smooth muscle cells when compared with normal and atherosclerotic aortas.[26-27] As smooth muscle cells are depleted, the normal deposition and maintenance of the aorta's normal extracellular matrix are disrupted. Inflammatory cells also alter the expression of various prostaglandins, most notably prostaglandin-E_2 (PGE_2). In human aortic aneurysm tissue, there is expression of cyoloxygenase-2 (Cox-2), localizing primarily to infiltrating macrophages. Cox-2 is thought to be responsible for the increased PGE_2 levels found in human aortic aneurysm tissue as well as the increased levels of PGE_2 in conditioned media from aortic tissue culture.[28-29] PGE_2 has the ability to alter matrix metalloproteinase (MMP) activity, cytokine expression, and smooth muscle cell viability. The large influx of inflammatory cells also increases the number of reactive oxygen species present within the aortic wall. Reactive oxygen species combined with increased oxidative damage are noted to be markedly increased in human aortic aneurysm tissue when compared with normal tissue.[30-31] Finally, the invading inflammatory cells produce proteases as well as induce the surrounding mesenchymal cells to produce proteases. These proteases have the ability to destroy the extracellular matrix structures necessary for maintaining aortic wall integrity. Through the disruption of aortic wall integrity, there is a decrease in both the tensile strength of the aortic wall and the elasticity inherent in the structure of the wall.

Proteolytic Degradation in the Aortic Wall Connective Tissue

Collagen and elastin combine both tensile strength and elasticity in the aortic wall, allowing the effective transport of blood and the transmission of pulsatile energy. Collagen is present within both the aortic media and the adventitia, and it is responsible primarily for imparting tensile strength to the aorta.[32] Elastin comprises approximately 50% of the dry weight of a normal aorta.[33] It is responsible for the aorta's viscous and elastic properties.[34] Disruption of these two proteins is necessary for aortic aneurysm pathogenesis, and a substantial amount of research has been dedicated to studying the enzymes capable of destroying these two connective tissues.

The MMPs are a family of structurally related enzymes capable of digesting various components of the extracellular matrix. The normal physiologic function of these enzymes is thought to be extracellular matrix remodeling. However, they also contribute to cell motility and cell signaling. MMP-9 is one of the most extensively studied MMPs in aortic aneurysm research. It has the ability to degrade both elastin as well as collagen that has been partially hydrolyzed. MMP-2 also possesses the ability to degrade elastin and intact fibular collagen.[35] MMP-12 is also seen to be elevated in human aortic aneurysm tissue when compared with normal controls.[36] There are alterations in other MMPs within aortic aneurysms. However, a definitive role has not been delineated for these enzymes. The cysteine protease, cystatin C, could also play a role in aortic aneurysm development, because it appears to be reduced in human aortic aneurysm tissue.[37] Research has also been devoted to studying the serine proteases, particularly neutrophil elastase. The role of this protease, as well as those proteases from the plasminogen activator family, has not had its exact role in aortic aneurysm formation determined.[38]

Biomechanical Wall Stress

The infrarenal abdominal aorta is the most common location for aneurysm development throughout the arterial tree. This portion of the aorta is subject to unique flow patterns, primarily related to the reflection of pressure waves from the aortic bifurcation and the presence of both large renal and splenic artery takeoffs resulting in disturbed flow patterns.[39] Furthermore, the elastin-to-collagen ratio decreases as one moves distally down the aorta. This translates into increased stiffness in the distal aspect of the aorta.[40] Furthermore, there is an absence of the vasa vasorum in the abdominal aortic media, which when combined with the presence of a thick intraluminal thrombus (as frequently seen in aortic aneurysms), results in impaired oxygen and nutrient delivery to the aortic wall.[41]

Aortic wall stress is one of the key factors involved in the rupture of aortic aneurysms. The simplistic approach would be to utilize the law of Laplace in which wall tension is directly proportional to the product of the radius (AAA diameter) and its intraluminal pressure (patient blood pressure). However, because AAAs are often asymmetric and thick-walled and come in a variety of shapes, researchers are currently developing new methods to noninvasively determine the wall stress distribution and correlate this with rupture risk.[42-43] Furthermore, the unique conditions present in the infrarenal abdominal aorta resulting in abnormal hemodynamic flow patterns may also impact the expression of MMPs and reactive oxygen species as well as macrophage infiltration and antioxidative gene expression.[44-47]

PHARMACOLOGIC TREATMENT OF ABDOMINAL AORTIC ANEURYSMS

Each of the previously mentioned theories for AAA development and progression has a corresponding medical treatment to address offending elements (Tables 45–1 and 45–2). In conjunction with the addition of various medical treatments to reduce aneurysm growth, smoking cessation remains a hallmark in attempting to decrease aneurysm development and expansion. Smoking confers a 2.5 times greater risk for AAA development than coronary artery disease.[48] Furthermore, greater than 90% of all aortic aneurysm patients relate a history of smoking.[49] Smoking is also consistently demonstrated to be a factor positively associated with aneurysm growth in studies looking at risk factors for aneurysm development.[50]

Beta Blockers

The most studied of the various pharmaceutical therapies have been beta blockers. Studies have included the medications propranolol, atenolol, and metoprolol. There have been three randomized controlled trials as well as five prospective cohort studies.[50-57] Beta blockers are believed to have beneficial effects in decreasing aneurysm disease due to the biochemical effects of beta blockade of matrix proteins within the aortic wall and alteration of the hemodynamic properties in the infrarenal abdominal aorta. However, the three randomized controlled trials failed to demonstrate a significant difference in growth rates on either an individual trial basis or a meta-analysis of all subjects in these trials. Beta blockers in cohort studies did demonstrate a significant reduction in growth rate when the results of the five trials were pooled together. Individually, only two of the trials demonstrated a statistically significant reduction of growth rates in aortic aneurysms when compared with the control population of interest within the trials.[58] Of note, when looking at the effect of beta blockers on aneurysm growth, there is some question about the compliance of the subjects within the trial owing to the fact that beta blockade has been demonstrated to negatively affect the quality of life.

Angiotensin Converting Enzyme Inhibitors and Angiotensin Receptor Blockers, Antihypertensives

Angiotensin converting enzyme (ACE) inhibitors have the ability to both stimulate as well as inhibit matrix metalloproteinases, depending on the cell type. Angiotensin receptor blockers (ARBs) do not have a direct effect on MMPs. In animal models, ACE inhibitors (captopril) do demonstrate the ability to prevent aneurysm formation.[59] In a single prospective cohort trial, patients treated with ACE inhibitors did not have the statistically significant difference in aneurysm growth rates when compared with controls.[54] However, there was a trend toward decreased growth rates. In animal studies, the ARB losartan demonstrated the prevention of aneurysm formation.[60-62] No human trials have yet been done with this agent. There have also been prospective cohort trials done for diuretics and calcium channel blockers.[51] Treatment with either of these agents failed to demonstrate any statistically significant decrease in aneurysm growth rates.

Statins and Anti-inflammatory Agents

Statins are suspected of decreasing aneurysm growth rates based on their anti-inflammatory properties. There is evidence suggesting that statin therapy inhibits inflammatory cell

TABLE 45-1. Description of Included Studies

First Author, Year	Study Design	Agent (Number of Participants)	Type of Control (Number of Controls)	Dosage (SD)	Device	Mean Follow-up Duration in Months	
						Intevention	Control
Beta blockers							
Lindholt [21] 1999	RCT	Propanolol (30)	Placebo (24)	40 mg/bid	US	24	24
PATI [22] 2002	RCT	Propanolol [276]	Placebo (272)	20–240 mg/d	US	30	30
Wilmink [33] 2000	RCT	Propanolol (256)	No propanolol (221)	40 mg/d	US†	34‡	33‡
Wilmink [23] 2002	Cohort†	Beta blockers* (77)	No beta blockers (255)	NR	US	48	48
Lindholt [24] 2001	Cohort	Beta blockers* (25)	No beta blockers (112)	NR	US	28	28
Gadowski [25] 1994	Cohort	Propanolol (21), Atenolol (10), Metoprolol (7)	No beta blockers (83)	Propanolol 92 mg/d (38), Atenolol 68 mg/d (30), Metoprolol 80 mg/d (21)	US	43	43
Leach [26] 1988	Cohort	Propanolol (6), Selective beta blockers* (6)	No beta blockers (15)	Propanolol 20–80 mg/d	US	27	38
Biancari [27] 2002	Cohort	Beta blockers* (17)	No beta blockers (24)	NR	US	87	87
Other antihypertensive agents							
Wilmink [23]†2002	Cohort†	diuretics* (54)	No diuretics (278)	NR	US	48	48
Wilmink [23] 2002	Cohort†	ACE inhibitors* (24)	No ACE inhibitors (308)	NR	US	48	48
Wilmink [23] 2002	Cohort†	Ca channel blockers* (48)	No Ca channel blockers (284)	NR	US	48	48
Brady [34] 2004	Cohort	antihypertensive* (932)	No antihypertensive (765)	NR	US	NR	NR

(Continued)

TABLE 45-1. Description of Included Studies *(Continued)*

First Author, Year	Study Design	Agent (Number of Participants)	Type of Control (Number of Controls)	Dosage (SD)	Device	Mean Follow-up Duration in Months	
						Intevention	Control
Antibiotics							
Mosorin [28] 2001	RCT	Doxycycline (17)	Placebo (15)	150 mg/d	US	18	18
Vammen [29] 2001	RCT	Roxithromycin (40)	Placebo (44)	300 mg/d	US	18	18
Anti-inflammatory agents							
Schouten [30] 2006	Cohort	Simvastatin (24), atorvastatin (19), fluvastatin (11), pravastatin (5)	No statins (91)	.NR	US	34	38
Sukhija [31] 2006	Cohort	Simvastatin (31), atorvastatin (44)	No statins (55)	20–80 mg/d	CT	23	24
Walton [32] 1999	Cohort	NSAID* (15)	No NSAID (63)	NR	US	>12	>12

*Without precision
†Same cohort study
‡Data provided directly by the authors
NR Not reported
doi:10.1371/journal.pone.0001895.t001

TABLE 45-2. Annual Growth Rate and Growth Rate Difference

First Author, Year	Study Design	Growth Rate (SD) in mm/year		Growth Rate Difference (mm/year)	95% CI	
		Intervention	Control			
Beta blockers						
Lindholt [21] 1999	RCT	3.12 (2.5)†	2.84 (2.4)†	0.28	−0.65	1.21
PATI [22] 2002	RCT	2.2 (2.9)	2.6 (3.0)	−0.40	−0.89	0.09
Wilmink [33] 2000	RCT	0.06 (0.6)	0.1 (0.6)	−0.04	−0.16	0.08
Wilmink [23] 2002	Cohort*	0.8 (2.6)	0.7 (3.2)	0.10	−0.62	0.82
Lindholt [24] 2001	Cohort	1.6 (1.2)	2.5 (2.1)	−0.90‡	−1.54	−0.26
Gadowski [25] 1994	Cohort	3.0 (3.9)	4.4 (4.2)	−1.40	−2.93	0.13
Leach [26] 1988	Cohort	1.7 (2.7)	4.4 (5.0)	−2.70	−5.69	0.29
Biancari [27] 2002	Cohort	1.56 (1.8)†	2.27 (1.9)†	−0.71‡	−1.42	0.00
Other antihypertensive agents						
Wilmink [23] 2002 (diuretic)	Cohort*	0.8 (2.6)	0.7 (3.4)	0.10	−0.71	0.91
Wilmink [23] 2002 (ACEI)	Cohort*	0.02 (1.6)	0.8 (2.6)	−0.78	−1.58	0.02
Wilmink [23] 2002 (Calcium blockers)	Cohort*	0.5 (2.1)	0.8 (2.5)	−0.30	−0.97	0.37
Brady [34] 2004 (antihypertensives)	Cohort	NR	NR	−0.11	−0.34	0.12
Antibiotics						
Mosorin [28] 2001 (doxycycline)	RCT	1.5 (2.2)	3.0 (4.3)	−1.50	−3.93	0.93
Vammen [29] 2001 (roxithromycin)	RCT	1.56 (3.6)	2.75 (4.3)	−1.19	−3.25	0.87
Anti-inflammatory agents						
Schouten [30] 2006 (statins)	Cohort	2.0 (1.9)	3.6 (2.9)	−1.60‡	−2.38	−0.82
Sukhija [31] 2006 (statins)	Cohort	−0.52 (3.0)	4.0 (3.0)	−4.52‡	−6.10	−2.94
Walton [32] 1999 (NSAIDS)	Cohort	2.5 (2.2)†	3.8 (2.4)†	−1.30‡	−2.59	−0.01

*Same cohort study
†Data provided directly by the authors
‡p value<0.05
NR Not reported
doi:10.1371/journal.pone.0001B95.t002
Idris G, Daniel P, Diane L, Jacques C, Ghali WA. The efficacy of pharmacotherapy for decreasing the expansion rate of abdominal aortic aneurysms: a systematic review and meta-analysis. PloS one 2008;3(3)e1895.

activation. It also acts through reduction in matrix metalloproteinase activity. Combining these elements with the known ability of statin therapy to reduce progression of atherosclerosis and improve overall outcomes in cardiovascular disease, it stands to reason that statins could influence aneurysm formation and progression. Two cohort trials utilizing simvastatin, atorvastatin, pravastatin, and fluvastatin demonstrated a statistically significant decrease in aneurysmal growth rates when compared with controls that lacked statin treatment.[63-64] In human aortic aneurysm specimens exploited for organ culture, the addition of cerivastatin was able to greatly reduce the tissue levels of both total and active MMP-9 in a concentration-dependent manner.[65] Furthermore, in patients pretreated with simvastatin prior to undergoing open aneurysm repair tissue, sampling demonstrated decreased levels of MMP-9.[66] And in animal models, there was noted to be a reduction in aneurysm development as well as aneurysm size when subjects were treated with simvastatin.[67]

There has been one single trial, a prospective cohort trial, evaluating the action of nonsteroidal anti-inflammatory drugs (NSAIDs) on aneurysm growth rates. Theoretically, the addition of NSAIDs would impact PGE_2 levels, thus having an indirect effect on matrix metalloproteinase activity, cytokine expression, as well as smooth muscle cell viability. In the prospective cohort evaluating the efficacy of NSAIDs, there was noted to be a statistically significant decrease in aneurysm growth rates favoring the NSAID group over the control group.[68] Indomethacin, a nonspecific cyclo-oxygenase inhibitor, has been shown to reduce PGE_2 in aortic tissue cultures as well as decrease the size of experimental aneurysm formation in an elastase infusion model of aneurysm development.[69]

Antibiotics

Macrolides. Macrolides were initially suggested as a means of reducing aortic aneurysm growth as well as preventing the development of AAAs based on the belief that AAA progression is enhanced by secondary infection within the aortic wall by *Chlamydia pneumoniae*. The belief was that secondary treatment of the chlamydial infection could slow both the progression of atherosclerosis as well as the damage within the aortic wall and subsequent aneurysm growth. There has been one randomized controlled trial investigating this hypothesis[70] in which 40 patients received roxithromycin and 44 patients received a placebo agent. There was no statistical significance found between the two patient groups; however, there was a trend toward decreased aneurysm growth in the patients receiving roxithromycin. Interestingly, there was no correlation between the chlamydial titers and roxithromycin's ability to inhibit aneurysm expansion noted in this trial.

Tetracyclines. Tetracyclines have been studied because of their known inhibitory properties of the matrix metalloproteinases. The tetracycline, doxycycline, was demonstrated to suppress aortic wall MMP activity, elastin degradation, and aneurysm development in the elastase-induced rat model as well as in a murine aneurysm model utilizing calcium chloride.[71-72] In human studies, patients receiving doxycycline prior to open repair were demonstrated to have a statistically significant decrease in the MMP-9 levels in the aortic wall when compared with untreated patients.[73] Furthermore, patients treated with doxycycline were also demonstrated with have a statistically significant decrease in their plasma MMP-9 levels when compared with their baseline pretreatment levels.[74] In a small randomized controlled trial in which 17 patients were treated with doxycycline and 15 patients were given a placebo, there was noted to be a decrease in the aneurysm growth rates.[75] However, this did not achieve statistical significance. It should be noted, though, that based on the randomized control of trials of the macrolides and tetracyclines, Level B evidence does exist, suggesting that these agents will decrease the rate of aneurysm expansion (Table 45–3).

TABLE 45-3. RESULTS OF INTERVENTIONS ON ABDOMINAL AORTIC ANEURYSM GROWTH

Intervention	Reference(s)	Effect on AAA Growth	Level of Evidence	Class of Recommendation
Beta blockers	50–58	No inhibition	A	III
Macrolides	70	Inhibition	B	IIa
Tetracycline*	71–75	Inhibition	B	IIa
Statins	63–67	Inhibition	B	IIb
ACE inhibitors	54, 59	No inhibition	B and C	IIb
AR blockers	60–62	Animal data	C	IIb

*Inhibition at 6 and 12 months after 3 months of treatment.
Idris G, Daniel P, Diane L, Jacques C, Ghali WA. The efficacy of pharmacotherapy for decreasing the expansion rate of abdominal aortic aneurysms: a systematic review and meta-analysis. PloS one 2008;3(3)e1895.

CONCLUSION

As our knowledge of aneurysm development and progression increases, the ability to design an algorithm for the medical treatment of AAAs should become clearer. Currently, the medical treatments for small AAAs have involved the utilization of existing drugs not originally designed for halting aneurysm progression. Furthermore, the theories behind the utilization of these agents have been to nonspecifically target a broad area believed responsible for aneurysm development. Although there has been mixed success with these agents, the eventual hope is to develop a medication to specifically inhibit one or several of the seminal steps toward aneurysm development and progression. Thus, high-risk individuals could be treated prior to aneurysm formation and those persons found with a small aneurysm could begin pharmacologic treatment in an effort to stave off operative therapy.

REFERENCES

1. Johnston KW, Rutherford RB, Tilson MD, et al. Suggested standards for reporting on arterial aneurysms. Subcommittee on Reporting Standards for Arterial Aneurysms, Ad Hoc Committee on Reporting Standards, Society for Vascular Surgery and North American Chapter, International Society for Cardiovascular Surgery. J Vasc Surg 1991;13:452–8.
2. Wilmink TB, Quick CR, Hubbard CS, et al. The influence of screening on the incidence of ruptured abdominal aortic aneurysms. J Vasc Surg 1999;30:203–8.
3. Lederle FA, Johnson GR, Wilson SE, et al. The Aneurysm Detection and Management Study Screening Program: validation cohort and final results. Aneurysm Detection and Management Veterans Affairs Cooperative Study Investigators. Arch Intern Med 2000;160: 1425–30.
4. Ashton HA, Buxton MJ, Day NE, et al. The Multicentre Aneurysm Screening Study (MASS) into the effect of abdominal aortic aneurysm screening on mortality in men: a randomised controlled trial. Lancet 2002;360:1531–9.
5. Lawrence-Brown MM, Norman PE, Jamrozik K, et al. Initial results of ultrasound screening for aneurysm of the abdominal aorta in Western Australia: relevance for endoluminal treatment of aneurysm disease. Cardiovasc Surg 2001;9:234–40.
6. Wilmink AB, Quick CR. Epidemiology and potential for prevention of abdominal aortic aneurysm. Br J Surg 1998;85:155–62.
7. Lindholt JS, Juul S, Fasting H, et al. Hospital costs and benefits of screening for abdominal aortic aneurysms. Results from a randomised population screening trial. Eur J Vasc Endovasc Surg 2002;23:55–60.

8. Kent KC, Zwolak RM, Jaff MR, et al. Screening for abdominal aortic aneurysm: a consensus statement. J Vasc Surg 2004;39:267–9.
9. Lederle FA, Johnson GR, Wilson SE, et al. Prevalence and associations of abdominal aortic aneurysm detected through screening. Aneurysm Detection and Management (ADAM) Veterans Affairs Cooperative Study Group. Ann Intern Med 1997;126:441–9.
10. Chang JB, Stein TA, Liu JP, et al. Risk factors associated with rapid growth of small abdominal aortic aneurysms. Surgery 1997;121:117–22.
11. Brewster DC, Cronenwett JL, Hallett JW Jr, et al. Guidelines for the treatment of abdominal aortic aneurysms. Report of a subcommittee of the Joint Council of the American Association for Vascular Surgery and Society for Vascular Surgery. J Vasc Surg 2003;37:1106–17.
12. United Kingdom Small Aneurysm Trial Participants. Long-term outcomes of immediate repair compared with surveillance of small abdominal aortic aneurysms. N Engl J Med 2002;346:1445–52.
13. Lederle FA, Wilson SE, Johnson GR, et al. Immediate repair compared with surveillance of small abdominal aortic aneurysms. N Engl J Med 2002;346:1437–44.
14. Beckman EN. Plasma cell infiltrates in atherosclerotic abdominal aortic aneurysms. Am J Clin Pathol 1986;85:21–4.
15. Bobryshev YV, Lord RS, Parsson H. Immunophenotypic analysis of the aortic aneurysm wall suggests that vascular dendritic cells are involved in immune responses. Cardiovasc Surg 1998;6:240–9.
16. Koch AE, Haines GK, Rizzo RJ, et al. Human abdominal aortic aneurysms. Immunophenotypic analysis suggesting an immune-mediated response. Am J Pathol 1990;137:1199–213.
17. Freestone T, Turner RJ, Coady A, et al. Inflammation and matrix metalloproteinases in the enlarging abdominal aortic aneurysm. Arterioscler Thromb Vasc Biol 1995;15:1145–51.
18. Brophy CM, Reilly JM, Smith GJ, et al. The role of inflammation in nonspecific abdominal aortic aneurysm disease. Ann Vasc Surg 1991;5:229–33.
19. Juvonen J, Juvonen T, Laurila A, et al. Demonstration of *Chlamydia pneumoniae* in the walls of abdominal aortic aneurysms. J Vasc Surg 1997;25:499–505.
20. Kalayoglu MV, Libby P, Byrne GI. *Chlamydia pneumoniae* as an emerging risk factor in cardiovascular disease. JAMA 2002;288:2724–31.
21. Koch AE, Kunkel SL, Pearce WH, et al. Enhanced production of the chemotactic cytokines interleukin-8 and monocyte chemoattractant protein-1 in human abdominal aortic aneurysms. Am J Pathol 1993;142:1423–31.
22. Colonnello JS, Hance KA, Shames ML, et al. Transient exposure to elastase induces mouse aortic wall smooth muscle cell production of MCP-1 and RANTES during development of experimental aortic aneurysm. J Vasc Surg. 2003;38:138–46.
23. Szekanecz Z, Shah MR, Pearce WH, et al. Human atherosclerotic abdominal aortic aneurysms produce interleukin (IL)-6 and interferon-gamma but not IL-2 and IL-4: the possible role for IL-6 and interferon-gamma in vascular inflammation. Agents Actions 1994;42:159–62.
24. Newman KM, Jean-Claude J, Li H, et al. Cytokines that activate proteolysis are increased in abdominal aortic aneurysms. Circulation 1994;90:II224–7.
25. Juvonen J, Surcel HM, Satta J, et al. Elevated circulating levels of inflammatory cytokines in patients with abdominal aortic aneurysm. Arterioscler Thromb Vasc Biol 1997;17:2843–7.
26. Henderson EL, Geng YJ, Sukhova GK, et al. Death of smooth muscle cells and expression of mediators of apoptosis by T lymphocytes in human abdominal aortic aneurysms. Circulation 1999;99:96–104.
27. Lopez-Candales A, Holmes DR, Liao S, et al. Decreased vascular smooth muscle cell density in medial degeneration of human abdominal aortic aneurysms. Am J Pathol 1997;150:993–1007.
28. Holmes DR, Wester W, Thompson RW, et al. Prostaglandin E2 synthesis and cyclooxygenase expression in abdominal aortic aneurysms. J Vasc Surg 1997;25:810–5.

29. Walton LJ, Franklin IJ, Bayston T, et al. Inhibition of prostaglandin E2 synthesis in abdominal aortic aneurysms: implications for smooth muscle cell viability, inflammatory processes, and the expansion of abdominal aortic aneurysms. Circulation 1999;100:48–54.
30. Li PF, Dietz R, von Harsdorf R. Reactive oxygen species induce apoptosis of vascular smooth muscle cell. FEBS Lett 1997;404:249–52.
31. Rajagopalan S, Meng XP, Ramasamy S, et al. Reactive oxygen species produced by macrophage-derived foam cells regulate the activity of vascular matrix metalloproteinases in vitro. Implications for atherosclerotic plaque stability. J Clin Invest 1996;98:2572–9.
32. Dobrin PB, Baker WH, Gley WC. Elastolytic and collagenolytic studies of arteries. Implications for the mechanical properties of aneurysms. Arch Surg 1984;119:405–9.
33. Parks WC, Pierce RA, Lee KA, et al. Elastin. Adv Mol Cell Biol 1993;6:133–82.
34. Boucek R. Contributions of Elastin and Collagen Organization to Passive Mechanical Properties of Arterial Tissue. Boca Raton, FL: CRC Press: 1988.
35. Aimes RT, Quigley JP. Matrix metalloproteinase-2 is an interstitial collagenase. Inhibitor-free enzyme catalyzes the cleavage of collagen fibrils and soluble native type I collagen generating the specific 3/4- and 1/4-length fragments. J Biol Chem 1995;270:5872–6.
36. Curci JA, Liao S, Huffman MD, et al. Expression and localization of macrophage elastase (matrix metalloproteinase-12) in abdominal aortic aneurysms. J Clin Invest 1998;102: 1900–10.
37. Shi GP, Sukhova GK, Grubb A, et al. Cystatin C deficiency in human atherosclerosis and aortic aneurysms. J Clin Invest 1999;104:1191–7.
38. Carmeliet P, Moons L, Lijnen R, et al. Urokinase-generated plasmin activates matrix metalloproteinases during aneurysm formation. Nat Genet 1997;17:439–44.
39. Moore JE Jr, Ku DN, Zarins CK, et al. Pulsatile flow visualization in the abdominal aorta under differing physiologic conditions: implications for increased susceptibility to atherosclerosis. J Biomech Eng 1992;114:391–7.
40. Peterson L, Jensen RE, Parnell J. Mechanical properties of arteries in vivo. Circ Res 1960;8: 622–33.
41. Vorp DA, Lee PC, Wang DH, et al. Association of intraluminal thrombus in abdominal aortic aneurysm with local hypoxia and wall weakening. J Vasc Surg 2001;34:291–9.
42. Vorp DA, Raghavan ML, Webster MW. Mechanical wall stress in abdominal aortic aneurysm: influence of diameter and asymmetry. J Vasc Surg 1998;27:632–9.
43. Raghavan ML, Vorp DA, Federle MP, et al. Wall stress distribution on three-dimensionally reconstructed models of human abdominal aortic aneurysm. J Vasc Surg 2000;31:760–9.
44. Sho E, Sho M, Hoshina K, et al. Hemodynamic forces regulate mural macrophage infiltration in experimental aortic aneurysms. Exp Mol Pathol 2004;76:108–16.
45. Nakahashi TK, Hoshina K, Tsao PS, et al. Flow loading induces macrophage antioxidative gene expression in experimental aneurysms. Arterioscler Thromb Vasc Biol 2002;22: 2017–22.
46. Grote K, Flach I, Luchtefeld M, et al. Mechanical stretch enhances mRNA expression and proenzyme release of matrix metalloproteinase-2 (MMP-2) via NAD(P)H oxidase-derived reactive oxygen species. Circ Res 2003;92:e80–6.
47. Howard AB, Alexander RW, Nerem RM, et al. Cyclic strain induces an oxidative stress in endothelial cells. Am J Physiol 1997;272:C421–7.
48. Lederle FA, Nelson DB, Joseph AM. Smokers' relative risk for aortic aneurysm compared with other smoking-related diseases: a systematic review. J Vasc Surg 2003;38:329–34.
49. Powell JT, Worrell P, MacSweeney ST, et al. Smoking as a risk factor for abdominal aortic aneurysm. Ann N Y Acad Sci 1996;800:246–8.
50. Lindholt JS, Heegaard NH, Vammen S, et al. Smoking, but not lipids, lipoprotein(a) and antibodies against oxidised LDL, is correlated to the expansion of abdominal aortic aneurysms. Eur J Vasc Endovasc Surg 2001;21:51–6.
51. Brady AR, Thompson SG, Fowkes FG, et al. Abdominal aortic aneurysm expansion: risk factors and time intervals for surveillance. Circulation 2004;110:16–21.

52. Propranolol Aneurysm Trial Investigators. Propranolol for small abdominal aortic aneurysms: results of a randomized trial. J Vasc Surg 2002;35:72–9.
53. Wilmink AB, Hubbard CS, Day NE, Quick CR. Effect of propranolol on expansion of abdominal aortic aneurysms: a randomized study abstract. Br J Surg 2000;87:499.
54. Wilmink AB, Vardulaki KA, Hubbard CS, et al. Are anti-hypertensive drugs associated with abdominal aortic aneurysms? J Vasc Surg 2002;36:751–7.
55. Gadowski GR, Pilcher DB, Ricci MA. Abdominal aortic aneurysm expansion rate: effect of size and beta-adrenergic blockade. J Vasc Surg 1994;19:727–31.
56. Leach SD, Toole AL, Stern H, et al. Effect of beta-adrenergic blockade on the growth rate of abdominal aortic aneurysms. Arch Surg 1988;123:606–9.
57. Biancari F, Mosorin M, Anttila V, et al. Ten year outcome of patients with very small abdominal aortic aneurysm. Am J Surg 2002;183:53–5.
58. Guessous I, Periard D, Lorenzetti D, et al. The efficacy of pharmacotherapy for decreasing the expansion rate of abdominal aortic aneurysms: a systematic review and meta-analysis. PLoS ONE 2008;3: e1895.
59. Liao S, Miralles M, Kelley BJ, et al. Suppression of experimental abdominal aortic aneurysms in the rat by treatment with angiotensin-converting enzyme inhibitors. J Vasc Surg 2001;33:1057–64.
60. Neptune ER, Frischmeyer PA, Arking DE, et al. Dysregulation of TGF-beta activation contributes to pathogenesis in Marfan syndrome. Nat Genet 2003;33:407–11.
61. Habashi JP, Judge DP, Holm TM, et al. Losartan, an AT1 antagonist, prevents aortic aneurysm in a mouse model of Marfan syndrome. Science 2006;312:117–21.
62. Recruiting comparison of two medications aimed at slowing aortic root enlargement in individuals with Marfan syndrome. Available at: http://clinicaltrials.gov/ct/search?term=marfans+syndrome
63. Schouten O, van Laanen JH, Boersma E, et al. Statins are associated with a reduced infrarenal abdominal aortic aneurysm growth. Eur J Vasc Endovasc Surg 2006;32:21–6.
64. Sukhija R, Aronow WS, Sandhu R, et al. Mortality and size of abdominal aortic aneurysm at long-term follow-up of patients not treated surgically and treated with and without statins. Am J Cardiol 2006;97:279–80.
65. Nagashima H, Aoka Y, Sakomura Y, et al. A 3-hydroxy-3-methylglutaryl coenzyme A reductase inhibitor, cerivastatin, suppresses production of matrix metalloproteinase-9 in human abdominal aortic aneurysm wall. J Vasc Surg 2002;36:158–63.
66. Evans J, Powell JT, Schwalbe E, et al. Simvastatin attenuates the activity of matrix metalloprotease-9 in aneurysmal aortic tissue. Eur J Vasc Endovasc Surg 2007;34:302–3.
67. Steinmetz EF, Buckley C, Shames ML, et al. Treatment with simvastatin suppresses the development of experimental abdominal aortic aneurysms in normal and hypercholesterolemic mice. Ann Surg 2005;241:92–101.
68. Walton LJ, Franklin IJ, Bayston T, et al. Inhibition of prostaglandin E2 synthesis in abdominal aortic aneurysms: implications for smooth muscle cell viability, inflammatory processes, and the expansion of abdominal aortic aneurysms. Circulation 1999;100: 48–54.
69. Miralles M, Wester W, Sicard GA, et al. Indomethacin inhibits expansion of experimental aortic aneurysms via inhibition of the cox2 isoform of cyclooxygenase. J Vasc Surg 1999;29:884–92.
70. Vammen S, Lindholt JS, Ostergaard L, et al. Randomized double-blind controlled trial of roxithromycin for prevention of abdominal aortic aneurysm expansion. Br J Surg 2001;88:1066–72.
71. Petrinec D, Holmes DR, Liao S, et al. Suppression of experimental aneurysmal degeneration with chemically modified tetracycline derivatives. Ann N Y Acad Sci 1996;800: 263–5.
72. Longo GM, Xiong W, Greiner TC, et al. Matrix metalloproteinases 2 and 9 work in concert to produce aortic aneurysms. J Clin Invest 2002;110:625–32.

73. Curci JA, Mao D, Bohner DG, et al. Preoperative treatment with doxycycline reduces aortic wall expression and activation of matrix metalloproteinases in patients with abdominal aortic aneurysms. J Vasc Surg 2000;31:325–42.
74. Baxter BT, Pearce WH, Waltke EA, et al. Prolonged administration of doxycycline in patients with small asymptomatic abdominal aortic aneurysms: report of a prospective (Phase II) multicenter study. J Vasc Surg 2002;36:1–12.
75. Mosorin M, Juvonen J, Biancari F, et al. Use of doxycycline to decrease the growth rate of abdominal aortic aneurysms: a randomized, double-blind, placebo-controlled pilot study. J Vasc Surg 2001;34606–10.

46

Abdominal Aortic Aneurysm Disease and Exercise

Maureen M. Tedesco, M.D., Julie J. White, B.S., and Ronald L. Dalman, M.D.

Rupture of unrecognized or untreated abdominal aortic aneurysms (AAAs) is a common cause of death for many older Americans. After reviewing evidence that AAA screening may reduce related mortality by 43% in men aged 65 to 75 years, this benefit was added to the "Welcome to Medicare" physical examination beginning at age 65. Through such screening and related public awareness campaigns, thousands of unsuspecting and otherwise healthy patients have become aware of AAAs early in the course of their disease. Indeed, more than 90% of AAAs detected through screening fall below the 4.5-to 5.5-cm intervention thresholds currently recommended for women and men, respectively.[1-2]

Evidence-based recommendations for early AAA treatment or suppression are currently limited to smoking cessation and possibly statin therapy.[3] Most early AAA disease patients are offered no disease-specific therapy at the time of diagnosis. Diagnosis is usually followed by recommendations to stop smoking, with subsequent serial surveillance examinations determined by aortic diameter and rate of enlargement.[3-4] The potential therapeutic impact of even modestly effective medical therapy for early disease is substantial: a 50% reduction in annual growth rate for a 4.0-cm AAA could extend the time to surgical repair by 5 years or more, eliminating the need for intervention altogether in many older or high-risk patients.[4] To date, nonsurgical inhibition strategies have proven minimally effective in preventing progression of AAA disease at early or late time points, and no validated algorithms exist to guide therapy.

The predilection for aortic aneurysms to form distal to the renal arteries may provide a unique insight into potentially effective therapies for early disease. Compared with the more proximal aorta, hemodynamic conditions distal to the renal arteries are characterized by increased peripheral resistance, increased oscillatory WSS, and reduced antegrade flow. These "resistive" aortic hemodynamic conditions are also found following major limb amputation, chronic spinal cord injury (SCI), and severe peripheral vascular disease, conditions all associated with increased AAA risk.[5-7] Resistive hemodynamic conditions promote proinflammatory, pro-oxidative mural conditions by inactivating endogenous antiproteases, increasing expression of proinflammatory transcription factors, chemokines, and cytokines and stimulating apoptosis.[8] Lower extremity exercise obliterates resistive hemodynamic conditions and, ultimately, may limit AAA progression via upregulation of antioxidant gene expression.

One example of a redox-related gene differentially expressed under variable flow conditions is heme oxygenase-1 (HO-1). HO-1 is an antioxidant stress-response gene linked to human AAA disease susceptibility.[9] We recently investigated the effects of extremity exercise on aortic WSS, HO activity, and AAA disease progression growth in murine models of aortic aneurysm disease. AAAs were induced in hyperlipidemic mice via chronic infusion of angiotensin II. Some mice were provided free access to exercise wheels (exercise group), and aortic diameters at late time points were measured and compared with those in mice without access to exercise wheels (usual activity group). Suprarenal aortic WSS was consistently greater in the exercise group during serial ultrasound examinations over a 1-month period. The exercise group demonstrated consistently smaller average suprarenal aortic diameters at all time points, and exercising mice in a separate experiment demonstrated increased HO-1 activity. These results suggest that exercise-induced increases in aortic WSS promotes HO expression and activity, limiting progression of experimental AAA.

The effect of chronic SCI on aortic diameter and aneurysm susceptibility provides further support for the relationship between lower extremity activity and AAA risk. SCI was considered specifically as an extreme example of sedentary existence. After controlling for all other known variables related to risk of AAA progression (e.g., age, smoking status, gender, race) in a retrospective review of patients who were at least 5 years out from their injury, AAAs were more prevalent in SCI patients than in age- and traditional risk factor–matched ambulatory control subjects. In addition, SCI patients had larger average aortic diameters and smaller average common iliac artery diameters. Whereas diminished iliac artery diameter was expected in SCI patients as a result of inward remodeling in response to sustained blood flow reductions, the combination of enlarged aortas and diminished iliac diameters was unique and unexpected. On the basis of these observations, we concluded that sedentary existence and chronically reduced/asymmetric aortic flow may represent a novel and independent risk factor for AAA disease.[10]

MR flow imaging and computational flow modeling clearly delineate the ability of lower extremity exercise to reduce proinflammatory hemodynamic conditions in the infrarenal aorta.[11-12] Using a custom MR-compatible exercise cycle in an open GE 0.5 T magnet, transitioning from rest to exercise significantly increased WSS in both the supraceliac and the infrarenal aortas. Moderate exercise (as defined by a 50% increase in resting heart rate) disproportionately increases infrarenal more than supraceliac flow and WSS, suggesting that lower extremity hyperemia occurs in part at the expense of visceral and renal perfusion. Throughout the infrarenal aorta, proinflammatory resting hemodynamic conditions (retrograde and oscillating diastolic flow) are obliterated during exercise. Using three-dimensional finite element methods to model flow conditions, the infrarenal aortic velocity field becomes more unidirectional and ordered under exercise conditions.

The potential mechanism(s) of aneurysm resistance derived from intermittent periods of exercise are not limited to the local effects of increased time-averaged aortic WSS. Intermittent periods of moderate to vigorous exercise produce sustained systemic cardiovascular benefits, including marked reductions in all-cause mortality and vascular-related complications in patients with cardiovascular disease.[13] In a meta-analysis of 8940 patients undergoing cardiac rehabilitation compared with usual care, exercise training resulted in marked reductions in all-cause mortality. Further meta-analysis of 30 cohort studies involving more than 2 million person-years of observation demonstrated nearly linear declines in the risk of coronary heart disease with increasing levels of physical activity.[14] Even single episodes of exercise produce sustained increases in human circulating progenitor cells,[15] anti-inflammatory trends in redox-related gene expression, and when repeated over long intervals, conduit artery remodeling and disease resistance.[16]

Exercise training and increased levels of physical fitness are also highly effective in reducing systemic markers of inflammation relevant to AAAs. Serum high-sensitivity C-reactive protein (hsCRP) levels are increased in patients with AAA disease, correlate with increasing AAA diameter, and originate in part from within aneurysm tissue itself.[17-19] Exercise training reduces a wide range of serum inflammatory markers including hsCRP level: 2.5 h/wk for 6 months reduced mononuclear production of atherogenic cytokines by 58% ($P<.001$), while production of atheroprotective cytokines rose by 36% ($P<.001$). Changes in cytokine production were proportionate to the time spent performing repetitive lower-body motion exercises ($P<0.02$), suggesting a dose-response relationship.[19]

Although exercise testing has proven generally safe and effective in stratifying perioperative risk in surgical candidates[20] and as potentially improving overall fitness for surgical repair,[21] the consequences of sustained exercise training on progression of early AAA disease has not been evaluated in a systematic fashion. Safety considerations aside, given their advanced age and concomitant conditions, the ability of AAA patients to reach exercise targets is uncertain, as is their interest and commitment to the sustained participation necessary to effect meaningful change. Recent data support a role for exercise training in patients with AAAs. Anaerobic thresholds, a marker of surgical high risk in AAA patients, improved significantly in patients participating in a short-term, 7-week exercise programs in contrast to those participants who continued their usual activity.[21]

Based on our prior observations in animal models and in patients with chronic ACI, we are conducting a randomized, prospective longitudinal trial to test the ability of supervised exercise training to modify AAA biology and early disease progression. Our hypothesis is that increased activity reduces the prevalence and progression of small AAA disease. Following recruitment, aortic diameter is measured via transabdominal ultrasound, and samples are collected for markers of systemic inflammation and relevant comorbid conditions (such as diabetes and smoking).

The expected treatment effect of supervised exercise training is a reduction in the population average AAA growth rate. Standardized medical examinations are performed prior to testing and medications are continued as prescribed. Symptom-limited exercise testing is performed at baseline, 3, 12, 24, and 36 months on all exercise trial participants using an individualized treadmill protocol as previously described.[22-23] Exercise capacity in metabolic equivalents (METs) is estimated from peak treadmill speed and grade based on published algorithms.[24]

Exercise training is performed at either our on-site training facility, at home, or a combination of both, depending on individual requirements. The goal of training is to achieve a mean energy expenditure of 2000 kcal/wk. This amounts to approximately 1 hour of moderate exercise/day. The initial intensity target is 60% of heart rate reserve estimated from baseline testing, increasing to 80% as tolerated.[25] In addition to measured response to training, total daily activity is estimated from a 7-day activity recall questionnaire. Estimates of recreational energy expenditure are obtained from weekly telephone interviews. These interviews recognize and record study-related complications as well as monitor compliance with exercise prescriptions.

Eligible small AAA participants also undergo magnetic resonance imaging (MRI) and arteriography (MRA) in the supine position at 1.5T using an 8-channel cardiac coil. A three dimensional gadolinium-enhanced MRA sequence is used to acquire thoracic and abdominal aorta and branch artery geometry. Cardiac-gated phase contrast sequences (PC-MRI) are acquired through plane aortic flow velocity at the supraceliac (SC) and infrarenal (IR) levels. Brachial systolic and diastolic blood pressures are measured immediately following the scan.

Three-dimensional patient-specific geometric models are constructed from MRA data and separated into finite-element meshes. PC-MRI images are segmented at 24 reconstructed time points during the cardiac cycle and assembled into patient-specific SC and IR volumetric flow waveforms.[25-27] To simulate exercise, the resistance values, inflow SC waveforms, cardiac cycle lengths, and target pressures are scaled to simulate aortic response associated with a 50% increase in heart rate. Specifically, participant-specific mean resting IR flows are increased by 5.44-fold[28] and upper branch flows are decreased by 21%.[29] Diastolic inflow SC waveforms are truncated to achieve a 50% increase in heart rate and then increased 2.54±0.27-fold to achieve target exercise IR and branch vessel flows. Target exercise systolic and diastolic pressures are calculated by linear interpolation of data for hypertensive and normotensive patients.[29] Iliac artery resistance is reduced to simulate exercise-induced downstream vasodilation.[30] The Navier-Stokes equations are then solved using the aforementioned rest and exercise inlet and outlet boundary conditions and assuming rigid walls.

While the trial is ongoing, interim analysis of our experience to date suggests that exercise training at our target levels is safe and well tolerated in small aneurysm patients for periods over 1 year. No participants in training experienced AAA-related symptoms, exercise-related clinical events, or excessive aneurysm growth rates. Nearly half of small AAA patients identified through this study are potentially able to participate in exercise training, at least within the context of a controlled trial. The amount of training provided has reduced weight, body mass index, and waist and hip circumference for participants completing 1 year in the study. Computational modeling based on comparable target heart rate increases demonstrates tangible hemodynamic benefits associated with lower extremity exercise of similar intensity.

At the 3-year interval in a planned 5-year study, insufficient observations exist to determine whether increasing activity levels as outlined in the study protocol will limit aneurysm progression or effectively reduce serum or plasma markers associated with AAA disease. No prior data exist to guide development of AAA disease–specific exercise protocols or measurement instruments. Exercise training and the provision of participant-specific exercise prescriptions appear effective in achieving presumed exercise targets in many patients with small AAA disease, as demonstrated by our experience to date. If ultimately proven to limit disease progression, exercise training and efforts to increase patient fitness may play a substantial role in the management of patients with early AAA disease.

REFERENCES

1. Lederle FA, Johnson GR, Wilson SE, et al. The Aneurysm Detection and Management Study Screening Program: validation cohort and final results. Aneurysm Detection and Management Veterans Affairs Cooperative Study Investigators. Arch Intern Med 2000;160:1425–30.
2. Brewster D, Cronenwett J, Hallett J, et al. Guidelines for the treatment of abdominal aortic aneurysms. Report of a subcommittee of the Joint Council of the American Association for Vascular Surgery and Society for Vascular Surgery. J Vasc Surg 2003;37:1106–17.
3. Baxter BT, Terrin MC, Dalman RL. Medical management of small abdominal aortic aneurysms. Circulation 2008;117:1883–9.
4. Powell JT, Brady AR. Detection, management, and prospects for the medical treatment of small abdominal aortic aneurysms. Arterioscler Thromb Vasc Biol 2004;24:241–5.
5. Vollmar JF, Paes E, Pauschinger P, et al. Aortic aneurysms as late sequelae of above-knee amputation. Lancet 1989;2:834–5.
6. Gordon IL, Kohl CA, Arefi M, et al. Spinal cord injury increases the risk of abdominal aortic aneurysm. Am Surg 1996;62:249–52.
7. Sandgren T, Sonesson B, Ryden A, Lanne T. Arterial dimensions in the lower extremities of patients with abdominal aortic aneurysms—no indications of a generalized dilating diathesis. J Vasc Surg 2001;34:1079–4.
8. Lum H, Roebuck KA. Oxidant stress and endothelial cell dysfunction. Am J Physiol Cell Physiol 2001;280:C719–41.
9. Schillinger M, Exner M, Mlekusch W, et al. Heme oxygenase-1 gene promoter polymorphism is associated with abdominal aortic aneurysm. Thromb Res 2002;106:131–6.
10. Yeung JJ, Kim HJ, Abbruzzese TA, et al. Aortoiliac hemodynamic and morphologic adaptation to chronic spinal cord injury. J Vasc Surg 2006;44:1254–65.
11. Cheng C, Herfkens R, Taylor C. Abdominal aortic hemodynamic conditions in healthy subjects aged 50–70 at rest and during lower limb exercise: in vivo quantification using MRI. Atherosclerosis 2003;168:323–31.
12. Masuda H, Zhuang Y-J, Singh TM, et al. Adaptive remodeling of internal elastic lamina and endothelial lining during flow-induced arterial enlargement. Arterioscler Thromb Vasc Biol 1999;19:2298–307.
13. Bassuk S, Manson J. Physical activity and the prevention of cardiovascular disease. Curr Atheroscler Rep 2003;5:299–307.
14. Thompson P. Additional steps for cardiovascular health. N Engl J Med 2002;347:755–6.
15. Rehman J, Li J, Parvathaneni L, et al. Exercise acutely increases circulating endothelial progenitor cells and monocyte-/macrophage-derived angiogenic cells. J Am Coll Cardiol 2004;43:2314–8.
16. Green D, Maiorana A, O'Driscoll G, Taylor R. Effect of exercise training on endothelium-derived nitric oxide function in humans. J Physiol 2004;561:1–25.
17. Powell JT, Muller BR, Greenhalgh RM. Acute phase proteins in patients with abdominal aortic aneurysms. J Cardiovasc Surg 1987;28:528–30.
18. Norman P, Spencer CA, Lawrence-Brown MM, Jamrozik K. C-reactive protein levels and the expansion of screen-detected abdominal aortic aneurysms in men. Circulation 2004;110:862–66.
19. Vainas T, Lubbers T, Stassen FRM, et al. Serum C-reactive protein level is associated with abdominal aortic aneurysm size and may be produced by aneurysmal tissue. Circulation 2003;107:1103–5.
20. Carlisle J, Swart M. Mid-term survival after abdominal aortic aneurysm surgery predicted by cardiopulmonary exercise testing. Br J Surg 2007;94:966–69.
21. Kothmann E, Batterham AM, Owen SJ, et al. Effect of short-term exercise training on aerobic fitness in patients with abdominal aortic aneurysms: a pilot study. Br J Anaesth 2009 Oct; 103:505–10.

22. Myers J, Do D, Herbert W, et al. A nomogram to predict exercise capacity from a specific activity questionnaire and clinical data. Am J Cardiol 1994;73:591–6.
23. Myers J, Buchanan N, Walsh D, et al. Comparison of the ramp versus standard exercise protocols. J Am Coll Cardiol 1991;17:1334–42.
24. Froelicher VF, Myers JN. Research as part of clinical practice: use of Windows-based relational data bases. Veterans Health System J 1998.
25. Lippincott, Williams & Wilkins. American College of Sports Medicine. Guidelines for Exercise Testing and Prescription. Baltimore; 2006.
26. Womersley JR. Method for the calculation of velocity, rate of flow and viscous drag in arteries when the pressure gradient is known. J Physiol 1955;127:553–63.
27. Moore JE Jr, Ku DN. Pulsatile velocity measurements in a model of the human abdominal aorta under resting conditions. J Biomech Eng 1994;116:337–46.
28. He X, Ku DN. Pulsatile flow in the human left coronary artery bifurcation: average conditions. J Biomech Eng 1996;118:74–82.
29. Montain SJ, Jilka SM, Ehsani AA, Hagberg JM. Altered hemodynamics during exercise in older essential hypertensive subjects. Hypertension 1988;12:479–84.
30. O'Rourke MF. Vascular impedance in studies of arterial and cardiac function. Physiol Rev 1982;62:570–623.

47

Can Patient-Specific Biomechanical Evaluation of Abdominal Aortic Aneurysm Be Used To Predict Rupture?

David A. Vorp, Ph.D., David E. Schmidt, Ph.D., and Michel S. Makaroun, M.D.

INTRODUCTION

Abdominal aortic aneurysm (AAA) rupture is the 13th leading cause of death in the United States. This condition is more prevalent among the older population, with approximately 150,000 new cases diagnosed each year. Rupture can occur without warning, because the characterizing focal dilation in the aortic wall is asymptomatic. Clinicians attempt to avoid rupture by performing elective repair. However, the risks associated with the repair dictate that the surgery should be recommended only when the potential for rupture outweighs the risks of the interventional procedure. At present, metrics to guide surgical intervention are incomplete. Given the rapid evolution of patient-specific analysis techniques, researchers and clinicians are looking toward biomechanical evaluation to extend such metrics. With validated new markers, we can therefore ponder: can patient-specific biomechanical evaluation of abdominal aortic aneurysm be used to predict rupture?

Most patients with AAAs are elderly and/or have comorbid conditions. These considerations, coupled with the potential for complications that are associated with current repair techniques, present a clinical dilemma, that is, balancing the risks of AAA rupture and an appropriate repair procedure. At present, no common measurement to characterize the potential for AAA rupture has been accepted. However, researchers have presented several quantitative predictors in the literature. These include the estimation of wall cyclic strain or compliance,[1] intraluminal thrombus (ILT) volume,[2] wall diameter,[3] enlargement rate,[4,5] and biomechanical conditions.[6] Among clinicians, the most common metric focuses on the assessment of maximum aortic transverse diameter.[7] This "maximum diameter criterion" establishes a threshold (typically 5 or 5.5 cm) delineating the point at which the risk of rupture warrants repair.[3] However, this criterion is only a general rule-of-thumb and has been shown to be unreliable.[8,9,10] Autopsy studies have revealed that relatively small AAAs can rupture[10] in contrast to those in a population considered to be large that will not rupture given the life expectancy of the patient.[8] Therefore, a diameter-based intervention may be offered too late or may be unwarranted for a particular patient. Biomechanical analysis based on patient-specific data holds the potential to frame the risk on an individual basis as opposed to a "one-criterion-fits-all" approach.

Based on recognition that AAA rupture occurs when the acting wall forces exceed the mechanical capacity of the degenerated AAA wall, we and others have advocated the use of biomechanical principles to assess AAA rupture risk.[1,6,11] For example, we reported noninvasive-based methods to estimate wall stress[11] and strength[12] distributions in patient-specific AAA computational models. These techniques provided the foundation for the development of a clinically relevant "Rupture Potential Index" (RPI),[13] a biomechanical metric based on the localized ratio of wall stress to strength. An RPI-based risk assessment may exhibit increased fidelity compared with other methodologies because it leverages patient-specific information and casts failure conditions in terms of fundamental biomechanical mechanisms.

PATIENT-SPECIFIC MODELING

Using computed tomography (CT) images, a patient-specific three-dimensional (3D) model of the AAA wall and ILT can be generated. Segmentation of the CT image set with respect to the lumen and wall serves as the foundation for the construction of a high-fidelity wall surface geometry. This 3D geometry can subsequently be used to form the basis for a computational model (Figure 47–1).

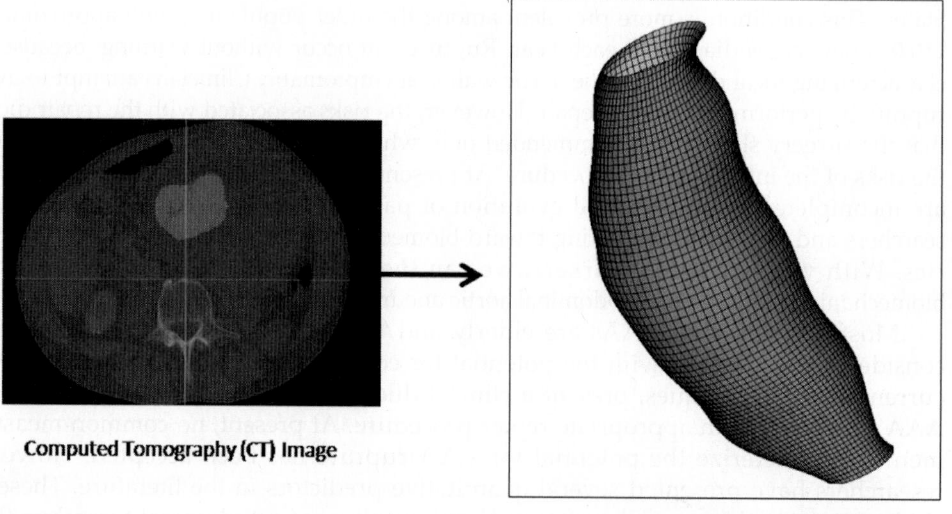

Figure 47-1. Three-dimensional reconstruction of an AAA from patient CT data. The resulting solid model provides a high-fidelity geometric description of the AAA wall as well as the contained ILT.

Noninvasive patient-specific assessment of the surface geometry of AAAs may be beneficial for a number of reasons. For example, knowledge of the spatial variations in wall curvature will identify regions of high wall tension based on the generalized law of Laplace, which states that wall tension is proportional to the inverse of mean curvature. Moreover, detailed analysis of AAA wall curvature will aid in the determination of localized blebs in the aneurysm wall.[14] We previously performed noninvasive assessment of the curvature of in situ AAAs[15] and found the existence of distinct features within individual AAAs and clear variations between AAAs.

MOTIVATION FOR BIOMECHANICAL EVALUATION

An AAA is typically composed of two primary structures – the diseased and dilated aortic wall and an ILT, which is a large, stationary blood clot incorporated with blood cells, platelets, blood proteins, and cellular debris.[16] Because ILT is contained in most AAAs,[17] it is prudent to consider the biomechanical behavior of both this material and the AAA wall as well as in vivo studies that evaluated the biomechanical behavior of the entire AAA structure in situ. The consideration of the coupled ILT and AAA response is central to the development of an RPI to evaluate the need for surgical intervention. By extending concepts relating wall stress to rupture risk presented in the literature, an RPI approach seeks to provide a comprehensive biomechanical evaluation. A detailed description of the RPI metric is presented below.

Hall et al.[18] described the relationship between aortic wall stress predicted using the law of Laplace (i.e., based on maximum AAA diameter) and risk of AAA rupture. In their study of 40 AAA patients, they suggested that there exists a threshold tension of 2.8×10^5 N/m^2 after which rupture was imminent. However, it has been shown by our laboratory[11,19-21] and others[6,22-24] that the stresses acting on an AAA are not evenly distributed and cannot be adequately described by the law of Laplace. In fact, the stresses acting on the wall of an aneurysm are highly dependent on the shape (e.g., profile, tortuosity, and asymmetry) of the specific AAA.[19,25-26] Therefore, AAAs with equivalent diameters and pressures (and thus Laplace-predicted wall stress) could have largely different actual stress distributions. It is clear that like the "maximum diameter criterion," the law of Laplace cannot effectively describe an aneurysm's risk of rupture on a patient-specific basis.

More recently, the use of peak wall stress as a potential predictor of AAA rupture was explored.[23-24] Fillinger, Raghavan, et al. found that the peak wall stress for AAAs that either ruptured or were symptomatic was significantly greater than that for electively repaired AAAs.[23] In a subsequent study,[6] this same group concluded that peak wall stress is a more superior measure than maximum diameter for predicting patients with an unfavorable outcome. A more recent study found similar results, while also showing that the location of AAA rupture correlated with the location of peak wall stress.[24] Although this is at least a step in the right direction with regard to incorporating biomechanical principles into considering AAA severity, this approach considers only one of the two biomechanical factors that govern AAA rupture.

As stated above, AAA rupture occurs when the stresses acting on an AAA exceed its wall strength. That is, the rupture risk of a given AAA would increase with an increase in peak wall stress only if the wall strength is unchanged. Not only is wall strength different from patient to patient, but it also varies significantly within the same aneurysm as shown by us[20,27] and others.[28] In addition, we have recently shown that the strength of AAA wall from ruptured AAAs is significantly less than that for electively repaired AAAs.[29] Taken alone, much like the peak wall stress correlation to rupture risk, these data might suggest that AAA wall strength on its own is predictive of aneurysm rupture. However, based on the principles of material failure, consideration of neither AAA wall stress nor wall strength alone is sufficient to assess rupture potential, but rather knowledge of both is necessary. Therefore, we are motivated to seek biomechanical evaluation of AAA rupture risk potential in terms of coupled stress and strength characteristics.

BIOMECHANICAL BEHAVIOR OF ABDOMINAL AORTIC ABEURYSM TISSUES

Abdominal Aortic Abeurysm Wall Behavior

To perform stress analysis on individual AAAs, the material parameters specific to each aneurysmal wall should be employed. However, the only way to accurately determine these parameters currently is to perform ex vivo, destructive mechanical testing, which of course is not possible in a presurgical situation. Instead, the group mean values of the material parameters as assessed for a large number of AAAs and ILT specimens[20,30] have typically been used.[6,23-24,31] We evaluated this approach by performing parametric analyses to demonstrate that "biologically reasonable" deviations in the actual values of the material parameters for an individual AAA and ILT from the mean values determined for a large AAA population will not significantly affect the estimated wall stress distribution.[30,31] This was accomplished by repeated finite element stress analysis on a hypothetical, 3D, asymmetric AAA model. Differences in AAA wall stresses from patient to patient have been shown to be driven more by the differences in surface geometry than by material properties.

Vande Geest and associates[32] have reported a population-wide biaxial constitutive relation for human AAA and nonaneurysmal abdominal aortic (AA) tissue. In brief, 26 AAA tissue samples and 8 age-matched (>60 years) AA tissue samples were obtained and tested within a well-validated biaxial tensile testing system.[15,33] Both types of tissue exhibited an anisotropic exponential response.

Intraluminal Thrombus

Using noninvasive, ultrasound-based measures of ILT, we have determined that the ILT undergoes nonlinear strains in vivo and is incompressible.[34] This work supported the idea that the ILT may be "mechanically protective," providing a stress shielding or cushioning effect for the AAA wall,[35] Furthermore, recent studies suggest that the ILT is nonlinearly elastic, inhomogeneous, and isotropic.[36] In a biomechanical modeling context, the ILT can be characterized as a hyperelastic material.[36] Planar biaxial mechanical testing supports this assumption.[32]

Abdominal Aortic Abeurysm Wall Strength

Structural remodeling characteristics common among AAAs lead to a significant weakening of the aortic wall. Uniaxial tensile testing performed on freshly excised specimens has demonstrated that AAA wall tissue is approximately 50% weaker than control (nonaneurysmal) abdominal aorta.[37-38] Studies have also revealed that AAA wall strength varies throughout the dilated region,[28, 39-40] possibly due to cellular hypoxia associated with the presence of ILT.[41-43] The strength characteristics reported were invariant to orientation (circumferential and longitudinal). Ruptured AAA wall is weaker that nonruptured AA wall.[44] Additionally, it has been shown that the wall of infected AAAs is weaker that of noninfected AAA wall.[13] The potential mechanisms of these trends of AAA wall degeneration are discussed in a recent review.[45]

A strong inverse correlation between local ILT thickness and adjacent wall thickness exists. Work performed in our laboratory suggested that the presence of ILT tends to decrease local wall strength in an ILT-thickness–dependent manner[39] and that this inverse relationship is due to ILT's serving as a barrier to oxygen flux from the lumen to the inner layers of the aortic wall, thereby inducing hypoxic conditions and wall degeneration.[19,39] This seemingly negative effect of ILT on the AAA wall is opposite to the positive effect that it has in terms of AAA wall stress,[46] In this way, the ILT is sort of a "Jekyll and Hyde" in that it is both good and bad in terms of AAA biomechanics. What remains to be determined is which effect is dominant, and this may be patient-specific itself.

Given the above observations, wall strength estimations must be cast in a localized manner. Apart from diameter and ILT, our studies have demonstrated that patient age, sex, and family history influence AAA wall strength properties. In consideration of these variables, we recently utilized multiple-linear regression techniques to derive the following mathematical model to estimate wall strength.[27]

$$\begin{aligned} \mathit{Strength} = 71.9 - 37.9\,(\mathit{ILT}^{\frac{1}{2}} - .81) - 15.6(\mathrm{Nord} - 2.46) \\ - 21.3^{*}\,\mathit{Hist} + 19.3^{*}\,\mathit{Sex} \end{aligned} \tag{1}$$

Here, Strength (dependent variable) is the AAA wall strength at any given point (in units of N/cm^2), and the independent variables are ILT (the local thickness of intraluminal thrombus in centimeters), Nord (the diameter of the AAA at that location, normalized by the nondilated aorta proximal to the AAA), HIST, and Sex. The last two are binary variables that account for the patient's family history and gender, respectively. Inspection of Equation 2 provides several insights as to its physical meaning:

- For two patients with the same gender and identical AAAs, the one with family history has an AAA that is globally weaker by 21.3 N/cm^2 compared with the one without a family history.
- For two patients with the same family history and identical AAAs, a female will have an AAA that is globally weaker by 19.3 N/cm^2 compared with a male.
- For any two points within any given AAA with the same NORD, an increase in $ILT^{1/2}$ of 1.0 results in a corresponding decrease in strength of 37.9 N/cm^2.
- For any two points within any given AAA with the same $ILT^{1/2}$, an increase in NORD of 1.0 results in a corresponding decrease in strength of 15.6 N/cm^2.

Computational Analysis

The biomechanical evaluation techniques presented above can be put into a computation framework such as the finite element method.[47] This approach provides a means to fully leverage 3D geometric reconstructions prepared from patient-specific CT scans. Additionally, this methodology is suitable for translation into a clinical environment because patient-specific models can be quickly developed and evaluated.

Rupture Potential Index

As suggested above, a comprehensive AAA rupture risk assessment should consider the coupled nature of stress and strength. As established by Vande Geest et al.,[12] an RPI can be defined as the ratio of the local wall stress to the wall strength, that is,

$$RPI_i = \frac{\text{Stress}_i}{\text{Strength}_i} \tag{2}$$

The subscript i denotes the local position in terms of the local coordinates within the AAA wall. In practice, RPI is computed at each "node" point within the patient-specific finite element model. Point-wise AAA wall stress, strength, and RPI can be mapped to a patient-specific computational model (Figure 47–2). This example highlights the location of rupture recorded by the surgeon overlaid on the RPI distribution. The peak RPI for this AAA was .70, which can be interpreted as the corresponding location on this AAA being at 70% of its capacity to withstand mechanical wall stress. In this case, the CT scan used to develop the model and perform the biomechanical evaluation was obtained approximately 1 month before rupture.

EVALUATION OF AAA RUPTURE RISK POTENTIAL

The biomechanical characteristics of AAAs change over time, and the examination of these properties can demonstrate the predictive nature of biomechanical indices with respect to rupture potential. By leveraging CT scans at varied time points, patient-specific simulations can be developed to evaluate temporal changes in the key biomechanical indices such as peak RPI and wall stress and minimum wall strength.

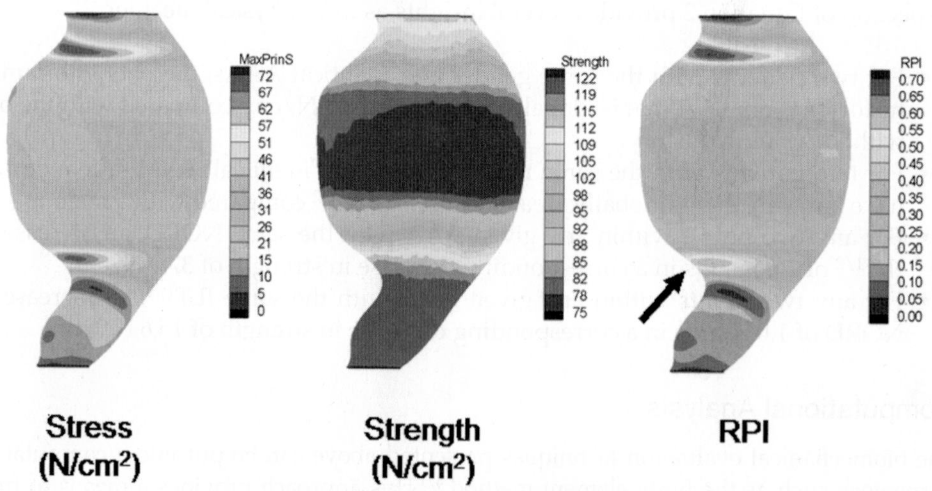

Figure 47-2. Distributions of stress, strength, and RPI on a ruptured AAA. The location of rupture recorded by the surgeon is denoted by the arrow and corresponds to a region of elevated RPI. The CT scan used to develop the model and perform the biomechanical evaluation was obtained approximately 1 month before rupture.

Data from a representative patient highlights this concept (Figure 47–3). Comparison of stress, strength, and RPI between two time points shows distinct differences in the adopted metrics. Data from a small cohort of patients to date (n=25) demonstrate results consistent with previous findings in that the maximum diameter and peak wall stress of AAAs significantly increase over time but also reveal that the peak RPI increases while strength characteristics decrease. Figure 47–4 summarizes these findings in a comparison between evaluations based on two CT scan dates. These

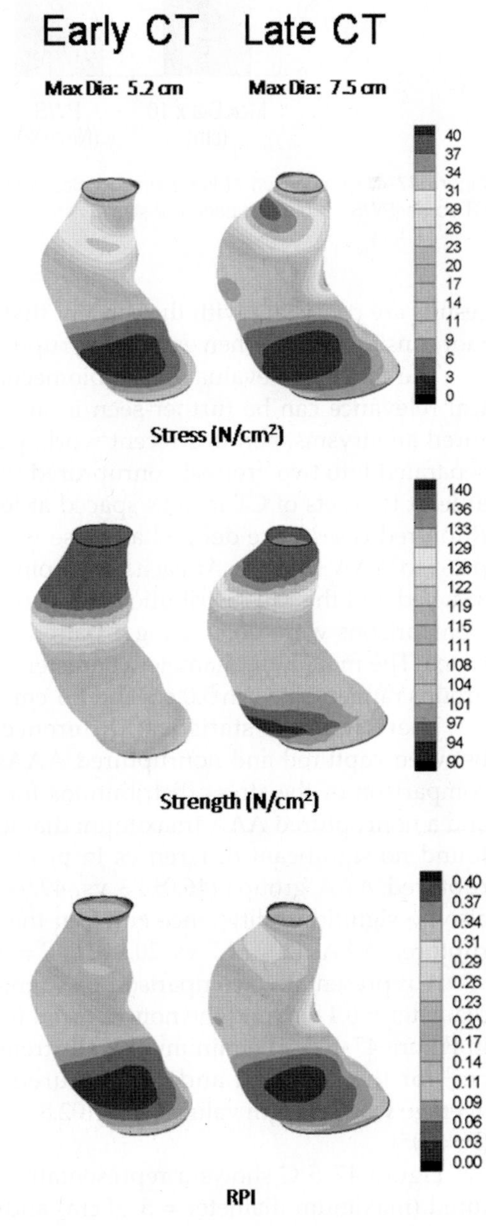

Figure 47-3. Representative stresses, strength, and RPI distributions for one nonruptured AAA. For this case, the time period between CT scans (denoted as "early" and "late") was 980 days.

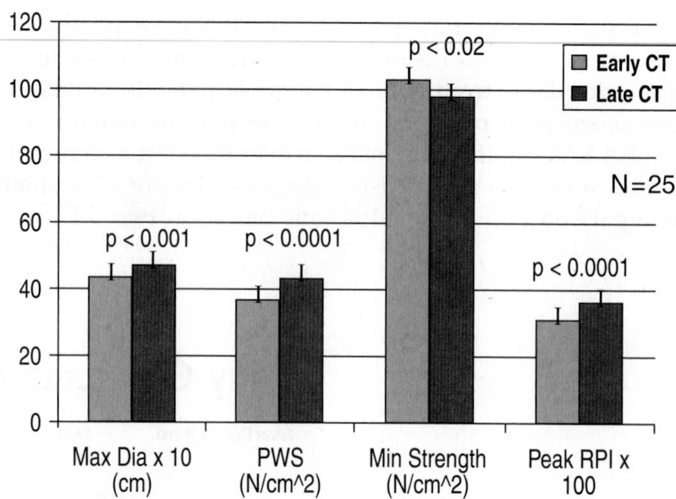

Figure 47-4. Comparison of key biomechanical indices between AAA models derived from early and late CT scans. PWS denotes the peak wall stress.

results are consistent with the concept that stress and strength distributions are important considerations when evaluating rupture potential.

The concept of evaluations in biomechanical properties of AAAs in relation to clinical relevance can be further seen in an analysis comparing nonruptured with ruptured aneurysms.[48] In this recent work, patient-specific simulations of 13 AAAs were separated into two groups: nonruptured (n=5) and ruptured (n=8) repairs . In all cases, at least two sets of CT images spaced at least 1 year apart were available for analysis. Ruptured cases were defined as those with CT scans completed no more than 1 year prior to AAA rupture. At each time point, each AAA was three-dimensionally reconstructed and the RPI distribution was estimated using the techniques described above. Comparisons were done using a paired Student *t*-test, with P=.05, indicating significance. The maximum diameter characterizing the dilated state of the aorta across both groups ranged between 5.0 cm and 8.1 cm.

There were no statistical differences in the maximum transverse diameters between ruptured and nonruptured AAAs (6.8±.3 vs. 6.1±.5, P=.26). A representative comparison of the stress distributions for a ruptured (maximum diameter = 7.0 cm) and a nonruptured AAA (maximum diameter = 6.7 cm) is shown in Figure 47–5 A. We found no significant differences in peak stresses between the nonruptured and the ruptured AAA groups (46.0±4.3 vs. 49.9±4.0 N/cm^2, respectively; P=.62). There was also no significant difference between the mean stresses for the nonruptured and the ruptured AAAs (20.4±1.7 vs. 20.7±2.6; P =.95).

A representative comparison of strength distributions for a ruptured (maximum diameter = 6.1 cm) and the nonruptured (maximum diameter = 5.8 cm) AAA is shown in Figure 47–5 B. The minimum wall strength values were 81.2±3.9 and 108.3±10.2 N/cm^2 for the ruptured and nonruptured AAA models, respectively (P=.045). The average wall strength values were 102.8±3.4 and 124.5±5.8 N/cm^2 for these two groups (P =.005).

Figure 47–5 C shows a representative comparison of RPI distribution for a ruptured (maximum diameter = 5.20 cm) and a nonruptured (maximum diameter = 5.23 cm) AAA of nearly equivalent maximum diameter. Although the differences between

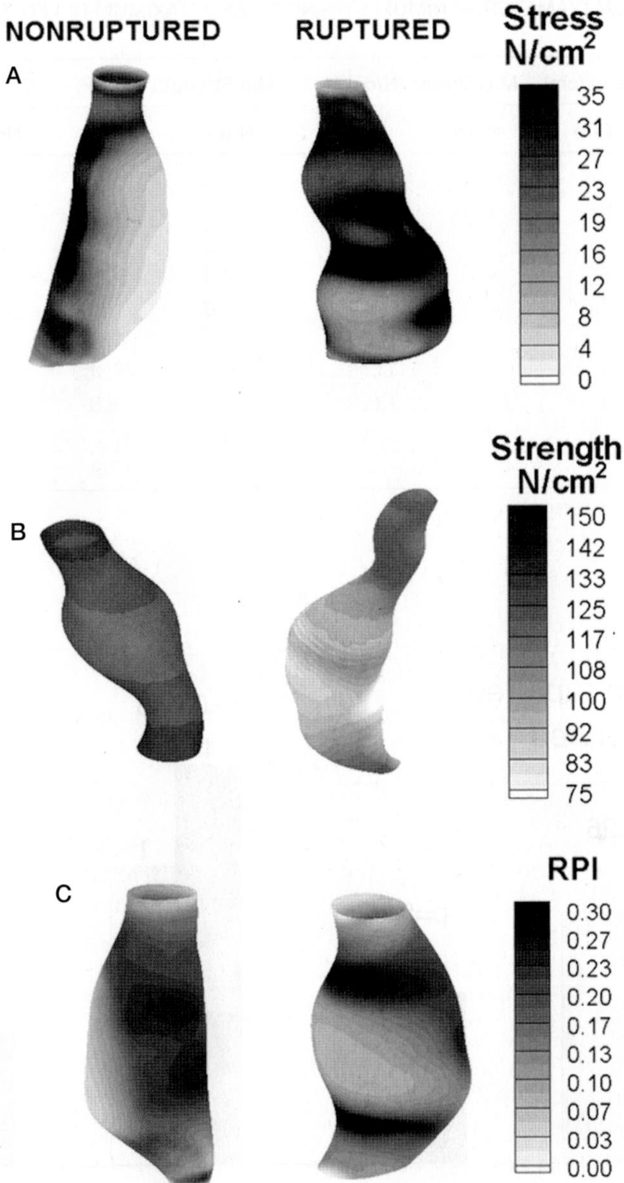

Figure 47-5. Representative comparison of the stress (A), strength (B), and RPI (C) between a representative electively repaired (nonruptured) AAA and a representative ruptured AAA.

ruptured and nonuptured peak RPI values (0.48±.05 vs. 0.36±.03, respectively; P=.10) did not reach statistical significance for the small numbers of AAAs studied here, the P value for the peak RPI comparison was lower than that for both the maximum diameter (P=.26) and the peak wall stress (P=.62) comparisons. This result suggests that the peak RPI may be better able to identify those AAAs at high risk of rupture than maximum diameter or peak wall stress alone. The results for maximum transverse diameter, peak wall stress, minimum wall strength, and RPI between the ruptured and the nonruptured groups are summarized in Table 47–1 and Figure 47–6.

TABLE 47-1. MAXIMUM DIAMETER, MINIMUM STRENGTH, AND MAXIMUM RPI FOR ALL AAAs IN THIS STUDY

	Max Diameter (cm)		Max Stress (N/cm^2)		Min Strength (N/cm^2)		RPI	
	Nrup	Rup	Nrup	Rup	Nrup	Rup	Nrup	Rup
	7.9	7.1	53.0	33.5	90.6	89.5	0.41	0.31
	5.8	6.6	41.4	54.5	130.7	85.1	0.31	0.64
	5.0	7.7	58.9	64.0	132.8	95.7	0.44	0.51
	5.2	8.1	36.5	55.1	104.6	68.8	0.27	0.55
	6.7	6.7	40.1	44.4	82.9	68.5	0.38	0.57
		7.0		67.3		70.5		0.60
		5.2		42.3		92.4		0.38
		6.1		34.3		78.8		0.28
MEAN	6.1	6.8	46.0	49.9	108.3	81.2	0.36	0.48
SEM	0.5	0.3	4.3	4.0	10.2	3.9	0.03	0.05

NRUP – nonruptured; RUP – ruptured.

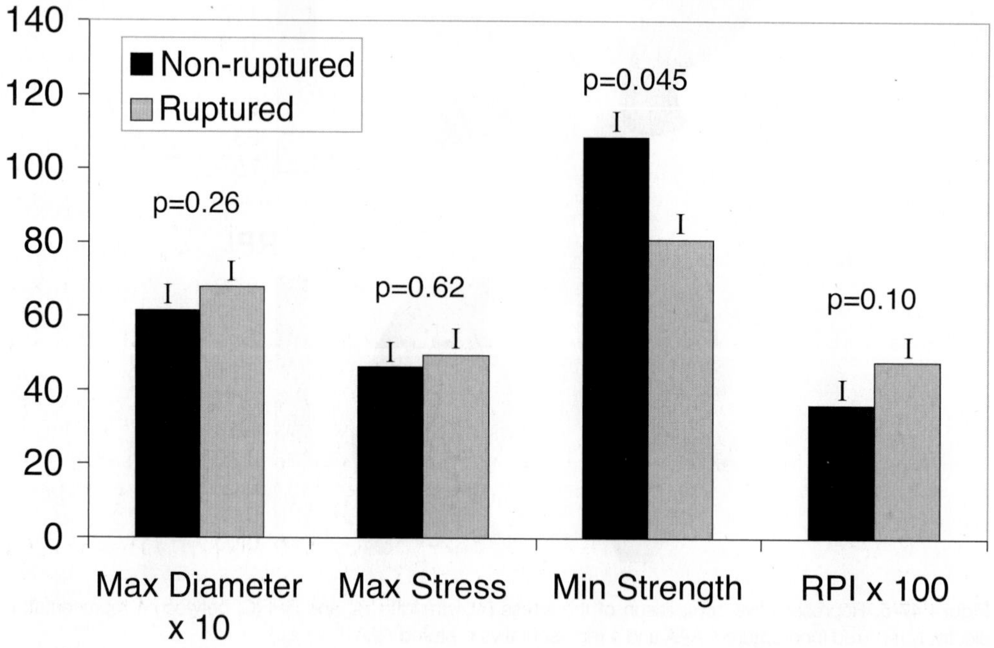

Figure 47-6. Comparison of group mean peak diameter, peak wall stress, and RPI between ruptured (n=8) and nonruptured AAAs (n=5).

SUMMARY

Current clinical assessment methods to evaluate AAA rupture potential are unreliable. In general, an enlarging AAA is accompanied by both an increase and a decrease in wall strength, and both of these parameters are critical and need to be taken into account, because the instant of AAA rupture occurs when the former exceeds the latter. For these reasons, research has been focused over recent years on the biomechanics of AAAs, particularly with regard to wall stress assessment. The law of Laplace has been erroneously applied and is not reliable for the analyses of the complexly shaped AAA. Rather, more established and accurate methods such as finite element analysis are required. The methodology presented leverages patient-specific data to develop a computational predictive model that can be used to track the biomechanical response of the AAA.

Clearly, the ability to reliably evaluate the susceptibility of a particular AAA to rupture could vastly improve the clinical management of these patients. Although the application of biomechanics in this regard is in its infancy, it is clear from the above studies that it holds much promise. However, validation of biomechanics-based rupture prediction will require carefully planned retrospective and prospective studies.

Acknowledgments

This work was funded in part by grants from the National Institutes of Health (# R01 HL60670 and # R01 HL 079313) awarded to DAV. The authors would like to acknowledge the contributions of Jonathan Vande Geest, Ph.D., and Samarth Shah in this work.

REFERENCES

1. Sonesson B, Sandgren T, Lanne T. Abdominal aortic aneurysm wall mechanics and their relation to risk of rupture. Eur J Vasc Endovasc Surg 1999;18:487–93.
2. Hans SS, Jareunpoon O, Balasubramaniam M, Zelenock GB. Size and location of thrombus in intact and ruptured abdominal aortic aneurysms. J Vasc Surg 2005;41:584–8.
3. Dryjski M, Driscoll RC, Blair MA, et al. The small abdominal aortic aneurysm: the eternal dilemma. J Cardiovasc Surg 1994;35:95–100.
4. Lobato AC, Puech-Leao P. Predictive factors for rupture of thoracoabdominal aortic aneurysm. J Vasc Surg 1998;27:446–53.
5. Vardulaki KA, Prevost TC, Walker NM, et al. Growth rates and risk of rupture of abdominal aortic aneurysms. Br J Surg 1998;85:1674–80.
6. Fillinger MF, Marra SP, Raghavan ML, Kennedy FE. Prediction of rupture risk in abdominal aortic aneurysm during observation: wall stress versus diameter. J Vasc Surg 2003;37: 724–32.
7. Long-term outcomes of immediate repair compared with surveillance of small abdominal aortic aneurysms. N Engl J Med 2002;346:1445–52.
8. Darling RC, Messina CR, Brewster DC, Ottinger LW. Autopsy study of unoperated abdominal aortic aneurysms. Circulation 1977;56:161–64.
9. Geroulakos G, Nicolaides A. Infrarenal abdominal aortic aneurysms less than five centimeters in diameter: the surgeon's dilemma. Eur J Vasc Surg 1992;6:661–22.
10. Choksy SA, Wilmink AB, Quick CR. Ruptured abdominal aortic aneurysm in the Huntingdon district: a 10-year experience. Ann R Coll Surg Engl 1999;81:27–31.
11. Raghavan ML, Vorp DA, Federle MP, et al. Wall stress distribution on three-dimensionally reconstructed models of human abdominal aortic aneurysm. J Vasc Surg 2000;31: 760–69.
12. Vande Geest JP. Towards an improved rupture potential index for abdominal aortic aneurysms: anisotropic constitutive modeling and noninvasive wall *strength* estimation: Ph.D Thesis. Pittsburgh: University of Pittsburgh; 2005.

13. Vande Geest JP, Di Martino ES, Bohra A, et al. A biomechanics-based rupture potential index for abdominal aortic aneurysm risk assessment: demonstrative application. Ann N Y Acad Sci 2006;1085:11–21.
14. Hunter GC, Leong SC, Yu GSM, et al. Aortic blebs: possible site of aneurysm rupture. J Vasc Surg 1989;10:93–9.
15. Sacks MS, Vorp DA, Raghavan ML, et al. In vivo three-dimensional surface geometry of abdominal aortic aneurysms. Ann Biomed Eng 1999;27:469–79.
16. Adolph R, Vorp DA, Steed DL, Webster MW, et al. Cellular content and permeability of intraluminal thrombus in abdominal aortic aneurysm. J Vasc Surg 1997;25:916–26.
17. Harter LP, Gross BH, Callen PW, Barth RA. Ultrasonic evaluation of abdominal aortic thrombus. J Ultrasound Med 1982;1:315–8.
18. Hall AJ, Busse EFG, McCarville DJ, Burgess JJ. Aortic wall tension as a predictive factor for abdominal aortic aneurysm rupture: improving the selection of patients for abdominal aortic aneurysm repair. Ann Vasc Surg 2000;14:152–7.
19. Vorp DA, Raghavan ML, Webster MW. Mechanical wall stress in abdominal aortic aneurysm: influence of diameter and asymmetry [published erratum appears in J Vasc Surg 1998;28: 272]. J Vasc Surg 1998;27:632–9.
20. Wang DHJ, Makaroun MS, Webster MW, Vorp DA. Effect of intraluminal thrombus on wall stress in patient-specific models of abdominal aortic aneurysm. J Vasc Surg 2002;36: 598–604.
21. Raghavan ML. Mechanical wall stress in abdominal aortic aneurysm: towards the development of a clinical tool to predict rupture. Ph.D. Thesis. Pittsburgh: University of Pittsburgh; 1998.
22. Stringfellow MM, Lawrence PF, Stringfellow RG. The influence of aorta-aneurysm geometry upon stress in the aneurysm wall. J Surg Res 1987;42:425–33.
23. Fillinger MF, Raghavan ML, Marra SP, et al. In vivo analysis of mechanical wall stress and abdominal aortic aneurysm rupture risk. J Vasc Surg 2002;36:589–97.
24. Venkatasubramaniam AK, Fagan MJ, Mehta T, et al. A comparative study of aortic wall stress using finite element analysis for ruptured and non-ruptured abdominal aortic aneurysms. Eur J Vasc Endovasc Surg 2004;28:168–76.
25. Elger DF, Blackketter DM, Budwig RS, Johansen KH. The influence of shape on the stresses in model abdominal aortic aneurysms. J Biomech Eng 1996;118:326–32.
26. Doyle BJ, Callanan A, Burke PE, et al. Vessel asymmetry as an additional diagnostic tool in the assessment of abdominal aortic aneurysms. J Vasc Surg 2009;49:443–54.
27. Vande Geest JP, Wang DHJ, Wisniewski SR, et al. A noninvasive method for determination of patient-specific wall strength distrubtion in abdominal aortic aneurysms. Ann Biomed Eng (in press)(2006).
28. Vallabhaneni SR, Gilling-Smith GL, How TV, et al. Heterogeneity of tensile strength and matrix metalloproteinase activity in the wall of abdominal aortic aneurysms. J Endovasc Ther 2004;11:494–502.
29. DiMartino ES, Bohra A, VandeGeest JP, et al. Biomechanical properties of ruptured versus electively repaired abdominal aortic aneurysm wall tissue. J Vasc Surg 2006;43:570–6.
30. Raghavan ML, Vorp DA. Toward a biomechanical tool to evaluate rupture potential of abdominal aortic aneurysm: identification of a finite strain constitutive model and evaluation of its applicability. J Biomech 2000;33:475–82.
31. Di Martino ES, Vorp DA. Effect of variation in intraluminal thrombus constitutive properties on abdominal aortic aneurysm wall stress. Ann Biomed Eng 2003;31:804–9.
32. Vande Geest JP, Sacks MS, Vorp DA. A planar biaxial constitutive relation for the luminal layer of intra-luminal thrombus in abdominal aortic aneurysms. J Biomech (in press). 2006.
33. Sacks MS. Biaxial mechanical evaluation of planar biological materials. J Elasticity 2001; 61:199–246.
34. Vorp DA, Mandarino WA, Webster MW, Gorcsan J 3rd. Potential influence of intraluminal thrombus on abdominal aortic aneurysm as assessed by a new non-invasive method. Cardiovasc Surg 1996;4:732–9.

35. Inzoli F, Boschetti F, Zappa M, et al. Biomechanical factors in abdominal aortic aneurysm rupture. Eur J Vasc Surg 1993;7:667–74.
36. Wang DHJ, Makaroun MS, Webster MW, Vorp DA. Mechanical properties and microstructure of intraluminal thrombus from abdominal aortic aneurysm. J Biomech Eng 2001;123: 536–9.
37. Raghavan ML, Webster MW, Vorp DA. Ex vivo biomechanical behavior of abdominal aortic aneurysm: assessment using a new mathematical model. Ann Biomed Eng 1996;24: 573–82.
38. Vorp DA, Raghavan ML, Muluk SC, et al. Wall strength and stiffness of aneurysmal and nonaneurysmal abdominal aorta. Paper presented at Proceedings in Volume 800 in the Annals of the New York Academy of Sciences; 1996 Nov 18, 1996; United States.
39. Vorp DA, Lee PC, Wang DHJ, Makaroun MS, et al. Association of intraluminal thrombus in abdominal aortic aneurysm with local hypoxia and wall weakening. J Vasc Surg 2001;34: 291–9.
40. Thubrikar MJ, al-Soudi J, Robicsek F. Wall stress studies of abdominal aortic aneurysm in a clinical model. Ann Vasc Surg 2001;15:355–66.
41. Vorp DA, Wang DH, Webster MW, Federspiel WJ. Effect of intraluminal thrombus thickness and bulge diameter on the oxygen diffusion in abdominal aortic aneurysm. J Biomech Eng 1998;120:579–83.
42. Vorp DA, Lee PC, Wang DHJ, et al. Association of intraluminal thrombus in abdominal aortic aneurysm with local hypoxia and wall weakening. J Vasc Surg 2001;34:291–9.
43. Vorp DA, Federspiel WJ, Webster MW. Does laminated intraluminal thrombus within abdominal aortic aneurysm cause anoxia of the aortic wall? J Vasc Surg 1996;23:540–1.
44. DiMartino ES, Bohra A, VandeGeest JP, et al. Biomechanical properties of ruptured versus electively repaired abdominal aortic aneurysm wall tissue. J Vasc Surg 2006;43:570–6.
45. Vorp DA, Vande Geest JP. Biomechanical determinants of abdominal aortic aneurysm rupture. Arterioscler Thromb Vasc Biol 2005;25:1558–66.
46. Wang DHJ, Makaroun MS, Webster MW, Vorp DA. Effect of intraluminal thrombus on wall stress in patient-specific models of abdominal aortic aneurysm. J Vasc Surg 2002;36: 98–604.
47. Vande Geest JP, Wang DH, Wisniewski SR, et al. Towards a noninvasive method for determination of patient-specific wall strength distribution in abdominal aortic aneurysms. Ann Biomed Eng 2006;34:1098–106.
48. Vande Geest JP, Dillavou ED, Di Martino ES, et al. Gender-related differences in the tensile strength of abdominal aortic aneurysm. Ann N Y Acad Sci 2006;1085:400–2.

48

The Natural History of Abdominal Aortic Aneurysm

Frank A. Lederle, M.D.

Management of abdominal aortic aneurysms (AAAs) is determined to a considerable extent by natural history, particularly rupture rate and enlargement rate.

RUPTURE

When AAA rupture occurs, only about half of the patients make it to the operating room and operative mortality remains at about 50%; therefore, total mortality is higher than 75%.[1] AAA rupture causes 9000 deaths per year in the United States.[2] Elective repair of AAAs can prevent rupture but is expensive, carries some risk of morbidity, and itself causes more than 1400 deaths per year in the U.S.[3] Furthermore, evidence from autopsy studies indicates that most AAAs never rupture,[4] and therefore, elective repair is reserved for patients at high rupture risk.

The only widely accepted and commonly used predictor of rupture risk is the maximum AAA diameter. Two randomized clinical trials, UK Small Aneurysm Trial (UKSAT) and ADAM, compared open repair with surveillance for AAAs smaller than 5.5 cm in diameter in patients at low operative risk and found that repair did not reduce mortality compared with the less invasive and less expensive strategy of surveillance.[5-6] In the surveillance strategy, patients with unrepaired AAAs who are potential operative candidates undergo periodic AAA measurement, usually ultrasound every 6 months, with repair reserved for those whose AAAs enlarge to 5.5 cm or become symptomatic.

Many risk factors for rupture other than diameter have been proposed, including both aneurysm-related factors (such as shape, estimated stress, compliance, and amount of thrombus) and patient factors (such as gender and various measures of patient size). However, none of these have been persuasively confirmed and widely adapted to clinical use, with the possible exception of gender (discussed below). Thus, although it is unlikely that AAA diameter is the best possible predictor of rupture, it is the only one in widespread use and virtually all natural history and randomized trial data are based on AAA diameter.

The rupture rate for patients with AAAs 4.0 to 5.5 cm was 1.0% per year in UKSAT[5] and 0.7% per year in ADAM.[7] A surveillance interval of 6 months was shown to be safe for AAAs 4.0 to 5.4 cm in the ADAM trial.[6] Longer intervals of 2 to 3 years have been proposed for smaller AAAs.[8] Natural history data are generally limited for AAAs larger than 5.5 cm because the great majority of patients with aneurysms of this size have AAA repair. Presumably as a result, substantial disagreement among experts has been documented regarding risk of rupture of large AAAs.[9]

Of the few studies available on the natural history of large AAAs, most predate the introduction of accurate measurement techniques. In 1966, Szilagyi et al. reported rupture in 61 of 141 AAAs ≥7 cm followed for a mean of 17 months, a crude rate of 30.5% per year.[10] Thirty-five years later, Powell et al. observed a very similar 0.28 ruptures per patient-year in 100 patients with AAAs >5.5 cm.[11]

The VA Natural History of Large Abdominal Aortic Aneurysms (NHLA) Study enrolled 198 patients with AAAs ≥5.5 cm for whom elective repair was not expected in the next 6 months because of medical contraindications to surgery or patient refusal.[12] All patients but 1 were male, and nearly all had a history of smoking. In addition to initial diameter, attained AAA diameter was obtained by follow-up imaging measurements (primarily ultrasound) every 6 months. The study duration was 5 years and mean follow-up was 1.5 years. Outcome ascertainment was complete for all patients, and autopsy was performed on 52 of 112 deaths (46%): 45 patients had probable AAA rupture. The 1-year incidence of probable rupture by initial AAA diameter was 9.4% for AAAs 5.5 to 5.9 cm, 10.3% for AAAs 6.0 to 6.9 cm (20% for the subgroup of 6.5 to 6.9 cm), and 29.5% for AAAs ≥7.0 cm. Much of the increased risk associated with initial diameters of 6.5 to 7.9 cm was related to an increased likelihood that the AAA would reach 8.0 cm during follow-up, after which more than one fourth ruptured within 6 months. AAA diameter was the strongest predictor of rupture in terms of variance explained. Other studies have also reported rupture rates generally consistent with those reported here.[13-15]

These findings can inform decision making in high–operative risk male patients but might not apply to good–operative risk patients. The 9.4% 1-year probable rupture rate observed for AAAs with initial diameters of 5.5 to 5.9 cm is tenfold higher than the rates described above from the two randomized trials for AAAs 4.0 to 5.4 cm.[5-6] Whereas some of this difference likely results from the slightly larger AAA diameters, much of it probably reflects a difference in rupture rates between these mostly high–operative risk patients with severe comorbidities and the healthier patients randomized into the trials. Several pieces of evidence support this interpretation:[1] in a study from Kingston, Ontario, rupture rates in men were the same (0.8%/yr) for AAAs 5.5 to 5.9 cm as for those 5.0 to 5.4 cm[16], and[2] ineligible (and presumably sicker) patients followed outside UKSAT had a higher rupture rate than randomized patients with comparable AAA diameters.[11]

In recent years, many patients who are not medically fit for open repair have been treated with endovascular repair. The United Kingdom Endovascular Aneurysm Repair trial 2 (EVAR-2) was a randomized trial designed to evaluate this practice by comparing endovascular repair with observation in 338 patients with AAAs ≥5.5 cm who were candidates for endovascular repair but judged medically unfit for open repair.[17] Natural history data were obtained on the 172 patients randomized to observation. These patients had a mean AAA diameter of 6.3 cm (IQR 6.0 to 7.0). There were 23 ruptures in the observation group, resulting in a crude rupture rate of 9.0 per 100 person years (95% CI 6.0-13.5), a rate similar to that observed in the VA NHLA study for AAAs with initial diameters of 5.5 to 6.9 cm.[12]

Recently, much attention has been paid to the influence of gender on rupture rate. In patients evaluated for the UKSAT, the rate of AAA rupture was three times higher in women than in men after adjustment for age, body size, and initial AAA diameter and the mean AAA diameter preceding rupture was 6.0 cm in men but only 5.0 cm in women.[18] In the 8-year report of the UKSAT,[19] which included 188 women, the hazard ratio for rupture for women versus men was 4.0 (95% CI 2.0-7.9, P<0.001), although there was still no benefit from early repair in women (HR=.99). In a recent meta-analysis by the same U.K. authors, no gender difference could be demonstrated for rupture risk of AAAs >5.5 cm.[20] The Kingston study reported that AAAs 5 to 5.9 cm ruptured four times as often in women as in men, although this finding was based on only five ruptures in women, and there were no ruptures in either gender in AAAs less than 5 cm.[16]

A rapid rate of AAA enlargement rate (usually >1.0 cm/yr) has occasionally been considered to increase rupture risk (and has therefore been proposed as an independent indication for repair of small AAAs), but it is difficult to find evidence to support this view. Sharp and Collin[21] observed no ruptures in 50 patient-years of follow up on 32 AAAs <5.5 cm that had enlarged 0.5 cm or more in the previous 6 months. In the VA NHLA study described above,[12] prior rate of AAA enlargement was not a significant predictor of rupture when adjusted for current AAA diameter, although there was a trend in that direction. For AAAs <5.5 cm that grew 1.0 cm or more in the Multicentre Aneurysm Screening Study,[22] two ruptures occurred in 256 patient-years of follow-up, a rate of 0.8%/yr that is similar to that observed in all patients with small AAAs in ADAM and UKSAT. These data do not offer much support to the concept that rapid enlargement rate increases rupture risk.

ENLARGEMENT

Because AAA diameter is the most important known predictor of rupture and is the usual reason for elective repair, the factors that influence AAA enlargement are important to AAA management. These are of course related to the factors associated with the presence of AAAs in the first place. These latter factors have been examined in numerous screening studies, the largest of these being the ADAM screening program, which collected data prior to ultrasound to detect AAAs on 126,196 veterans 50 to 79 years old.[23] In that study, age, smoking, family history of AAAs, and atherosclerotic diseases were the principal positive associations with AAAs, whereas female sex, diabetes, and black race were the principal negative associations.

A few studies have examined the incidence of AAAs by looking for the development of new AAAs after an initial negative screening test. In the ADAM study, 2622 mostly male veterans aged 50 to 79 years who had aortic diameters <3.0 cm on an initial ultrasound screen had repeat ultrasound after 4 years.[24] On the second screening, 2.2% had AAAs >3.0 cm, but these aneurysms were small: 95% of them were less than 4.0 cm and none were larger than 5.0 cm. Similarly, in the Chichester, U.K. screening study, 4308 men aged 65 years with aortic diameters <3.0 cm on an initial ultrasound had repeat ultrasound every 2 years,[25] and after a mean follow-up time of 5 years, 2.2% had AAAs >3.0 cm. Not surprisingly, larger aortic diameter on the first ultrasound (i.e., ≥2.5 cm) increased the likelihood of an AAA on follow-up in both studies.

Several longitudinal studies that used computed tomography have stressed that AAA enlargement is often irregular and unpredictable.[26-27] Furthermore, variations in

AAA measurement up to 0.5 cm are common.[28] Several studies have found that increasing AAA diameter is associated with cardiovascular and all-cause mortality,[29–30] suggesting that larger AAA diameter may be a marker for poor health.

In the ADAM trial, AAAs 4.0 to 5.5 cm enlarged at a mean rate of 0.3 cm/yr.[6] Smaller AAAs 3.0 to 3.9 cm followed outside of the trial expanded at a slower median rate of 0.11 cm/yr.[8] In the VA NHLA study of patients unfit for repair,[12] AAAs >5.5 cm enlarged at a median rate of 0.43 cm/yr. Because AAA enlargement expressed in the usual way as centimeters per year increases with AAA diameter, it may be more generalizable to express enlargement as percent per year, with 6%/yr being the most accurate figure.

AAA enlargement rate has been reported to be associated with several factors, including initial AAA diameter,[6,31-33] smoking,[34-36] age,[31-35] and absence of diabetes.[6,36]

Hypertension and lipid levels were not associated with rapid enlargement in these studies. Whereas there have been a few isolated reports of associations of various manifestations of occlusive vascular disease with increased AAA enlargement rate (e.g., low ankle-brachial pressure index,[36] severe cardiac disease and previous stroke,[35] other studies have reported no associations with these factors. AAA enlargement rate has been reported to be both faster and slower in women than in men,[37] and rates did not differ by gender in patients followed by the UKSAT group.[36]

CONCLUSION

There is now sufficient published evidence to describe with confidence much but not all of the natural history of AAAs. AAAs of 4.0 to 5.5 cm in diameter have a rupture rate of 0.7 to 1.0%/yr, and for AAAs <4.0 cm this rate is even lower. Women appear to have a higher rupture rate than men for small AAAs, but there is no evidence of this for AAAs >5.5 cm. Rupture rates of AAAs >5.5 cm in fit individuals are unknown and unlikely to be known in the future. However, for unfit individuals with AAAs >5.5 cm, the rupture rate is high, starting at about 10%/yr and increasing by severalfold in the largest AAAs.

Median enlargement rate of AAAs 4.0 to 5.5 cm is about 0.3 cm/yr. Enlargement rate is influenced by AAA diameter, being approximately half this rate for AAAs 3.0 to 4.0 cm and half again faster for AAAs >5.5 cm. There is, however, considerable individual variability in enlargement rates, and a variety of diseases and conditions appear to influence these rates. The search is on for drugs to favorably alter this natural history, and if successful, it will doubtless shed much light on the pathophysiology of AAA enlargement.

REFERENCES

1. Adam DJ, Mohan IV, Stuart WP, et al. Community and hospital outcome from ruptured abdominal aortic aneurysm within the catchment area of a regional vascular surgical service. J Vasc Surg 1999;30:922–8.
2. Gillum RF. Epidemiology of aortic aneurysm in the United States. J Clin Epidemiol 1995;48: 1289–98.
3. McPhee JT, Hill JS, Eslami MH. The impact of gender on presentation, therapy, and mortality of abdominal aortic aneurysm in the United States, 2001–2004. J Vasc Surg 2007;45:891–9.

4. Bengtsson H, Bergqvist D, Sternby NH. Increasing prevalence of abdominal aortic aneurysms: a necropsy study. Eur J Surg 1992;158:19–23.
5. The UK Small Aneurysm Trial Participants. Mortality results for randomised controlled trial of early elective surgery or ultrasonographic surveillance for small abdominal aortic aneurysms. Lancet 1998;352:1649–55.
6. Lederle FA, Wilson SE, Johnson GR, et al. for the Aneurysm Detection and Management (ADAM) Veterans Affairs Cooperative Study Group. Immediate repair compared with surveillance of small abdominal aortic aneurysms. N Engl J Med 2002;346:1437–44.
7. Lederle FA. Small abdominal aortic aneurysms—reply. N Engl J Med 2002;347:1114.
8. Santilli SM, Littooy FN, Cambria RA, et al. Expansion rates and outcomes for the 3.0-cm to the 3.9-cm infrarenal abdominal aortic aneurysm. J Vasc Surg 2002;35:666–71.
9. Lederle FA. Risk of rupture of large abdominal aortic aneurysms: disagreement among vascular surgeons. Arch Intern Med 1996;156:1007–9.
10. Szilagyi DE, Smith RF, DeRusso FJ, et al. Contribution of abdominal aortic aneurysmectomy to prolongation of life. Ann Surg 1966;164:678–99.
11. Powell JT, Brown LC. The natural history of abdominal aortic aneurysms and their risk of rupture. Acta Chir Belg 2001;101:11–6.
12. Lederle FA, Johnson GR, Wilson SE, et al. for the Veterans Affairs Cooperative Study #417 Investigators. Rupture rate of large abdominal aortic aneurysms in patients refusing or unfit for elective repair. JAMA 2002;287:2968–72.
13. Reed WW, Hallett JW Jr, Damiano MA, Ballard DJ. Learning from the last ultrasound. A population-based study of patients with abdominal aortic aneurysm. Arch Intern Med 1997;157:2064–8.
14. Jones A, Cahill D, Gardham R. Outcome in patients with a large abdominal aortic aneurysm considered unfit for surgery. Br J Surg 1998;85:1382–4.
15. Conway KP, Byrne J, Townsend M, Lane IF. Prognosis of patients turned down for conventional abdominal aortic aneurysm repair in the endovascular and sonographic era: Szilagyi revisited? J Vasc Surg 2001;33:752–7.
16. Brown PM, Zelt DT, Sobolev B. The risk of rupture in untreated aneurysms: the impact of size, gender, and expansion rate. J Vasc Surg 2003;37:280–4.
17. EVAR trial participants. Endovascular aneurysm repair and outcome in patients unfit for open repair of abdominal aortic aneurysm (EVAR trial 2): randomised controlled trial. Lancet 2005;365:2187–92.
18. Brown LC, Powell JT. Risk factors for aneurysm rupture in patients kept under ultrasound surveillance. Ann Surg 1999;230:289–96.
19. United Kingdom Small Aneurysm Trial Participants. Long-term outcomes of immediate repair compared with surveillance of small abdominal aortic aneurysms. N Engl J Med 2002;346:1445–52.
20. Powell JT, Brown LC, Greenhalgh RM, Thompson SG, EVAR Trial Participants. The rupture rate of large abdominal aortic aneurysms: is this modified by anatomical suitability for endovascular repair? Ann Surg 2008;247:173–9.
21. Sharp MA, Collin J. A myth exposed: fast growth in diameter does not justify precocious abdominal aortic aneurysm repair. Eur J Vasc Endovasc Surg 2003;25:408–11.
22. Scott RA, Kim LG, Ashton HA, Multi-centre Aneurysm Screening Study Group. Assessment of the criteria for elective surgery in screen-detected abdominal aortic aneurysms. J Med Screen 2005;12:150–4.
23. Lederle FA, Johnson GR, Wilson SE, et al. The Aneurysm Detection and Management Study screening program: validation cohort and final results. Arch Intern Med 2000;160: 1425–30.
24. Lederle FA, Johnson GR, Wilson SE, et al, and the ADAM VA Cooperative Study Investigators. Yield of repeated screening for abdominal aortic aneurysm after a four-year interval. Arch Intern Med 2000;160:1117–21.
25. Hafez H, Druce PS, Ashton HA. Abdominal aortic aneurysm development in men following a "normal" aortic ultrasound scan. Eur J Vasc Endovasc Surg 2008;36:553–8.

26. Kurvers H, Veith FJ, Lipsitz EC, et al. Discontinuous, staccato growth of abdominal aortic aneurysms. J Am Coll Surg 2004;199:709–15.
27. Vega de Céniga M, Gómez R, Estallo L, et al. Analysis of expansion patterns in 4-4.9 cm abdominal aortic aneurysms. Ann Vasc Surg 2008;22:37–44.
28. Lederle FA, Wilson SE, Johnson GR, et al, for the Abdominal Aortic Aneurysm Detection and Management Veterans Administration Cooperative Study Group. Variability in measurement of abdominal aortic aneurysms. J Vasc Surg 1995;21:945–52.
29. Brady AR, Fowkes FG, Thompson SG, Powell JT. Aortic aneurysm diameter and risk of cardiovascular mortality. Arterioscler Thromb Vasc Biol 2001;21:1203–7.
30. Norman P, Le M, Pearce C, Jamrozik K. Infrarenal aortic diameter predicts all-cause mortality. Arterioscler Thromb Vasc Biol 2004;24:1278–82.
31. Couto E, Duffy SW, Ashton HA, et al. Probabilities of progression of aortic aneurysms: estimates and implications for screening policy. J Med Screen 2002;9:40–2.
32. McCarthy RJ, Shaw E, Whyman MR, et al. Recommendations for screening intervals for small aortic aneurysms. Br J Surg 2003;90:821–6.
33. Norman P, Spencer CA, Lawrence-Brown MM, Jamrozik K. C-reactive protein levels and the expansion of screen-detected abdominal aortic aneurysms in men. Circulation 2004;17; 110:862–6.
34. MacSweeney STR, Ellis M, Worrell PC, et al. Smoking and growth rate of small abdominal aortic aneurysms. Lancet 1994;344:651–2.
35. Chang JB, Stein TA, Liu JP, Dunn ME. Risk factors associated with rapid growth of small abdominal aortic aneurysms. Surgery 1997;121:117–22.
36. Brady AR, Thompson SG, Fowkes FG, et al. UK Small Aneurysm Trial Participants. Abdominal aortic aneurysm expansion: risk factors and time intervals for surveillance. Circulation 2004;110:16–21.
37. Smart CJ, Fisher RK. Influence of sex on expansion rate of abdominal aortic aneurysms. Br J Surg 2007;94:1041–2.

49

Investigating the Unique Relationship of Tobacco Smoke and Abdominal Aortic Aneurysms

John A. Curci, M.D.

EPIDEMIOLOGY OF ABDOMINAL AORTIC ANEURYSMS AND SMOKING

Although awareness of the impact of abdominal aortic aneurysms (AAAs) on the health of the nation has been increasing, it remains underappreciated that 3 to 10% of the male population over the age of 55 are affected by this disease, resulting in about 1% of the annual deaths in this population. As the country ages owing to improved care for other concomitant vascular diseases and malignancies, this proportion is likely to increase. The effects of the disease are typically limited to the infrarenal segment of the abdominal aorta, although it often extends into the iliac vasculature as well. The fusiform dilation of the aorta and iliac vessels in this location is difficult to detect on physical examination and is nearly always asymptomatic. Because of this, the exact prevalence of disease is unknown, and most aneurysms are found serendipitously during evaluation for other abdominal pathology. Increasing appreciation for the significance of the disease has resulted in recent legislation the Screening Abdominal Aortic Aneurysms Very Efficiently (SAAAVE) Act that provides reimbursement for AAA screening of males older than 65 with a history of tobacco smoking.

Tobacco smoke exposure (TSE) is widely acknowledged to be the most potent environmental toxin to which individuals are exposed on a chronic basis. Notwithstanding the effects on smokers themselves, the vascular and cardiac effects of environmental TSE (aka second-hand smoke) cause 35,000 deaths annually in the United States alone.[1] Although smoking prevalence has decreased in the United States over the past 20 years, it still remains near one-fifth of the population, and worldwide smoking is expected to increase for the foreseeable future.[2] Tobacco smoke (TS) may be as dangerous to vascular health as a high-fat/high-cholesterol diet. However, relative to our scientific mechanistic understanding of lipid and cholesterol metabolism on the evolution of vascular disease, the understanding of the effects of TSE on the vascular tree is quite meager.

Among TS-related vascular diseases, the incidence of death from an AAA is increased dramatically among those with past or ongoing smoke exposure, with relative risks reaching 5- to 10-fold compared with nonsmokers.[3-4] Although other vascular diseases are also significantly affected by exposure to TS, the effect is dramatically lower. The effect of TS on the overall incidence of death from coronary disease, for example, is only in the relative risk range of 1.5 to 2.0, based on a systematic review of the epidemiologic literature.[5] Although AAA incidence is correlated with the presence of risk factors for atherosclerotic vascular disease,[4] careful evaluation of the predisposing factors makes it clear that atherosclerotic disease and aneurysmal disease are products of distinct disease processes.[5-7]

The only diseases more closely related to TSE are pulmonary diseases such as lung cancer and chronic obstructive pulmonary disease (COPD).[5] There is even a strong epidemiologic overlap of COPD and AAA, but this is likely to be primarily coincidental to the common effects of cigarette smoking rather than a direct effect of diminished pulmonary function on aneurysm development.[8] The large increases in risk of lung cancer and COPD can be reasonably understood in the context of the direct exposure of the lung to the inhaled TS. Unlike these pulmonary diseases, however, the infrarenal aortic tissue most prone to aneurysmal development is never directly exposed to the inhaled TS components. This makes the effect of smoke on the incidence of AAA even more remarkable.

The natural history of the AAA disease is progressive dilation with eventual compromise of the integrity of the structural elements of the aortic wall to the point of failure.[9] Subsequent exsanguination from aortic rupture is nearly always fatal. More rapid growth of an aneurysm has been related to hypertension,[10] although this finding has been inconsistent.[11] It is clear, however, that ongoing TSE also promotes more rapid growth of the aneurysm compared with individuals who have stopped smoking.[8,12]

Available treatments for large (>5.5 cm) AAAs currently rely on the physical exclusion of the abnormal arterial segments. However, these therapies have shown no benefit in the treatment of small aortic aneurysms (3-5.5 cm in maximal diameter), which have a very low risk of rupture.[13-14] Whereas appropriate treatment of the patient's hypertension and encouragement of smoking cessation are advised in these patients, the effects of these interventions are small, and the AAA will continue to grow. Because the majority of aneurysms identified by screening are smaller than 5.5 cm, there is currently no effective treatment to offer these patients, and management is limited to serial imaging of the aneurysm until the threshold for surgical treatment is met. This asymptomatic interval of this disease offers an important opportunity for medical intervention to alter the natural history of the disease. Research over the past several years has begun to determine the mechanisms of the disease and potential therapeutic targets to alter disease progression. However, there are currently no agents demonstrated to be effective in limiting disease progression or death. Furthermore, no agents have been evaluated in the setting of TSE. Therefore, there remains tremendous opportunity to impact the lives of people affected by this disease.[15-18]

SMOKING AND ABDOMINAL AORTIC ANEURYSMS PATHOLOGY

The most striking feature of AAA histology is the loss of normal medial arterial structure and, in particular, the near-complete absence of a normal lamellar elastin matrix, a feature that it has in common with COPD.[19] In the aorta, these matrix changes are attributed to three general features that are believed to be interrelated: (1) elaboration of high levels of proteases, (2) chronic inflammatory infiltration, and (3) loss/dysfunction of parenchymal cells central to matrix deposition and repair.

How TSE interacts with the matrix or cellular functions of the aorta to cause the development of an AAA is unknown. The lack of a disease-specific model involving TSE has been a major limitation, but there are studies that support TSE involvement in all three of these general features. The vast majority of studies that have investigated the disease-causing effects of TSE on vascular biology have relied primarily on gross extracts or purified specific components of TSE applied in vivo or to tissues or cells. These are techniques successfully used to define similar pathologic processes induced by TSE in the lung.[20-26] Many of these studies are focused primarily on the vascular pathology as it relates to disease pathways previously defined to influence the development of atherosclerosis or thrombosis. Although these studies do offer some clues to the effects of TSE on AAA development, it must be acknowledged that they are severely limited by two inherent assumptions: First, it is assumed that the toxin or toxin mixture applied to the cells in culture is similar to the milieu to which in vivo cells are exposed. Second, it is assumed that TS or TS component exposure will activate known pathways of disease. Neither of these assumptions has been rigorously investigated or validated.

Experimentation into the effects of inhaled TSE on AAA development is particularly complicated by the indirect exposure of the vascular tree to the toxins contained in TS. There are an enormous number of compounds with toxic potential in both primary and environmental TS. Which of these compounds or secondary phenomena play a key role in aneurysm development and growth is unknown and, in the absence of disease models, extremely difficult to study. Figure 49–1 emphasizes the potentially complicated relationship between smoke inhalation and the toxic effects of TS on the vasculature and the development of aortic aneurysms. Because of the complex makeup of TS and the variety of intermediaries that may be involved, the clinical effects could be occurring through alterations of the inflammatory response, the function of resident smooth muscle cells, or the vessel matrix itself. Recent successes in developing a specific mouse model of AAA development as described below is a key initial step to understanding the alterations in vascular biology that accompany increased aneurysm development in the setting of TSE.

Detailing the pathophysiology of TS on AAA and vascular disease will provide benefits to the care and prevention of patients afflicted with these diseases in a variety of ways. First, the mechanisms and means to understand the underlying causes of this particular inhaled environmental toxin may be extrapolated to other potentially disease-causing inhaled agents. Second, novel mechanisms for disease initiation and progression may be specifically enhanced by TSE that may be important to our understanding of all causes of vascular disease. Third, mechanisms initiated by TSE may not be limited to the acute exposure period but may persist and cause disease long after the exposure has concluded. Specific therapies will need to be developed to ameliorate the long-term consequences, particularly for children and others exposed involuntarily to TS.

Effect of Smoking on Matrix Degrading Enzymes and Elastin Damage in abdominal aortic aneurysms

Under normal conditions, aortic elastin is thought to be extremely durable, with a half-life approximating the lifetime of the individual.[27] Therefore, the elastin loss characteristic of

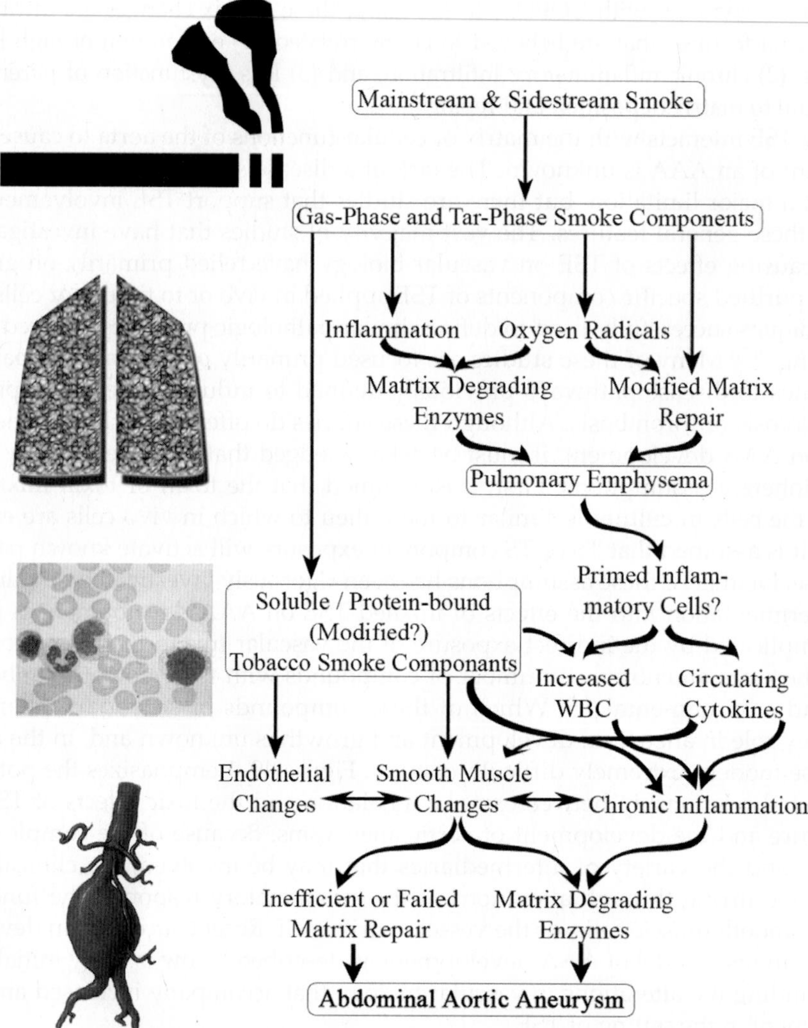

Figure 49-1. Diagrammatic representation of the potential interaction pathways between inhaled tobacco smoke (TS) and the development of aortic aneurysm. The relationship between TS inhaled in the lungs and its action on the aorta to promote abdominal aortic aneurysms (AAA) development has a potentially complicated network of intermediaries. In the absence of an in vivo model of abdominal aortic aneurysms development that depends on TS, it is impossible to predict which of these pathways or intermediaries is most relevant.

AAA is particularly remarkable. Because enzymatic degradation of lamellar elastin depends on a relatively small subset of appropriately specific proteases, considerable research has focused on characterizing the elastolytic activities in aneurysms. Studies of human tissue demonstrate dramatically increased expression and/or activity of elastolytic matrix metalloproteases (MMPs): MMP-2,[28] MMP-3,[29-30] MMP-9,[31-33] MMP-7,[34] and MMP-12.[35-36] Corresponding findings in murine models of AAA have also been seen, particularly with respect to MMP-9.[37-38] There is increasing evidence that inhibition of these enzymatic activities with doxycycline results in favorable alterations in AAA biology, although thorough clinical testing has not yet been performed.[18] More recently, there has been accumulating evidence that several other protease groups have been shown to be upregulated in the aneurysm wall of both diseased human tissue and laboratory models. A strong association between elastolytic cysteine protease activity, including cathepsin S and cathepsin L, and aneurysm progression has been demonstrated in both human AAA and animal models.[39-40] Depressed levels of the specific cysteine protease inhibitor, cystatin C, has also been associated with AAA growth in models and humans.[41-42] It has been suggested that these enzymes may work cooperatively with members of the MMP family of enzymes to produce matrix damage.[43] The recent findings regarding the cathepsin dipeptidyl protease I and neutrophil recruitment into model AAAs has brought new attention to the potential role of the serine proteases in the elastin loss seen in AAA.[44]

It is now well recognized that TSE results in upregulation of expression and activity of multiple MMPs in pulmonary disease. Much of the data comes from studies of MMP production in the lungs of mice exposed to TS. In these studies, MMP-12 was somewhat uniquely elevated, and the development of pulmonary emphysema was significantly inhibited in animals deficient in this single enzyme.[45] Other elastolytic enzymes of MMP, serine and cysteine proteinase families, are also elevated in response to TSE in model and human pulmonary emphysema and may play important roles.[22]

To date, studies of MMP expression specifically within the arterial wall related to TSE are very meager. For example, in rabbits exposed to TS, one study demonstrated a significant increase in aortic elastase activity,[46] although it should be noted that even any remote physical injury in these rabbits also resulted in increased aortic elastase activity.[47] A study of microdissected lung determined that MMP-12 was increased in the lung vasculature of smokers and might be causally related to the development of TSE-induced pulmonary hypertension.[48] There is some evidence that the carotid plaque taken from individuals who were actively smoking at the time of carotid endarterectomy had increased levels of MMP-12 and decreased levels of tissue inhibitor of metalloprotenases-1 compared with nonsmokers.[49] Components of TS that may be in circulation have also been shown to increase MMP production by macrophages that are involved in atherosclerotic lesion development.[50]

Effect of Tobacco Smoke Exposure on Vascular Parenchymal Cells

The vascular smooth muscle cell (VSMC) must be centrally positioned in aneurysm pathobiology. It is the most populous cell of the aortic media, and it is capable of (1) matrix synthesis, (2) proteinase (and inhibitor) elaboration, and (3) cytokine release/inflammatory cell recruitment. There is evidence that VSMC derived from aneurysmal tissue is characterized by apoptosis and poor in vitro propagation[51-54] and has reduced matrix-producing capabilities.[51-53,55-56] There is also evidence that these cells can produce significantly more proteolytic enzymes[57-58] and increased MCP-1 possibly via a protein kinase Cδ pathway.[59] It may be possible, based on direct and indirect evidence, that TSE can alter any of these three principal function activities of medial VSMC to promote AAA pathology. There are certainly other resident cells that may participate in the vascular injury characteristic of aneurysm, but the numbers of those cells are relatively small, particularly within the media, and they are unlikely to have much of an effect in the absence of abnormalities of the VSMCs.

The responses of VSMCs to TSE in vivo are poorly understood. Exacerbation of intimal disease processes that may be dependent on VSMC activity can be induced in animals exposed to TS.[60-63] In these studies, increased lesion size, including significant increases in intimal proliferation of smooth muscle cells, occurs in response to periarterial cuff placement or in hypercholesterolemic mice. The mechanisms most frequently studied in these models relate to increased oxidative stress and alterations in endothelial function that may promote disease activity.[60,64] Altered cholesterol trafficking and proinflammatory alterations in endothelial function have been described.[65] However, these effects may have limited applicability to the development of AAAs, because the typical alterations seen in aneurysms are of reduced VSMC activity, not the increased proliferation and matrix deposition seen with intimal hyperplasia or atherosclerosis. Moreover, the effect was limited to the intima of the vessels, not the media.

Smoking can impair matrix repair through several described mechanisms. Smoke exposure and smoke extracts have been shown to result in cellular apoptosis and oxidative stress.[25,66-67] TSE also results in abnormal tissue repair of bronchial epithelium and cultured fibroblasts.[68-69] In addition to the local effects of smoke on the lung, there are also systemic effects that suggest impairment of normal repair mechanisms at remote locations. For example, normal acute wound healing has been shown in several studies to be significantly impaired in the face of continued cigarette smoking.[70-74] This would suggest that cigarette smoking may impede normal repair to injury within the vascular tree.

Other studies have used lipid or water-soluble cigarette smoke extracts (CSE) and assayed the in vitro effects of TSE on MMP production on parenchymal cell types that may participate in aneurysm development, such as fibroblasts[75-78] and endothelium,[79-80] but not on VSMC. The increase in MMP activity in the lung associated with TSE has been primarily ascribed to the effects on infiltrating pulmonary monocytes/macrophages. However, there has been little direct investigation into the potential for these cells to participate in disease outside the lung, although their ability to act remotely to promote aneurysm disease has been hypothesized.[8] TSE-induced immune alterations of antibody responses to oxidized low density lipoprotein (LDL) have also been identified and further suggest that systemic leukocyte alterations can impact vascular disease.[81]

MODELING THE EFFECTS OF TS ON ABDOMINAL AORTIC ANEURYSMS DEVELOPMENT AND GROWTH

Over the past 20 years, much of the progress in understanding AAA biology has resulted from sophisticated models of aneurysm disease. Although there are several different models of AAAs that are actively being studied, the oldest and most well-characterized model is the elastase perfusion model. In this model, a brief elastase perfusion to the infrarenal aorta has minimal effect on the structure of the aorta initially but induces the production of proteases within the wall that subsequently cause extensive medial matrix damage that is maximal at 14 days following perfusion.[37] The loss of stainable medial elastic fibers is temporally correlated with the onset of aortic wall inflammation, including the increase in lymphocytes and tissue macrophages. The elastase-perfused murine model of aneurysm disease was developed in rats and later was extended to mice and has confirmed the role of MMP-9 in the development of aneurysms utilizing mice with targeted genetic deletions.[37-38] This model also recapitulates the inadequate reparative capacity of the aortic mesenchymal cells once the aneurysm cycle is established.[82] Overall, there is a loss of smooth muscle cells and impaired production of normal elastin and collagen fibers. Thus, histologically and physiologically, this model closely mirrors the process seen in human tissue.

The potential for modeling the effects of TSE on the arterial tree has been considered since the development of models of COPD in mice after in vivo smoke exposure. However, based on the phenotype of these animals, smoke exposure of adult mice has been known to not have an appreciable effect on the arterial tree. Even after the long duration of TSE necessary for this model (>24 wk), there have been no significant effects of TS on large vessel gross appearance or function.[83]

With this background, attempts were made to combine elastase perfusion of the aorta with concomitant exposure to TS. The mice were exposed via a mechanical device to a regimen of TS of two unfiltered research cigarettes (University of Kentucky) per day for 6 days per week, as previously described.[45] The experimental animals were started on this regimen beginning 4 weeks prior to elastase perfusion and continued with TS until harvest. This protocol failed to significantly alter the development of the subsequent aortic aneurysm when the animals were harvested at the standard interval of 2 weeks following perfusion.[84] However, in these same experiments, there were the first glimmers of some very weak effects of TSE on the size of aneurysms at very late time points following elastase perfusion.[84] Although encouraging, this was not likely to be an adequate model of TSE in aneurysms. Not only were these effects rather small, but these studies were done in the SvEv background mice, which have been recognized as having a different aneurysm development compared with the more commonly studied C57Bl/6 background mice.[85] Further, the late onset of the difference suggested that the changes seen may be related primarily to stabilization of the dilated aorta rather than to development of the aneurysm.

Additional refinement of the model was necessary, and it was hypothesized that the initial elastin injury established by elastase perfusion may result in essentially complete elastin degradation by 2 weeks and therefore near-maximal aneurysm diameter. Therefore, the effect of TSE was phenotypically unobserved in the standard model of AAA development. By making a relatively small modification to the model, that is, reducing elastase concentration in the perfusate, the histologic damage to elastin was clearly less substantial, and there was ultimately a smaller aneurysm that had a less severe degree of damage to the medial elastin fiber network.[86]

In the setting of this modified or low-dose elastase perfusion of the mouse aorta, TSE of the mice has now been shown to result in a significantly greater increase in aortic dilation.[86] As shown in Figure 49–2, the increase in aortic diameter was present even when the elastase was heat-inactivated prior to perfusion. The mice in this study were exposed to TS beginning 2 weeks prior to elastase perfusion and continuing through harvest. Compared with the months of TSE that are required to induce the development of pulmonary emphysema, this is a remarkably short duration of smoke exposure. It is also a considerably shorter period compared with models of TSE-enhanced atherosclerosis development in hyperlipidemic mice.[62-63]

There are several other remarkable features of this model. First, the histology (Figure 49–3) demonstrates that the elastin damage to the aorta is also substantially worse at 14 days in the smoke-exposed versus the room air–exposed animals. However, immediately after perfusion, there were no significant differences in the matrix histology of the aortas, nor was there any difference in the acute dilation of the aorta during the elastase perfusion. Further, there was no clear alteration in the degree of inflammation between the aortas from TSE mice compared with the roomair–exposed mice. Second, the increased aneurysm formation occurred in the absence of

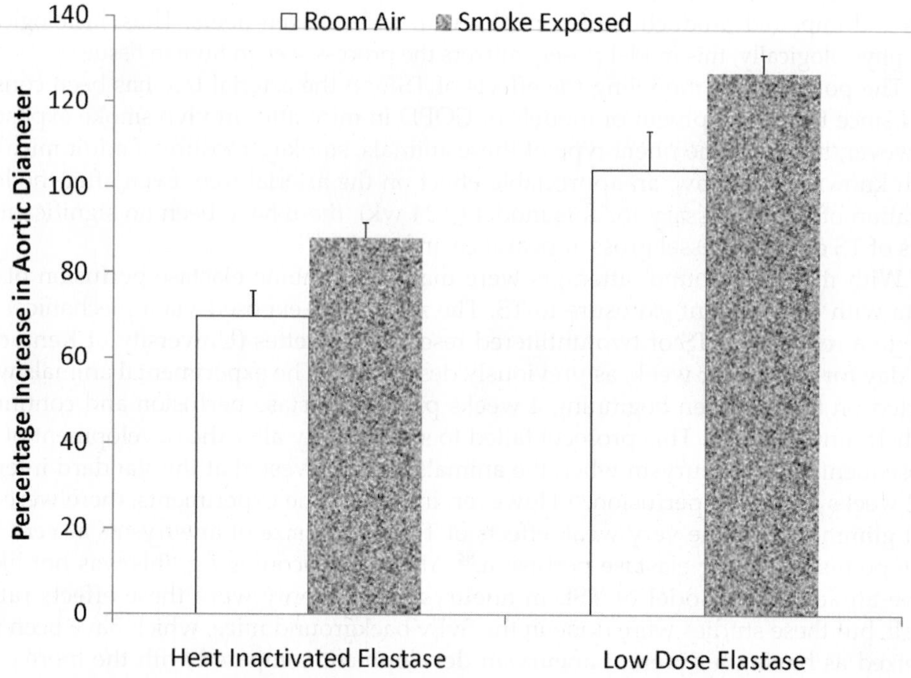

Figure 49-2. Effect of smoke exposure on the development of model abdominal aortic aneurysms in mice. Littermate mice were randomly allocated into smoke-exposure (n=37) or room air–exposure (n=48) groups and were exposed to TS in specialized chambers for 2 weeks at a dose used to induce pulmonary emphysema. Aortic diameters were measured before perfusion and then were perfused with active (n=23 smoke and n=24 nonsmoke) or heat-inactivated (n=14 smoke and n=24 nonsmoke) elastase at a dose significantly lower than the standard perfusion model. Fourteen days later, the aortic diameter was measured under physiologic pressure prior to sacrifice. The percentage increase in aortic diameter represents the change in aortic diameter over that 2-week interval. Note that regardless of the activity of the elastase infusion, the subsequent aortic dilatation is significantly larger in mice exposed to TS than in those exposed to room air alone.

any alteration in systemic blood pressure in response to TSE. Finally, there was no significant increase in the production of either MMP-9 or MMP-12 by quantitative polymerase chain reaction analysis.

FUTURE DIRECTIONS

Currently, the effects of TSE on the vasculature of an intact animal have been rather cursorily investigated. We have moderate evidence for alterations in certain cellular activities after in vitro exposure of the cells to CSE, including diminished nitric oxide, increased MMP production, increased oxidation stress, and increased cytokine production. Most of the data are from pulmonary disease, and the relevance of CSE on the actual pathology of arterial diseases remains mostly speculative, although some limited in vivo studies have been done to confirm alterations in recognized pathways of disease. In general, these studies presume that TSE affects arterial disease development via pathways that have already been defined in relation to atherosclerosis.

The strong relationship between TSE and AAA offers a unique opportunity to identify disease pathogenesis. Given the variety of different mechanisms, both known

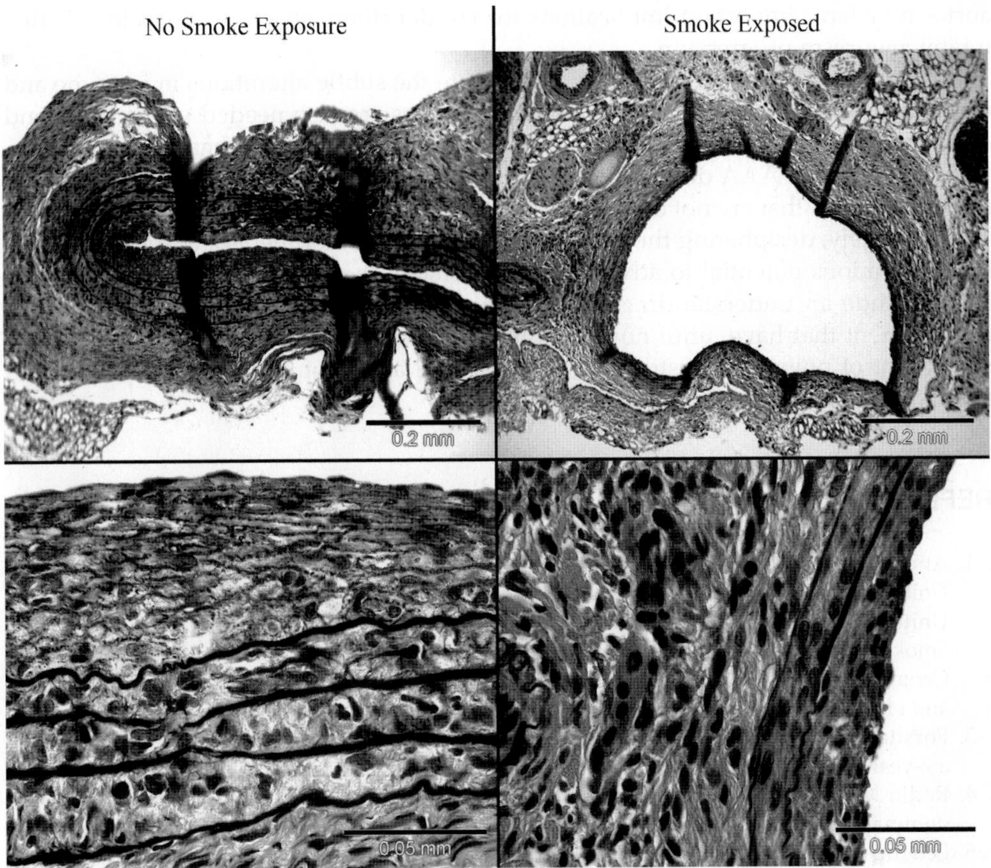

Figure 49-3. Elastin-specific staining of aortic tissue 14 days following perfusion with low-dose elastase. Note that the tissues taken from animals that had been exposed to TS had dramatically less stainable elastic fibers remaining in the medial layer at harvest than the aortas taken from mice exposed to room air only. Top row of images taken at 200X magnification and the lower row taken at 1000X magnification.

and unknown, for TSE to potentially influence aneurysm development, it is essential to have an in vivo model to begin to evaluate the specific contribution of these alterations in vessel wall biology. Dissecting the mechanisms of TSE on AAAs may also have significant important benefits for overall understanding of the pathophysiology of environmental toxins on the vascular tree.[87-88] The availability of this novel model also allows the opportunity to evaluate the durability of the effects of TSE, a particularly important question in the setting of the apparent long interval between smoke exposure and clinical AAA development.

Certainly, further evaluations of the interaction of metalloproteinases and TSE need to be conducted to define the interrelationship. Although there was no significant increase in aortic MMP expression with TSE during aneurysm development, MMPs have multiple other means of regulation that may be altered in the setting of TSE. Because of the important contributions of MMP-12 to TSE-induced pulmonary emphysema, it remains reasonable to hypothesize that there is an important contribution of these enzymes to TSE-induced AAA. Conversely, the potential for an alternative mechanism to play an important role in the elastin matrix destruction seen in these aortas may have important implications for the development of pharmaceuticals that inhibit aneurysm progression.

Other lines of investigation need to evaluate the subtle alterations in immune and vascular wall function that accompany TSE. Studies are also needed of the DNA and epigenetic alterations that may impact the function of the parenchymal and inflammatory cells active in AAA development. There may also be injury or changes in the matrix of the vessel that are not evident on standard histologic stains.

Ultimately, deciphering the effects of TSE on the development of aortic aneurysms has tremendous potential to advance our understanding of arterial disease. This may even include an understanding of the initiating/precipitating events of aneurysm development that have, until now, been impossible to study. This may allow the development of novel diagnostic techniques as well as the opportunity to intervene in aneurysm development at a far earlier stage.

REFERENCES

1. Annual smoking-attributable mortality, years of potential life lost, and productivity losses — United States, 1997–2001. MMWR. Morb Mortal Wkly Rep 2005;54:625–8.
2. United States Department of Health and Human Services. The Health Consequences of Smoking: A Report of the Surgeon General. In: Department of Health and Human Services Centers for Disease Control and Prevention, National Center for Chronic Disease Prevention and Health Promotion, Office of Smoking and Health; 2004.
3. Forsdahl SH, Singh K, Solberg S, et al. Risk factors for abdominal aortic aneurysms: a 7-year prospective study: the Tromso Study, 1994–2001. Circulation 2009;119:2202–8.
4. Rodin MB, Daviglus ML, Wong GC, et al. Middle age cardiovascular risk factors and abdominal aortic aneurysm in older age. Hypertension 2003;42:61–8.
5. Lederle FA, Nelson DB, Joseph AM. Smokers' relative risk for aortic aneurysm compared with other smoking-related diseases: a systematic review. J Vasc Surg 2003;38:329–34.
6. Shteinberg D, Halak M, Shapiro S, et al. Abdominal aortic aneurysm and aortic occlusive disease: a comparison of risk factors and inflammatory response. Eur J Vasc Endovasc Surg 2000;20:462–5.
7. Blanchard JF, Armenian HK, Friesen PP. Risk factors for abdominal aortic aneurysm: results of a case-control study. Am J Epidemiol 2000;151:575–83.
8. Lindholt JS, Jorgensen B, Klitgaard NA, et al. Systemic levels of cotinine and elastase, but not pulmonary function, are associated with the progression of small abdominal aortic aneurysms. Eur J Vasc Endovasc Surg 2003;26:418–22.
9. Glimaker H, Holmberg L, Elvin A, et al. Natural history of patients with abdominal aortic aneurysm. Eur J Vasc Surg 1991;5:125–30.
10. Naydeck BL, Sutton-Tyrrell K, Schiller KD, et al. Prevalence and risk factors for abdominal aortic aneurysms in older adults with and without isolated systolic hypertension. Am J Cardiol 1999;83:759–64.
11. Vardulaki KA, Walker NM, Day NE, et al. Quantifying the risks of hypertension, age, sex and smoking in patients with abdominal aortic aneurysm. Br J Surg 2000;87:195–200.
12. MacSweeney ST, Ellis M, Worrell PC, et al. Smoking and growth rate of small abdominal aortic aneurysms. Lancet 2004;344:651–2.
13. Greenhalgh RM, Forbes JF, Fowkes FG, et al. Early elective open surgical repair of small abdominal aortic aneurysms is not recommended: results of the UK Small Aneurysm Trial. Steering Committee [editorial]. Eur J Vasc Endovasc Surg 1998;16:462–4.
14. Anonymous. Mortality results for randomised controlled trial of early elective surgery or ultrasonographic surveillance for small abdominal aortic aneurysms. The UK Small Aneurysm Trial Participants. Lancet 1998;352:1649–55.

15. Baxter BT. Could medical intervention work for aortic aneurysms? Am J Surg 2004;188: 628–32.
16. Mosorin M, Juvonen J, Biancari F, et al. Use of doxycycline to decrease the growth rate of abdominal aortic aneurysms: a randomized, double-blind, placebo-controlled pilot study. J Vasc Surg 2001;34:606–10.
17. Thompson RW, Liao S, Curci JA. Therapeutic potential of tetracycline derivatives to suppress the growth of abdominal aortic aneurysms. Adv Dent Res 1998;12:159–65.
18. Baxter BT, Pearce WH, Waltke EA, et al. Prolonged administration of doxycycline in patients with small asymptomatic abdominal aortic aneurysms: report of a prospective (Phase II) multicenter study. J Vasc Surg 2002;36:1–12.
19. Snider GL. Distinguishing among asthma, chronic bronchitis, and emphysema. Chest 1985; 87:35S–39S.
20. Shapiro SD. The pathogenesis of emphysema: the elastase:antielastase hypothesis 30 years later. Proc Assoc Am Physicians 1995;107:346–52.
21. Shapiro SD. Evolving concepts in the pathogenesis of chronic obstructive pulmonary disease. Clin Chest Med 2000;21:621–32.
22. Shapiro SD. Proteinases in chronic obstructive pulmonary disease. Biochem Soc Trans 2002;30:98–102.
23. Finlay GA, O'Driscoll LR, Russell KJ, et al. Matrix metalloproteinase expression and production by alveolar macrophages in emphysema. Am J Respir Crit Care Med 1997;156: 240–7.
24. Finlay GA, Russell KJ, McMahon KJ, et al. Elevated levels of matrix metalloproteinases in bronchoalveolar lavage fluid of emphysematous patients. Thorax 1997;52:502–6.
25. Segura-Valdez L, Pardo A, Gaxiola M, et al. Upregulation of gelatinases A and B, collagenases 1 and 2, and increased parenchymal cell death in COPD. Chest 2000;117:684–94.
26. Betsuyaku T, Nishimura M, Takeyabu K, et al. Neutrophil granule proteins in bronchoalveolar lavage fluid from subjects with subclinical emphysema. Am J Respir Crit Care Med 1999;159:1985–91.
27. Shapiro SD, Endicott SK, Province MA, et al. Marked longevity of human lung parenchymal elastic fibers deduced from prevalence of D-aspartate and nuclear weapons-related radiocarbon. J Clin Invest 1991;87:1828–34.
28. McMillan WD, Patterson BK, Keen RR, et al. In situ localization and quantification of seventy-two-kilodalton type IV collagenase in aneurysmal, occlusive, and normal aorta. J Vasc Surg 1995;22:295–305.
29. Higashikata T, Yamagishi M, Sasaki H, et al. Application of real-time RT-PCR to quantifying gene expression of matrix metalloproteinases and tissue inhibitors of metalloproteinases in human abdominal aortic aneurysm. Atherosclerosis 2004;177:353–60.
30. Carrell TW, Burnand KG, Wells GM, et al. Stromelysin-1 (matrix metalloproteinase-3) and tissue inhibitor of metalloproteinase-3 are overexpressed in the wall of abdominal aortic aneurysms. Circulation 2002;105:477–82.
31. Hovsepian DM, Ziporin SJ, Sakurai MK, et al. Elevated plasma levels of matrix metalloproteinase-9 in patients with abdominal aortic aneurysms: a circulating marker of degenerative aneurysm disease. J Vasc Interv Radiol 2000;11:1345–52.
32. McMillan WD, Patterson BK, Keen RR, et al. In situ localization and quantification of mRNA for 92–kD type IV collagenase and its inhibitor in aneurysmal, occlusive, and normal aorta. Arterioscler Thromb Vasc Biol 1995;15:1139–44.
33. Elmore JR, Keister BF, Franklin DP, et al. Expression of matrix metalloproteinases and TIMPs in human abdominal aortic aneurysms. Ann Vasc Surg 1998;12:221–8.
34. Fontaine V, Jacob M-P, Houard X, et al. Involvement of the mural thrombus as a site of protease release and activation in human aortic aneurysms. Am J Pathol 2002;161:1701–10.
35. Annabi B, Shedid D, Ghosn P, et al. Differential regulation of matrix metalloproteinase activities in abdominal aortic aneurysms. J Vasc Surg 2002;35:539–46.
36. Curci JA, Liao S, Huffman MD, et al. Expression and localization of macrophage elastase (matrix metalloproteinase-12) in abdominal aortic aneurysms. J Clin Invest 1998;102:1900–10.

37. Pyo R, Lee JK, Shipley JM, et al. Targeted gene disruption of matrix metalloproteinase-9 (gelatinase B) suppresses development of experimental abdominal aortic aneurysms. J Clin Invest 2000;105:1641–9.
38. Longo GM, Xiong W, Greiner TC, et al. Matrix metalloproteinases 2 and 9 work in concert to produce aortic aneurysms. J Clin Invest 2002;110:625–32.
39. Sukhova GK, Shi G-P. Do cathepsins play a role in abdominal aortic aneurysm pathogenesis? Ann N Y Acad Sci 2006;1085:161–9.
40. Gacko M, Glowinski S. Cathepsin D and cathepsin L activities in aortic aneurysm wall and parietal thrombus. Clin Chem Lab Med 1998;36:449–52.
41. Lindholt JS, Erlandsen EJ, Henneberg EW. Cystatin C deficiency is associated with the progression of small abdominal aortic aneurysms. Br J Surg 2001;88:1472–5.
42. Shi GP, Sukhova GK, Grubb A, et al. Cystatin C deficiency in human atherosclerosis and aortic aneurysms. J Clin Invest 1999;104:1191–7.
43. Said A, Kevin GB, Matthew W, et al. Cysteine protease activity in the wall of abdominal aortic aneurysms. J Vasc Surg 2007;46:1260–6.
44. Pagano MB, Bartoli MA, Ennis TL, et al. Critical role of dipeptidyl peptidase I in neutrophil recruitment during the development of experimental abdominal aortic aneurysms. Proc Natl Acad Sci U S A 2007;104:2855–60.
45. Hautamaki RD, Kobayashi DK, Senior RM, et al. Requirement for macrophage elastase for cigarette smoke-induced emphysema in mice. Science 1997;277:2002–4.
46. Cohen JR, Sarfati I, Wise L. The effect of cigarette smoking on rabbit aortic elastase activity. J Vasc Surg 1989;9:580–2.
47. Cohen JR, Schroder W, Mandell C, et al. Activation of rabbit aortic elastase by nonaortic intraabdominal surgery. Ann Vasc Surg 1988;2:133–7.
48. Wright JL, Tai H, Wang R, et al. Cigarette smoke upregulates pulmonary vascular matrix metalloproteinases via TNF-alpha signaling. Am J Physiol Lung Cell Mol Physiol 2007;292: L125–L133.
49. Kangavari S, Matetzky S, Shah PK, et al. Smoking increases inflammation and metalloproteinase expression in human carotid atherosclerotic plaques. J Cardiovasc Pharmacol Ther 2004;9:291–8.
50. O'Toole TE, Zheng Y-T, Hellmann J, et al. Acrolein activates matrix metalloproteinases by increasing reactive oxygen species in macrophages. Toxicol Appl Pharmacol 2009;236: 194–201.
51. Henderson EL, Gang YJ, Sukhova GK, et al. Death of smooth muscle cells and expression of mediators of apoptosis by T lymphocytes in human abdominal aortic aneurysms. Circulation 1999;99:96–104.
52. Holmes DR, Lopez-Candales A, Liao S, et al. Smooth muscle cell apoptosis and p53 expression in human abdominal aortic aneurysms. Ann N Y Acad Sci 1996;800:286–7.
53. Lopez-Candales A, Holmes DR, Liao S, et al. Decreased vascular smooth muscle cell density in medial degeneration of human abdominal aortic aneurysms. Am J Pathol 1997;150:993–1007.
54. Jacob T, Hingorani A, Ascher E. Examination of the apoptotic pathway and proteolysis in the pathogenesis of popliteal artery aneurysms. Eur J Vasc Endovasc Surg 2001;22:77–85.
55. Liao S, Curci JA, Kelley BJ, et al. Accelerated replicative senescence of medial smooth muscle cells derived from abdominal aortic aneurysms compared to the adjacent inferior mesenteric artery. J Surg Res 2000;92:85–95.
56. Thompson RW, Liao S, Curci JA. Vascular smooth muscle cell apoptosis in abdominal aortic aneurysms. Coron Artery Dis 1997;8:623–31.
57. Tung WS, Lee JK, Thompson RW. Simultaneous analysis of 1176 gene products in normal human aorta and abdominal aortic aneurysms using a membrane-based complementary DNA expression array. J Vasc Surg 2001;34:143–50.
58. Pearce WH, Sweis I, Yao JS, et al. Interleukin-1 beta and tumor necrosis factor-alpha release in normal and diseased human infrarenal aortas. J Vasc Surg 1992;16:784–9.

59. Schubl S, Tsai S, Ryer EJ, et al. Upregulation of protein kinase C (delta) in vascular smooth muscle cells promotes inflammation in abdominal aortic aneurysm. J Surg Res 2009;153: 181–7.
60. Anazawa T, Dimayuga PC, Li H, et al. Effect of exposure to cigarette smoke on carotid artery intimal thickening: the role of inducible NO synthase. Arterioscler Thromb Vasc Biol 2004;24:1652–8.
61. Matsumoto M, Dimayuga PC, Wang C, et al. Exogenous heat shock protein-70 inhibits cigarette smoke-induced intimal thickening. Am J Physiol Regul Integr Comp Physiol 2008; 295:R1320–7.
62. Kunitomo M, Yamaguchi Y, Kagota S, et al. Biochemical evidence of atherosclerosis progression mediated by increased oxidative stress in apolipoprotein e-deficient spontaneously hyperlipidemic mice exposed to chronic cigarette smoke. J Pharmacol Sci 2009; 110:354–61.
63. von Holt K, Lebrun S, Stinn W, et al. Progression of atherosclerosis in the Apo E-/- model: 12–month exposure to cigarette mainstream smoke combined with high-cholesterol/fat diet. Atherosclerosis 2009;205:135–43.
64. Orosz Z, Csiszar A, Labinskyy N, et al. Cigarette smoke-induced proinflammatory alterations in the endothelial phenotype: role of NAD(P)H oxidase activation. Am J Physiol Heart Circ Physiol 2007;292:H130–H139.
65. Barbieri SS, Weksler BB. Tobacco smoke cooperates with interleukin-1beta to alter beta-catenin trafficking in vascular endothelium resulting in increased permeability and induction of cyclooxygenase-2 expression in vitro and in vivo. FASEB J 2007;21:1831–43.
66. Carnevali S, Petruzzelli S, Longoni B, et al. Cigarette smoke extract induces oxidative stress and apoptosis in human lung fibroblasts. Am J Physiol Lung Cell Mol Physiol 2003;284: L955–63.
67. Yokohori N, Aoshiba K, Nagai A, et al. Increased levels of cell death and proliferation in alveolar wall cells in patients with pulmonary emphysema. Chest 2004;125:626–32.
68. Wang H, Liu X, Umino T, et al. Cigarette smoke inhibits human bronchial epithelial cell repair processes. Am J Respir Cell Mol Biol 2001;25:772–9.
69. Wong LS, Green HM, Feugate JE, et al. Effects of "second-hand" smoke on structure and function of fibroblasts, cells that are critical for tissue repair and remodeling. BMC Cell Biol 2004;5:13.
70. Sorensen LT, Karlsmark T, Gottrup F. Abstinence from smoking reduces incisional wound infection: a randomized controlled trial. Ann Surg 2003;238:1–5.
71. Sorensen LT, Horby J, Friis E, et al. Smoking as a risk factor for wound healing and infection in breast cancer surgery. Eur J Surg Oncol 2002;28:815–20.
72. Sorensen LT, Friis E, Jorgensen T, et al. Smoking is a risk factor for recurrence of groin hernia. World J Surg 2002;26:397–400.
73. Sorensen LT, Jorgensen T, Kirkeby LT, et al. Smoking and alcohol abuse are major risk factors for anastomotic leakage in colorectal surgery. Br J Surg 1999;86:927–31.
74. Manassa EH, Hertl CH, Olbrisch RR. Wound healing problems in smokers and nonsmokers after 132 abdominoplasties. Plast Reconstruct Surg 2003;111:2082–7; discussion 2088–9.
75. Zhang W, Song F, Windsor LJ. Cigarette smoke condensate affects the collagen-degrading ability of human gingival fibroblasts. J Periodontal Res 2009;44:704–13.
76. Philips N, Burchill D, O'Donoghue D, et al. Identification of benzene metabolites in dermal fibroblasts as nonphenolic: regulation of cell viability, apoptosis, lipid peroxidation and expression of matrix metalloproteinase 1 and elastin by benzene metabolites. Skin Pharmacol Physiol 2004;17:147–52.
77. Yin L, Morita A, Tsuji T. Skin aging induced by ultraviolet exposure and tobacco smoking: evidence from epidemiological and molecular studies. Photodermatol Photoimmunol Photomed 2001;17:178–83.
78. Ning W, Dong Y, Sun J, et al. Cigarette smoke stimulates matrix metalloproteinase-2 activity via EGR-1 in human lung fibroblasts. Am J Respir Cell Mol Biol 2007;36:480–90.

79. Nordskog BK, Blixt AD, Morgan WT, et al. Matrix-degrading and pro-inflammatory changes in human vascular endothelial cells exposed to cigarette smoke condensate. Cardiovasc Toxicol 2003;3:101–17.
80. Nordskog BK, Blixt AD, Zieske AW, et al. MMP-1 polymorphic expression in aortic endothelial cells: possible role in lesion development in smokers and nonsmokers. Cardiovasc Toxicol 2004;4:75–83.
81. Tani S, Dimayuga PC, Anazawa T, et al. Aberrant antibody responses to oxidized LDL and increased intimal thickening in apoE-/- mice exposed to cigarette smoke. Atherosclerosis 2004;175:7–14.
82. Huffman MD, Curci JA, Moore G, et al. Functional importance of connective tissue repair during the development of experimental abdominal aortic aneurysms. Surgery 2000;128: 429–38.
83. Wright JL, Churg A. Effect of long-term cigarette smoke exposure on pulmonary vascular structure and function in the guinea pig. Exp Lung Res 1991;17:997–1009.
84. Buckley C, Wyble CW, Borhani M, et al. Accelerated enlargement of experimental abdominal aortic aneurysms in a mouse model of chronic cigarette smoke exposure. J Am Coll Surg 2004;199:896–903.
85. Thompson RW, Curci JA, Ennis TL, et al. Pathophysiology of abdominal aortic aneurysms. Insights from the elastase-induced model in mice with different genetic backgrounds. Ann N Y Acad Sci 2006;1085:59–73.
86. Bergoeing MP, Arif B, Hackmann AE, et al. Cigarette smoking increases aortic dilatation without affecting matrix metalloproteinase-9 and -12 expression in a modified mouse model of aneurysm formation. J Vasc Surg 2007;21:328–38.
87. Ramos C, Cisneros J, Gonzalez-Avila G, et al. Increase of matrix metalloproteinases in woodsmoke-induced lung emphysema in guinea pigs. Inhal Toxicol 2009;21:119–32.
88. Montaño M, Beccerril C, Ruiz V, et al. Matrix metalloproteinases activity in COPD associated with wood smoke. Chest 2004;125:466–72.

SECTION XI

Abdominal Aortic Aneurysm II

50

Salvage Procedures for Late Endovascular Failures

Jon S. Matsumura, M.D.

INTRODUCTION

Abdominal aortic aneurysm is a leading cause of death in adults, responsible for approximately 13,800 deaths in the United States in 2005.[1] Parodi first inserted an endograft for definitive treatment of abdominal aortic aneurysm, which he reported in 1991.[2] Also in 1991, Volodos from the Soviet Union described a self-fixing synthetic prosthesis for repair of both thoracic and abdominal aneurysms.[3]

Endovascular aneurysm repair has become an option to repair aneurysms with proven lower perioperative mortality. In the Endovascular Aortic Repair trial 1, a randomized trial of 1082 patients with large aneurysms, in-hospital mortality was 2.1% with endovascular repair versus 6.2% with open repair.[4] Four-year survival rate was similar. In the Dutch Randomized Endovascular Aneurysm Management Trial, 351 patients were randomized to endovascular versus open repair, and combined mortality and severe complications totaled 4.7% with endovascular repair compared with 9.8% with open repair.[5] There were equivalent 2-year survival rates, although oral presentations have suggested that a worse late hazard may be associated with endovascular repair. The Open Versus Endovascular Repair trial, which randomized 881 Veterans Affairs patients, and the French Aneurysme Chirurgie de l'aorte contre Endoprothese trial are due to report 2-year results soon. In a propensity-score risk-adjusted analysis of the Nationwide Inpatient Sample, endovascular repair was associated with lower perioperative mortality compared with open repair (1.2% vs. 4.8%).[6] Late survival is similar for the two techniques. Taken together, the literature demonstrates that endovascular repair is associated with lower perioperative mortality, but concern remains about late events and mitigation of these early benefits. The degree of mitigation is partially dependent on the ability to identify late failure modes and effectively retreat them with risks. This chapter focuses on reoperative procedures after late endovascular failures.

LATE COMPLICATIONS

Treatment of late endovascular complications requires identification and understanding of the mechanisms of failure of endovascular repair. The major failure modes are covered in another chapter and include device migration, graft material failure (holes), graft ultrafiltration, limb occlusion, infection, neck dilation, metallic fatigue fracture, endoleak, and rupture.[7-23] Often, multiple failure modes are combined, such as migration leading to endoleak (Figure 50–1). In early series, vascular surgeons frequently proceeded with open conversion as a standard approach to endovascular complications. This was highly effective but may have been overtreatment for some problems and was associated with high mortality rates.[24] As knowledge of the late failure modes was gained, less invasive and effective approaches have been developed for retreatment.

COMPLETE EXPLANT

Complete removal of the endograft is favored when there is unsuitable anatomy for an endovascular salvage or the graft is infected (see Figure 50–1). Familiar "tricks" derived from reoperative procedures for subsequent proximal aneurysms and open prosthetic graft infections can be used in these conversions. These include mobilization of the left renal vein or transaction of the left renal vein medial to the left adrenal and lumbar veins in a transperitoneal approach. Often, a retroperitoneal approach or supraceliac clamp is necessary to remove the endograft, particularly if there is a suprarenal component. Placement of ureteral stents can accelerate pelvic dissection when there are extensive iliac aneurysms and previously placed devices in the pelvis. Various methods to disengage hooks and barbs can be used but have in common the radial compression of the device before applying downward traction so as to minimize injury to the pararenal aorta. The graft can be snared, twisted, stents fragmented with wire cutters, digitally collapsed, or cooled to assist

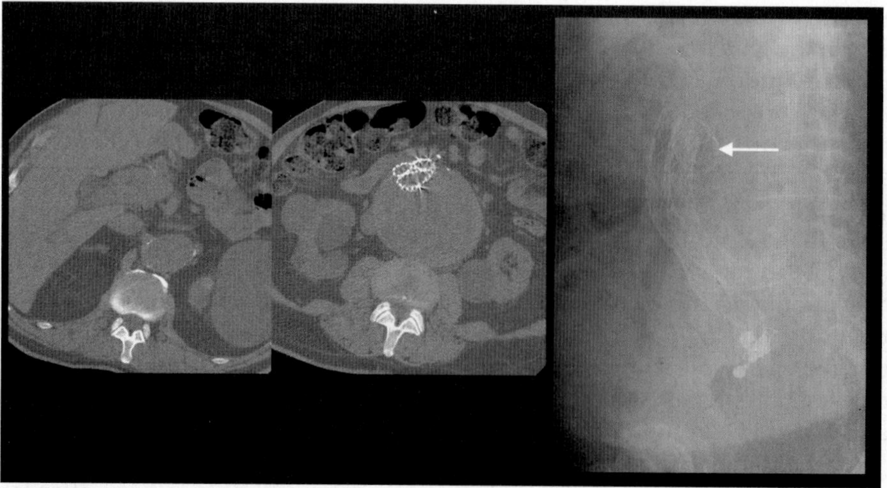

Figure 50-1. This patient presented 6 years after endovascular repair with an AneuRx device (Medtronic, Inc., Santa Rosa, CA). He had acute limb ischemia from iliac occlusion and a pulsatile aneurysm on physical examination. Computed tomography (CT) scan (left and middle) and abdominal radiograph (right) show the device has migrated out of the proximal neck and kinked (arrow). He had successful conversion and explant.

in removal. Often, an endarterectomy of the aortic cuff accompanies these maneuvers, and felt reinforcement of the proximal suture line is needed. Rarely, thoracoabdominal aortic reconstruction becomes necessary.

PARTIAL CONVERSION

An attractive alternative when infection is absent are partial explantations. If the retained components have not failed, then leaving an embedded suprarenal stent or iliac component can reduce the risk of vascular injury with complete explantation. Self-expanding stents can often be compressed with vascular clamps and still remain patent after unclamping. Other systems are relatively noncompressible, and balloon occlusion may assist in vascular control. Suturing to endografts is complicated by the presence of metallic stents that may cut the suture line or the surgeon. This problem can be minimized by careful selection of the transection point of the endograft between major stent elements; or for sinusoidal wireforms, cutting the wire in a single location and unwinding it to the point of transection, hence leaving a single wire termination that can be bent into a benign position. Suture retention attributes may have been sacrificed in favor of thinner materials and smaller introducer systems, and felt reinforcement is useful. When leaving parts of the endograft, suturing the surgical graft to the native wall and the endograft provides excellent fixation and isolates the retained segment from the main aneurysm should later failure occur in the retained portion.

Another form of partial conversion is to perform an extra-anatomic bypass, such as a femoral-femoral crossover bypass for limb occlusion. These procedures fall under the familiar domain of vascular surgeons' treating similar complications after open aortic repair.

RELINING

Relining an endograft is considered when the failure mode includes threatened or actual fabric holes (Figures 50–2 and 50–3), transgraft ultrafiltration (Figure 50–4), kinking of unsupported segments, stent compression/fracture, or component separation.[25-26] The main consideration is if the entire previous endograft needs relining rather than a more limited portion that is exposed to the aneurysm sac (Figure 50–5).[25] Sometimes, there may

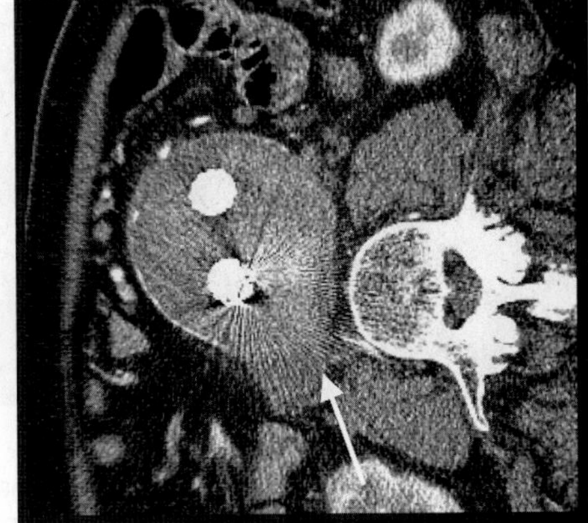

Figure 50-2. This patient presented with back pain 6 years after endovascular repair with an AneuRx device. White arrow points to aneurysm rupture diagnosed with CT scan.

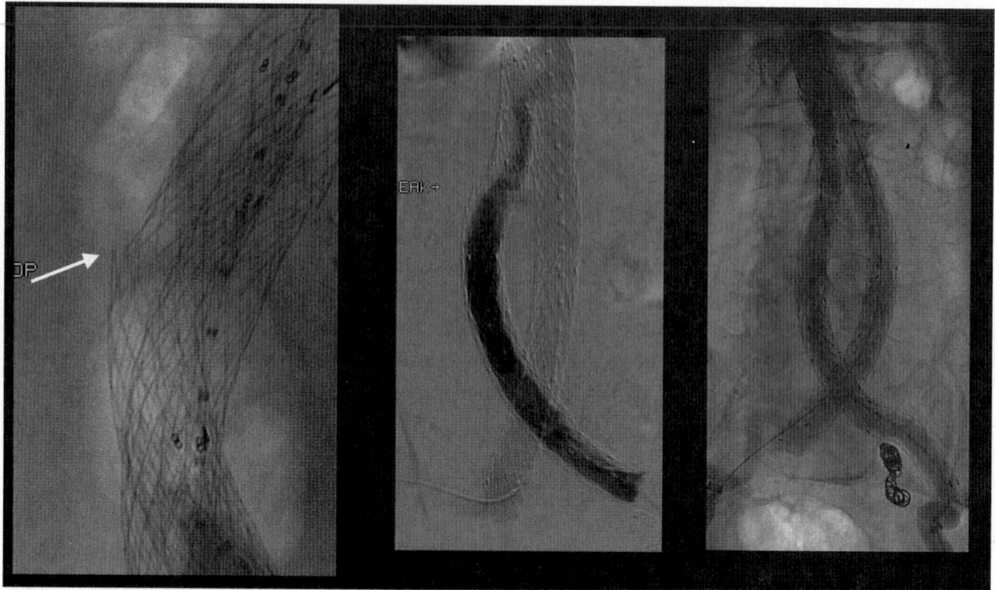

Figure 50-3. Same patient as Figure 50–2. Left panel is radiograph showing suture pop and stent displacement (white arrow). Middle panel is arteriogram showing fabric defect at the same location. Right panel shows completion angiogram after successful relining.

be a temptation to address only the most clinically significant fabric defect or fracture if it occurs in a single iliac limb, but the forces that led to failure of that portion are likely to lead to failure in other parts after a short latency period. It seems reasonable to reline as much as is anatomically feasible if failure is evident in part of the device. Exceptions may be a focal kink leading to late limb occlusion or an intercomponent junction that was never sufficiently overlapped.

EXTENSIONS

Extensions are useful when there is suitable residual anatomy for an endovascular approach after the device fixation has failed (i.e., migration) or in the small fraction of

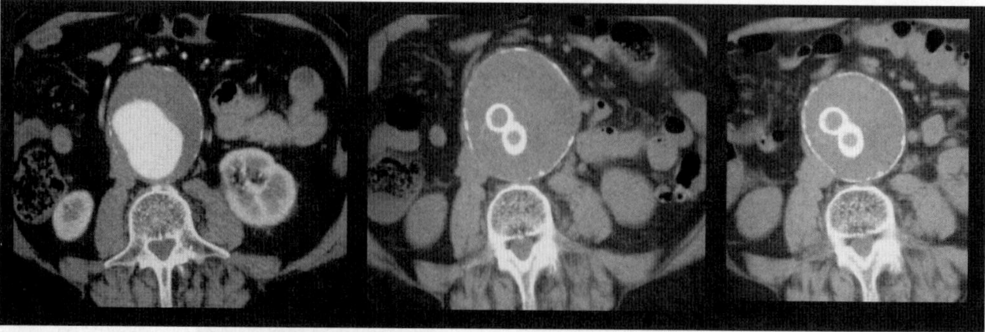

Figure 50-4. This patient had endovascular repair of a 7.0-cm aneurysm (left panel) with the original Excluder (WL Gore & Associates, Flagstaff, AZ) endoprosthesis made with expanded polytetrafluoroethylene. The aneurysm grew 9 mm in the first 8 months after repair (middle panel). After relining, the aneurysm shrunk 20 mm over the subsequent 7 months (right panel).

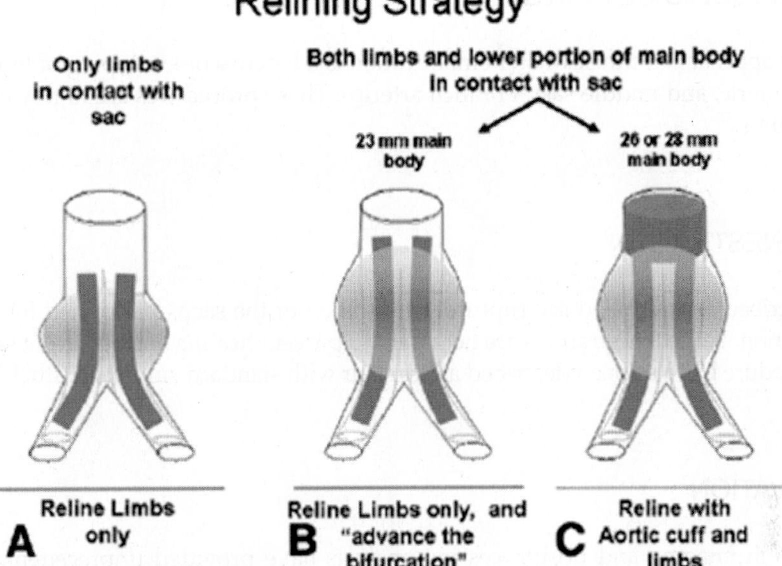

Figure 50-5. Options for complete or partial relining of endograft in contact with sac. (With Permission from Goodney PP, Fillinger MF J Vasc Surg 2007;45:686–93.)

patients who experience clinically important dilation of the native aorta.[7-12,20] Extension to the external iliac artery (with embolization of the hypogastric artery) is not an uncommon procedure for patients long after an initial endovascular repair (Figure 50–6).[27] This enlargement and late endoleak may happen 8 or more years after initial treatment, just as subsequent aneurysms are known to form decades after an open repair.

EMBOLIZATION

The armamentarium of devices, delivery catheters, techniques, and imaging systems continues to expand the capabilities of embolization (see Figure 50–6). Using the latest-generation coils and liquid embolic agents, triaxial and microcatheter systems, modern rotational angiography, and road mapping with blended CT fluoroscopy has greatly extended treatment of endoleaks and reduced procedure times. Needle tracking, robotic navigation, and morphing of catheters and wires are less impressive, and it is not clear if these innovations are useful adjuncts or superfluous technology.

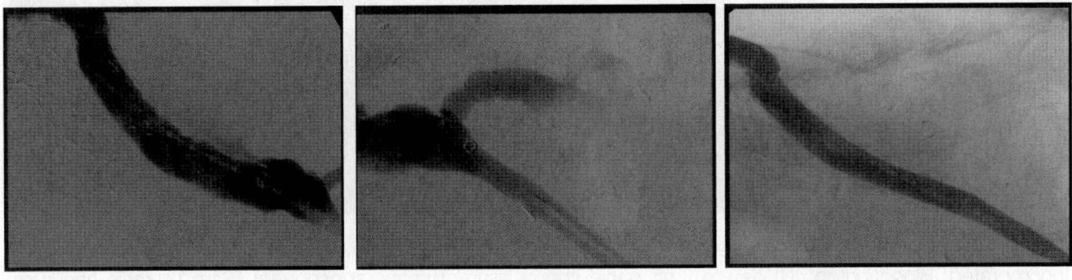

Figure 50-6. Late distal iliac artery dilation with type I endoleak (left panel). Middle panel shows embolic device occluding proximal hypogastric artery and preserving collateral pathways. Right panel is completion arteriogram with extension to external iliac artery.

LAPAROSCOPIC CLIPPING

A variant approach to transcatheter embolization is a laparoscopic clipping of lumbar, inferior mesenteric, and middle sacral branch arteries. These procedures are highly effective in skilled hands.[28]

SAC FENESTRATION

Also described as controlled sac rupture, fenestration of the sac is performed for transgraft ultrafiltration. Large fenestrations are necessary to prevent healing and recurrent sac growth. This procedure has also been described after repair with standard surgical grafts.[28-29]

OBSERVATION

Advances in imaging and postprocessing analysis have provided unprecedented resolution and new quantification such as volumetric analysis or sac pressure. Like subsegmental pulmonary emboli and calf muscle deep vein thrombosis, the high-quality evidence to guide clinical management has lagged behind the technology. Many findings like small endoleaks, minor growth of aneurysm volume, and suture pops can be imaged and identified, but what should be done? Clinical judgment and discretion are needed to avoid overtreatment.[30-31] Even with large type I endoleaks or threatened component separation, an observational course may be preferred in fragile patients similar to abstaining from primary treatment of aortic aneurysms in unfit patients (Figure 50–7).

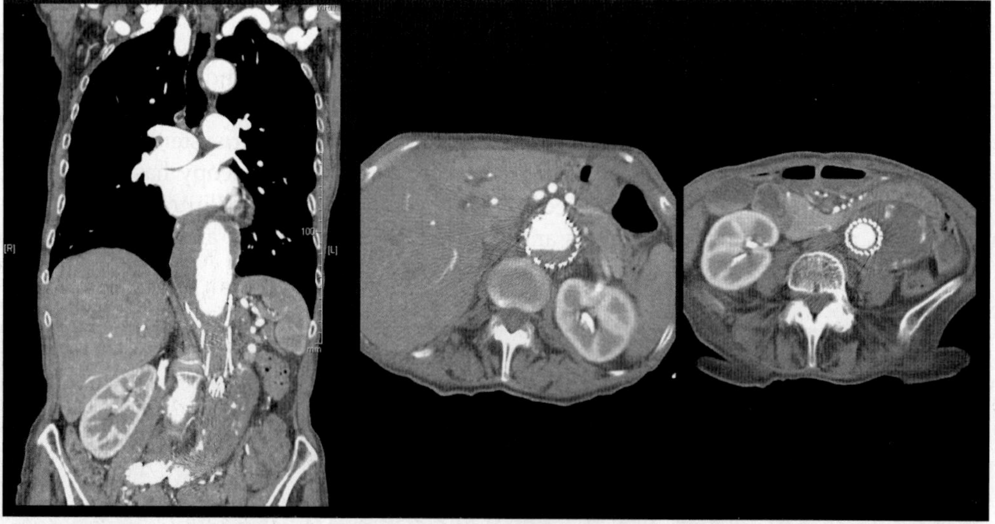

Figure 50-7. CT of a fragile octogenarian patient with a branched endovascular repair with a Zenith (Cook Incorporated, Bloomington, IN) device. Left panel shows asymptomatic subsequent 6-cm thoracic aneurysm above bare topstent component. Middle panel shows patent branch grafts. Right panel shows large excluded abdominal aneurysm. Observation is recommended.

CONCLUSION

Endovascular aneurysm repair has clearly improved perioperative mortality and initial treatment of abdominal aortic aneurysms. Late device failure modes have been identified in clinical trials and by astute physicians, and device engineering solutions are emerging. Because of the many years before recognition of late complications and the slow product development cycle, clinicians have and will continue to encounter patients with these difficult late problems. Learning to recognize and treat these problems should reduce late mortality until device innovation addresses more of the shortcomings of currently used devices.

REFERENCES

1. Kung HC, Hoyert DL, Xu JW, Murphy SL. National Vital Statistics Report. National Center for Health Statistics; Hyattsrille, MD 2008.
2. Parodi JC, Palmaz JC, Barone HD. Transfemoral intraluminal graft implantation for abdominal aortic aneurysms. Ann Vasc Surg 1991;5:491–9.
3. Volodos NL, Karpovich IP, Troyan VI, et al. Clinical experience of the use of self-fixing synthetic prostheses for remote endoprosthetics of the thoracic and the abdominal aorta and iliac arteries through the femoral artery and as intraoperative endoprosthesis for aorta reconstruction. Vasa Suppl 1991;33:93–5.
4. Greenhalgh RM, Brown LC, Kwong GP, et al. Comparison of endovascular aneurysm repair with open repair in patients with abdominal aortic aneurysm (EVAR trial 1), 30-day operative mortality results: randomised controlled trial [see comment]. Lancet 2004; 364:843–8.
5. Blankensteijn JD, de Jong SE, Prinssen M, et al. Two-year outcomes after conventional or endovascular repair of abdominal aortic aneurysms.[see comment]. N Engl J Med 2005; 352:2398–405.
6. Schermerhorn ML, O'Malley AJ, Jhaveri A, et al. Endovascular vs. open repair of abdominal aortic aneurysms in the Medicare population [see comment]. N Engl J Med 2008;358: 464–74.
7. Ebaugh JL, Eskandari MK, Finkelstein A, et al. Caudal migration of endoprostheses after treatment of abdominal aortic aneurysms. J Surg Res 2002;107:14–7.
8. Cao P, Verzini F, Zannetti S, et al. Device migration after endoluminal abdominal aortic aneurysm repair: analysis of 113 cases with a minimum follow-up period of 2 years. J Vasc Surg 2002; 35:229–35.
9. Zarins CK, Bloch DA, Crabtree T, et al. Stent graft migration after endovascular aneurysm repair: importance of proximal fixation. J Vasc Surg 2003;38:1264–72; discussion 1272.
10. Sternbergh WC 3rd, Money SR, Greenberg RK, et al. Influence of endograft oversizing on device migration, endoleak, aneurysm shrinkage, and aortic neck dilation: results from the Zenith Multicenter Trial. J Vasc Surg 2004;39:20–6.
11. Azizzadeh A, Sanchez LA, Rubin BG, et al. Aortic neck attachment failure and the AneuRx graft: incidence, treatment options, and early results. Ann Vasc Surg 2005;19:516–21.
12. Fulton JJ, Farber MA, Sanchez LA, et al. Effect of challenging neck anatomy on mid-term migration rates in AneuRx endografts. J Vasc Surg 2006;44:932–7; discussion 937.
13. Brown KE, Heyer KS, Matsumura JS, Eskandari MK. Late type III endoleak and graft failure of an Ancure stent graft. JVIR 2008;19:1506–8.
14. Bertges DJ, Chow K, Wyers MC, et al. Abdominal aortic aneurysm size regression after endovascular repair is endograft dependent. J Vasc Surg 2003;37:716–23.
15. Peterson BG, Matsumura JS, Brewster DC, Makaroun MS, Excluder Investigators. Five year report of a multicenter controlled clinical trial of open versus endovascular treatment of abdominal aortic aneurysms. J Vasc Surg 2007;45885–90.

16. Tang G, Fillinger M, Matsumura JS. Original excluder component overlap from proximal or distal extension during initial repair not correlated with aneurysm sac shrinkage. J Vasc Surg 2009.
17. Cornelissen SA, Verhagen HJ, Prokop M, et al. Visualizing type IV endoleak using magnetic resonance imaging with a blood pool contrast agent. J Vasc Surg 2008;47:861–4.
18. Carroccio A, Faries PL, Morrissey NJ, et al. Predicting iliac limb occlusions after bifurcated aortic stent grafting: anatomic and device-related causes. J Vasc Surg 2002;36:679–84.
19. Heyer KS, Modi PK, Morasch MD, et al. Secondary infection of thoracic and abdominal aortic endografts. JVIR 2009;20:173–9.
20. Matsumura JS, Chaikof EL. Continued expansion of aortic necks after endovascular repair of abdominal aortic aneurysms. EVT Investigators. J Vasc Surg 1998;28:422–30; discussion 430–1.
21. Bernhard VM, Mitchel RS, Matsumura JS, et al. Ruptured abdominal aortic aneurysm after endovascular repair. J Vasc Surg 2002;35:1155–62.
22. White GH, May J, Waugh RC, et al. Type III and type IV endoleak: toward a complete definition of blood flow in the sac after endoluminal AAA repair. J Endovasc Surg 1998;5: 305–9.
23. White GH, Yu W, May J, et al. Endoleak as a complication of endoluminal grafting of abdominal aortic aneurysms: classification, incidence, diagnosis, and management. J Endovasc Surg 1997; 4:152–68.
24. May J, White GH, Yu W, et al. Conversion from endoluminal to open repair of abdominal aortic aneurysms: a hazardous procedure. Eur J Vasc Endovasc Surg 1997;14:4–11.
25. Goodney PP, Fillinger MF. The effect of endograft relining on sac expansion after endovascular aneurysm repair with the original-permeability Gore Excluder abdominal aortic aneurysm endoprosthesis. J Vasc Surg 2007;45:686–93.
26. Kougias P, Lin PH, Dardik A, et al. Successful treatment of endotension and aneurysm sac enlargement with endovascular stent graft reinforcement. J Vasc Surg 2007;46:124–7.
27. Rhee RY, Muluk SC, Tzeng E, et al. Can the internal iliac artery be safely covered during endovascular repair of abdominal aortic and iliac artery aneurysms? Ann Vasc Surg 2002; 16:29–36.
28. Van Sambeek MRHM, Hendriks JM, Tseng L, et al. Sac enlargement without endoleak: when and how to convert and technical considerations. Semin Vasc Surg 2004;17:284–7.
29. Risberg B, Delle M, Lonn I, et al. Management of aneurysm sac hygroma. J Endovasc Ther 2004;11:191–5.
30. Mennander A, Pimenoff G, Heikkinen M, et al. Nonoperative approach to endotension. J Vasc Surg 2005;42:194–9.
31. Thoo CHC, Bourke BM, May J. Symptomatic sac enlargement and rupture due to seroma after open abdominal aortic aneurysm repair with polytetrafluoroethylene graft: implications for endovascular repair and endotension. J Vasc Surg 2004;40:1089–94.

51

Late Failure of Endovascular Abdominal Aortic Aneurysm Repair

Donald T. Baril, M.D. and Michel S. Makaroun, M.D.

INTRODUCTION

The treatment of abdominal aortic aneurysms (AAAs) has changed radically over the past 15 years since the introduction of endovascular abdominal aortic aneurysm repair (EVAR). EVAR has been shown to lead to decreased early mortality, shorter hospital stays, and lower perioperative complications.[1-2] However, despite these early benefits, the long-term durability of EVAR has been in question since it was first reported, and studies have shown no survival benefit for patients undergoing EVAR over patients undergoing open repair after 1 year.[3]

EVAR is associated with its own unique complications, both early and late, which differ from those of conventional open repair. Although certain devices, particularly the early-generation stent grafts, have been associated with higher rates of both early and late complications, most have been described with nearly all devices.[4] Along with improved device technology, EVAR failures have also decreased over time with physician experience and improved preoperative planning. Despite advances in device technology and operator experience, however, a number of late failure modes continue to plague the long-term durability of EVAR. These late failures include endoleaks, graft migration, limb occlusions, landing zone degeneration, material fatigue and failure, and graft infection. Although many of these late failures can be treated with secondary endovascular interventions, particularly when patients are monitored appropriately, they carry their own inherent risks and potential for significant morbidity and mortality.

FAILURE MODES

Endoleaks

Endoleaks, first described as the "persistence of blood flow outside the lumen of the endoluminal graft but within an aneurysm sac,"[4] continue to complicate the long-term effectiveness of EVAR. Endoleaks are classified into those that result from inadequate seal at either the proximal or the distal stent-graft attachment site (type I); those that originate through retrograde flow in the collateral side-branch arteries of the aneurysm, typically lumbar and inferior mesenteric arteries (type II); those arising from antegrade flow into the aneurysm at a junction point between graft components or a graft defect (type III); and those with inflow related to the porosity of the graft itself (type IV). Additionally, endotension, often referred to as type V endoleak, has been defined as "persistent or recurrent pressurization of the aneurysm sac following endovascular repair" without a demonstrable leak on imaging studies.[5-6]

Type I and III endoleaks, which have incidences of 8.2 to 18% and 0.7 to 8% following EVAR, respectively,[7-8] carry the greatest risk of aneurysm rupture and should almost all uniformly be treated. Conversely, the natural course of type II endoleaks, which have a reported incidence of 8 to 45% following EVAR,[9-10] is less well understood, because many spontaneously thrombose. However, aneurysm expansion has been reported with type II endoleaks, and at the very least, close clinical observation is warranted. Type IV endoleaks typically resolve without intervention. Type V endoleaks often pose the greatest diagnostic and therapeutic dilemma and require intervention if aneurysm growth persists. Endoleaks may be managed with graft extension or cuff insertion, coil embolization, laparoscopic ligation of the feeding vessels, conversion to standard open repair, or simply observation in the correct clinical setting (Figure 51–1).

Migration

Stent-graft fixation may be either passive or active. Passive fixation relies on friction generated by the radial strength of the stent, which is oversized to the artery in which it is being deployed. Active fixation relies on not only friction but additionally some form of hook or other anchoring mechanism that is embedded in the stent-graft itself and engages the arterial wall.

Migration is a result of failure of the fixation mechanism of the stent-graft related to the device itself or degeneration of the landing zone, leading to either caudal movement of the device >10 mm at the proximal neck or cranial movement at the iliac attachments relative to anatomic landmarks or any degree of movement associated with a clinically adverse event. Although some migrations may not necessarily be clinically significant so long as the aneurysm remains excluded, many lead to loss of the proximal or distal seal and subsequent pressurization of the aneurysmal sac. In addition to loss of aneurysm exclusion, migration may lead to graft kinking and occlusion or graft disconnection. Migration typically occurs at least 1 year following deployment but has been reported at any time from days following implantation to 4 to 5 years later.

Preoperative assessment and planning for EVAR will help minimize migration, because appropriately sizing an endograft to a healthy segment of aorta or iliac artery is vital to successful long-term aneurysm exclusion. A number of specific anatomic factors have been shown to be associated with migration over time, including severely angulated aortic necks, conical neck shapes, wide necks, short necks, and necks containing large amounts of thrombus or those with heavy calcification.[11-12] In addition to anatomic factors related to the proximal attachment zone, distal iliac fixation is also important in preventing migration. Secure fixation to the iliac bifurcation helps to minimize the risk of migration by providing support along the longitudinal axis of the stent graft.[13] Based on this, extension of both iliac limbs to cover the entire common iliac artery to the iliac bifurcation may contribute to endograft stability.

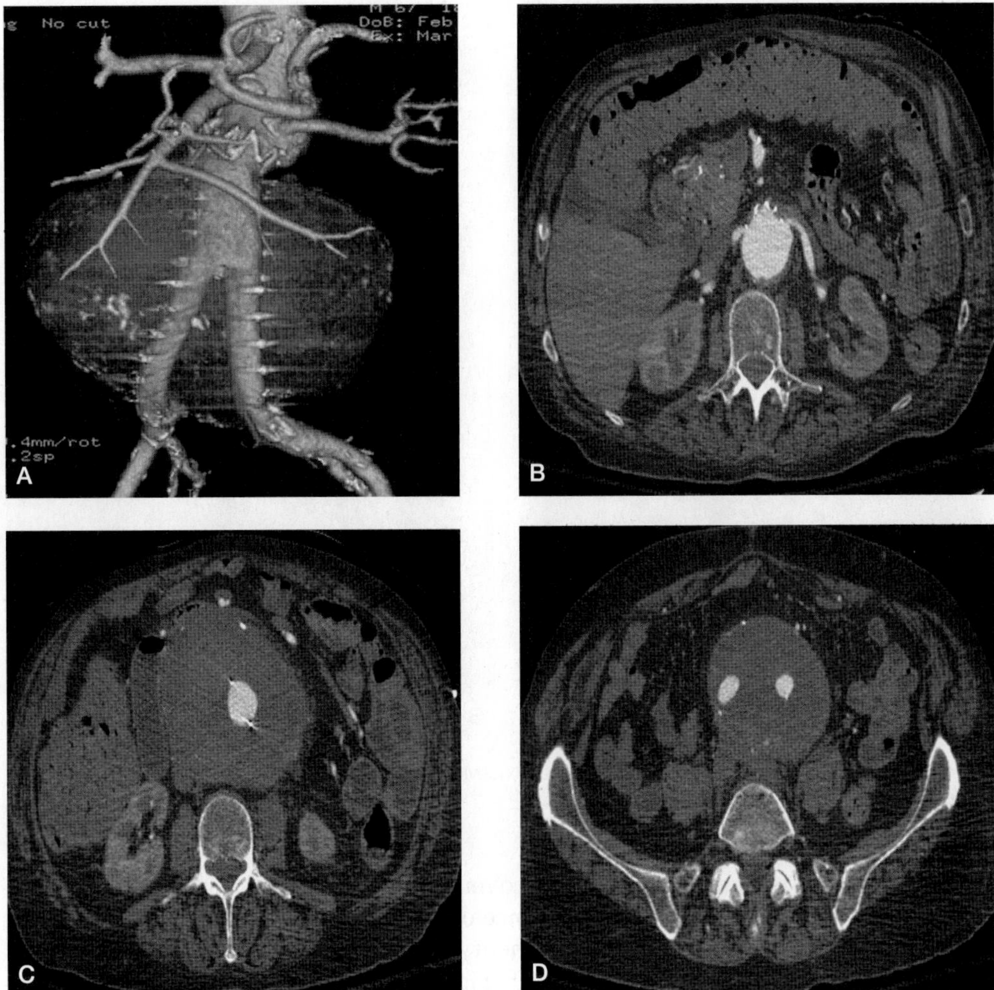

Figure 51-1. A. A 3-D CT angiogram demonstrating a 12-cm AAA 9 years following initial Ancure placement. B-D. Axial cuts demonstrating the same AAA without gross evidence of an endoleak. The patient went on to open conversion, at which time several type II lumbar endoleaks were discovered.

Device-related causes of migration may, however, be more important. Design of the device, lack of flexibility, and the mechanism of passive fixation may all contribute to the migration. Moreover, inherent failure of the device itself, including hook fractures, stent fractures, or separation of the stent from the graft, may also be at fault. Although migration has been described with nearly every endograft, including those with active fixation in the absence of graft failure, the AneuRx device has demonstrated higher rates of migration compared with other devices (up to 32% at 36 months).[12,14] Conversely, endografts with active proximal fixation mechanisms, including the Excluder and the Zenith devices, have been associated with much lower rates of migration.[15-16] Additional factors that may contribute to migration include the degree of oversizing of the endograft to the landing zone vessel and the type of stents used in the construction of the endograft.

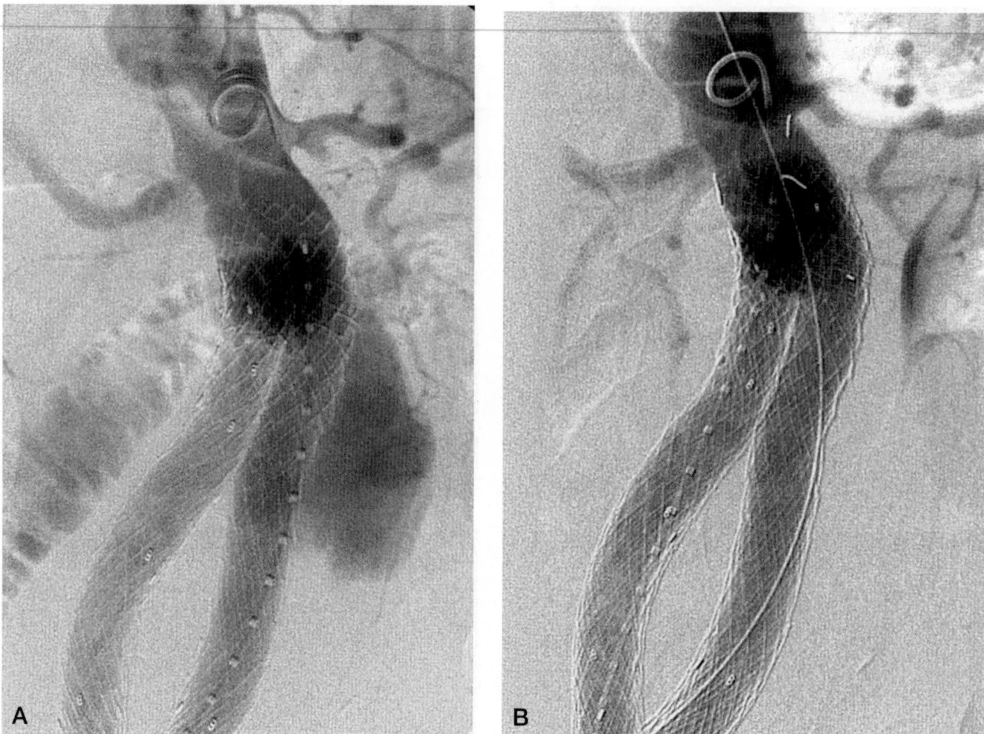

Figure 51-2. A. Aortogram of distal migration of AneuRx device and proximal type I endoleak. B. Successful AAA exclusion following aortic cuff extension.

In patients in whom migration is discovered, intervention is warranted when the seal zone is 5 mm or less or there is evidence of a clinically or radiographically significant event such as a type I endoleak or aneurysm enlargement. Treatment options include placement of a proximal aortic cuff (Figure 51–2), placement of an entire new aortic endograft (Figure 51–3), or open conversion (Figure 51–4).

Landing Zone Enlargement

Landing zone enlargement, either proximal or distal, may occur following EVAR. Although this may often be clinically insignificant, landing zone enlargement may ultimately lead to the development of stent-graft migration, type I endoleak, and subsequent repressurization of the aneurysm sac. Despite a large amount of literature regarding this entity, there is a great deal of variability in the data due in large part to the variance in the methods used to measure the aortic neck and the timing of these measurements.

Proximal neck dilation may occur following both EVAR and open repair, although the rates appear to be lower with EVAR. The occurrence of aortic neck dilation following open repair implies that the aorta in the setting of an infrarenal AAA probably is diseased throughout and hence will dilate over time. Although most aortic necks remain stable after EVAR, approximately 20 to 30% demonstrate some degree of enlargement at 2 years.[15] This phenomenon does not appear to be device-related among devices with similar deployment methods, although select studies have demonstrated higher rates of aortic neck dilation in patients treated with self-expanding devices.

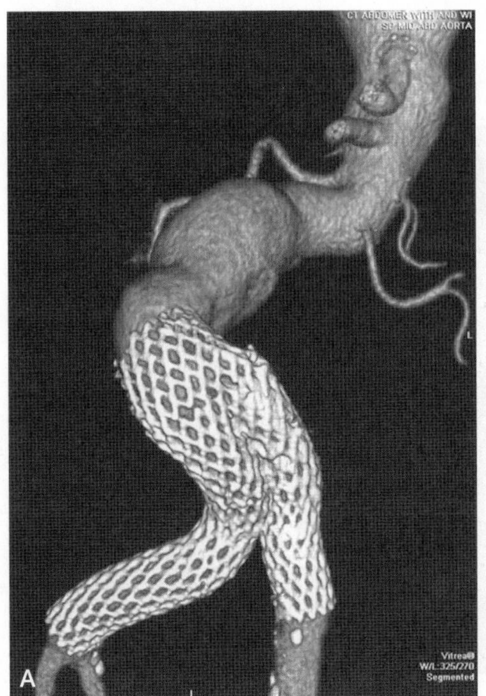

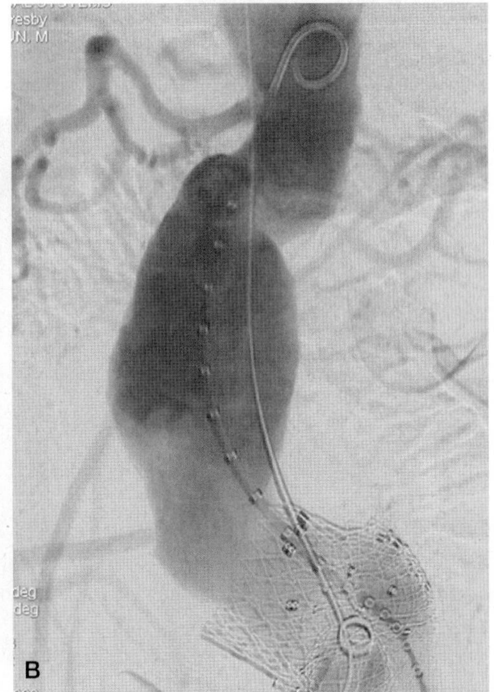

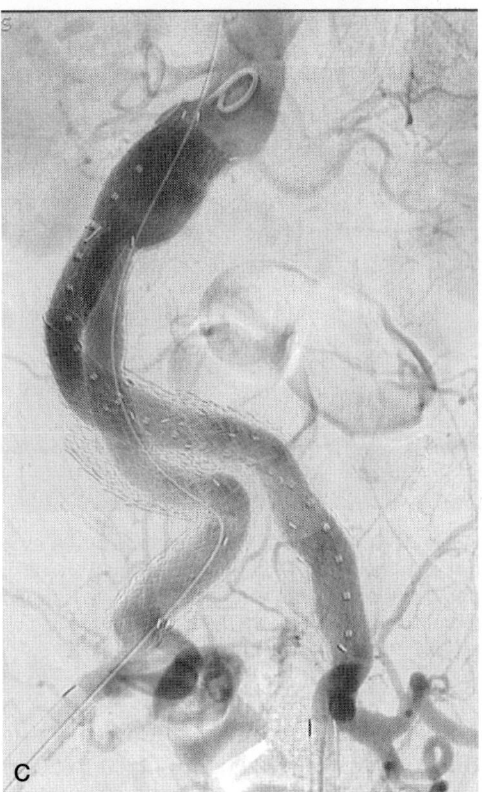

Figure 51-3. a-b. CT angiogram and aortogram of distal migration of Aneurx device. c. Successful AAA exclusion following placement of entire secondary endograft.

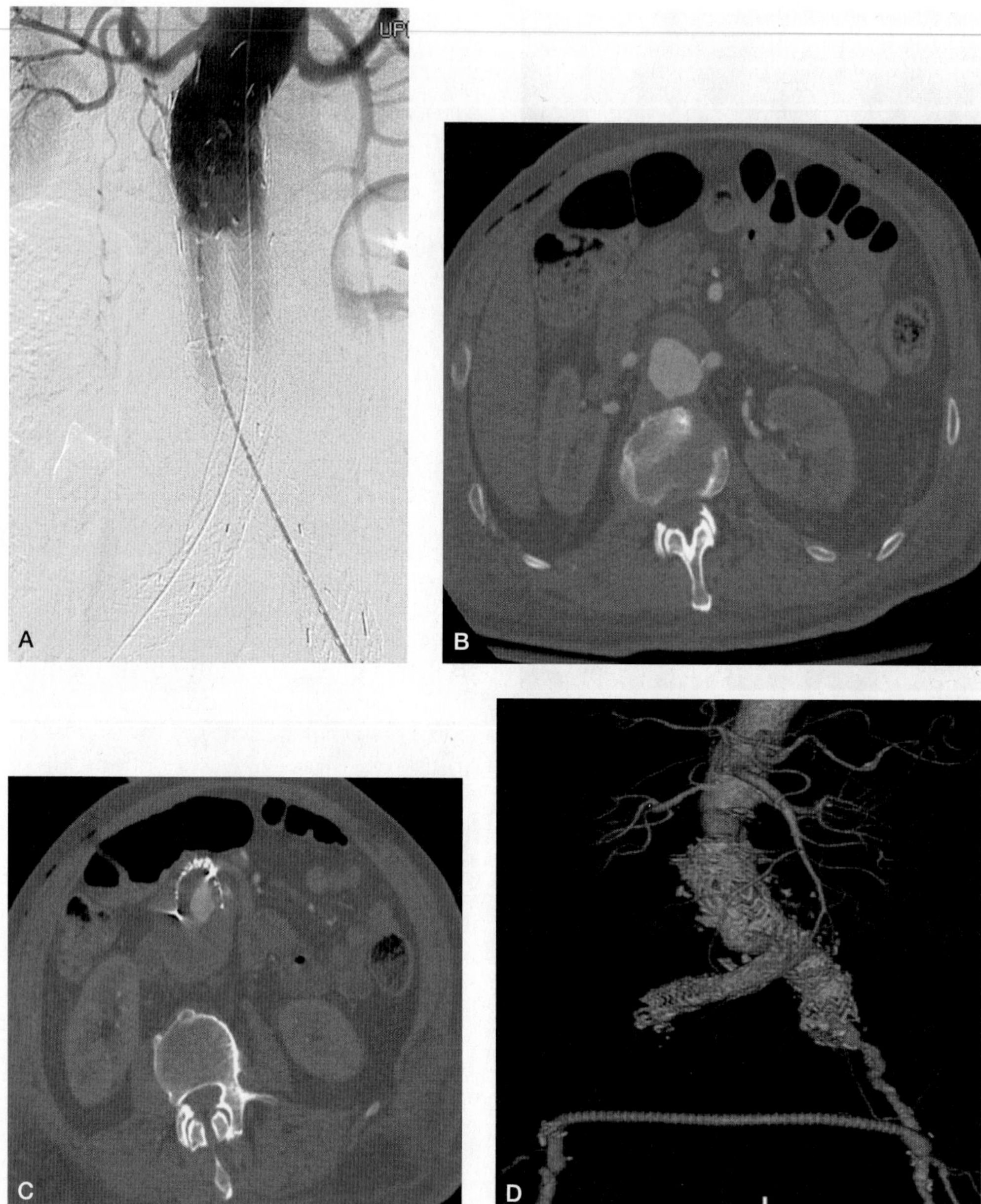

Figure 51-4. A. Completion aortogram with AAA exclusion following Gore Excluder placement along with aortic cuff extension. B-D. CT angiogram obtained 4 years later in a patient who was lost to follow-up and developed limb occlusion requiring femorol-femoral bypass following an emergent coronary bypass. CT demonstrates distal migration and neck dilation. The patient was treated with conversion using an aortobifemoral bypass following recovery from his coronary bypass.

In addition to device type, device sizing appears to have an impact on aortic neck dilation, and an oversizing of 10 to 20% appears to be most appropriate. Oversizing up to 30% has been associated with a higher incidence of aortic neck dilation. Specific anatomic factors that may have an impact on aortic neck dilation include

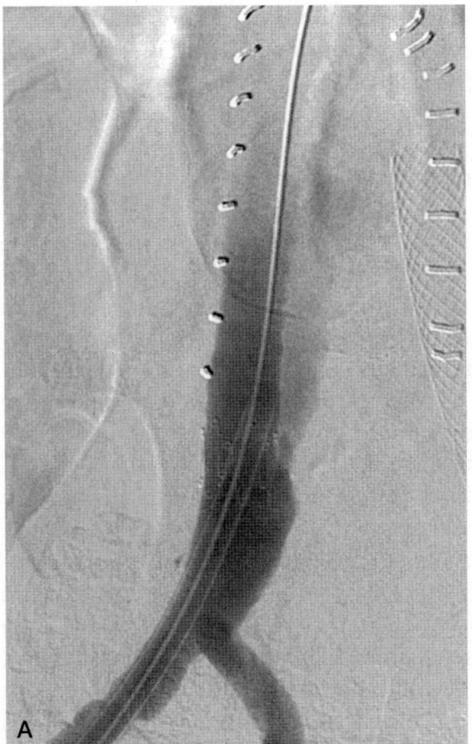

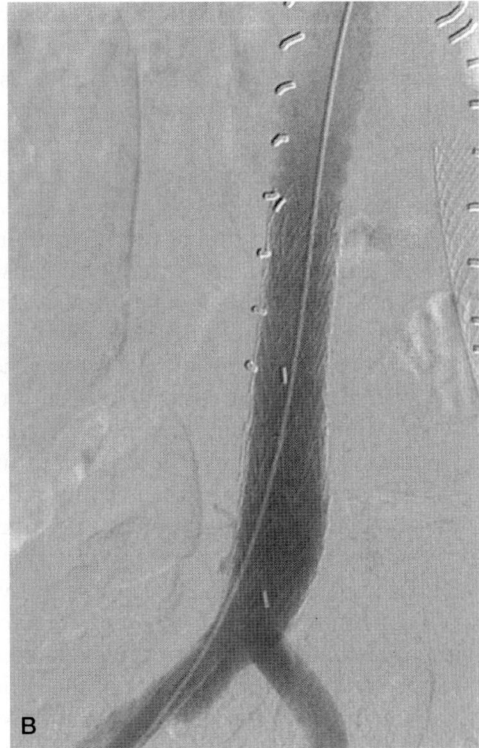

Figure 51-5. A. Distal type I endoleak secondary to dilation at iliac landing zone. B. Completion angiogram following treatment with iliac limb extension.

initial aortic neck size and aneurysm diameter. In particular, patients with larger aortic necks, larger overall AAA diameters, and those with circumferential thrombus at the level of the aortic neck are at higher risk for aortic neck dilation over time (Figure 51–5).

Distal landing zone degeneration in the iliac arteries may occur as well, leading to graft migration and distal type I endoleaks (Figure 51–5). As with the proximal neck, anatomic factors contributing to this phenomenon include large initial iliac size and the presence of circumferential thrombus.

Limb Occlusions

Limb occlusions are rare and most commonly reported within the first 90 days following implantation in grafts with unsupported limbs. However, limb occlusion may also occur in supported grafts and this has been documented as a late occurrence in all endografts. It has been postulated that conformational changes that occur over time with aneurysm remodeling may impact the patency of endograft limbs in supported devices. Aneurysm sac shrinkage occurs in many patients following EVAR, which may introduce kinks into the iliac limbs of some endografts, because some limb designs are less able to conform to changes in aneurysm sac anatomy. This presents a potentially adverse outcome in that sac shrinkage, a desired outcome of EVAR, may predispose patients to graft limb occlusion if kinks occur as a result of aneurysm remodeling.

The etiology of limb occlusions may be divided into anatomic factors and graft-related factors. The most common anatomic factors leading to limb occlusion include tortuous iliac artery anatomy and preexisting iliac stenosis. These anatomic characteristics may lead to kinking and narrowing of the endograft limbs. Similarly, a narrow aortic bifurcation can compress the iliac graft limbs because it must accommodate two limbs that are each equal to or greater than one half the size of the main body portion of the endograft.[17]

Dissection of the femoral or iliac arteries that is either preexisting or created at the time of graft implantation may also cause endograft limb occlusion due to poor outflow. There is also an association between small size of the iliac artery and graft limb occlusion. Women are at higher risk of graft limb occlusion than men, which is presumably because of the smaller size of the iliac arteries. Extending the stent-graft into the external iliac artery has also been found to contribute to limb occlusion, because there is commonly some degree of angulation at the origin of the external iliac artery in an area susceptible to atherosclerotic disease and calcifications.[18]

Furthermore, this extension limits the runoff by eliminating internal iliac artery flow and ends the limb in a smaller-diameter vessel.

Endograft-related charateristics are also a major causative factor in the development of graft limb occlusion. Excessive oversizing of the endograft can be a significant cause of limb or occlusion secondary to infolding of the graft material within the lumen. The most significant graft-related cause of limb occlusion, however, is the lack of support within the structure of the endograft. Limb occlusion with the Ancure graft was not infrequent secondary to either external compression or twisting of the limbs arising from the unibody construction and lack of limb support. Twisting of the graft limbs usually occurs during deployment of the endograft, narrows the lumen, and predisposes to thrombosis (Figure 51–6).

Patients who develop limb occlusion will typically complain of acute onset of pain and paresthesias in the affected extremity, but occasionally present only late after they notice the development of claudication. The femoral pulse is always absent and they manifest varying degrees of sensory dysfunction. The majority of patients do not present with threatened extremities that would necessitate expeditious surgical revascularization. Options for treatment include either endovascular or open surgical approaches. Endovascular approaches include thrombolysis, pharmacomechanical thrombectomy, or angioplasty and stenting (with either bare metal stents or additional endografts). Surgical options include conventional thrombectomy or extra-anatomic bypass.

Thromboembolectomy may be problematic in the EVAR population due to the potential for disruption or damage to the graft. Mechanical thrombectomy with a balloon catheter is hazardous, because it might dislodge the endograft that, in many cases, is held in place by radial force or self-expanding stents. Likewise, standard surgical thrombectomy may cause component separation due to traction of the balloon on the endograft. This concern about potential hazards of mechanical or surgical thrombectomy has led many to advocate extra-anatomic bypass for extremity reperfusion in cases of graft limb thrombosis.

Although open surgical repair has its proponents, many prefer an endovascular approach to graft limb occlusion. Pharmacomechanical thrombectomy along with simple thrombolysis may prove to be beneficial, because both are able to debulk the thrombus load and may uncover a kink in the graft limb or a previously unrecognized area of stenosis in the iliac artery.

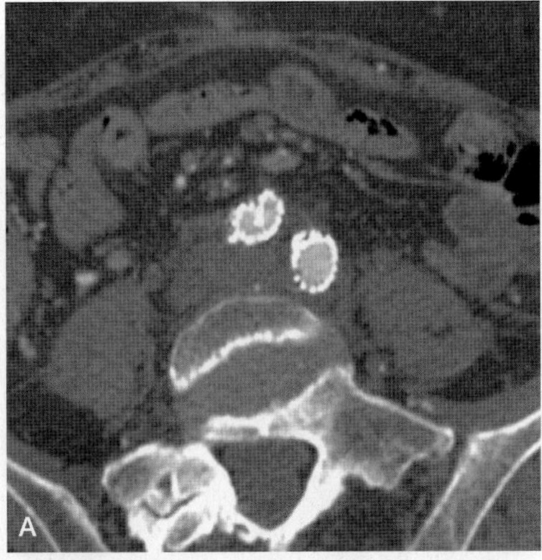

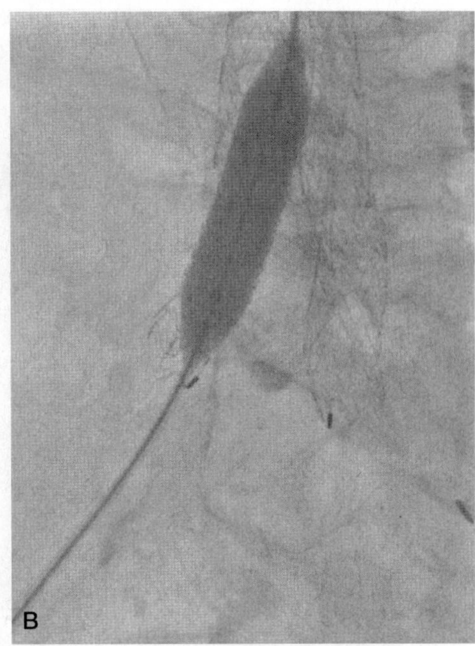

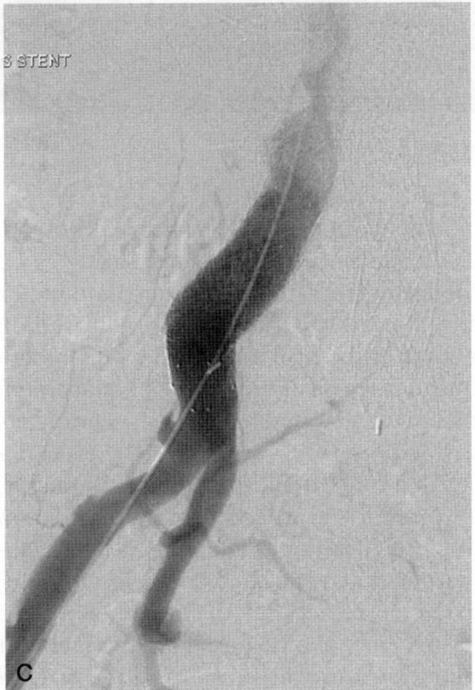

Figure 51-6. A. Right iliac limb endograft inflowing due to oversizing. B-C. Angiogram showing infolding treatment with angioplasty and stenting.

Material Failure

Material failure remains one of the most concerning modes for potential late EVAR failure, encompassing the breakdown of the intrinsic mechanical parts of the stent graft. It is often difficult to identify material failure because patients typically are asymptomatic at the time of presentation. Many of the first identified stent fractures were initially recognized within explanted stent graft devices that had been removed for evidence of aneurysm expansion or recovered at autopsy. The difficulty in identifying device failure limits a true understanding of the magnitude of the problem, because patients are rarely imaged closely enough during

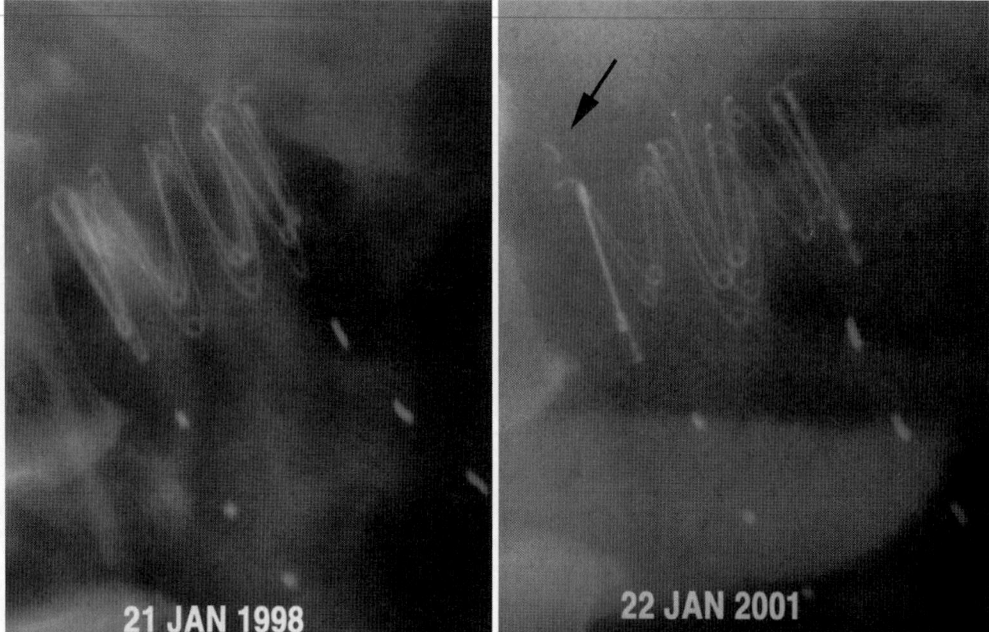

Figure 51-7. Attachment hook separation 3 years following initial EVAR.

their follow-up examinations to identify all the potential material breakdowns. Furthermore, the clinical significance of many identified device failures is unknown.[19]

Material failures may occur in the form of metal fractures, suture breakdown, or fabric erosion. Metal fractures can occur at any point throughout the graft, including the proximal or distal attachments, along the graft body, or involving the attachment hooks. Early-generation devices that suffered from fracture of the proximal attachment hooks were associated with distal migrations and development of type I endoleaks (Figure 51–7), The impact of mid-body stent fractures is less clear, but the risk of a sharp metal edge puncturing the fabric leading to a type III endoleak exists. Similarly, suture breaks leading to separation of the stent from the graft and subsequent friction between metal and fabric may occur, again ultimately leading to fabric tears. Such fabric tears have been seen in patients in whom bare metal stents have been placed in unsupported portions of endografts leading to the aforementioned phenomenon and resultant type III endoleak (Figure 51–8). In addition to the potential for the metal of the stent wearing on the fabric, potential exists for sharp calcifications in the arterial wall to compromise the fabric.

Patients who develop material fatigue may be asymptomatic or may present with new endoleaks and aneurysm enlargement. The majority of these may be treated with subsequent relining or, in select cases, endograft extension, but some patients will go on to require open conversion.

Component Separation

Component separation occurs primarily as a result of inadequate overlap between endografts at junction points. Following EVAR, there is typically some change in the anatomy of the AAA sac and its adjacent structures that contributes to changes or forces exerted on the

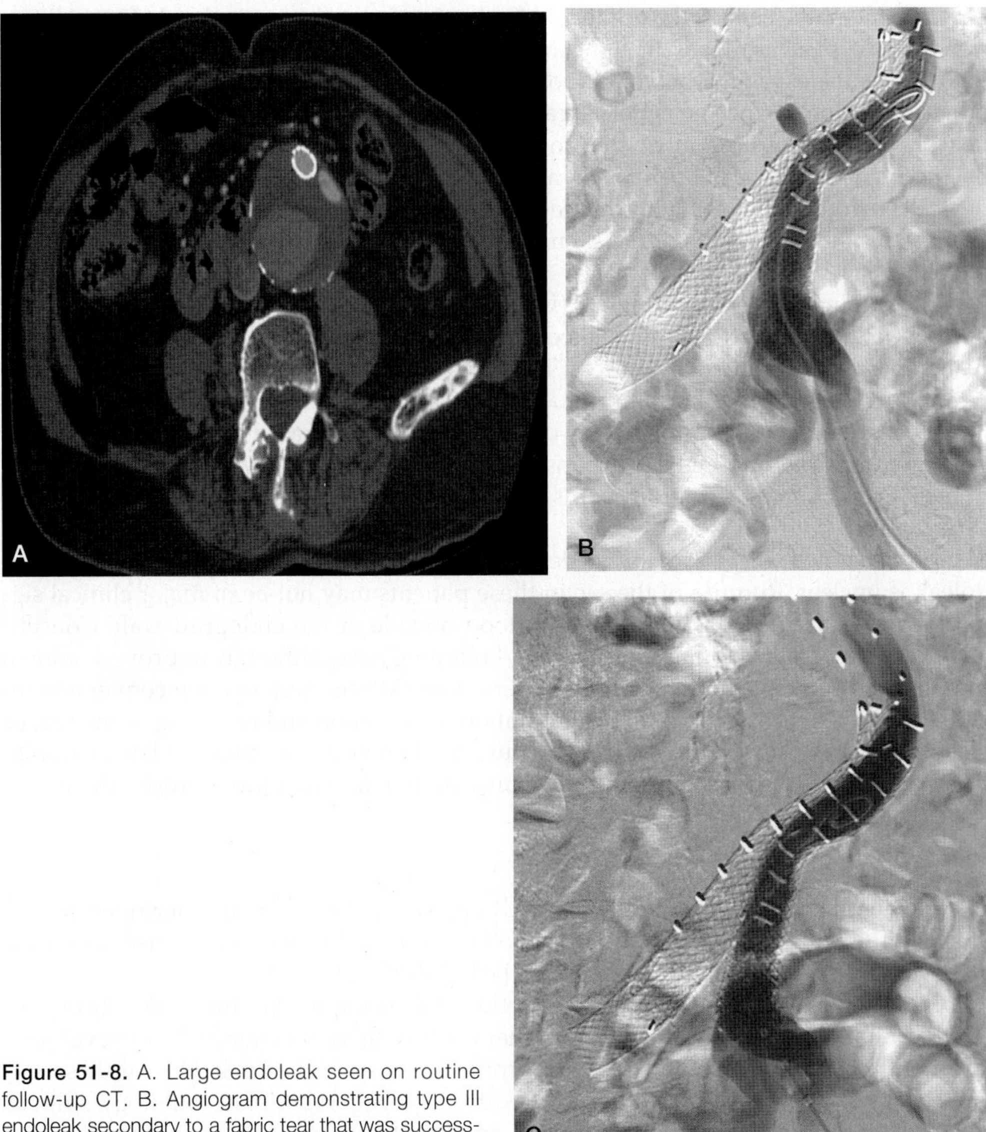

Figure 51-8. A. Large endoleak seen on routine follow-up CT. B. Angiogram demonstrating type III endoleak secondary to a fabric tear that was successfully treated with placement of an iliac limb (C).

endograft, possibly leading to component separation. This has become a relatively rare complication owing to improved device design along with operator experience. Furthermore, appropriate surveillance helps to avoid failure prior to its occurrence by careful examination of the position of the endograft components. When component separation does occur, patients typically develop a type III endoleak that may commonly be managed using endovascular techniques via a bridging endograft.

Hygroma and Endotension

Graft porosity can lead to a type IV endoleak in the early postoperative period. These endoleaks tend to seal spontaneously following reversal of anticoagulation. However, in certain stent grafts, namely the original Excluder device, graft porosity has led to endotension in some patients; this is thought to be the result of transmural movement of serous fluid across the expanded polytetrafluoroethylene (PTFE) material, thus resulting in hygroma formation.[20] When no endoleak can be identified after aggressive evaluation, continued sac growth has been attributed to endotension. Aneurysm sac hygroma has been documented at the time of open repair, and in vitro studies demonstrate that the particular device construct correlates with the degree of plasma permeability. Apparent endotension has resulted in rupture of the aneurysm wall following EVAR, often without clinical sequelae.

The original Excluder endograft (W. L. Gore & Associates, Inc, Flagstaff, AZ) was noted in clinical trials to be associated with less sac regression and more sac growth than some other commercial devices. However, since that time, a modified endograft with a low-permeability layer to reduce fluid flow across the graft material has been introduced. Patients with this newer device have demonstrated significant aneurysm sac regression and minimal sac expansion, implying that the low-porosity fabric used in the construction of endograft seems to be an important factor in early aneurysm sac shrinkage.[21]

The treatment of patients who demonstrate sac expansion in the absence of endoleak is unclear. Rupture of the sac in these patients may not be of major clinical significance, because there is no egress of blood outside of the endograft wall. Concern about short necks becoming effaced with enlarging sacs, although unproved, adds a theoretical disadvantage to long-term observation. Alternatives to open conversion include emptying the sac by means of aspiration, exploration and reclosing of the sac, or performing a window in the sac laparoscopically. However, the simplest has proven to be an endovascular relining of the endograft with the modified low-porosity device.

Infection

The incidence of infection following EVAR appears to be less than after open repair. Although the incidence of graft infections following EVAR is not well-defined, given the low overall reported incidence, it appears to be less than 0.5%.

Given the low incidence of graft infections following EVAR, there have been few significant statistical analyses of factors that contribute to infection.[22-23] However, certain risk factors have been postulated to contribute to a higher risk. One of these factors has been performing the initial procedure in an interventional radiology suite as opposed to performing the procedure in an operating room. The hypothesis is that sterile technique is followed less stringently and the use of periprocedure antibiotics less well regulated than in the operating room. An additional factor that has been repeatedly identified is the performance of concomitant endovascular procedures at the time of endograft implantation, primarily coil embolization. The relationship here is unclear, but it has been hypothesized that these procedures add additional time and steps (including wire, catheter, and sheath exchanges) to the implantation, allowing for greater potential for breaks in sterile technique. Other factors that may contribute to late graft infections include an immunocompromised state, bacterial infection leading to bacteremia, and postoperative infection at the femoral access site.

Given the low incidence of these infections, their treatment remains ill-defined, but surgical treatment has been performed for most cases. Following the established surgical principle involving graft infections after conventional open aortic aneurysm repair, the widespread use of surgical treatment is in accordance with the premise that an infected prosthesis should always be completely removed if the patient's medical condition allows. Overall mortality appears to be low, however, when compared with mortality reported for graft infection after open repair (18% vs. 40 to 70%). Options, as with infection following open repair, include graft excision and thorough débridement with extra-anatomic bypass or in situ replacement, either in a staged fashion or at the same setting. In situ replacement has been performed using Dacron prostheses, PTFE grafts, and autologous vein grafts. For select high-risk patients without evidence of overwhelming sepsis, long-term suppressive antibiotics with surgical drainage may be the treatment of choice, although this will likely not fully eradicate the infection (Figure 51–9).

Aortoenteric Fistula (AEF)

Primary aortoenteric fistulas have a reported incidence of 0.04 to 0.07%, whereas the development of secondary aortoenteric fistulas complicates 0.36 to 1.6% of all aortic operations.[24] Although the overall incidence of aortoenteric fistula seems to be decreasing and the diagnostic delays are shorter than they were historically, morbidity and mortality after repairs remain high. Aortoenteric fistula most commonly occurs at the third and fourth parts of the duodenum, usually coinciding with the anastomosis of the proximal aorta; however, aortoenteric fistulas have been reported throughout the length of the gastrointestinal tract. More recently, secondary aortoenteric fistulas have been reported following EVAR. The true incidence of aortoenteric fistula complicating EVAR is unknown but is assumed to be lower than the incidence in patients who have undergone open surgery of the aortoiliac region, because endografts have neither the suture line of an aortic anastomosis nor any other graft material in direct contact with the digestive tract. It has been

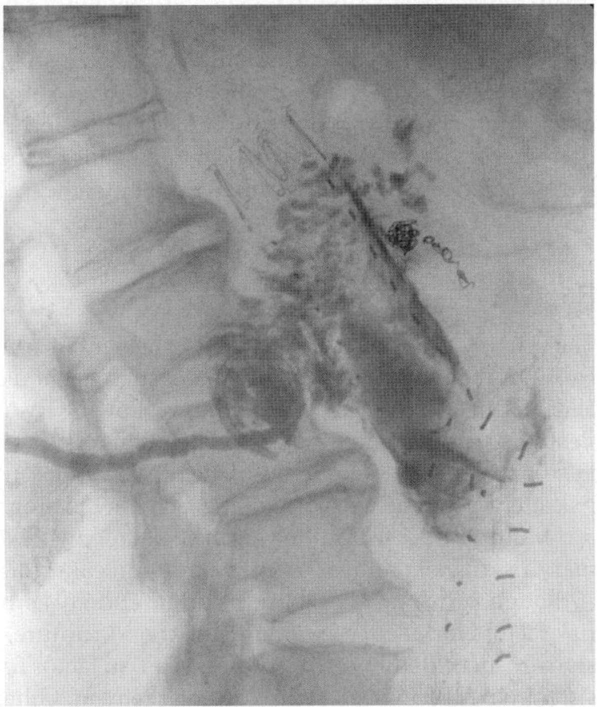

Figure 51-9. Infected endograft with a large perigraft collection that was drained percutaneously.

postulated that aortoenteric fistulas complicating EVAR are related to erosion of the aneurysm wall, migration, or endoleak. However, there have been several cases of aortoenteric fistula post-EVAR in patients without any evidence of endoleak or migration. An additional possible cause or contributory factor to the development of aortoenteric fistula in post-EVAR patients is infection whereby the presence of inflammatory periaortic tissue may contribute to adhesion of the duodenum to the aortic wall and subsequent fistula development. This may result because either the initial aneurysm was mycotic in origin or a low-virulent microbial infection of the endograft subsequently developed. Endotension has also been suggested as a possible source for erosion of the bowel by an aneurysm following EVAR as a consequence of mechanical pressure exerted on the digestive tract by the aorta.

Despite technological advances, the cornerstone of diagnosing an aortoenteric fistula continues to be clinical suspicion. Initial bleeding is usually minor and is often self-limited, and this may lead to a delay in definitive diagnosis. Additionally, the time from the "herald bleed" to massive rebleeding may be hours to months. CT scanning has been advocated as the preferred initial diagnostic test. Findings suspicious for aortoenteric fistula include the presence of periaortic gas more than 2 weeks after open surgery, periaortic inflammatory tissue or fluid, loss of fat between the aorta and the bowel, a defect in the aortic wall, pseudoaneurysm, and extravasation of intravenous contrast medium into the bowel lumen. Esophagogastroduodenoscopy (EGD) has less sensitivity than CT scanning but should be performed in patients with equivocal CT findings. Angiography should be reserved for patients in whom the diagnosis of aortoenteric fistula is unclear to help determine a source of bleeding.

For stable patients with minimal comorbidities and significant life expectancies, surgical management of aortoenteric fistula following EVAR via staged extra-anatomic bypass followed by graft excision is optimal because it provides definitive management, limits lower extremity ischemia, and allows for patient recovery between operations. Simultaneous repair of extra-anatomic bypass followed immediately by graft excision is an acceptable alternative that has also been shown to be feasible, with acceptable morbidity and mortality. Additional surgical options include graft excision alone, graft excision with in situ replacement, and primary repair, all of which should be reserved for select patients. Management of the intestinal portion of fistulas has been demonstrated to have acceptable outcomes with simple bowel repair, although resection may be necessary for certain patients.

Rupture

The primary goal of AAA treatment, whether performed via conventional open repair or EVAR, is the prevention of rupture and subsequent death. Unfortunately, despite its overall excellent effectiveness, rupture rates following EVAR are reported in up to 1.2% per patient per year, depending on the type of endograft and degree of follow-up.[25] Given the increasing survival times of this patient population, AAA rupture is a small but significant risk after EVAR and a major limiting factor in the prognosis of patients over time.

Multiple risk factors for rupture following EVAR have been identified. The primary risk factors appear to be major endoleaks, migration, and the type of endograft. Although proximal type I and type III endoleaks have been reported as the greatest risk factors for aneurysm enlargement and rupture, type II endoleaks have been occasionally identified in select studies as a risk factor for rupture as well, particularly persistent type II endoleaks with sac enlargement. Other factors that contribute to rupture include larger initial aneurysm size, poor sealing zones, female gender, stent-graft infection, and the presence of aortoenteric fistula.

Ruptures following EVAR have been reported at all time periods, from the immediate perioperative period (<30 days) up to 5 years following initial implantation, emphasizing the need for strict follow-up of patients. Patients who develop rupture after EVAR typically present with the same signs and symptoms as patients with rupture of native AAAs, including abdominal and back pain along with associated hypotension. However, patients with rupture after EVAR are less likely to be hemodynamically unstable, because there may be some protective effect by the endograft (Figure 51–10).

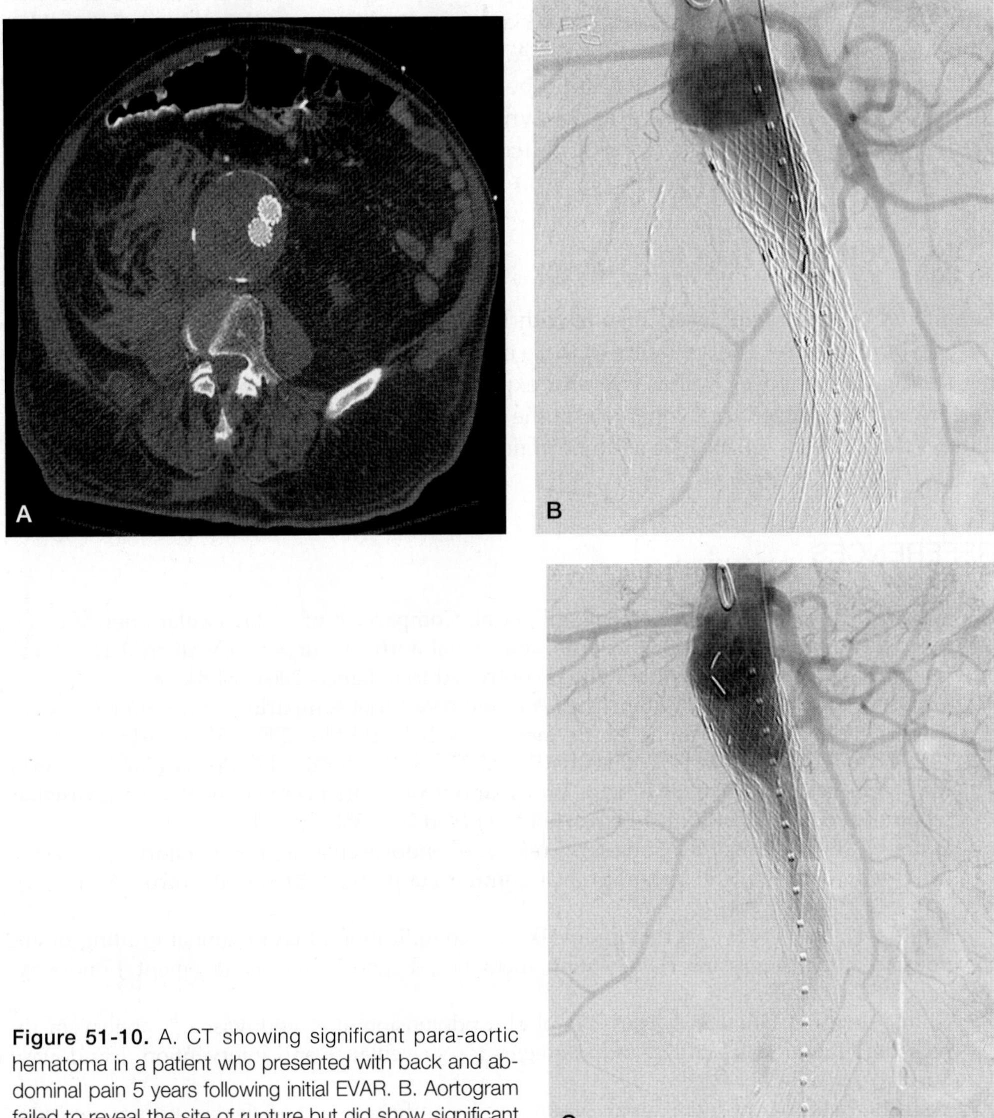

Figure 51-10. A. CT showing significant para-aortic hematoma in a patient who presented with back and abdominal pain 5 years following initial EVAR. B. Aortogram failed to reveal the site of rupture but did show significant migration treated with proximal aortic cuff extension (C).

Treatment of ruptured AAAs following EVAR is associated with relatively high morbidity and mortality rates, although these have been reported to be lower than repair following primary rupture. Endovascular means can easily be employed to correct the defect that led to the rupture, but on occasion, an open conversion is the only remaining option. Both retroperitoneal and transabdominal approaches have been reported.[26] In removing an endograft, technical challenges may arise related to incorporation of stents from endografts into the vessel wall, the presence of external stents or barbs, and periaortic inflammation. Depending on the location of the rupture, complete endograft removal may not be needed, and it may be necessary to transect an endograft. Despite early concerns regarding the use of a transected endograft as a part of the anastomosis and the development of pseudoaneurysms over time, there have been no reported anastomotic complications using this technique.

Data on outcomes for patients who develop rupture after EVAR are limited, although the presence of an endograft appears to be somewhat protective when compared with rupture in a native AAA.[27] However, as with patients who present with rupture of a native AAA, it should be expected that for patients with rupture following EVAR, those who have hemodynamic instability, delays in treatment, and greater comorbidities will have worse outcomes.

CONCLUSION

Despite very encouraging early results with EVAR, the technique continues to be plagued by long-term failures. The incidence of these complications may be decreasing with improving stent-graft design as well as operator experience in selecting appropriate patients and performing the procedure. Nonetheless, the persistent and unpredictable nature of these failures dictate that vigilant follow-up be maintained to avoid potentially fatal outcomes.

REFERENCES

1. Greenhalgh RM, Brown LC, Kwong GP, et al. Comparison of endovascular aneurysm repair with open repair in patients with abdominal aortic aneurysm (EVAR trial 1), 30-day operative mortality results: randomised controlled trial. Lancet 2004;364:843–8.
2. Prinssen M, Verhoeven E, Buth J, et al. A randomized trial comparing conventional and endovascular repair of abdominal aortic aneurysms. N Engl J Med 2004;351:1607–18.
3. Blankensteijn, JD, de Jong SE, Prinssen M, et al. Dutch Randomized Endovascular Aneurysm Management (DREAM) Trial Group. Two-year outcomes after conventional or endovascular repair of abdominal aortic aneurysms. N Engl J Med 2005;352: 2398–405.
4. Leurs LJ, Buth J, Laheij RJ. Long-term results of endovascular abdominal aortic aneurysm treatment with the first generation of commercially available stent grafts. Arch Surg 2007;142:33–41.
5. White GH, Yu W, May J, et al. Endoleak as a complication of endoluminal grafting of abdominal aortic aneurysms: classification, incidence, diagnosis, and management. J Endovasc Surg 1997;4:152–68.
6. Gilling-Smith G, Brennan J, Harris P, et al. Endotension after endovascular aneurysm repair: definition, classification, and strategies for surveillance and intervention. J Endovasc Surg 1999;5:305–7.
7. Veith FJ, Baum RA, Ohki T, et al. Nature and significance of endoleaks and endotension: summary of opinions expressed at an international conference. J Vasc Surg 2002;35:1029–35.

8. Faries PL, Cadot H, Agarwal G, et al. Management of endoleak after endovascular aneurysm repair: cuffs, coils, and conversion. J Vasc Surg 2003;37:1155–61.
9. Rhee SJ, Ohki T, Veith FJ, et al. Current status of management of type II endoleaks after endovascular repair of abdominal aortic aneurysms. Ann Vasc Surg 2003;17:335–44.
10. Silverberg D, Baril DT, Ellozy SH, et al. An 8-year experience with type II endoleaks: natural history suggests selective intervention is a safe approach. J Vasc Surg 2006;44:453–9.
11. Hobo R, Kievit J, Leurs LJ, et al. Influence of severe infrarenal aortic neck angulation on complications at the proximal neck following endovascular AAA repair: a EUROSTAR study. J Endovasc Ther 2007;14:1–11.
12. Sampaio SM, Panneton JM, Mozes G, et al. AneuRx device migration: incidence, risk factors, and consequences. Ann Vasc Surg 2005;19:178–85.
13. Benharash P, Lee JT, Abilez OJ, et al. Iliac fixation inhibits migration of both suprarenal and infrarenal aortic endografts. J Vasc Surg 2007;45:250–7.
14. Tonnessen BH, Sternbergh WC 3rd, Money SR. Mid- and long-term device migration after endovascular abdominal aortic aneurysm repair: a comparison of AneuRx and Zenith endografts.J Vasc Surg 2005 Sep;42:392–400.
15. Sternbergh WC III, Money SR, Greenberg RK et al. Influence of endograft oversizing on device migration, endoleak, aneurysm shrinkage, and aortic neck dilation: results from the Zenith Multicenter Trial. J Vasc Surg 2004;39:20–6.
16. Kibbe MR, Matsumura JS, Excluder Investigators, The Gore Excluder US multi-center trial: analysis of adverse events at 2 years. Semin Vasc Surg 2003;16:144–50.
17. Dillavou ED, Muluk S, Makaroun MS. Is neck dilatation after endovascular aneurysm repair graft dependent? Results of 4 US Phase II trials. Vasc Endovasc Surg 2005;39:47–54.
18. Cao P, Verzini F, Parlani G. et al. Predictive factors and clinical consequences of proximal aortic neck dilatation in 230 patients undergoing abdominal aorta aneurysm repair with self-expandable stent-grafts. J Vasc Surg 2003;37:1200–05.
19. Woody JD, Makaroun MS. Endovascular graft limb occlusion. Semin Vasc Surg 2004; 17:262–7.
20. Carroccio A, Faries PL, Morrissey NJ, et al. Predicting iliac limb occlusions after bifurcated aortic stent grafting: anatomic and device-related causes. J Vasc Surg 2002;36:679–84.
21. Jacobs TS, Won J, Gravereaux EC, et al. Mechanical failure of prosthetic human implants: a 10-year experience with aortic stent graft devices. J Vasc Surg 2003;37:16–26.
22. Cho JS, Dillavou ED, Rhee RY, Makaroun MS. Late abdominal aortic aneurysm enlargement after endovascular repair with the Excluder device. J Vasc Surg 2004;39:1236–41.
23. Haider SE, Najjar SF, Cho JS, et al. Sac behavior after aneurysm treatment with the Gore Excluder low-permeability aortic endoprosthesis: 12-month comparison to the original Excluder device. J Vasc Surg 2006;44:694–700.
24. Sharif MA, Lee B, Lau LL, et al. Prosthetic stent graft infection after endovascular abdominal aortic aneurysm repair. J Vasc Surg 2007;46:442–8.
25. Ducasse E, Calisti A, Speziale F, et al. Aortoiliac stent graft infection: current problems and management. Ann Vasc Surg 2004;18:521–6.
26. del Moral L, Alonsoa SF, Kiuri SS, et al. Aortoenteric fistula arising as a complication of endovascular treatment of abdominal aortic aneurysm. Ann Vasc Surg 2009;23:255.e13–7.
27. Schlösser FJ, Gusberg RJ, Dardik A, et al. Aneurysm rupture after EVAR: can the ultimate failure be predicted? Eur J Vasc Endovasc Surg 2009;37:15–22.
28. Kelso RL, Lyden SP, Butler B, et al. Late conversion of aortic stent grafts. J Vasc Surg 2009; 49:589–95.
29. Coppi G, Gennai S, Saitta G, et al. Treatment of ruptured abdominal aortic aneurysm after endovascular abdominal aortic repair: a comparison with patients without prior treatment. J Vasc Surg 2009;49:582–8.

52

The Cost of Endovascular Peripheral Interventions and Endovascular Aneurysm Repair

Britt H. Tonnessen, M.D., W. Charles Sternbergh III, M.D., and Samuel R. Money, M.D., M.B.A.

COST AND ENDOVASCULAR PROCEDURES

Hospitals and providers are increasingly feeling the strain of a financially overburdened health care system. Yet, as medical technology develops, there is substantial pressure from the public and industry to offer the most minimally invasive and "cutting-edge" techniques. From a physician's perspective, these techniques should be offered if they are proven to provide clinical benefit and the increased cost is commensurate with improved care and recovery. Endovascular aneurysm repair (EVAR) and endovascular treatment of peripheral arterial disease (PAD) are prime examples of technological advances that have improved patient care. However, technology is expensive. Third-party payers have failed to correspondingly increase reimbursement to adequately meet these technologically driven expenses. Ultimately, a physician's ability to even offer EVAR and other endovascular techniques may be restricted by fiscally motivated hospital policies.

The term "cost" refers to the actual expense that is incurred by the hospital itself. This somewhat nebulous concept for physicians is far more practical in the day-to-day activities of department managers, administrators, and the hospital accounting department. Cost can be broken down into direct cost and indirect cost. Direct cost includes supplies, equipment, salaries, and facility use. Indirect cost includes cost from departments not directly involved with the patient's care (e.g., cafeteria, finance, computer services) as well as institutional overhead. Charges are then generated by a cost-to-charge ratio and submitted to the third-party payers. Reimbursement is defined as the actual money received and is generally substantially less than the actual charge. The balance between the actual cost and the reimbursement determines whether a profit margin is generated.

The largest cost drivers for EVAR and endovascular interventions are usually the devices (endografts, stents). In addition, vigorous surveillance regimens after these procedures add to the overall expense. The durability of many endovascular techniques is more limited than traditional open techniques and may require additional maintenance procedures, further draining the health care system. The purpose of this chapter is to review the literature on the cost of endovascular interventions, focusing on lower extremity revascularization procedures and EVAR.

THE COST OF LOWER EXTREMITY ENDOVASCULAR INTERVENTIONS

The emergence and exponential growth of endovascular interventions for the lower extremities has significantly altered the treatment algorithms for PAD. Current guidelines recommend endovascular procedures as the first-line therapy for shorter-segment lesions in the iliac and superficial femoral arteries (SFAs).[1] Preprocedure imaging, the initial procedure, postprocedure surveillance, and reinterventions are all factors that contribute to the overall cost of endovascular and open interventions. Concern about the durability of endovascular procedures and lack of standard surveillance protocols may lead to aggressive and expensive follow-up.

Stoner et al. retrospectively examined the cost of revascularization for femoral-popliteal segments, comparing endovascular (n=198) and open (n=183) procedures.[2] Using the model proposed by these authors, cost-efficacy curves for endovascular interventions can be calculated on a cost-per-day basis (Figure 52–1). Importantly, this methodology incorporates overall patency and reintervention rates into the final analysis. Thus, a procedure that achieves long-term patency without reintervention has the lowest cost-per-day of patency, whereas a procedure that fails after a short duration would have the highest.

In this study, 12-month primary-assisted patency was 77% in the open femoral-popliteal bypass group vs. 65% for the endovascular group (P<.01). Although the initial cost of endovascular intervention was just over half as much as open bypass ($6739 vs. $12,389; P<.001), this benefit was offset by the cost of more reinterventions in the endovascular group by 1 year. At 12 months, the cost-per-day analysis found a compa-

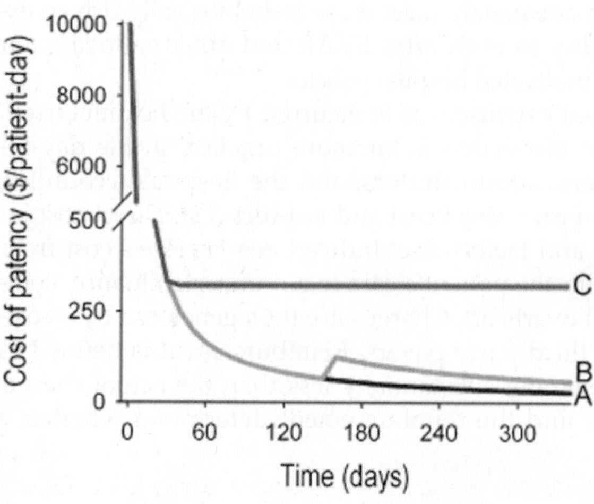

Figure 52-1. Hypothetical cost curves for the following revascularization scenarios. A. Successful initial revascularization without failure of patency or reintervention. B. Reintervention to maintain patency. C. Failure of patency without reintervention. (Used with permission from Stoner MC, deFreitas DJ, Manwaring MM, et al. Prophylatic use of the silver-acetate-coated graft in arterial occlusive disease. J Vasc Surg 2008;48:1489–96.)

rable cost of $229 for open bypass and $185 for endovascular intervention (P=.71). Interestingly, there was a trend toward greater cost-per-day for endovascular interventions in the critical limb ischemia group ($359 vs. $210; P=0.33), although statistically insignificant. Conversely, the subgroup of claudicants had a lower cost-per-day of $86 versus $259 with endovascular intervention (P=.31), with particularly lower cost if no stent was used. It is also noteworthy that only 21% of patients in the endovascular group of this study received stents. This pithiness in stent usage probably does not reflect most practice patterns, however. As such, this study may underestimate the cost of peripheral vascular intervention.

Although costs will vary somewhat by region and institution, certain aspects of this study can be applied broadly. Endovascular interventions on the SFA have patency rates inferior to femoral-popliteal bypass and therefore require more numerous (and costly) reinterventions. Stents are used with varying frequency in the SFA; greater stenting percentage translates to higher cost. Follow-up in the above-mentioned study was truncated at 1 year, but longer follow-up could reveal even greater divergence in the number of reinterventions and cost.

The type of endovascular intervention being performed also factors into the procedural cost. For example, atherectomy or stenting has higher direct cost than angioplasty alone in the lower extremities. When more than one stent is used, as is sometimes necessary, the cost additive from these devices is significant. From a purely costing perspective, selective stenting after angioplasty of the SFA is recommended until the clinical data conclusively demonstrate better patency for primary stenting. Lasers, cryoplasty, atherectomy, re-entry devices, and drug-eluting stents are examples of innovative technologies that are in various stages of development for treating lower extremity occlusive disease. Unless clinical superiority and durability can be demonstrated with a new technology, fiscally responsible endovascular interventionalists should proceed cautiously with adopting more costly technology.

The setting in which the procedure is performed (operating room or radiology suite, outpatient or inpatient) further influences both the cost and the reimbursement. In a study from Buffalo, New York, the authors grimly point out that net losses are seen for outpatient endovascular procedures, even more so for private pay insurers than for Medicare.[3] Costs are less in the catheterization laboratory than in the operating room and less for outpatient than inpatient procedures. The cost of an arterial stenting procedure in the catheterization laboratory was $3392 compared with $5844 in the operating room, largely due to greater expense of operating room personnel and medical supplies. However, reimbursement was worse for outpatient procedures. As a result, only inpatient procedures performed in the radiology suite earned profit. These findings argue for the use of the catheterization laboratory as the primary site for pure endovascular interventions. However, competition for catheterization laboratory time and space, as well as the inability to perform hybrid procedures in this setting, makes this a less attractive option. Given the increased patient satisfaction, safety, and efficiency of ambulatory endovascular procedures, a lower reimbursement rate is counterintuitive.

Coding guidelines also limit the reimbursement for ambulatory endovascular procedures and are based on the Current Procedural Terminology (CPT) for outpatient procedures and Diagnosis Related Group (DRG) for inpatients. Currently, outpatient procedures may have several components within a single procedure that can be coded, with each reimbursed at a lower tier. This system requires that each of the components is accurately listed. For example, endovascular treatment of the SFA may include components for the stenting, angioplasty, catheter placement, and the radiologic interpretation codes. However, a stent placed in the SFA can be coded as an additional component of the procedure only if it is documented to have been placed for a residual >20% stenosis or dissection or a ≥5 mm Hg gradient postangioplasty.[4] Multiple stents placed within the same vessel are coded as one procedure, and therefore, losses are incurred from the cost of multiple stents. Separate "carve-out" reimbursement for the cost of implantable devices is sometimes negotiated with private insurers and would help to defray some of these losses. Reimbursement within the DRG system is more global and based upon the patient's comorbid conditions and complications. A greater number of comorbid conditions and complications will reimburse at a higher DRG level. Therefore, meticulous documentation by health care providers of pre-existing conditions becomes a critical part of reimbursement.

THE COST OF ENDOVASCULAR ANEURYSM REPAIR

EVAR results in lower rates of perioperative morbidity and mortality compared with open repair, as shown in two randomized trials.[5-6] Nonetheless, the cost-effectiveness of this procedure is controversial. The cost of EVAR can be broken down into two categories. First, there is the initial cost of endograft placement that includes the device, operating room costs, and costs from the hospital stay. Intuitively, a lower complication rate and shorter hospital stay for EVAR would reduce hospital costs. However, these benefits have failed to translate into a cost-effective procedure when all cost components are considered. The largest cost component is the endograft device itself. Post-placement costs are incurred after the initial hospital stay and include surveillance imaging, follow-up visits, laboratory work, and secondary procedures. Indeed, these late costs increase the global cost of EVAR by 44%.[7]

PLACEMENT COSTS

In a retrospective cost analysis of EVAR performed on the U.S. Food and Drug Administration (FDA) Phase II multicenter AneuRx (Medtronic, Santa Rosa, CA) trial published in 2000, the initial placement costs for EVAR were significantly greater than those for open repair.[8] The largest cost component was the device, which accounted for 52% of the total placement cost of EVAR. Several other retrospective studies have confirmed the greater initial expense of EVAR compared with open repair.[9-11] In each of these studies, EVAR resulted in significantly shorter length of hospital stay, ICU admissions, and operating room time. In addition, a lower cost of floor nursing, pharmacy, and laboratory use in the EVAR group did not translate to overall lower costs. Because the cost of stent grafts exceeds that of open surgical grafts by 10 to 20 times, EVAR is the more expensive treatment.

Although prospective data have shown a lower mortality for EVAR, in these retrospective costing studies, mortality was not statistically different between the open and the EVAR groups. This point is important because in modeling analyses, the cost-effectiveness of EVAR hinges upon its potential to reduce morbidity and mortality compared to open repair.[12] Costs may also vary depending on the patient population being treated. Thus, patients with a greater number of comorbidities may require additional tests and hospital costs, although the reimbursement for these patients will be at a higher tier. In a Canadian prospective, nonrandomized observational study of

TABLE 52-1. ENDOGRAFT PLACEMENT

	Year	EVAR Cost	Open Cost	Device Cost
Patel[12]	1999	$20,083	$16,016	$8000
Sternbergh[8]	2000	$19,985	$12,546	$10,400
Clair[9]	2000	$7205	Greater for EVAR	$8976
Bosch[10]	2001	$20,716	$18,484	$7000
Dryjski[11]	2003	$17,539	$9042	$9475-9975
MEAN		$19,581	$14,022	$8820

In each of these studies, the initial cost of EVAR exceeded that for open repair. The largest cost driver is the cost of the device.

EVAR cost specifically looking at high-risk patients, initial hospital costs were comparable for EVAR versus open repair.[13] This study is of particular interest because two thirds of the patients in both groups were from the American Society of Anesthesiologists Class IV (severe systemic disease that is a constant threat to life). However, a median length of hospital stay of 6 days in the EVAR group, longer than in many studies, may have skewed these data.

The dominant cost component in all of these reports is the device, which accounts for 30 to 50% of initial placement cost. Current devices on the market retail for more than $13,000 per case. From these U.S. studies between 1999 and 2003, a mean initial hospital cost of $19,581 for EVAR is estimated (Table 52–I). Using the medical component of the Consumer Price Index, the estimated 2009 placement cost of EVAR would be $24,212.[14]

POST-PLACEMENT COSTS

Costs incurred after the initial endograft placement have been dubbed "post-placement costs." In a study from the Ochsner Clinic, the cumulative post-placement cost per patient at 5 years after EVAR was $11,351, thereby increasing the global cost of EVAR by 44%.[7] Post-placement costs include the cost of secondary procedures, surveillance imaging, outpatient visits, and laboratory work. Despite institutional and regional differences, there are certain trends in the post-placement costs. Consistently, secondary procedures and surveillance imaging are the number one and two contributors to post-placement costs, respectively (Figure 52–2).

Secondary procedures are defined as additional interventions after the original EVAR, such as treatment for endoleak, migration, or limb thrombosis. Secondary procedures are a time-dependent phenomenon and may be needed after EVAR in 10 to 20% of patients.[15-17] Secondary procedures are particularly costly, constituting 57.4% of the total post-placement costs in the Ochsner study. In fact, patients who undergo secondary procedures had 8.6 times higher costs compared with those patients who never underwent a secondary procedure. Although secondary procedures such as diagnostic angiograms and endocuffs are more common, the rare delayed open aneurysm conversion accounts for a significant proportion of secondary procedure cost.

Surveillance after EVAR has traditionally been vigilant owing to concern for migration and endoleak, potential sources of aneurysm-related morbidity. However, imaging performed with thin-slice helical CT scans is costly. A typical post-placement regimen includes a CT and abdominal radiographs at 1, 6, and 12 months after initial

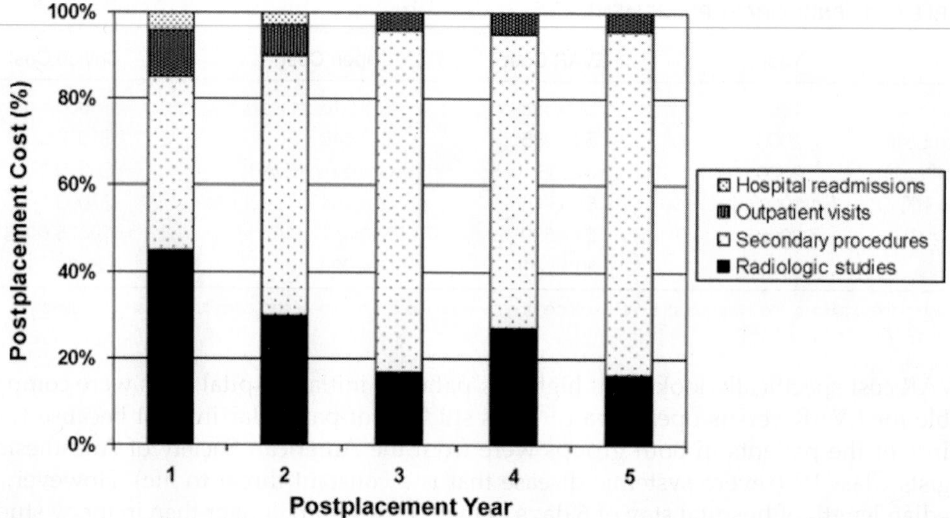

Figure 52-2. Yearly post-placement cost components. Secondary procedures and surveillance radiographic studies are the number one and two sources of post-placement costs, respectively. (Adapted with permission from Noll RE, Tonnessen BH, Mannava K, et al. Long-term postplacement cost offer endovascular aneurysm repair. J Vasc Surg 2007;46:9–15.)

implantation and then yearly thereafter. The frequency of imaging is even more intensive in patients identified with problems such as endoleaks. In contrast, surveillance after open aneurysm repair is recommended only every 3 to 5 years to detect late and infrequent complications such as anastomotic pseudoaneurysms.[18] Most practices rarely perform long-term radiographic follow-up after open repair.

COST-EFFECTIVENESS OF EVAR

Although the true cost of EVAR is greater than that of open repair, determining cost-effectiveness is less concrete. Markov modeling is one strategy by which a hypothetical cohort is subjected to either EVAR or open repair (Figure 52–3). As the model progresses, the probability of various outcomes is determined for each branch of the model. Using incidences derived from the medical literature, the model makes basic presumptions, such as risk of death, reintervention, and medical complications. The costs are then calculated for each branch within this theoretical framework. A major weakness of Markov modeling is that the outcome varies depending upon the initial hypothetical cohort inputted, that is, a healthy 70-year-old male with a 5.0-cm abdominal aortic aneurysm (AAA) is not representative of all patients. Also, the model hinges upon predetermining a number of variables, such as estimated mortality risk.

Once the Markov model is completed, quality-adjusted life-years (QALYs) can be calculated. This methodology evaluates the societal impact of a medical or surgical intervention, potentially providing a tool for determining the cost-effectiveness of a procedure. A QALY score of 1.0 indicates a year of perfect health, whereas death is scored as a 0.0. A surgical procedure that affects the patient's ability to function at a 1.0 level is scored between 0.0 and 1.0. The cost-effectiveness ratio of a particular surgical procedure or intervention can be determined by calculating a ratio of cost to QALY. Health care resources may potentially be allocated based upon lower cost-to-QALY ratios.

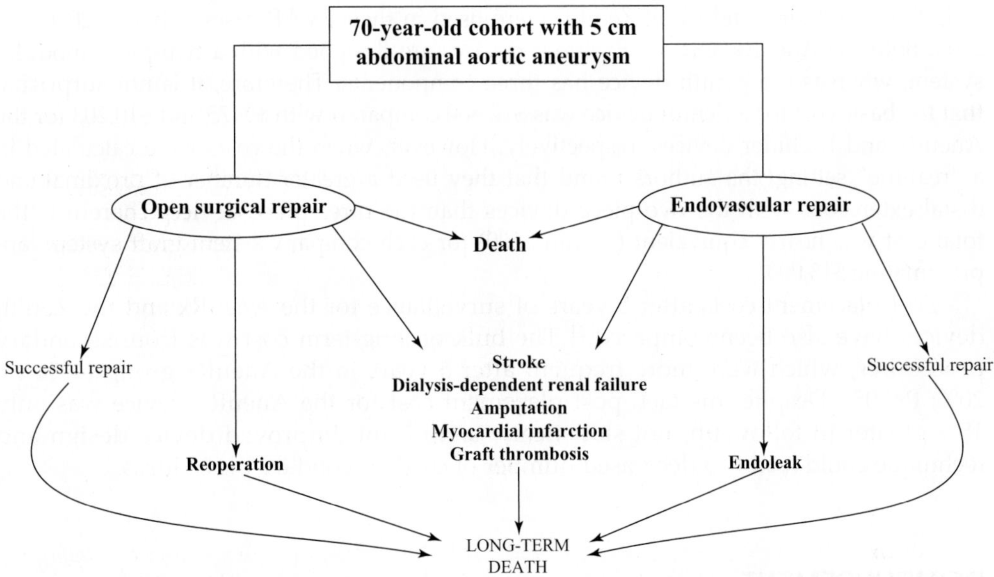

Figure 52-3. Simplified Markov decision analysis model. A hypothetical cohort with a 5-cm abdominal aortic aneurysm (AAA) may undergo either open surgical repair or endovascular repair. The outcomes of each strategy may be either successful repair or any of a number of complications. Each member of the cohort is followed until death. (With permission from Patel ST, Haser PB, Bush HL, et al. The cost-effectiveness of endovascular repair versus open surgical repair of abdominal aortic aneurysms: a decision analysis model. J Vasc Surg 1999;29: 958–72.)

In one such Markov modeling analysis, EVAR was found to be cost-effective even though the lifetime cost of EVAR exceeded that of open repair.[12] EVAR had a cost-effective ratio of $22,826, which is below the threshold of $60,000 that society is typically willing to pay for medical interventions. The authors used another example of the cost-effectiveness ratio for chronic hemodialysis being $54,400. However, cost-effectiveness in societal terms does not take into account day-to-day realities of hospital costs and reimbursement.

In the only randomized trial to examine "real-life" cost-effectiveness of EVAR, 340 patients were randomly assigned to either EVAR or open AAA repair.[19] When clinical outcomes were scrutinized in terms of cost, the initial placement costs for EVAR exceeded those for open repair significantly. Shorter length of stay and fewer complications could not substantially offset the endovascular device cost. At 1 year follow-up, patients who underwent EVAR or open repair had nearly equivalent QALY (0.72 vs. 0.73). When the higher cost of EVAR was balanced against the similar QALY scores for EVAR and open repair, open repair was determined to be the more cost-effective technique. This Dutch study likely underestimates the actual cost-effectiveness differential owing to limited 1-year follow-up and may also be difficult to apply to U.S. costs.

DEVICE DEPENDENCE

Given that the device cost dominates the initial cost of EVAR, it is relevant to consider the potential cost differences among device types. A retrospective review from the University of Florida looked at precisely this point.[20] Three different endografts (Medtronic AneuRx,

W.L. Gore Excluder, and Cook Zenith) were used in their EVAR cases between 2000 and 2006. Both the AneuRx and the Excluder devices are designed with a two-piece modular system, whereas the Zenith device has three components. Therefore, it is not surprising that the basic cost for a Zenith device was $12,800 compared with $9475 and $10,203 for the AneuRx and Excluder devices, respectively. However, when the costs were calculated in a "real-life" setting, the authors found that they used a greater number of proximal and distal extensions with the two-piece devices than the three-piece device. Therefore, the total cost was nearly equivalent (within $500) for each company's stent graft system, approximating $13,000.

Post-placement costs after 5 years of surveillance for the AneuRx and the Zenith devices have also been compared.[21] The bulk of long-term cost was from secondary procedures, which were more frequent after 5 years in the AneuRx group (49% vs. 20%; $P<.05$). Despite this fact, post-placement cost for the AneuRx device was only 15% greater in follow-up, not statistically significant. Improved device design and technique could lead to a decreased number of costly secondary procedures.

REIMBURSEMENT

AAA repairs are reimbursed through the Medicare system using a DRG-based code to standardize payment. Under this system, DRG 237 refers to a major cardiovascular procedure with comorbidities/complications, whereas DRG 238 refers to a major cardiovascular procedure without comorbidities/complications (Table 52–2). DRG 237 reimburses ~$32,440 versus ~$18,460 for DRG 238 (Arizona urban teaching hospital rate) – but these numbers vary somewhat by region and population density. Currently, only 38% of AAA repairs code to the higher-reimbursing DRG 237 (data from Thomson-Reuters, 2008). Using our 2009 estimated cost of EVAR of $24,212 and a mean weighted reimbursement of $23,772 per case, many hospitals may barely break even or sustain losses after EVAR (Table 52–3). Therefore, more stringent criteria that could place even more EVAR in the less complex DRG 238 group would be financially devastating for hospitals.

In a multicenter study published in 2003, a cross-section of three university and four community hospitals was examined with respect to actual EVAR reimbursement.[22] Ultimately, a net loss of $3898 per patient was seen for initial placement and hospital stay. Losses was greater for the lower-weighted DRG at $9198 per patient. Community hospitals fared the worst owing to lower reimbursement rates.

TABLE 52-2. EXAMPLES OF MAJOR COMORBIDITIES AND COMPLICATIONS THAT CODE TO DRG 237 (MAJOR CARDIOVASCULAR PROCEDURE)

Cardiac arrest
Acute congestive heart failure
Myocardial infarction
Pulmonary embolus
Acute respiratory failure
End-stage renal disease
Acute renal failure
Chronic renal failure
Pneumonia (including aspiration)

TABLE 52-3. ESTIMATED HOSPITAL COST AND REIMBURSEMENT FOR EVAR

Hospital Cost of EVAR		**$24, 212**
Cost of Endograft		~$13,000
% Cost of endograft		54%
Reimbursement for EVAR		
DRG 238	(62% of cases)	~$18,460
DRG 237	(38% of cases)	~$32,440
Weighted mean:		$23,772
Hospital net for EVAR		**–$440**

In a 2008 single-center study, Medicare and private insurance reimbursement were examined over 5 years of follow-up after EVAR.[23] Overall, an actual net institutional loss of $2235 per patient occurred. Losses were greater with Medicare than with capitated and commercial insurance. Overall, Medicare reimbursed only 68.5% of the total cost of surveillance (Figure 52–4). Patients who underwent secondary procedures (19.1% by 38.8 months) generated the greatest inequity in reimbursement rates, whereas patients with uncomplicated follow-up actually netted a slight profit for all third-party payers. The bottom line is that reimbursement for the post-placement costs of EVAR is currently inadequate to meet the true costs.

COST REDUCTION STRATEGIES

Standard surveillance regimens that include frequent and lifelong serial CT imaging emerged from early multicenter trials as a means to identify endoleak, migration, and sac expansion. One such regimen would include a CT and abdominal radiographs at 1, 6, and 12 months and yearly thereafter. Although these regimens were designed to prevent post-placement aneurysm-related morbidity, there is risk from cumulative exposure to radiation and iodinated contrast exposure. Furthermore, such vigorous regimens add significantly to the post-placement cost. More recent data from the multicenter Zenith trial suggest that a more "relaxed" surveillance regimen is feasible and safe in selected patients.[24] Absence of

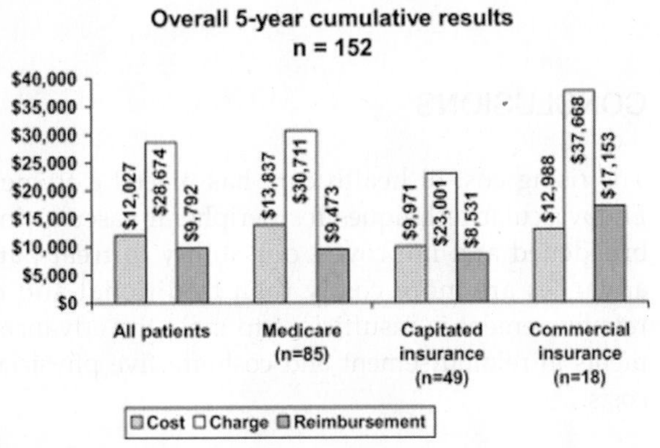

Figure 52-4. Five-year cumulative cost, charges, and reimbursement by payer for all patients after EVAR. Both Medicare and capitated insurance, which covered 88% of patients, were inadequate to cover the costs of follow-up after EVAR. (Adapted with permission from Kim JK, Tonnessen BH, Noll RE Jr, et al. Reimbursement of long-term post-placement cost after endovascular abdominal aortic aneurysm repair. J Vasc Surg 2008;48:1390–5.)

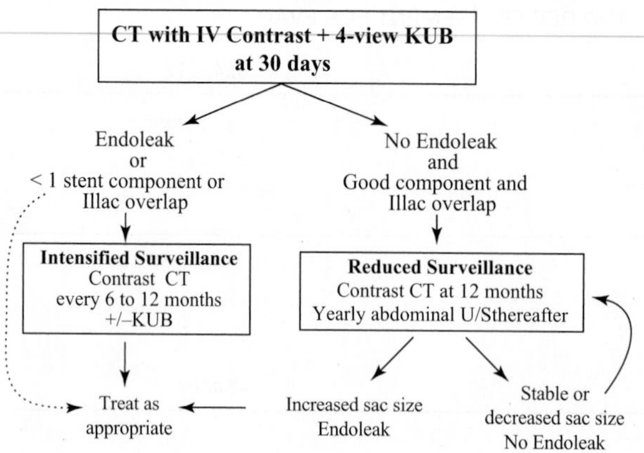

Figure 52-5. New surveillance protocol for Zenith endografts. CT, computed tomography; IV, intravenous; KUB, plain abdominal radiographs; U/S, ultrasound. (With permission from Sternbergh WC III, Greenbergh RK, Chuter TAM, et al. Zenith investigators. J Vasc Surg 2008;48:278–85.)

early endoleak at 30 days predicts a patient population at lower risk for aneurysm-related morbidity. Moreover, sac shrinkage ≥5 mm in combination with no endoleak at 1 year has only a 5.3% risk of subsequent aneurysm-related morbidity.

Duplex ultrasound has been used with increased frequency for surveillance after EVAR. From a cost standpoint, it is significantly less expensive. The major downside to this technique is that it is highly operator-dependent. Duplex ultrasound can accurately determine endoleak type and aneurysm sac size.[25] Based on the above data, Sternbergh et al.[23] suggested a surveillance regimen that eliminates the 6-month CT for patients with no endoleak at 30 days, and abdominal duplex ultrasound yearly for patients with no endoleak and stable sac size on the 1 year CT (Figure 52–5). However, the authors caution against extrapolating these data to patients whose aneurysms were treated outside the Instructions for Use (IFU) or with other devices until more data are available on those topics.

The frequency of secondary procedures after EVAR is the largest driver of post-placement cost. One strategy would be to minimize the need for and the number of secondary procedures. Earlier in the EVAR experience, most endoleaks were treated with trepidation and often intervention. Current evidence supports an expectant approach to type II endoleaks (that affect approximately 20% of EVAR), treating only if the endoleak is persistent and associated with sac growth of 5 mm or more.[26] Using these guidelines, only 1% of the original cohort of EVAR may require intervention for type II endoleaks. This management is also cost-effective. However, the presence of a type II leak at 30 days or beyond does greatly increase the need for a secondary procedure.[24]

CONCLUSIONS

The rising cost of health care has placed a tremendous burden on the U.S. economy. Endovascular techniques for peripheral vascular intervention and aneurysm repair have broadened and improved our ability to treat patients. However, these technological advances are more costly than traditional and often outdated techniques. Current reimbursement is insufficient to meet the advances in vascular care. Significant adjustments in reimbursement and cost-effective physician practices will help to balance these costs.

REFERENCES

1. Norgren L, Hiatt WR, Dormandy JA, et al. Inter-society consensus for the management of peripheral arterial disease (TASC II). J Vasc Surg 2007;45(Suppl S):S5–67.
2. Stoner MC, deFreitas DJ, Manwaring MM, et al. Cost per day of patency: understanding the impact of patency and reintervention in a sustainable model of healthcare. J Vasc Surg 2008;48:1489–96.
3. O'Brien-Irr MS, Harris LM, Dosluoglu HH, et al. Lower extremity endovascular interventions: can we improve cost efficacy? J Vasc Surg 2008;47:982–7.
4. Miller J. CMS withdraws CCI policy change. Endovasc Today 2008;7:71–3.
5. Prinssen M, Verhoven EL, Buth J, et al. A randomized trial comparing conventional and endovascular repair of abdominal aortic aneurysms. N Engl J Med 2004;351:1607–18.
6. Greenhalgh RM, Brown LC, Kwong GP, et al. Comparison of endovascular aneurysm repair with open repair in patients with abdominal aortic aneurysm (EVAR trial 1), 30 day operative mortality results: randomized controlled trial. Lancet 2004;364:843–8.
7. Noll RE, Tonnessen BH, Mannava K, et al. Long-term postplacement cost after endovascular aneurysm repair. J Vasc Surg 2007;46:9–15.
8. Sternbergh WC, Money SR. Hospital cost of endovascular versus open repair of abdominal aortic aneurysms: a multicenter study. J Vasc Surg 2000;31:237–44.
9. Clair DG, Gray B, O'Hara PJ, et al. An evaluation of the costs to health care institutions of endovascular aortic aneurysm repair. J Vasc Surg 2000;32:148–52.
10. Bosch JL, Lester JS, McMahon PM, et al. Hospital costs for elective endovascular and surgical repairs of infrarenal abdominal aortic aneurysms. Radiology 2001;220:494–7.
11. Dryjski M, O'Brien-Irr MS, Hassett J. Hospital costs for endovascular and open repair of abdominal aortic aneurysm. J Am Coll Surg 2003;197:64–70.
12. Patel ST, Haser PB, Bush HL, et al. The cost-effectiveness of endovascular versus open surgical repair of abdominal aortic aneurysms: a decision analysis model. J Vasc Surg 1999; 29:958–72.
13. Tarride JE, Blackhouse G, De Rose G, et al. Cost-effectiveness analysis of elective endovascular repair compared with open surgical repair of abdominal aortic aneurysms for patients at high surgical risk: a 1-year patient-level analysis conducted in Ontario, Canada. J Vasc Surg 2008;48:779–87.
14. http://www.cms.hhs.gov/MedicareProgramRatesStats/downloads/mktbskt-economic-index.pdf
15. Hobo R, Buth J; EUROSTAR collaborators. Secondary interventions following endovascular abdominal aortic aneurysm repair using current endografts. A EUROSTAR report. J Vasc Surg 2006;43:896–902.
16. Brewster DC, Jones JE, Chung TK, et al. Long-term outcomes after endovascular abdominal aortic aneurysm repair: the first decade. Ann Surg 2006;244:426–38.
17. Conners MS III, Sternbergh WC III, Carter G, et al. Secondary procedures after endovascular aortic aneurysm repair. J Vasc Surg 2002;35:992–6.
18. Hallett JW Jr, Marshall DM, Patterson TM, et al. Graft-related complications after abdominal aortic aneurysm repair: reassurance from a 36-year population-based experience. J Vasc Surg 1997;25:277–86.
19. Prinssen M, Buskens E, de Jong SE, et al. Cost-effectiveness of conventional and endovascular repair of abdominal aortic aneurysms: results of a randomized trial. J Vasc Surg 2007;46:883–90.
20. Feezor RJ, Huber TS, Berceli SA, et al. Impact of endograft design and product line on the device cost of endovascular aneurysm repair. J Vasc Surg 2008;47:499–503.
21. Noll RE, Tonnessen BH, Kim J, et al. Long-term postplacement cost comparison of AneuRx and Zenith endografts. Ann Vasc Surg 2008;22:710–15.
22. Bertges DJ, Zwolak RM, Deaton DH, et al. Current hospital costs and Medicare reimbursement for endovascular abdominal aortic aneurysm repair. J Vasc Surg 2003;37:272–9.

23. Kim JK, Tonnessen BH, Noll RE, et al. Reimbursement of long-term postplacement costs after endovascular abdominal aortic aneurysm repair. J Vasc Surg 2008;48:1390–5.
24. Sternbergh WC III, Greenberg RK, Chuter TAM, et al. Redefining postoperative surveillance after endovascular aneurysm repair: recommendations based on 5-year follow-up in the US Zenith multicenter trial. J Vasc Surg 2008;48:278–85.
25. Parent FN, Meier GH, Godziachvili V, et al. The incidence and natural history of type I and II endoleak: a 5-year follow-up assessment with color duplex ultrasound scan. J Vasc Surg 2002;35:474–81.
26. Steinmetz E, Rubin BG, Sanchez LA, et al. Type II endoleak after endovascular abdominal aortic aneurysm repair: a conservative approach with selective intervention is safe and cost-effective. J Vasc Surg 2004;39:306–13.

53

Role of Endovascular Aneurysm Repair For Ruptured Abdominal Aortic Aneurysms

Mark K. Eskandari, M.D.

INTRODUCTION

Ruptured abdominal aortic aneurysms (RAAAs) are the 13th leading cause of death in the United States, accounting for more than 15,000 deaths annually. The overall mortality rate for RAAAs is 80 to 90%, whereas survival ranges from 30 to 65% for those patients who reach the hospital alive.[1-4] Since the first repair of an RAAA, the mortality rate has decreased only 3.5% per decade to the current rate of 41%,[2] although this reduction may be due to selection and reporting bias. It is unlikely that the surgical technique for open repair will improve.

The high mortality rate during open repair of ruptured aneurysms is largely attributed to the significant systemic inflammatory response and subsequent multiorgan failure that develops.[5] The loss of both abdominal wall muscle tone[4] and compensated sympathetic activation[6] during the induction of general anesthesia can promote ongoing blood loss. Further blood loss from the retroperitoneal vasculature can occur during dissection through the hematoma. This is exacerbated by the fibrinolytic and acidotic state created by aortic cross-clamping, resultant ischemic-reperfusion injury, and coagulopathy that develops from hypothermia and large volume resuscitation.

Since the first published report of endovascular repair of a ruptured aortic aneurysm (rEVAR) in 1994,[7] several early reports documented the feasibility of this approach, and several retrospective studies and prospective trials have demonstrated its potential benefit over open repair. The ability to perform rEVAR under local anesthesia, with the maintenance of abdominal wall and vascular smooth muscle tone, may promote peritoneal tamponade of bleeding. The decreased aortic occlusion time, diminished blood loss, and better thermoregulation during rEVAR[6,8-9] may all contribute to improvements in surgical mortality.

MULTIDISCIPLINARY ALGORITHM

Personnel and Angiosuite

Paramount to the effective endovascular treatment of an RAAA is the development of a protocol that facilitates the synchronous passage of the patient through the emergency department and computed tomography (CT) scanner to the endovascular suite.[10] The group from Albany noted that the early diagnosis and treatment of RAAA by the emergency department staff and the increased comfort level of the operating room staff made the greatest contribution to the improvement in their ability to perform rEVAR.[11]

An on-call endovascular team of a radiologist, radiology technicians, transport personnel, anesthesiologist, operating room nurses, interventional radiologist, and/or a vascular surgeon with experience in both open and endovascular repair of RAAA must be readily available at all times. In one study, only 3 out of 24 procedures were performed during regular work hours,[12] and in several studies, endovascular repair was not performed in some patients owing to the unavailability of experienced personnel.[13-16]

The hospital should have a dedicated endovascular suite in which open repair can also be performed. This can be in the form of either a mobile imaging unit or preferably a fixed fluoroscopic imaging unit in an operating room. Equipment for both endovascular and open repair should be present. A "rupture kit"[17] for endovascular RAAA repair should be maintained, with an inventory of preferred stent grafts components. This kit should contain device components that the treating physician has prior experience with in elective cases. As a rough guide, large-diameter main body devices with short and long limb lengths should suffice in most emergent cases.

Imaging

Although ultrasonography can demonstrate an aortic aneurysm, it is not a sensitive modality for the detection of extraluminal blood. In addition, it has not been validated in its ability to assess aortic morphology.[18] Therefore, a preoperative CT scan should be obtained in all conscious, hemodynamically stable patients. The presence of a 64-bit multislice CT scanner in the emergency department can greatly facilitate rapid imaging. Although an intravenous contrast–enhanced scan is preferred, diagnosis of an RAAA and measurements for a stent grafts can be performed even with a noncontrast scan. In a 1998 report, 63 minutes were required for an emergent aortic CT scan.[19] Several current studies have shown that a CT scan can now be obtained in 10 to 15 minutes[14-15]

If rEVAR is to be pursued in patients who have not had preoperative imaging, intravascular ultrasound (IVUS)[20] has been used as an alternative imaging modality. Von Segesser has demonstrated IVUS to be as effective as digital subtraction angiography (DSA) in the endovascular treatment of nonruptured AAAs. In a study of 80 patients comparing nonruptured EVAR with either IVUS or DSA, no significant difference in mortality was noted between the groups, and early endoleaks and quantity of contrast material were significantly less with IVUS.[21]

Although Alsac has proposed the use of DSA as a means to reduce preoperative delay,[22] several studies have documented the inability of conventional angiography to evaluate the integrity of the aneurysm sac and to provide sufficient information for accurate stent grafts sizing.[23] In the Nottingham experience, angiographic calibration of aneurysm morphology was performed in three hypotensive patients. The authors noted that the angiogram did not reveal thrombus or atheroma at the graft landing zones, making graft sizing difficult.[10]

Concern has been raised over the deterioration of the patient during the time needed to obtain preoperative imaging. In one large study, 9% of patients died during transfer to the operating suite once the decision for emergent open surgery was made.[19] However, in a study by Lloyd et al., the median survival was almost 11 hours in patients managed nonoperatively, and 87.5% of patients survived longer than 2 hours after admission.[24] In a prospective study of 100 consecutive patients treated by open surgical repair, no difference in survival was observed between patients who underwent CT scans and those who did not, although a selection bias may have impacted these results because unstable patients were taken emergently to the operating room.[25]

Resuscitation

Approximately one quarter of patients with RAAA will arrive at the hospital hypotensive.[26] Permissive hypotension[9,27] should be practiced during the resuscitation of these patients.[17] Fluid should be restricted to an amount needed to maintain patient consciousness and a systolic blood pressure higher than 80 mmHg (50 to 100 mmHg).[12,28-29] The preferential use of blood products during these resuscitation efforts has been advocated.[28] The role of antihypertensive agents has not been universally defined, although several groups use sodium nitroprusside and nitroglycerin to treat systolic blood pressure higher than 100 mmHg.[30-31] Patients who are unconscious or unable to maintain a systolic blood pressure above 80 mmHg should be immediately transferred to the operating room. The decision to proceed with emergent open repair, placement of an aortic occlusion balloon, or invasive imaging studies will depend on the comfort level of the surgeon and the condition of the patient.

ENDOLUMINAL STRATEGIES

Anatomic Considerations

The anatomic suitability for rEVAR is commonly reported at 60% (18 to 83%).[13-15,32-36] The wide range (18 to 83%) quoted in the literature is due to the different stent grafts systems and anatomic criteria used. Many groups use the same anatomic criteria for rEVAR that is used in elective endovascular aneurysm repair (EVAR) patients. A neck length of greater than 15 mm with a diameter less than 30 to 32 mm and a neck angulation of less than 60 to 90 degrees are commonly reported anatomic limitations. In addition, a common iliac artery diameter less than 22 to 23 mm with an external iliac diameter greater than 7 mm is preferred. At thrombus, more than 40% of the aneurysm circumference and calcification of more than 80% of the aneurysm circumference have been listed as relative contraindications to rEVAR.[14]

More often, the belief is that the morbidity and mortality of delayed conversion to open repair are better than emergent open surgical repair and "therefore" an acceptance of more liberal criteria occurs particularly in regards to the proximal seal zone length. Some authors are even willing to proceed when there is a proximal neck length of >5 mm. Advocates of this more liberal anatomic criteria state that the primary goal is to save the patient's life,[17] whereas others feel that an unacceptable rate of type I endoleaks is seen. With newer stent grafts systems that utilize bare suprarenal stents, a greater number of RAAAs may be suitable for endovascular repair.

Anesthesia

It has been suggested that the improvement in morbidity and mortality seen with rEVAR is due to the use of local anesthesia, which, as stated earlier, promotes peritoneal tamponade. In a nonrandomized, retrospective study, the use of local anesthesia was associated with a shortened ICU stay and improved hemodynamic stability in elective EVAR.[37] The use of local anesthesia during the treatment of rEVAR has been well established.[15,38-39] Kapma et al. were able to avoid general anesthesia in 83% of patients,[13] and Lachat et al. performed bifurcated RAAA repair in 15 out of 21 patients under local anesthesia.[39] The use of local anesthesia in 28 out of 37 patients by the group from Zurich, as stated by Gerassimidis et al., may be the most important factor in avoiding hemodynamic disturbances and increasing the chance of survival.[36]

Pain from the aortic rupture, instrumentation of the aneurysm sac, and lower extremity ischemia have led some authors to recommend general anesthesia during the treatment of rEVAR.[22,30] Pain can cause the adverse physiologic response of hypertension and tachycardia, while the resultant restlessness can lead to motion artifact and inadequate stent positioning.[6,10,22] Alternatively, local anesthesia can be used to achieve femoral access and placement of a sheath, at which time general anesthesia can be instituted for the remainder of the procedure. This allows for access and the ability to place an aortic occlusion balloon if hemodynamic collapse occurs during anesthetic induction. Epidural anesthesia, with its autonomic sympathetic blockade, can exacerbate hemodynamic instability and should be avoided. Additionally, complications can arise from epidural placement in these coagulopathic patients.

Aortic Occlusion Balloon

The placement of an aortic occlusion balloon can be used to control hemodynamic instability from ongoing blood loss. However, aortic balloon occlusion risks renal and splanchnic ischemia, distal embolization, and ischemic-reperfusion injury and does not prevent ongoing blood loss from iliofemoral arteries.[40] Although carbon dioxide contrast injection can help delineate the aortic branches,[29] the loss of aortic blood flow can impact poorly on angiogram quality. For these reasons, several groups prefer definitive hemorrhage control with swift graft deployment.[22,34,36,40] Alternatively, Franks has reported achieving some degree of aortic occlusion through partial deployment of the Zenith or Talent stent grafts.[41]

Aortic occlusion balloons can be placed via either femoral or brachial access. The Montefiore group has demonstrated good success with brachial access, and Okhi routinely places a guidewire into the thoracic aorta through a 5-Fr (French) brachial artery sheath prior to the induction of general anesthesia.[8] Good stabilization of the occlusion balloon is achieved with brachial access; in addition, deflation of the balloon is not required during stent placement.[9,28] However, percutaneous brachial access is difficult in hypotensive patients[29] and brachial artery exploration is often required. Passage through the aortic arch risks cerebral embolization, while unfavorable angulation of the left subclavian artery orifice can make deployment difficult.[10]

The groups from Nottingham, Zurich, and Malmo and our own institution favor transfemoral balloon occlusion.[6,8,39,42] The femoral artery, while offering the largest access to the aorta, can also be catheterized under local anesthesia, and then utilized during the endovascular repair.[42] The sheath-over-balloon and balloon-ahead-of-sheath techniques of transfemoral aortic occlusion balloon placement have been described elsewhere.[8,43] During the sheath-over-balloon method, a second occlusion balloon can be inflated in the main body of the stent grafts[44] if the balloon and sheath are withdrawn prior to stent grafts deployment. Malina et al. prefer to withdraw the balloon through a sheath after graft deployment but recommend using only stent grafts with bare, barbed suprarenal stents to prevent dislodgement.[29] With either method, the balloon should be supported with the sheath, which is secured outside the body, and should be deflated slowly in unstable patients to prevent hemodynamic collapse.[29,43]

Stent Graft Systems

Both uni-iliac and bi-iliac devices have been used in the endovascular treatment of RAAAs. Aorto-uni-iliac (AUI) stent grafts have the advantages of allowing expeditious introduction and deployment, rapidly controlling bleeding by decreasing the intra-aneurysmal pressure more effectively than bi-iliac devices.[45] AUI stent grafts also may offer a broader applicability by requiring only favorable unilateral iliac anatomy[46-47] and by lowering the learning curve for deployment.[48] Exclusion of contralateral iliac aneurysms can be performed with AUI devices.[49] Several groups have found these qualities to favor the use of AUI devices in the treatment of RAAAs.[14-15] Brandt has even suggested that a reduced stock of components is required.[50] However, a femoro-femoral crossover graft is required with AUI stent grafts, preventing the use of local anesthesia, increasing the rate of wound infections, and creating the potential risk of graft occlusion.[51] It also prolongs the reconstitution of contralateral hypogastric artery blood flow,[52] raising the risk of spinal cord, splanchnic, and lower extremity ischemia.

The use of bi-iliac stent grafts has been supported by the groups from Zurich and Ulm.[39,53] Although the concern of longer operative times has been raised, with bifurcated grafts, this varies by reports.[22,39,14,12] If difficulty is encountered with contralateral limb deployment, a bi-iliac stent grafts can be converted to an AUI device with the placement of an aortic cuff (AneuRx, Excluder, or Zenith AUI converter) across the flow divider.[11,54] Again, it cannot be overemphasized that the devices used for RAAA should be systems that the operator uses routinely for elective EVAR and with which he or she has significant prior experience.

Technical Aspects of rEVAR

Technical success rates of 96 to 100% have been reported in multiple series.[12,34,39,42,54] The patient's chest, abdomen, and thighs should be prepared and draped. Access to the common femoral artery should be obtained either via a standard groin cutdown or percutaneously with an 18-gauge needle directed at the inferomedial aspect of the femoral head. A 6-Fr sheath can be placed into the common femoral artery after advancement of a 0.035-in J-wire into the aorta. Location of the puncture in the common femoral artery should be confirmed with fluoroscopic imaging in an ipsilateral oblique projection. If an occlusion balloon is to be used, a larger sheath should be placed, followed by percutaneous access of the contralateral limb. At our institution, the "preclose" technique is performed using a 10-Fr suture-mediated arterial closure device (Prostar, Abbot Vascular Devices, Redwood City, CA), which is deployed prior to placement of the larger sheaths. Alternatively, two 6-Fr Proglide devices can be used in a similar manner.

After advancing a pigtail catheter over a guidewire, renal artery location can be confirmed with DSA. Exchange of the catheter with a super-stiff guidewire is followed by positioning and by deployment of a stent grafts as is routinely done in elective situations. The stent grafts should be oversized by 10 to 20% to prevent graft migration and endoleaks. Sealing of a persistent type I endoleak can be accomplished with either a proximal aortic cuff or a large size Palmaz stent.[22,55]

rEVAR Outcomes

Mortality rates of 6.7 to 45% have been observed with rEVAR, with several studies reporting mortality rates of 20% or less.[13,15,17,29,33-34,39,41,53] Several studies have demonstrated a significant reduction in death with rEVAR when compared with open surgical repair.[13,22,41,56] In a systematic review of endovascular vs. open surgical repair of RAAAs, Visser et al. found a reduction in 30-day mortality rate for rEVAR after adjustment for hemodynamic conditions at presentation. This review of ten observational studies, composed of 478 patients, 148 of whom underwent endovascular repair, noted a 30-day mortality of 22% for rEVAR and 38% for open surgical repair.[57] Whereas some have attributed lower mortality rates in rEVAR to the avoidance of general anesthesia,[39] the wide variance may be due to selection bias.

Several groups have also reported a reduction in mortality after the introduction of a protocol that preferentially utilizes EVAR.[15,17,50] In Eindhoven, the mortality was 20% in patients treated preferentially with rEVAR, compared with 40% in the control group, and Lee et al. reported rates of 12% and 37%, respectively.[17]

In addition to improved mortality rates, several studies have demonstrated a significant reduction in the amount of blood loss during rEVAR as compared with open repair.[13,16,33,58-59] Reichart reported an average blood loss of 300 cc in 6 rEVAR vs. 4500 cc in 13 open repairs, whereas Kapma et al. reported 200 cc and 3500 cc, respectively. As a corollary to the decreased blood loss seen in rEVAR, the transfusion requirement in rEVAR has also been reportedly less when compared with that of open repair.[13,16,41,50,58] At our institution, rEVAR was performed on average with 6.6±4.7 units of blood given, whereas open repair required 11.0±5.3 units of blood. As with other reports, in a review of 37 patients treated for RAAA at our institution, Najjar noted a significantly decreased procedure time. On average, rEVAR was completed in 107±30 minutes as compared with 205±31 minutes for open repair.[42] In a systematic review, Visser et al. noted a shorter duration of endovascular procedures compared with open surgical repair (138 minutes vs. 181 minutes).[57] Several groups have also noted a significantly shorter ICU stay[13,15-16,22,33,41,59] and shorter overall hospital stay with rEVAR when compared with conventional repair.[13-15,42]

COMPLICATIONS

Abdominal Compartment Syndrome

Although several studies have shown a decreased rate of pulmonary, hemodynamic, and renal complications with rEVAR when compared with open surgery,[56] significant morbidity still exists. One study, in which an increased complication rate was seen in the endovascular group, suggested that these complications may have resulted in death if open surgery was performed.[52]

Abdominal compartment syndrome (ACS) has been seen in up to 20% of patients undergoing rEVAR.[17,54] The diagnosis is made based on clinical criteria: tense abdominal distention, oliguria, increased central venous pressure, decreased cardiac output, increased pulmonary capillary wedge pressure, increased peak airway pressure, and bladder pressure greater than 25 mmHg.[60-62] ACS can lead to respiratory, pulmonary, renal, and cardiac dysfunction. A significantly higher mortality rate is seen in patients who develop ACS.[11,54] Factors that have been associated with the development of ACS are the need for an aortic occlusion balloon, the presence of severe coagulopathy, massive transfusion requirements, and the conversion of a bifurcated stent grafts to an AUI device. Because of these findings, Mehta et al. have urged the avoidance of systemic heparinization to decrease the ongoing bleeding from collateral vessels. If one or more of ACS risk factors are present, they perform an on-table laparotomy.[11] In addition to routine, physiologic monitoring, patients who have undergone rEVAR should have hourly bladder pressures recorded to help in the early diagnosis of ACS.

Endoleaks

The development of both early and late endoleak after rEVAR has been reported. In a study of 37 patients, Hechelhammer et al. reported the freedom of endoleak to be 57±8.5% and 48.8±9% at 2 and 4 years. In this study, endoleak was responsible for 58.8% of secondary interventions.[34] Type I endoleaks have been observed in 5 to 25% of patients.[10,12,15,30,34,36,53] This range may be due to the different anatomic criteria in determining patient eligibility for rEVAR. The group from Ulm noted that the rate of type I endoleaks was comparable with that of patients undergoing elective EVAR. Use of a Palmaz stent, conversion to open repair, or/and packing of the aneurysm sac with a thrombogenic sponge or glue have been described as solutions to treat this complication.

The low rate of type II endoleaks seen in rEVAR may be due to the compression and subsequent thrombosis of lumbar arteries by periaortal hematoma.[12,53] However, 20% of patients in Zurich were noted to have late type II endoleak after resorption of the retroperitoneal hematoma. As with elective EVAR, intervention for type II endoleaks is indicated if an increase in size of the aneurysm sac is observed.[63]

End-Organ Ischemia

Spinal cord ischemia, which is seen in 1 to 2.8% of open surgical cases,[64-66] has been observed in up to 11.5% of patients undergoing rEVAR.[52] Higher postoperative mortality (50% vs. 19%)[52] is seen among patients who experience spinal cord ischemia. Hypogastric artery occlusion and prolonged functional aortic occlusion have been shown to be risk factors for cord ischemia. Although studies suggest that unilateral or bilateral internal iliac artery occlusion can be done safely during elective EVAR,[67-68] it has often been performed in a staged fashion, allowing collateral vessel formation. Peppelenbosch et al. have recommended the use of bell-bottom iliac device limbs to avoid hypogastric artery occlusion.[52]

Renal failure has been well documented in open RAAA[4] and is related to hypoperfusion, hypotension, and embolization. The associated mortality is 75%.[69] It has been reported in a similar number of patients (28 to 30%) undergoing rEVAR.[10,39] Its development may be potentially decreased by the use of dilute contrast, carbon dioxide angiography, or IVUS.[38,70] In the Nottingham study, renal failure developed in 6 of 21 patients. Two cases of acute tubular necrosis resolved spontaneously, 2 patients died from renal failure, and 2 with renal failure.[10] More often, this is due to either embolization or ischemia-reperfusion after placement of an aortic occlusion balloon. A similar mechanism may also be involved in the scattered cases of visceral ischemia after rEVAR.

CONCLUSION

EVAR has revolutionized the elective treatment of AAA and has the potential to change the management of RAAAs. Unlike elective repair, rEVAR requires a dedicated multidisciplinary approach as well as an operating room angiosuite and a readily available on-the-shelf supply of endografts. Allowing for more liberal anatomic criteria, particularly in regard to proximal neck length, will expand the application of rEVAR and potentially change the morbidity and mortality of RAAA. Adjuncts such as permissive hypotension, local anesthesia, aortic balloon occlusion, and avoidance of a laparotomy seem to improve the outcome of patients undergoing rEVAR; however, a unique complication of this therapy is the development of ACS. Several institutional centers have reported on the successful results of this approach and it is hoped that this review will provide some guidance in establishing a system applicable to the reader's site.

REFERENCES

1. Dardik A, Burleyson GP, Bowman H, et al. Surgical repair of ruptured abdominal aortic aneurysms in the state of Maryland: factors influencing outcome among 527 recent cases. J Vasc Surg 1998;28:413–20; discussion 420–1.
2. Bown MJ, Sutton AJ, Bell PR, Sayers RD. A meta-analysis of 50 years of ruptured abdominal aortic aneurysm repair. Br J Surg 2002;89:714–30.
3. Darling RC 3rd, Cordero JA Jr, Chang BB, et al. Advances in the surgical repair of ruptured abdominal aortic aneurysms. Cardiovasc Surg 1996;4:720–3.
4. Gloviczki P, Pairolero PC, Mucha P Jr, et al. Ruptured abdominal aortic aneurysms: repair should not be denied. J Vasc Surg 1992;15:851–57; discussion 857–9.
5. Bown MJ, Nicholson ML, Bell PR, Sayers RD. The systemic inflammatory response syndrome, organ failure, and mortality after abdominal aortic aneurysm repair. J Vasc Surg 2003;37:600–6.
6. Hinchliffe RJ, Braithwaite BD, Hopkinson BR. The endovascular management of ruptured abdominal aortic aneurysms. Eur J Vasc Endovasc Surg 2003;25:191–201.
7. Yusuf SW, Whitaker SC, Chuter TA, Wenham PW, Hopkinson BR. Emergency endovascular repair of leaking aortic aneurysm. Lancet 1994;344:1645.
8. Ohki T, Veith FJ. Endovascular grafts and other image-guided catheter-based adjuncts to improve the treatment of ruptured aortoiliac aneurysms. Ann Surg 2000;232:466–79.
9. Veith FJ, Ohki T. Endovascular approaches to ruptured infrarenal aortoiliac aneurysms. J Cardiovasc Surg (Torino) 2002;43:369–78.
10. Hinchliffe RJ, Yusuf SW, Macierewicz JA, et al. Endovascular repair of ruptured abdominal aortic aneurysm—a challenge to open repair? Results of a single centre experience in 20 patients. Eur J Vasc Endovasc Surg 2001;22:528–34.
11. Mehta M, Darling RC 3rd, Roddy SP, et al. Factors associated with abdominal compartment syndrome complicating endovascular repair of ruptured abdominal aortic aneurysms. J Vasc Surg 2005;42:1047–51.
12. Scharrer-Pamler R, Kotsis T, Kapfer X, et al. Endovascular stent grafts repair of ruptured aortic aneurysms. J Endovasc Ther 2003;10:447–52.
13. Kapma MR, Verhoeven EL, Tielliu IF, et al. Endovascular treatment of acute abdominal aortic aneurysm with a bifurcated stentgraft. Eur J Vasc Endovasc Surg 2005;29:510–5.
14. Reichart M, Geelkerken RH, Huisman AB, et al. Ruptured abdominal aortic aneurysm: endovascular repair is feasible in 40% of patients. Eur J Vasc Endovasc Surg 2003;26:479–86.
15. Peppelenbosch N, Yilmaz N, van Marrewijk C, et al. Emergency treatment of acute symptomatic or ruptured abdominal aortic aneurysm. Outcome of a prospective intent-to-treat by EVAR protocol. Eur J Vasc Endovasc Surg 2003;26:303–10.

16. Resch T, Malina M, Lindblad B, et al. Endovascular repair of ruptured abdominal aortic aneurysms: logistics and short-term results. J Endovasc Ther 2003;10:440–6.
17. Lee WA, Hirneise CM, Tayyarah M, et al. Impact of endovascular repair on early outcomes of ruptured abdominal aortic aneurysms. J Vasc Surg 2004;40:211–5.
18. Shuman WP, Hastrup W Jr, Kohler TR, et al. Suspected leaking abdominal aortic aneurysm: use of sonography in the emergency room. Radiology 1988;168:117–9.
19. Bradbury AW, Makhdoomi KR, Adam DJ, et al. Twelve-year experience of the management of ruptured abdominal aortic aneurysm. Br J Surg 1997;84:1705–7.
20. Peppelenbosch N, Geelkerken RH, Soong C, et al. Endograft treatment of ruptured abdominal aortic aneurysms using the Talent aortouniiliac system: an international multicenter study. J Vasc Surg 2006;43:1111–23; discussion 1123.
21. von Segesser LK, Marty B, Ruchat P, et al. Routine use of intravascular ultrasound for endovascular aneurysm repair: angiography is not necessary. Eur J Vasc Endovasc Surg 2002;23:537–42.
22. Alsac JM, Desgranges P, Kobeiter H, Becquemin JP. Emergency endovascular repair for ruptured abdominal aortic aneurysms: feasibility and comparison of early results with conventional open repair. Eur J Vasc Endovasc Surg 2005;30:632–9.
23. Hinchliffe RJ, Hopkinson BR. Ruptured abdominal aortic aneurysm. Time for a new approach. J Cardiovasc Surg (Torino) 2002;43:345–7.
24. Lloyd GM, Bown MJ, Norwood MG, et al. Feasibility of preoperative computer tomography in patients with ruptured abdominal aortic aneurysm: a time-to-death study in patients without operation. J Vasc Surg 2004;39:788–91.
25. Boyle JR, Gibbs PJ, Kruger A, et al. Existing delays following the presentation of ruptured abdominal aortic aneurysm allow sufficient time to assess patients for endovascular repair. Eur J Vasc Endovasc Surg 2005;29:505–9.
26. Lawrie GM, Morris GC Jr, Crawford ES, et al. Improved results of operation for ruptured abdominal aortic aneurysms. Surgery 1979;85:483–8.
27. Crawford ES. Ruptured abdominal aortic aneurysm. J Vasc Surg 1991;13:348–50.
28. Greenberg RK, Srivastava SD, Ouriel K, et al. An endoluminal method of hemorrhage control and repair of ruptured abdominal aortic aneurysms. J Endovasc Ther 2000;7:1–7.
29. Malina M, Veith F, Ivancev K, Sonesson B. Balloon occlusion of the aorta during endovascular repair of ruptured abdominal aortic aneurysm. J Endovasc Ther 2005;12:556–9.
30. Van Herzeele I, Vermassen F, Durieux C, et al. Endovascular repair of aortic rupture. Eur J Vasc Endovasc Surg 2003;26:311–6.
31. Lombardi JV, Fairman RM, Golden MA, et al. The utility of commercially available endografts in the treatment of contained ruptured abdominal aortic aneurysm with hemodynamic stability. J Vasc Surg 2004;40:154–60.
32. Rose DF, Davidson IR, Hinchliffe RJ, et al. Anatomical suitability of ruptured abdominal aortic aneurysms for endovascular repair. J Endovasc Ther 2003;10:453–7.
33. van Sambeek MR, van Dijk LC, Hendriks JM, et al. Endovascular versus conventional open repair of acute abdominal aortic aneurysm: feasibility and preliminary results. J Endovasc Ther 2002;9:443–8.
34. Hechelhammer L, Lachat ML, Wildermuth S, et al. Midterm outcome of endovascular repair of ruptured abdominal aortic aneurysms. J Vasc Surg 2005;41:752–7.
35. Veith FJ, Ohki T, Lipsitz EC, et al. Treatment of ruptured abdominal aneurysms with stent grafts: a new gold standard? Semin Vasc Surg 2003;16:171–5.
36. Gerassimidis TS, Papazoglou KO, Kamparoudis AG, et al. Endovascular management of ruptured abdominal aortic aneurysms: 6-year experience from a Greek center. J Vasc Surg 2005;42:615–23; discussion 623.
37. Bettex DA, Lachat M, Pfammatter T, et al. To compare general, epidural and local anaesthesia for endovascular aneurysm repair (EVAR). Eur J Vasc Endovasc Surg 2001;21:179–84.
38. Henretta JP, Hodgson KJ, Mattos MA, et al. Feasibility of endovascular repair of abdominal aortic aneurysms with local anesthesia with intravenous sedation. J Vasc Surg 1999;29: 793–8.

39. Lachat ML, Pfammatter T, Witzke HJ, et al. Endovascular repair with bifurcated stent grafts under local anaesthesia to improve outcome of ruptured aortoiliac aneurysms. Eur J Vasc Endovasc Surg 2002;23:528–36.
40. Schonholz C, Donnini F, Naselli G, et al. Acute rupture of an aortic false aneurysm treated with a stent grafts. J Endovasc Surg 1999;6:293–6.
41. Franks S, Lloyd G, Fishwick G, et al. Endovascular treatment of ruptured and symptomatic abdominal aortic aneurysms. Eur J Vasc Endovasc Surg 2006;31:345–50.
42. Najjar SF, Mueller KH, Ujiki MB, et al. Percutaneous endovascular repair of ruptured abdominal aortic aneurysms. Arch Surg 2007;142:1049–52.
43. O'Donnell ME, Badger SA, Makar RR, et al. Techniques in occluding the aorta during endovascular repair of ruptured abdominal aortic aneurysms. J Vasc Surg 2006;44:211–5.
44. Zarins CK, White RA, Schwarten D, et al. AneuRx stent grafts versus open surgical repair of abdominal aortic aneurysms: multicenter prospective clinical trial. J Vasc Surg 1999;29: 292–305; discussion 306–8.
45. Gawenda M, Heckenkamp J, Zaehringer M, Brunkwall J. Intra-aneurysm sac pressure—the holy grail of endoluminal grafting of AAA. Eur J Vasc Endovasc Surg 2002;24:139–45.
46. Armon MP, Yusuf SW, Latief K, et al. Anatomical suitability of abdominal aortic aneurysms for endovascular repair. Br J Surg 1997;84:178–80.
47. Moore WS, Brewster DC, Bernhard VM. Aorto-uni-iliac endograft for complex aortoiliac aneurysms compared with tube/bifurcation endografts: results of the EVT/Guidant trials. J Vasc Surg 2001;33:S11–20.
48. Forbes TL, DeRose G, Kribs SW, Harris KA. Cumulative sum failure analysis of the learning curve with endovascular abdominal aortic aneurysm repair. J Vasc Surg 2004;39:102–8.
49. Chuter TA, Faruqi RM, Reilly LM, et al. Aortomonoiliac endovascular grafting combined with femorofemoral bypass: an acceptable compromise or a preferred solution? Semin Vasc Surg 1999;12:176–81.
50. Brandt M, Walluscheck KP, Jahnke T, et al. Endovascular repair of ruptured abdominal aortic aneurysm: feasibility and impact on early outcome. J Vasc Interv Radiol 2005;16: 1309–12.
51. Walker SR, Braithwaite B, Tennant WG, et al. Early complications of femorofemoral crossover bypass grafts after aorta uni-iliac endovascular repair of abdominal aortic aneurysms. J Vasc Surg 1998;28:647–50.
52. Peppelenbosch N, Cuypers PW, Vahl AC, et al. Emergency endovascular treatment for ruptured abdominal aortic aneurysm and the risk of spinal cord ischemia. J Vasc Surg 2005;42:608–14.
53. Orend KH, Kotsis T, Scharrer-Pamler R, et al. Endovascular repair of aortic rupture due to trauma and aneurysm. Eur J Vasc Endovasc Surg 2002;23:61–7.
54. Mehta M. TJ, Spirig A., Sternbach Y., et al. EVAR Treatment of ruptured AAAs and TAAs. Endovasc Today 2007; 2007:5.
55. Dias NV, Resch T, Malina M, et al. Intraoperative proximal endoleaks during AAA stent grafts repair: evaluation of risk factors and treatment with Palmaz stents. J Endovasc Ther Jun 2001;8:268–73.
56. Greco G, Egorova N, Anderson PL, et al. Outcomes of endovascular treatment of ruptured abdominal aortic aneurysms. J Vasc Surg 2006;43:453–9.
57. Visser JJ, Bosch JL, Hunink MG, et al. Endovascular repair versus open surgery in patients with ruptured abdominal aortic aneurysms: clinical outcomes with 1-year follow-up. J Vasc Surg 2006;44:1148–55.
58. Vaddineni SK, Russo GC, Patterson MA, et al. Ruptured abdominal aortic aneurysm: a retrospective assessment of open versus endovascular repair. Ann Vasc Surg 2005;19: 782–6.
59. Yilmaz N, Peppelenbosch N, Cuypers PW, et al. Emergency treatment of symptomatic or ruptured abdominal aortic aneurysms: the role of endovascular repair. J Endovasc Ther 2002;9:449–57.

60. Kron IL, Harman PK, Nolan SP. The measurement of intra-abdominal pressure as a criterion for abdominal re-exploration. Ann Surg 1984;199:28–30.
61. Loftus IM, Thompson MM. The abdominal compartment syndrome following aortic surgery. Eur J Vasc Endovasc Surg 2003;25:97–109.
62. Ivatury RR, Diebel L, Porter JM, Simon RJ. Intra-abdominal hypertension and the abdominal compartment syndrome. Surg Clin North Am 1997;77:783–800.
63. van Marrewijk C, Buth J, Harris PL, et al. Significance of endoleaks after endovascular repair of abdominal aortic aneurysms: the EUROSTAR experience. J Vasc Surg 2002;35: 461–73.
64. Johnston KW. Ruptured abdominal aortic aneurysm: six-year follow-up results of a multicenter prospective study. Canadian Society for Vascular Surgery Aneurysm Study Group. J Vasc Surg 1994;19:888–900.
65. Noel AA, Gloviczki P, Cherry KJ Jr, et al. Ruptured abdominal aortic aneurysms: the excessive mortality rate of conventional repair. J Vasc Surg 2001;34:41–6.
66. Hans SS, Huang RR. Results of 101 ruptured abdominal aortic aneurysm repairs from a single surgical practice. Arch Surg 2003;138:898–901.
67. Mehta M, Veith FJ, Ohki T, et al. Unilateral and bilateral hypogastric artery interruption during aortoiliac aneurysm repair in 154 patients: a relatively innocuous procedure. J Vasc Surg 2001;33:S27–32.
68. Wolpert LM, Dittrich KP, Hallisey MJ, et al. Hypogastric artery embolization in endovascular abdominal aortic aneurysm repair. J Vasc Surg 2001;33:1193–8.
69. Barratt J, Parajasingam R, Sayers RD, Feehally J. Outcome of acute renal failure following surgical repair of ruptured abdominal aortic aneurysms. Eur J Vasc Endovasc Surg 2000; 20:163–8.
70. Yusuf SW, Whitaker SC, Hinwood D, et al. Carbon dioxide: an alternative to iodinated contrast media. Eur J Vasc Endovasc Surg 1995;10:156–61.

60. Kron IL, Harman PK, Nolan SP. The measurement of intra-abdominal pressure as a criterion for abdominal re-exploration. Ann Surg 1984;199:28–30.
61. Loftus IM, Thompson MM. The abdominal compartment syndrome following aortic surgery. Eur J Vasc Endovasc Surg 2003;25:97–109.
62. Ivatury RR, Diebel L, Porter JM, Simon RJ. Intra-abdominal hypertension and the abdominal compartment syndrome. Surg Clin North Am 1997;77:783–800.
63. van Marrewijk C, Buth J, Harris PL, et al. Significance of endoleaks after endovascular repair of abdominal aortic aneurysms: the EUROSTAR experience. J Vasc Surg 2002;35:461–73.
64. Johnston KW. Ruptured abdominal aortic aneurysm: six-year follow-up results of a multicenter prospective study. Canadian Society for Vascular Surgery Aneurysm Study Group. J Vasc Surg 1994;19:888–900.
65. Noel AA, Gloviczki P, Cherry KJ Jr, et al. Ruptured abdominal aortic aneurysms: the excessive mortality rate of conventional repair. J Vasc Surg 2001;34:41–6.
66. Hans SS, Huang RR. Results of 101 ruptured abdominal aortic aneurysm repairs from a single surgical practice. Arch Surg 2003;138:898–901.
67. Mehta M, Veith FJ, Ohki T, et al. Unilateral and bilateral hypogastric artery interruption during aortoiliac aneurysm repair in 154 patients: a relatively innocuous procedure. J Vasc Surg 2001;33:S27–32.
68. Wolpert LM, Dittrich KP, Hallisey MJ, et al. Hypogastric artery embolization in endovascular abdominal aortic aneurysm repair. J Vasc Surg 2001;33:1193–8.
69. Barratt J, Parajasingam R, Sayers RD, Feehally J. Outcome of acute renal failure following surgical repair of ruptured abdominal aortic aneurysms. Eur J Vasc Endovasc Surg 2000;20:163–8.
70. Yusuf SW, Whitaker SC, Hinwood D, et al. Carbon dioxide: an alternative to iodinated contrast medium. Eur J Vasc Endovasc Surg 1995;10:156–61.

54

Sac Pressure Measurement after Endovascular Aortic Aneurysm Repair

Colin M. Brady, M.D. and Ross Milner, M.D.

INTRODUCTION

Since the publication of the initial reports of the first endovascular repair of an abdominal aortic aneurysm (AAA) by Parodi et al. in 1991, endovascular aortic aneurysm repair (EVAR) has rapidly gained momentum as a viable alternative to open surgical intervention.[1] In its infancy, academicians utilized this minimally invasive modality primarily in the setting of those patients with significant medical comorbidities, which made the risks of conventional open repair prohibitive. In the intervening 2 decades, however, EVAR has enjoyed almost unparalleled success among novel surgical procedures, as conclusive evidence of its early efficacy in the minimization of periprocedural morbidity and potential mortality has been prolific. Encouraged by these reports, the vascular community at large has begun to utilize this modality in a broader patient population, including the young and those of adequate health status who would otherwise be candidates for traditional open repair. Despite relatively untainted early success, midterm analysis has brought to light a relevant incidence of modality-specific complications, including device failure, endoleaks, and endoluminal procedural limitations. With a 10% reintervention rate at a mean interval of 25.5 months from primary EVAR procedure out of a high-volume academic center, the need for safe and effective long-term surveillance modalities has never been clearer.[2]

SURVEILLANCE: THE GOLD STANDARD

The primary purpose of all AAA treatment modalities is the reduction of pressure within the aneurysm sac and the prevention of potentially fatal complications, such as aneurysm rupture. Total exclusion allows complete depressurization, whereas partial or inadequate sac exclusion results in exposure to persistent pressurization that can be as high as systemic pressure.[3-4] Given the potential mortality associated with incomplete exclusion, it is vital for the practitioner to have the means by which to evaluate procedural success in the intra-, peri-, and postoperative settings.

Currently, the gold standard for the evaluation of sac pressurization and efficacy of exclusion in the intraoperative setting is conventional angiography. In the peri- and postoperative settings, the standard is computed tomographic angiography (CTA). Current practice guidelines dictate that follow-up imaging after EVAR occurs at 1, 6, and 12 months for the first year and annually thereafter, assuming no interval symptoms or patient concerns. Although adjunct imaging modalities such as plain film radiography and conventional duplex ultrasonography have been employed to aid in the detection and characterization of endoleaks, postprocedural sac dimensions, and device placement, none has proven superior to CTA as a surveillance technology. The risks and limitations inherent in frequent use of this modality have been well-characterized and include (1) radiation exposure, (2) nephrotoxicity associated with iodinated contrast agents, (3) patient noncompliance, (4) potential inaccuracy, and (5) appreciable expense, with a recent study showing that >65% of postoperative EVAR follow-up costs are secondary to CT surveillance.[5] Attempts have been made to limit the contrast-associated nephrotoxicity associated with CTA by employing magnetic resonance angiography (MRA); however, with the recent press surrounding gadolinium-associated nephrogenic systemic fibrosis, the use of this modality has also been limited in the setting of acute or chronic renal insufficiency. To expand alternatives, investigators sought to further circumvent the limitations of CTA by exploring the surveillance sensitivities of duplex ultrasonography and its variants. Initial surveillance efforts in this realm centered on color duplex ultrasound, which disappointingly, revealed a lower sensitivity and positive predictive value in detecting postprocedural endoleaks when compared with CTA.[6] More recently, some early success has been reported with the use of non-nephrotoxic ultrasound contrast agents, which improve sensitivity by allowing improved blood flow echogenicity during duplex evaluation. This modality is referred to as contrast-enhanced ultrasound (CEUS), and in one study was even shown to characterize several endoleaks not identified on CTA.[7] Alhough the sensitivity of CEUS is inherently operator-dependent, this strategy could represent a plausible alternative to CTA while simultaneously improving patient compliance, obviating nephrotoxicity, and reducing follow-up costs. Table 54–1 compares and contrasts these primary and adjunctive periprocedural imaging modalities. With limited long-term data, however, the need for safe, effective, and economically feasible alternatives for endograft surveillance has never been greater.

REMOTE PRESSURE SENSORS: A POTENTIAL ANSWER TO THE CALL?

As previously emphasized, the ideal surveillance modality would be noninvasive, nontoxic, sensitive, and cost-effective while not requiring extensive training or expertise to obtain clinically useful information. A new wave of surveillance technology is remote pressure sensing—a technology that utilizes wireless sensors that are implanted into the excluded aneurysm sac at the time of endograft placement in order to obtain intrasac pressure measurements both intraoperatively and beyond.

How do pressure sensors answer the call as an effective surveillance measure? Complications following EVAR, whether via device failure, migration, or endoleak, all manifest a common feature: elevated pressures within the residual aneurysm sac. As

TABLE 54-1. COMPARISON OF CURRENT SURVEILLANCE MODALITIES

	CTA/MRA	CEUS7	Remote Pressure Sensing
Imaging Location	Hospital	Hospital	Office or home
Contrast Agents	Yes	Yes	No
Parameters Measured			
Aneurysm Diameter	Yes	Yes	No
Aneurysm Volume	Yes	Yes	No
Presence of Contrast	Yes	Yes	No
Mean Pressure	No	Yes	Yes
Pulsatility of Flow	No	Yes	Yes
Sensitivity	Moderate	High	High
Frequency	1-2/annum	1-2/annum	Flexible/PRN (hourly - monthly)
Risks and Limitations	1. Radiation exposure 2. Contrast-induced nephrotoxicity 3. Patient noncompliance 4. Expense	Operator-dependent	Risks: None Limitations: Lacks ability to measure change in diameter or volume

previously alluded to, the goal of EVAR is adequate sac exclusion. Incomplete or partial exclusion results in exposure of the sac to systemic pressures, placing the sac at risk of dilation and rupture. To this end, Sonesson et al. developed an experimental model in order to elucidate the association of significantly reduced sac pressures with successful exclusion of the sac following EVAR. The investigators performed direct translumbar puncture and resulting catheter pressure transduction after EVAR in patients who manifested sac shrinkage and had no evidence of endoleak. In this series, mean intrasac pressure was shown to diminish to 20% of mean arterial pressure. In patients with an endoleak, intrasac pressures were measured either by a similar translumbar approach or via cannulation of a patent superior or inferior mesenteric artery. In the presence of an endoleak, intrasac measurements were uniformly consistent with elevated and pulsatile sac pressures.[8] These findings provide fundamental proof of the concept supporting the utility of remote pressure sensors in confirming adequate sac exclusion in the acute intraoperative setting as well as lending credence to their use as a sensitive, noninvasive, nontoxic, and economically feasible modality for long-term surveillance after EVAR.

REMOTE PRESSURE SENSORS: THE NUTS AND BOLTS

The following discussion evaluates the two devices that have been utilized for the detection of intrasac pressures following aneurysm exclusion after EVAR.

Impressure Sensor. The first of the two devices is termed the Impressure AAA Sac Pressure Transducer (Remon Medical) and measures 3 mm x 9 mm x 1.5 mm in dimension (Figure 54–1). The device is constituted by a piezoelectric crystal that charges a capacitor

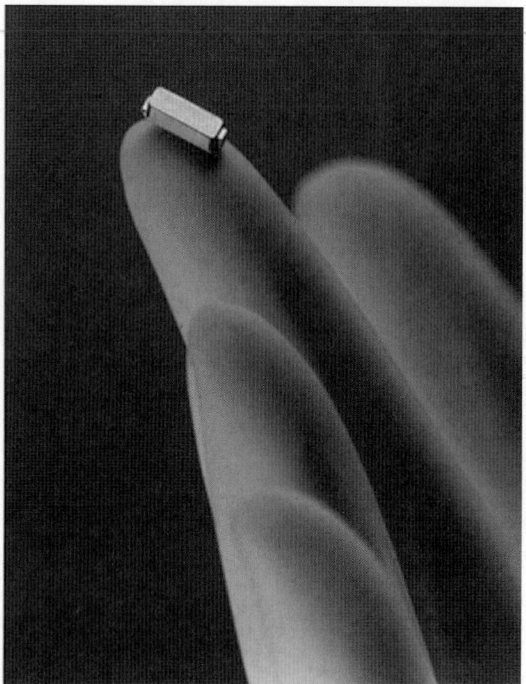

Figure 54-1. Impressure abdominal aortic aneurysm (AAA) sac pressure transducer (Remon Medical Tecnologies.)

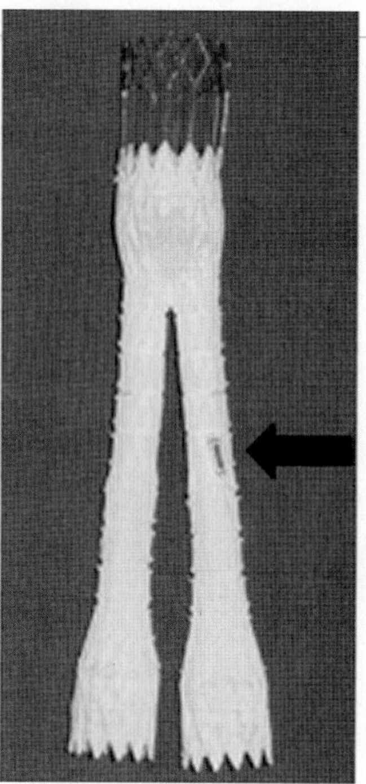

Figure 54-2. Impressure transducer sewn to contralateral limb of bifurcated endoprosthetic. The sensor is highlighted by the black arrow.

when actuated by a hand-held probe emitting ultrasonic waves. Once charged, ambient pressure measurements are obtained and the data are converted in a retrograde fashion from an electrical to an ultrasonic signal that is relayed to the probe. The pressure parameters are displayed on a monitor and can be downloaded and exported as a spreadsheet for documentation and further analysis. The sensor is hand-sewn to the stent graft device (Figure 54–2). In those receiving an aortouni-iliac device, the transducer is sewn 6 cm below the attachment system and then repacked in the delivery system. In the bifurcated variety, conversely, the device is sewn to the contralateral limb immediately below its exit from the main body gate before final packaging in the delivery system. It should be noted that the delivery sheath must be upsized to 20-Fr from its original 18-Fr diameter as a result of the presence of the pressure sensor.[9]

In 2004, Milner et al. performed in vivo pilot studies with the Impressure Transducer in a porcine experimental model. AAAs were surgically induced and excluded in an endovascular fashion and followed by intrasac implantation of the sensor. Pressure measurements were taken as described above, utilizing an external ultrasound probe, and results were compared with those of standard invasive catheter measurements. To evaluate the sensitivity of the device for detection of endoleaks, they allowed for an experimental design in which type II and III endoleaks were iatrogenically introduced. As expected, in the presence of an endoleak, the intrasac pressure increased accordingly, and transcutaneous measurements from the device were observed to correlate well with elevated invasive intrasac catheter readings.[10]

In the same year, Ellozy and associates published results of the first human experience with the Impressure device in a series of 14 patients with a mean follow-up of 2.6 months. Only a single case of nonfunction occurred at 2 months follow-up. Complete sac exclusion was confirmed intraoperatively by angiography and in follow-up by CTA. The investigators showed that in the presence of complete sac exclusion, there was (1) a significant difference in systemic and sac pressures postexclusion intraoperatively and at 1 month follow-up, (2) the ratio of systemic to sac pressures continued to increase over time, and (3) that sac pressures fell to ≤40 mm Hg by 3 months in four of six patients without angiographic evidence of endoleak. The authors attributed the persistently elevated surveillance pressure readings in the remaining two patients without endoleaks to endotension, a theoretical concept that is not well understood and is highly debated. In the setting of a type I endoleak at the time of initial endograft placement, the patient's transcutaneous sac pressures correlated with intrasac catheter readings, and following extension cuff repair, the pressures diminished appropriately. Three patients had angiographic evidence of type II endoleaks. Their intrasac pressures decreased over time, but not to the extent as in those patients without endoleaks. Alhough the series was small, reflecting the limited statistical power of the study, the investigators concluded that noninvasive sac pressure transduction with the Impressure device is a feasible and correlative alternative to CTA.[9] Further studies by the group attempted to further elaborate on two clinically significant relationships: (1) endoleak versus sac pressure, and (2) changes in sac dimension versus sac pressure. The investigators found that the interval between device deployment and surveillance measurement can influence the specificity of the transducer to detect angiographically evident endoleaks. In a series of 21 patients published in 2006, the presence or absence of endoleak could not be predicted by sac pressure at 1 month. With respect to sac pressures as they relate to changes in sac diameter, the authors reported that those aneurysms that continue to shrink following exclusion are associated with a greater diminution of intrasac pressures.[11] What is clear, regardless, is that further investigative efforts are required to elucidate the relationship of endoleak to sac pressure and, by extension, provide evidence to support the sufficiency of the Impressure transducer as both an acute and a chronically feasible surveillance modality.

Endosure Sensor

The second device is termed the CardioMems Endosure Wireless AAA Pressure Sensor (CardioMems, Inc., Atlanta, GA). The device is a 30 mm x 5 mm x 1.5 mm externally powered sensor that has a nitinol construct surrounding its electronic constituents (Figure 54–3). Preclinical longitudinal in vivo studies have touted the device's stability and functional accuracy over several years. The sensor consists of a hermetically sealed reference cavity surrounding a network of flexible plates bearing inductor windings. The plates are displaced in response to a change in ambient pressure, resulting in a shift of the device's capacitance and resonant frequency. Alterations in the resonant frequency are monitored via antenna, and the pressure measurements are output to an external monitor in real time, both numerically and graphically. In contrast to the Impressure device, the CardioMems sensor is placed in the aneurysm sac via its own 14-Fr delivery device (Figure 54–4). This device has already received U.S. Food and Drug Administration (FDA)-clearance for use in evaluating the efficacy of acute aneurysm exclusion following endograft deployment. However, further investigation is necessary before the device can be approved for use as a chronic surveillance measure.

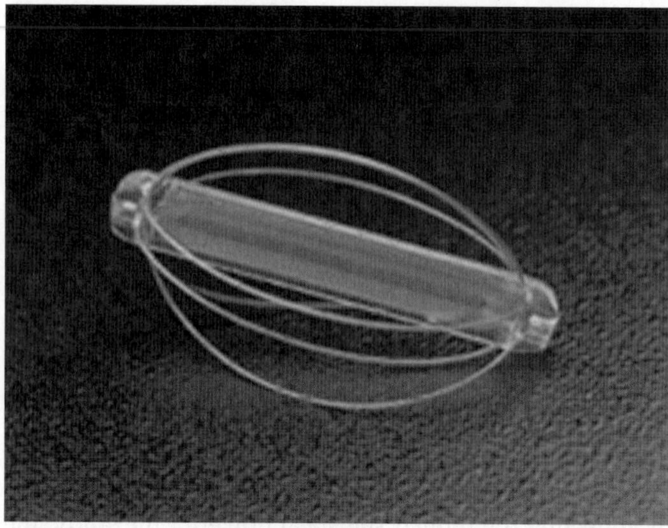

Figure 54-3. U.S. Food and Drug Administration (FDA)-approved CadioMems EndoSure Wireless AAA Pressure Sensor.

Recent FDA approval of the Endosure sensor as a short-term surveillance modality can in large measure be attributed to the 2007 publication of The APEX Trial—Acute Pressure Measurement to Confirm Aneurysm Sac Exclusion. The large multicenter prospective trial enrolled 90 patients over 12 sites, 76 of whom were available for analysis. Sac pulse pressures after the deployment of the main body but prior to deployment of the contralateral limb were simultaneously measured via catheter angiography and the CardioMems device. The timing of the initial pressure readings reflects the flow dynamics that would be seen in the sac in the presence of a type I endoleak. The pulse pressures were again recorded via both methods after completion of EVAR to evaluate sac exclusion. The authors reported the following findings: (1) excellent correlation between angiography and the Endosure sensor in all per-protocol patients at the time of type I endoleak equivalent, (2) 92.1% agreement between modalities in the determination of the presence or absence of type I and type III endoleaks at the completion of

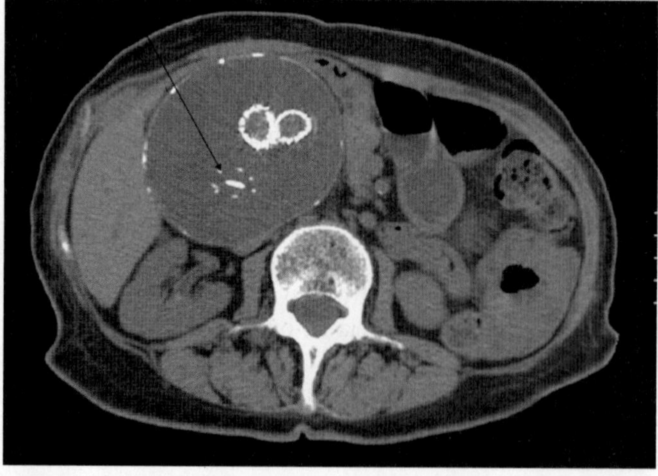

Figure 54-4. Computed tomographic image illustrating the EndoSure device within the excluded aneurysm sac. The black arrow highlights the sensor sitting within the mural thrombus independent from the two limbs of the endoprosthetic. The nitinol basket is easily visualized and demarcates the circumferential extent of the sensor.

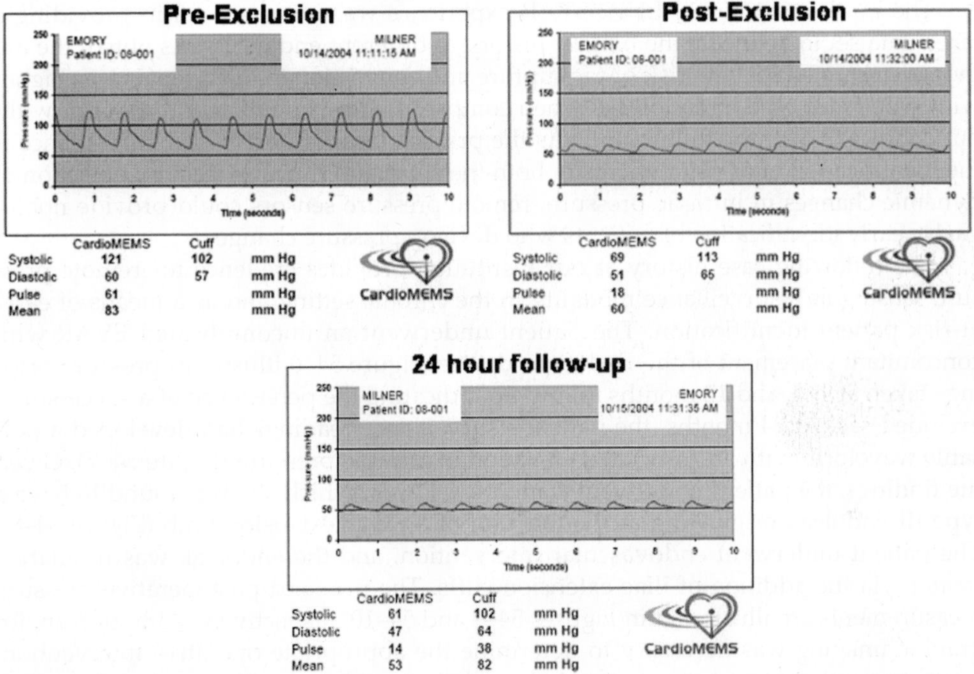

Figure 54-5. Perioperative pressure readings from the CarioMems EndoSure device at our institution. The intrasac pulse pressures can be seen to reduce appropriately following sac exclusion with an absolute decrement of 43 mm Hg. At 24 hours post-EVAR, the pulse pressure was 14 mm Hg, illustrating the persistence of an adequately excluded sac.

EVAR, and (3) in the presence of intraoperative type I and III endoleaks, intrasac pressure readings appropriately diminished in real time with interventional resolution of the endoleak.[12] The perioperative pressure measurements in a patient treated at our institution as part of the APEX trial are shown in Figure 54–5.

REMOTE PRESSURE SENSING AND THE QUESTION OF ENDOLEAKS

To reiterate, the goal of AAA repair, and specifically EVAR, is complete aneurysm sac exclusion from the systemic circulation. Endoleak is the most frequent phenomenon threatening successful exclusion and has the potential to occur at any and all junctures from the time of device placement through the life of the repair. Several authors have reported a statistic of 20% for the incidence of endoleak after EVAR. Because clinical management of the endoleak is type-specific, determination of not only the presence but also the type of endoleak is of clinical relevance. The accepted classification scheme discriminates endoleaks with respect to the origin of flow into the aneurysm sac. Flow into the sac from the proximal and distal ends of the endograft is termed type I. Flow via a branched artery is termed type II. Flow due to endoprosthetic leaks from the midgraft via fabric defects or seal failure at constituent element junctions is a type III leak. Though each type can potentially be clinically relevant, types I and III carry with them the most significant risk of potentially fatal sac rupture due to the development of systemic pressure.[13]

The multi-institutional EUROSTAR experience was instrumental in providing a large data set to delineate the natural history of different endoleaks. As noted, the authors determined that the risk of sac rupture and conversion to open repair was higher with type I and type III endoleaks when compared with patients with type II or without endoleaks over the follow-up.[13] As the primary goal of post-EVAR surveillance is the identification of at-risk patients in both the short and the long term by detection of dynamic changes in intrasac pressure, remote pressure sensors could provide noninvasive early identification of patients who develop pressure changes.

The following case history at our institution provides credence for remote pressure sensing as a surveillance modality in the chronic setting and as a means of early at-risk patient identification. The patient underwent an uncomplicated EVAR with concomitant placement of the EndoSure device. Figure 54–6 illustrates pressure readings taken at 1, 6, and 12 months follow-up indicating the persistence of a successfully excluded sac. At 24 months, the patient's surveillance readings had developed a pulsatile waveform with an associated elevation in intrasac pressure (Figure 54–7). Given the findings, the patient underwent standard CTA, on which she was found to have a type III endoleak originating at the junction of an iliac extension limb (Figure 54–8). The patient underwent endovascular intervention, and the endoleak was ultimately treated via the addition of iliac extension cuffs. The pre- and postoperative pressure measurements are illustrated in Figures 54–9 and 54–10, respectively. Although angiographic imaging was necessary to determine the appropriate operative intervention, pressure sensing alone served as an adequate long-term surveillance modality, alerting the practitioner to the presence of an at-risk patient.

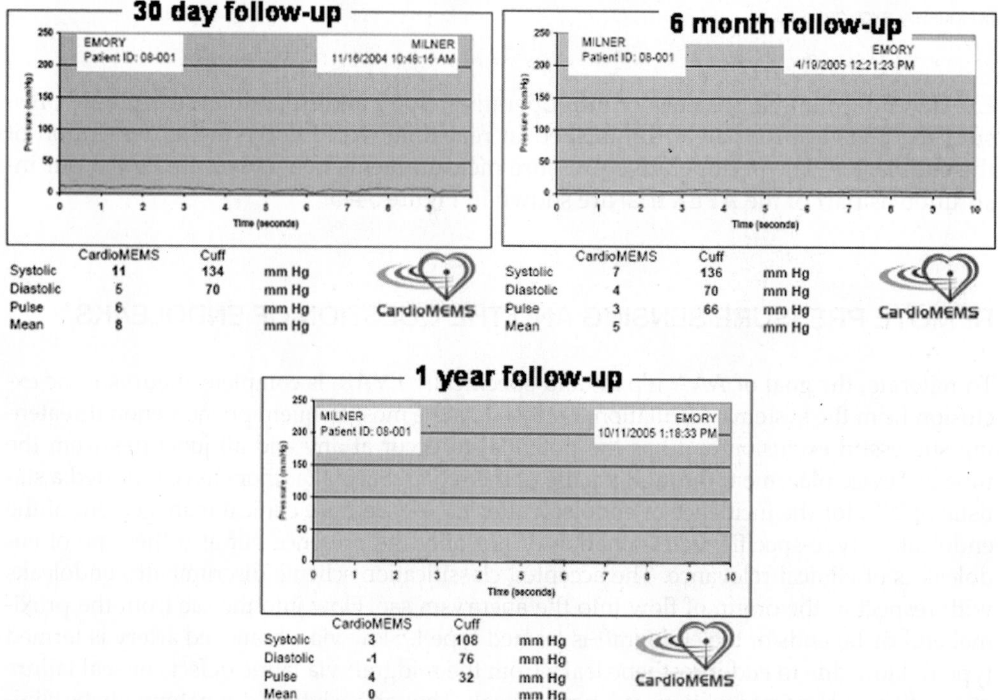

Figure 54-6. The patient's pulse pressure reading at 1, 6, and 12 months follow-up evidencing continued sac exclusion by a flat-line tracing and a pulse pressure of 6 mm Hg.

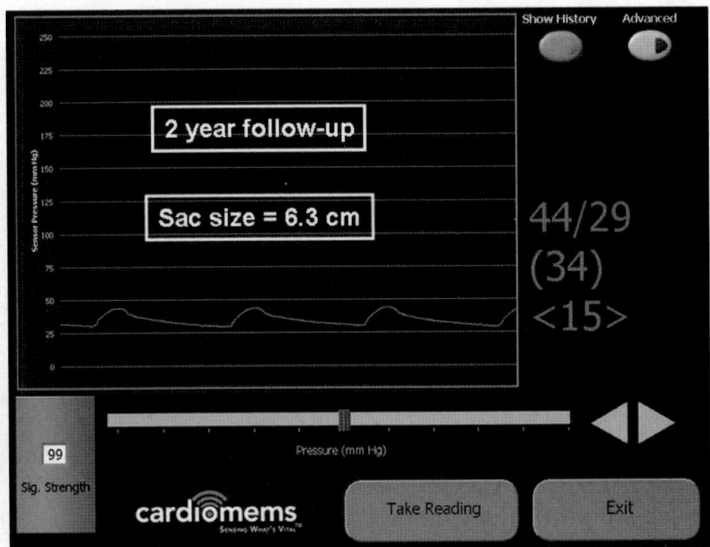

Figure 54-7. Surveillance measurements in the same patient at 24 months post-EVAR. One can appreciate the absolute elevation of intrasac pressure accompanied by a pulsatile waveform.

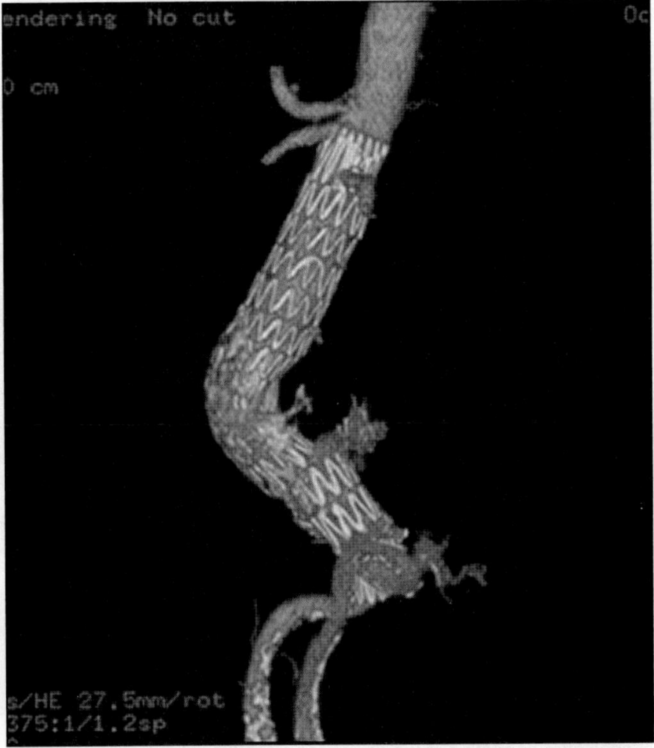

Figure 54-8. To elucidate the etiology of the pulsatile pressure readings, the patient underwent CTA shown here demonstrating a type III endoleak at the junction of the iliac extension limb.

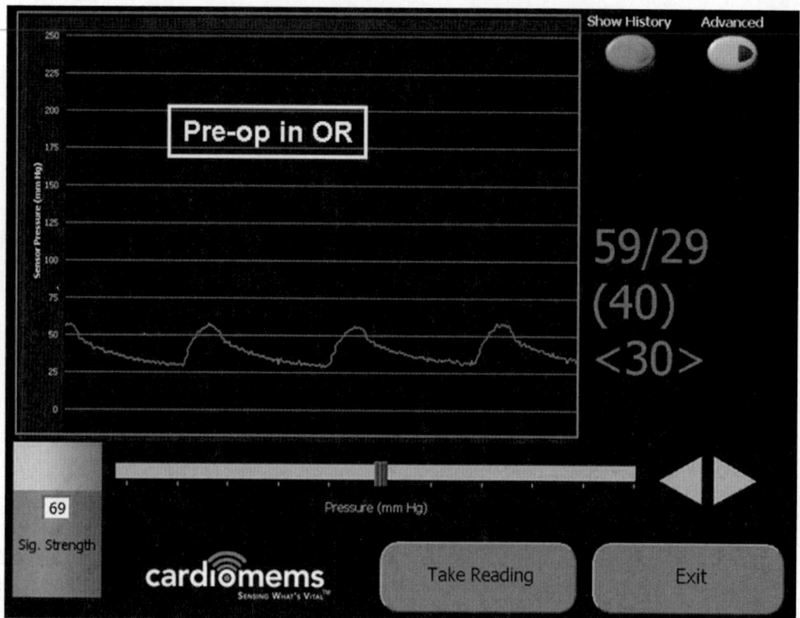

Figure 54-9. Intraoperative surveillance from the same patient prior to treatment of the confirmed type III endoleak. The pattern of elevated pulse pressure with a pulsatile waveform is again acknowledged.

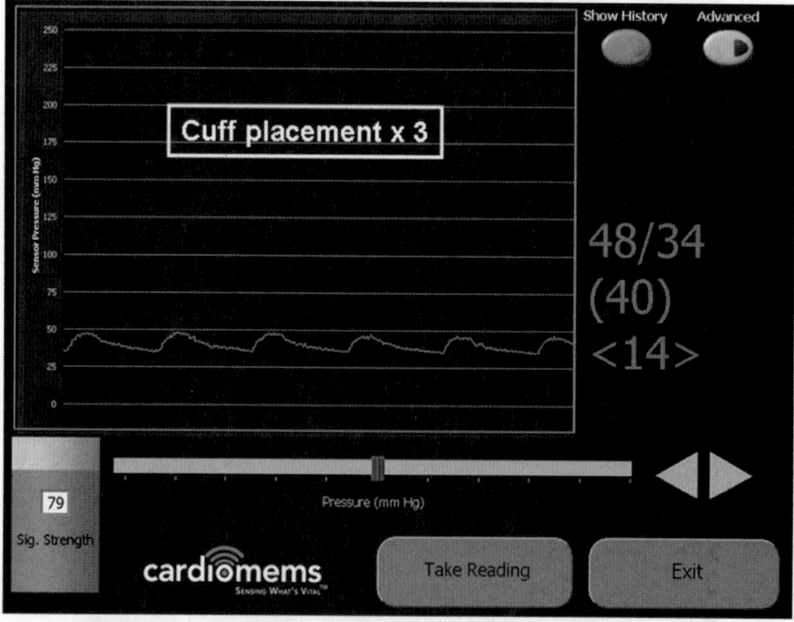

Figure 54-10. Surveillance after correction of the device failure by the addition of iliac extension limbs. Note that the pulse pressure has decreased by >50% and that pressure tracing reflects a dampened waveform indicating successful re-exclusion after repair.

As the risk of sac rupture is considerably smaller with type II endoleaks, the extent of their clinical relevance remains controversial. Chong et al.s used a computer-generated three-dimensional model of a real aneurysm to mathematically interpret the relationship between endoleak subset, flow rates, and intrasac pressures. In this model, when a type II endoleak was present, sac pressure was observed to be a function of inflow pressure.[14] Dias et al. corroborated these findings, noting that sac pressures in patients with type II endoleaks were dynamic entities.[15] The majority of intraoperative type II endoleaks spontaneously resolve secondary to the stasis-induced thrombosis of the aortic side branches. Although the extent of their clinical significance is not clear, it would be cavalier to assume that all type II endoleaks are benign entities. In a situation comparable with that of EVAR, severe symptoms and aneurysmal rupture predicating the need for a second surgical intervention have been reported in upward of 41% of individuals with retrograde collateral flow after conventional aortic exclusion without side branch ligation.[16] In part, it is the dynamic nature of type II endoleaks and their potential persistence or incidence during long-term follow-up that necessitate surveillance after EVAR in the chronic setting. In 2006, Gelfand et al. addressed the question of the clinical significance of type II endoleaks after EVAR.[17] This large, multi-institutional review reported the incidence of early and late endoleaks to be 6 to 17% and 1 to 8%, respectively. In 2617 patients, there were no incidents of type II-related ruptures. After reviewing the data from 10 separate trials, the authors emphasized the following guidelines for reintervention in the setting of type II endoleaks: (1) symptomatic or pulsatile sac, (2) persistence of endoleak >1 year, (3) aneurysmal sac pressure >20% of systolic pressure, or (4) sac enlargement >5 mm.[17] As a noninvasive surveillance modality, remote pressure sensing offers a feasible means by which to monitor the parameters set forth in treatment guidelines one through three.

REMOTE PRESSURE SENSING: THE LIMITATIONS

Despite promising preliminary results in a number of studies, the applicability of remote pressure sensing as a long-term self-sufficient surveillance tool has yet to be fully validated. To date, prospective trials have been limited by small sample sizes, lending less statistical power to the analysis. Furthermore, a number of questions have arisen during clinical trials of the pressure sensing devices. Will the sensors maintain long-term functional accuracy? Will the device migrate or will constituent parts degrade over time? How does the ability of the sensor to accurately record intrasac pressures change depending on (1) location within the sac, or (2) sac milieu (e.g., presence of thrombus)? Currently, limited data exist to adequately address the issue of sac compartmentalization raised in the last question. Experimental work by Pacanowski and associates demonstrated that in the excluded aneurysm laden with thrombus, the sac pressure reaches a maximum closest to the graft.[18] In their experience with the Impressure Transducer, Ellozy et al. observed in a single patient with type I endoleak that pressures obtained at the origin of the leak coincided with those obtained by the remote pressure transducer fixed to the device 7 cm away.[9] Further investigatory efforts will obviously be necessary to further elucidate this potentially significant issue.

In the setting of endoleaks, remote pressure sensing technology remains limited in terms of the experience in discriminating between pressure elevations caused by type I and type III endoleaks, which require more emergent intervention, and those, such as type II, that may be followed with conservative management. More clinical experience is necessary in order to better evaluate the pressure changes seen with type II endoleaks. It is clear that aneurysm sac behavior is different in the setting of a type II endoleak. More pressure sensing data are needed prior to determining the efficacy of pressure sensing concerning type II leaks. The PRICELESS trial by CardioMEMS is currently enrolling patients and will help answer this question.

Last, because the technology is currently still experimental as a chronic surveillance tool, device implantation at the time of EVAR is an additional expense that is covered by insurance companies, but with limited reimbursement. There is also limited reimbursement for surveillance with the sensor. The economic feasibility and cost-benefit ratios are thus yet to be determined for this modality.

CONCLUSION

With the rapid expansion of the indications for EVAR in recent years, the need for a safe, nontoxic, sensitive, and economically feasible long-term surveillance modality has never been more pressing. The current standard is CTA, which carries with it the significant limitations of radiation exposure, contrast-associated nephrotoxicity, and appreciable annual follow-up costs. The technology of remote pressure sensing has risen to the forefront in clinical trials as a promising alternative to angiographic imaging. Small clinical studies have proven the devices' ability to detect aneurysm sac pressures and endoleaks in the perioperative setting. Whether the devices will be consistently useful in the early detection of endoleaks and potential endoprosthetic migration and structural defects has yet to be determined. Furthermore, the devices offer a practical, noninvasive means for frequent pressure monitoring in the outpatient setting, leading to greater patient compliance with follow-up. If economically feasible, the technology inherently possesses the potential for portability, with patients recording and transmitting pressure readings to their physician without the need for frequent office visits. Highly anticipated prospective studies to determine the devices' utility as a primary surveillance tool in the long term are currently ongoing.

REFERENCES

1. Parodi JC, Palmaz JC, Barone HD. Transfemoral intraluminal graft implantation for abdominal aortic aneurysms. Ann Vasc Surg 1991;5:491–9.
2. Brewster DC, Jones JE, Chung TK, et al. Long-term outcomes after endovascular abdominal aortic aneurysm repair: the first decade. Ann Surg 2006;244:426–38.
3. Marston WA, Criado E, Baird CA, et al. Reduction of aneurysm pressure and wall stress after endovascular repair of abdominal aortic aneurysm in a canine model. Ann Vasc Surg 1996;10:166–73.
4. Sanchez LA, Faries PL, Marin ML, et al. Chronic intraaneurysmal pressure measurement: an experimental method for evaluating the effectiveness of endovascular aortic aneurysm exclusion. J Vasc Surg 1997;26:222–30.
5. Prinssen M, Wixon CL, Buskens E, et al. Surveillance after endovascular aneurysm repair: diagnostics, complications, and associated costs. Ann Vasc Surg 2004;18:421–7.
6. Raman KG, Missig-Carroll N, Richardson T, et al. Color-flow duplex ultrasound scan versus computed tomographic scan in the surveillance of endovascular aneurysm repair. J Vasc Surg 2003;38:645–51.

7. Henao EA, Hodge MD, Felkai DD, et al. Contrast-enhanced duplex surveillance after endovascular abdominal aortic aneurysm repair: improved efficacy using a continuous infusion technique. J Vasc Surg 2006;43:259–64; discussion 264.
8. Sonesson B, Dias N, Malina M, et al. Intra-aneurysm pressure measurements in successfully excluded abdominal aortic aneurysm after endovascular repair. J Vasc Surg 2003;37:733–8.
9. Ellozy SH, Carroccio A, Lookstein RA, et al. First experience in human beings with a permanently implantable intrasac pressure transducer for monitoring endovascular repair of abdominal aortic aneurysms. J Vasc Surg 2004;40:405–12.
10. Milner R, Verhagen HJ, Prinssen M, et al. Noninvasive intrasac pressure measurement and the influence of type 2 and type 3 endoleaks in an animal model of abdominal aortic aneurysm. Vascular 2004;12:99–105.
11. Ellozy SH, Carroccio A, Lookstein RA, et al. Abdominal aortic aneurysm sac shrinkage after endovascular aneurysm repair: correlation with chronic sac pressure measurement. J Vasc Surg 2006;43:2–7.
12. Ohki T, Ouriel K, Silveira PG, et al. Initial results of wireless pressure sensing for endovascular aneurysm repair: the APEX Trial–Acute Pressure Measurement to Confirm Aneurysm Sac EXclusion. J Vasc Surg 2007;45:236–42.
13. van Marrewijk C, Buth J, Harris PL, et al. Significance of endoleaks after endovascular repair of abdominal aortic aneurysms: the EUROSTAR experience. J Vasc Surg 2002;35: 461–73.
14. Chong CK, How TV, Gilling-Smith GL, et al. Modeling endoleaks and collateral reperfusion following endovascular AAA exclusion. J Endovasc Ther 2003;10:424–32.
15. Dias NV, Ivancev K, Malina M, et al. Intra-aneurysm sac pressure measurements after endovascular aneurysm repair: differences between shrinking, unchanged, and expanding aneurysms with and without endoleaks. J Vasc Surg 2004;39:1229–35.
16. Resnikoff M, Darling RC 3rd, Chang BB, et al. Fate of the excluded abdominal aortic aneurysm sac: long-term follow-up of 831 patients. J Vasc Surg 1996;24:851–5.
17. Gelfand DV, White GH, Wilson SE. Clinical significance of type II endoleak after endovascular repair of abdominal aortic aneurysm. Ann Vasc Surg 2006;20:69–74.
18. Pacanowski JP, Stevens SL, Freeman MB, et al. Endotension distribution and the role of thrombus following endovascular AAA exclusion. J Endovasc Ther 2002;9:639–51.

SECTION XII

Vascular Laboratory

55

Some Business Aspects of the Noninvasive Vascular Laboratory

Amir Azarbal, M.D. and Gregory L. Moneta, M.D.

INTRODUCTION

The noninvasive vascular laboratory is an essential component to the practice of vascular surgery. The role of the noninvasive vascular laboratory has evolved since its initial emergence in the 1950s. Technological advances and dedicated research efforts by investigators have made noninvasive vascular imaging the first-line and often definitive test for multiple pathologic processes. Carotid duplex ultrasonography is often the only imaging study required prior to carotid endarterectomy and has reduced the number of angiography-related complications. Venous duplex studies have generally replaced venography for the detection and surveillance of deep vein thromboses.

Participating in and running a noninvasive vascular laboratory is an exciting and rewarding enterprise where physicians can provide quality patient care. However, running a vascular laboratory can be a complex endeavor with multiple facets and potential pitfalls. Many sets of special skills such as administrative, medical, technical, and financial must be integrated in order for a vascular laboratory to be successful. The current need to decrease costs while providing expanded services to a growing population demands that a vascular laboratory be run as efficiently as possible to survive.

This chapter aims to highlight effective concepts in the setup and operation of a vascular laboratory. The focus is on running the business side of the laboratory. Not all business aspects of the vascular laboratory can be covered. Nevertheless, we attempt to point out some of the salient aspects of managing a vascular laboratory. Physical layout and up-to-date equipment acquisition, including newer image acquisition and computer storage systems Picture Archiving and Computer Storage (PACS), are important first steps. There must also be recruitment, training, and retention of a qualified and efficient staff that is educated in the mission of the vascular laboratory. The laboratory must be committed to providing high-quality patient care in line with the national standards published by the Intersocietal Commission for the Accreditation of Vascular Laboratories (ICAVL). Finally, there must be an informed and organized administrative staff that can deal effectively with complex coding, billing, and legal issues.

EFFICIENCY OF THE VASCULAR LABORATORY

Efficiency is of paramount importance. The current climate of reduced reimbursements in the face of expanding services mandates that the vascular laboratory function as efficiently as possible. Efficiency will depend on an interplay of staff, equipment, and patient factors. The vascular laboratory must be able to recruit and retain high-quality and efficient individuals. Laboratory equipment and setup must be conducive to providing patient care without wasted time and resources. Finally, ways to overcome patient factors of absenteeism and tardiness must be assessed.

RECRUITMENT OF STAFF

Recruitment of staff occurs in a multitude of ways: advertisements in journals and newsletters, Internet postings on ultrasound society sites, direct mailings, sponsorship and attendance at local and national meetings, and involvement in ultrasonography schools. For larger laboratories, involvement with a vascular ultrasound program is particularly attractive because it could allow both the laboratory and the student to become familiar with each other prior to graduation through clinical rotations and internships.

Once a potential pool of staff has been created, the selection process needs to be able to match a potential staff member with a position. Unfortunately, hiring managers often rely on their intuition or a loose and subjective set of criteria and interviews to make decisions regarding new hires. The interview needs to be a focused and standardized process that allows the manager to determine which applicant has the key characteristics needed to excel in that particular laboratory. This requires the manager to do a thorough and realistic assessment of what key characteristics are needed for any given position (i.e., communication skills, critical thinking, customer service). The interview process must then be focused on assessing those key characteristics without wasting time on irrelevant questions. It must be standardized so that each applicant for a given position is asked the same or similar questions. An organized team approach, in which multiple members of the laboratory staff are involved in the interview process, will likely lead to a hire that is a better fit for the laboratory as a whole.[1]

Questions during the interview process should ideally be "experience-based." Avoid presenting the applicant with hypothetical situations. Instead ask for specific examples of how interviewees have reacted to and handled past situations relevant to the position. This will help separate good employees from those who simply have good interviewing skills. Last, taking extensive notes on standardized forms helps ensure that selection will not be left to memory. Research has suggested that first candidates interviewed from a large field are often forgotten. [2]

Finally, the interview process should include a technical component, such as a carotid or venous scan, on one of the current staff. This helps assess the proficiency and efficiency of a potential staff member with the specific tasks that he or she will spend the majority of time doing.

RETENTION OF STAFF

The costs of new employee orientation and training is substantial within a vascular laboratory. Therefore, the laboratory must be able to retain its staff. Furthermore, a satisfied cohesive staff will be more likely to further recruit new talent to that laboratory. Salary and compensation are obviously factors in the retention of staff. Surprisingly, however, they may not be as important as one might think. Glenn Tobe and Associates and others have published a survey of employee satisfaction that lists money as fourth or lower on a list of factors of employee satisfaction. This list of factors is shown in Table 55–1.[3]

The majority of these factors are controlled by managers and, therefore, managers likely represent the largest single factor in employee retention. Sullivan et al. have indicated the six main expectations workers have of their managers:[4]

1. Honest and frequent two-way communication
2. Challenging and exciting work
3. Continuing opportunities to learn and grow professionally
4. Recognition of performance
5. Some degree of control over the job (e.g., hours)
6. Knowing their work makes a difference.

Vascular laboratory managers should strive to achieve the above expectations. Effective communication begins with making sure that every new hire understands the mission of the laboratory and is properly oriented. Regular, structured, and standardized feedback will provide employees with a gauge of their performance while minimizing the personal connotation of random sporadic feedback. Finally, growth in the form of training in new vascular procedures and participation in continuing medical education can provide employees with new, challenging, and exciting work while giving them opportunities to grow professionally, an asset to both the individual and the laboratory.[1]

TABLE 55-1. LIST OF FACTORS IDENTIFIED BY EMPLOYEES AS MOST IMPORTANT IN THEIR CAREER SATISFACTION

1. Recognition
2. Work environment
3. Hours
4. Salary
5. Benefits
6. Respect
7. Quality work
8. Management support
9. Opportunity for growth
10. Continuing education

From a survey by Glenn Tobe and associates.[3]

ON-CALL COVERAGE

One particular factor associated with technologist dissatisfaction and "burnout" has been demanding on-call schedules. Patient care demands that there will be times when a vascular laboratory study needs to be done during on-call hours. However, overly demanding on-call coverage schedules can have deleterious effects on staff morale and satisfaction. Vascular studies performed during on-call coverage can also be financially burdensome to the vascular laboratory. There are several different technologist compensation practices for on-call coverage. A thorough investigation of the on-call scanning practices of a laboratory should be done by the laboratory manager to find the coverage schedule and compensation practice that are best suited to lower costs and enhance staff satisfaction.

The most expensive option for call coverage is to pay existing full-time staff overtime pay, which is usually 1.5 times their normal salary. Most laboratories provide compensation for a minimum of 3 hours for each on-call study. Therefore, a full-time staff that is receiving overtime pay is paid for 4.5 hours for just one study.

Alternative strategies could include longer business hours with staggered shifts. For example, there could be a 7 AM to 3 PM shift and a separate 11 AM to 7 PM shift. Staggered shifts also have the benefit of providing flexibility and some degree of control for the staff. Alternatively, it may be beneficial for the laboratory to hire part-time staff for weekends and late shifts rather than having full-time staff cover those hours. Generally, as the number of studies that are performed during on-call hours exceeds ten per week, it becomes important to analyze alternative coverage strategies.[5]

EQUIPMENT

The equipment within any vascular laboratory depends on the resources and mission of that particular laboratory. However, certain principles can be applied rather broadly. First, every effort should be made to maximize the use of scanning equipment, because scanning is usually the rate-limiting factor in delivery of care. The laboratory should be set up such that all nonscanning work, such as chart review, patient interaction, and scan interpretation, is done outside of the scanning area so as to not tie up scanning time. Vascular technologist time should also be allocated mainly to scanning and performance of studies, not to other areas of patient care. Patient transport, calling report, and answering phone calls can be performed by other office personnel.

Last, a system of capital budgeting should exist whereby the need and priority for obtaining new equipment are constantly assessed. It is often difficult to undertake acquisition of new equipment because of the substantial upfront costs. However, replacing old equipment in a timely manner will avoid lost revenue from equipment down time and breakdown, poor performance by and dissatisfaction of vascular technologists, and increased maintenance costs.

Furthermore, as technological advancements progress, more efficient equipment can increase the productivity of a vascular laboratory. Ultrasound scanners are now available that have preset and adjustable protocol settings for the common tests performed by vascular laboratories. This allows the vascular technologists to make only some minor adjustments prior to starting each examination and maximize scanning time. Similarly, there are scanners with automatic reporting worksheets that are automatically populated with data from the examination for streamlining the reporting process. These worksheets can then be checked, finalized, and transmitted directly to the laboratory's image storage system (PACS) along with the examinationimages, where the interpreting provider can access them. This innovation eliminates the cumbersome practice of filling out worksheets by hand and manually scanning them into the image storage system. Therefore, vascular laboratory managers must be well educated and informed about technologic advances in order to properly weigh new equipment costs against the increased revenue generated by increased efficiency.

PACS SYSTEMS

The use of PACS systems in the vascular laboratory has proved to be an improvement over the older system of film handling in almost every facet. PACS systems are advantageous from the perspective of patient care, physician and technologist productivity, economics, and research.

PACS systems allow vascular laboratories to provide prompter, more efficient, and more comprehensive care to patients. It is estimated that by eliminating the need for film handling, videotaping, and file retrieval, technologist and physician productivity increases by 10 to 15% a day. This translates into about one extra laboratory study per technologist per day, which could substantially reduce patient waiting times.[6]

PACS systems allow easy and prompt retrieval of a patient's old studies and make them available for side-by-side comparison with new studies without the need to retrieve old studies from a film library. Interfacing of vascular laboratory PACS systems with larger hospital databases allows the images and reports from the vascular laboratory to be instantaneously disseminated to referring physicians and other providers at a hospital. Interfacing with larger hospital information systems also allows long-term storage of vascular laboratory data in the patient's medical file. Because of the nature of digital image storage, study images will remain high quality and can be viewed with the same clarity as the day they were created. The images can be annotated multiple times without affecting or altering the original image. Furthermore, remote access options for most PACS systems allow access to images from almost any location with an Internet connection, thereby streamlining delivery of care.

PACS systems and the image retrieval systems designed to search the databases of digital images will also aid in clinical research. Automated text searches of study reports for particular diagnoses enable the physician to compare large numbers of similar abnormal studies with each other or with normal controls. In addition to text searches and image retrieval that rely on exact and sometimes variable wording by the reader, more efficient alternatives exist and are being developed. Image recognition software will allow for programs that automatically recognize the image characteristics of a particular pathologic process, for example, proximal internal carotid artery stenosis greater than 70%. The software can then search the databases of all images for other images that meet the criteria for internal carotid artery stenosis and retrieve these studies for further examination.[7]

The initial costs of a PACS and data handling system can be substantial. Although the actual cost is quite variable, based on the equipment provider and the needs of the laboratory, prices can range from $300,000 for a more limited PACS system to well over a million dollars for large PACS systems integrated with a hospital image database. However, maintenance costs are low, with minimal update costs and additional memory storage is available at relatively inexpensive prices. There are also cost savings as a result of decreased spending on film and film handling. However, the majority of the cost benefit stems from increased technologist and physician productivity. In one particular vascular laboratory, implementation of a PACS system allowed volume to grow from 10,500 studies in 1999 to 17,500 studies in 2002 with the addition of only two additional technologists. The center estimated that the initial cost expenditure of the PACS system was recovered in 12 months.[6]

MISSED APPOINTMENTS

Absenteeism, or "no shows," occur independent of medical specialty. No shows lead to lost revenue and inefficient scheduling, which hurt providers, patients, and taxpayers.[8] Owing to its large impact on the efficiency of health care delivery, many systems to reduce or overcome absenteeism have been studied. These measures can be classified into two broad groups. First, there are measures designed to reduce the number of missed appointments. The second group of measures deals with different ways to overbook appointments so as to minimize the effect of missed appointments.

Studies of missed outpatient appointments have found rates anywhere between 8 and 39%. One particular study of vascular laboratory appointments found an absenteeism rate of 12%. Analysis of a vascular laboratory that performs approximately 750 laboratory studies a year shows that a 12% no show rate causes a loss of nearly $90,000 per year. Reducing this missed appointment rate to 5% would save the laboratory approximately $51,000 a year.[9]

Reducing Missed Appointments

Automated telephone reminders, personal calls, and reminder cards are some of the different methods that have been studied to reduce absenteeism. The results of these studies are mixed. There have been prospective randomized trials of outpatient clinics indicating that patient reminder calls result in lower missed appointment rates and higher cancellation rates that can be used to schedule other patients.[10] There have also been studies of vascular laboratories that have shown patient telephone reminders to actually be associated with decreased appointment compliance rates. However, other studies based on procedural appointments, such as outpatient pulmonary function tests, suggest improved compliance with appointments if a patient is contacted either in person or with a message on an answering machine.[11] Although the data are somewhat mixed, some type of patient reminder system should be considered in a vascular laboratory. For larger laboratories and hospital-based laboratories, an automated telephone service can be relatively inexpensive and its cost can be shared among several departments.[9]

Overbooking

Overbooking a vascular laboratory schedule can be a somewhat complex process that must take into account the absenteeism rate, the category of patients (inpatient, outpatient, or mixed), the size of the laboratory, and the cost of overbooking due to overtime pay for staff. In addition, intangible factors such as patient satisfaction and staff "burnout "should be considered.

In general, the higher the absenteeism rate is within a vascular laboratory, the higher the benefits of overbooking. Laboratories that serve inpatients or a mixed group of patients have less incentive to overbook, because there is a pool of inpatient requests that can be substituted for missed appointments. The third factor in overbooking is the size of the laboratory. In general, larger laboratories have a larger revenue benefit from overbooking than smaller laboratories, probably owing to the decreased costs of providing overbooked studies.

Complex mathematical models of overbooking have been developed and extrapolated from service industries such as airlines. In general, however, these models are ill suited to patient care. A rough idea of the extent of overbooking and its benefits can be gained from a relatively simple mathematical model based on endoscopy appointments at the Portland Oregon Veterans Hospital.[12] This purely mathematical study determined the optimal number of patients that must be scheduled for a varying number of procedure slots over a range of patient appointment compliance rates and the cost of adding on extra studies. Table 55–2 is from the study and can be easily adapted to vascular laboratory overbooking.

CODING AND BILLING

Coding and billing in the vascular laboratory are ever-changing and complex targets. The Society of Vascular Surgery (SVS) provides periodic courses on vascular laboratory coding and reimbursement. These courses, conducted by Drs. Sean Roddy and Robert Zwolak, are an excellent introduction to the complexities of coding and billing in the vascular laboratory. Information about attending an SVS-sponsored coding and reimbursement course is available on the vascular web site sponsored by the SVS: http://www.vascularweb.org

In recent years, there has been an extensive movement toward expanding medical services while reducing costs. The reimbursement offices of Medicare and Medicaid have trimmed the indications and situations under which they will reimburse a physician for a medical service or test. This is of particular importance in the vascular laboratory, where decreased reimbursements have already resulted in a very narrow profit margin.

Coding and billing will differ based on whether the laboratory is office- or hospital-based. In addition, each vascular laboratory procedure will be billed as two separate components. The technical component addresses the performance of the actual test and the professional component addresses the interpretation of the study. In hospital-based systems, the technical component is billed according to an Ambulatory Payment Schedule (APC) that is assigned to a given test and reimbursed according to the "hospital outpatient prospective payment system" (HOPPS). It is important to note that within the APC system, no difference is made between a limited unilateral examinationand a complete bilateral exam. The professional component is billed according to the Current Procedural Terminology (CPT) code. In the office-based setting, the technical and professional components are both billed according to CPT codes and reimbursed according to the Medicare fee schedule. Unilateral and limited exams within this system are reimbursed at different rates than complete bilateral exams by Medicare/Medicaid.

Most vascular laboratories perform the majority of their services on Medicare beneficiaries, and therefore, Medicare billing is emphasized in this section. Billing Medicare for a service is tedious. Approximately 4 weeks after a claim is submitted for a service, the provider and beneficiary both receive an "Explanation of Medical

TABLE 55-2. OPTIMAL OVERBOOKING OF PROCEDURAL APPOINTMENT SLOTS AS A FUNCTION OF PATIENT ATTENDANCE RATES, COST OF OVERBOOKING, AND NUMBER OF AVAILABLE SLOTS

	Patient attendance rate				
No. endoscopy slots	**0.6**	**0.7**	**0.8**	**0.9**	**0.95**
Cost of overbooking equals 0.5× benefit of procedure					
5	9	8	7	6	5
10	17	15	13	11	11
15	26	22	19	17	16
20	35	30	26	23	21
25	44	37	32	28	27
30	52	44	39	34	32
35	61	52	45	40	37
40	69	59	51	45	43
45	78	66	58	51	48
50	86	74	64	56	53
Cost of overbooking equals benefit of procedure					
5	8	7	6	5	5
10	16	14	12	11	10
15	25	21	18	16	16
20	33	28	25	22	21
25	41	35	31	28	26
30	50	43	37	33	31
35	58	50	43	39	37
40	66	57	50	44	42
45	75	64	56	50	47
50	83	71	62	55	52
Cost of overbooking equals 1.5× benefit of procedure					
5	7	6	6	5	5
10	15	13	12	11	10
15	23	20	18	16	15
20	32	27	24	22	21
25	40	34	30	27	26
30	48	41	36	33	31
35	56	49	43	38	36
40	65	56	49	44	42
45	73	63	55	49	47
50	81	70	61	55	52

Benefits (EOMB)" that indicates Medicare's decision regarding the claim. "Full payment" by Medicare is actually 80% of the "Medicare Fee Schedule." The remaining 20% is then submitted to a secondary insurer. This is important because the profit margin of a vascular laboratory is well below 20% for each test. In general, secondary insurers will not deny claims that Medicare has accepted and will rarely pay claims that Medicare has denied.

Therefore, it is of paramount importance to understand why Medicare will or will not reimburse for a certain exam. Not infrequently, the denial is based on a clerical error. However, most commonly, the denial is based on the absence of proof that the test is indicated. A recent review of Medicare denials in Florida showed that the top three reasons for Medicare denials are diagnosis not payable for service billed (i.e., test not proven to be indicated), diagnosis reference code not indicated, and missing Unique Physician Identifier Number (UPIN).[13] It is no longer sufficient for a physician to order a test simply because he or she feels that it is indicated. Rather, physicians must show that the test is of "medical necessity." To meet the criteria for medical necessity, the test must be associated with an ICD-9 code that is on a pre-established list of diagnoses that Medicare/Medicaid feels indicates that the given test is appropriate. The situation is complicated by the fact that the list of acceptable diagnoses is determined on a regional level. Therefore, each physician's office or vascular laboratory must contact their local Medicare carrier and review the "Local Medical Review Policy (LMRP)" for noninvasive vascular testing in order to determine which diagnoses are acceptable for billing of vascular laboratory studies.

In addition, Medicare/Medicaid will reimburse for medically necessary tests only on a predetermined schedule. For example, a patient who undergoes a carotid duplex ultrasound and then develops new transient ischemic attack (TIA) symptoms 4 months later would not be reimbursed automatically for a repeat carotid ultrasound owing to the fact that not enough time has elapsed since his or her last carotid ultrasound. Most physicians would argue that this test is indicated to assess for progression of disease. In fact, Medicare would likely end up reimbursing for this test. However, the physician's office should be prepared to have the claim rejected based on an automatic and often computerized review of the testing schedule and then prove that the test was indeed indicated. This may require an appeals process or a request for the claim to be reviewed by a higher level of the review process. The appeal must be done in a timely manner in order to avoid forfeiture of the claim.

Many Medicare claims are denied on their first submission. Studies of vascular laboratory tests have shown that upto 20 to 40% of first-time claims are denied. Again, the number one reason for denial is an ICD-9 code that was not accepted by the regional Medicare carrier as indicating "medical necessity."[14] A review of noninvasive vascular tests that were denied by Medicare showed that in the majority of cases, the tests yielded an abnormal result, and quite commonly, the result could cause in a change in clinical management.[15] Furthermore, systematic review and resubmission of denied Medicare claims showed that ultimately 88% of denied claims would be accepted upon resubmission and appropriate coding and clerical corrections. This seems to suggest two paths of action. First and most important, the coding and billing staff should be intimately familiar with the ICD-9 codes that are reimbursed by their regional provider. It is also absolutely necessary for each vascular laboratory to have a systematic review process of denied claims and to resubmit claims in a timely manner so as to not forfeit payment. Hospitals and other specialties have shown that implementing formal denied claims management protocols can greatly reduce the denial rate and increase revenue.[15]

Second, the fact that a large number of denied vascular imaging studies yield abnormal results indicates that the pre-existing lists of medically necessary ICD-9 codes are too narrow. One problematic solution to this problem has been to use "Advance Beneficiary Notices" that inform the patient that Medicare may not deem their test medically necessary and that they may be responsible for the payment. This is not an ideal solution for the patient or the physician, who does not want to miss a chance to treat a patient secondary to billing issues. Patients often feel trapped by such agreements and most vascular laboratories do not use this practice. Therefore, the usual course of action is for vascular laboratories to perform tests when they are indicated, even if they will not be reimbursed by an insurer. This becomes a financial burden to the laboratory and is not a viable long-term option. The ultimate but time-intensive option then becomes for vascular surgeons and other physicians to look for opportunities to petition and influence their local Medicare providers to expand their list of ICD-9 codes so that opportunities to treat patients are not compromised secondary to billing issues. This is not an easy task and certainly takes dedicated time that most physicians do not have. Luckily, support of professional organizations such as the SVS and the Society for Vascular Ultrasound can help bring about these changes through the work of government relation committees.[16]

ACCREDITATION AND QUALITY ASSURANCE

A system of quality assurance is of paramount importance to the vascular surgeon, technologist, referring physician, and most of all, the patient. The vascular laboratory provides a large number of services for a multitude of indications. Many of the results and interpretations of these studies are operator-dependent. Therefore, a minimal standard of quality and uniformity must be established for a laboratory to provide reliable and clinically relevant data and for data to be valid from one laboratory to the next. Fortunately, the ICAVL has established protocols for the equipment, technique, test components, indications, interpretation, and reporting of various noninvasive studies. Minimal volume criteria for a given test as well as correlation and confirmation of vascular laboratory studies with gold standard tests are also mandated. For example, the minimal number of annual visceral duplex ultrasounds that must be performed in order to maintain proficiency is 100 studies. The results of noninvasive studies must then be compared with those of available gold standard tests—angiography in most cases—to ensure accurate testing and acceptable sensitivities and specificities for detecting pathologic processes within a given vascular laboratory. These quality assurance checks are usually performed quarterly. In addition, the ICAVL sets minimum requirements for vascular laboratory personnel in terms of studies that directors and technologists must have performed. The ICAVL has set requirements for vascular laboratory organizations as well as intracranial cerebrovascular, extracranial cerebrovascular, peripheral arterial, peripheral venous, visceral vascular, and screening studies. Such standardized protocols have helped improve delivery of consistent, high-quality noninvasive testing to patients and reliable clinical information to providers. In the recent era of performance-driven practice, reimbursement is often tied to laboratory and technologist accreditation. Information on accreditation of a vascular laboratory is available on the ICAVL web site at http://www.icavl.org[17]

LEGAL ASPECTS

A thorough review of the legal aspects that govern the billing, referrals to, and compensation of a vascular laboratory is beyond the scope of this chapter. There are, however, several laws and regulations that must be well understood by any physician planning to own or participate in a vascular laboratory.

The "Ethics in Patient Referrals Act," known most commonly as the Stark Laws, was passed in 1988 and has undergone a series of revisions since its inception. These laws govern referrals, ownership, billing, and compensation pertaining to physicians who refer Medicare and Medicaid patients for "designated health services (DHS)". DHS is a broad term that encompasses clinical laboratory, imaging, vascular laboratory, home health, radiation therapy, inpatient, outpatient, physical, and occupational therapy services as well as medical supplies and supplements. The spirit of the law is to keep physicians from referring patients to services or centers that they or their immediate family have a financial interest in. The entire Stark system of laws is a complex and at times cumbersome series of rules, the complete understanding of which would require a great deal of time and effort. There are several exceptions to the Stark Laws that are important for vascular surgeons, especially those in group practices, to be familiar with.

The "In-Office Ancillary Services Exception" allows physicians to order ancillary services such as vascular laboratory studies, provided that such services are located in the same building as the physician's office or the office of one of the group's partners. The physician must be present at that building for a certain number of hours a week, and a portion of that time must be unrelated to the ancillary services, that is, the vascular laboratorystudies that are being ordered.

The "personal services arrangement" exception pertains to the physician-hospital relationship. This means that a physician can be an employee of a hospital (e.g., the director of the vascular laboratory) and make referrals to that hospital's vascular laboratory. He may even receive bonuses based on profits from that laboratory. However, his compensation is subject to regulations in terms of amount compared with similar services by other physicians and the amount of bonuses can in no way be related to the number or value of the referrals that the physician makes.[18-19]

There are certain other exceptions that usually do not affect the operations of a vascular laboratory but may deal with employees in academic settings, physicians in rural practices, and several other situations. As mentioned, the Stark Laws have undergone several changes and are subject to further revisions. Even as this chapter is being written, there is proposed legislation at the federal level to alter several of the exceptions to the Stark Laws, including the owning of medical equipment by physicians. Often, expert legal advice is necessary in the setup of a noninvasive vascular laboratory and to ensure compliance with a changing legal system. However, a basic understanding of the Stark Laws and several of its exceptions is necessary for every practitioner in an academic, managed care, or private practice setting.

CONCLUSION

Running or participating in a noninvasive vascular laboratory is a multifaceted, challenging, and rewarding experience. It requires the physician to use many different areas of expertise in addition to medical knowledge and to provide high-quality patient care. Administrative, business, legal, and leadership skills are all necessary for a vascular laboratory to run smoothly and efficiently. With such a wide variety of skills required for the success of the laboratory, the recruitment, training, and retention of a high-quality staff is of paramount importance. Appropriate delegation of responsibility by the laboratory director as well as flexibility and innovative thinking by the laboratory management will allow the laboratory to adjust to ever-changing technological advancements, legal issues, staff needs, and reimbursement practices. At each step of staff recruitment (e.g., staff training and retention), efforts should be made to present and promote the guiding mission of the vascular laboratory. This will allow for the development of a cohesive staff with a clear uniform goal for quality and cost-efficient care.

REFERENCES

1. Theisen P. The skill of hiring "the right" people. J Vasc Ultrasound 2004;28:124–6.
2. Sampson M, Schwebler M. Recruitment and retention: staffing for quality in the vascular laboratory. J Vasc Ultrasound 2994;28:127–30.
3. Glenn Tobe and Associates Survey. The working communicator. Lawrence Ragan Communications, Inc. The Winners Circle.
4. Sullivan J. Getting managers to own retention. Employ Manag Today 2000;5:1–3.
5. Kupinski A. Managing today's vascular laboratory: patients, personnel, and policies. J Vasc Ultrasound 2004;28:138–40.
6. Bendick P. Digital archiving (PACS) in the vascular laboratory: improving efficiency and decreasing costs. J Vasc Ultrasound 2004;28:149–51.
7. Muller H, Michoux N, Geissbuhler A. A review of content-based image retrieval systems in medical applications—clinical benefits and future directions. Int J Med Inform 2004;73:1–23.
8. Macharia W, Leon G, Rowe B, Stephenson B. An overview of interventions to improve compliance with appointment keeping for medical services. JAMA 1992;267:1813–7.
9. Satiani B, Miller S, Patel D. No-show rates in the vascular laboratory: analysis and possible solutions. J Vasc Interv Radiol 2009;20:87–91.
10. Hashim M, Franks P, Fiscell K. Effectiveness of telephone reminders in improving rate of appointments kept at an outpatient clinic: a randomized controlled trial. J Am Board Fam Pract 2001;14:193–6.
11. Haynes J, Sweeny E. The effect of telephone appointment-reminder calls on outpatient absenteeism in a pulmonary function laboratory. Respir Care 2006;51: 36–9.
12. Sonnenberg A. How to overbook procedures in the endoscopy unit. Gastrointest Endosc 2009;69:710–5.
13. Schroedter W, Zwolak R, Olmsted K. Survival tactics for the vascular laboratory: coding and billing issues, J Vasc Ultrasound 2004;28:161–7.
14. Passman M, Guzman R, Pierce R, Naslund, TC. Impact of Medicare denials on noninvasive vascular diagnostic testing. J Vasc Surg 2001;34:846–560
15. Hodges J. Effective claims denial management enhances revenue. Health Care Financ Manag 2002;Aug:40–50.
16. Jones A, Schroedter, W. The Society for Vascular Ultrasound government relations committee: Impact on practice, standards and reimbursement. J Vasc Ultrasound 2004;28:168–70.
17. The Inter-Societal Association for the Accreditation of Vascular Laboratories official web site. http://www.ICAVL.org
18. Satiani B. Exceptions to the Stark Law: practical considerations for surgeons. Plast Reconstruct Surg 2006;117:1012–22.
19. Gosfield J. The stark truth about the Stark Law. Fam Pract Manag 2003;Nov-Dec:27–33.

56

Criteria for Carotid Stenosis and Plaque Characteristics

Timothy Wu, M.D. and Hisham S. Bassiouny, M.D.

OVERVIEW

Approximately 500,000 people in the United States suffer a first-time stroke each year, resulting in nearly 200,000 annual deaths and carrying a prevalence of 1 million disabled. The annual direct and indirect cost of stroke in the United States was estimated to be about $40 billion in the late 1990s, a figure that is likely much higher in 2009. The earliest link between stroke and carotid artery disease is credited to Gowers,[1] who reported a case of left monocular symptoms in the setting of right hemiplegia due to occlusion of the left internal carotid artery (ICA) and bilateral subclavian artery occlusions found on postmortem examination. Reports in subsequent decades increasingly linked carotid artery occlusive disease to stroke and what would later come to be called transient ischemic attacks (TIAs). Today carotid artery occlusive disease is an important risk factor in the development of stroke, and reconstruction of the carotid artery has been shown to decrease risk of stroke and, by inference, stroke-related death. Carotid artery occlusive disease accounts for 15 to 20% of all ischemic strokes.[2]

In 1937, Moniz[3] developed carotid arteriography and ushered in an era of understanding of carotid artery occlusive disease and its anatomy. Arteriography is still considered the gold standard for diagnosing luminal stenosis against which other modalities in carotid artery imaging are to be compared. A movement toward noninvasive carotid imaging culminated in investigations by Strandness[4] at the University of Washington, which resulted in criteria for the estimation of carotid stenosis utilizing velocity measurements obtained by duplex ultrasound, followed by further refinement of these criteria by other investigators in the years that followed. Stenosis of the ICA as estimated by duplex ultrasound, however, is only a part of the equation in determining whether or not carotid artery occlusive disease would eventually cause symptoms. How else can we explain, for example, why an ulcerated plaque is an ominous finding on carotid arteriography given two plaques of equal stenoses as measured by either duplex ultrasound or arteriography?

Validation of criteria for carotid stenosis, intervention, and risk of cerebrovascular events has been shown through several large carotid endarterectomy trials, namely, the North American Symptomatic Carotid Endarterectomy Trial (NASCET),[5] European Carotid Surgery Trial (ECST),[6] and the Asymptomatic Carotid Atherosclerosis Study (ACAS).[7] These form the basis on which our current indications for carotid intervention are based. It should be noted, however, that the evidence for interventions in patients with asymptomatic carotid stenosis is marginal, given that approximately 20 procedures need to be performed for the prevention of a single stroke based on ACAS data.[7] Beyond stenosis, however, morphology and histobiochemical composition of carotid plaques are emerging as increasingly important considerations in determining which carotid stenoses, particularly in asymptomatic patients, demand intervention. Imaging modalities commonly employed in the diagnosis of carotid artery occlusive disease include duplex ultrasound, computed tomographic angiography (CTA), and magnetic resonance angiography (MRA). In some cases, positron emission tomography (PET) scanning is being investigated for its utility in carotid plaque characterization and to identify vulnerable plaques at risk for disruption. Information accrued from such studies will help develop a paradigm shift in selecting asymptomatic ICA stenoses truly in need of an intervention.

ARTERIOGRAPHY

Introduced in 1937, arteriography remains the gold standard in diagnosing carotid artery occlusive disease. Two landmark carotid surgery trials, the NASCET[5] and the ECST,[6] utilized arteriography as the standard in determining luminal stenosis in carotid artery occlusive disease. It was from these two trials that carotid stenosis became the most important factor in defining stroke risk. NASCET and ECST utilized different methods in estimation of luminal stenosis by arteriography, however, and this caused some confusion as to which methodology would be the basis for determining the threshold stenosis for intervention.

The NASCET estimated ICA stenosis by utilizing a ratio between the minimal lumen diameter within the ICA bulb (A) and the diameter of the normal distal ICA (B). Similarly, the ECST calculated a ratio between the narrowest luminal diameter within the ICA bulb (A) and the estimated maximum diameter of the ICA bulb (C). Few studies attempting to correlate stenosis measurements between the two trials failed to find an agreement (Figure 56–1).

Alexandrov et al.[8] prospectively analyzed 45 patients undergoing carotid arteriography to compare NASCET and ECST measurements of carotid stenosis versus duplex ultrasound and direct visualization of the pathologic specimens that were removed intact and underwent computer analysis. They found significant differences between NASCET and duplex ($P<.0001$), ECST and duplex ($P<.01$), and even between NASCET and ECST measurements ($P<.006$). They further found that NASCET ($P<.0007$) and ECST ($P<.007$) significantly underestimated the true anatomic stenosis of the carotid plaque at the bulb as measured by their computer analysis.

Clearly the noninvasive measurement of carotid stenosis can underestimate true luminal reduction, but perhaps stenosis is not the only plaque characteristic that renders it symptomatic. Beyond characterization of the degree of stenosis of the internal carotid artery and quantification of stroke risk based on the NASCET and ECST data,

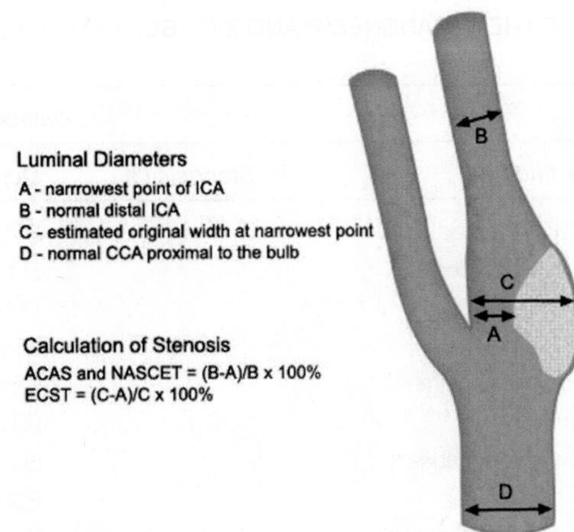

Figure 56-1. Illustration of method for NASCET and ECST measurements of carotid stenosis.

arteriography also provides data on plaque surface morphology. It has previously been reported that plaque surface ulceration as seen on arteriography can be predictive of a high risk of subsequent stroke in asymptomatic as well as symptomatic plaques.[9] Arteriography is an excellent tool to detect carotid plaque ulceration based on standardized criteria[10] and has been shown to have good interobserver as well as intraobserver reliability,[11-12] good histopathologic validity,[10-11] and to be associated with adherence of thrombus noted at the time of operation.[10] Eliasziw[13] et al. studied 659 patients with severe (70 to 99%) carotid stenosis from the NASCET trial and found that ipsilateral stroke at 24 months for medically treated patients with ulcerated plaques increased from 26.3 to 73.2% as the degree of stenosis increased from 75 to 95%, while patients without ulcerations had a risk of stroke that remained flat at 21.3% for all degrees of stenosis.

To date, while arteriography remains a reliable gold standard in determining the degree of luminal carotid stenosis based on the NASCET and ECST trials, less invasive modalities such as CTA offer distinct advantages over arteriography because of added information on the plaque burden and structural nature of the plaque

DUPLEX ULTRASONOGRAPHY

Velocity Measurements

Duplex ultrasonography has emerged as the screening and diagnostic study of choice in carotid occlusive disease as well as the most studied modality in this setting because of its relatively low cost and noninvasiveness. A variety of studies developed specific velocity criteria for the diagnosis of carotid occlusive disease, but the two most commonly used are those developed by Strandness[4] and Zwiebel.[14-15] Zwiebel additionally stressed the importance of velocity ratios in better categorizing the degree of carotid occlusive disease (Table 56–1).[14]

A recent meta-analysis showed that ultrasonography was best for more critical lesions, those at least 70% or greater, carrying a sensitivity of 89% and a specificity of 84%. For lesions between 50 and 69%, however, the sensitivity and specificity were

TABLE 56-1. SUMMARY OF THE STRANDNESS[4] AND ZWIEBEL[14–15] DUPLEX CRITERIA FOR ICA STENOSIS

Strandness		Zwiebel	
Stenosis (%)	*Duplex findings*	*Stenosis (%)*	*Duplex findings*
0	PSV < 125 cm/sec	0	PSV < 110 cm/sec
	No spectral broadening		EDV < 40 cm/sec
	Bulb flow reversal		PSV ICA/CCA < 1.8
1-15	PSV < 125 cm/sec		EDV ICA/CCA < 2.4
	No or minimal spectral		Spectral broadening < 30 cm/sec
	Broadening	1-39	PSV < 110 cm/sec
	Bulb flow reversal absent		EDV < 40 cm/sec
16-49	PSV > 125 cm/sec		PSV ICA/CCA < 1.8
	Marked spectral broadening		EDV ICA/CCA < 2.4
50-79	PSV > 125 cm/sec		Spectral broadening < 40 cm/sec
	EDV < 140 cm/sec	40-59	PSV < 130 cm/sec
80-99	PSV > 125 cm/sec		EDV < 40 cm/sec
	EDV > 140 cm/sec		PSV ICA/CCA < 1.8
100	No flow		EDV ICA/CCA < 2.4
			Spectral broadening < 40 cm/sec
		60-79	PSV > 130 cm/sec
			EDV > 40 cm/sec
			PSV ICA/CCA > 1.8
			EDV ICA/CCA > 2.4
			Spectral broadening > 40 cm/sec
		80-99	PSV > 250 cm/sec
			EDV > 100 cm/sec
			PSV ICA/CCA > 3.7
			EDV ICA/CCA > 5.5
			Spectral broadening > 80 cm/sec
		100	No flow

quite poor, that is, 36 and 91%, respectively.[16] AbuRahma[17] found the Strandness criteria to be less reliable and that they required modification in the presence of contralateral stenosis greater than 70% or for complete occlusion because of compensatory flow through the ipsilateral carotid artery. His group identified 356 carotid arteries with duplex ultrasound evidence of greater than 50% stenosis. Arteriography as the diagnostic gold standard for these vessels found the Strandness criteria to be less reliable in the setting of occlusion, high-grade contralateral stenosis, or less than 70% ipsilateral stenosis.[17] Fujitani et al. [18] modified the Strandness criteria based on 154 patients with unilateral ICA occlusion on angiogram and found these to be 97.5% accurate in detecting 80 to 99% stenosis and 96.9% accurate in detecting 50 to 79% stenosis. The results of both AbuRahma's and Fujitani's studies are comparable.

Because the major clinical trials for carotid endarterectomy were based on arteriographic categorization of stenosis, several authors have tried to correlate duplex findings with the results of the NASCET and ECST studies. Moneta et al. [19] reviewed 184 internal carotid arteries that were subjected to duplex ultrasonography within 1 week of arteriographic measurements by the NASCET method. Of several measures noted in their study, they found the best predictor of stenoses greater than 70% to be an ICA/CCA ratio of 4.0 or above.

In an analysis of the Strandness criteria for ICA ECST (ie bulb) stenosis the Univeristy of Chicago group (Shaalan, et al) correlated velocity measurements with CT angiogram measurements of ICA ECST stenosis. The underlying rationale was to better outline the outer boundary of the ICA plaque by CT rather than relying on an estimated imaginary line on arteriography as had been used to develop the Strandness criteria. 219 internal carotid arteries with a stenosis of 50 to 79% and 62 with a stenosis of 80 to 99% were included in the study. Generally, 80-99% ICA ECST stenoses are considered equivalent to ≥ 70% NASCET stenosis. Patients with a contralateral internal carotid artery occlusion or severe calcification were excluded from our study. Utilizing receiver operating characteristic (ROC) analysis, the optimal threshold velocities to identify at least a 50% stenosis of the internal carotid artery were a PSV of 155 cm/s and an ICA/CCA ratio of at least 2.0.[20] Additionally velocity criteria for a stenosis of at least 80% were found to be PSV >370 cm/s, EDV >140 cm/s, and an ICA/CCA ratio of at least 6.0 (Table 56–2).[20]

B-MODE IMAGING

The agreement between B-mode ultrasound imaging and CT angiogram measurements of ECST ICA stenosis is good.[20] In our research 74 carotid studies were reviewed with a range of stenoses: less than 50% (n = 29), 50 to 79% (n = 23), and 80 to 99% (n = 22). Two examiners measured the ICA stenosis on CT angiogram axial images with good interobserver and intraobserver agreement—κ = 0.8, 0.9, respectively. On regression analysis of the mean measurements of stenosis noted by the two examiners and the B-mode ultrasound measurements, we found there to be strong agreement between the two modalities (r = 0.9, P = 0.002).[20]

TABLE 56-2. SUMMARY OF SHAALAN[20] CRITERIA FOR CAROTID STENOSIS OF AT LEAST 50% AND 80%

≥50% ICA Stenosis	PSV≥155 cm/sec
	Sensitivity 82%, Specificity 88%, PPV 78%, NPV 90%
	Accuracy 84%
	ICA/CCA Ratio≥2.0
	Sensitivity 80%, Specificity 84%, PPV 73%, NPV 89%
	Accuracy 81%
≥80% ICA Stenosis	PSV≥370 cm/sec
	Sensitivity 87%, Specificity 90%, PPV 82%, NPV 93%
	Accuracy 89%
	EDV≥140 cm/sec
	Sensitivity 84%, Specificity 91%, PPV 83%, NPV 91%
	Accuracy 90%
	ICA/CCA Ratio≥6.0
	Sensitivity 82%, Specificity 91%, PPV 83%, NPV 91%
	Accuracy 89%

The role of direct B-mode image measurement of maximal ICA stenosis in improving the accuracy of Duplex velocity measurements was investigated at our institution.[21] The images and records of 192 patients who underwent both arteriography and duplex ultrasonography (DU) of 375 carotid arteries from January 1995 to November 2000 were reviewed. All DUs were performed by registered vascular technologists (n=6). Maximum arteriographic stenosis was determined according to the NASCET study design. With arteriography as the "gold standard," B-mode image (BMI) measurement of the maximal ICA luminal narrowing relative to the carotid bulb (n=162)as well as the peak systolic velocity in the internal carotid artery (PSVICA) (n=330), end-diastolic velocity in the internal carotid artery (EDV(ICA)) (n=198), and the ratio of the PSVs in both the ICA and the CCA (PSVICA/CCA) ratio (n=319) were subjected to (ROC) curves for 3 clinically relevant stenoses thresholds: 50-99%, 60-99%, and 70-99%. A strong correlation was found between B-mode image (BMI) and the NASCET arteriographic measures of carotid stenosis ($r = 0.80$; $p < 0.001$) and was similar among the 6 technologists ($r = 0.74$-0.89;$p > 0.2$). The overall accuracy of BMI measurement to diagnose 50%, 60%, and 70% arteriographic carotid stenosis was 85.3%, 82.2%, and 87%, respectively. BMI measurement was similar to the most accurate PSV(ICA), EDV(ICA), and PSV(ICA/CCA) ratio at all 3 threshold stenoses levels ($p > 0.3$). When combined with the velocity criteria, BMI measurement improved the positive predictive value (PPV) for all arteriographic stenoses thresholds by an average of 12.6% for PSV(ICA), 21.2% for EDV(ICA), and 14.2% for PSV(ICA/CCA) ratio. BMI measurement of carotid bifurcation stenosis is as reliable as duplex-derived velocity criteria in evaluating clinically relevant threshold ICA stenoses. The routine use of B-mode ultrasound in conjunction with the velocity parameters enhances the PPV of carotid DU. Our experience suggests that with current refinements in B-mode resolution, BMI stenosis measurements are accurate of stenosis[22-23] among experienced technologists and are a useful adjunct to duplex-derived velocity parameters provided that there is minimal calcification and acoustic shadowing. As noted above, plaque ulceration was noted in data from NASCET to be particularly ominous in determining stroke risk. While biplanar arteriography has showed good results in detecting plaque ulceration, several large studies of ultrasonography in detecting plaque ulceration and intraplaque hemorrhage have showed wide variations in both sensitivity and specificity.[24-28] Moreover, in up to 37% of cases it is not possible to evaluate the plaque surface for ulceration due to acoustic shadowing or a high degree of stenosis.

GSM ANALYSIS

Other useful anatomic information that B-mode ultrasound imaging has offered us is derived from data of plaque echolucency, which is becoming a critical determinant of plaque risk. Echogenicity refers to overall plaque structure, its relative composition of lipid, intraplaque hemorrhage, calcium, and core necrosis. Calcium specifically is highly contributory in producing an echodense (e.g., high calcium content, excessive fibrosis) plaque versus an echolucent (low calcium content) plaque. Initial studies[29-30] into plaque echolucency were based on highly subjective visual analyses between observers, and as might be expected, interobserver variation was unacceptably high and without agreement with subsequent histologic analysis.[31] Two common methods of computer-aided analysis of plaque echolucency are the gray scale median (GSM) and pixel distribution analysis (PDA), and these have helped to advance carotid imaging. GSM analysis is most commonly performed using Adobe Photoshop (Adobe Systems, Inc., San Jose, CA) to analyze a digitized image of the artery, with blood (GSM = 0) and adventitia (GSM = 180-190) as reference points and measuring the median grayness of the B-mode image after normalization of the image. From this a GSM score is derived, and this method has been found to be highly reproducible with low interobserver variation and reliability between scanners.[32-33] PDA is similar in that it also involves use of a digitized B-mode carotid image, uses blood and adventitia as reference points, but provides further mapping of the carotid plaque with pixel by pixel normalization and complete plaque structure, a kind of "virtual histology."

EX VIVO GSM ANALYSIS OF CAROTID PLAQUES

To identify features on B-mode ultrasonography (US) prevalent in symptomatic plaques and correlate these findings with histopathologic markers of plaque instability. we investigated carotid endarterectomy (CEA) plaques from symptomatic and asymptomatic patients with critical stenoses (>70%).[34] Plaques were qualitatively assessed using preoperative B-mode US for echolucency and calcific acoustic shadowing. US echolucency was quantitated ex vivo using computerized techniques for gray-scale median (GSM) analysis. Histopathologic correlates for US plaque echolucency (percentage of necrotic core area) and acoustic shadowing (percentage of calcification area) were determined. Using ex-vivo B-mode US and GSM analysis, symptomatic plaques were more echolucent (41 +/− 19) than asymptomatic plaques (60 +/−13), $P < .03$. A strong inverse correlation was found between the percent plaque necrotic area core and GSM ($R = -0.9$, $P < .001$). Percentage of calcification area in plaques with acoustic shadowing was 66% and only 27% in those without acoustic shadowing ($P < .05$). Using B-mode US, symptomatic plaques are more echolucent and less calcified than asymptomatic plaques and are associated with a greater degree of histopathologic plaque necrosis. Such features are indicative of plaque instability and should be considered in the decision-making algorithm when selecting patients with high-grade asymptomatic carotid stenosis for intervention.

IN VIVO GSM ANALYSIS OF CAROTID PLAQUES

The Imaging in Carotid Angioplasty and Risk of Stroke (ICAROS) trial also found that echolucent plaques (GSM < 25) had a 7.1% risk of stroke in the intraoperative and immediate postoperative period, whereas those with GSM scores higher than 25 had only a 1.5% risk.[35] There is very obviously clinical utility in GSM analysis of carotid occlusive disease, and this has formed the basis of one of our ongoing efforts in carotid disease imaging research.

We reviewed 448 carotid artery duplex studies from 250 patients who had greater than 50% stenosis of the ICA. Plaque morphologic characteristics were subjectively evaluated by duplex ultrasonography, and each plaque was graded predominantly (>50% area of plaque images) as echolucent (hypoechoic) or echodense (hyperechoic). The presence of acoustic shadowing and interference with pulsed Doppler sampling was indicative of a calcific plaque. Highly calcific plaques were excluded from the study and images were analyzed only if greater than 50% of the plaque depicted acoustic information. Multiple longitudinal views of carotid plaques were utilized to assess GSM and values were averaged.

Based on B-mode imaging 92 (21%) plaques were excluded owing to calcific acoustic shadowing, leaving 356 plaques from 223 patients in the core study population. The mean GSM value for the entire group was 50.7±1.20. Of the 356 plaques in which GSM values were assessed, 46 (13%) had a history of TIA, stroke, or amaurosis fugax, and 310 were asymptomatic. The GSM differed significantly between symptomatic and asymptomatic plaques (symptomatic 32, asymptomatic 54; [{P< 0.001}]). Of all demographic and atherosclerotic risk factors, only sex was significantly associated with the GSM. Mulitvariate Generalized Estimating Equation (GEE) modeling of symptomatic status using GSM and all the risk factors indicated that only GSM was a significant predictor of symptoms. In regard to symptom status and risk factors, in symptomatic plaques, none of the factors can predict GSM. Consistent with the difference in GSM of asymptomatic plaques between females and males, plaques without GSM values owing to heavy calcification were predominantly in females (63%, P=0.01 from a binomial test, assuming plaques from females and males have the same probability of heaving calcification).

ROC analysis of the relationship between symptoms and GSM value shows an area under the curve of 0.82 (95% CI: 0.76-0.88), with a sensitivity and specificity of 85% and 76% for an optimal cutoff GSM value of 40. In a multivariate GEE analysis for GSM, sex was found to be the only significant risk factor (P=.001). Sex was again found to be statistically significant with females: 57.3±1.53 and males: 47.6±2.01; P< 0.001. When diabetic patients were separated into male and female categories, regardless of the presence of diabetes, female sex was still shown to have a significantly higher GSM (P=.0241 with diabetes and P=0.0013 without diabetes).

GSM analysis is a valuable measure of plaque vulnerability. A GSM of 40 or lower is predictive of symptomatic plaque with reasonable accuracy. Older age was demonstrated to have a higher GSM value. Increased GSM with age may suggest that asymptomatic patients older than 75 years tend to have more stable plaques. This is consistent with observations that plaques become more fibrocalcific with age. In addition, asymptomatic females have significantly higher GSM values than men. Prospective randomized trials comparing interventions for asymptomatic patients should consider incorporating GSM as an independent variable to identify plaque risk in addition to severity of stenosis. Based on our series, asymptomatic patients of 75 years harboring minimally or no calcified critically stenotic (≥80%) ICA plaques with a GSM of 40 are considered for intervention. (submitted to Joural of Vascular Surgery)

COMPUTED TOMOGRAPHY

CT scanning is a versatile technology that has found diagnostic applicability in many areas. With the introduction and advancement of high-resolution multidetector CT (MDCT) scanners, which allow us to perform CTA, investigators have been looking into its utility in carotid occlusive disease. Early studies in the evaluation of carotid occlusive disease by CT scanners utilized single-slice scanners with much lower resolution than the current state of the art. As a result, for internal carotid stenosis less than 70%, sensitivity was found to be 79 to 87% with a specificity of 88 to 90%.[36] For carotid stenosis greater than 70%, however, sensitivity and specificity were found to be 100%.[37] Beyond the question of whether or not there is a stenosis present and to what degree, evolving clinical studies examining plaque composition are providing us with a clearer understanding of the role of CTA in determining overall plaque risk.

With MDCT scanning technology, a recent investigation of eight patients found a 72.6% agreement between plaque composition as determined by CT compared with histologic examination. The greater the amount of calcification, the better the overall sensitivity and specificity, approaching 100% with a high degree of calcification.[36] For noncalcified components of the carotid plaque, however, such as necrotic core, lipid volume, intraplaque hemorrhage, and connective tissue, there was significant overlap seen that confounded the ability of CT to determine plaque composition.[38] In fact it appears that calcification is the only histologic component that is reliably delineated by CT.[39-41] To illustrate how important MDCT technology is to its role as a kind of virtual histology, single-slice scanners have an overall poor detection of plaque morphology such as ulceration with a sensitivity of 50 to 94% and a specificity of 74 to 99%[42] and poor correlation with postoperative histology.[43] Two recent studies showed that single-slice CT could not depict plaque composition for the purposes of virtual histology.[40,43] A few groups have studied plaque calcification on CT and its correlation with symptoms, partially borrowing the premise for GSM analysis that highly calcified plaques are relatively stable and, therefore, less likely to be symptomatic, and the results have been mixed.[41,44] This is probably because the sample sizes were quite small, the largest of all studying just 14 patients.[45] Our group has begun studying carotid plaque calcification on CTA and correlating this with symptoms.

MAGNETIC RESONANCE IMAGING

MRA has yet to prove its clinical usefulness as compared with CTA, which has emerged as a reliable technology in peripheral vascular imaging, producing high-quality studies; in some institutions, it has supplanted the need for conventional diagnostic arteriography. Its role in carotid imaging, however, is unclear. Although in comparison to CT imaging of carotid plaque calcification MR technology appears similar with sensitivities of 76 to 98% and specificities of 86 to 98%,[46-48] it appears to have a superior ability to distinguish the various carotid plaque components.[49]

Intraplaque hemorrhage, through a technique of T1-shortening, can identify histologically confirmed carotid plaque hemorrhage and distinguish hemorrhage of varying ages with moderate agreement (κ=.44 to 0.66).[50] Overall the sensitivity in the detection of intraplaque hemorrhage ranges from 82 to 92% and the specificity from 74 to 100% in different studies.[47,48,50,51]

The ability of MR to distinguish the lipid component of a carotid plaque is similarly superior to that of CT, with sensitivities reported to be 84 to 98% and specificities of 65 to 100%.[46-48,51,52] MR measurements of the lipid component of carotid plaque did not differ significantly compared with histologic examination (correlation $r=.75$, $P<.001$),[48] with an even better correlation with the use of gadolinium-enhanced images ($r=.87$, $P<.001$).[52]

Despite these advantages in carotid plaque imaging and the elimination of ionizing radiation offered by MR technology, the disadvantages of this modality may ultimately render it a noncontender. Current MR scan times are noted to be much longer than CT, which leads to a high failure rate for obtaining proper imaging of anywhere between 8% and 28% secondary to motion artifact.[49] The risk of gadolinium-induced nephrogenic systemic fibrosis is a very real complication of contrast-enhanced magnetic resonance imaging (MRI) and can occur in up to 3% of patients with renal insufficiency.[53] Finally interobserver disagreement was found to be up to 20% when MR was used to image carotid plaques. In a small observational study, 30 time-of-flight images along with T1, T2, and proton density images were obtained, and findings were compared between two reviewers in three different rounds of image analysis of the common carotid artery through the ICA with 6-mm slices. One of the limitations of MR that was identified by this study was that normal values for the different measures performed in the carotid artery have yet to be standardized, and therefore, interobserver agreement was not ideal. Intraobserver correlation, however, was found to be acceptable and good.[54]

FUTURE TRENDS IN THE ASSESSMENT OF THE CAROTID PLAQUE

Current modalities in carotid plaque imaging seek to provide anatomic information that may be of use in indirectly determining plaque risk. Above all anatomic markers, carotid plaque risk is probably better stratified by an assessment of the cellular and molecular processes underlying its structural composition. Inflammation is an important component in risk stratification for cardiovascular events, and although measurement of serum markers of inflammation, such as C-reactive protein, may be useful, these may not be specific to the carotid plaque and more likely constitute a systemic risk.[55] The area of functional molecular imaging is a developing one and may provide us with greater insight into carotid plaque risk by correlating anatomic findings with molecular and cellular processes.

THERMOGRAPHY

Catheter-based temperature sensors have been developed to measure subtle temperature differences in coronary plaque, based on the principle that atherosclerosis is an inflammatory process and that an increase in temperature is suggestive of the fact that activated macrophages are producing heat.[56] Thermography would be able to provide us with a metabolic functional characterization of atherosclerotic plaques and, potentially, provide data on which plaques may be at higher risk to becoming symptomatic. Coronary plaques subjected to thermography have shown increases in temperature and a wider range of temperature variations across the entire plaque in patients with ischemic heart disease when compared with patients who are asymptomatic from their coronary disease. These differences were accentuated in patients who were found to have "severe" disease, for example, acute myocardial infarction versus stable angina.[57] Similar findings on the luminal surfaces of carotid plaque specimens studied ex vivo after carotid endarterectomy with a needle thermistor were also found.[58] The application of thermography, however, is invasive, and further trials to determine its true clinical applicability need to be evaluated.

PET/SPECT IMAGING

Positron emission tomography (PET) and single photon emission computed tomography (SPECT) are nuclear imaging techniques that are capable of visualizing metabolic activity and molecular processes. Spatial resolution with PET is superior to SPECT, offering two to three times better imaging results. However, this still renders PET most useful for the imaging of larger arteries. Combining PET with CT or MRI improves the spatial resolution and allows for acceptable imaging quality for the carotid artery. The most widely available tracer for use in PET/SPECT imaging of carotid artery inflammation is ^{18}F-fluorodeoxyglucose (FDG), which accumulates in macrophage-rich areas of carotid plaques. Symptomatic, unstable atherosclerotic lesions tend to accumulate more FDG than asymptomatic lesions.[59] Whereas FDG-PET has shown a clear reduction in inflammation with use of statin therapy,[60] there is still no conclusive evidence that quantification of inflammation has a direct causal relationship with plaque symptoms.

NEAR-INFRARED SPECTROSCOPY

Near-infrared spectroscopy (NIRS) emits light into tissue and measures the range of wavelengths of reflected light to determine the chemical composition of tissue quantitatively and qualitatively.[61] Ex vivo analyses of fresh carotid endarterectomy specimens showed significantly different absorption spectra between asymptomatic and symptomatic plaques.[62] Current work with NIRS is ongoing in coronary plaque imaging.[61] NIR fluororescence (NIRF) has been shown to image molecular processes like atherosclerosis.[63] With devices such as MMPSense, a "smart activatable probe," activated MMPs such as MMP-2 and MMP-9, which are considered important biomarkers in vulnerable plaques,[64] can be visualized in vivo. In the coming years, research into this technique may prove its efficacy and provide us with another imaging modality for the assessment of carotid plaque risk.

CONCLUSION

Our understanding of carotid artery occlusive disease has evolved over a number of decades and its diagnosis has been greatly refined by state-of-the-art imaging technologies. Whereas still newer technologies in imaging and characterization of the carotid plaque are on the horizon and promise to make risk stratification a priority, allowing us to better select patients (particularly those who have asymptomatic carotid occlusive disease and who would benefit from carotid interventions), the continued evolution of criteria for already established modalities, such as duplex ultrasonography and CT, will better refine and improve our decision making for carotid occlusive disease.

REFERENCES

1. Gowers W. On a case of simultaneous embolism of central retinal and middle cerebral arteries. Lancet 1875;2:794.
2. Chaturvedi S, Bruno A, Feasby T, et al. Carotid endarterectomy—an evidence-based review: report of the Therapeutics and Technology Assessment Subcommittee of the American Academy of Neurology. Neurology 2005;65:794–801.
3. Moniz E, Lima A, deLacerda R. Hemiplegies par thrombose de la carotide interne. Presse Med 1937;45:977.
4. Strandness D Jr. Extracranial arterial disease. In: Duplex Scanning in Vascular Disorders. 2nd ed. New York: Raven Press; 1993.

5. Beneficial effect of carotid endarterectomy in symptomatic patients with high-grade carotid stenosis. North American Symptomatic Carotid Endarterectomy Trial Collaborators. N Engl J Med 1991;325:445–53.
6. MRC European Carotid Surgery Trial: interim results for symptomatic patients with severe (70-99%) or with mild (0-29%) carotid stenosis. European Carotid Surgery Trialists' Collaborative Group. Lancet 1991;337:1235–43.
7. Study design for randomized prospective trial of carotid endarterectomy for asymptomatic atherosclerosis. The Asymptomatic Carotid Atherosclerosis Study Group. Stroke 1989; 20:844–9.
8. Alexandrov AV, Bladin CF, Maggisano R, Norris JW. Measuring carotid stenosis. Time for a reappraisal. Stroke 1993;24:1292–6.
9. Moore WS, Boren C, Malone JM, et al. Natural history of nonstenotic, asymptomatic ulcerative lesions of the carotid artery. Arch Surg 1978;113:1352–9.
10. Streifler JY, Eliasziw M, Fox AJ, et al. Angiographic detection of carotid plaque ulceration. Comparison with surgical observations in a multicenter study. North American Symptomatic Carotid Endarterectomy Trial. Stroke 1994;25:1130–2.
11. Rothwell PM, Gibson R, Warlow CP. Interrelation between plaque surface morphology and degree of stenosis on carotid angiograms and the risk of ischemic stroke in patients with symptomatic carotid stenosis. On behalf of the European Carotid Surgery Trialists' Collaborative Group. Stroke 2000;31:615–21.
12. Rothwell PM, Villagra R, Gibson R, et al. Evidence of a chronic systemic cause of instability of atherosclerotic plaques. Lancet 2000;355:19–24.
13. Eliasziw M, Streifler JY, Fox AJ, et al. Significance of plaque ulceration in symptomatic patients with high-grade carotid stenosis. North American Symptomatic Carotid Endar - terectomy Trial. Stroke 1994;25:304–8.
14. Zwiebel WJ. Spectrum analysis in carotid sonography. Ultrasound Med Biol 1987;13: 625–36.
15. Zwiebel WJ. Introduction to Vascular Ultrasonography. Philadelphia: WB Saunders; 1992.
16. Wardlaw JM, Chappell FM, Best JJ, et al. Non-invasive imaging compared with intraarterial angiography in the diagnosis of symptomatic carotid stenosis: a meta-analysis. Lancet 2006;367:1503–12.
17. AbuRahma AF, Richmond BK, Robinson PA, et al. Effect of contralateral severe stenosis or carotid occlusion on duplex criteria of ipsilateral stenoses: comparative study of various duplex parameters. J Vasc Surg 1995;22:751–61; discussion 61–2.
18. Fujitani RM, Mills JL, Wang LM, Taylor SM. The effect of unilateral internal carotid arterial occlusion upon contralateral duplex study: criteria for accurate interpretation. J Vasc Surg 1992;16:459–67; discussion 67–8.
19. Moneta GL, Edwards JM, Chitwood RW, et al. Correlation of North American Symptomatic Carotid Endarterectomy Trial (NASCET) angiographic definition of 70% to 99% internal carotid artery stenosis with duplex scanning. J Vasc Surg 1993;17:152–7; discussion 7–9.
20. Shaalan WE, Wahlgren CM, Desai T, et al. Reappraisal of velocity criteria for carotid bulb/internal carotid artery stenosis utilizing high-resolution B-mode ultrasound validated with computed tomography angiography. J Vasc Surg 2008;48:104–12; discussion 12–3.
21. MacKenzie KS, French-Sherry E, Burns K, Pooley T, Bassiouny HS. B-mode ultrasound Measurement of carotid bifurcation stenoses: Is it reliable? Vasc Endovasc Surg 2002, 36:123–35.
22. Denzel C, Balzer K, Muller KM, et al. Relative value of normalized sonographic in vitro analysis of arteriosclerotic plaques of internal carotid artery. Stroke 2003;34:1901–6.
23. Gronholdt ML, Wiebe BM, Laursen H, et al. Lipid-rich carotid artery plaques appear echolucent on ultrasound B-mode images and may be associated with intraplaque haemorrhage. Eur J Vasc Endovasc Surg 1997;14:439–45.
24. Barry R, Pienaar C, Nel CJ. Accuracy of B-mode ultrasonography in detecting carotid plaque hemorrhage and ulceration. Ann Vasc Surg 1990;4:466–70.

25. Denzel C, Fellner F, Wutke R, et al. Ultrasonographic analysis of arteriosclerotic plaques in the internal carotid artery. Eur J Ultrasound 2003;16:161–7.
26. O'Donnell TF, Jr., Erdoes L, Mackey WC, et al. Correlation of B-mode ultrasound imaging and arteriography with pathologic findings at carotid endarterectomy. Arch Surg 1985; 120:443–9.
27. Ratliff DA, Gallagher PJ, Hames TK, et al. Characterisation of carotid artery disease: comparison of duplex scanning with histology. Ultrasound Med Biol 1985;11:835–40.
28. Reilly LM, Lusby RJ, Hughes L, et al. Carotid plaque histology using real-time ultrasonography. Clinical and therapeutic implications. Am J Surg 1983;146:188–93.
29. Geroulakos G, Ramaswami G, Nicolaides A, et al. Characterization of symptomatic and asymptomatic carotid plaques using high-resolution real-time ultrasonography. Br J Surg 1993;80:1274–7.
30. Gray-Weale AC, Graham JC, Burnett JR, et al. Carotid artery atheroma: comparison of preoperative B-mode ultrasound appearance with carotid endarterectomy specimen pathology. J Cardiovasc Surg (Torino) 1988;29:676–81.
31. Arnold JA, Modaresi KB, Thomas N, et al. Carotid plaque characterization by duplex scanning: observer error may undermine current clinical trials. Stroke 1999;30:61–5.
32. Elatrozy T, Nicolaides A, Tegos T, et al. The effect of B-mode ultrasonic image standardization on the echodensity of symptomatic and asymptomatic carotid bifurcation plaques. Int Angiol 1998;17:179–86.
33. Sabetai MM, Tegos TJ, Nicolaides AN, et al. Reproducibility of computer-quantified carotid plaque echogenicity: can we overcome the subjectivity? Stroke 2000;31:2189–96.
34. Grogan JK, Shaalan WE, Cheng H, Gewertz B, Desai T, Schwarze G, Glagov S, Lozanski L, Griffin A, Castilla M, Bassiouny HS. B-mode ultrasonographic characterization of carotid atherosclerotic plaques in symptomatic and asymptomatic patients. J Vasc Surg 2005, 42:435–41.
35. Biasi GM, Froio A, Diethrich EB, et al. Carotid plaque echolucency increases the risk of stroke in carotid stenting: the Imaging in Carotid Angioplasty and Risk of Stroke (ICAROS) study. Circulation 2004;110:756–62.
36. Cinat M, Lane CT, Pham H, et al. Helical CT angiography in the preoperative evaluation of carotid artery stenosis. J Vasc Surg 1998;28:290–300.
37. Randoux B, Marro B, Koskas F, et al. Carotid artery stenosis: prospective comparison of CT, three-dimensional gadolinium-enhanced MR, and conventional angiography. Radiology 2001;220:179–85.
38. Wintermark M, Jawadi SS, Rapp JH, et al. High-resolution CT imaging of carotid artery atherosclerotic plaques. Am J Neuroradiol 008;29:875–82.
39. Denzel C, Lell M, Maak M, et al. Carotid artery calcium: accuracy of a calcium score by computed tomography—an in vitro study with comparison to sonography and histology. Eur J Vasc Endovasc Surg 2004;28:214–20.
40. Gronholdt ML, Wagner A, Wiebe BM, et al. Spiral computed tomographic imaging related to computerized ultrasonographic images of carotid plaque morphology and histology. J Ultrasound Med 2001;20:451–8.
41. Nandalur KR, Baskurt E, Hagspiel KD, et al. Carotid artery calcification on CT may independently predict stroke risk. Am J Roentgenol 2006;186:547–52.
42. Oliver TB, Lammie GA, Wright AR, et al. Atherosclerotic plaque at the carotid bifurcation: CT angiographic appearance with histopathologic correlation. Am J Neuroradiol 1999; 20:897–901.
43. Walker LJ, Ismail A, McMeekin W, et al. Computed tomography angiography for the evaluation of carotid atherosclerotic plaque: correlation with histopathology of endarterectomy specimens. Stroke 2002;33:977–81.
44. Culebras A, Otero C, Toledo JR, Rubin BS. Computed tomographic study of cervical carotid calcification. Stroke 1989;20:1472–6.
45. de Weert TT, Ouhlous M, Meijering E, et al. In vivo characterization and quantification of atherosclerotic carotid plaque components with multidetector computed

tomography and histopathological correlation. Arterioscler Thromb Vasc Biol 2006;26: 2366–72.
46. Clarke SE, Hammond RR, Mitchell JR, Rutt BK. Quantitative assessment of carotid plaque composition using multicontrast MRI and registered histology. Magn Reson Med 2003; 50:1199–1208.
47. Puppini G, Furlan F, Cirota N, et al. Characterisation of carotid atherosclerotic plaque: comparison between magnetic resonance imaging and histology. Radiol Med 2006;111: 921–30.
48. Saam T, Ferguson MS, Yarnykh VL, et al. Quantitative evaluation of carotid plaque composition by in vivo MRI. Arterioscler Thromb Vasc Biol 2005;25:234–9.
49. Kampschulte A, Ferguson MS, Kerwin WS, et al. Differentiation of intraplaque versus juxtaluminal hemorrhage/thrombus in advanced human carotid atherosclerotic lesions by in vivo magnetic resonance imaging. Circulation 2004;110:3239–44.
50. Chu B, Kampschulte A, Ferguson MS, et al. Hemorrhage in the atherosclerotic carotid plaque: a high-resolution MRI study. Stroke 2004;35:1079–84.
51. Yuan C, Mitsumori LM, Ferguson MS, et al. In vivo accuracy of multispectral magnetic resonance imaging for identifying lipid-rich necrotic cores and intraplaque hemorrhage in advanced human carotid plaques. Circulation 2001;104:2051–6.
52. Cai J, Hatsukami TS, Ferguson MS, et al. In vivo quantitative measurement of intact fibrous cap and lipid-rich necrotic core size in atherosclerotic carotid plaque: comparison of high-resolution, contrast-enhanced magnetic resonance imaging and histology. Circulation 2005;112:3437–44.
53. Issa N, Poggio ED, Fatica RA, et al. Nephrogenic systemic fibrosis and its association with gadolinium exposure during MRI. Cleve Clin J Med 2008;75:95–7, 103–4, 6 passim.
54. Chu B, Phan BA, Balu N, et al. Reproducibility of carotid atherosclerotic lesion type characterization using high resolution multicontrast weighted cardiovascular magnetic resonance. J Cardiovasc Magn Reson 2006;8:793–9.
55. de Ferranti SD, Rifai N. C-reactive protein: a nontraditional serum marker of cardiovascular risk. Cardiovasc Pathol 2007;16:14–21.
56. Madjid M, Naghavi M, Malik BA, et al. Thermal detection of vulnerable plaque. Am J Cardiol 2002;90:36L–9L.
57. Stefanadis C, Diamantopoulos L, Vlachopoulos C, et al. Thermal heterogeneity within human atherosclerotic coronary arteries detected in vivo: A new method of detection by application of a special thermography catheter. Circulation 1999;99:1965–71.
58. Casscells W, Hathorn B, David M, et al. Thermal detection of cellular infiltrates in living atherosclerotic plaques: possible implications for plaque rupture and thrombosis. Lancet 1996;347:1447–51.
59. Rudd JH, Warburton EA, Fryer TD, et al. Imaging atherosclerotic plaque inflammation with [18F]-fluorodeoxyglucose positron emission tomography. Circulation 2002;105:2708–11.
60. Tahara N, Kai H, Ishibashi M, et al. Simvastatin attenuates plaque inflammation: evaluation by fluorodeoxyglucose positron emission tomography. J Am Coll Cardiol 2006;48: 1825–31.
61. Caplan JD, Waxman S, Nesto RW, Muller JE. Near-infrared spectroscopy for the detection of vulnerable coronary artery plaques. J Am Coll Cardiol 2006;47(8 Suppl):C92–6.
62. Wang J, Geng YJ, Guo B, et al. Near-infrared spectroscopic characterization of human advanced atherosclerotic plaques. J Am Coll Cardiol 2002;39:1305–13.
63. Chen J, Tung CH, Mahmood U, et al. In vivo imaging of proteolytic activity in atherosclerosis. Circulation 2002;105:2766–71.
64. Papaspyridonos M, Smith A, Burnand KG, et al. Novel candidate genes in unstable areas of human atherosclerotic plaques. Arterioscler Thromb Vasc Biol 2006;26:1837–44.

Index

D

P

Q

R

S

T

W